Surgery of the Peripheral Nerve

Susan E. Mackinnon, M.D., F.R.C.S. (C)

Associate Professor of Plastic Surgery
University of Toronto
Director of Peripheral Nerve Program
Toronto Hospital
Toronto General Division
Toronto, Ontario, Canada

A. Lee Dellon, M.D. F.A.C.S.

Associate Professor of Plastic Surgery
and Neurosurgery
Johns Hopkins University
Baltimore, Maryland

1988
Thieme Medical Publishers, Inc., New York
Georg Thieme Verlag, Stuttgart · New York

Thieme Medical Publishers, Inc.
381 Park Avenue South
New York, New York 10016

Cover design by Bermedica Production

SURGERY OF THE PERIPHERAL NERVE
Susan E. Mackinnon
A. Lee Dellon

Library of Congress Cataloging-in-Publication Data

Mackinnon, Susan E., 1949–
Surgery of the peripheral nerve / Susan E. Mackinnon, A. Lee Dellon.
Bibliography: p. 595
Includes index.
ISBN 0-86577-283-5
1. Nerves, Peripheral—Wounds and injuries—Surgery. 2. Nerves, Peripheral—Wounds and injuries. I. Dellon, A. Lee (Arnold Lee), 1944– II. Title.
[DNLM: 1. Peripheral Nerves—surgery. WL 500 N158s]
RD595.M23 1988
617'.483—dc19
DNLM/DLC
for Library of Congress

88-24791
CIP

Important note: Medicine is an ever-changing science. Research and clinical experience are continually broadening our knowledge, in particular our knowledge of proper treatment and drug therapy. Insofar as this book mentions any dosage or application, readers may rest assured that the authors, editors, and publishers have made every effort to ensure that such references are strictly in accordance with the state of knowledge at the time of production of the book. Nevertheless, every user is requested to carefully examine the manufacturers' leaflets accompanying each drug to check on his own responsibility whether the dosage schedules recommended therein or the contraindications stated by the manufacturers differ from the statements made in the present book. Such examination is particularly important with drugs that are either rarely used or have been newly released on the market.

Some of the product names, patents, and registered designs referred to in this book are in fact registered trademarks or proprietary names even though specific reference to this fact is not always made in the text. Therefore, the appearance of a name without designation as proprietary is not to be construed as a representation by the publisher that it is in the public domain.

References in this volume were updated and a second Foreword added in December, 1990, at the time of the second printing.
Printed in the United States of America
5 4 3 2

TMP ISBN 0-86577-283-5
GTV ISBN 3-13-728701-4

This book is dedicated with love and appreciation to

our parents

Elizabeth J. and Donald L. Mackinnon

and

Irene J. and Alfred L. Dellon

Contents

Forewords

This book is the collaborative effort of Dr. Susan Mackinnon of Toronto and Dr. Lee Dellon of Baltimore, who have combined to commit their wide experience and the results of their clinical and investigative skills to a book that is a valuable addition to a growing list of publications on nerve injuries and their management.

In recent years, both authors have contributed consistently to the literature on nerve injury and repair, Dr. Mackinnon in particular on nerve allografting and Dr. Dellon on sensation and sensory mechanisms. Because of their experimental studies combined with a wide and diversified clinical experience, they are well equipped to undertake the task of writing a text on peripheral nerve surgery.

World War II provided an impetus to peripheral nerve research that greatly increased our knowledge of the neurobiological background of nerve injury and repair. From this emerged many important advances in the clinical management of these injuries. It is essential that the momentum created by these advances be maintained because despite all the new knowledge of improved techniques, and the best efforts of skilled and experienced surgeons, the results of nerve repair continue at times to fall short of expectations, even to the point of being decidedly bad. The failure to improve the results of nerve repair on a broader front is also partly due to the failure to exploit information that is already available. The inevitable result is a widening gap between what is known and what is practiced.

The authors are mindful of these considerations. The essential value of this contribution to the literature on nerve injuries and their repair is that it provides an informative record of the current state of the art based as it is on the wide personal experience of the two authors. Because of the authors' direct involvement with the growing edges of the subject, the reader is also exposed to the latest developments. All this sets an authoritative seal on the contents of the book.

The book will repay all who have an interest and involvement in nerve injury and nerve repair. Those who are not specialists in this field will find the book a reliable guide to the subject, and for the specialist, it is a repository of factual material of considerable interest and value.

The value of the book is greatly enhanced by the inclusion of a wealth of illustrations and diagrams that reflect the wide range of the authors' personal experiences, both in the clinic and the laboratory. They are outstanding features of the book and are worthy of careful study.

Though some of the authors' views on certain topics may not meet with universal acceptance, they cannot fail to prompt the reader to further thought and study. Disagreement is the spur to further effort and provides the key that ultimately opens the locked doors of ignorance.

Writing this book has obviously been an assignment of immense labor, and we are indebted to the authors for having undertaken so demanding a task and for having brought it to so admirable a conclusion.

Sir Sydney Sunderland
Professor Emeritus of Experimental Neurology
University of Melbourne, Australia

Everyone who has followed the recent literature on peripheral nerves has witnessed the regular appearance of extremely interesting papers written by a pair of authors—A. Lee Dellon and Susan E. Mackinnon. Each of these papers covers a selected anatomic, clinical, or research problem in an exhaustive way. It could be expected that from the continuous cooperation between Toronto and Baltimore, a textbook on peripheral nerve surgery would be born. Both authors are extremely well suited to produce such a textbook. A. Lee Dellon has accumulated worldwide recognition by his studies on sensibility testing and sensory reeducation. Susan E. Mackinnon has attracted attention by her numerous experimental studies on nerve allografting. Together they have developed the areas of nerve compression and neuroma treatment.

The general chapters in this volume cover todays knowledge about normal anatomy, physiology, and classification of nerve injuries. Problems according to the special field of interest of the authors, such as nerve entrapment syndromes, and painful sequelae of nerve injuries are presented. These are completely discussed and presented in detail. In particular, the chapter Sensory Rehabilitation After Nerve Injury reflects the enormous experience of the authors in this field.

Peripheral nerve surgery has developed into such a complex entity that one person cannot cover the entire field. Therefore, the usual textbooks are editions collaborated upon by many authors. While each of them may be a top level specialist in their field, the result nevertheless is an accumulation of individual chapters of varying quality which may or may not be controversial. This volume by Doctors Mackinnon and Dellon represents the approach and the way of thinking of two highly qualified specialists who think and write as one. The authors have restricted themselves only to subjects to which they have contributed personally with clinical or research studies. It is this fact which makes *Surgery of the Peripheral Nerve* so valuable. In addition, it is of extreme interest to read how the two authors, who are in the frontline of research in peripheral nerve surgery, think about the future developments of this field.

Certainly, this book represents a milestone in the literature on surgery of peripheral nerves.

Prof. Dr. Hanno Millesi
Vienna, Austria
March 1988

Preface

The purpose of this volume is to present our approach to the management of peripheral nerve injuries. This approach is systematic, and encompasses the current concept of neural function, including the response to injury and nerve regeneration. It includes the clinical manifestations of this response to nerve injury. The unique modifications of this response will be determined by the individual peripheral nerves and their unique sensory and motor components. This systematic approach includes the techniques for evaluating sensibility and motor function, thereby diagnosing the peripheral nerve injury. Finally, this approach includes both nonoperative and operative modes of treatment for the nerve injury. The system we present diverges in many ways from traditional surgical teaching.

The history of surgery teaches us that the past has relied too heavily on anecdotal teaching. Surgical teaching based solely on the experience of a single authoritative figure might suffice for solutions to a variety of problems but, in general, has stifled the creativity of the questioning minds of many surgical preceptees.* The history of surgery teaches that solid contributions to patient care must be based on observations and techniques that are reproducible, and generally this results from questions put to the test in an experimental, that is, scientific, method. These abstract concepts are better visualized by considering the relationship of the teachings of Galen and Vesalius. In A.D. 200, Galen published works that presented a systematic view of the anatomy and physiology of the human body and that permitted therapeutic intervention based on this system. His ideas came from detailed anatomic investigations, which form the first experimental medicine. His experimental technique consisted essentially of cutting away parts of the body to learn the results of that part's function. His unified approach was translated into all the teaching languages of his time. His system, based on his science and his authority,

*Robert F. Buckman, M. D., lecture: "Does the history of surgery teach us anything?", 7/9/86, Johns Hopkins Hospital.

persisted over the next 13 centuries. It was not until the 15th century that Vesalius seriously questioned Galen's concepts. Vesalius' questions were based on additional anatomic studies and research. Furthermore, although Vesalius was not the only surgeon and anatomist nor his writing the only anatomy textbook of his time, his work, *De humani corporis fabrica,* was widely acclaimed in its time and persists to the present generation. Vesalius asked Jan Stephan van Kalkar, an artist who had studied with Titian, to illustrate his anatomic dissections. Vesalius' teachings demonstrate that it is not enough to have recognition as a surgeon and for one's science, but to be able to popularize and clearly convey one's ideas it is necessary to utilize the techniques of medical illustration.

It is our hope that this volume combines more than our anecdotal experience for the reader: It is our goal to unite our combined clinical experience in managing patients with nerve injuries, our combined years of peripheral nerve research, including both basic and clinical science, with the best medical illustrators of our time. Toward this end, we have sought to review in each chapter the historical works, and where those have not been available in English, we have had them translated. We have derived much of the joy of learning from reading the original thoughts of earlier investigators, seeing the world as they saw it at their time and with the understanding of the instruments they had at their disposal to dissect the problem at hand. Toward this end, we have incorporated within our volume the best illustrations from the works of others and have had created for this work many new ones to illustrate our own operative technique. We have written only about areas in which we have directly worked, where we have carried out investigations and where we feel that we have been able to make significant contributions. The Contents will therefore reflect areas where some might feel the book is less than comprehensive because a particular nerve or particular area has been omitted. Any subject omitted has been by deliberate design in that this book is meant to contain material about which we have posed and answered questions ourselves. We have used both basic science and experimental and clinical investigational techniques. Although this may limit somewhat the scope of the book, we feel the advantage of a book on a subject in which the authors have carried out scientific investigations to add to their own surgical experience represents the height of surgical scholarship.

This volume will challenge many existing dogmas in the neurosciences. Sir Charles Bell, the founder of experimental neurology, believed that the complexity of the nervous system was such that it virtually dissuaded researchers from attempting to solve its problems. His research techniques were similar to those of Galen. He would cut a nerve and attempt to learn the results of that action. In this manner, in 1821, he identified that it was the seventh cranial nerve that was responsible for facial motor function, whereas the fifth cranial nerve was responsible for facial sensation. Our experimental techniques are only slightly more sophisticated. We still carry out a surgical manipulation on a peripheral nerve and attempt to learn its effects. Traditionally, however, attempts to treat one of the most common peripheral nerve problems, nerve entrapment, have been restricted to simply decompressing external forces about the nerve. The traditional concepts have been that operations performed within the nerve, itself, would create more scarring, if not cause ischemia within the nerve and thereby worsen neural function. This problem stimulated the development of an experimental model for chronic nerve compression. Experience with this model led to the understanding that an intraneural dissection could be done safely by people appropriately trained in microsurgery. The guidelines for the use of this surgical technique came through careful experimental work and in clinical studies of nerve compression. These have led to guidelines for noninvasive techniques for determining when a nerve is under appropriate compression to require decompression and when it is appropriate to carry out internal neurolysis. The classic testing instruments have been used in new ways. The standard tuning fork will evaluate peripheral nerve vibratory thresholds. A newly developed sensory testing instrument, the Disk-Criminator,™ will measure peripheral nerve innervation density.

There are other areas in which this volume presents a departure from tradition. The clinical problem of the painful neuroma was investigated in the laboratory. Models were defined to create neuromas in primates. Evaluation by electrophysiologic recordings defined the neurophysiologic mechanisms of pain from neuromas. Subsequently, the classic neuroma formation was modified by implantation of nerve into muscle. These experimental models were then evaluated clinically. The technique of nerve implantation into muscle was incorporated into an overall systematic approach to the management of the painful neuroma.

Our extensive clinical experience with patients with pain due to peripheral nerve injury has resulted in a surgical approach to this problem. A pain evaluation scale defines surgical candidates by determining functional and organic components of the pain syndrome. The long standing problem of reflex sympathetic dystrophy (RSD) has been reevaluated in light of our understanding of pain, nerve injury, and sympathetic dysfunction.

Wherever clinical confusion in diagnosis of nerve problems occurred, this problem was taken to the gross anatomy laboratory. Dissections of the upper and lower extremities were carried out in order to answer specific anatomic questions raised from our clinical practices. Thus, the traditional picture of a peripheral nerve's anatomic relationships, as given in the leading anatomy texts, could be modified to include a statistical analysis of the variations of these nerves in the areas for which surgical intervention was required.

When the clinical problem was one in which insufficient nerve tissue was available to reconstruct a localized anatomic nerve problem, the problem of reconstruction of the nerve deficit was studied. Hanno Millesi, one of the most courageous of surgical researchers of our time, had already set the stage for challenging the traditional approach for nerve reconstruction. He represents the combination of science and authority that has permitted the use today of autogenous interfascicular interposition nerve grafting for this problem. However, occasions arise when insufficient autogenous material exists. We have investigated the basic host response to nerve allografts and the effect of manipulating this reaction by various immunosuppressive techniques. Currently, techniques to add nerve allografting to the clinical armamentarium continue to be investigated. For the short nerve gap situation, another alternative has been explored. The current concepts of neurotrop(h)ism have led to an appreciation that the neural regenerative capacity is best able to find its own distal course, rather than having a course imposed on the nerve by the microsurgeon's attempt to do precise fascicular alignments. This area was investigated in the laboratory with studies in primate regeneration utilizing Lundborg's pseudosynovial sheath as a two-stage technique and finally by advancing to one-stage biodegradable nerve tubes. This basic investigation has demonstrated that the peripheral nerve can regenerate through a biodegradable tube with a facility similar to that through which it regenerates through an autogenous interposition, interfascicular nerve graft. This work has now been brought into clinical usefulness, so that the future may find the bioabsorbable nerve tube being used not only to reconstruct short nerve gaps but also to be used for primary or secondary nerve repair, to manage the painful neuroma and neuroma in-continuity situations.

William Stewart Halsted had written that the operating rooms should be surgical laboratories of the highest order. By this monograph, we hope to have demonstrated that by taking the questions from the clinical situation, which largely have come from our failures surgically to improve the patient's problem, to the laboratory and submitting them to the rigors of scientific investigation, solid advances can be made in the clinical care of our patients with peripheral nerve injury. At the time of writing this volume, the traditional concept that diabetic neuropathy is progressive and irreversible is being investigated. The hypothesis being tested is that much of the symptomatology of this metabolic neuropathy is due to multiple superimposed nerve compression syndromes. Again, our pattern of addressing clinical problems with a systematic detailed approach that combines basic science experimental studies with anatomic studies has yielded rewarding clinical results. An experimental model to create nerve compression in diabetic rats was subsequently evaluated in the nonhuman primate. Previous investigations of internal neurolysis have been supplemented with anatomic studies (for example, the radial sensory nerve in the forearm, the lateral sural and deep peroneal nerve in the leg). This has enabled a technique to be brought into clinical use, the relief of symptoms of diabetic neuropathy through internal neurolysis of multiple compressed peripheral nerves.

In terms of organization, the volume begins with the fundamentals for understanding the neuroscience of the peripheral nerve. This forms the basis for the clinical observation and physical diagnosis for peripheral nerve injuries and forms the basis for techniques used in surgery of the peripheral nerve. Individual chapters follow on those peripheral nerves for which we have found our approaches to have the most relevance, including the brachial plexus. A chapter on the management of the painful sequelae of peripheral nerve injury, which are frequent complications with which the peripheral nerve surgeon must deal, not only of his own making but commonly patients referred for secondary or tertiary opinions is included, as well as a chapter on nerve tumors. A chapter on rehabilitation of the patient with an injured nerve follows. We conclude with a chapter that outlines the direction that we believe nerve repair may take in the very near future. This direction combines the neurobiology of nerve regeneration with refinements in microneurosurgical technique. Appendices are included of patient information materials which we have found most useful in our clinical practice. Finally, there is a combined bibliography so that the student of peripheral nerve injury may find in one place, the references scattered throughout the chapters of this book.

Acknowledgments

The most essential support for our research and the preparation of this book has been that of our families. Thank you Marge and Evan, Glenn and Brian Dellon, and Alec Patterson, and Lachlan, Megan, Brendan, and Caitlan Mackinnon-Patterson. Your willingness to allow us to pursue answers to our questions and record our observations has given us the confidence and security essential to the creative spirit.

Three men have influenced our work significantly and stimulated our productivity. These surgeons have taught us by example to challenge surgical dogma and we are indebted to them for their inspiration. Raymond M. Curtis, M. D., of Baltimore, a President of The American Society for Surgery of the Hand, was there in the beginning for both of us. He established the Hand Center at Union Memorial Hospital where, though five years apart, we both obtained our training in hand surgery, and where we together in 1981 began our research collaboration. We thank Alan R. Hudson, M. B., Professor and Chairman of the Division of Neurosurgery, University of Toronto, for his refinement of our ideas, criticism of our results and support of our laboratory efforts. We thank James F. Murray, M. D., of Toronto, also a President of The American Society for Surgery of the Hand, who continues to challenge us with ever increasing complex clinical problems.

Our laboratory efforts would have been impossible without the daily attention of William (David) A. Seiler, IV, Chief of the Microsurgery Laboratory at the Curtis Hand Center in Baltimore, and Daniel A. Hunter, who, in the Peripheral Nuerosurgical Laboratory at the University of Toronto, Saint Michael's Hospital in Toronto, may be the finest and hardest working neurohistologist and morphometric assessor of our time.

We thank our medical illustrators, all of whom have been in the direct lineage of Max Broedel's School of Art as Applied to Medicine at Johns Hopkins University. Susan P. Clow, of Toronto, not only contributed her own illustrations, but coordinated those of our other illustrators: From the Johns Hopkins Medical Institutions, these included David Jonah, Marge Gregorman, Dona Cavi and Michael Leonard, while from the University of Toronto, where the founder of medical illustration, Maria Wishart, trained with Max Broedel from 1924 to 1926, are included Leila Lax, Elise Burrows and Terry Watkinson.

The preparation of this book and our research has been supported by two main sources: The Dellon Foundation and the Medical Research Council of Canada. Additional major contributions toward research have come from our peer review groups, such as Physicians Services Incorporation of Ontario, the Sunnybrook Medical Research Trust, and The Raymond M. Curtis Research Foundation, The Educational Foundation of The American Society for Plastic and Reconstructive Surgery, and The American Society for Surgery of the Hand.

We thank Phyllis Morrow of Baltimore, and Gayle Burke of Toronto for their superb job of manuscript preparation. We apologize to them for their multiple nerve entrapments and multiple trigger fingers that developed after hours of repetitive work with their word processors. Special thanks to Elizabeth (Betsy) Tait for careful and diligent preparation of the combined bibliography. We thank Berta Steiner of Bermedica Production, for carefully guiding the final production of this book and finally Hilary Evans, Editor-In-Chief, of Thieme Medical Publishers for literally years of support and enthusiasm.

Thank you all.

1

Anatomy and Physiology of the Peripheral Nerve

A prerequisite to the understanding of both the timing and the technique of nerve repair is a clear understanding of the pathophysiologic aspects of nerve injury. In order to discuss nerve injury and regeneration, it is equally important to appreciate the normal anatomy of the peripheral nerve. The surgeon should be able to reconstruct, in his mind, the gross surgical anatomy of the peripheral nerve and the complexity of the internal anatomy of the nerve with its changing internal fascicular patterns. The surgeon should be able to picture the myelinated and unmyelinated fibers both in a unidimensional and 3-dimensional sense. Equally important is an appreciation of the currently accepted nomenclature for the components of the peripheral nerve and its various intraneural arrangements.

The morphologic consequences of nerve injury can then be described based on description of the normal nerve. The response of sensory receptors and the muscle to denervation and reinnervation will be critical in determining the final result after nerve repair. Finally, recent concepts in nerve sprouting, axonal elongation, and the influence of neurotropism on nerve regeneration may significantly alter our current thoughts on nerve repair and regeneration.

Nerve Fibers

The peripheral nerve is composed of motor, sensory, and sympathetic nerve fibers. The cell body of the motor nerve fibers lies in the anterior horn of the spinal cord and the motor nerve fiber terminates at the neuromuscular junction in the muscle. The cell body of the presynaptic sympathetic nerve fibers lies in the anterior horn, since these are effector nerves. The cell body of the sensory nerve fibers lies in the dorsal root ganglia. These sensory nerve fibers terminate in the skin as free nerve endings or end in a number of specialized receptors (Fig. 1-1).

The metabolic activities of the cell occur in the cell body and products are then transported the length of the axon as required. This is quite remarkable when the relationships in size between the cell body and the axon are recalled. A striking analogy is presented by Ducker: "If the central cell body were the height of an average man, its axon would be one or two inches in width and would extend more than two miles."[1]

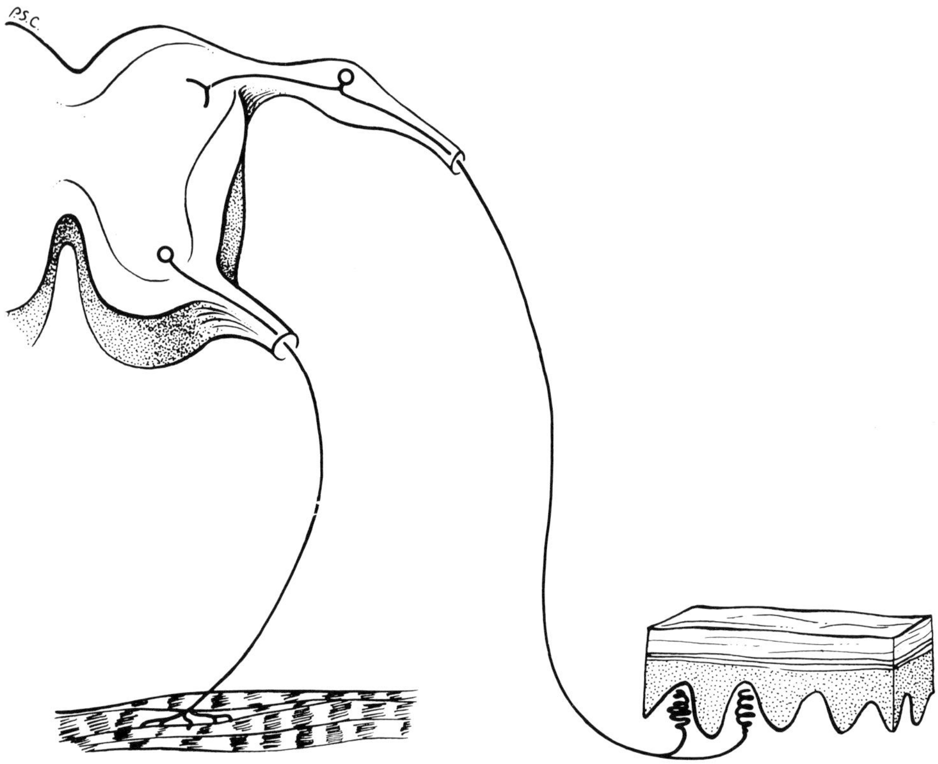

Figure 1-1. Schematic diagram of the basic composition of the peripheral nerve.

Nerve fibers will be either myelinated or unmyelinated (Fig. 1-2a). Sensory and motor nerves contain both unmyelinated and myelinated nerve fibers in a ratio of 4 to 1. Postganglionic sympathetic nerve fibers originate in the neurons of the ganglion located from T_1 to T_7. These unmyelinated fibers will innervate the skin, blood vessels, and hair follicles. Unmyelinated fibers are composed of several axons, wrapped by a single Schwann cell (Fig. 1-2b). The axons of myelinated nerve fibers are enveloped individually by a single Schwann cell (Fig. 1-2b). The membrane of the Schwann cell wraps around the axon to form a multilaminated myelin sheath. The double basement membrane of the Schwann cell can only be identified on electron microscopy. Individual myelinated nerve fibers and groups of unmyelinated fibers will be surrounded by this double membrane of basal lamella. The endoneurial sheath refers to the basal lamina outside the Schwann cell.

Along the length of a myelinated nerve fiber, the axon will relate to many schwann cells. The length of the axon that a single schwann cell relates to is called the internode. For a short distance between internodes, that is, between Schwann cell processes, the axon is not myelinated. This is the node of Ranvier. The larger the fiber diameter, the longer the internode length (0.1 to 1.8 mm) (Fig. 1-3).

Surrounding the individual myelinated nerve fibers or the groups of unmyelinated nerve fibers are the thin collagen fibers of the endoneurium.

Many nerve fibers collect together to form a fascicle (termed by Sunderland "funicle").[2] These fascicles are bound by the perineurium, which is a connective tissue sheath consisting of several layers of perineurial cells. Thus, a fascicle is a group of nerve fibers or a bundle of nerve fibers surrounded by perineurium.

The fascicular patterns can be of three basic types: a monofascicular pattern with just one large fascicle; an oligofascicular pattern consisting of a few fascicles; and a polyfascicular pattern consisting of many fascicles of varying sizes.[3] This polyfascicular pattern can be arranged with or without groupings of fascicles (Fig. 1-4). The connective tissue that surrounds the individual fascicles or the intrafascicular portion of the nerve is termed the internal or interfascicular epineurium. The connective tissue that surrounds the entire nerve is termed the external or extrafascicular epineurium. The epineurium generally makes up 50% of the cross-sectional area of the nerve. As the nerve crosses a joint, the connective tissue content increases. The amount of connective tissue is greater in the proximal regions of the extremities. The amount of cross-sectional area composed of neural tissue in the brachial plexus (roots,

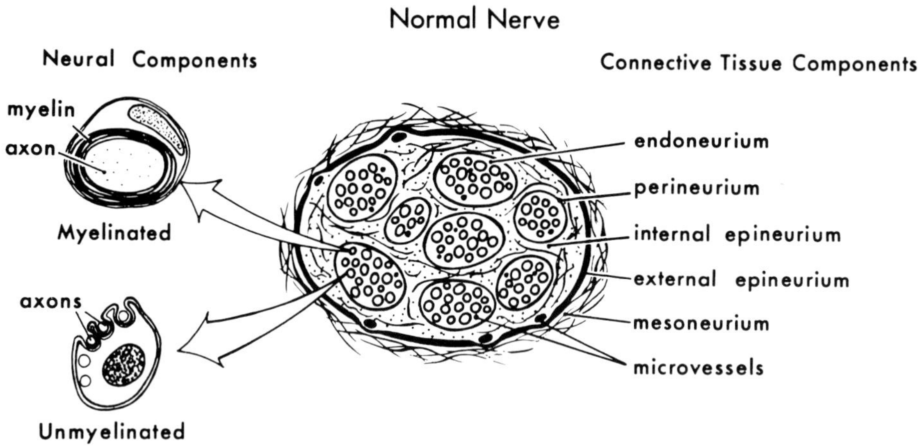

a

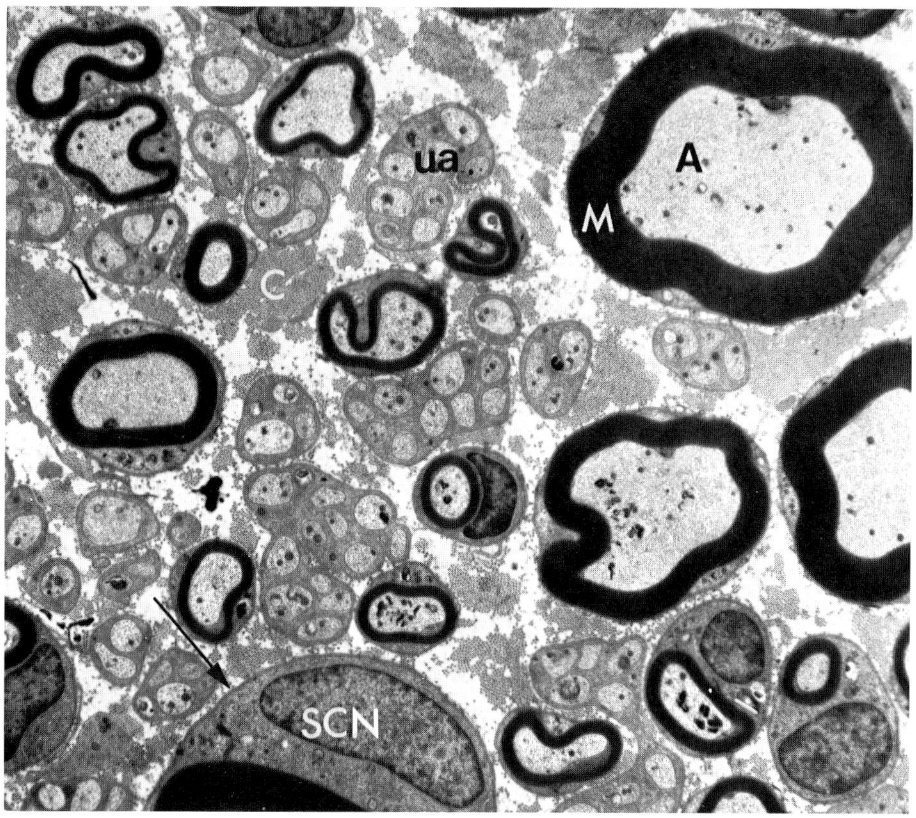

b

Figure 1-2a. The normal peripheral nerve is composed of connective tissue and neural tissue components. The nerve fibers may be myelinated or unmyelinated. **b.** A population of myelinated and unmyelinated nerve fibers are seen. The basement membrane of the Schwann cell is a double basement membrane that can only be identified by electron microscopy. (See also Fig. 1-15.) M: myelin; A: axon; SCN: Schwann cell nucleus; arrow: double basement membrane; C: endoneurial collagen; ua: unmyelinated axon. (Uranyl acetate, ×4760.)

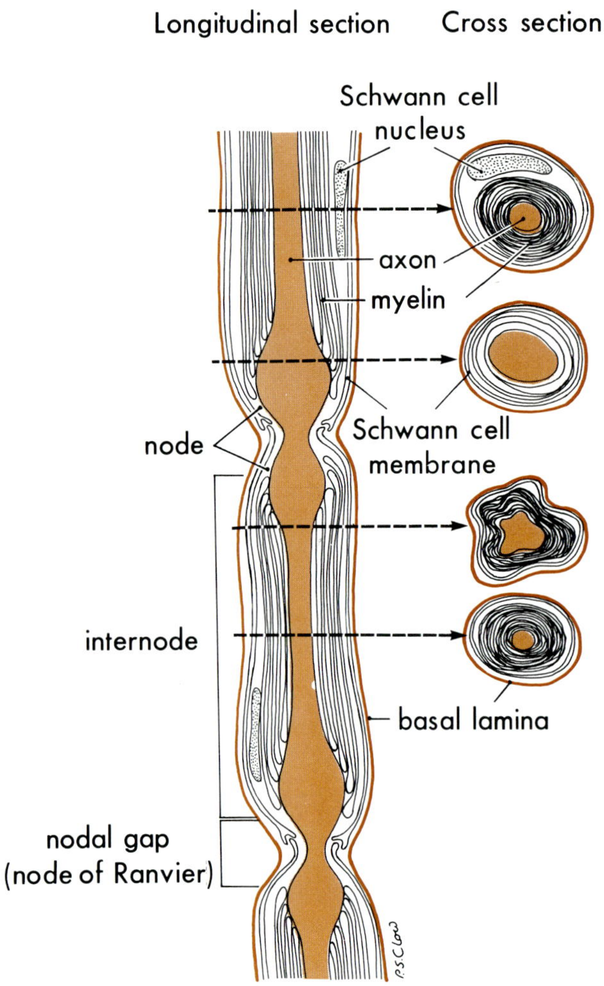

Figure 1-3. Schematic diagram of a single nerve fiber demonstrating the variations that will be seen in a single fiber at different points along the nerve fiber.

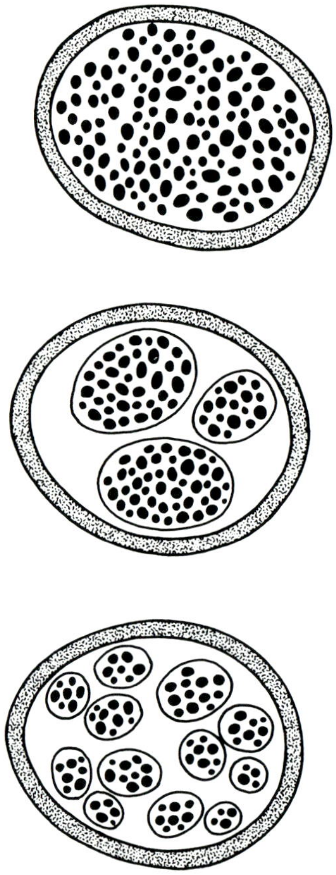

Figure 1-4. The three basic fascicular patterns are monofascicular, oligofascicular, and polyfascicular.

trunks, cords) is one-third, and in the lower extremity it is even less (sciatic nerve, 25%).[4]

The mesoneurium makes up a loose areolar tissue around the outside of the nerve, which extends from the epineurium to the surrounding tissue. It is continuous with the epineurium and is critical in maintaining longitudinal excursion of the peripheral nerve. Segmental blood supply enters the nerve via the mesoneurium. After surgery, nerve repair, or with nerve compression, the epineurium thickens and adhers to the surrounding tissue. This will prevent gliding of the nerve, and because of relative tethering at this point of injury, secondary and superimposed traction injury may occur.

It is fair to note that some investigators have disputed the existence of the mesoneurium,[2,5] but its existence has been supported by most,[6-8] including ourselves.

Millesi[8] has stressed the importance of the mesoneurium in facilitating this gliding of the nerve in its tissue bed as the extremity moves through its range of movement. For example, as the arm moves to full extension, the median nerve must elongate by 4.5%. With elbow flexion, the median nerve must slacken by 14.5% of its length.[8] Millesi[8] has reported the excursion of median and ulnar nerves during maximal flexion and maximal extension of the elbow and wrist. He noted that from maximal flexion and extension, the median nerve moved 2 to 3 cm distally and the ulnar nerve 1 cm proximally.[8] He also emphasized that motion between individual fascicles was facilitated by the interfascicular epineurium. Fibrosis at this level, as seen with chronic nerve compression, will inhibit this longitudinal gliding. (See Chapters 2 and 5.)

The peripheral nerve is supplied by a segmental, external blood supply as well as an intrinsic longitudinal blood supply.[9,10] An extensive longitudinal blood supply exists in the epineurium, perineurium, and endoneurium. Although large vessels are found within the epineurium and perineurium, only capillaries are found within the endoneurial environment of the nerve fascicles. Recent studies have demonstrated the very extensive nature of the intrinsic blood supply, suggesting that previous dye injection studies have vastly underestimated the longitudinal extent of the intrinsic blood supply.[11] We are dependent on the intrinsic blood supply when we elevate and mobilize peripheral nerves over a long distance, such as during an ulnar nerve transposition.

A classification for the external blood supply to the peripheral nerve based on the potential for free vascularized nerve grafts has been recently presented.[11] A dramatic plexus arrangement exists between the extrinsic and intrinsic vascular network linking the vascular systems in the epineurium, perineurium, and endoneurium. (see Chapter 4.)

Since first noted in 1781,[12] the cross-striations on the peripheral nerves have been considered to be related to an optical phenomenon relating to the relaxation of the nerve fascicles.[13,14] It has been noted that, with tension or traction on the nerve, these bands disappear. Fontana[12] was the first to suggest that these spirals were due to the undulating course of the nerve fibers rather than the nerve fascicles. The indirect or undulating course of the nerve fibers allows the nerve to accommodate to the longitudinal excursion that nerve and nerve fibers must make as the extremity moves from flexion to extension.

We have noted that in areas of nerve compression, these bands are not visible. After appropriate neurolysis, the bands of Fontana reappear. Return of the appearance of these bands is a good indication that the appropriate degree of neurolysis has been carried out (see Chapter 5). Recently, Greenberg[15] has described the dynamic variation in the volume of the axon and has noted the swelling or varicosities in the axons that change in location with time. These varicosities relate to transport substances. This variation in axon diameter has direct relevance to morphometric measurements of axon diameter (Fig. 1-5).

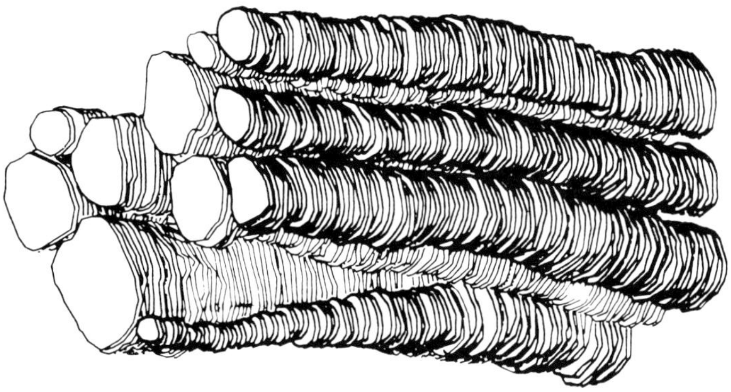

a

Figure 1-5a. A computerized serial electron microscopic reconstruction of single unmyelinated nerve fibers with a single Schwann cell unit demonstrating the variations in axon diameter that can be related to mitochondrial swellings. Not only are the axons at any cross-section of different sizes, but some axons undergo dramatic changes in caliber. **b.** Reconstruction of the same group of axons illustrates visual appearance of an axon with different maximum or minimum ratios. (Reproduced with permission from Greenberg et al.[15])

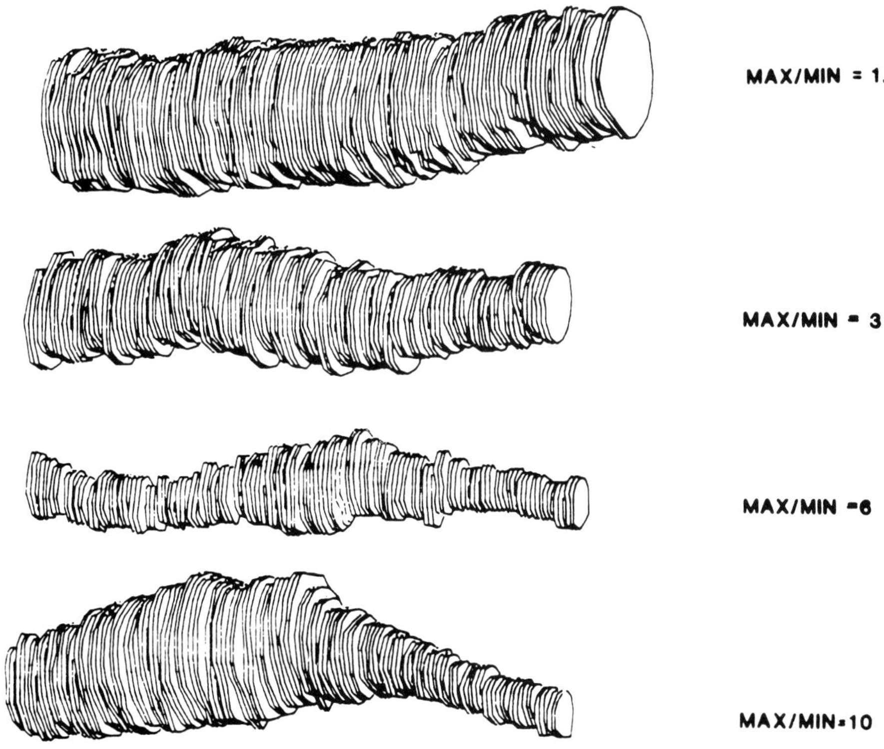

b

Internal Topography of the Peripheral Nerve

The relationship between the fascicles within the peripheral nerve is constantly changing along a longitudinal course in the extremity. Studies by Chow et al,[16] Jabalay et al,[17] Williams and Jabalay[18] and Shizhen et al[19] have expanded Sunderland's[20] classic work and provide the important information necessary to align motor and sensory fascicles at various levels in the extremity. Sunderland's classic diagram of the musculocutaneous nerve outlining the 3-dimensional reconstruction demonstrates marked changes in the fascicular arrangement over very short distances of the nerve (Fig. 1-6). Sunderland noted that the maximum length of nerve with a constant pattern was: "15 mm. in general, however, the pattern is altered so rapidly that transverse sections of the nerve taken more than a few millimeters apart fail to present precisely the same pattern."[2]

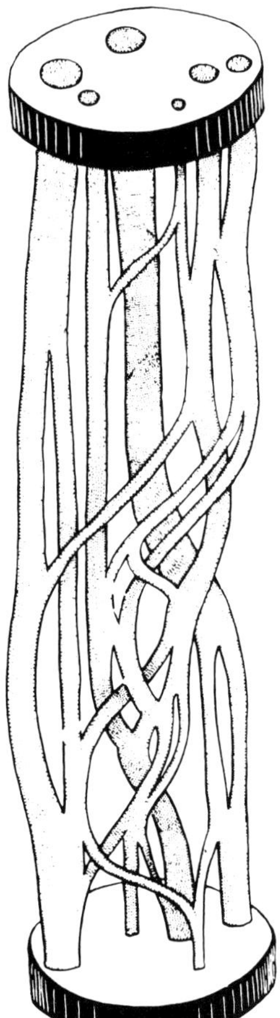

Figure 1-6. Sunderland's classic reconstruction of the internal topography of the musculocutaneous nerve demonstrating the marked plexus formation that is present in the musculocutaneous nerve. (Reproduced with permission from S. Sunderland.[2])

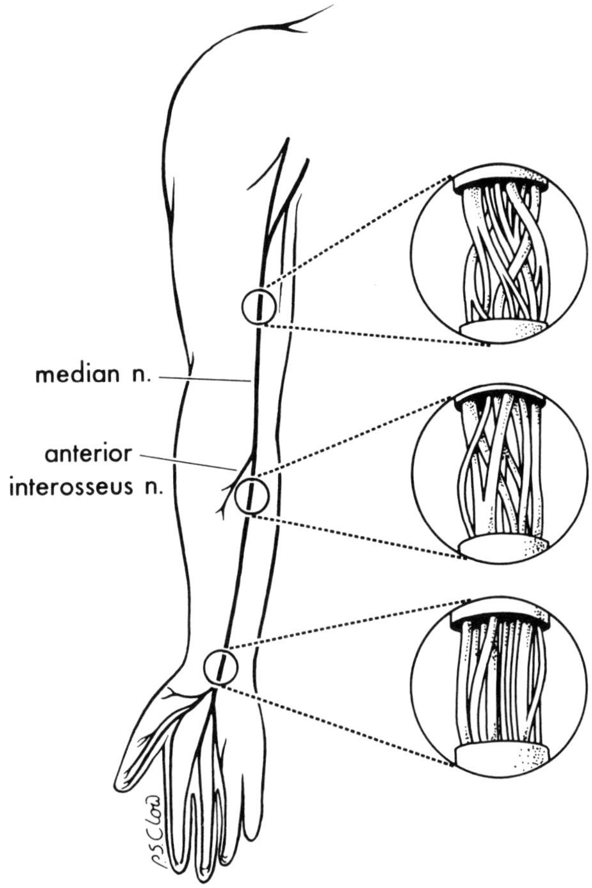

Figure 1-7. A schematic diagram of the internal topography of the median nerve. The degree of plexus formation that occurs between fascicles decreases in the distal portion of the median nerve.

Fortunately for the peripheral nerve surgeon, Sunderland's classic diagram outlining the 3-dimensional reconstruction of the musculocutaneous nerve is true for only the initial course of nerves in the proximal portion of the extremity (Fig. 1-7). These changes in the fascicular organization facilitate a sorting out of motor and sensory fibers. By the time the nerve has reached the forearm, the majority of this sorting is complete and long fascicular segments are noted without any intercommunications between fascicles. Studying fresh cadaver extremities, Jabalay et al[17] noted that in the distal portion of the extremity fascicles could be dissected for long distances before merging with other bundles. The recurrent motor branch of the median nerve could be dissected for more than 70 mm before it fused with adjacent fascicles.[17] At the level of the medial epicondyle, they noted that the anterior interosseous nerve had no interconnections with other fascicles of the median nerve for a distance of 59 mm. Similar dissections of the ulnar nerve in the forearm demonstrated that fascicular components of the nerve traveled over long distances without demonstrating interconnections to adjacent fascicles. In particular, it was noted that the dorsocutaneous branch of the ulnar nerve traveled as a separate group of fascicles for 209 mm and that no communications were noted between the motor branch of the ulnar nerve and the sensory fascicles for a length of 81 mm. Combining his work with Jabalay et al's initial dissections, Williams[18] has stressed that, although there is complex interfascicular relationships between some fascicles in the median and ulnar nerves in the forearm and hand, there are several groups of fascicles that can be dissected over a long distance without any plexus formation with adjacent fascicles. These investigators, in particular, stressed that the recurrent branch of the median nerve, branches to the lumbricals, and the motor, sensory, and dorsocutaneous branches of the ulnar nerve are bundles of fascicles that traverse long distances without interconnections or plexus formation.

Dissections of fresh cadaver upper extremity nerves in the arm and forearm demonstrate that the number of plexus formation and intercommunication between fascicles varies indirectly with the distance from the brachial plexus to the termination of the nerve. In the proximal portion of the peripheral nerve there is marked plexus formation. In the distal portion of the nerve much less is noted. We have demonstrated, for example, that the thoracodorsal nerve can be split proximally to give separately innervated slips of latissimus dorsi muscle.[21] As well, a greater degree of plexus formation is noted in nerves that carry both sensory and motor function or innervate multiple muscles or have a large sensory distribution (Fig. 1-8).

A detailed computerized study by Terzis et al[22] of the intraneural topography of the median nerve reconstructed the route of individual fascicles as they moved in a proximodistal direction along the extremity. Using a retrograde tracer technique (horseradish peroxidase),

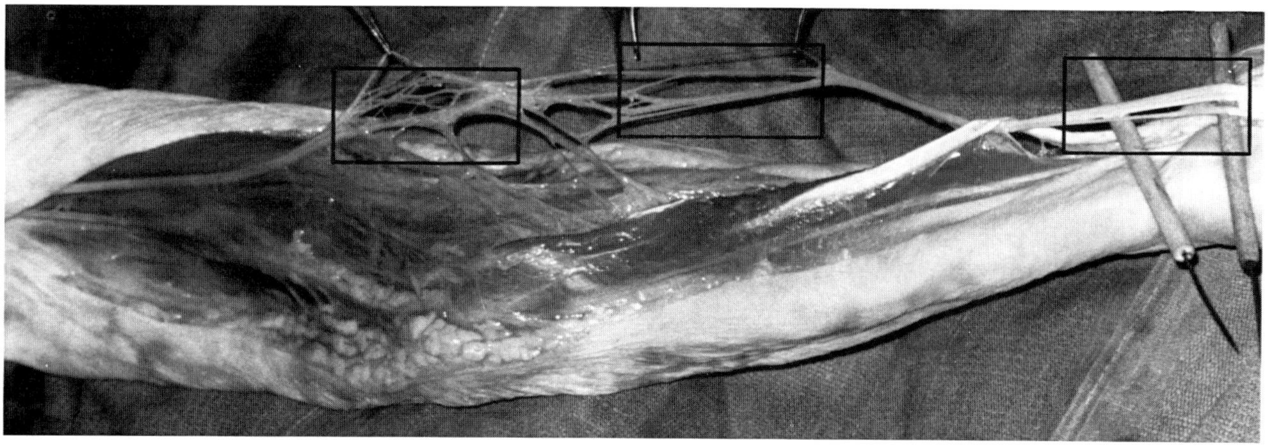

a

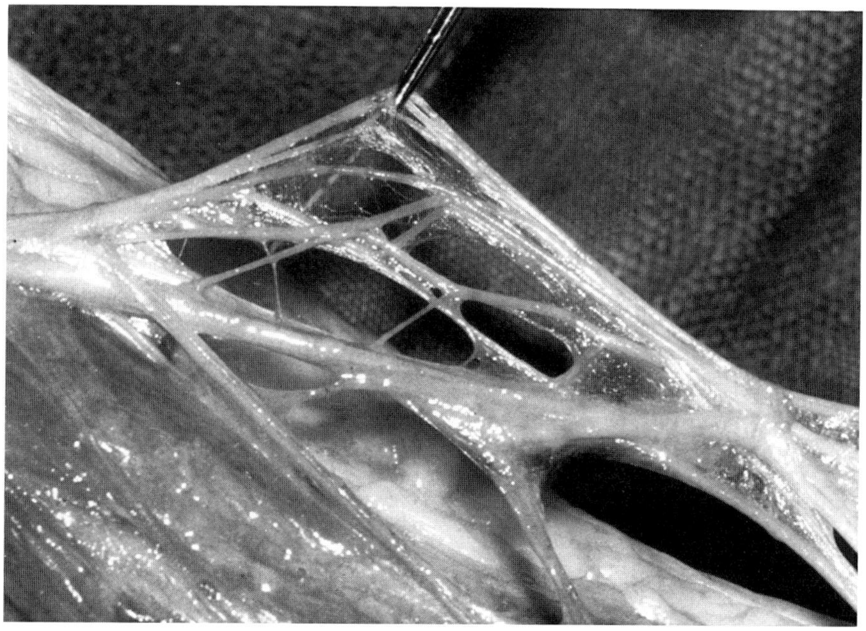

b

Figure 1-8a. A cadaver dissection of the left median nerve, with hand toward right and axilla toward left. The internal fascicles of the median nerve have been dissected by means of microneurosurgical techniques. **b.** A closer view of the intraneural topography within the most proximal rectangular box demonstrates a marked plexus formation between the fascicles of the median nerve in the distal arm. (*Figure continues.*)

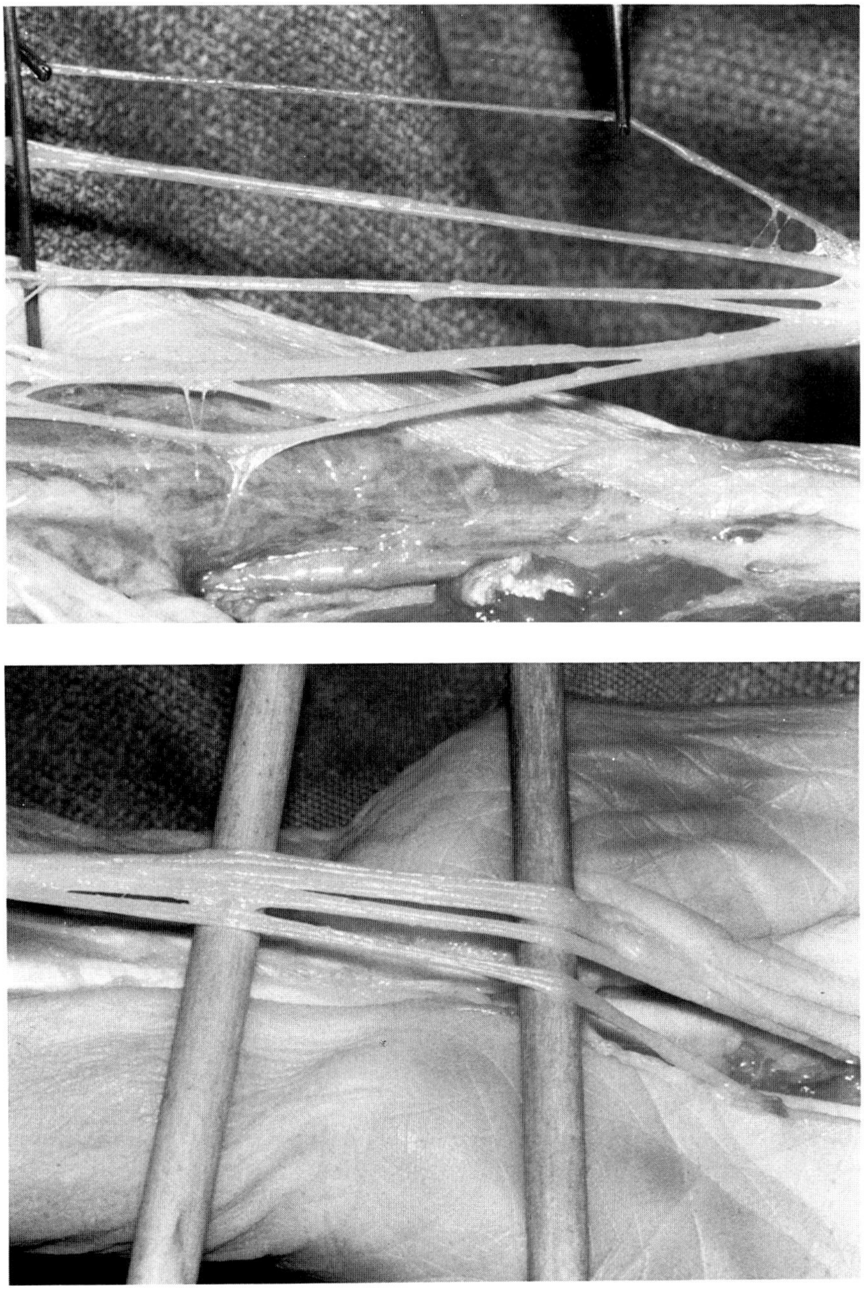

c

d

Figure 1-8 (*continued*) **c.** A closer view of the internal anatomy of the median nerve in the proximal forearm demonstrates less plexus formation. **d.** In the median nerve, just proximal to the wrist, there is little plexus formation and the fascicles run parallel to each other with few interfascicular communications.

Brushart[23] followed the course of digital nerve fibers in a distoproximal direction along the extremity. These two studies demonstrated that fibers were well localized over long distances. These microanatomic studies combined with the neuroanatomic studies support the feasibility of operating within the nerve at least in the distal part of the extremity and provide the anatomic basis for internal neurolysis (Chapter 5) and for improved results after nerve repair in the distal portion of the extremities.

Physiology of the Peripheral Nerve

Blood–Nerve Barrier

There exists in the peripheral nerve a barrier system that functions similarly to the blood–brain barrier. There are two anatomic sites for this barrier, the internal layers of the perineurium and the endothelial cells of these endoneurial microvessels.[24] Tight junctions exist between these endothelial cells and unlike endothelial cells of the capillaries in the epineurium and perineurium are impermeable to many substances. This barrier is permeable to simple sugars. (See Chapter 14

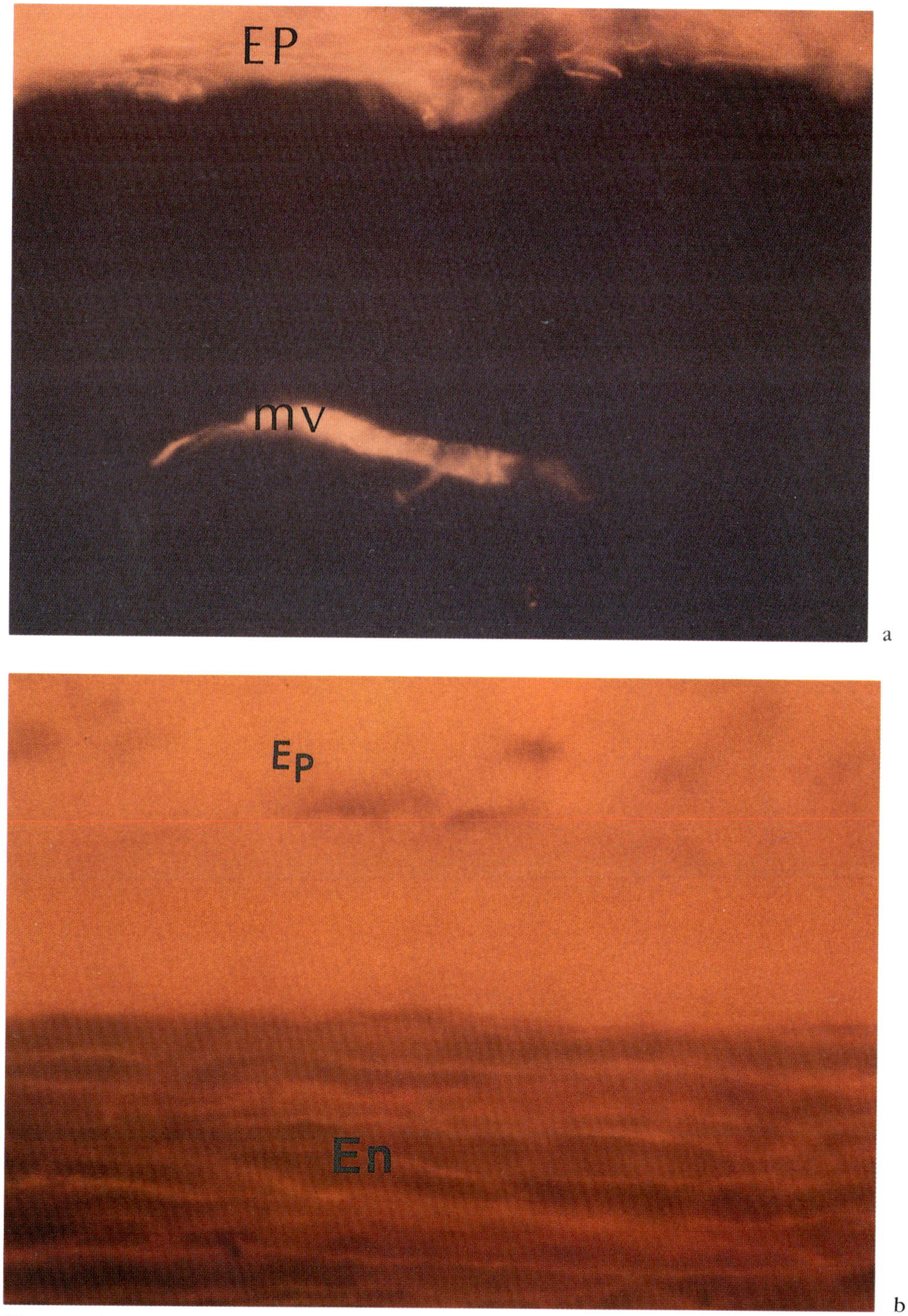

Figure 1-9a. Longitudinal section of the sciatic nerve after intravenous injection of Evans blue albumin. Bovine albumin is mixed with 1% Evans blue. The Evans blue albumin complex emits a bright red fluorescence, permitting histologic localization of the tracer. In this normal sciatic nerve, the fluorescence tracer is confined to the microvessel (mv). EP: epineurium. (×704.) **b.** Nerve injection injury. A breakdown in the blood–nerve barrier is noted. The fluorescence tracer has passed from the epineurium (EP) through the perineurium and through the endoneurial (EN) microvessels into the endoneurial environment. Nerve fibers are outlined by the fluorescence tracer within the endoneurium. (×704.)

for relevance of this point to diabetic neuropathy.) This blood–nerve barrier maintains the internal environment of the peripheral nerve fibers. Breakdown of the blood–nerve barrier at either of these two anatomic sites will result in loss of the normal homeostatic mechanisms.

Barrier function can be studied using fluorescence techniques and protein enzyme tracers.[24,25] If Evans blue albumin is injected intravenously, it fluoresces in a red color. This red fluorescence is normally noted outside of the outer layers of the perineurium and within the confines of the endoneurial microvessels. With breakdown in the blood–nerve barrier, the red fluorescent tracer is noted between the individual nerve fibers in the endoneurial environment (Fig. 1-9). Similarly, the protein tracer, horseradish peroxidase, when injected intravenously, is also normally noted outside the endoneurial environment and located within the endoneurial capillaries or the outer layers of the perineurium. With a breakdown in the blood–nerve barrier, the tracer is noted to leak between the endothelial cells of the endoneurial microvessels and pass between all layers of the perineurium and into the endoneurium (Fig. 1-10). The perineurium appears to be the more resistant of the two anatomic structures of the blood–nerve barrier.[26] Thus, with ischemia or trauma to the peripheral nerve, the blood–nerve barrier may leak initially at the site of the endothelial cells of the endoneurial microvessels and fluid may leak into the endoneurial space between the endothelial cells of the endoneurial capillaries. This will result in endoneurial edema and an increase in the endoneurial fluid pressure. As the intrafascicular edema increases, so does the intrafascicular endoneurial fluid pressure and a type of compartment syndrome may develop within the environment of the peripheral nerve. Such a scenario has been suggested in several neuropathies and with nerve compression (See chapter 14, "Diabetic Neuropathy"). Thus, nerve compression develops from the inside out as well as the outside in.

Studies of blood–nerve barrier function have demonstrated a breakdown in the blood–nerve barrier after nerve repair and nerve grafting techniques,[27] with nerve injection injuries,[28–31] acute and chronic nerve compression[32,33] and transiently (up to 3 days) after internal neurolysis. The role of the blood–nerve barrier as a potential barrier for immunologic reactions has recently been suggested.[34] Association between disease proc-

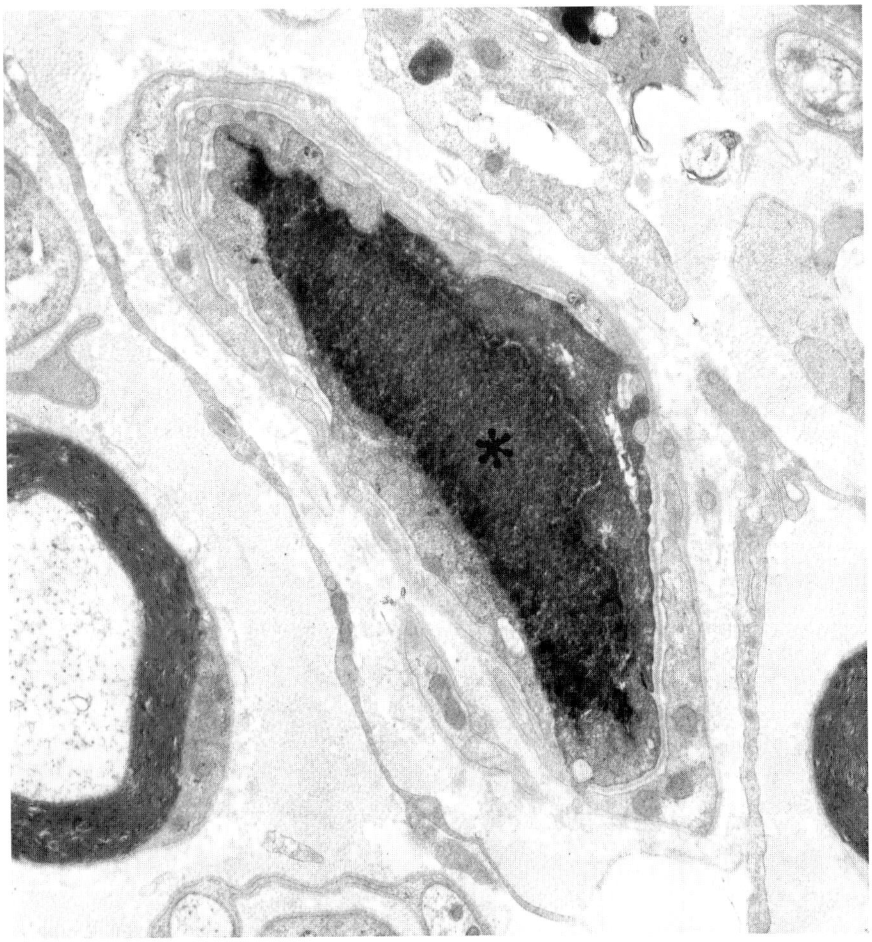

Figure 1-10a. Transverse section of normal rat sciatic nerve. The horseradish peroxidase produces a black reaction product that is electron dense and can be seen by electron microscopy. In these sections uranyl acetate is not used in counterstaining of the tissues so that the enzyme granules can be well seen against the background tissues. The horseradish peroxidase is confined to the lumen of the endoneurial microvessel (*). (Uranyl acetate, × 10,468.) a (*Figure continues.*)

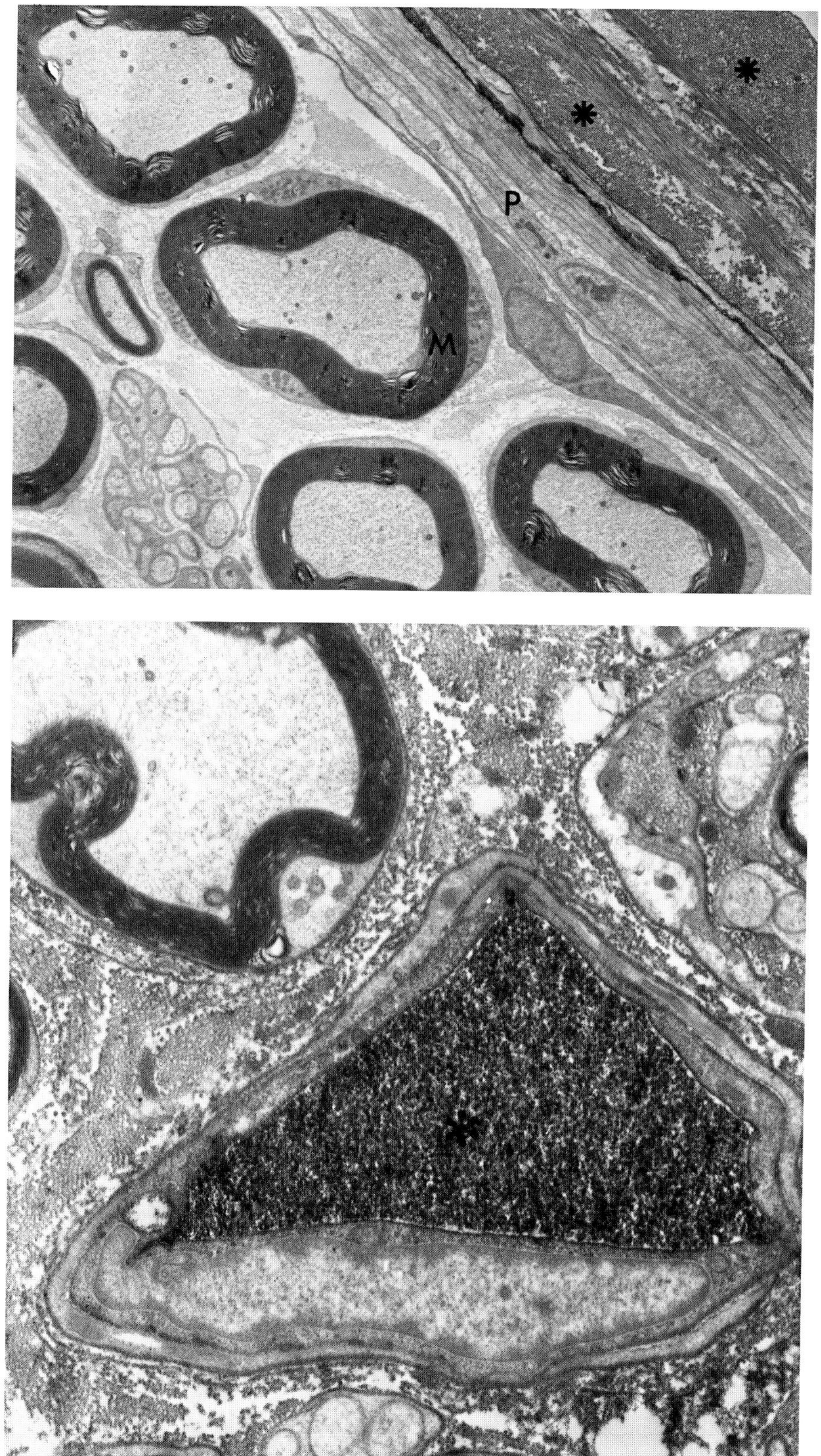

b

c

Figure 1-10 (*continued*) **b.** Transverse section of normal rat sciatic nerve after intravenous injection of horseradish peroxidase. The horseradish peroxidase is noted to be outside the outer layers of the perineurium (*) P: perineurium; M: myelin. (×8139.) **c.** Transverse section after nerve injury demonstrating a breakdown in the blood–nerve barrier. The horseradish perioxidase is no longer confined to the lumen of the microvessels (*) but now is seen staining the collagen in the endoneurium between the nerve fibers (compare the endoneurial collagen staining with Figure 1-10a.) (×10,468.)

esses and disturbances of the immune system is well documented in the central nervous system. Experimental allergic encephalomyelitis is the prototype of the immune disorders.[35] Normally, the central nervous system has no lymphoid structures and the blood–brain barrier prevents antibody or antigen entering into the nervous system. If the blood–brain barrier is broken (for example, with inflammation or injury), components that facilitate both humoral and cellular response are allowed access to the central nervous system. An imbalance between T-cell (cellular immunity) and B-cell (humoral immunity) function has now been shown to be responsible for many neurologic disorders (for example, multiple sclerosis, Guillain-Barré polyneuritis, viral encephalitis, poliomyelitis, and myasthenia gravis).[36]

The potential role of the immune system in nerve regeneration remains to be evaluated. During nerve injury and repair, the blood–nerve barrier is breached and possibly an immunologic barrier is breached as well. Although there is a lymphatic capillary network present in the epineurium, it is not in communication with the perineurial and endoneurial spaces. The epineurial lymphatic network is drained by channels that accompany the arteries making up the extrinsic blood supply. There are no true lymphatic capillaries inside the perineurial confines of the nerve fascicles or within the endoneurial spaces. The perineurium provides a strong barrier function to disease and infective processes.[37]

It is postulated that with a breakdown in the blood–nerve barrier an immunologic response may be directed at the components of the peripheral nerve, thus inhibiting nerve repair and regeneration. It is suggested that nerve regeneration must always occur through an environment of immunologically reactive cells and that recovery that does occur is in spite of this immunologic response. The modification of immune or inflammatory processes by cyclosporine or other immunomodulants may potentiate nerve regeneration. This hypothesis has been investigated experimentally. Animals that had received allograft or syngeneic nerve grafts with or without cyclosporine treatment were assessed using a functional walking tract assay.[38] Significantly improved functional testing in the early postoperative period was noted in the syngeneic nerve graft group who had received cyclosporine when compared with all other groups[34] (Fig. 1-11). This improvement could be due to a primary effect of cyclosporine on

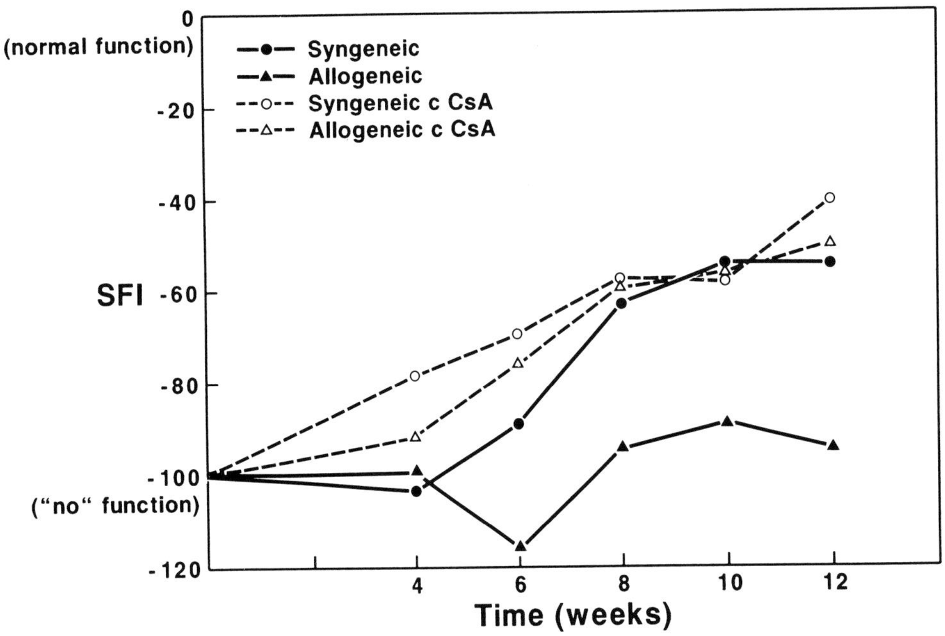

Figure 1-11. A walking track evaluation was used to assess function after various nerve grafting techniques. The sciatic function index (SFI) was calculated with −100 representing no function and zero representing normal function. In the first few weeks after the nerve grafting techniques, it was the syngeneic graft treated with cyclosporine that demonstrated the best recovery of sciatic nerve function, significantly better than that demonstrated with syngeneic grafts treated without cyclosporine (syngeneic represents a graft from an inbred strain of rat to another rat of the same immunologic make-up; thus, it is akin to an autograft situation). An allograft represents a graft from one inbred strain to an entirely different inbred strain. In this instance, the inbred strains were histoincompatible. (Reproduced with permission from Bain et al.[34])

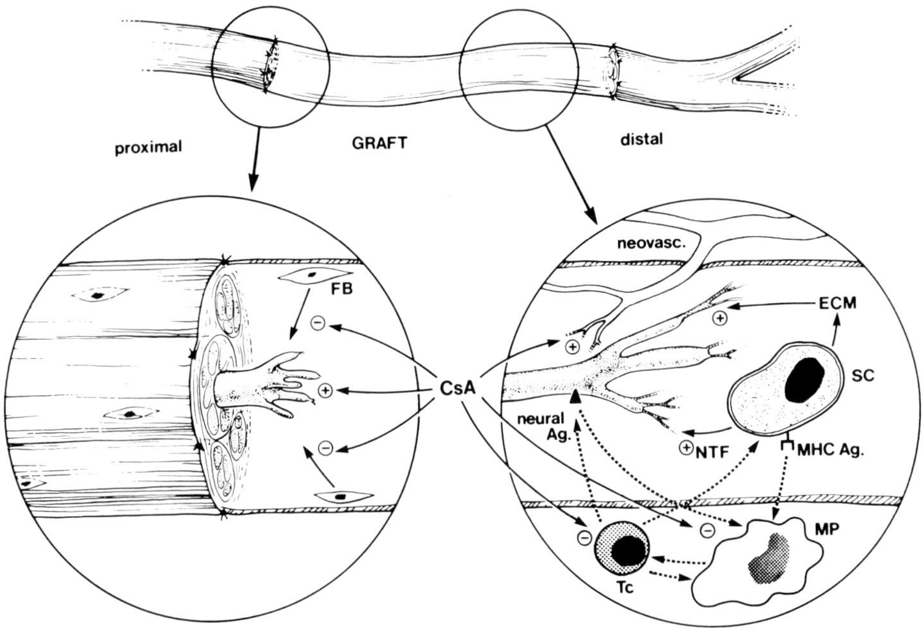

Figure 1-12. Possible sites of action of cyclosporine on nerve regeneration across allogeneic and syngeneic nerve grafts. Cyclosporine may promote nerve regeneration across the suture lines by inhibiting wound healing and fibroblasts migration. In the nerve graft cyclosporine prevents rejection of the allogeneic nerve graft by blocking the activation and proliferation of T cells sensitized to the foreign major histocompatibility complex (MHC) antigens, which mediated allograft rejection. Cyclosporine may prevent sensitization of the syngeneic nerve graft recipient to "unseen" neural antigens liberated by nerve injury, and subsequent subclinical damage to regenerating fibers. In addition, cyclosporine may promote revascularization of the nerve graft. CsA: cyclosporine; Tc: T lymphocyte; SC: Schwann cell; FB: fibroblast; MP: macrophage; ECM: extracellular matrix; NTF: neuronotrophic factor; MHC Ag: major histocompatibility complex class I antigens; neural AG: neural antigens. (Reproduced with permission from Bain et al.[34])

nerve regeneration or other factors inhibiting or promoting nerve regeneration. Cyclosporine may remove a potential inhibitory effect of the immune system on nerve regeneration by blocking the activation of a population of T cells sensitized to neural antigens not "seen" by the immune system before nerve injury.[39] Similarly, cyclosporine may have a potentiating effect on nerve regeneration by modulating the microenvironment through which the nerve is regenerating (Fig. 1-12).

Axoplasmic Transport

We have all seen clinical examples of the bidirectionally active process of axoplasmic transport, as is evident from the swelling of the nerve proximal and distal to an area of circumferential pressure. Similarly, when repairing a peripheral nerve, the outflow of axoplasm from the proximal freshly cut end of a peripheral nerve has been noted.

Although the concept of axoplasmic transport is relatively new, the suggestion that substances were transported along the axon to and from the cell body was made in the early 1900s.[40] Bodian and Howe,[41,42] in 1941, suggested that the mechanism of infection of the anterior motor horn cell by the poliomyelitis virus was via a retrograde axonal transport system. In the late 1940s, Weiss,[43,44] placing ligatures around nerves, demonstrated increasing buildup of axoplasmic materials at the ligature site with time and suggested that this corresponded to a transport rate of 1 to 2 mm/day. Weiss actually went on to suggest that such flow was responsible for supplying synaptic terminals with transmitter substances and providing the necessary material to facilitate outgrowth of axons. In a more sophisticated autoradiographic study, Droz and Leblond,[46] in 1963, followed the distribution of a labeled amino acid compound along the axon and suggested that proteins in the nucleus of the nerve cells were moved along the axons at the same rate of 1 to 1.5 mm/day.[44,45] This was followed by reports of proximodistal enzyme transfer mechanisms involving many enzymes at varying rates of transport Lubinska and Niemierko[47] and Miani[48] described a bidirectional flow along the axon at much greater rates than those described previously. It is now well established that fast and slow transport systems

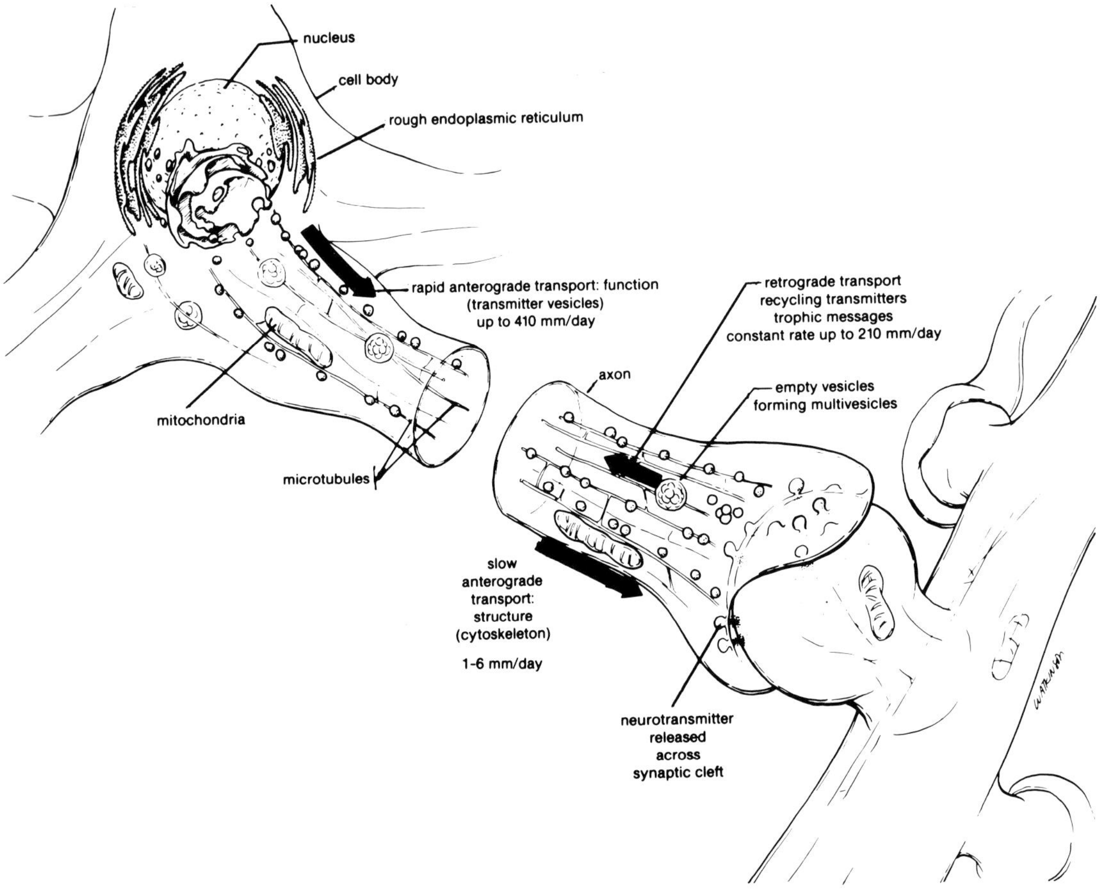

Figure 1-13. A schematic diagram of the axoplasmic transport system. Fast and slow transport systems operate in an anterograde direction. A fast transport system acts in a retrograde direction. The slow anterograde transport system plays a structural role carrying building blocks for the cytoskeleton, whereas the fast transport system is involved with transmission of vesicles carrying neurotransmitters and substances that play a functional role. Recycled neurotransmitters are transported in a retrograde fashion. It is postulated that tropic factors are also transmitted along the axon with this retrograde transport mechanism.

operate in a proximodistal or anterograde direction and a fast transport system in a distoproximal, or retrograde direction (Fig. 1-13).[49]

Anterograde transport moves at two rates. The slow axonal transport system carries proteins and provides the major structural skeleton for axon (tubulin, microtubules, neurofilaments, microfilaments, and actin).[50] Material synthesized in the cell body that has a structural function moves at this slow rate of about 1 to 6 mm/day. Materials that have a functional role at the nerve fiber terminals, such as neurotransmitters, or are necessary to reconstitute plasma membrane (lipids or glycoproteins) move at a rapid transport rate of up to 410 mm/day.[51]

The rate of retrograde transport is constant and generally less than that described for anterograde transport (up to 240 mm/day).[47,51,53] Recycled neurotransmitter vesicles are transported from the axon terminals. Ochs[54] has suggested that this retrograde transport system serves as a feedback mechanism to control the level of activity of the cell body. It is postulated that "trop(h)ic" factors are also transmitted along the axon.

Two theories have been postulated to account for the mechanism of axonal transport. Droz has suggested that movement occurs along a continuous system of smooth endoplasmic reticulum.[51]

Ochs[54] and Schmitt and Sampson[55] have suggested a second mechanism of transmission involving microtubules as a transport filament. They suggest that mitochondria, small molecular proteins, and enzyme synaptic vesicles attach to the filaments and are transported along the axon using ATP-dependent metabolism. It is generally held that it is the second microtubule mechanism that is operative in axonal transport.[54] Vesicles containing neurotransmitter substance are manufactured in the Golgi apparatus of the cell body. These vesicles then attach themselves to the microtubules and are transmitted along the microtubules. Distally at the synaptic terminal after the transmitters have been released, the surplus membrane is organized into larger vesicle packages and transported in a proximal direction for degradation by lysosomes in the cell body. A single microtubule is capable of transmitting substances in both an anterograde and retrograde direction. This movement is adenosine triphosphate (ATP)-energy dependent. Mitochondria move at a noncontinuous rate in both directions along the microtubule to meet the energy requirements of transport.

It has been postulated that sidearm ATPase proteins along the microtubule surface are capable of changing shape or position, attaching to the vesicle, and moving the vesicle along the microtubule.[50]

During nerve regeneration, it is not clear whether the actual rate of axonal transport is increased. Varying studies have suggested an increase, decrease, and no change in axonal transport rate with nerve regeneration. It is more likely that the actual amount of material transported increases or the composition of the transported protein changes during regeneration rather than that the actual rate of transport is altered.[56]

The role of axoplasmic transport in the transmission of "trophic" substances has been suggested by several investigators. Black[57] has demonstrated trophic factors in the development of the sympathetic cervical ganglion and Levi-Montalcini's Nobel Prize winning work (1986 award) suggested trophic interactions in the development of the ciliary ganglion.[58]

The importance of axonal transport has been established for maintenance of the structure of the nerve fiber and also for the functional aspects of neurotransmission. It is most likely that the mechanism for the trophic effects of nerve on sensory and motor target end organs is dependent on axonal transport. Demonstration of the release of materials along the axon as well as at axonal terminals suggests a role in nerve fiber-to-nerve fiber communication as well.[59]

Neurotrop(h)ism, Contact Guidance

In 1898, Forssman[60] noted that peripheral nerves would regenerate across small gaps. He attributed this influence to neurotropism. The concept was popularized by Ramón y Cajal,[61] who postulated that chemical agents, possibly myelin or Schwann cells from the distal stump, would "attract" nerve sprouts from the proximal stump. The work of Weiss[62,63] in the 1940s placed the concept of neurotropism into disrepute in favor of contact guidance.

Weiss agreed that nerves would regenerate across short nerve gaps but suggested that this was not due to any attraction of the distal stump from the proximal stump or any neurotropic effects. He suggested that this was related to the ability of regenerating nerve fibers to reach the distal nerve stump because of contact guidance along the tissues that surrounded the nerve ends and not because of chemical or tropic factors released distally from the nerve. In a series of classic multiple choice experiments using Y-shaped arteries (abdominal aorta with the iliac bifurcation) Weiss showed that "in no cases were the regenerating nerves attracted towards the peripheral nerve fragment but the fiber stream divided itself more or less evenly regardless of the kind of destination awaiting them." This work was further presented to support the concept of contact guidance rather than neurotropism. It is interesting to note that the silver stain used to assess nerve regeneration in Weiss and Taylor's[62] work was not appropriate for either quantitative or ultrastructural assessment of nerve regeneration. As well, most certainly the presence of the aortic allografts used as the Y channels obscured nerve regeneration because of the immunologic response directed at the vascular allografts.

Very recent work has demonstrated conclusively that neurotropism does exist and that there is a high degree of specificity associated with this neurotropism. Target-specific nerve regeneration has been documented at various levels of tissue, fascicular, and end-organ specificity. The proximal stump of a peripheral nerve will discriminate between nerve and other tissue (tissue specificity, such as nerve versus tendon). This has been demonstrated in both the rat and the primate model[64,65] (Fig. 1-14). Studies to investigate end-organ specificity (such as motor nerve regeneration toward sensory versus motor nerve) have demonstrated that this degree of specificity also exists.[66] Seckel et al[67] have demonstrated that a fascicle mediating sensory and motor function to one anatomic region can discriminate between a distal fascicle specific to that region and a fascicle specific to another region (fascicular specificity, for example, posterior tibial versus peroneal nerve). The peroneal nerve, when placed in the proximal limb of a Y chamber, will grow preferentially by a ratio of 2 to 1 to the appropriate distal peroneal fascicle when presented with distal nerve choices of peroneal and posterior tibial nerve.

It has been demonstrated that a critical distance must exist between the proximal and distal nerve segments in order to appreciate the influence of neurotropism. At a very short distance (2 mm), motor tropism is not demonstrated. Axonal behavior is independent of the nature of the distal stump. With a distance of 5 mm between the proximal and distal nerves, neurotropism is demonstrated with evidence of preferential growth of motor nerve toward the distal motor nerve.[66]

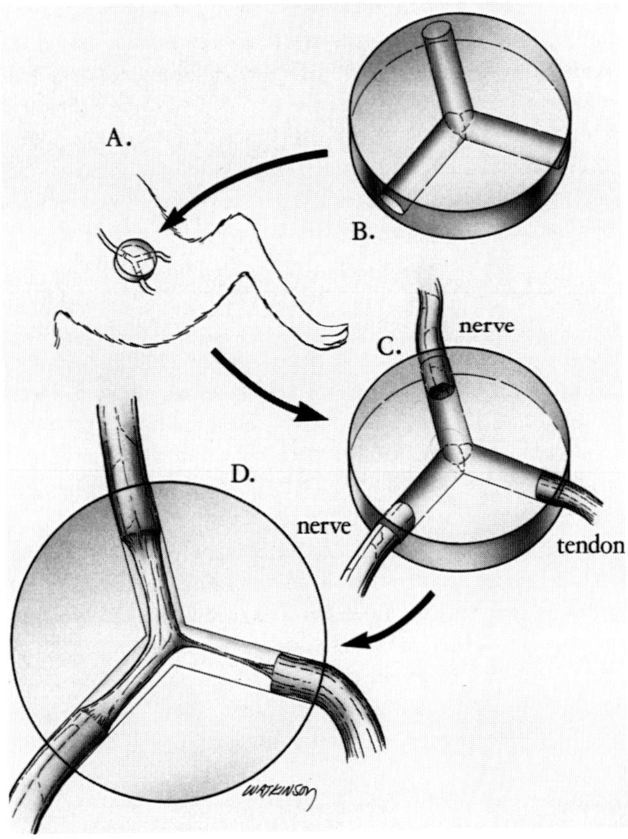

Figure 1-14. In the rat model, tissue specificity has been clearly demonstrated. In an in vivo study, when the proximal sciatic nerve is given the choice of distal nerve or tendon, it grows specifically toward the distal nerve. (Adapted with permission from Lundborg et al.[64])

Some work has also demonstrated that contact guidance is important in determining quality of axonal elongation. Williams[68] has emphasized the importance of longitudinal fibrin matrix within a nerve conduit. In an isolated chamber model of nerve regeneration, Williams demonstrated that axons would elongate along a linear fibrin matrix much more effectively than through either a randomly oriented fibrin matrix pattern or an empty chamber. Clot was first noted to impede nerve regeneration in 1915. Thus, although certainly neurotropic effects can be utilized to influence nerve regeneration, contact guidance is also important in directing fiber elongation.

The ideal nerve repair would maximize neurotropic and neurotrophic effects (neurotrophism implies an ability to influence maturation of the nerve, neurotropism, to influence direction of nerve regeneration). We coin the term "neurotrop(h)ism" to suggest influences that both facilitate fiber maturation and appropriate direction of regeneration.[69]

In standard nerve grafting or nerve repair techniques, it is the surgeon who determines the topography of the proximal and distal nerve fascicles and aligns these as he deems most appropriate. It is possible that the fascicular alignment he chooses may not be correct. Millesi[70] has stated "we always talk about the necessity to produce an exact fascicular coaptation but we also know that in many cases it is not possible at all, for example in the case of the coaptation between a fascicle group of four fascicles and a nerve graft consisting of six fascicles. After such a procedure, one is always left a little disappointed." Brushart's[66] important work has demonstrated that a critical distance must exist between the proximal and distal ends of the nerve in order to allow neurotropism to exert its effect. We may see, in the future, that our surgical repairs make use of the properties of nerve regeneration described herein (Chapter 20).

Nerve Injury and Regeneration

After simple division of a peripheral nerve, complex changes occur in the nerve cell body, in the proximal segment of the nerve, at the site of the nerve injury, in the distal segment of the nerve, and in the distal endings of both muscle end-plates and sensory receptors. Basic understanding of these various changes is critical for both the timing and the technique of nerve repair. No doubt a better understanding of the intricacies of nerve regeneration would produce improved functional results after nerve repair.

Nerve Cell

After interruption of its axon, the nerve cell responds in a predictable fashion. The responses seen in the dorsal root ganglion cell body or the anterior horn cell are identical. Changes are noted in the cell body as early as several hours after the injury. The process of chromatolysis has been well described and consists of a slight increase in the size of the cell body as it assumes a more rounded appearance. Breaking up of the Nissl substance is noted and the nucleus migrates from the center of the cell to the periphery. An increase in ribonucleic acid (RNA) occurs. Protein metabolism is altered so that protein components required for regeneration of the axon are increased (such as tubulin). By contrast, production of materials required for neurotransmitter function is decreased because the efforts of the cell body are directed toward repair of the cytoskeleton of the axon.

Biochemical studies have demonstrated that after division of the axon there is a shift of the metabolic pathways away from the citric acid cycle and toward the pentose phosphate pathway.[71]

A significant increase is noted in lipid synthesis after axonal injury. This will be used to reconstitute the Schwann cell plasma membrane.

These metabolic changes will be directed toward replenishing the cytoskeleton of the damaged axon. The substances manufactured in the cell body will be transported to the level of injury, and both slow and fast components of axoplasmic transport will be utilized.[72] Although rates of these systems are not altered, the amount of material transported is increased and altered.

After nerve injury, actual death of some of the central neurons may occur.[73,74] This appears to be directly related to the proximity of the lesion to the cell body. As well, after sensory nerve division, reorganization of the somatosensory cortex of adult experimental animals has been noted.[75,76] Short-term reversible cortical changes have been noted after epidural nerve block.[76]

Proximal Nerve Segment

In 1850, Waller[77] described changes in the distal nerve of the glossopharyngeal and hypoglossal nerves of the frog after nerve transection; these changes are now called Wallerian degeneration. The identical changes occur in the proximal segment of the nerve after nerve injury and occur for a varying distance along the proximal portion of the nerve. The distance will vary directly with the severity of the injury and may extend far more proximally than one node of Ranvier. Some lesions will result in death of the cell body.[73,74] This degeneration pattern appears histologically to be identical to that seen with Wallerian degeneration but is termed "traumatic degeneration" (Fig. 1-15a,b).

Site of Nerve Injury

At the level of the nerve injury, the axons will sprout into regenerating units as early as the first 24 hours after injury. A single axon will produce multiple axons limited by the perineurium.[78] This regenerating unit appears to be the minimum functional unit for regeneration (Fig. 1-15c). Initially, the regenerating units contain only unmyelinated fibers even when the parent axon is a myelinated fiber. With time, these unmyelinated fibers become myelinated and then, as time progresses, the number of nerve fibers within each regenerating unit decreases. The decline in the number of fibers within the regenerating unit probably relates to whether or not the axon has made successful contact with a distal target end organ.[79]

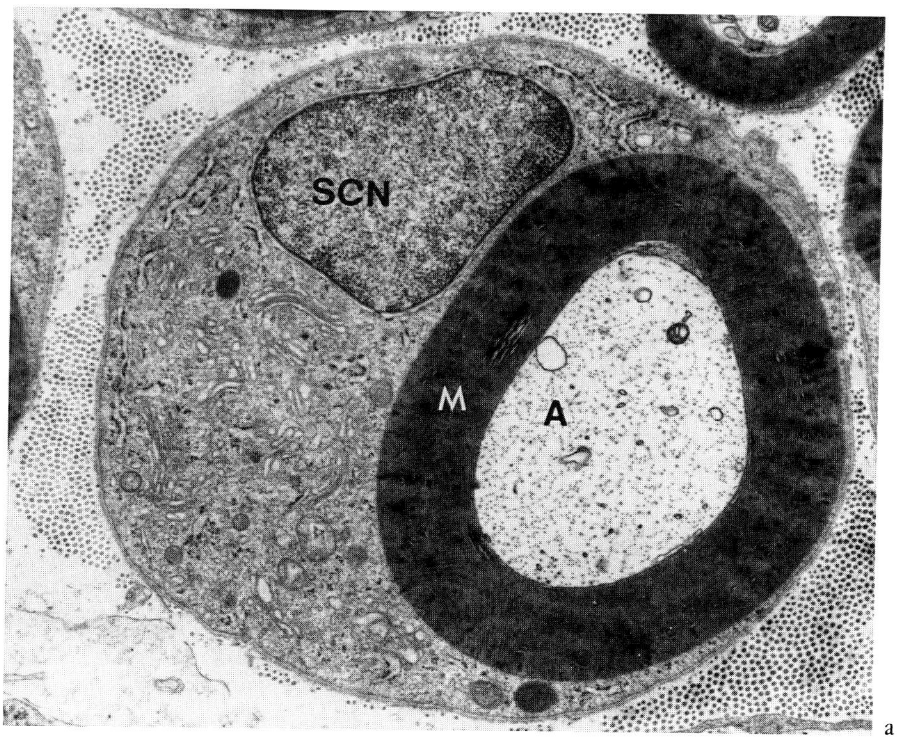

Figure 1-15a. A normal myelinated nerve fiber is noted (M: myelin; A: axon; SCN: Schwann cell) (Reproduced courtesy of Alan R. Hudson, M.B.) (Uranyl acetate lead citrate, ×13,000.) (*Figure continues.*)

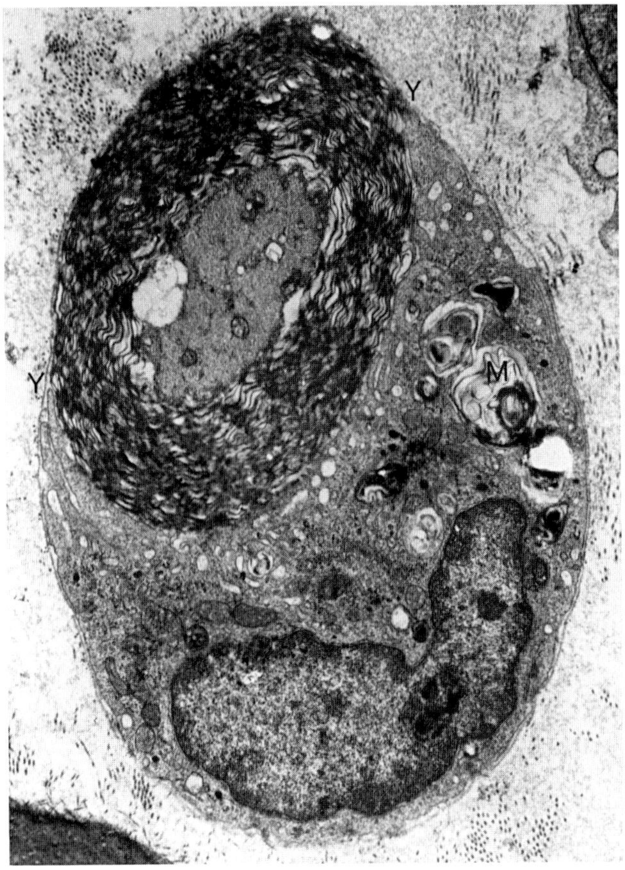

b

Figure 1-15 (*continued*) **b.** After nerve injury, Wallerian degeneration occurs. The Schwann cells proliferate and become phagocytic. Myelin and axonal degeneration are noted as well as frank areas of myelin debris. M: myelin debris; Y: endoneurium. (×20,000.) (Reproduced courtesy of Alan R. Hudson, M.B.) **c.** A classic regenerating unit containing myelinated and unmyelinated fibers surrounded by perineurium. **d.** The process of regeneration and degeneration will occur simultaneously in the distal stump. A regenerating unit is noted on the right and ongoing Wallerian degeneration with myelin debris is noted on the left.

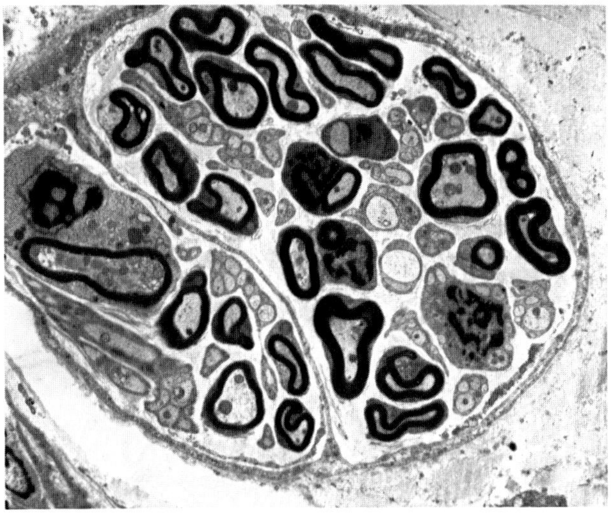

c

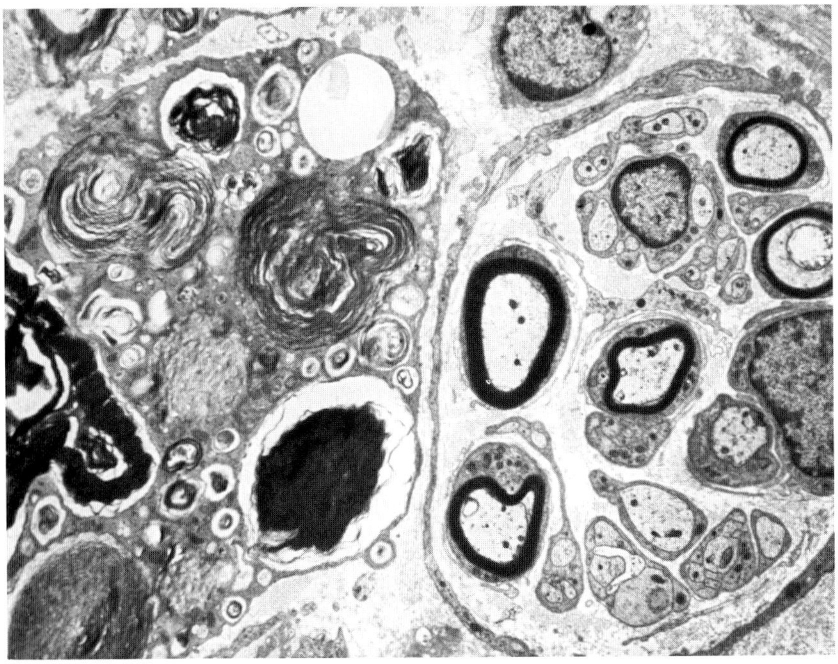

d

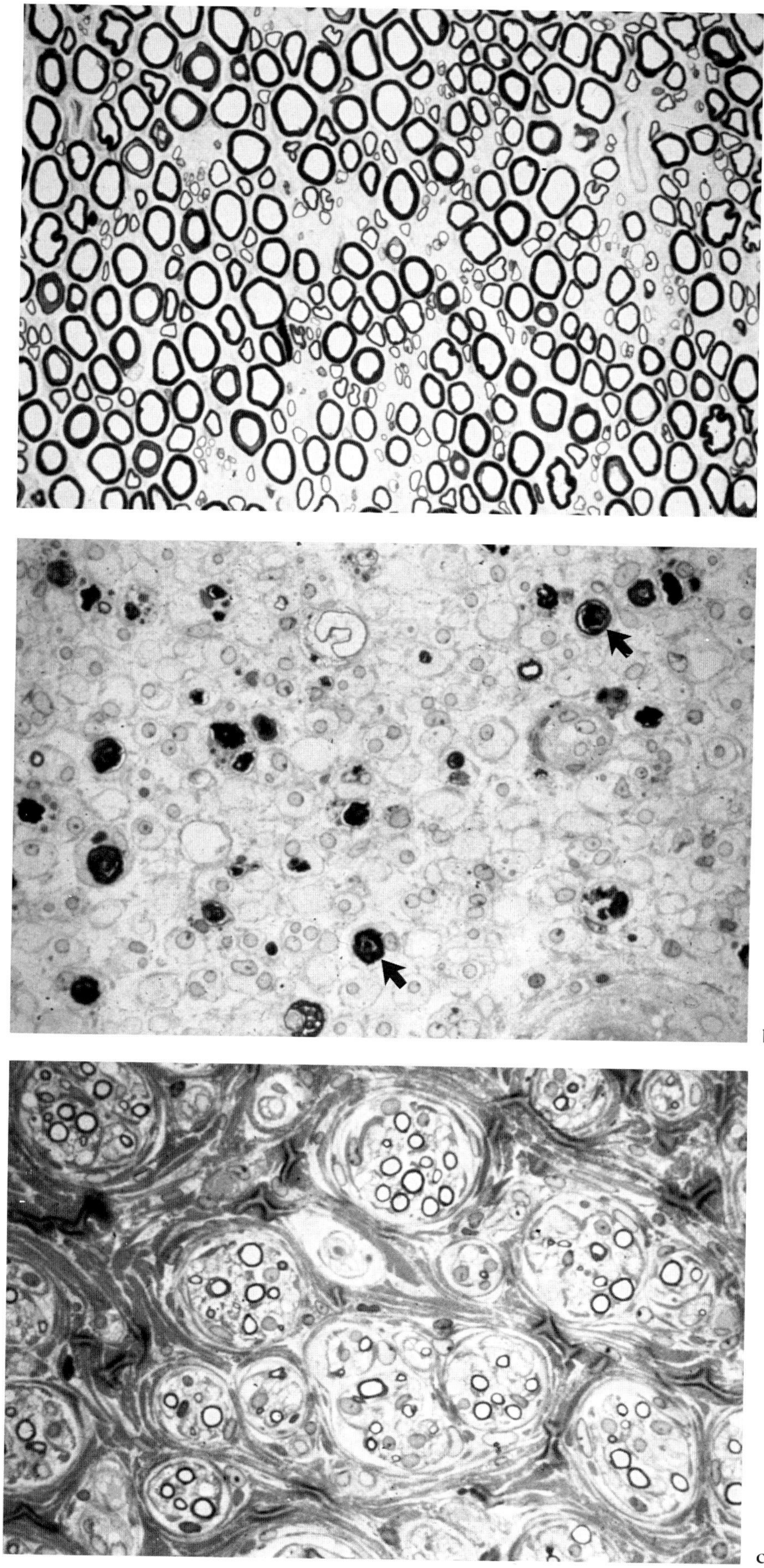

a

b

c

Figure 1-16a. A similar sequence of events is noted with light microscopy. A population of well-myelinated fibers is noted in the proximal normal nerve. (Toluidine blue, ×588.) **b.** After nerve transection, Wallerian degeneration is noted in the distal nerve, with areas of myelin debris (arrows) noted within a population of cells, which are determined by electron microscopy to be Schwann cells. (Toluidine blue, ×588.) **c.** Each nerve fiber will sprout into a regenerating unit. A field of regenerating units is noted. (Toluidine blue, ×588.) *(Figure continues.)*

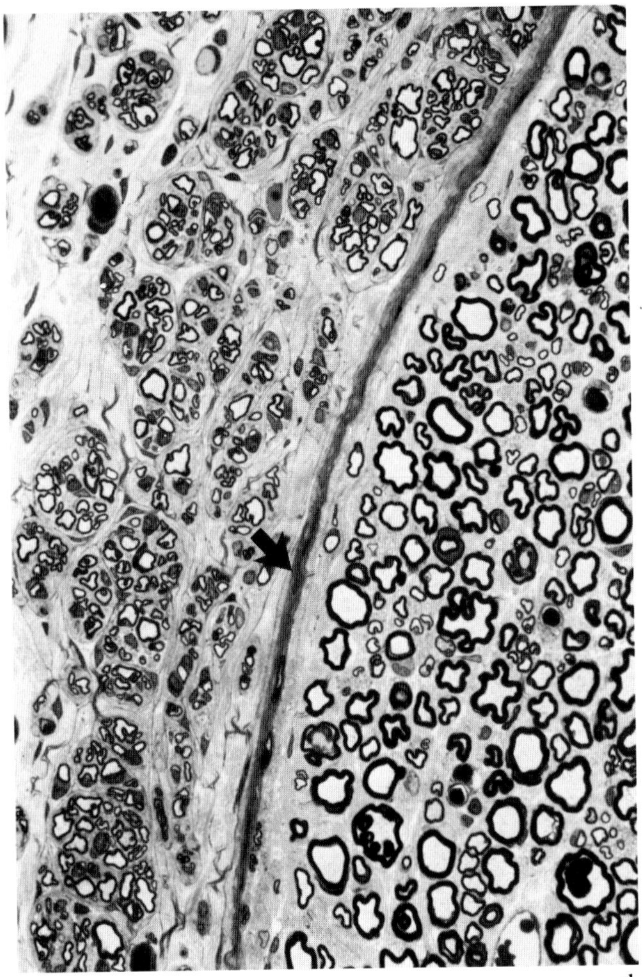

d

Figure 1-16 (*continued*) **d.** Just distal to a nerve repair, a population of well myelinated fibers is noted within the nerve (right). In the extraepineurial space (left), a population of regenerating units is noted. These units represent both lost function and potential pain as a suture line neuroma. Arrow: epineurium. (Toluidine blue, ×588.)

When these regenerating units reach the distal nerve and appropriate distal receptors, functional recovery may be realized. If the regenerating units are lost in the extraepineurial environment, then a neuroma will be formed (Fig. 1-16). This neuroma will represent potential lost function and may well be a source of neuromatous type pain.

In the distal portion of each axon sprout there is a growth cone that consists of filopodia rich in actin.[80] The tips of these filopodia will explore the distal environment and retract back into the body of the growth cone if they make no contact with a physical substrate. By contrast, if they contact a substrate to which they can adhere, they will attach to this structure and draw the entire growth cone distally toward this attachment site.[81–86] Letourneau has presented videos of growth cones that show these filopodia reaching out into an empty space making no contact, pulling back, and advancing again toward a more appropriate substrate. By this process of contact guidance, the entire growth cone is advanced along a grid of laminin. Letourneau has demonstrated that these growth cones prefer to advance along such substances as fibronectin and laminin, which are components of the basal lamina of the Schwann cell. Thus, axons will not grow into an environment that does not have some solid structures within the environment onto which the filopodia of the growth cone can attach. It would appear that the more "adhesive" the substrate is, the greater will be the number of axons that will arise from each single nerve fiber (Fig. 1-17).

It is not known how many of the fibers in each regenerating unit will potentially reinnervate distal targets and how many will deteriorate. It is not known whether the potential for maturation of nerve fibers varies in the sensory and motor systems. It is known that early on in the regeneration period, the number of nerve fibers, either in the nerve graft or in the distal nerve across the simple nerve repair, is much higher than in the parent nerve.[87] This is explained by the concept of sprouting and regenerating units, as already discussed. The previous perception that there was an actual loss of nerve fibers across a nerve repair is inaccurate.[88] Although there is certainly loss of regenerating units at the site of the repair in the extraepineurial environment because of the dramatic increase in the total nerve fibers due to the sprouting effect, there is actually an overall increase in nerve fibers that cross the nerve repair.[89] Similarly, if the number of nerve fibers are counted across a simple nerve repair, initially, an increased number of fibers are noted in the distal nerve but with time and the passage of many months, the number of nerve fibers returns to normal.[89] This would be explained by the process of sprouting and distal target contact with maturation of nerve fibers that make distal contact and deterioration of others that do not.

Distal Nerve Segment

After nerve transection, the nerve distal to the transection undergoes Wallerian degeneration. (The term "Wallerian degeneration" in actual fact pertains to the changes only in the myelinated fibers in the distal nerve). After nerve division, Schwann cells proliferate, the myelin breaks down, and the myelin debris is phagocytosed by the Schwann cells. It may take 1 to 3 months for the Schwann cells to phagocytose all cellular debris completely. Endoneurial tubes (the basal lamina of the Schwann cells) now collapse because of the phagocytosis of the myelin and axonal components inside these tubes. These endoneurial tubes are now seen as stacked processes of the Schwann cell and have been

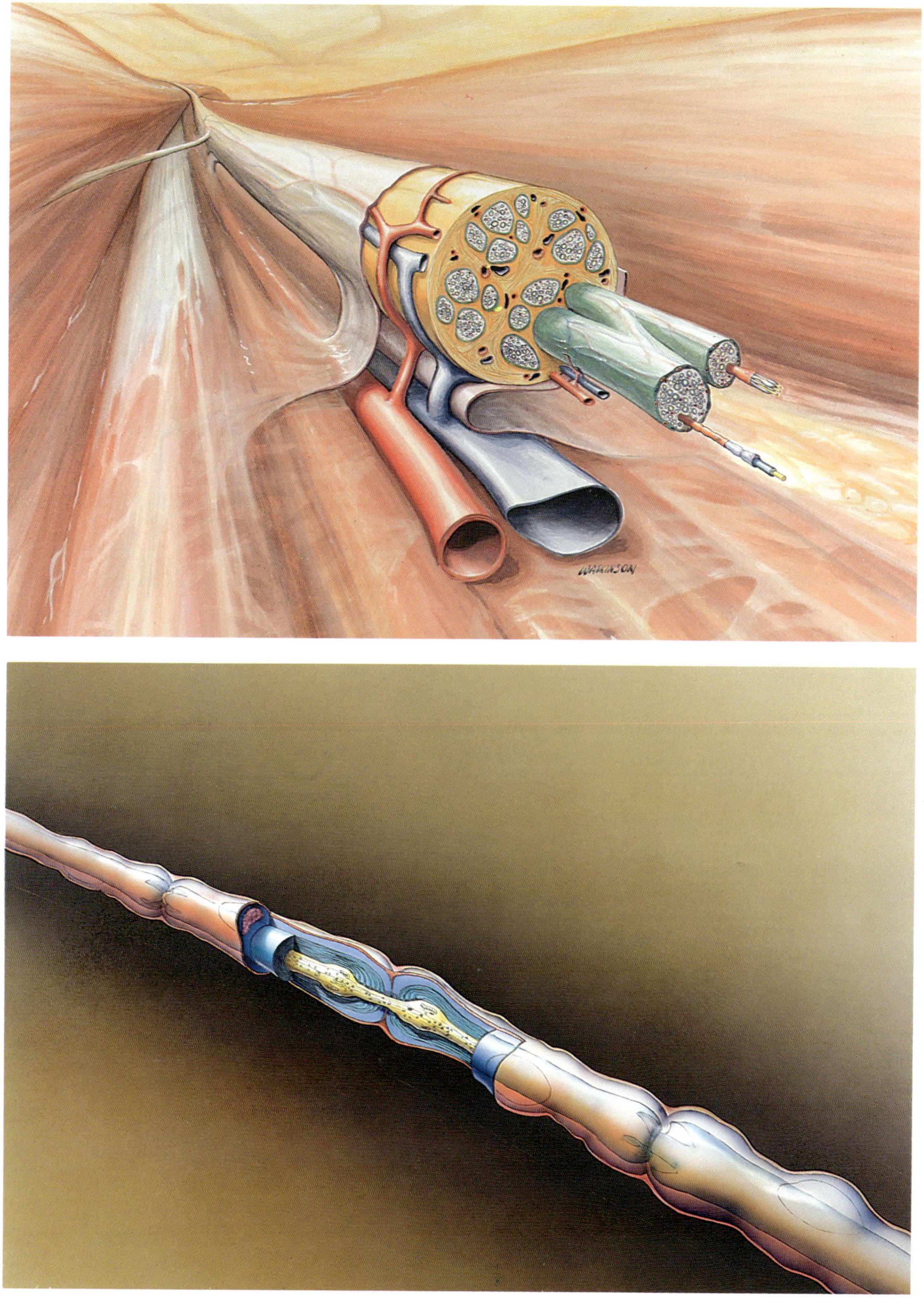

a

b

Figure 1-17. Conceptualization of the changes that occur after nerve division. **a.** The primary unit of the peripheral nerve is the nerve fiber. The segmental extrinsic blood supply and the mesoneurium are emphasized. In the extreme lower right, a single nerve fiber is shown protruding from the nerve fascicle. Plexus formation between these two fascicles is seen. **b.** A cut-away view of a single nerve fiber. Note the swelling of the axon on either side of the node of Ranvier. Axon: yellow; myelin: blue; basal lamina: orange. (*Figure continues.*)

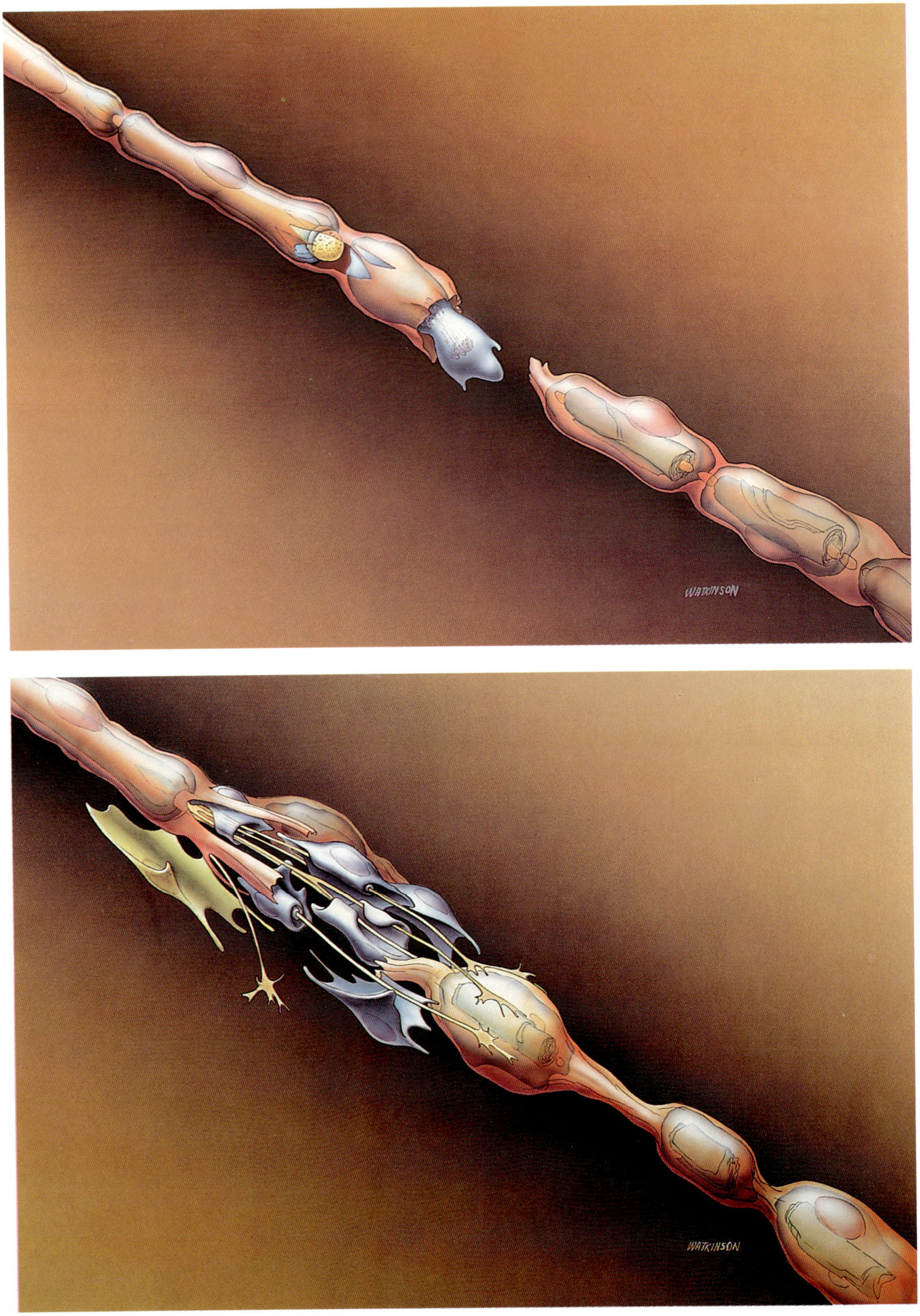

c

d

Figure 1-17 (*continued*) **c.** After division of the same single nerve fiber, Wallerian degeneration occurs distal to the division. Degeneration will also occur for a variable distance proximal to the nerve division. **d.** Although Wallerian degeneration continues distally in the nerve fiber, an attempt at regeneration occurs proximally. The single nerve fiber will "sprout" to form a regenerating unit. At the tip of each sprout is a growth cone with multiple filopodia. These filopodia will adhere to the basal lamina of the Schwann cell. The Schwann cells are intimately associated with the regenerating fibers. Schwann cells: blue; fibroblast: green; regenerating sprouts: yellow; basal lamina: orange. (*Figure continues.*)

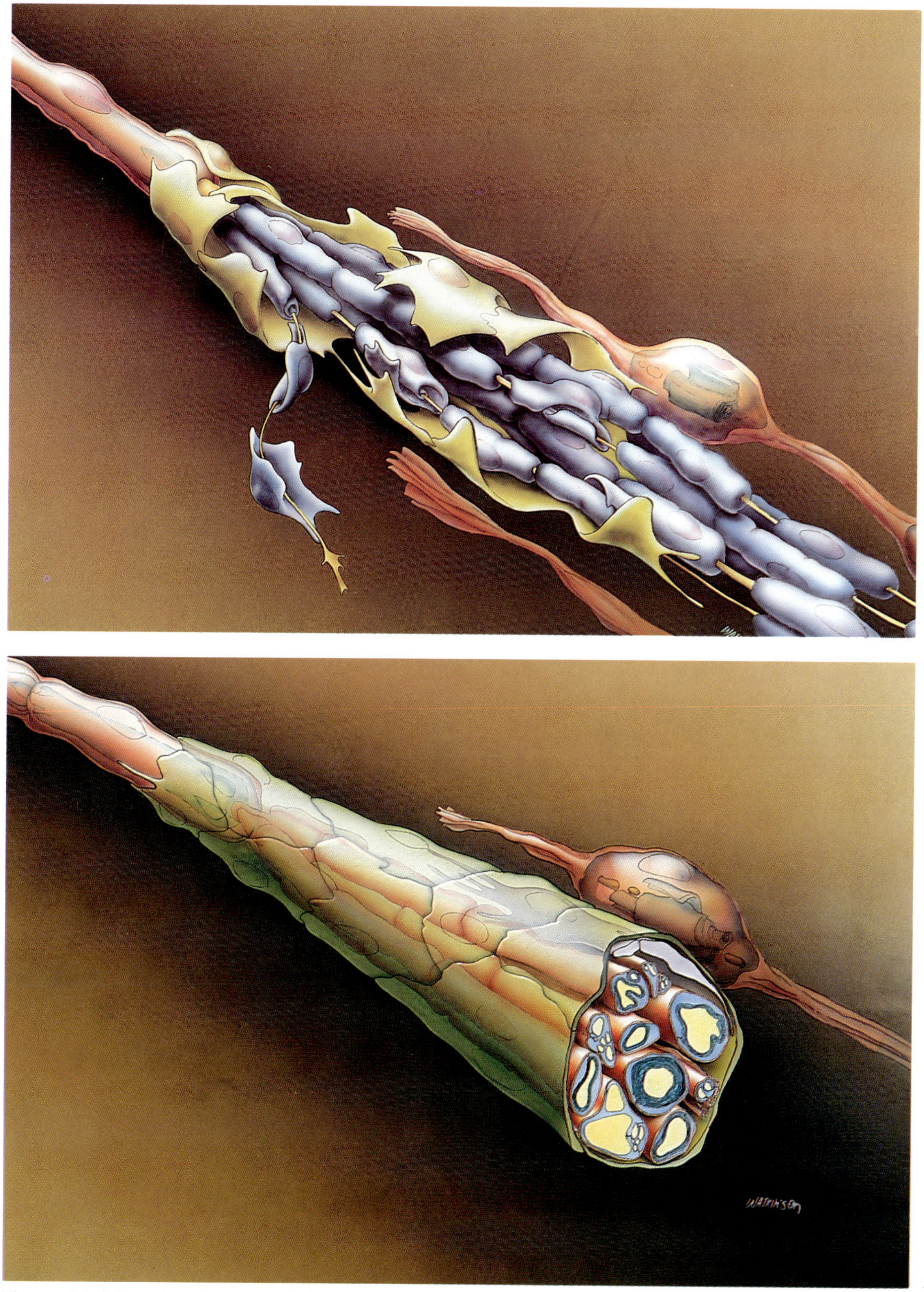

e

f

Figure 1-17 (*continued*) **e.** As the regenerating unit matures, the individual sprouts become myelinated. Regeneration occurs along the basal lamina of the Schwann cells. **f.** The "parent" single nerve fiber is noted proximally and a cut-away of the mature regenerating unit that has "sprouted" from that single fiber is seen to contain well-myelinated fibers. Basal lamina adjacent to this regenerating unit represents an area of degeneration without regeneration. (Bands of Büngner.)

called "bands of Büngner." The proliferating Schwann cells organize themselves into columns. As the axon sprouts from the proximal stump regenerate into the environment of the distal nerve, they associate themselves with these Schwann cells and regenerate between the layers of basal lamina of the Schwann cell processes. These endoneurial tubes should be considered potential tubes rather than thought of as actual empty tubes into which the nerve sprouts will grow. If the regenerating sprouts enter or travel along inappropriate tubes (for example, sensory into motor) there will be misdirection of growth, and the final functional result will not be good. The final result will depend on the number of axon sprouts that associate themselves with the appropriate Schwann cell columns and reinnervate appropriate end organs. Bands of Büngner in the distal nerve segment represent these potential endoneurial tubes that have not been re-innervated.

After nerve repair, Wallerian degeneration will occur in the distal nerve. This process will last several weeks. Fiber regeneration from the proximal stump across the repair will occur within several hours to days of the injury. In the distal nerve these two processes must be thought of as occurring concurrently (Fig. 1-15d). The axonal sprouts will regenerate down the distal segment at rates varying between 1 and 4 mm/day.

Distal Receptors

Muscle and Motor End Plates

After denervation, muscle fibers undergo atrophy. This is usually apparent several weeks after the injury. Target cells are the pathognomonic sign of neurogenic atrophy.[90] These are seen histologically to be alternating zones of dark and light staining present within the type 1 fibers. Histologically, the atrophic muscle fibers will appear in cross-section as round structures, with alterations in the location of the nucleus from its normal peripheral position to a central position.

Histochemical staining in normal muscle will demonstrate a random checkerboard arrangement of types I and II fibers, that is, a mix of physiologically fast and slow fibers. With reinnervation and collateral axonal sprouting, there will be a conversion of an entire group of muscle fibers to one histochemical fiber type rather than a mix. Thus, rather than a random mixture of types I and II fibers, there will be groupings of either type I or type II fibers noted. This grouping of one type of muscle fibers together is indicative of reinnervation.

After denervation, while the muscle fibers atrophy, the postsynaptic part of the muscle at the motor end plate is not altered. The synaptic folds are present for more than 1 year after denervation. The distribution of the acetylcholine receptors changes markedly after denervation.[91] Normally, the receptors are located in the

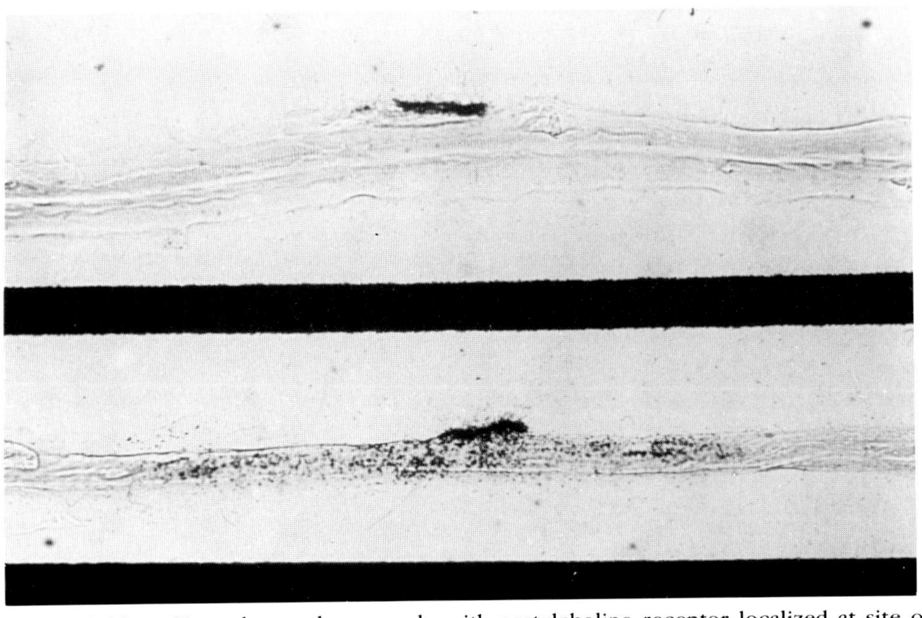

a

Figure 1-18a. Normal rat soleus muscle with acetylcholine receptor localized at site of normal neuromuscular junction. Bottom: extrajunctional sites of increased receptor activity as seen after denervation. (Alpha-bungarotoxin stain ^{125}I autoradiography.) (*Figure continues.*)

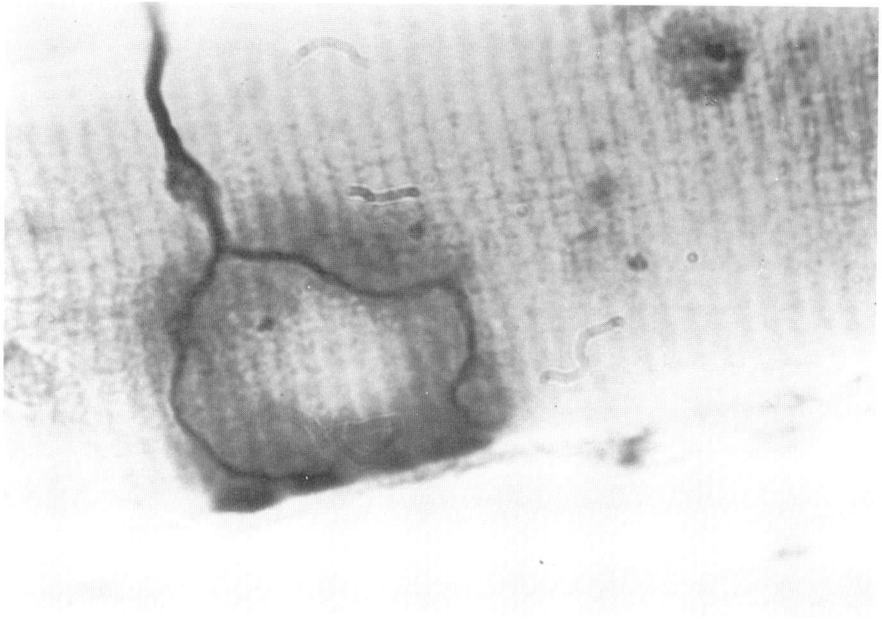

b

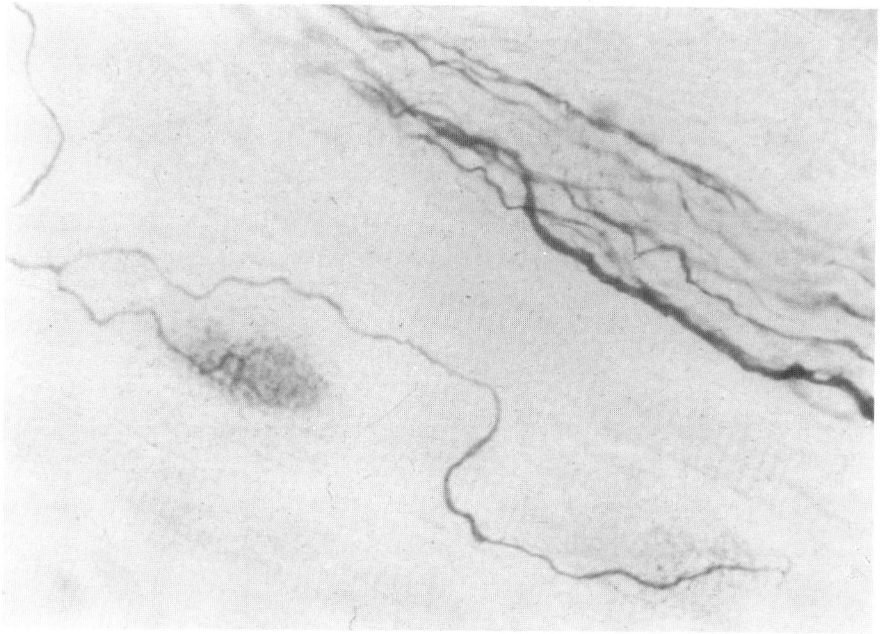

c

Figure 1-18 (*continued*) **b.** Nerve fiber innervating a normal motor end plate. **c.** A typical reinnervation pattern: thin sprouts reinnervate a former neuromuscular junction. Other sprouts approach a site of increased receptor sensitivity. For b and c: silver stain for axon, cholinesterase stain for receptor. (Reproduced courtesy of Alan Pestrunk, M.D., Baltimore.)

midportion of the muscle fiber. After denervation, there is a supersensitivity to acetylcholine along the entire length of the muscle. With reinnervation, sprouting axons will follow the original Schwann cells to reinnervate the original denervated motor end plates reforming the neuromuscular junctions. As well, axons close to the original end plates will sprout collaterally to reinnervate several muscle fibers. This will give the new picture histologically of groups of muscle fibers all of the same histochemical staining type. It is apparent, then, that it is the type of nerve that will determine the muscle type, not the converse. Thus, if a previous type I predominant muscle is reinnervated only with type II axons, the muscle will be converted to a type II muscle and vice versa.

Collateral axons will sprout to make contact with new motor end plates (Fig. 1-18). Sprouting and synapse formation will be followed by a process of synapse regression in which redundant reinnervation may be modified in favor of a predominant end-plate connection.

Skepticism remains regarding the possibility of reinnervating a denervated muscle by simply implanting the transected end of a motor nerve into the muscle (neurotization). A recent study has demonstrated that recovery of motor function will occur after this procedure, but it is not as satisfactory as that which occurs after either repair or nerve grafting of the motor nerve.[92]

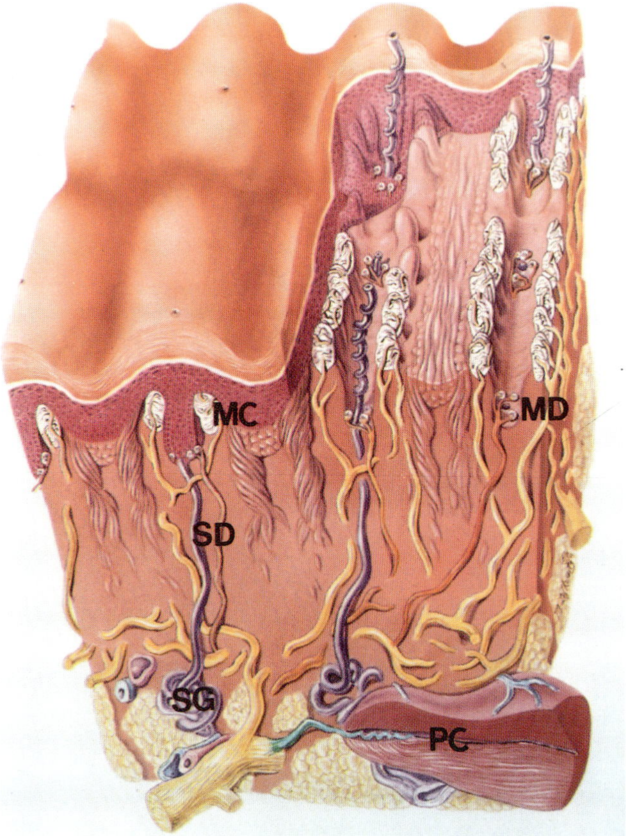

Figure 1-19. A model of distal glaborous human skin. MC: Meissner corpuscle; MD: Merkel cell-neurite complex; PC: Pacinian corpuscle; SG; sweat gland; SD: sweat duct. Note multiple innervation for Meissner corpuscles. Single innervation for Pacinian corpuscle and Merkel cell-neurite complex. Note overlapping peripheral nerve receptive fields.

Nerve regeneration is significantly altered by the environment into which axons elongate. There is no doubt that trophic factors are released by the muscle to influence nerve regeneration. If a divided sensory nerve is placed into a muscle, the axons will sprout and grow within the muscle fibers if the muscle is denervated (functional motor reinnervation does not occur).[93] If, on the other hand, the muscle is innervated, then sensory axonal growth is inhibited almost completely[94] (see Chapter 17).

Sensory Receptors

A model of distal glabrous human skin has been presented (Fig. 1-19).[95] Pacinian and Meissner corpuscles are quickly adapting fiber receptors mediating moving touch and vibration, varying from each other only in sensitivity to different vibration frequencies. The Merkel cell neurite complex is a slowly adapting fiber receptor mediating constant touch and pressure. Histologic studies have evaluated changes in sensory receptors after denervation and after reinnervation.[96,97] After denervation, these receptors undergo progressive changes (Figs. 1-20, 1-21). The non-nervous components will survive denervation for a long period of time and may be reinnervated many years after denervation (Fig. 1-22). Unlike the motor system, in which fibrosis between the motor fibers develops after 12 to 24 months and limits functional reinnervation, recovery of protective sensibility is possible even years after nerve injury. The critical time period, after which reinnervation of tactile receptors is no longer possible, has not been determined, but it has been suggested that functional sensation (two-point discrimination) decreases with a delay in repair longer than 6 months.[98,99]

In the nonglabrous hairy skin, sensory receptors for touch are located at the base of the hair folicles. The pattern of recovery of sensation in transplanted skin flaps has been documented in great detail in classic works by Davis[100] and Kredel and Evans.[101] With detailed serial examinations over many years, these investigators independently reported a pattern of recovery that would suggest that pain, touch, and temperature sensation will indeed recover to various degrees after distant transfer of noninnervated skin flaps in which all original vascular and nerve connections have been severed. They document that recovery begins proximally and proceeds distally, moving from the edges of the transferred skin into the center of the flap. These investigators were careful to distinguish between soft tissue coverage for skin flaps versus skin grafts in order to determine both the rate of recovery and the degree to which sensation recovered in skin grafts versus skin flaps. The relationship of the type of tissue to be innervated and the recipient tissue bed itself has been extensively investigated.[102,103]

Considerable work has been done on the innervation of transplanted skin flaps. There has been little work on sensory recovery in transplanted reinnervated free flaps. Review of results of toe to thumb transfers provides the largest source of material with which to evaluate the potential for sensory recovery in transplanted innervated tissue.[104] The report of sensation recovered in these toe to thumb transfers can be excellent (5 to 10 mm of static two-point discrimination). It would appear that sensory recovery will be influenced by many factors; the donor nerve, the recipient nerve in the free flap, the type and quantity of sensory end organs in the transferred tissue, and the exposure of the patient to sensory reeducation (see Chapter 18) can all potentially influence sensory recovery.

Review of a clinical case provides an interesting perspective on recovery of sensibility. In 1966, at age 26, a young man had a degloving injury to the central three digits of his right hand. At that time, it was elected to treat the injury with a flap fashioned from the hairy skin of the anterior chest wall (Fig. 1-23). When evaluated 21 years later, in 1987, he had pain-free functional sensation in the flap. The flap had been reinnervated by

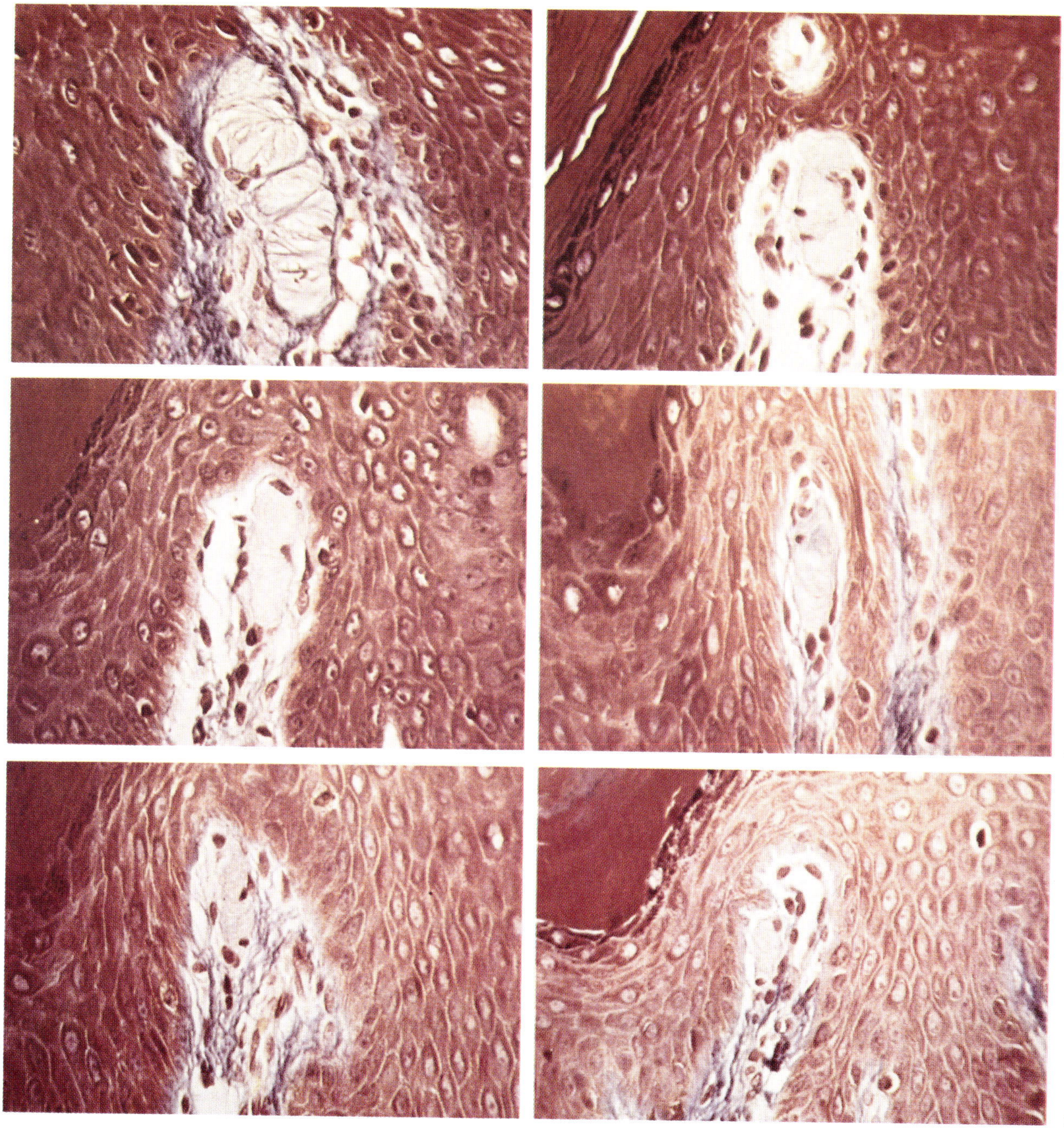

a b c d e f

Figure 1-20. Histologic analysis of denervated Meissner corpuscle. Masson trichrome stain ×160. **a.** normal. Other sections are the following intervals after denervation, **b,** 48 hours; **c,** 6 weeks; **d,** 3 months; **e,** 6 months; **f,** 9 months. **a.** The Meissner corpuscle demonstrates segmentation into multiple lobules, each of which contain lamellar arrangement of pink staining axoplasma division.

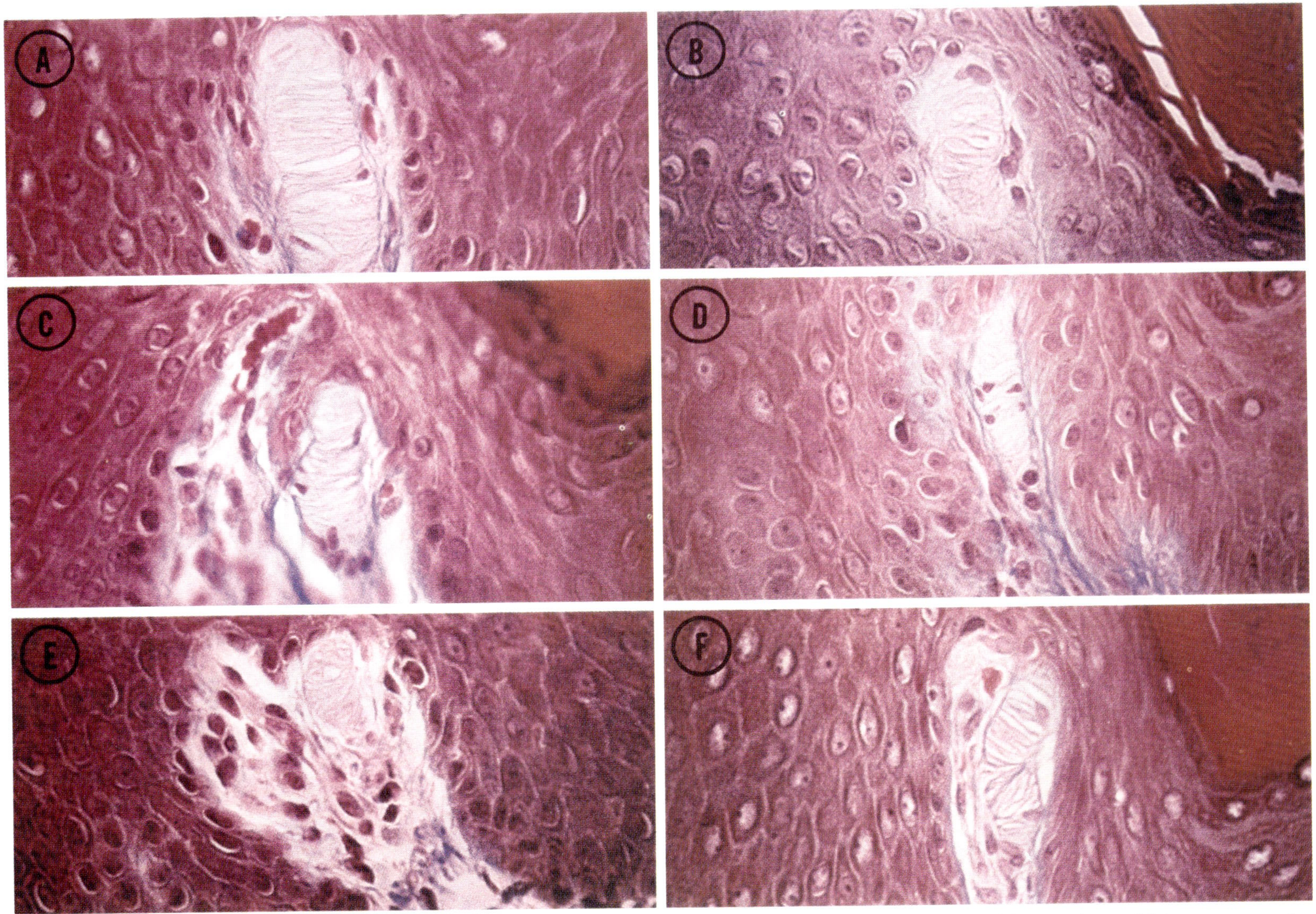

a b c d e f

Figure 1-21. Sequential histologic analysis of Meissner corpuscles after nerve repair: **a:** Preoperative control biopsy (note: Meissner corpuscle lobulated appearance and plump lamellar cells containing pink-staining material); after nerve repair (**b**) at 2 days early degeneration: loss of lobulations and lamellar detail; **c:** at 6 weeks progressive degeneration: bluish coloration as lamellar cells diminish and pink-staining material is absent; **d:** at 3 months progressive degeneration: further decrease in corpuscle size; **e:** at 6 months early reinnervation: lamellar cells become plump and pink-staining material is present; **f:** at 9 months Meissner corpuscle appears relatively normal after reinnervation process is completed. (Masson trichrome stain; original magnification, $\times 160$.) (Reproduced with permission from Dellon.[97])

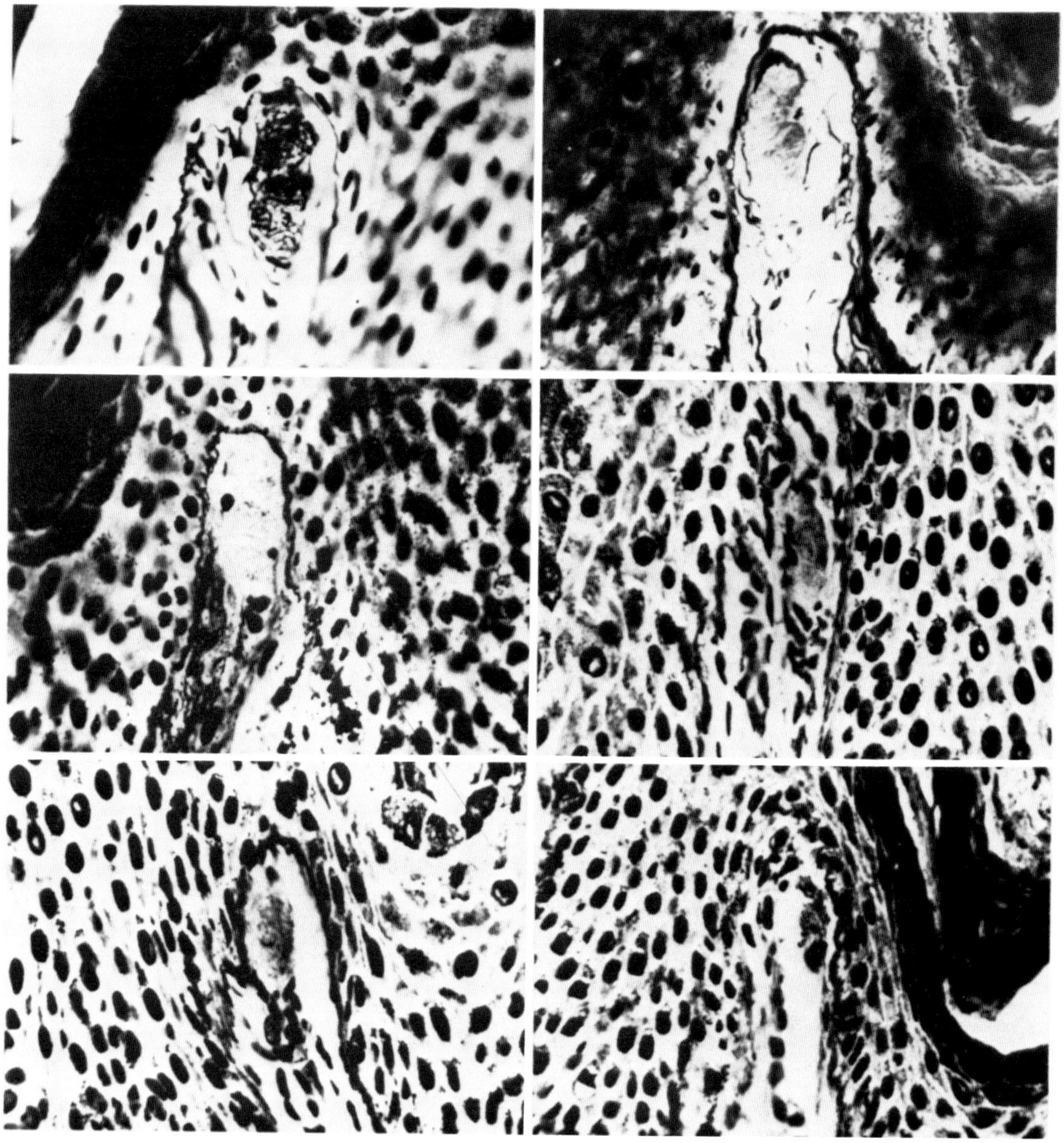

Figure 1-22. Progressive changes in the Meissner corpuscle after denervation. *Above left:* A representative normal Meissner corpuscle from a control fingertip; note the fine meshwork of nerve terminals within the corpuscle. The other photographs are of denervated Meissner corpuscle. *Above right:* Axonal fragments remain within the Meissner corpuscle at 72 hours after denervation. *Center left:* At 2 weeks. *Center right:* At 4 months. *Below left:* At 7 months. *Below right:* At 9 months after denervation, nerve terminals are absent from the Meissner corpuscle and there is a progressive decrease in the size of the Meissner corpuscle. In the last photograph (*below right*) the Meissner corpuscle remnant is adjacent to a capillary. (Silver stain, 160×.) (Reproduced with permission from Dellon, et al.[96])

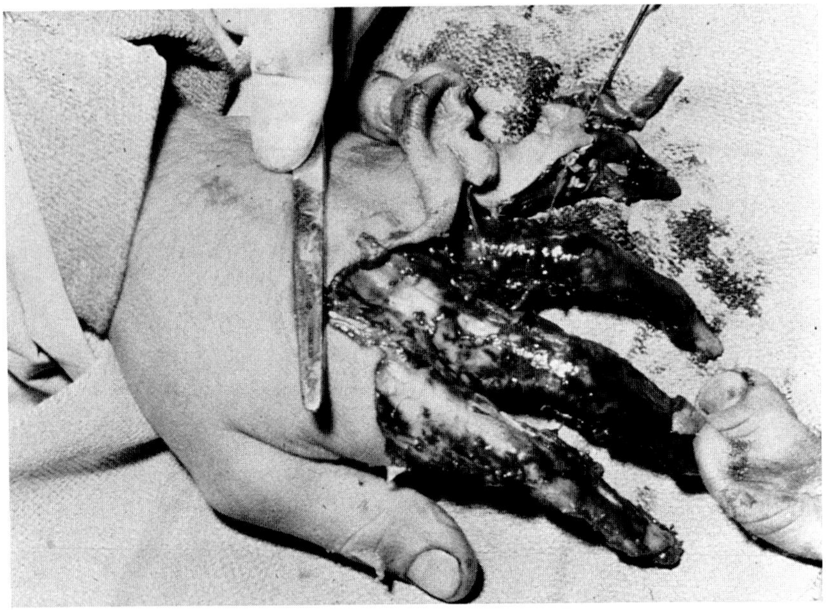

a

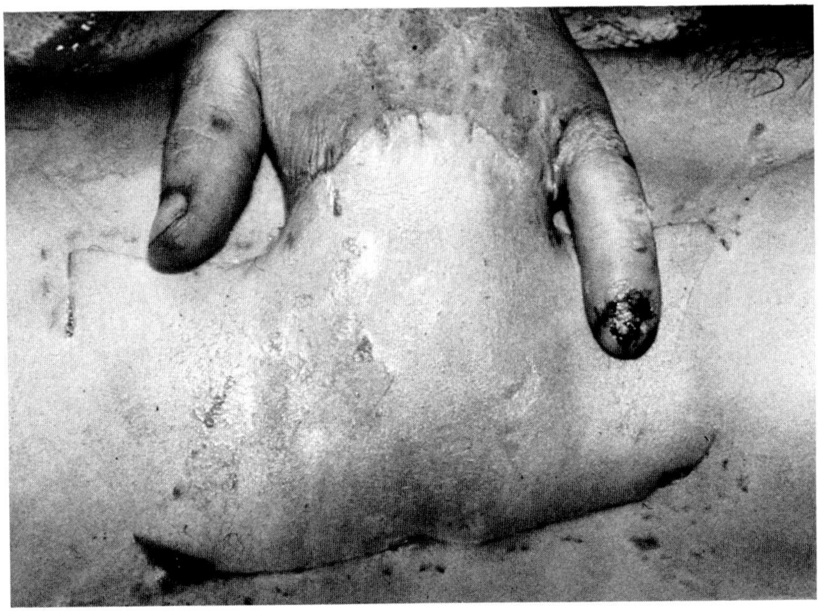

b

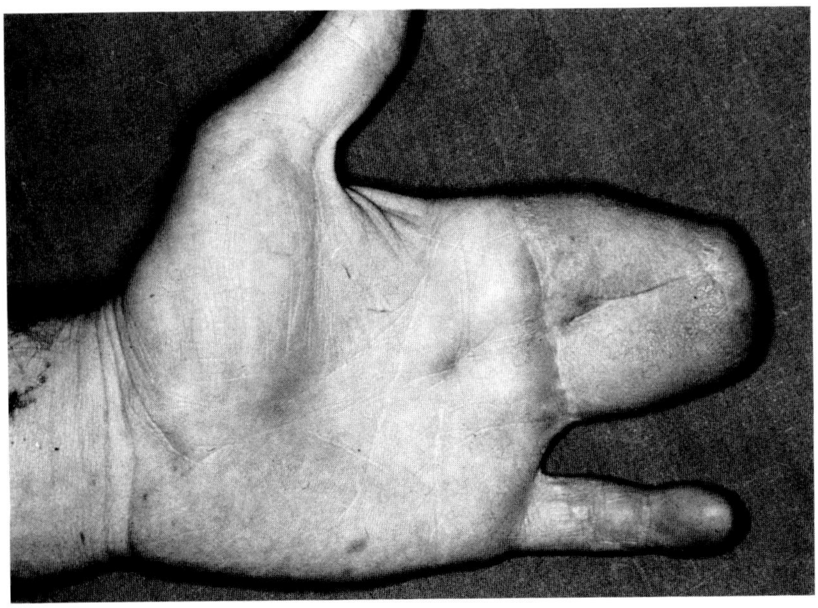

c

Figure 1-23a. In 1966, this man had a degloving injury to the right hand. **b.** This injury was managed with a chest wall flap to resurface the three central digits. **c.** When evaluated 21 years later, he had recovered excellent sensibility in the flap.

the digital nerves that previously innervated the glabrous skin of the hand. His moving two-point discrimination on the volar aspect of the flap was 8 mm compared with a moving and static two-point discrimination in the thumb of 3 and 4 mm and 5 and 6 mm in the little finger. His perception of Semmes-Weinstein monofilaments was equal to that of the normal thumb, as was his vibration thresholds. Anterior chest skin contains no Meissner corpuscles or Merkel cell-neurite complexes, the slowly and quickly adapting receptors that these digital nerves normally innervate. The functional sensation this patient recovered is mediated through reinnervation of the quickly and slowly adapting receptors (lancinate and Ruffini end organs, respectively) that exist about the base of the hair follicle, the receptor systems of the hairy skin.

References

1. Ducker TB: Pathophysiology of peripheral nerve trauma. In Omer GE, Spinner M, eds: Management of Peripheral Nerve Problems. WB Saunders, Philadelphia, 1980, p 476.
2. Sunderland S: Nerve and Nerve Injury. Churchill, Livingstone, Edinburgh, 1978, p 31.
3. Millesi H, Terzis JK: Nomenclature in peripheral nerve surgery. Clin Plast Surg 11:3–8, 1984.
4. Slingluff CL, Terzis JK, Edgerton MT: The quantitative microanatomy of the brachial plexus in man—reconstructive relevance. In Terzis JK, ed: Microreconstruction of Nerve Injuries. WB Saunders, Philadelphia, 1987, pp 285–324.
5. Lundborg G: A method for long term *in vivo* studies on the microcirculation of a peripheral nerve. Adv Microcirc 3:91, 1970.
6. Kline DG, Hackett ER, Davis GD, Myers MB: Microcirculation of peripheral nerves. J Neurosurg 42:114, 1975.
7. Noble W: Observations on the microcirculation of peripheral nerves. Bibl Anat 10:316, 1968.
8. Millesi H: The nerve gap. Hand Clin 2:651–663, 1986.
9. Lundborg G, Branemark PI: Microvascular structure and function of peripheral nerves. Vital microscopic studies of the tibial nerve in the rabbit. Adv Microcirc 1:66, 1968.
10. Lundborg G, Rydevik B: Effects of stretching the tibial nerve of the rabbit. A preliminary study of the intraneural circulation and the barrier function of the perineurium. J Bone Joint Surg 55B:390, 1973.
11. Breidenbach WB, Terzis JK: The blood supply of vascularized nerve grafts. J Reconstr Microsurg 3:43, 1986.
12. Fontana F: Taite sur le venin de la vipere sur la poisons, Americains, vol 2. Florence, 1798.
13. Clarke E, Bearn JG: The spiral bands of Fontana. Brain 95:1, 1972.
14. Sunderland S: The connective tissues of peripheral nerves. Brain 88:841, 1965.
15. Greenberg M, Leitao C, Stevens JK: Irregular geometries in normal unmyelinated axons: A 3D serial EM analysis. Exp Neurol 1988. In press.
16. Chow JA, Sunderland S, Van Beek AL: Surgical significance of the motor fascicular group of the ulnar nerve in the forearm. J Hand Surg [Am] 9:605, 1985.
17. Jabaley ME, Wallace WH, Heckler FR: Internal topography of major nerves of the forearm and hand. A current view. J Hand Surg [Br] 51:1, 1980.
18. Williams HB, Jabaley ME: The importance of internal anatomy of the peripheral nerves to nerve repair in the forearm and hand. Hand Clin 2:689–707, 1986.
19. Shizhen Z, Xiangluo T, Muzhil L: The microsurgical anatomy of peripheral nerves. In Shizhen Z, Yongjian M, Wencyun Y, eds: Microsurgical Anatomy. MTP Press, Lancaster, England, 1985, pp 299–350.
20. Sunderland S: The intraneural topography of the radial, median and ulnar nerves. Brain 68:243, 1945.
21. Dellon AL, Mackinnon SE: Segmentally innervated latissimus dorsi muscle—microsurgical transfer for facial reanimation. J Reconstr Microsurg 2:7–12, 1985.
22. Terzis JK, Feeker BL, Sismour EN: A computerized study of the intraneural organization of the median nerve. J Hand Surg [Am] 9:605, 1984.
23. Brushart TM: The central course of primate digital nerve axons. American Society for Surgery of the Hand, Scientific Session, 1985.
24. Olsson Y, Reese T: Permeability of vasa nervorum and perineurium in mouse sciatic nerve studies by fluorescence and electronmicroscopy. J Neuropathol Exp Neurol 30:105–119, 1971.
25. Olsson Y, Kristensson K, Klatzo J: Permeability of blood vessels in connective tissue sheaths in the peripheral nervous system to exogenous proteins. Acta Neuropathol [Suppl] (Berl) 5:61, 1971.
26. Lundborg G: Mechanical effects on circulation and nerve function. In Gorio A, Mellesi H, Mingerino S, eds: Posttraumatic Nerve Regeneration. Raven Press, New York, 1981, pp 157–158.
27. Bain JR, Hudson AR, Mackinnon SE, Gentili F, Hunter DA: Restoration of the blood-nerve barrier following nerve grafting techniques. Plast Reconstr Surg 1988. In press.
28. Mackinnon SE, Hudson AR, Gentili F, Kline DG, Hunter DA: Peripheral nerve injection injuries with steroid agents. Plast Reconstr Surg 69:482–490, 1982.
29. Mackinnon SE, Hudson AR, Llamas F, Dellon AL, Kline DG, Hunter DA: Peripheral nerve injury by chymopapain injection. J Neurosurg 61:1–8, 1984.
30. Mackinnon SE, Hudson AR, Bojanowski V, Hunter DA, Maraghi E: Peripheral nerve injury with purified bovine collagen—an experimental model in the rat. Ann Plast Surg 14:428–436, 1985.
31. Gentili F, Hudson AR, Hunter DA, Kline DG: Nerve injection injury with local anesthetic agents. A light and electron microscopic, fluorescent microscopic and horseradish peroxidase study. Neurosurgery 6:263–272, 1980.
32. Ryvevik B, Lundborg G: Permeability of intraneural microvessels in perineurium following acute graded ex-

perimental nerve compression. Scand J Plast Reconstr Surg 11:179, 1977.
33. Mackinnon SE, Dellon AL, Hudson AR, Hunger DA: Chronic nerve compression—an experimental model in the rat. Ann Plast Surg 13:112–120, 1984.
34. Bain JR, Mackinnon SE, Hudson AR, Falk RE, Hunter DA: The nerve allograft response in the rat immunosuppressed with Cyclosporin A. Plast Reconstr Surg 82:1052—1064, 1988.
35. Behan PO, Currie S: In Behan PO, Currie S, eds: Clinical Neuroimmunology. WB Saunders, London, 1978.
36. Arnason BGW: Idiopathic polyneuritis and experimental allergic neuritis in comparison. In Rowland LP, ed: Immunological Disorders of the Nervous System, vol. 49. Williams & Wilkins, Baltimore, 1971.
37. Larson DL, Rodin AE, Robertson DK, O'Steen WK, Rapperport AS, Lewis SR: Perineural lymphatics: Myth or fact. Am J Surg 12:488, 1966.
38. Bain JR, Mackinnon SE, Hunter DA: Functional evaluation of complete sciatic, peroneal and posterior tibial nerve lesions in the rat. Plast Reconstr Surg 1988. In press.
39. Cohen DJ, Loertscher R, Rubin MF, Tilney NL, Carpenter CB, Strom TB: Cyclosporine: A new immunosuppressive agent for organ transplantation. Ann Intern Med 101:677–682, 1984.
40. Scott FH: On the relation of nerve cells to fatigue of their nerve fibres. J Physiol (Lond) 34:145, 1906.
41. Bodian D, Howe HA: Experimental studies of intraneural spread of poliomyelitis virus. Bull Johns Hopkins Hosp 68:248–267, 1941.
42. Bodian D, Howe HA: The rate of progression of poliomyelitis virus in nerve. Bull Johns Hopkins Hosp 69:79–85, 1941.
43. Weiss P: Damming of axoplasm in constrictive nerve. A sign of perpetual nerve growth in the nerve fibres. Anat Rec 88 (Suppl):48, 1944.
44. Weiss P: Evidence of perpetual proximal-distal growth of the nerve fibres. Biol Bull 87:160, 1944.
45. Droz B, Leblond CP: Migration of proteins along the axons of the sciatic nerve. Science 137:1047, 1962.
46. Droz B, Leblond CP: Axonal migration of proteins in the central nervous system and peripheral nerves as shown by radio autography. J Compar Neurol 121:325, 1963.
47. Lubinska L, Niemierko S: Velocity and intensity in bidirectional migration of acetylcholinesterase in transected nerves. Brain Res 27:329–342, 1971.
48. Miani N: Proximal-distal movement along the axon of protein perikaryon of regenerating neurons. Nature 185:541, 1960.
49. Smith BH, Kornblith PL: Axoplasmic transport in neurological surgery. Neurosurgery 10:268–276, 1982.
50. Lasek JR, Shelanski ML, Brinkely BR, Condeelis JS, Ellisman MH, Goldman RD, Solomon F, Taylor EW: Cytoskeletons and the architecture of nervous systems. Neurosci Res Program Bull 19:1–153, 1981.
51. Droz B, Rambourg A, Koenig HL: The smooth endoplasmic reticulum. Structure and role in the renewal of axonal membrane and synaptic vesicles by fast axonal transport. Brain Res 93:1–13, 1975.
52. Edstrom A, Hanson M: Retrograde axonal transport of proteins in vitro in frog sciatic nerves. Brain Res 61:311–320, 1973.
53. Stockel K, Schwab M, Thoenen H: Specificity of retrograde transport of nerve growth factor (NGF) and sensory neurons. A biochemical and morphological study. Brain Res 89:1–14, 1975.
54. Ochs S: Basic properties of axonplasmic transport. In Dyck PJ, Thomas PK, Lambert EH, Bunge R, eds: Peripheral Neuropathy, 2nd ed. WB Saunders, Philadelphia, 1984.
55. Schmidt FO, Sampson FE: Neuronal fibres proteins. Neurosci Res Program Bull 6:113–219, 1968.
56. Lasek RJ, McQuarrie IG, Wujek JR: The central nervous system regeneration problem. Neuron and environment. In Gorio A, Millesi H, Miringo S, eds: Posttraumatic Peripheral Nerve Regeneration. Raven Press, New York, 1981, pp 59–70.
57. Black IB: Growth and development of cholinergic and adrenergic neurons in a sympathetic ganglion. In Fuxe K, Olson L, Zotterman Y, eds: Dynamics of Degeneration in Growth in Neurons. Proceedings of the International Symposium, Stockholm, May, 1973. Pergamon Press, New York, 1974, pp 455–467.
58. Levi-Montalcini R, Hamburger V: Selective growth stimulating effects of sarcoma on sensory and sympathetic nervous system of the chick embryo. J Exp Zool 116:321, 1951.
59. Schmidt FO, Dev P, Smith BH: Electronic processing of information by brain cells. Science 193:114–120, 1976.
60. Forssman J: Ueber de Ursachen welche die Wachstufstrichtung der peripheren Nervenfasern vie der Regeneration bestimmen. Beitr Pathol Anat 24:55, 1898.
61. Ramón y Cajal SR: Mechanismo de la degeneracion y regeneration de nervos. Trab Lab Inbest Biol (Madrid) 9:119, 1905.
62. Weiss P, Taylor AC: Further experimental evidence against neurotropism in nerve regeneration. J Exp Zool 95:233–257, 1944.
63. Weiss P: The technology of nerve regeneration. A review of sutureless tibulation and related methods of nerve repair. J Neurosurg 1:400, 1944.
64. Lundborg G, Danielson N, Dahlin LB, Nachensson A, Polloryd P: Tissue specificity in nerve regeneration. Scand J Plast Surg 1988. In press.
65. Mackinnon SE, Dellon AL, Lundborg G, Hudson AR: A study of neurotropism in the primate model. J Hand Surg [Am] 11:888–894, 1986.
66. Brushart TM: Selective reinnervation of distal motor stumps by peripheral motor axons. Exp Neurol 97:289–300, 1987.
67. Seckel BR, Ryan SE, Gagne JR, Tin Ho Chiu CST, Watkins E: Target specific nerve regeneration through a nerve guide in the rat. Plast Reconstr Surg 78:793–798, 1986.
68. Williams LR: Exogenous fibrin matrix precursor stimulate the temporal progress of nerve regeneration within a silicone chamber. Neurochem Res 1988. In press.
69. Mackinnon SE, Dellon AL: Reply to T. Brushart's letter on The study of neurotrophism in a primate model. J Hand Surg 12A:809, 1987.

70. Millesi H: Conclusions: Clinical science. In Gorio A, Millesi H, Mingrino S, eds: Posttraumatic Peripheral Nerve Regeneration. Raven Press, New York, 1981, p 626.
71. Ducker PB: The central body in axonal regeneration. In Gorio A, Millesi H, Mingrino S, eds: Posttraumatic Peripheral Nerve Regeneration. Raven Press, New York, 1981, pp 7–11.
72. Ochs S: Regeneration of nerve in relation to axoplasmic transport. An analysis. In Gorio A, Millesi H, Mingrino S, eds: Posttraumatic Peripheral Nerve Regeneration. Raven Press, New York, 1981, pp 115–128.
73. Horch K: Central responses of cutaneous sensory neurons to peripheral nerve crush in the cat. Brain Res 151:581–586, 1978.
74. Kristensson K: Retrograde signalling of nerve cell body resp onse to trauma. In Gorio A, Millesi H, Mingrino S, eds: Posttraumatic Peripheral Nerve Regeneration. Raven Press, New York, 1981, pp 27–34.
75. Rasmusson M: Reorganization of racoons somatosensory cortex following removal of the fifth digit. J Compar Neurol 205:313–326, 1982.
76. Metzler J, Marks PS: Functional changes in cat somatosensory-motor cortex during short term reversible epidural blocks. Brain Res 177:379–383. 1979.
77. Waller AV: Experiments on the glossopharyngeal and hypoglossal nerves of the frog and observations produced thereby in the structure of their primative fibres. Phil Trans R Soc Lond 140:423, 1850.
78. Morris J, Hudson A, Weddell G: A study of degeneration and regeneration in the divided rat sciatic nerve based on electron microscopy. Z Zellforsch Mikrosk Anat 124:76, 1972.
79. Sanders FK, Young JZ: The influence of peripheral connections on the diameter of regenerating nerve fibres. J Exp Biol 22:203–212, 1946.
80. Yamada KM, Spooner BS, Wessells NK: Ultrastructure and function of the growth cones and axons of cultured nerve cells. J Cell Biol 49:614–635, 1971.
81. Letourneau PC: Cell-to-substratum adhesion and guidance of axonal elongation. Dev Biol 44:92–101, 1975.
82. Letourneau PC: Chemotactic response of nerve fibre elongation to nerve growth factor. Dev Biol 66:183–196, 1978.
83. Letourneau PC: Cell-substratum adhesion of neurite growth cones and its role in neurite elongation. Exp Cell Res 124:127–138, 1979.
84. Letourneau PC, Wessels MK: Migratory cell locomotion versus nerve axon elongation. J Cell Biol 44:92–101, 1974.
85. Letourneau PC: Neurite extension by peripheral and central nervous system neurons in response to substratum bound fibronectin and laminin. Dev Biol 95:212, 1983.
86. Letourneau PC: Distribution of laminin in the developing nervous system of the chick. Dev Biol 98:212, 1986.
87. Mackinnon SE, Hudson AR, Trued S, Hunter DA: Nerve regeneration in the rat model. Peripheral Nerve Repair Regeneration. 1:41–48, 1986.
88. Gutmann E: Factors effecting recovery of motor function after nerve lesions. J Neurol Neurosurg Psychiatry 5:81–95, 1942.
89. Dellon AL, Mackinnon SE, O'Brien JP: Change in nerve fibre counts with time after sciatic nerve repair in the rat. Muscle and Nerve. Submitted 1989.
90. Cancilla PA: General reactions of muscle to injury. In Heffner RR, ed: Muscle Pathology. Contemporary Issues in Surgical Pathology. Churchill Livingstone, New York, 1984, pp 15–30.
91. Gorio A, Carmignoto G: Reformation, maturation and stabilization of neuromuscular junctions in peripheral nerve regeneration. In Gorio A, Millesi H, Mingrino S, eds: Posttraumatic Peripheral Nerve Regeneration. Raven Press, New York, 1981, pp 481–492.
92. McNamara MJ, Garrett WE, Seaber AV, et al: Neurorrhaphy nerve grafting and neurotization: A functional comparison of nerve reconstruction techniques. J Hand Surg [Am] 12:354–361, 1987.
93. Karpati G, Carpenter S, Sharron L: Experimental reinnervation attempts of skeletal muscle cells by nonmotor nerves. In Gorio A, Millesi H, Mingrino S, eds: Posttraumatic Peripheral Nerve Regeneration. Raven Press, New York, 1981, pp 495–506.
94. Mackinnon SE, Dellon AL, Hudson AR, Hunter DA: Alteration of neuroma formation by manipulation of neural environment in primates. Plast Reconstr Surg 76:345–352, 1985.
95. Dellon AL: Evaluation of sensibility and re-education of sensation in the hand. Williams & Wilkins, Baltimore, 1981.
96. Dellon AL, Witebsky FG, Terrill RE: The denervated Meissner corpuscle. A sequential histologic study following nerve division in the Rhesus monkey. Plast Reconstr Surg 56:182–193, 1975.
97. Dellon AL: Reinnervation of denervated Meissner corpuscles. A sequential histological study in primates following interfascicular nerve repair. J Hand Surg [Am] 1:98–109, 1976.
98. Kirklin JW, Murphy F, Berkson J: Suture of peripheral nerves; factors affecting prognosis. Surg Gynecol Obstet 88:719–730, 1949.
99. Oester VT, Davis L: Recovery of sensory functions. In Woodhall B, Beebee GW, eds: Peripheral Nerve Regeneration, U.S. Government Printing Office, Washington, D.C., 1956, pp 241–310.
100. Davis L: The return of sensation to transplanted skin. Surg Gynecol Obstet 59:533–543, 1934.
101. Kredel FE, Evans JP: Recovery of sensation in denervated pedicles and free skin grafts. J Neurol Neurosurg Psychiatry 19:1203–1221, 1933.
102. Adeymo O, Wyburn GN: Innervation of skin grafts. Trans Bull 4:152–153, 1957.
103. Mannerfelt L: Evaluation of functional sensation of skin grafts in the hand area. Br J Plast Surg 15:136–154, 1962.
104. Dellon AL: Sensory recovery in replanted digits and transplanted toes. A review. J Reconstr Microsurgery 2:123–129, 1986.

2

Classification of Nerve Injuries as the Basis for Treatment

In 1943, Sir Herbert Seddon[1] described three types of nerve injury; neurapraxia, axonotmesis, and neurotmesis. In 1951, Sir Sydney Sunderland[2] expanded Seddon's classification to include not only first degree injury (neurapraxia), second degree injury (axonotmesis), and fifth degree injury (neurotmesis), but also two types of intermediate nerve injury patterns. We describe a sixth degree injury pattern that combines, in the single nerve, nerve injury of various degrees. Thus, from fascicle to fascicle, a mixed combination of Sunderland's five degrees of injury may be found (Tables 2-1, 2-2; Fig. 2-1).

Table 2-1. Classification of Nerve Injury

Seddon	*Sunderland (degree)*	
Neurapraxia	I	VI (combination of any of Sunderland (I - V))
Axonotmesis	II	
	III	
	IV	
Neurotemesis	V	

Table 2-2. Classification of Nerve Injuries

	Histopathologic Changes					*Tinel Sign*	
Degree of Injury	*Myelin*	*Axon*	*Endoneurium*	*Perineurium*	*Epineurium*	*Present*	*Progresses Distally*
I Neurapraxia	+/−					−	−
II Axonotmesis	+	+				+	+
III	+	+	+			+	+
IV	+	+	+	+		+	−
V Neurotmesis	+	+	+	+	+	+	−
VI	Various fibers and fascicles demonstrate various pathologic changes					+	+/−

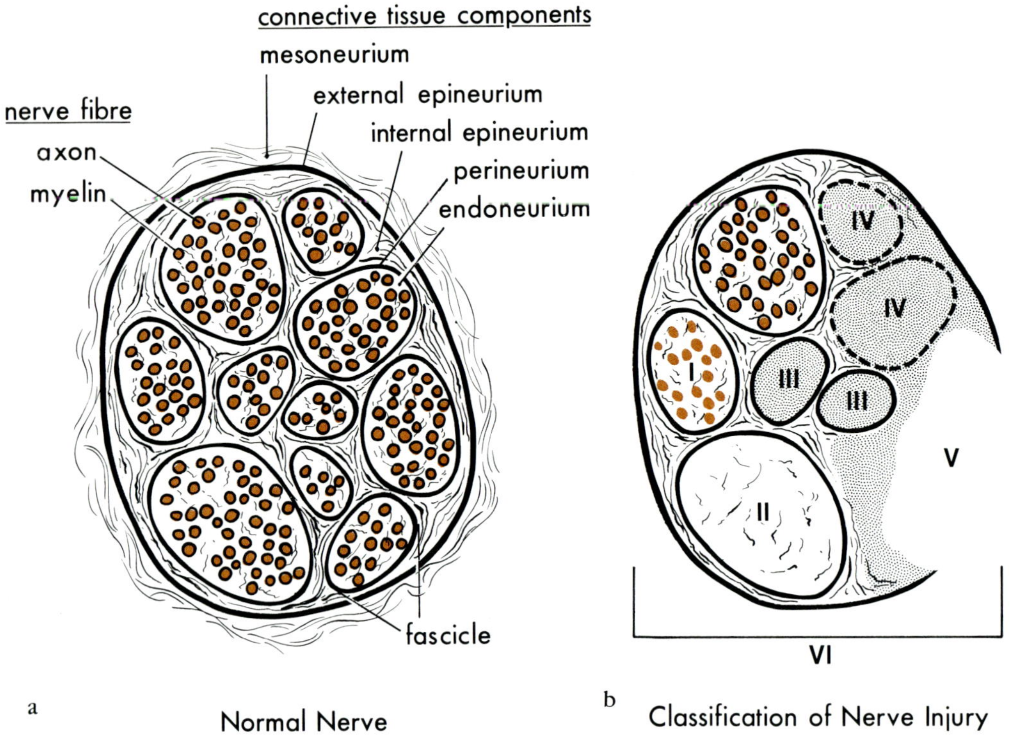

Figure 2-1a. Diagrammatic representation of the cross-section of a normal peripheral nerve demonstrating the connective tissue and nerve tissue components. **b.** The cross-section of the peripheral nerve demonstrates a mixed, or sixth degree, injury pattern. This fascicle at 11 o'clock is normal. Moving counterclockwise, the adjacent fascicle demonstrates a first degree injury (neurapraxia) with segmental demyelination. The next fascicle demonstrates a second degree injury (axonotmesis). This injury involves both the axon and the myelin. The endoneurial tissue is not damaged. The central two fascicles demonstrate a third degree injury, with injury to the axon, myelin, and endoneurium. The perineurium is intact and normal. The fascicles demonstrate at 12 and 1 o'clock a fourth degree injury with marked scarring across the nerve, with only the epineurium being intact. In a fifth degree injury pattern, the nerve is not in-continuity but is transected. The surgeon will separate the fourth and fifth degree injury patterns, which will require reconstruction from the normal fascicles and the fascicles demonstrating first, second, and third degree injury patterns. These latter patterns of injury require, at most, neurolysis.

Conduction Block (Neurapraxia)

Neurapraxia involves a local conduction block at a discrete area along the course of the nerve. The nerve is in-continuity and there is no Wallerian degeneration. The recovery that occurs is complete, but the time for recovery may vary from minutes or days to several weeks. The pathophysiologic extent of this injury involves an area of the nerve fiber that demonstrates a local block to nerve conduction. To the naked eye, the nerve may look entirely normal. If there is any histopathologic change, it is segmental areas of demyelination. Because there is no axonal abnormality, there will be no nerve regeneration involved in the recovery of function of the nerve. When the local conduction block restores itself, the nerve recovery should be immediate. A gradual or progressive recovery is more in keeping with a greater degree of injury. Because there is no axonal damage or subsequent regeneration, there will be no Tinel sign at the site of the lesion. There is therefore no advancing Tinel sign noted in a neurapraxia, or first degree type of injury. This type of injury will show recovery by 12 weeks. Examples of this type of injury are: tourniquet palsy or other localized pressure palsy, such as the radial nerve paralysis of the "Saturday night drinking palsy." This occurs when the alcoholic falls asleep with the arm resting on the back of a chair or other hard object. Compression of the radial nerve occurs because the inebriated person does not shift his weight off the compressed nerve and because the nerve of the chronic alcoholic is more susceptible to acute compression. In very early nerve entrapment syndromes, the degree of injury is a neurapraxia, or first degree injury.

Axonotmesis (Second Degree Injury)

The basis of axonotmesis is axonal damage to the extent that Wallerian degeneration will occur distal to the second degree injury. Proximal to the injury, an attempt will be made to regenerate, and axon sprouting will occur. The endoneurium and the perineurium are intact. Because actual nerve regeneration must occur in order to repair this degree of injury, a Tinel sign will be apparent at the level of the injury and with time the Tinel sign will advance distally. Recovery will occur after an axonotmetic type of injury, but the recovery will be at the classic rate of nerve regeneration (approximately 1 inch/month, or 1 to 1.5 mm/day).[4,5] The recovery of neurologic function will follow a serial progression as proximal then distal nerve divisions are innervated in a progressive anatomic order. In axonotmesis, because the endoneurium is not injured, the axonal sprouts do not have to regenerate through any degree of scar tissue. Because the injury is purely axonal in nature, the basal lamina of the Schwann cells, which makes up the endoneurial tubes, has not been violated and, thus, regeneration will restore full and original sensory and motor function. The diagnosis of second degree injury can only be made "after the fact" of recovery from the nerve injury.

After closed stretch injuries, if full recovery occurs within the first 3 months of the injury, the degree of injury is called a neurapraxia, or first degree injury. If the recovery is full but recovery occurs at the rate of 1 inch/month with an advancing Tinel sign present, then the injury is labeled an axonotmesis, or second degree injury. If the recovery is incomplete but follows the same time course as an axonotmetic type of injury, then it is called a third degree Sunderland injury. Thus, the differentiation between an axonotmesis and a Sunderland III degree injury will be based on the degree of recovery (Fig. 2-2).

By definition axonotmesis excludes metabolic or toxic axonopathies (see Chapter 14).

Third Degree Injury

Sunderland has very appropriately expanded Seddon's initial classification of nerve injury to include third degree injury patterns. In this situation there is scarring in the endoneurium so that the axons must regenerate through some degree of scar tissue. The regeneration then is often incomplete because some of the regenerating fibers do not make contact with distal receptors or end organs because they are lost within the scarring in the endoneurium. The basal lamina of the Schwann cell is violated with this type of injury; thus, there can be some mismatching of nerve fibers with regeneration of nerve fibers to inappropriate distal receptors. The perineurium is intact in a third degree type of injury, and whatever nerve fibers are within the confines of the perineurium will remain with regeneration within that fascicle. If the injury occurs relatively proximal in the extremity where motor and sensory nerves are adjacent to each other in the same fascicle, abnormal sensory and motor recovery is likely. With a third degree injury occurring more distal in the extremity, the nerve fibers within the fascicle bounded by that particular injury pattern may, indeed, be entirely motor or sensory and the recovery then may be much better even though the injury itself is the same. A third degree injury in the median nerve at the wrist would, at worst, demonstrate abnormal localization of sensation in the median nerve-innervated digits. The recurrent motor branch, at this level, is in its own perineurial confined fascicle, thus, recovery of thenar function would be, at worst, incomplete. The same injury in the ulnar nerve in the proximal arm where sensory and motor fibers are found in the same fascicle could result in a very poor degree of recovery because a mixing of sensory and motor regenerating fibers would likely occur.

In a Sunderland third degree injury, recovery occurs at the same rate as that after an axonotmesis, which would be approximately 1 inch/month. The advancing Tinel sign will demonstrate the level of the regeneration. Unlike an axonotmesis, however, the degree of recovery will not be full and complete. The variation of recovery is broadest in the Sunderland III injury and can vary from almost complete recovery to almost no recovery, depending on how pure or mixed is the fascicle involved and the degree of endoneurial scarring present.

Fourth Degree Injury

Sunderland's fourth degree injury describes a situation in which the nerve is physically in-continuity but not functioning. At the level of the fourth degree injury, the nerve continuity is maintained only with scar tissue. A Tinel sign will be present at the level of the injury, but no progression of the Tinel sign will be noted distal to the injury because regenerating nerve fibers are blocked by this scar tissue. Wallerian degeneration will occur in the nerve distal to the injury. Proximal to the injury, regenerating nerve units trapped in scar tissue will be noted. These injuries will never show any sensory or motor recovery. If any recovery is to occur, then surgical intervention with nerve repair, nerve grafting (see Chapter 4), or nerve conduit technique (see Chapter

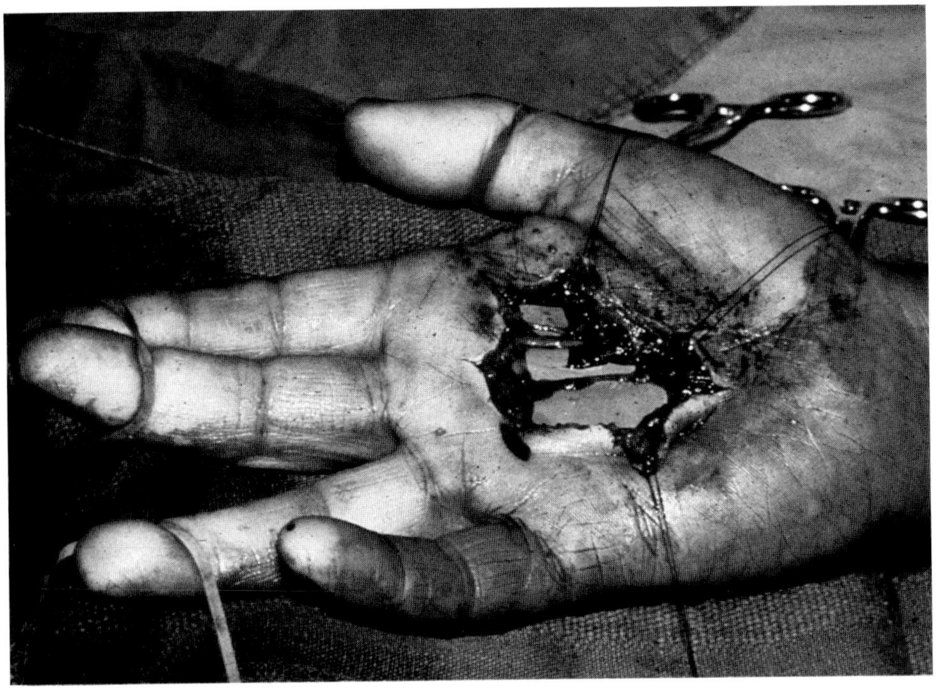

a

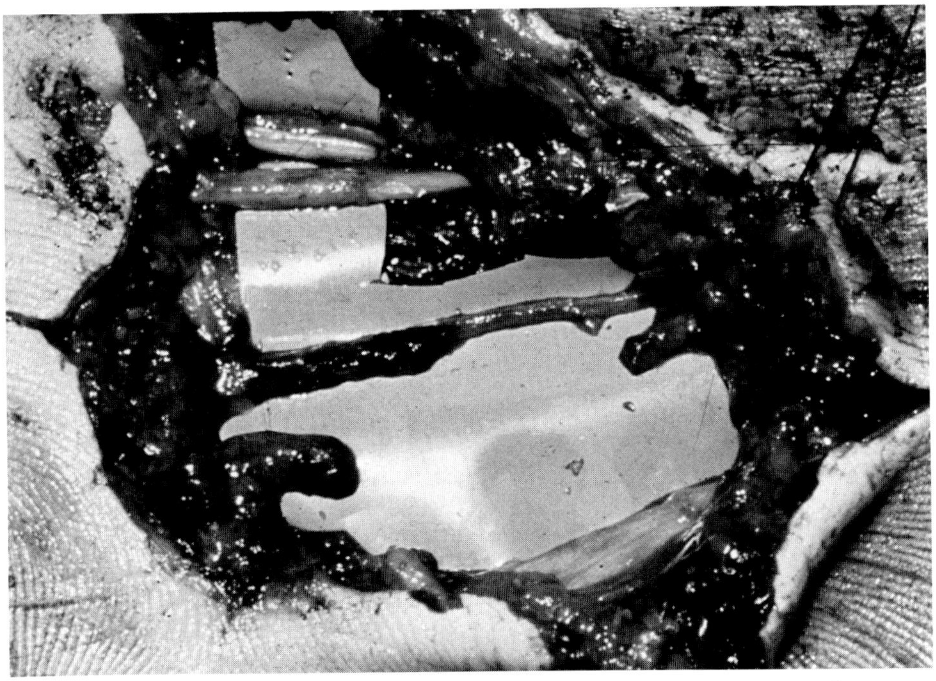

b

Figure 2-2a. After an injury sustained to the right hand while cleaning a gun, this patient demonstrated no sensation in the median nerve distribution. Thus, all the digits innervated by the median nerve presented with the same loss of sensibility. At exploration, it is interesting to note the different patterns of injury that occurred to the different fascicles of the median nerve. **b.** The common digital nerve to the long and ring fingers has been completely divided (fifth degree injury). The common digital to the index and long fingers was markedly contused over a long distance (query: I, II, III, or IV) The digital nerve to the radial side of the index finger looks relatively normal (neurapraxia). One year after this injury, the patient demonstrated normal sensibility and normal two-point discrimination in the distribution of the radial digital nerve to the index finger and diminished but present sensibility in the distribution of the common digital nerve to the index and long fingers with diminished two-point discrimination. In retrospect, then, the injury to this common digital nerve was a Sunderland third degree injury. The common digital nerve to the long and ring fingers was reconstructed secondarily with a nerve graft.

20) will be necessary. If there was some mechanism of identifying this fourth degree type of injury at the time of the initial nerve injury, then immediate repair, grafting, or nerve conduit technique could be carried out. Unfortunately, these injuries are usually the result of very severe stretch or traction injuries and a period of approximately 3 months is recommended after these injuries before any surgical intervention. It is during this 3-month period that first, second, and third degree injuries will recover or start to demonstrate an orderly progression of recovery that can be identified clinically or electrodiagnostically. By a process of exclusion, function that does not show evidence of recovery by 3 months is considered to be a Sunderland fourth degree injury and is considered for surgical management. The most common example of fourth degree injury occurs from a traction or stretch type of injury that produces such severe scarring in the nerve that no regeneration occurs. After a failed primary nerve repair in which no recovery occurs across the repair site, the degree of injury could be classified as a fourth degree injury in that the nerve is in-continuity after the initial repair but no function has occurred across the scar at the site of the unsatisfactory nerve repair. Nerve injection injuries can produce a similar type of picture.

Neurotmesis (Fifth Degree Injury)

Transection of a peripheral nerve constitutes a neurotmesis, or a fifth degree injury. These injuries are relatively easy to diagnose because all are open injuries with associated peripheral nerve deficit. Early surgical exploration of the wound will facilitate both the diagnosis and early management of these injuries.

Sixth Degree Injury (Neuroma in-Continuity)

We have previously emphasized the sixth degree injury pattern.[6] As peripheral nerve surgeons dealing with nerve-injured patients, we soon realize that the most challenging of nerve injuries is the type that combines all or many of Sunderland's five degrees of injury. It is this mixed, or sixth degree injury that we believe constitutes the surgical dilemma of the neuroma in-continuity injury. This injury will involve a mixed pattern of injury in the various fascicles of the peripheral nerve with, perhaps, normal function through some fascicles and varying degrees of injury (I,II,III,IV,V) in other fascicles (Table 2-2, Fig. 2-3). In a sixth degree injury the pattern of recovery will be mixed. No recovery will be seen in those fascicles with fourth or fifth degree injury patterns. Partial recovery will be noted in those fascicles with a third degree injury and complete recovery will be demonstrated in the involved fascicles that have a first or second degree injury. Electrodiagnostic tests will differentiate between first degree (neurapraxia) and other lesions (degrees II to VI). These tests will not distinguish between the lesions that will demonstrate eventual recovery (I,II,III) and those that will not (IV,V). It becomes the responsibility of the surgeon to evaluate the patient clinically to identify the degree of function in the extremity that corresponds to the degree of injury in the various fascicles of the peripheral nerve in question.

The surgeon then preoperatively makes a detailed clinical assessment of function in each fascicle or group of fascicles of the nerve to be explored. Through this clinical examination, the surgeon will be making a mental picture of the injury pattern within the nerve (corresponding to Figure 2-1b). Recognizing that first, second, and third degree injuries offer spontaneous recovery superior to that provided by surgical grafting techniques, the surgeon must take great care not to injure these fascicles or normal fascicles. It is the fourth and fifth degree injury patterns that will require surgical reconstruction (Fig. 2-3).

Three-Dimensional Injury Patterns

The degree of injury will vary from fascicle to fascicle and can be easily depicted with a cross-sectional diagram of the peripheral nerve. The injury, however, may also vary in a longitudinal nature along the length of the nerve. In traction injuries especially, "skip" lesions can be seen along the length of the nerve. We have, unfortunately, seen similar conditions after iatrogenic injury to the nerve. A detailed clinical examination supplemented with careful electrodiagnostic assessment will allow the surgeon to determine "the worst" degree of injury in any given fascicle. Although lesser degrees of injury patterns may be noted at other points along the nerve fascicle, it will be the greatest degree of injury that will determine the clinical presentation and the type of surgery required.

Chronic Nerve Compression

Chronic nerve compression or entrapment neuropathy is such a common clinical problem that a discussion of the pathophysiologic changes associated with this entity is indicated. The pathologic process of chronic nerve

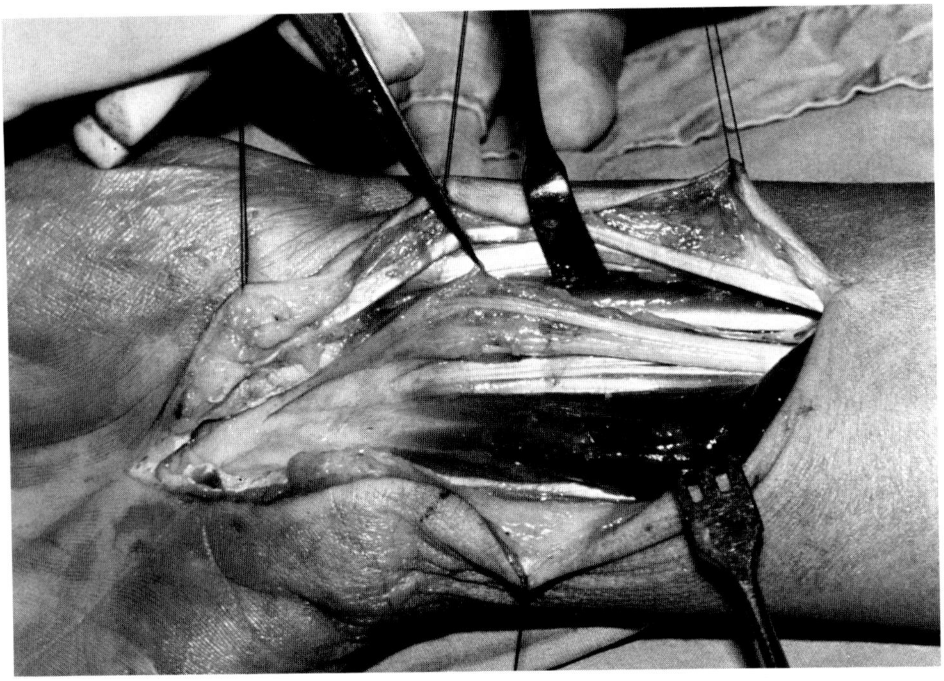

a

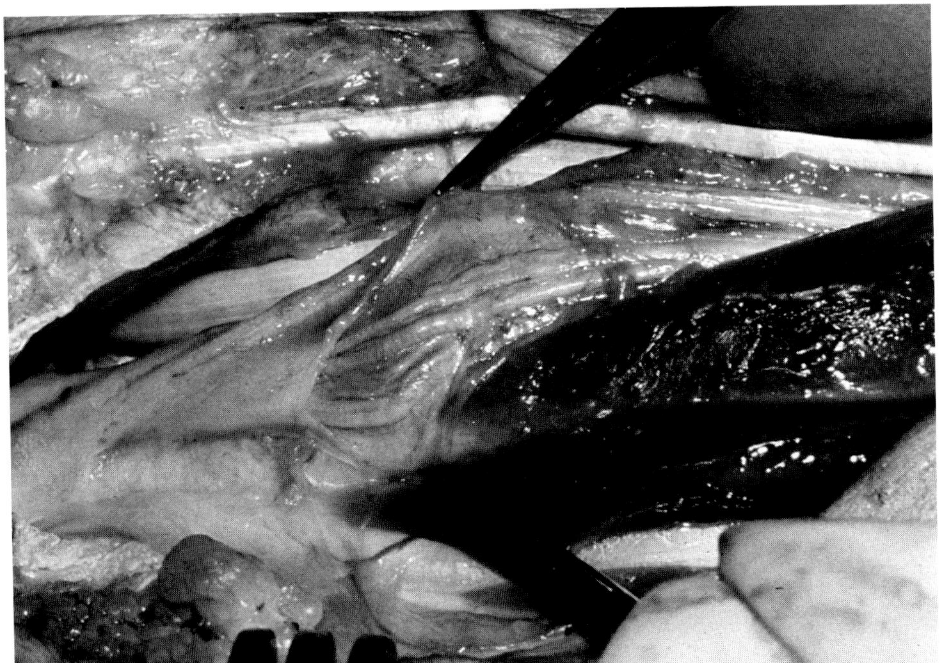

b

Figure 2-3a. Median nerve, sixth degree injury secondary to previous laceration and crush injury. The injured nerve is noted with the hand toward the left. **b.** After internal neurolysis. **c.** The nature of the mixed sixth degree injury is apparent. The palmar cutaneous nerve has been completely divided (fifth degree injury) (arrow). The fascicles to the thumb are in-continuity only with scar tissue, demonstrating no clinical or electrical function (fourth degree injury; double arrow). Fascicles to the index finger clinically demonstrated diminished but present sensation (*; third degree injury). **d.** The fourth degree injury will be repaired with a nerve graft (graft between arrows).

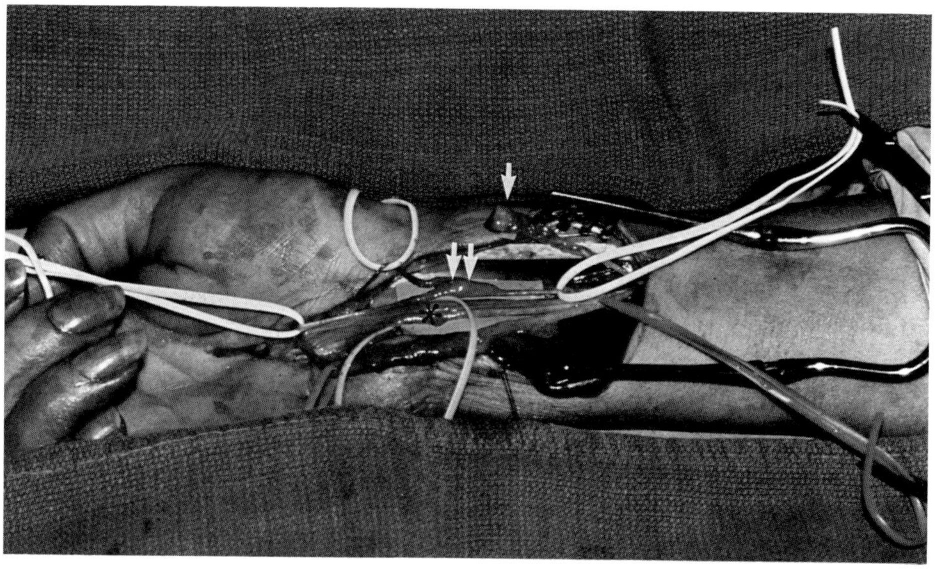

c

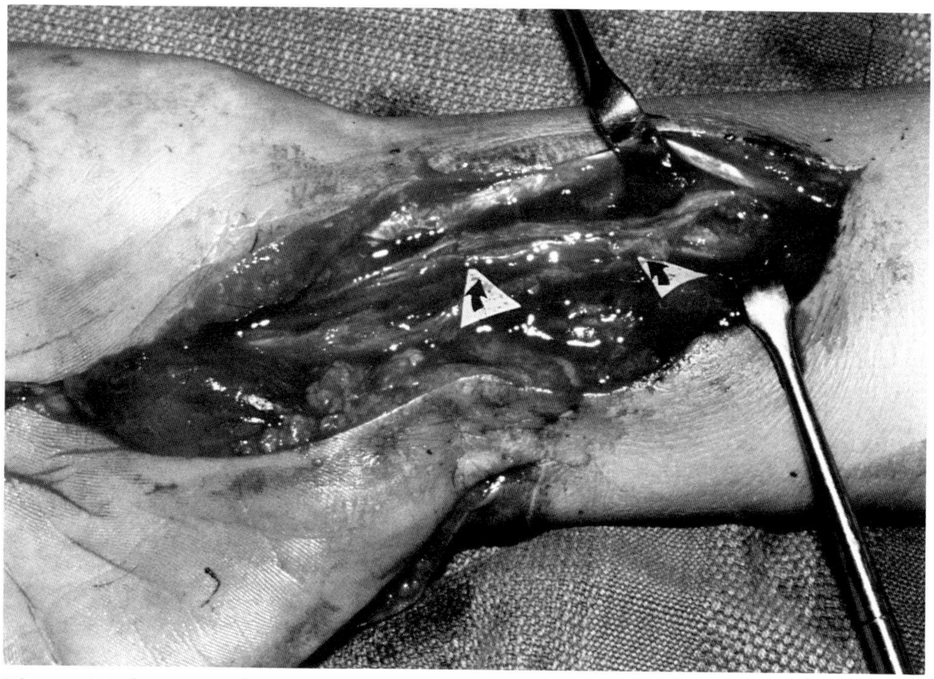

d

Figure 2-3 (*continued*).

compression will be reflected in the patient's symptoms and clinical findings. The histopathologic alterations of chronic nerve compression present a broad spectrum that progresses from blood–nerve barrier changes and transient ischemia to severe Wallerian degeneration.[7–9] Essentially, the pathologic changes seen with chronic nerve compression include the entire spectrum of nerve injury as has just been described (Fig. 2-4). Initially, the patient's symptoms are in response to periodic ischemia secondary to transient compromise of local blood flow. The earliest histologic changes will be a breakdown in the blood–nerve barrier with resulting subperineurial and endoneurial edema (Fig. 2-5). Eventually, connective tissue changes will be seen, with thickening of both the external and internal epineurium[10] (Fig. 2-6). When nerve fiber changes are finally noted, they initially involve only the peripheral fibers of the peripheral fascicles of the nerves. The fascicles in the center of the nerve or those away from direct pressure appear normal. Large myelinated fibers demonstrate segmental demyelination. All of the histopathologic changes just described are those of first degree injury, or neurapraxia.

The unmyelinated fibers undergo degeneration and demonstrate evidence of regeneration before similar changes are apparent in the large myelinated fibers. The presence of a new population of very small unmyelinated fibers attests to the fact that degeneration

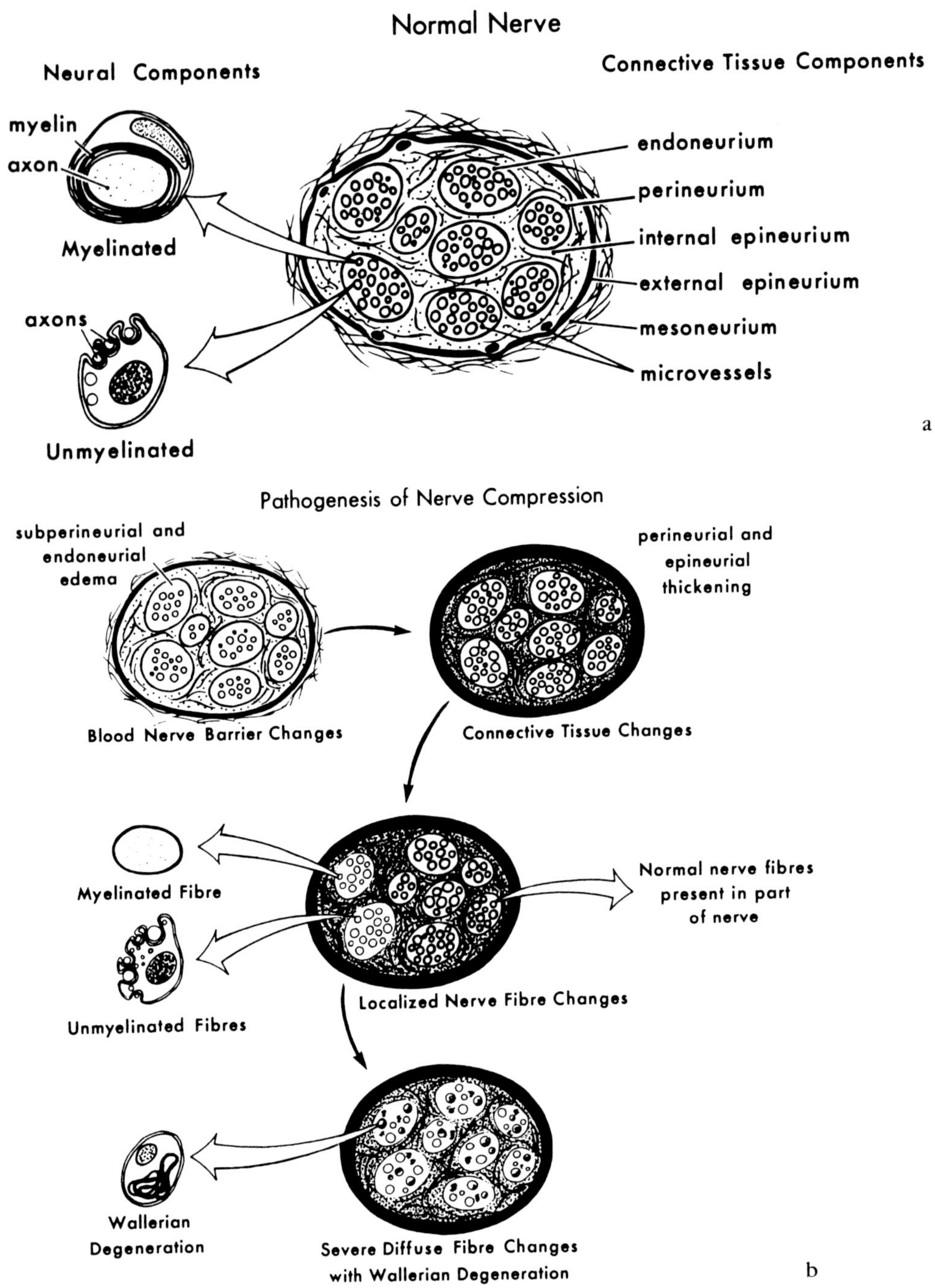

Figure 2-4. Schematic diagram outlining pathogenesis of chronic nerve compression. **a.** The normal nerve is drawn for comparison. **b.** The changes with chronic nerve compression are noted. The initial changes involve just the blood–nerve barrier: endoneurial and subperineurial edema will be seen relating to increased endoneurial fluid pressure. The next histologic changes to occur are those involving the connective tissue layers. Increased perineurial and epineurial thickening will be noted. Localized nerve fiber changes will then occur. Some fascicles will appear entirely normal, others will demonstrate segmental demyelination of the large fibers. The unmyelinated fibers will show evidence of regeneration with a new population of very small unmyelinated fibers noted. Central fascicles or the central fibers within a given fascicle are usually spared. With progression of either the degree of compression or the duration of the nerve compression, diffuse fiber changes will be noted across all fascicles and degeneration will be apparent in both the myelinated as well as unmyelinated nerve fibers.

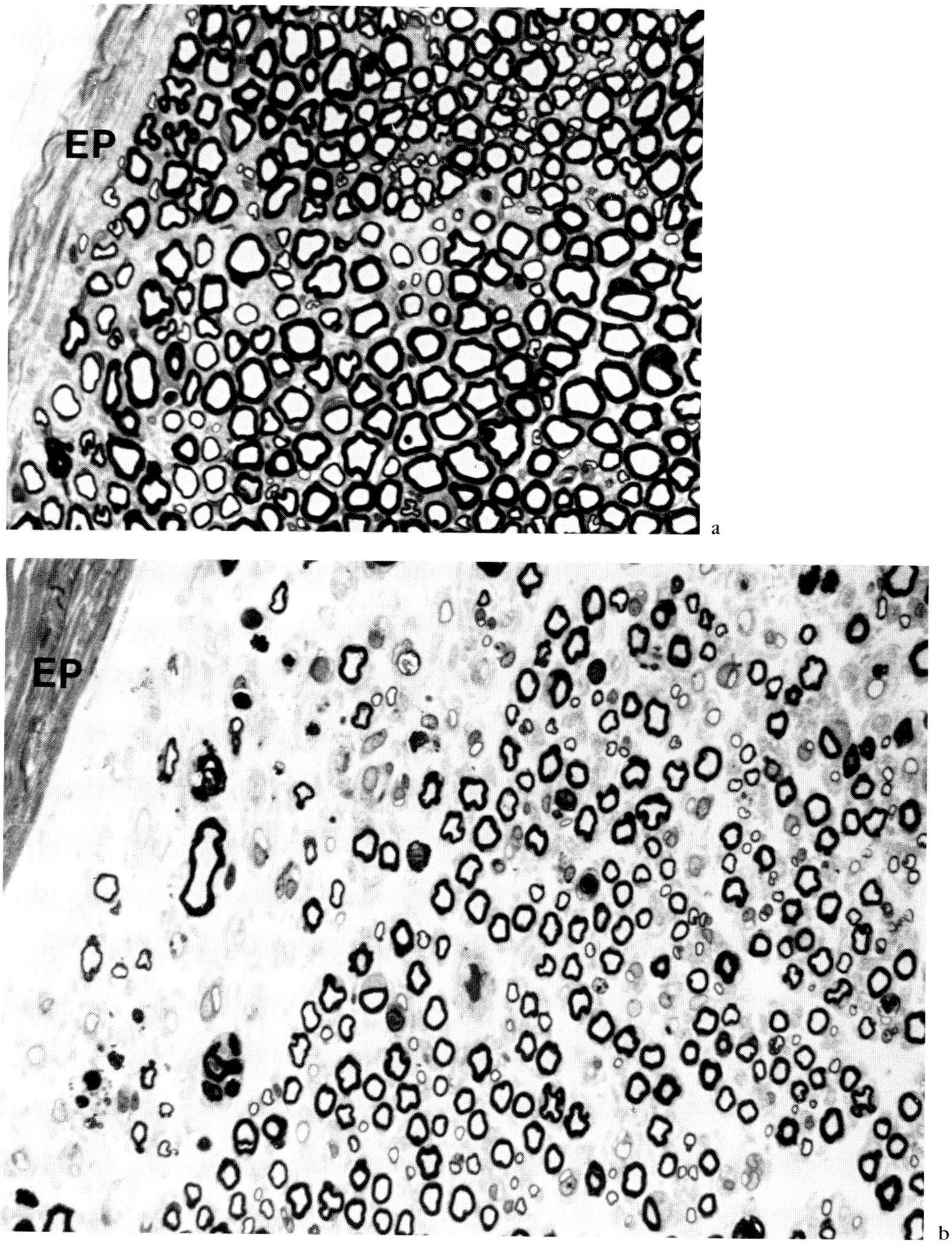

Figure 2-5. Transverse section of sciatic nerve of rat. (Toluidine blue.) **a.** After 2 months of compression with a 1.5 mm internal diameter silicone tube, the nerve looked essentially normal. (×345). **b.** After 2 months of compression with a 1.1 mm internal diameter tube, subperineurial edema is noted. A fallout in the large myelinated fiber group is noted at the periphery of the fascicle. EP: epineurium. (×322.) (Reproduced with permission from Mackinnon et al.[8])

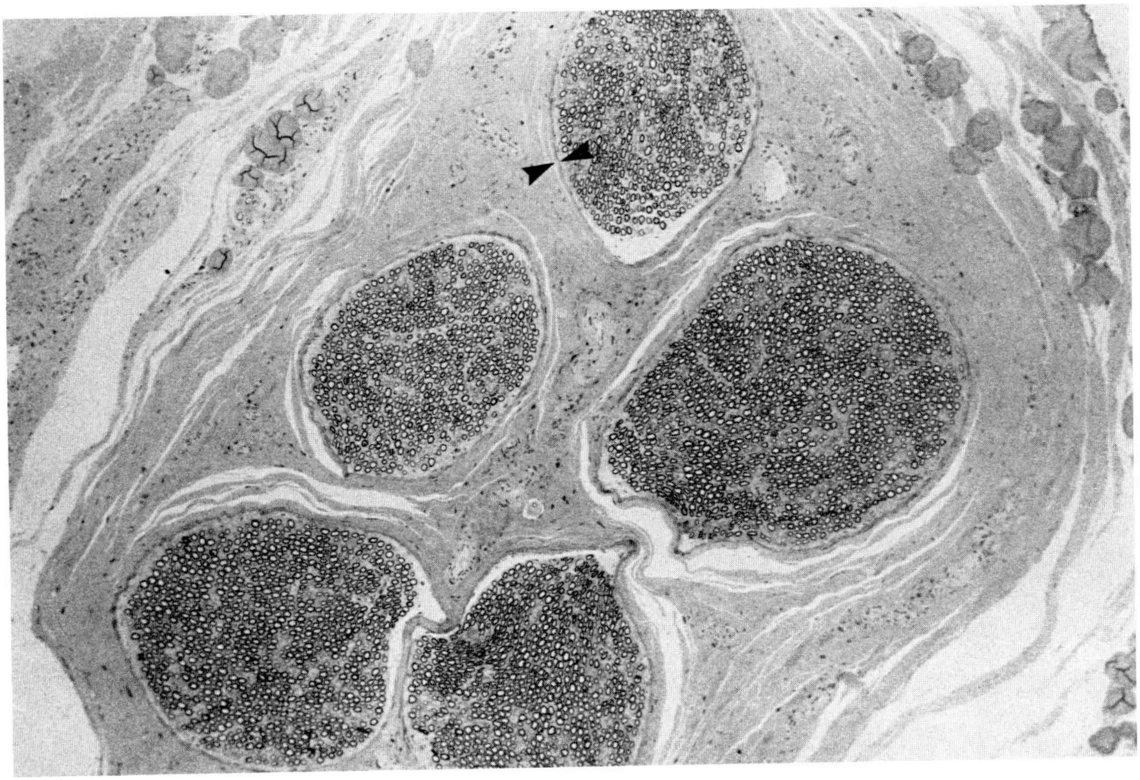

a

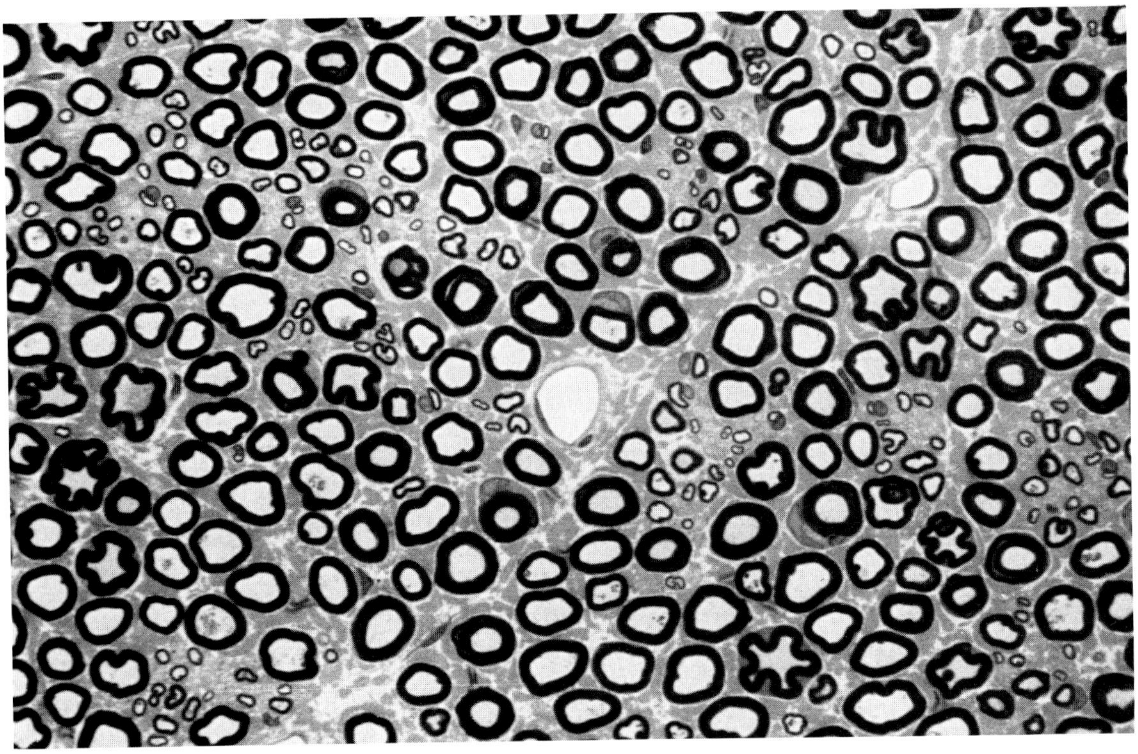

b

Figure 2-6. Transverse section of primate median nerve (Toluidine blue.) **a.** Transverse section of normal median nerve. The perineurium is thin (arrows). (×92.) **b.** At a higher magnification, a population of normal nerve fibers is seen. (× 588.) (*Figure continues.*)

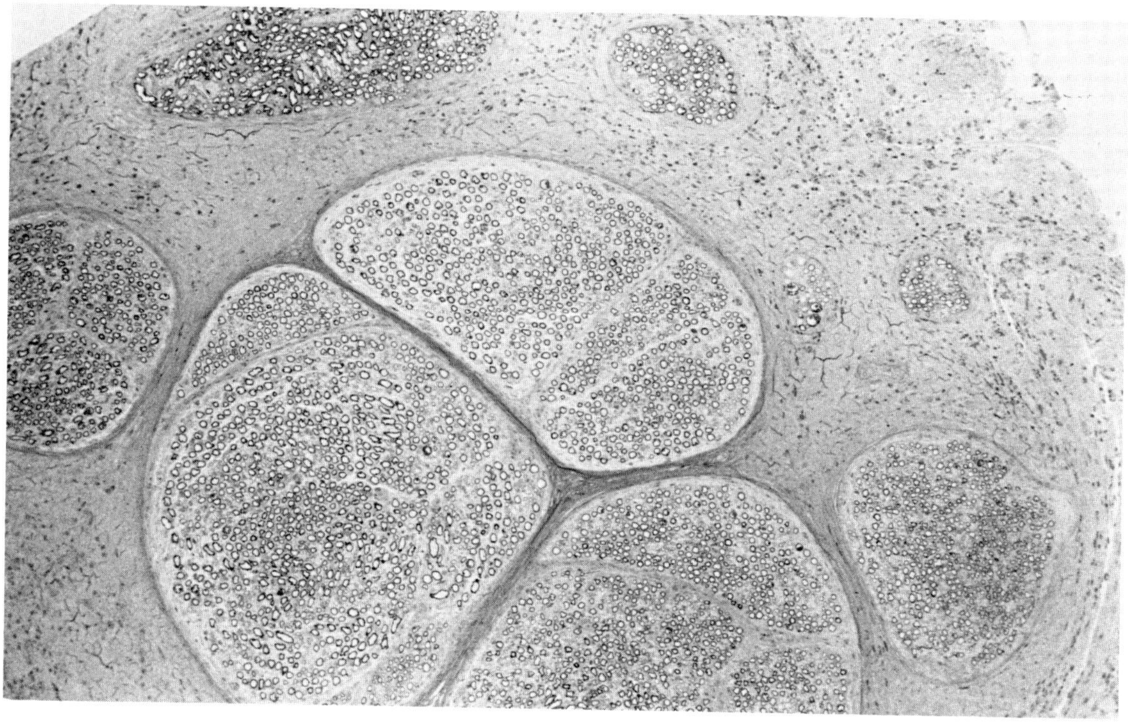

c

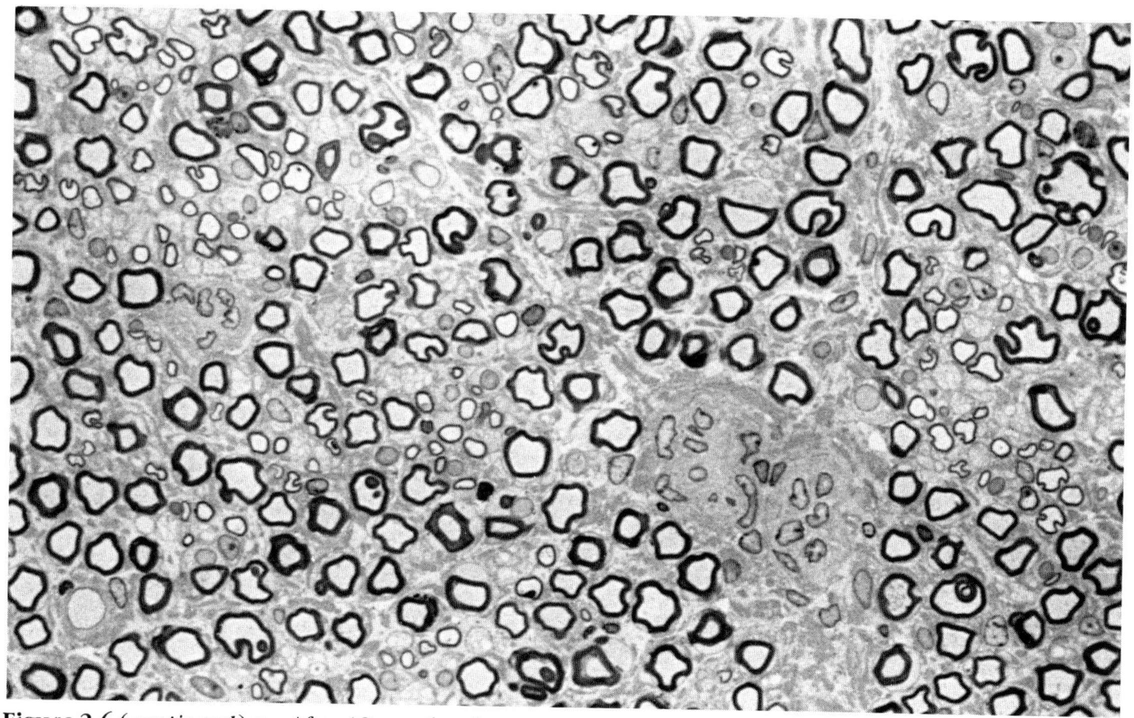

d

Figure 2-6 (*continued*) **c.** After 12 months of nerve compression, thickening of the internal epineurium and the perineurium is noted. (× 92.) **d.** At a higher magnification, nerve fiber changes with thinning of the myelin is seen. (× 588.) (Reproduced with permission from Mackinnon and Dellon.[10])

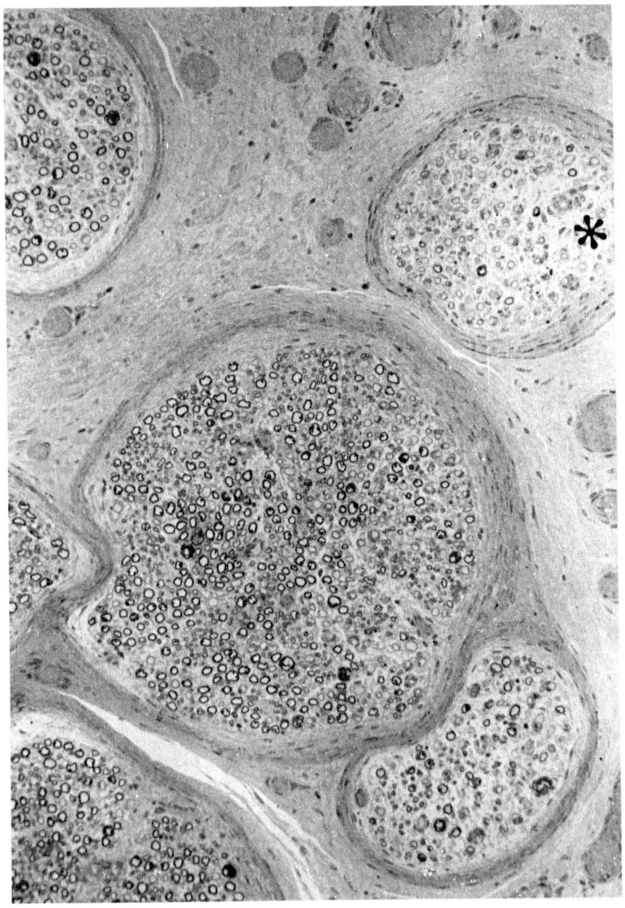

a

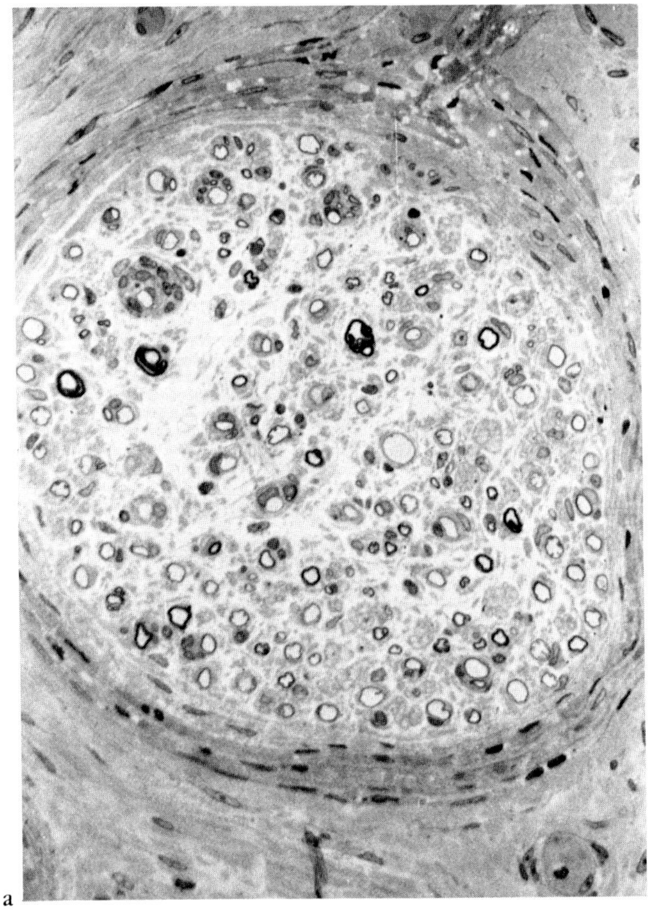

b

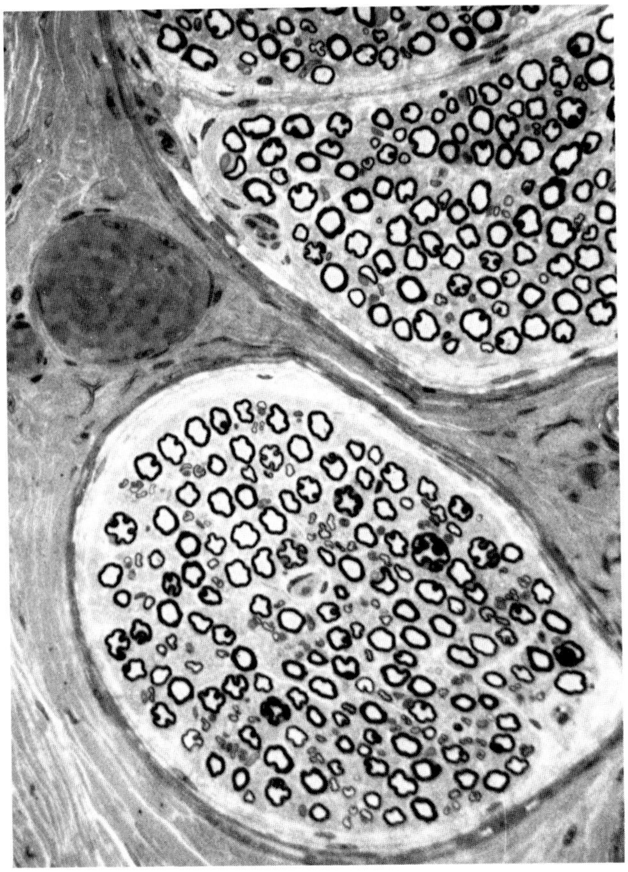

c

Figure 2-7. Toluidine blue-stained transverse section after 5 months of nerve compression in the primate median nerve. **a.** A compressed fascicle with thickened perineurium and a fallout of the large myelinated fibers is noted in the periphery of this nerve (*). A second larger fascicle does not demonstrate quite as severe a picture of nerve fiber damage. (×137.) **b.** At higher magnification, the details of histologic changes from the damaged fascicles are noted. The perineurium is markedly thickened (×344). **c.** Two fascicles from within the center of the same nerve demonstrate normal nerve architecture. The perineurium is much thinner than that noted in the damaged fascicles (Figure 2-7b). (Reproduced with permission from Mackinnon et al.[7])

has occurred and represents the regenerative potential of the unmyelinated fibers (see Fig. 2-17).

With progression of the degree or duration of the nerve compression, Wallerian degeneration will be noted in the large myelinated fibers. This injury pattern will initially be apparent only in the peripheral fascicles of the nerve (Fig. 2-7).

Eventually, diffuse fiber changes will be seen through the entire nerve, and Wallerian degeneration (which by definition relates only to myelinated nerve fibers) will be present. Both connective tissue and nerve fiber pathologic states increase directly with the amount of compression and the duration of time the compression is present.

Chronic Human Nerve Compression

Despite the common occurrence of nerve compression syndromes, the reports of the histopathologic characteristics of chronic nerve compression in man are scarce due primarily to the difficulty of obtaining suitable human material for study. Postmortem investigations from fresh, human cadavers with obvious muscle wasting have evaluated two median nerves from the wrist[11,12] and one ulnar nerve from the elbow.[13] "Survey" type of investigations of nerve compression from fresh, human cadavers have reported the incidence of disease in 12 median and ulnar nerves[14] and ten lateral femoral cutaneous nerves.[15] One posterior tibial nerve and two ulnar nerves with severe chronic nerve compression from patients with documented sensory and motor clinical findings as well as electrophysiologic studies have been reported.[16,17] A review of the histopathologic findings of four patients with chronic compression of the superficial branch of the radial nerve clearly describes the histopathologic characteristics of chronic human nerve compression.[18]

Clinical Data

All four nondiabetic patients with entrapment of the radial sensory nerve complained of similar symptoms of severe pain and burning sensation in the distribution of the radial sensory nerve. They all demonstrated altered sensibility in this area. Details of the patients' history are outlined in Table 2-3.

A brief explanation of the source of this biopsy material is indicated. A resection of the radial sensory nerve is not indicated as the initial treatment management for entrapment of this nerve (see Chapter 10). The four patients described in this series included three who had been labeled as "chronic Workers' Compensation Board" patients and a fourth who had had complaints of 15 years' duration. In these cases, based on good response to resection of the radial sensory nerve and implantation of the proximal end into the brachioradialis muscle in patients with neuromas of the radial sensory nerve[19] (see Chapter 17), it was elected to resect the nerve. This definitive method of treatment ensured that if neurolysis failed in these four very challenging and difficult patients, another procedure to resect the nerve would not be required.

Table 2-3. Clinical Data of Patients with Radial Sensory Nerve Entrapment

	Case 1	*Case 2*	*Case 3*	*Case 4*
Age (yr) sex	32 F	24 F	44 M	62 M
Precipitating factor	Excessive writing	Crush injury	Crush injury	Forearm fracture
WCB*	+	+	+	–
Duration of symptoms (yr)	7	1	3	15
Previous surgery	DQR*	—	DQR	—
Sensory examination (SBR)*				
M2PD* (mm)				
Compressed SBR	12	15	20	25
Contralateral SBR	8	10	6	10
Tinel sign	+	+	+	+
256 cps vibratory perception	↓	↓	↓	↓
Provocative test	+	+	+	+
NCS*	NA*	NA	N*	AB*

*SBR: Superficial branch of radial nerve; WCB: Worker's Compensation Board case; DQR: De Quervain's release; M2PD: moving two-point discrimination; NCS: nerve conduction studies; NA: not performed; N: normal; AB: abnormal; ↓: decreased

Gross Findings

In all cases, the radial nerve appeared to be compressed in the region of the intersection between the brachioradialis and extensor carpi radialis longus tendons. Intraoperatively, pronation of the forearm caused increased compression on the nerve as the two tendons tightened together. Swelling of the nerve proximal and distal to the area of compression was noted (Fig. 2-8).

Histologic Findings

In three cases, the nerve proximal and distal to the area of compression appeared entirely normal and histologic changes were restricted to the area of compression. In one case, the nerve appeared normal proximal to the area of compression but changes were noted in the region of the area of compression and distally as well (Fig. 2-9).

Endoneurial Microvessels

Electron microscopy demonstrated marked thickening of the endoneurial microvessels in all cases (Fig. 2-10).

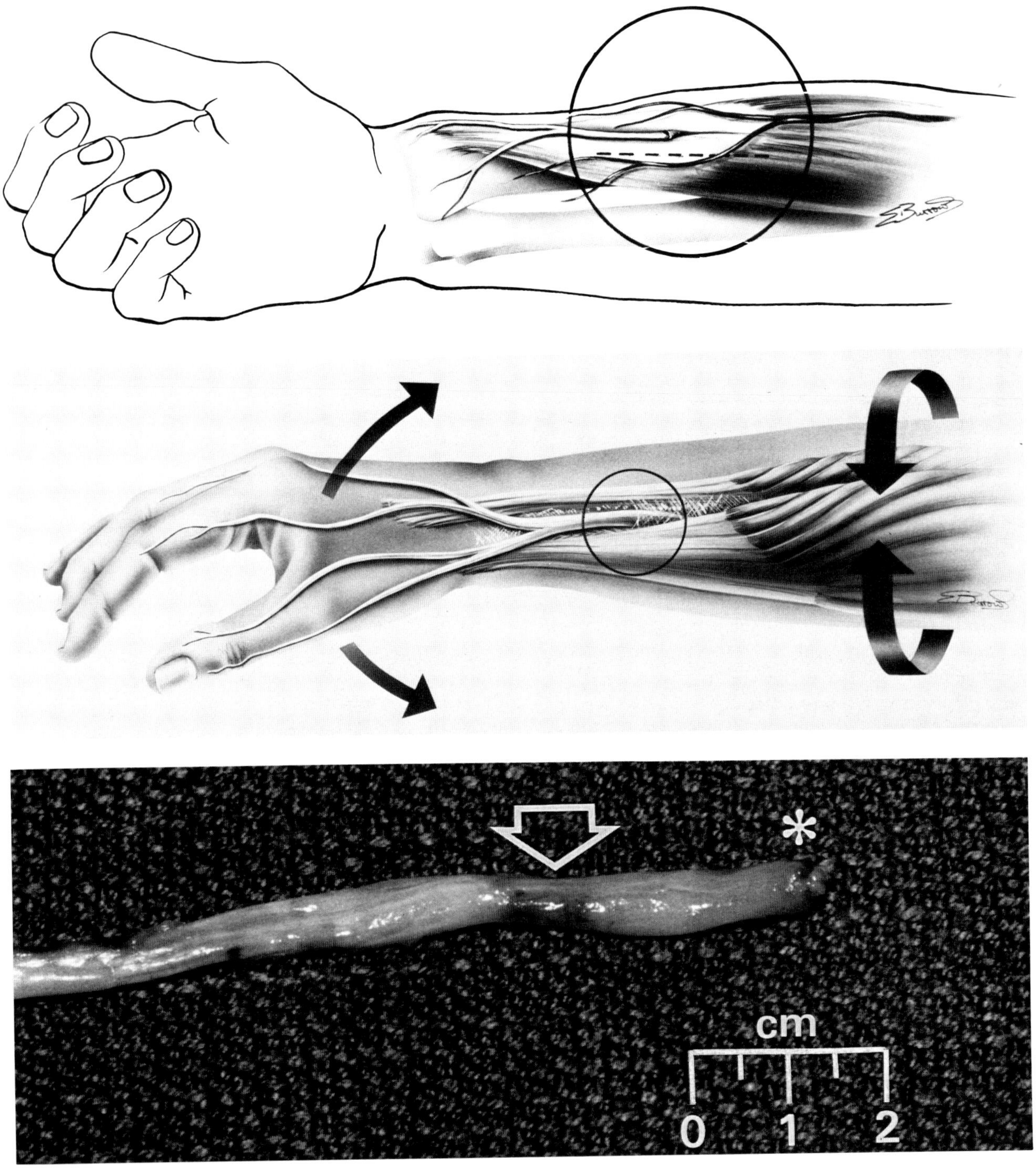

Figure 2-8. a, b. Schematic diagram showing location of the superficial radial nerve between the brachioradialis and the extensor carpi radialis longus tendons. At this intersection point, forearm pronation causes these two tendons to come closer together and entrap the nerve (**a**). Volar ulnar flexion causes increased traction or pull on the nerve so that compression and traction forces effect the SBR at this intersection area (**b**). (Reproduced with permission from Mackinnon et al.[18]) **c.** SBR nerve (case 2, proximal nerve;*)—area of compression demonstrating narrowing and hyperemia (arrow bar: 1 cm). (Reproduced with permission from Mackinnon et al.[18])

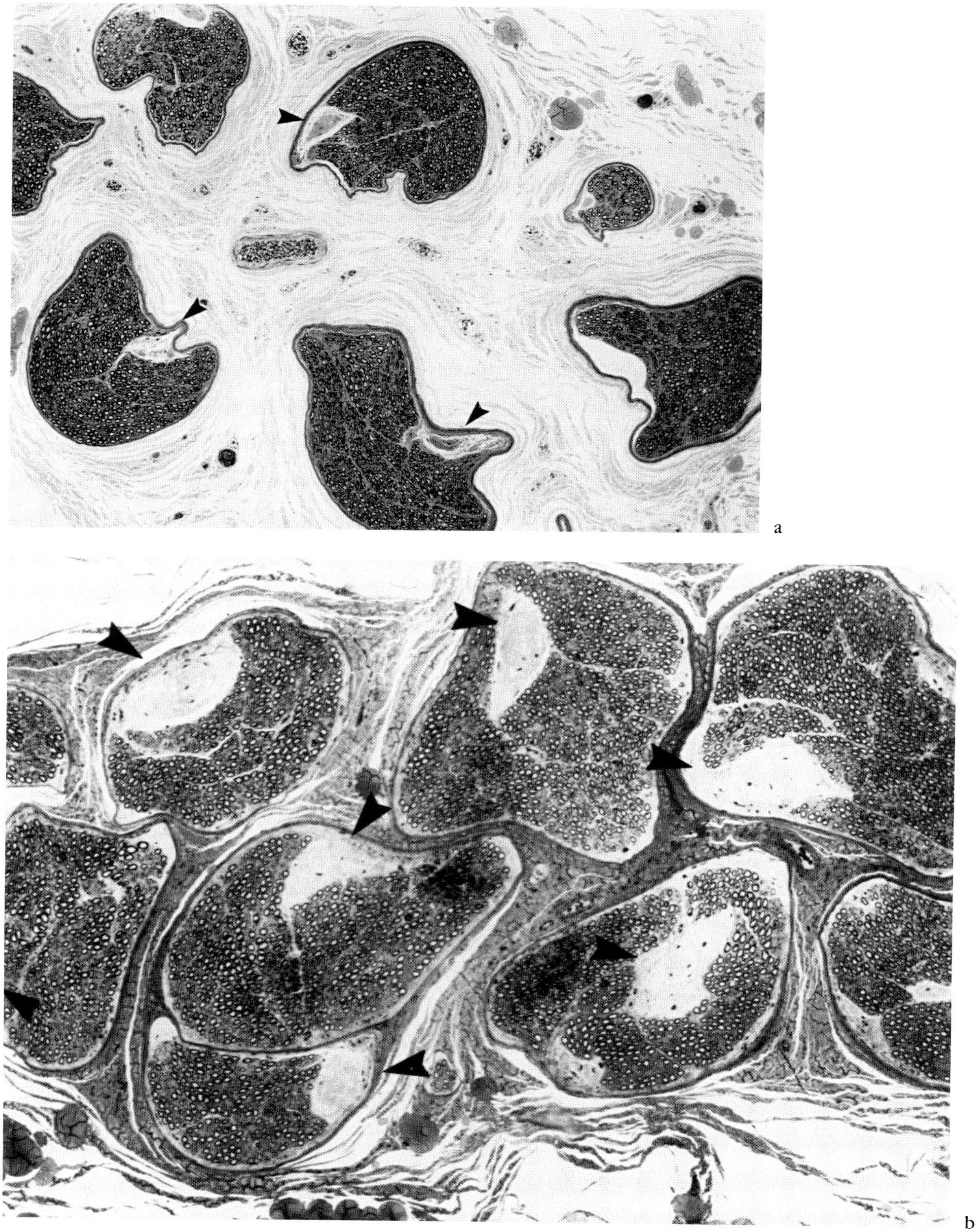

Figure 2-9. Transverse section, SBR, from the level of compression. (Toluidine blue, ×78.) a. Case 1, Renaut bodies were noted in all fascicles. The nerve is otherwise normal. b. Case 2, Renaut bodies were noted in all fascicles, many in the central position within the fascicles (arrows). The internal epineurium is markedly thickened and condensed. c. Case 4, a Renaut body is evident (arrow). There is marked increased thickening in the internal epineurium and the perineurium. Note the peripheral fascicles demonstrating pathologic fiber changes of varying degree. Normal fascicles are seen adjacent to fascicles demonstrating significant fiber disease. (Reproduced with permission from Mackinnon et al.[18]) (*Figure continues.*)

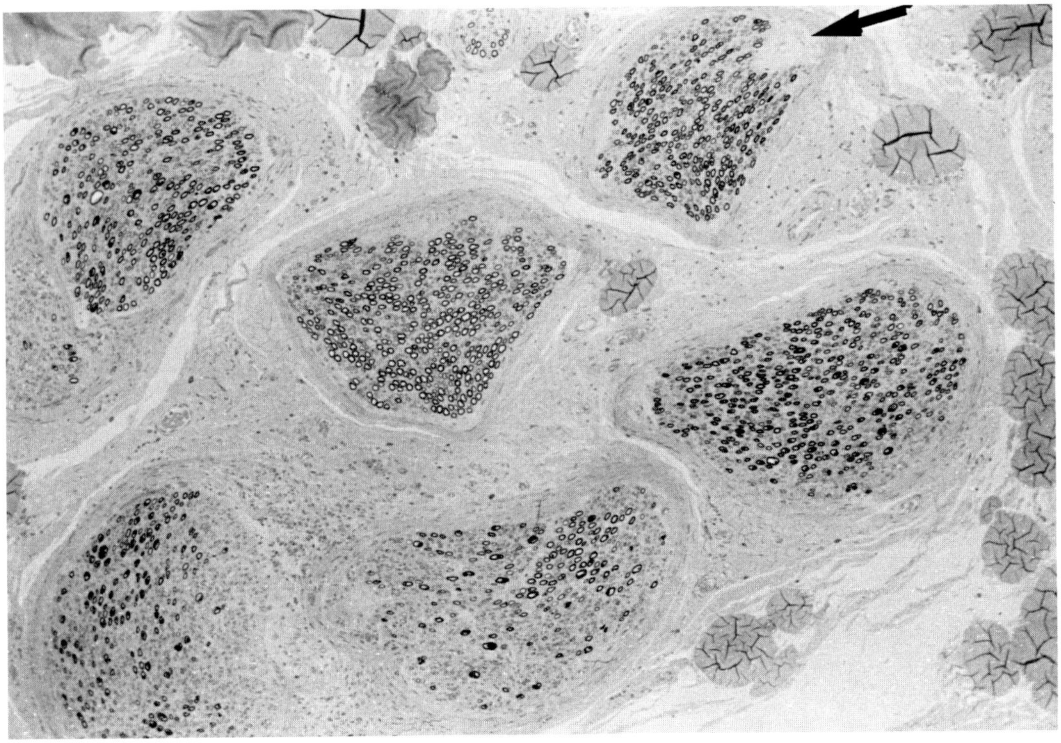

Figure 2-9 (*continued*) **c.**

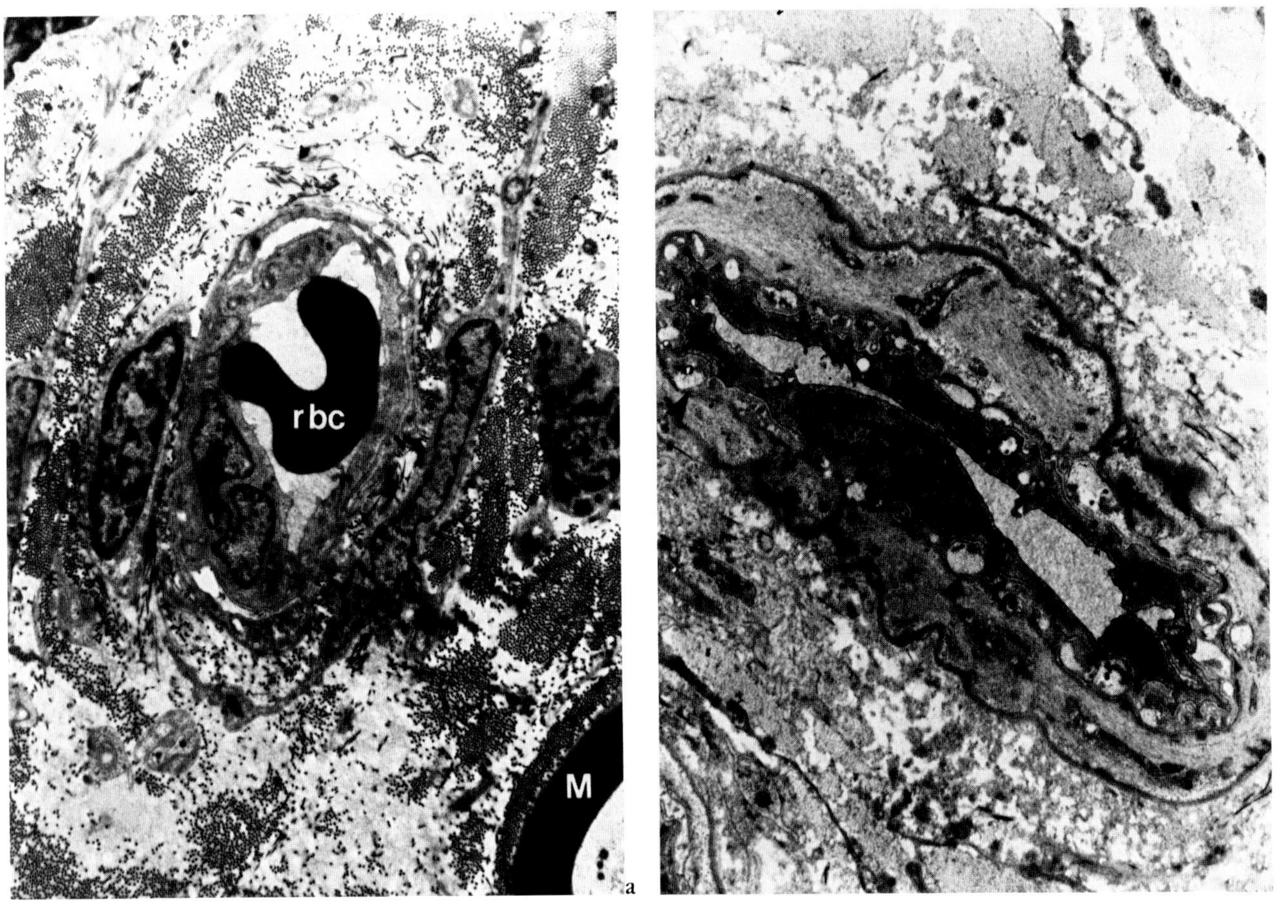

Figure 2-10. Transverse section SBR, case 1. (Uranyl acetate, ×14,136.) **a.** Proximal to the area of compression, the endoneurial microvessels appear normal. RBC: red blood cell, M: myelin. **b.** Endoneurial microvessels in the region of compression demonstrate marked thickening of the intima and media. Pockets of collagen are noted in the basement lamella (arrow). (Reproduced with permission from Mackinnon et al.[18])

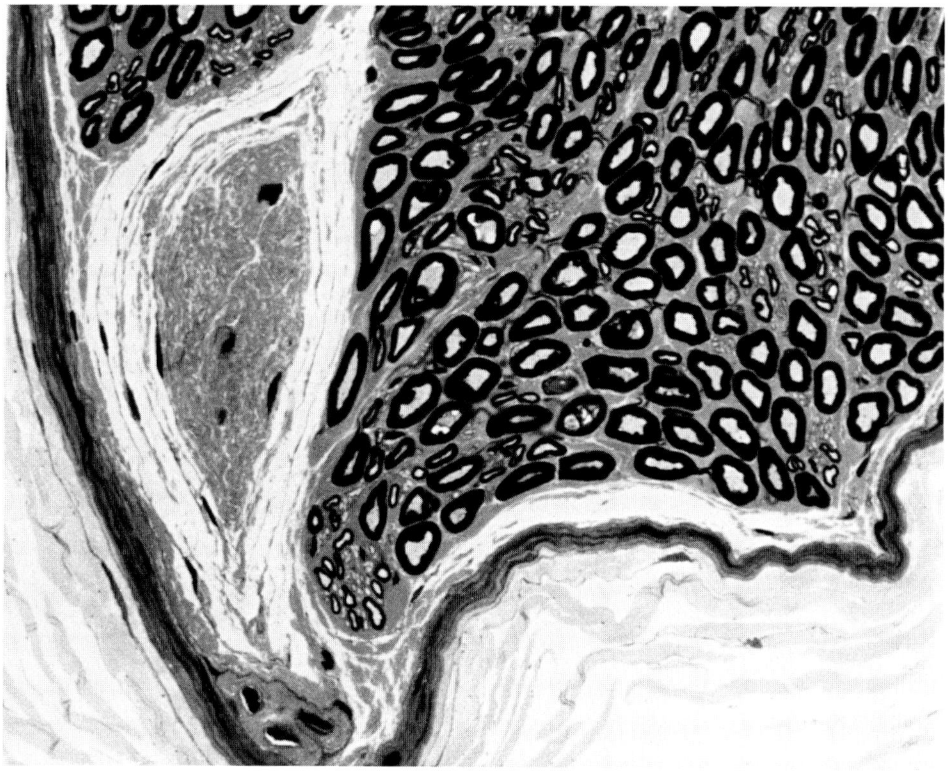

Figure 2-11. Transverse section of a Renaut body from case 1. This structure in the subperineurial space demonstrates an occasional cell nucleus in an amorphous connective tissue background. (Toluidine blue, ×500) (Reproduced with permission from Mackinnon et al.[18])

Renaut Bodies

In all cases, Renaut bodies were noted at the level of the area of compression (Figs. 2-9, 2-11). No Renaut bodies were noted proximal or distal to the area of compression and no Renaut bodies were noted in ten normal cadaver nerve biopsies of the radial sensory nerve. Since first described by Renaut,[20] these bodies have been noted in both experimental[21] and clinical[22] cases of nerve entrapment. It has been suggested that Renaut bodies are normal structures of the peripheral nerve.[23,25]

In reviewing autopsy studies of subclinical nerve entrapment, Jefferson and Eames[15] noted Renaut bodies in 60% of the nerves when the biopsies were taken from regions with a strong predilection for nerve entrapment. None of the control sections of the same nerve demonstrated Renaut bodies. No correlation between the number of Renaut bodies and the severity of nerve fiber changes was noted. Although the cause of these structures remains unclear, they do seem to be a marker for nerve entrapment. Bergouignan and Vital[24] noted their frequency in only 2% of the superficial peroneal nerve biopsies. This finding of Renaut bodies in a percentage of patients of underlying peripheral neuropathy would raise the question as to whether or not these patients had superimposed nerve entrapment to account for their presence (see Chapter 14, "Diabetic Neuropathy").

In our experimental models of chronic nerve compression in the rat,[8,9] we have not noted Renaut bodies in the sciatic nerves that have been subjected to compression with silicone tubes for up to 2 years. In the same animals, however, we have demonstrated Renaut bodies present in the medial and lateral plantar nerves in the foot. In the primate models of chronic nerve compression, we have seen Renaut bodies in the median nerve in the carpal tunnel but have not noticed these structures in the median nerve in the mid-forearm.[7] It is our impression that Renaut bodies are not normal structures in the peripheral nerve and represent a response of the nerve to a traction-type of injury. Direct compression without repetitive movement and traction does not result in the formation of these bodies, as is apparent in the 2-year nerve compression studies of the rat sciatic nerve in which no Renaut bodies were found compared with the findings in these same animals of frequent Renaut bodies in the medial and lateral plantar nerves in the foot.

Connective Tissue

Thickening of the epineurium and perineurium was noted in three cases (Fig. 2-12). In one instance, numerous myofibroblasts were noted in the epineurium.

Nerve Fibers

Proximal to the area of compression in all cases, the nerve fibers appeared normal. In two cases, in the

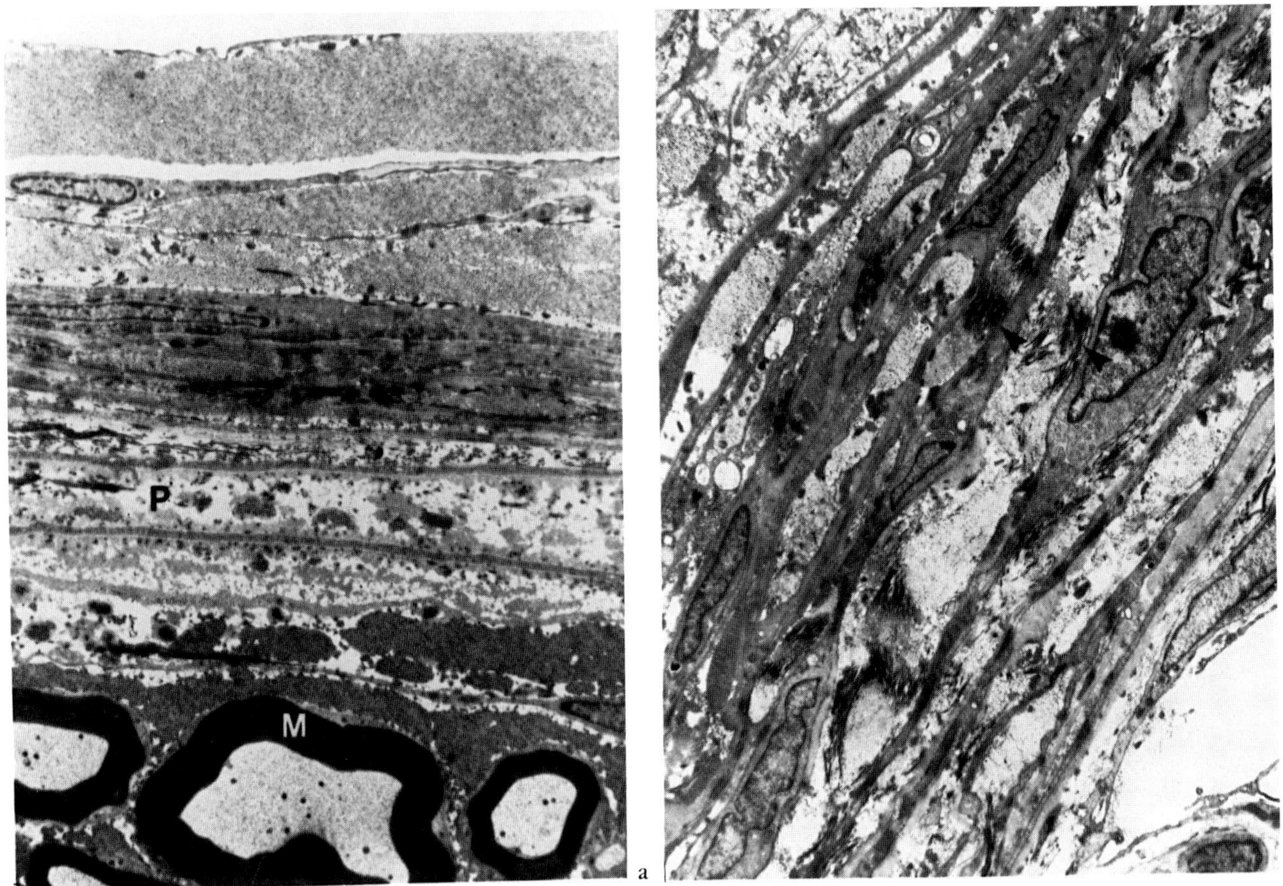

a b

Figure 2-12. Transverse section, SBR, case 2. (Uranyl acetate, ×98985.) **a.** The perineurium distal to the area of compression is normal. P: perineurium; M: myelin. **b.** In the region of the area of compression, the layers of the perineurium are markedly thickened. The perineurial cells are separated by an increased number of collagen fibers (arrow). (Reproduced with permission from Mackinnon et al.[18])

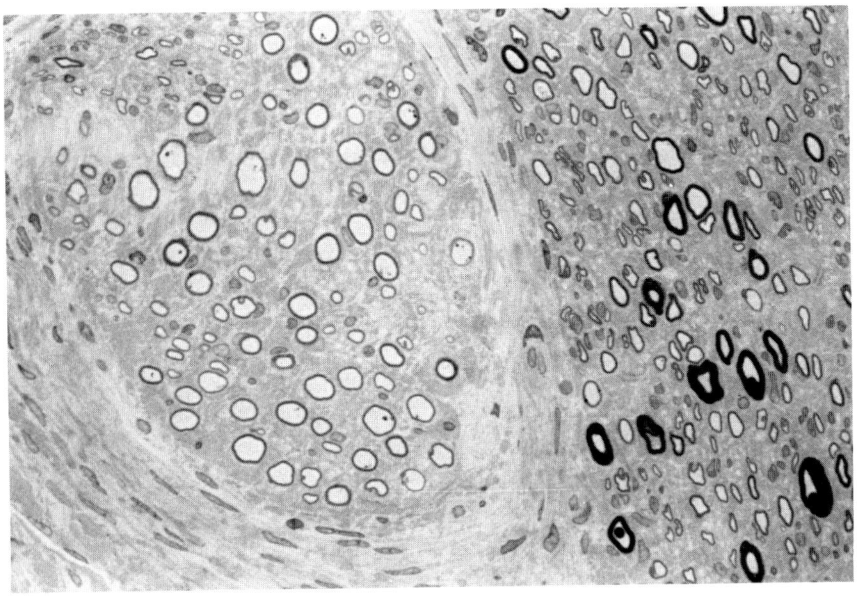

Figure 2-13. Transverse section, SBR, case 4. Marked thinning of the myelin is noted in one fascicle adjacent to a second fascicle that still contains several normally myelinated fibers. (Toluidine blue, ×500.) (Reproduced with permission from Mackinnon et al.[18])

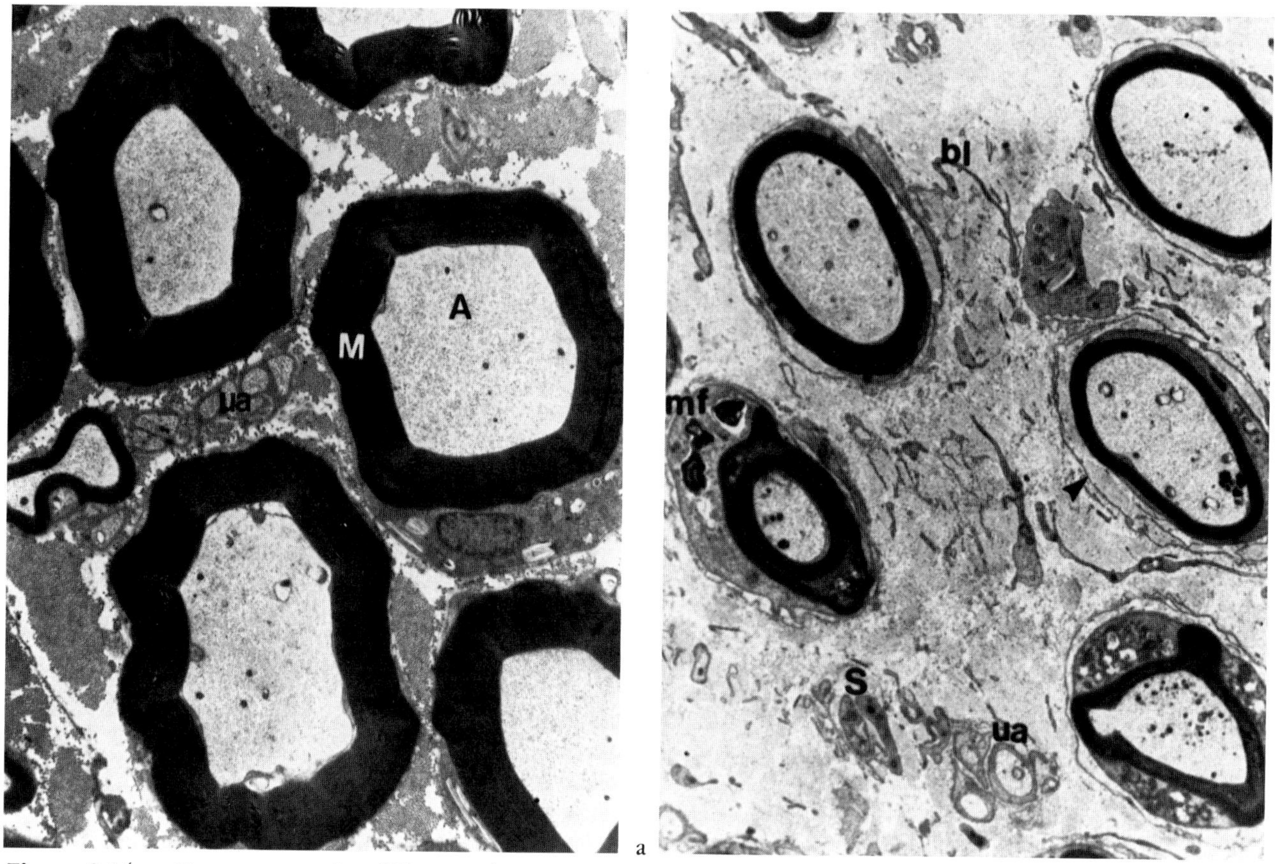

a b

Figure 2-14a. Transverse section, SBR, case 4, proximal area of nerve compression demonstrating normal detail of myelinated fibers. M: myelin; A: axon; ua: unmyelinated axons. (Uranyl acetate, ×9895.) **b.** Transverse section, SBR, case 4 in the area of nerve compression. The increase in the axon to myelin ratio due to myelin thinning is apparent. Evidence of active Wallerian degeneration is seen in the fiber whose Schwann cell cytoplasm contains myelin debris. Evidence of previous Wallerian degeneration is offered by the presence of the stacked Schwann cell processes. bl: basement lamina; mf: myelin fragments within Schwann cell cytoplasm; S: Schwann cell profile within band of Büngner; ua: unmyelinated axons; redundant basement membrane (arrow) (Uranyl acetate, ×9895.) (Reproduced with permission from Mackinnon et al.[18])

area of nerve compression, no nerve fiber abnormalities were seen. In the third case, a single fascicle demonstrated marked thinning of the myelin in the large myelinated fibers. In a fourth case, although some of the fascicles in the area of compression appeared quite normal, other more peripheral fascicles showed significant fiber damage consisting of marked thinning of the myelin (Fig. 2-13). This thinning of the myelin was apparent on both light and electron microscopy (Figs. 2-14, 2-15). Schwann cell processes devoid of axons (bands of Büngner) were also noted, suggesting that Wallerian degeneration had occurred without regeneration.

Light Microscopic Morphometric Assessment

The results of the morphometric assessment are noted in Table 2-4 with the data being presented from the case demonstrating the most significant fiber morphologic findings. Mean fiber diameter was significantly decreased in the area of compression. This was due to thinning of the myelin rather than axonal changes so that the axon to myelin and axon to fiber ratios increased. In Figures 2-14 and 2-15 the histologic findings corresponding to the data outlined in Table 2-4 are compared.

Electron Microscopic Morphologic Assessment

In three cases, the normal unimodal distribution of unmyelinated fibers was noted. The mean fiber diameter was approximately 0.7 μm and approximately 20% of the unmyelinated axons had a mean fiber diameter of less than 0.5 μm (Fig. 2-16). The ratio of unmyelinated

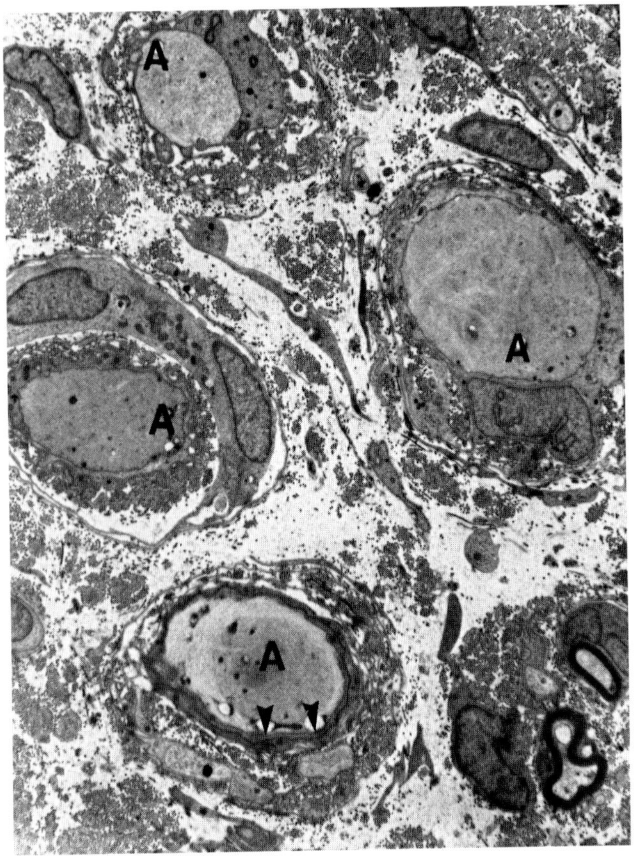

Figure 2-15. Transverse section, SBR, case four in area of compression. Single, very large axons (diameter 6 to 8 μm) represent previously myelinated fibers that have undergone demyelination. One axon is surrounded by two or three layers of myelin and may represent the final stages of demyelination or the early stages of remyelination. A: axon; layers of myelin (arrows). (Uranyl acetate, ×5107.) (Reproduced with permission from Mackinnon et al.[18])

to myelinated fibers was 4 to 1. In the case with the most significant fiber disease in the region of maximum compression, there was a shift in the fiber histogram to the left with a flattening of the unimodal peak suggestive of a tendency toward a bimodal distribution with peaks at 0.4 and 0.8 μm. The total number of unmyelinated axons less than 0.5 μm increased to 40% and the ratio of unmyelinated to myelinated fibers was 8 to 1 (Fig. 2-17). In this case, in the region proximal to the area of compression, a normal unimodal histogram was noted with a ratio of unmyelinated to myelinated fibers of 5 to 1. In the normal cadaver nerves, the mean unmyelinated fiber diameter was 1.0 μm and 9% of the unmyelinated axons had a mean diameter of less than 0.5 μm. The ratio of unmyelinated to myelinated fibers was 4 to 1.

Clinical Implications

All four patients complained of similar symptoms (marked pain and burning in the distribution of the radial sensory nerve). The fiber histologic findings, however, varied considerably from normal in one case to markedly abnormal in another. Thus, it is concluded that it is possible to have significant symptoms of nerve origin without nerve fiber changes. These findings of normal nerve fibers would correlate with the clinical circumstances in which the surgical patient notes almost immediate postoperative improvement in sensory complaints after surgical release of the compressed nerve. This rapid improvement of symptoms suggest that surgical decompression has alleviated a source of neural ischemia. Clinical improvement many weeks or months postoperatively would correspond to regeneration of a nerve with structural damage.

Table 2-4. Light Microscopic Morphometric Assessment of the Superficial Radial Nerve (SBR) of Case 4*

	Proximal	*Region of Compression*	*Distal*	*Control Cadaver SBR*
Mean fiber diameter† (μm) ±SD	8·12 ± 1·94	4·90 ± 1·78‡	3·85 ± 1·82‡	7·81 ± 3·02
Mean axon diameter† (μm)	4·32 ± 1·25	3·58 ± 1·68‡	2·18 ± 0·90‡	4·82 ± 1·91
Axon: fiber ratio (G) (diameter)	0·53	0·73	0·56	0·61
Mean fiber area (μm^2)	64·7 ± 2·26	32·1 ± 2·29†	22·3 ± 1·58†	66·3 ± 3·25
Mean axon area (μm^2)	20·7 ± 0·86	20·3 ± 1·70§	9·0 ± 0·48§	26·5 ± 1·26
Mean myelin area (μm^2)	43·7 ± 1·60	11·7 ± 0·65‡	13·3 ± 1·17‡	39·8 ± 2·12
Myelin (%)	67	36	60	60
Axon:myelin ratio (areas)	0·47	1·77	0·67	0·66
Axon: fiber ratio (areas)	0·32	0·63	0·40	0·40

*Reprinted with permission from Mackinnon et al.[18]

†Measuring shortest diameter.

‡ = $P < 0.001$.

§ = $P < 0.0001$.

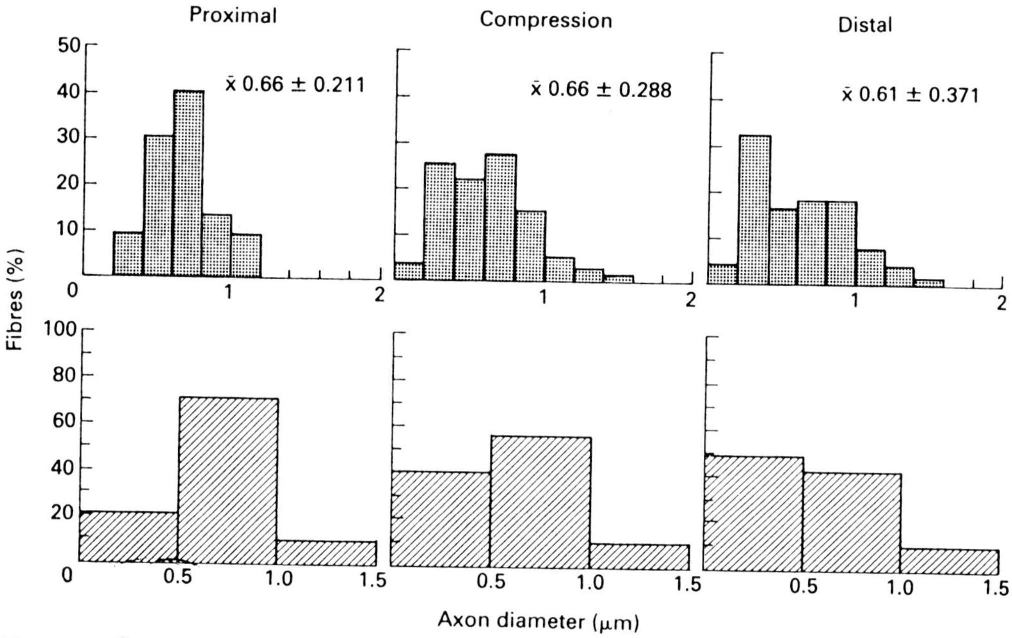

Figure 2-16. Histograms of fiber diameters (μm) of the unmyelinated axons of the superficial radial nerve from case 4. Histograms from the area of compression as well as proximal and distal to the area were noted. The histogram bars above demonstrate the percentage of fibers at 0;2 μm increments. The histogram bars below demonstrate the percentage of fibers at 0;2 μm increments. In the region of compression and distal to the region of compression, there is an increased population of small unmyelinated fibers (<0;5μm). (Reproduced with permission from Mackinnon et al.[18])

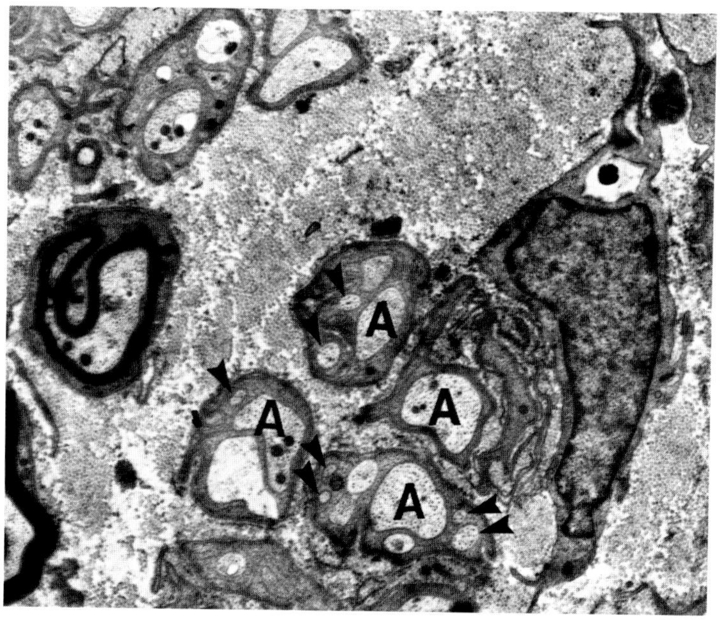

Figure 2-17. A transverse section, SBR, case four in area of nerve compression. A new population of very small unmyelinated fibers (mean fiber diameter less than 0.5 μm) (arrows) is seen adjacent to the unmyelinated axons of normal size (A). (Mean fiber diameter, 0.66 μm.) These very small axons are thought to be regenerating sprouts of unmyelinated axons. (Uranyl acetate, × 10,214.)(Reproduced with permission from Mackinnon et al.[18])

Varying pathologic conditions from fascicle to fascicle has also been noted in a compressed human nerve[13] but has, otherwise, not been emphasized. This varying distribution of fiber disease would account for the frequent paradox of the patient who presents with marked symptoms but normal electrodiagnostic findings. Although the pathologic changes in the worst fascicles would represent the patient's most severe symptoms, the normal large myelinated fibers in the best fascicles would provide the basis for normal nerve conduction studies (see also Chapter 3).

The histopathologic findings of chronic human nerve compression present a very broad spectrum. The surgeon should make an attempt to stage the degree of compression neuropathy and should expect patients to demonstrate both symptoms and clinical signs across a wide spectrum of severity. Any reports of treatment of chronic human nerve compression must take into account the number of patients in varying stages of nerve compression. (See also chapters on individual nerves for specific examples of stages, such as Chapter 6 for carpal tunnel syndrome and Chapter 9 for cubital tunnel syndrome)

Mild or Early Nerve Compression

In the early stages of nerve compression, symptoms may only be elicited with provocative tests used to render the nerve locally ischemic by manipulation of the extremity (that is, wrist flexion for median nerve compression at the wrist, elbow flexion for ulnar nerve compression at the elbow, or local pressure over the nerve at the anatomic site of compression). At this stage, the patient's symptoms are transient and are usually brought on by some abnormal positioning of the extremity either during sleep or during repetitive movements of the extremity or by abnormal sustained positioning of the extremity.

Moderate Nerve Compression

Patients may describe weakness and abnormal sensibility, but persistent paresthesia, is not yet present. Intraneural fibrosis is present; Wallerian degeneration is not.

Severe Nerve Compression

Persistent sensory change may be present. Muscle wasting and abnormal or two-point discrimination will be present only if there is advanced nerve compression with actual loss of nerve fibers, as occurs with Wallerian degeneration. The Tinel sign indicates some degree of neural regeneration and varies in incidence, depending on the stage of compression. In very early compression, it is negative, but in the very late compression it is also negative because regeneration has ceased.[24]

Acute Nerve Compression

The symptoms of transient ischemic nerve block after acute nerve compression is familiar to everyone that is, nocturnal paresthesia in the arms, the experience of the leg going to sleep in the movie theatre or after a long automobile ride. An interesting experience that no peripheral nerve surgeon should be without is that of a blood pressure cuff on the arm for 30 to 45 minutes.

Elegant experimental and clinical studies have investigated the effect of acute compression on the peripheral nerve. These studies have used both histologic and physiologic parameters to interprete the outcome of acute nerve compression. Experimental studies have utilized pressure cuffs placed directly over the nerve[26] as well as tourniquet paralysis models of acute compression.[27] Psychomotor studies using awake primates have correlated neurophysiologic and psychomotor responses to acute nerve compression.[28] Similar studies have been repeated in human subjects.[29]

The nerve injury associated with acute compartment syndromes has been evaluated in experimental and clinical situations. It will be important to review the findings of these studies.

Seddon's neurapraxia describes a form of acute nerve compression that is highlighted by a profound motor deficit with mild to moderate sensory changes. The nerve proximal and distal to the area of acute nerve compression remains electrically normal. Clinical examples of this include "Saturday night paralysis" and tourniquet palsy. The histologic effect of local, acute nerve compression, using both direct pressure from a clip and indirect pressure by a tourniquet, was to produce selective injury to the myelin sheaths, demonstrated by Denny-Brown and Brenner in the 1940s.[30,31]

In a series of experiments in the 1970s, from Queen's Square, a similar tourniquet paralysis model was developed in the baboon. Investigators Ochoa and colleagues[32–34] described several important histologic findings associated with acute compression:

1. Pathologic processes affected the large myelinated fibers but spared the small diameter fibers.
2. The nerve fiber defects were concentrated under the area of compression. The nerve fibers in the center of the nerve were spared.
3. The important pathologic processes involved local demyelination.
4. Significant classic nodal pathologic changes were seen. At the normal node position, the nodal gap disappeared due to an intussusception of myelin at the

location of the true node. A pseudonode was formed by indentation of the Schwann cell processes away from the area of injury.

These investigators postulated that the pathologic changes with acute compression is due to mechanical injury to the nerve so that a longitudinal driving force is generated along that nerve. Because of the varying attachments of axon, myelin, and Schwann cell, the nodes of Ranvier are dislocated away from the area of acute compression, causing the typical intussusception picture. Small fibers in this model would be spared because more force is required to displace the content of the smaller diameter fibers. Their studies would not necessarily be applicable to the injury seen with acute compartment syndromes because their experimental models investigating the effects of direct mechanical stimulation are clinically comparable to injuries that result in acute, direct pressure over the nerve.

Using a small transparent cuff, Rydevik et al[26] were able to observe directly the circulation of the nerve. With external pressures of 20 to 30 mmHg, a reduction in intraneural microcirculation at the epineurial venular level was noted. At 40 mmHg, a reduced flow was noted at the capillary level as well. With pressures between 60 and 80 mmHg, complete cessation of flow in the microcirculation was noted. These blood flow changes were immediately reversible with pressures between 20 to 80 mmHg for up to 2 hours. The same investigators studied the effect of higher pressures on the nerves and found that after application of 50 mmHg pressure for 2 hours, "epineurial" edema developed after release of the pressure cuff. The endoneurial vessels were not involved and functioned normally. At higher pressures (200 to 400 mmHg) "epineurial" edema developed but at these pressures the capillaries within the fascicles were also injured, with subsequent development of endoneurial edema. After 400 mm of compression for 2 hours, the injury was irreversible and the nerve fibers did not recover function.

Clinical and neurophysiologic studies of acute nerve compression have reported the important relationship between nerve compression and the function of the large group A beta fibers.[28,29,35–39] These fibers have been found to be the most sensitive to ischemic changes, possibly because of diminished oxygen delivery related to their size. Thus, compromised light touch and vibration sensation mediated by the group A beta fibers would be anticipated with abnormal function of this fiber system. Vibratory threshold tests are a measure of the quickly adapting group A beta fiber system. An animal and human model of the acute median nerve compression demonstrated that changes in vibration perception were the earliest tests indicating decrease in nerve function secondary to increased acute pressure on the nerve.[28,29] Human volunteers subjected to pressures of 50 mmHg in the carpal tunnel were found to have changes in cutaneous vibratory thresholds and changes in perception of a 256 cps vibratory stimulus as the earliest sensory test to indicate a decrease in nerve function.[29]

Nerve Injury in Acute Compartment Syndrome

Acute nerve compression, exerted over a prolonged period of time, has devastating sequelae. The type of nerve injury associated with acute compartment syndrome is similar to that seen with acute nerve compression. In acute compartment syndromes, however, the effects are largely due to ischemia of the nerve due to diminished flow within the compartment at risk. The pathophysiologic characteristics of compartment syndromes has been well described.[40] Increases in local tissue pressure will result in increased venous pressure leading to a decrease in the local arteriovenous gradiant. This diminished flow will result in decreased oxygen delivery to the tissue in the compartment, including the nerve. Experimental studies would suggest that when tissue pressures reach 30 mmHg, ischemic changes occur in both nerve and muscle.[26,38,41] The reversibility of these changes will be determined by both the amount of tissue pressure and the duration of the pressure. In an experimental study, Rorabeck et al[42] have defined the irreversibility of muscle damage at these pressures to occur at 6 hours compared with the irreversibility of neural function that occurred after 10 hours of acute compartment syndrome.

A clinical and experimental study reported the use of vibratory sensory testing in acute compartment syndromes.[38] Invasive and noninvasive diagnostic testing was correlated in 11 patients with forearm injuries that were clinically believed to have acute compartmental syndromes in the forearm. Sensory examination included light touch, pinprick stimuli, and moving and static two-point discrimination measurements in the median and ulnar nerve distributions bilaterally. The patient's perception of vibration was measured with the 256 cps tuning fork. Using a wick catheter technique, tissue pressures in the volar forearm were measured.[43]

In 9 of the 11 patients, compartment pressures were found to be elevated. These nine patients also had diminished or absent perception to 256 cps vibratory stimulation. In these patients, forearm fasciotomies were carried out. In two patients with normal response to 256 cps tuning fork examination, compartment pressures were not elevated. Table 2-5 outlines the clinical findings in the 11 patients studied. The findings of this clinical study, which had suggested that the 256 cps

Table 2-5. Clinical Data in Patients with Compartment Syndrome*

Case	Age/Sex	Injury	*Sensory Tests†* M2PD	S2PD	LT	PP	256	Systolic Blood Pressure (mmHg)	Compartment Pressure (mmHg)
1	48/F	Forearm puncture	N	N	N	N	↓	120	46
2	50/M	Forearm crush	0	0	N	N	↓	90	40
3	24/M	Drug injection	0	0	N	N	Absent	122	100
4	60/M	Arterial line	0	0	N	N	↓	90	30
5	47/M	Forearm puncture	N	N	N	N	↓	110	46
6	24/M	Postoperative ORIF† fracture radius	N	N	N	N	↓	120	38
7	26/M	Forearm crush	N	N	N	N	↓	120	52
8	58/M	Electrical hand burn	↑	0	↓	N	↓	130	68
9	42/M	Forearm crush	N	N	N	N	↓	125	40
10	21/M	Forearm laceration	N	N	N	N	N	120	15
11	22/M	Drug injection	N	N	N	N	N	120	12

*Reprinted with permission from Phillips et al.[38]

†N: normal; M2PD: moving two point discrimination; ↓ : decreased from; S2PD: moving and static two-point discrimination; LT: light touch; PP: pinprick; 256: 256-cps vibration; ORIF: open reduction, internal fixation.

tuning fork could be used as a noninvasive diagnostic test in the evaluation of patients with suspected acute compartment syndromes, were further evaluated in 12 adult, male volunteers. In these volunteers, elevated compartment pressures were created in the anterior tibial compartment of the leg. A decrease in perception to 256 cps vibratory stimulus was the earliest sensory abnormality to occur with elevated tissue compartment pressures. Analysis of variance showed significantly that 256 cps vibration was the most reliable and earliest sensory modality to change at pressures of 30 to 40 mmHg. The schemata of the experimental design are demonstrated in Figure 2-18 and the clinical data are outlined in Table 2-6.

A wick catheter was placed in the right anterior compartment of the leg of six subjects and in the left anterior compartment of six subjects. A pneumatic antishock garment (PASG) will provide a reliable method of producing experimental compartment syndromes.[44] Iatrogenic compartment syndrome has been documented clinically after inappropriately prolonged use of PASG for resuscitation.[45] A PASG was applied and inflated to produce compartment pressures of 35 to 40 mmHg. From time 0 before inflation and every 5 minutes after inflation, the subjects responses to sensory testing in the area innervated by the deep peroneal nerve was compared with testing in the contralateral foot. Sensory testing in the superficial peroneal nerve

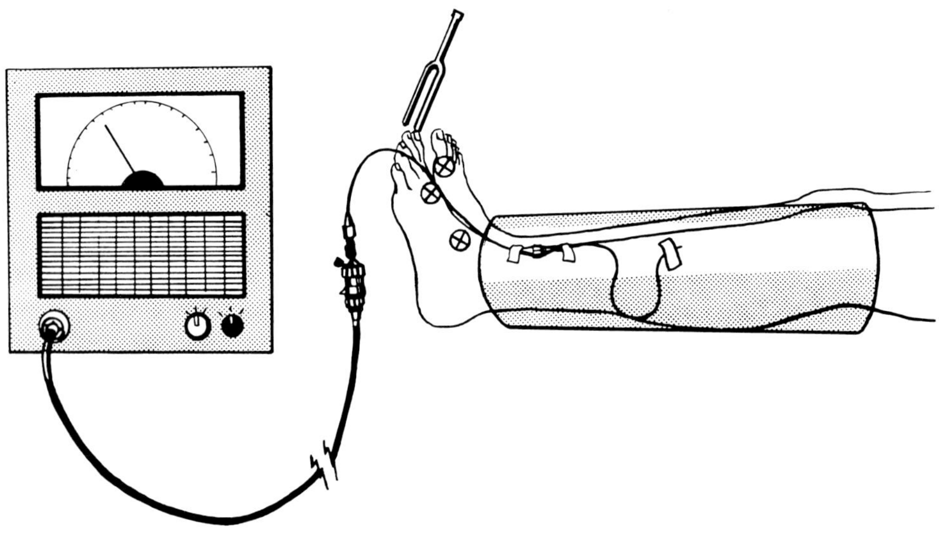

Figure 2-18. Schemata of experimental design. Sensory testing was carried out in the distribution of the deep peroneal nerves in both feet and the superficial peroneal nerve in the experimental foot. (Reproduced with permission from Phillips et al.[38])

Table 2-6. Clinical Data in 12 Adult Volunteers*

Volunteer	Vibration (cps) 256	128†	30†	Vibrometer†	L.T.†§	M2PD†§	S2PD†§	S.W.†§
1	30 ‖	55	‡	‡	40	‡	‡	‡
2	30	‡	‡	‡	‡	‡	‡	‡
3	35	‡	‡	‡	55	‡	‡	‡
4	25	30	†	25	‡	‡	‡	‡
5	40	†	‡	45	55	‡	‡	‡
6	35	45	‡	45	50	‡	‡	‡
7	25	‡	‡	‡	35	‡	‡	‡
8	10	15	20	15	15	‡	‡	15
9	35	50	‡	‡	‡	‡	‡	‡
10	50	‡	‡	‡	‡	‡	‡	‡
11	40	60	‡	‡	‡	‡	‡	‡
12	40	‡	‡	‡	50	‡	‡	‡

*Reprinted with permission from Phillips et al.[38]

†$p < 0.005$ sign test for differences from vibration 256.

‡Test still remains negative after 60 minutes.

§LT = light touch; M2PD = moving and static two-point discrimination; SW = Semmes-Weinstein pressure test.

‖ Time in minutes at which test became positive.

that was not in the compartment at risk for compartment syndrome but was directly under the pneumatic tourniquet and thus could be subject to acute direct compression from the tourniquet was used as a control test to differentiate the effects of pure ischemia that was affecting the deep peroneal nerve and acute pressure to the superficial peroneal nerve from the tourniquet cuff. Cutaneous vibratory threshold tests using 30, 125, and 256 cps tuning forks as well as an amplitude variable frequency fixed (120 cps) vibrometer was carried out. Tests of innervation density evaluating static and moving two-point discrimination were measured and cutaneous threshold tests of pressure were evaluated with Semmes-Weinstein monofilaments. Light touch perception was documented using the examiner's finger as a stimulus.

In all subjects, a decrease in 256 cps vibratory sensation was noted in the experimental leg in the distribution of the deep peroneal nerve. In each subject, abnormal perception at 256 cps vibration stimulus preceded other changes of vibration perception (30, 120, and 256 cps). It has been suggested that at frequencies less than 300 cps, the threshold of vibration sense is more sensitive to higher frequencies.[46,47] This may explain the finding that abnormal perception of 256 cps vibration preceded changes at lower frequencies. Once again, group A beta fibers, which are the most sensitive to ischemic changes, mediate vibratory perception as measured quantitatively with the 120 cps vibrometer and qualitatively with the 256 cps tuning fork. Other tests of innervation density and light touch often remained normal. Following normalization of compartment pressures after 60 minutes, all sensory testing returned to normal.

In the early stages of acute compartment syndrome, the histologic findings in the peripheral nerve would be anticipated to be normal. After 8 hours, irreversible Wallerian degeneration within the nerve would be expected.

Nerve Injection Injuries

The devastating sequelae of sensory and motor loss after injection of various agents into various peripheral nerves has been well-documented.[48] Detailed experimental studies have demonstrated the type of nerve injury that is associated with this clinical problem.[49–53] All experimental studies have demonstrated that the site of injection is critical in determining the degree of nerve injury (Fig. 2-19). In order to exert any compromise to the peripheral nerve, the substance must be injected in an intrafascicular position. Extrafascicular injections of the same substance causes no nerve injury (Fig. 2-20). The severity of the injury has a definite drug-dose relationship. A detailed study of the effects of many injectable steroid agents reported significant damage to the nerve fibers, with a breakdown in the blood–nerve barrier and Wallerian degeneration occurring with intrafascicular injection of most of the agents (Fig. 2-21). Dexamethasone was the only agent that caused minimal damage even with intrafascicular injection (Table 2-7). A similar study investigated the effect of various local anesthetics on nerve function.[49] The effect of many other commonly injected therapeutic agents has been studied.[49–53] Diazepam and penicillin have been found to evoke a very severe injury as has chymopapain. In many instances, it is believed that, although the drug itself may not be neurotoxic, the carrier agents that are combined with the drug may cause severe damage to the nerve when injected within the

Table 2-7. Results of Nerve Fiber Morphology (Light and Electron Microscopy)*

Agent	*Degree of Nerve Fiber Damage†*	
	EF Injection	*IF Injection*
Dexamethasone (Decadron)	No damage	Minimal damage
Triamcinolone acetonide (Kenalog)	No damage	Moderate damage
Methylprednisolone (Depo-Medrol)	No damage	Moderate damage
Hydrocortisone (Solu-Cortef)	No damage	Severe damage
Triamcinolone hexacetonide (Aristospan)	No damage	Severe damage
Normal saline (0.9%)	No damage	No damage

*Reprinted with permission from Mackinnon et al.[49]

†EF = extrafascicular injection; IF = intrafascicular injection.

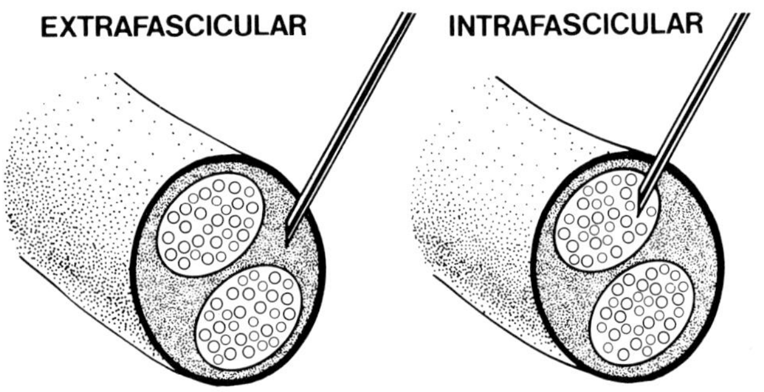

Figure 2-19. Schematic diagram of the sites of nerve injection. If the substances are injected in the extrafascicular location, nerve fiber damage rarely if ever occurs. By contrast, if the substances are injected intrafascicularly within the nerve, nerve injury is likely. (Reproduced with permission from Mackinnon et al.[52])

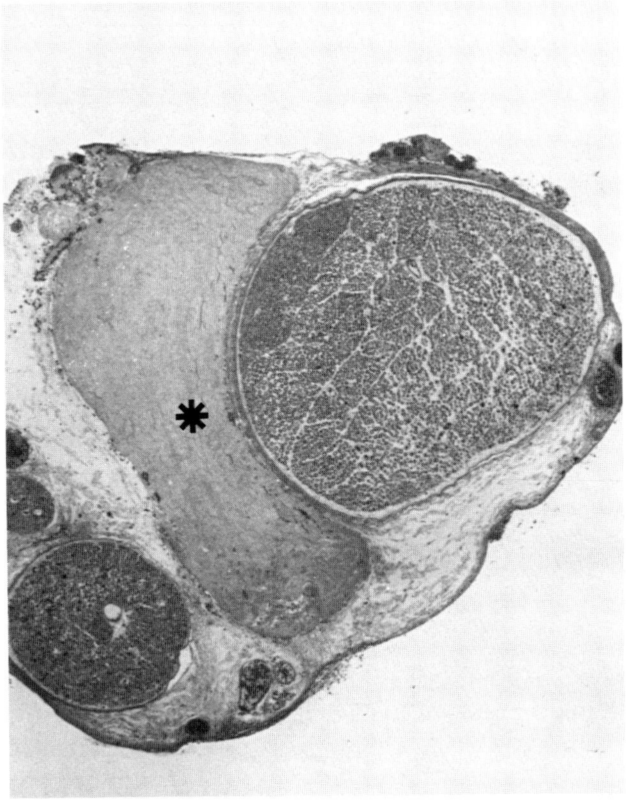

a

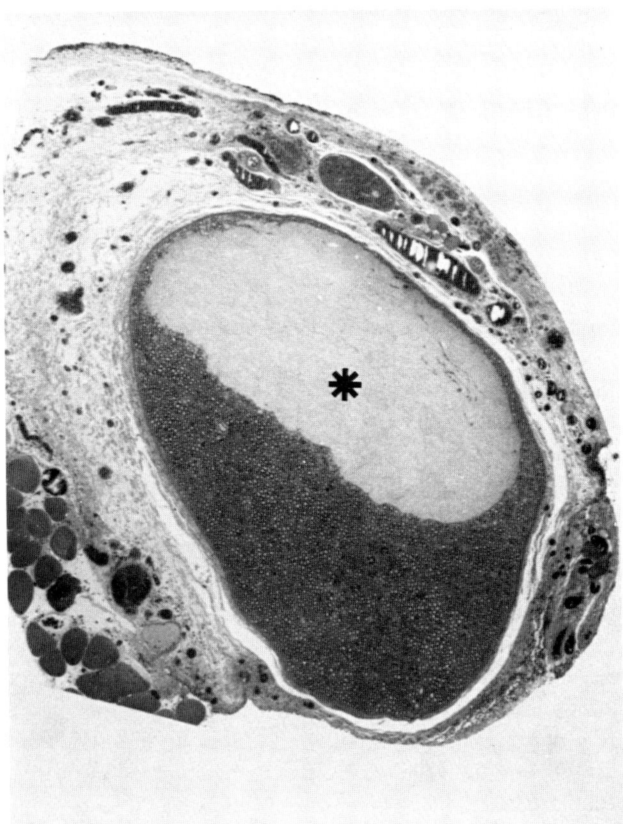

b

Figure 2-20. Toluidine blue transverse section of rat sciatic nerve. Zyderm (bovine collagen) can be seen as a homogeneous material (*) and easily located at the extrafascicular site (**a**) or at the intrafascicular site (**b**). (×60.) (Reproduced with permission from Mackinnon et al.[52])

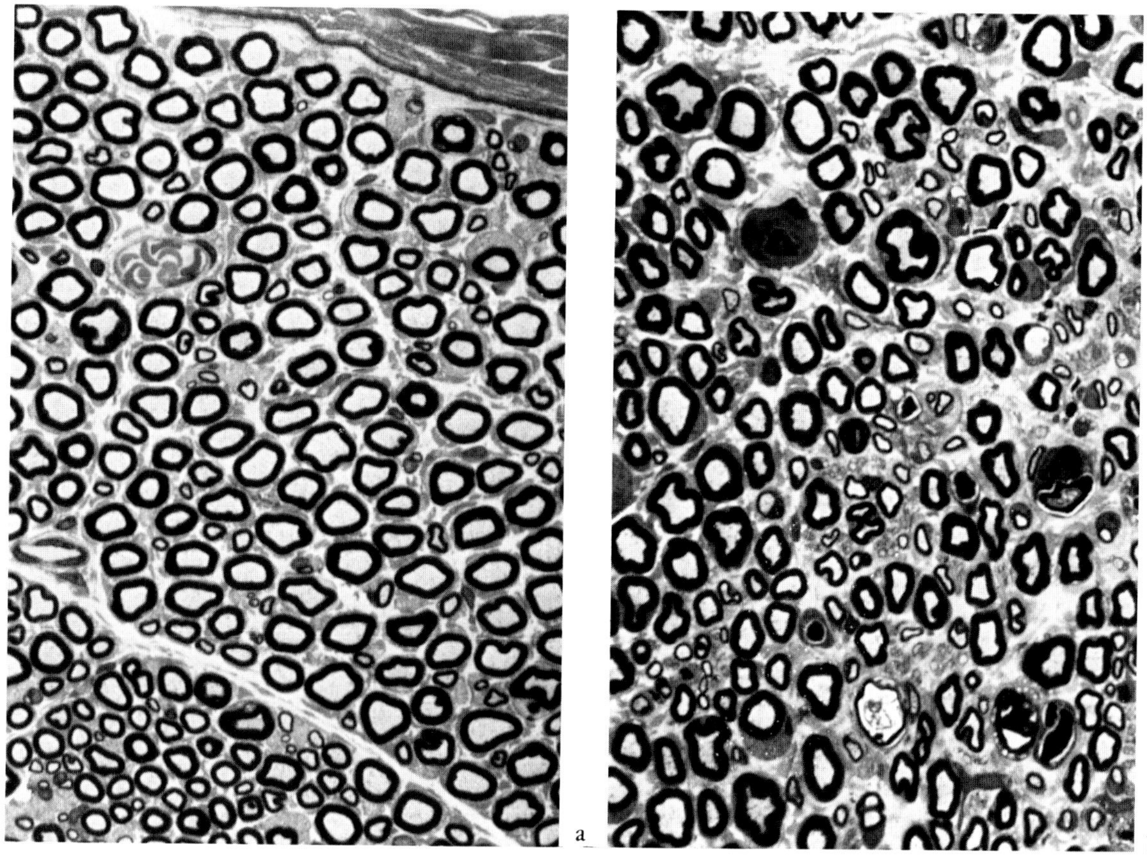

a b

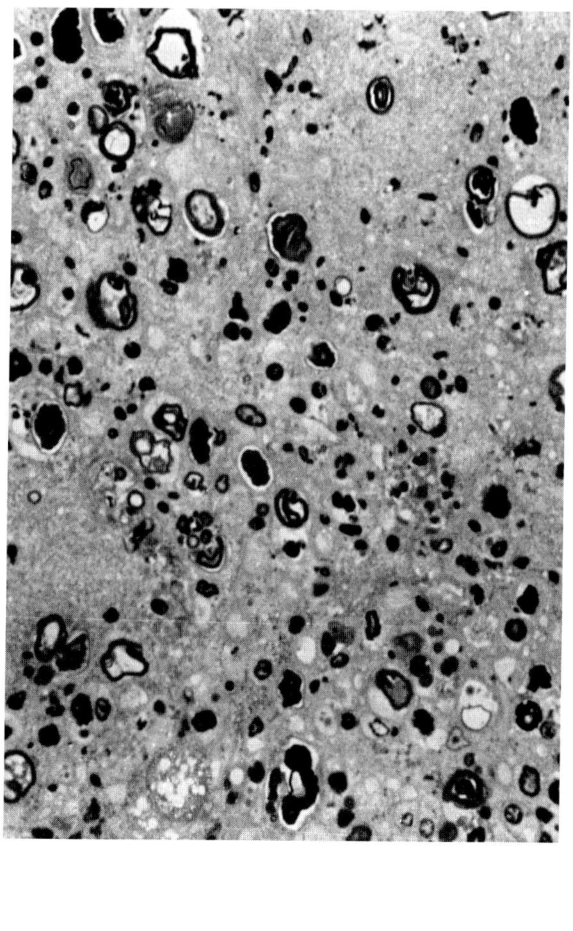

c

Figure 2-21. **a.** Cross-section of normal sciatic nerve. **b.** 12 days after intrafascicular injection of dexamethasone. **c.** 12 days after intrafascicular injection of triamcinolone hexacetonide. The section in **b** shows minor damage and the section in **c** shows severe widespread axonal and myelin degeneration. (Toluidine blue, ×336.) (Reproduced with permission from Mackinnon et al.[49])

nerve substance. Unfortunately, these carrier agents have not been separated from the therapeutic agent and are often necessary for the drug's therapeutic effect. These experimental studies demonstrated that a needle insertion and control saline injections do not cause damage to the nerve.

Based on these experimental studies of nerve injection injuries, considerable can be learned about the management of the clinical problem.[54,55] The history that the patient gives after a nerve injection injury is characteristic of one involving direct injection into the nerve. The patient will complain of severe, immediate pain not only at the site of the injection but radiating into the precise distribution of the nerve involved. Eventual clinical recovery of nerve function will be directly related to the type and amount of agent used. Unfortunately, early exploration of the nerve is not helpful. Failure to recover electrical or clinical function in an appropriate anatomic serial fashion after 3 months is an indication for surgical exploration and management of the injury, as one would manage a neuroma in-continuity. The only instance in which early surgical exploration and neurolysis (see Chapter 5) is recommended would be in those cases in which the injection injury has occurred in an area of known potential for nerve compression, such as the carpal tunnel or antecubital crease. The common nerves to be injected are the sciatic and radial nerve and these injection sites are usually well out of the area of any known anatomic location of nerve compression.

Certainly, the key to nerve injection is prevention. A knowledge of the surface anatomy is critical and, most importantly, injection should never be carried out into the nerve itself. The cooperation of the awake patient is required in order to communicate to the person carrying out the injection any symptoms of paresthesia. When paresthesia is evoked, the needle should be immediately withdrawn until the paresthesia has subsided. When the person injecting has the opportunity of choosing between various drugs with various toxicities, the least neurotoxic should be chosen. When injecting the substance, if the patient describes severe pain confined to a nerve distribution, the injection should immediately be discontinued. Long-term sequela of pain in the injected nerve are occasionally improved with microneurosurgical neurolysis. Unfortunately, these complaints are frequently influenced by malpractice litigation.

References

1. Seddon HJ: Three types of nerve injury. Brain 66:237, 1943.
2. Sunderland S: A classification of peripheral nerve injuries producing loss of function. Brain 74:491, 1951.
3. Seiler WA, Dellon AL, Mackinnon SE: Increased susceptibility of the alcoholic rat sciatic nerve to nerve compression: an electrophysiological study. Submitted. Ann Plast Surg.
4. Seddon HJ, Medawar PB, Smiths H: Rate of regeneration of peripheral nerves in man. J Physiol (Lond) 102:191–201, 1943.
5. Sunderland S: Rate of regeneration of I: sensory nerve fibers and II: motor fibres. Arch Neurol Psychiatry 58:1–14, 251–256, 1947.
6. Mackinnon SE: New directions in peripheral nerve surgery. Ann Surg 22:257—273, 1989.
7. Mackinnon SE, Dellon AL, Hudson AR, Hunter DA: A primate model for chronic nerve compression. J Reconstr Microsurg 1:185–194, 1985.
8. Mackinnon SE, Dellon AL, Hudson AR, Hunter DA: Chronic nerve compression: An experimental model in the rat. Ann Plast Surg 13:112–120, 1984.
9. O'Brien JP, Mackinnon SE, McLean A, Hudson AR, Dellon AL, Hunter DA: A model of chronic nerve compression in the rat. Ann Plast Surg, 19:430–435, 1987.
10. Mackinnon SE, Dellon AL: Evaluation of microsurgical internal neurolysis in a primate median nerve model of chronic nerve compression. J Hand Surg 13A:345–351, 1988.
11. Marie P, Foix C: Atrophie isolee de l'eminence thenar d'origine nervitique Role du ligament annulaire anterieur de carpe dans la pathogenie de la lesion. Rev Neurol (Paris) 26:647–648, 1913.
12. Thomas PK, Fullerton PM: Nerve fibre size in the carpal tunnel syndrome. J Neurol Neurosurg Psychiatry 26:520–527, 1963.
13. Neary D, Eames RA: The pathology of ulnar nerve compression in man. Neuropathol Appl Neurobiol 1:69–88, 1975.
14. Neary D, Ochoa J, Gilliatt RW: Subclinical entrapment neuropathy in man. J Neurol Sci 24:283–298, 1975.
15. Jefferson D, Eames RA: Subclinical entrapment of the lateral femoral cutaneous nerve. An autopsy study. Muscle Nerve 2:145–154, 1979.
16. Mackinnon SE, Dellon AL, Daneshvar A: Histopathology of the tarsal tunnel syndrome. An examination of the human tibial nerve. Contemp Orthop 9:43–48, 1984.
17. Dellon AL, Mackinnon SE: Human ulnar nerve compression at the elbow: Clinical, histologic and electrodiagnostic correlations. J Reconstr Microsurg 4:179–187, 1988.
18. Mackinnon SE, Dellon AL, Hudson AR, Hunter DA: Chronic human nerve compression. A histological assessment. Neuropathol Appl Neurobiol 12:547–565, 1986.
19. Mackinnon SE, Dellon AL: Results of treatment of recurrent dorsoradial wrist neuromas. Ann Plast Surg 19:54–61, 1987.
20. Renaut A: Recherches sur quelques points particuliers d'histologie des nerfs. Arch Physiol 8:180–190, 1881.
21. Ortman JA, Zarife S, Mendell JR: The experimental production of Renaut bodies. J Neurol Sci 62:233–241, 1983.
22. Jefferson D, Neary D, Eames RA: Renaut body distribution at sites of human peripheral nerve entrapment. J Neurol

Sci 49:19–29, 1981.

23. Asbury AK: Renaut bodies—a forgotten endoneurial structure. J Neuropathol Exp Neurol 32:334–343, 1973.
24. Bergouignan FX, Vital C: Occurrence of Renaut bodies in a peripheral nerve. Arch Pathol Lab Med 108:230–233, 1984.
25. Dellon AL: Tinel or not Tinel. J Hand Surg [Br] 9:216, 1984.
26. Rydevik B, Lundborg G, Bagge U: Effects of graded compression on interneural blood flow. J Hand Surg 6:3, 1981.
27. Ochoa J, Fowler TJ, Gilliatt RW: Anatomical changes in peripheral nerves compressed by a pneumatic tourniquet. J Anat 113:413–433, 1972.
28. Dellon AL, Schneider RJ, Burke R: Effect of acute compartmental change on response to vibratory stimuli in primates. Plast Reconstr Surg 72:208, 1983.
29. Szabo RN, Gilberman RH, Williamson RV, Dellon AL, Yaru NC, Dimick MP: Vibratory sensory testing in acute peripheral nerve compression. J Hand Surg [Am] 9:104, 1984.
30. Denny-Brown D, Brenner C: Paralysis of nerve induced by direct pressure and by tourniquet. Arch Neurol Psychol 51:119, 1944.
31. Denny-Brown D, Brenner C: Division in peripheral nerve resulting from compression by a spring clip. Arch Neurol Psychiatry 52:1, 1944.
32. Ochoa J, Danta G, Fowler TJ, Gilliatt RW: Nature of the nerve lesion caused by a pneumatic tourniquet. Nature 233:265, 1971.
33. Ochoa J, Gilliatt RW, Fowler TJ: Tourniquet paralysis in a baboon. Transam Neurolog Assoc 97:52, 1972.
34. Rudge P, Ochoa J, Gilliatt RW: Acute peripheral nerve compression in the baboon. Anatomical and physiological findings. J Neurol Sci 23:403, 1974.
35. Gregg EC: Absolute measurements of the vibratory threshold. Arch Neurol 66:403, 1951.
36. Dellon AL: Evaluation of Sensibility and Re-education of the Sensation in the Hand. Williams & Wilkins, Baltimore, 1981, pp 160, 164.
37. Lundborg G, Gelberman RH, Minteer-Convery M, Lee YF, Hargens AR: Median nerve compression in the carpal tunnel—functional response to experimentally induced controlled pressure. J Hand Surg 7:252, 1982.
38. Phillips JH, Mackinnon SE, Beatty SE, Dellon AL, O'Brien JP: Vibratory sensory testing in acute compartment syndromes—a clinical and experimental study. Plast Reconstr Surg 79:796–801, 1987.
39. Dellon AL: Clinical use of vibratory stimuli to evaluate peripheral nerve injury and compression neuropathy. Plast Reconstr Surg 65:466, 1980.
40. Matsen FA, Crugmire RB: Compartmental syndromes. Surg Gynecol Obstet 147:943, 1978.
41. Hargens AR, Romine JS, Sipe JC, et al: Peripheral nerve conduction block by high muscle-compartment pressure. J Bone Joint Surg 61A:192, 1979.
42. Rorabeck CH, Cassell GS, Hardie R, Logan J: Compartmental pressure measurements—an experimental investigation using the slit catheter. J Trauma 21:466, 1981.
43. Muburak SJ, Hargens AR, Owen CA, et al: The wick catheter technique for measurement of intramuscular pressure—a new research and clinical tool. J Bone Joint Surg 58A:1016, 1976.
44. Chisholm CD, Clark DE: Effect of pneumatic antishock garment on intramuscular pressure. Ann Emerg Med 13:8, 1984.
45. McLellan B, Phillips JH, Hunter GA, et al: Bilateral lower extremity amputation after prolonged application of pneumatic antishock garment: a case report. Can J Surg 30:55–56, 1987.
46. Cosh JA: Studies on the nature of vibration sense. Clin Sci 12:131, 1953.
47. Mountcastle VB, Talbot WH, Darian-Smith I, Kornhuber HH: Neural basis for the sense of flutter-vibration. Science 155:597, 1967.
48. Hudson AR, Kline D, Gentili F: Peripheral nerve injection injury. In Omer G, Spinner M, eds: Management of Peripheral Nerve Problems. WB Saunders, Philadelphia, 1980, pp 639–653.
49. Mackinnon SE, Hudson AR, Gentili F, et al: Peripheral nerve injection injury with steroid agents. Plast Reconstr Surg 69:482–489, 1982.
50. Gentili F, Hudson AR, Hunter DA, et al: Nerve injection injury with local anesthetic agents—a light and electron microscope fluorescent microscopic and horseradish peroxidase study. Neurosurgery 6:263, 172, 1980.
51. Mackinnon SE, Hudson AR, Llamas F, Dellon AL, Kline DG, Hunter DA: Peripheral nerve injury by chymopapain injection. J Neurosurg 61:1–8, 1984.
52. Mackinnon SE, Hudson AR, Bojanowski V, Hunter DA, Maraghi E: Peripheral nerve injury with purified bovine collagen—an experimental model in the rat. Ann Plast Surg 14:428–436, 1985.
53. Gentili F, Hudson AR, Kline D, et al: Peripheral nerve injection injury. Neurosurgery 4:244, 1979.
54. Yaffe B, Pri-chen S, Lin E, Engel J, Modan M: Peripheral nerve injection injury. An experimental pilot study of treatment modalities. J Reconstr Microsurg 3:33–37, 1986.
55. Rayan GM, Pitha JV, Wisdom P, Brentlinger A, Kopta A: Histologic and electrophysiologic changes following subepineurial hematoma induction in rat sciatic nerve. Clin Orthop 229:257–264, 1988.

Diagnosis of Nerve Injury

3

The appropriate management of a peripheral nerve injury is critically dependent on the initial careful examination of the nerve-injured patient. The diagnosis of a peripheral nerve injury can be made in almost all instances based on a detailed physical examination of the patient. In this chapter, and again specifically in the chapters devoted to individual nerve problems, the basic physical examination findings and key factors in the differential diagnosis will be reviewed to permit the examiner in most instances to arrive at the correct diagnosis, usually without the need for electrodiagnostic studies. The indications for electrodiagnostic studies and their application will be reviewed in this chapter, and their appropriate role in the management of peripheral nerve injuries delineated.

The essence of the approach to the diagnosis of peripheral nerve injury is the understanding of the behavior of the motor and sensory nerve fiber after injury. The normal anatomy of the peripheral nerve has been described in Chapter 1 and the response of the nerve to injury and the pathophysiologic characteristics of the injured nerve have been described in Chapter 2. The correlation of the pathophysiologic findings of the injured nerve with the physical examination is described in this chapter for individual mixed nerves, but is based on the firm grounding in the research work described in Chapter 2 and the more recent work in the rat,[1–3] primate,[4,5] and human upper[6–8] and lower extremities.[9]

Correlation of Degree of Nerve Injury with Physical Findings

In nerve compression the functions of the nerve are still maintained to some degree but are diminished both qualitatively and quantitatively, depending on the degree and duration of the nerve compression. Abnormalities in the motor system have been better described than those in the sensory system. For the muscle, the first manifestation of injury to its nerve is weakness. We can measure weakness by manual muscle testing[10] (Figs. 3-1 through 3-8) and quantitate this weakness with assessment of pinch and grip strength. (Examination of the hand is compromised in the office setting if a measurement of pinch and grip is not done.) Increasingly, techniques for this are being standardized.[11,12] When the measurement has been made for pinch and grip strength (with consideration of hand dominance and age, sex, and occupation of the patient), the diagnosis of weakness can be made. The nerve that supplies the muscles for lateral key pinch and for grip strength is primarily the ulnar nerve. Weakness is the first indication of ulnar motor nerve dysfunction.

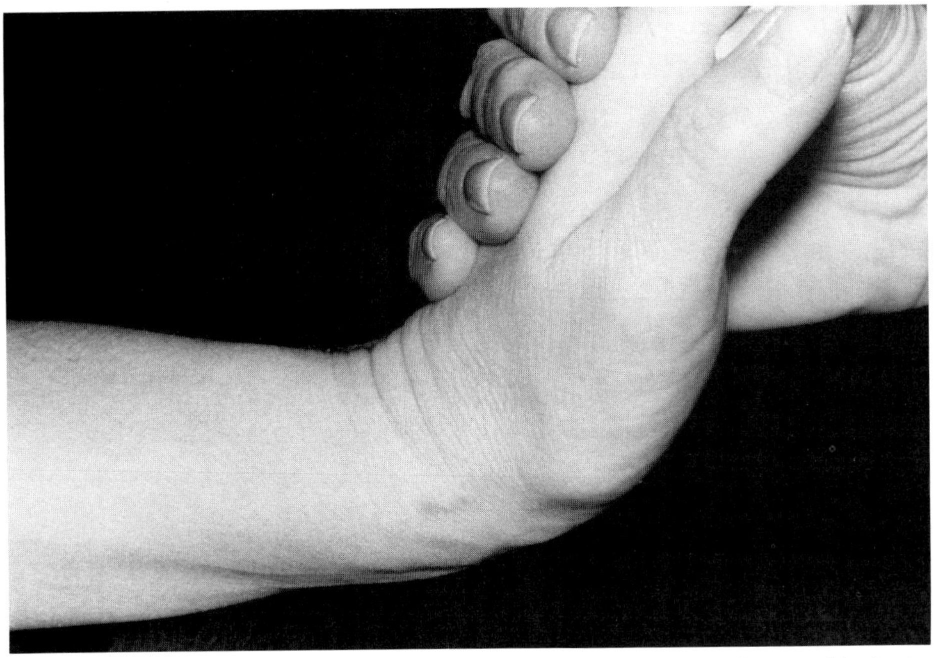

Figure 3-1. Examination of radial nerve extrinsic muscle function can be tested by having the patient hold the wrist in extension using the examiner's hand to test the strength by which the patient can resist this wrist dorsiflexion.

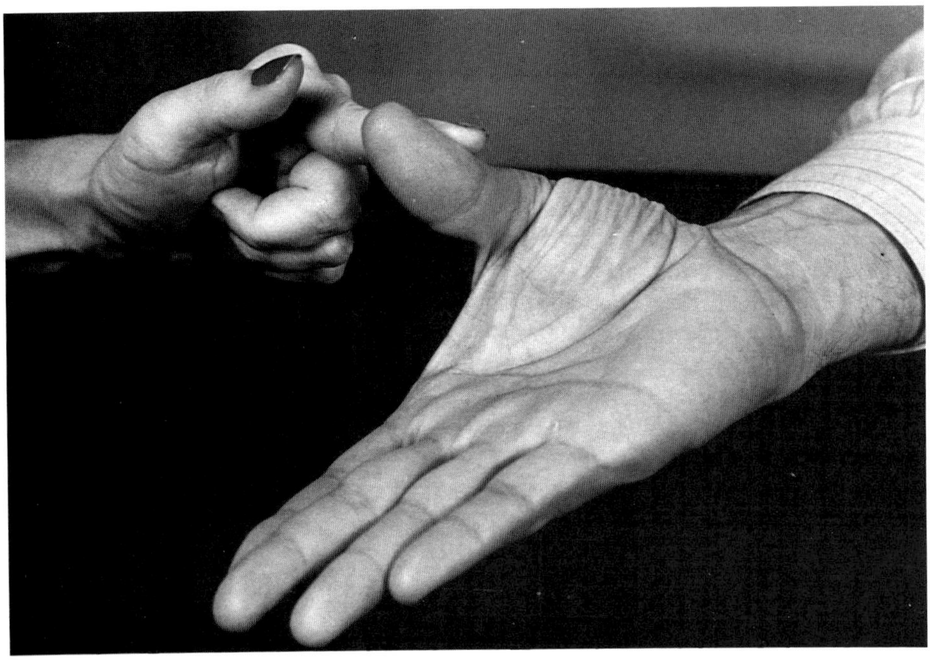

Figure 3-2. Assessment of median nerve intrinsic muscle function is best tested by having the patient abduct the thumb at 90° from the palm of the hand. The examiner then asks the patient to keep the thumb in this position and resist this movement. The contracting abductor pollicis brevis muscle belly which can be seen and palpated.

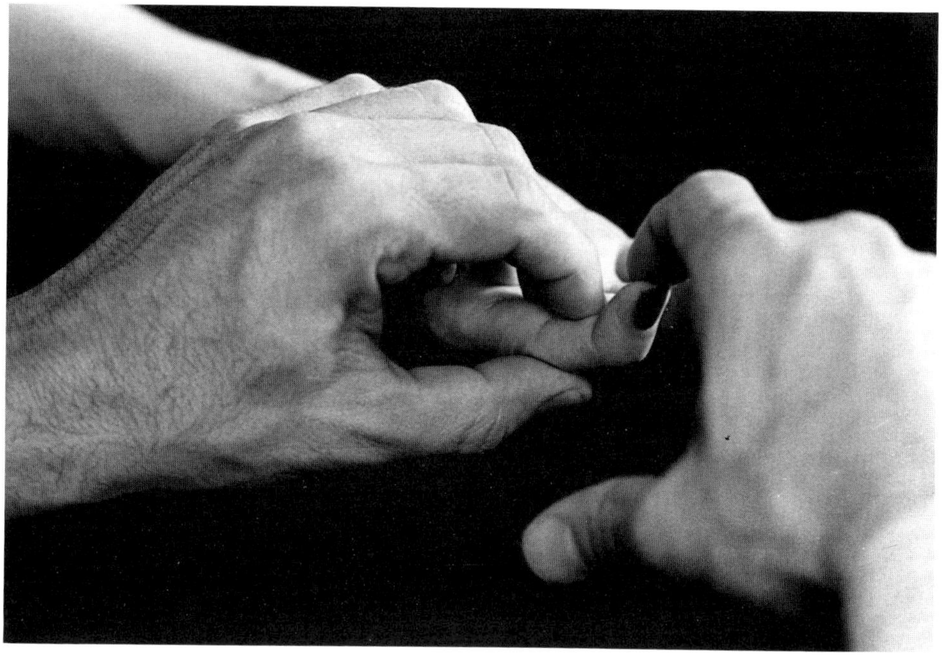

Figure 3-3. Median nerve extrinsic function can be assessed by asking the patient to flex the distal interphalangeal joint of the index finger and keep the joint in this position. The examiner then resists this movement with his own digit.

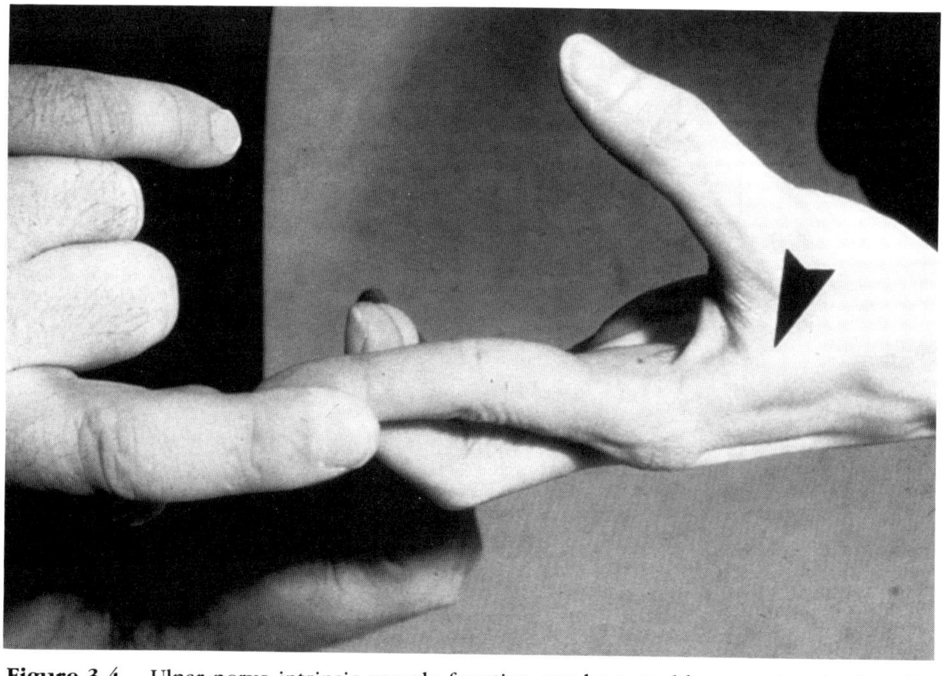

Figure 3-4. Ulnar nerve intrinsic muscle function can be tested by assessing the function in the first dorsal interosseous muscle by having the patient demonstrate a lateral key pinch and noting contraction in this muscle or, as is shown, resisting abduction of the index finger and noting a contraction of the first dorsal interosseous muscle (arrow). (Photo courtesy of T. R. Sullivan, M.D.)

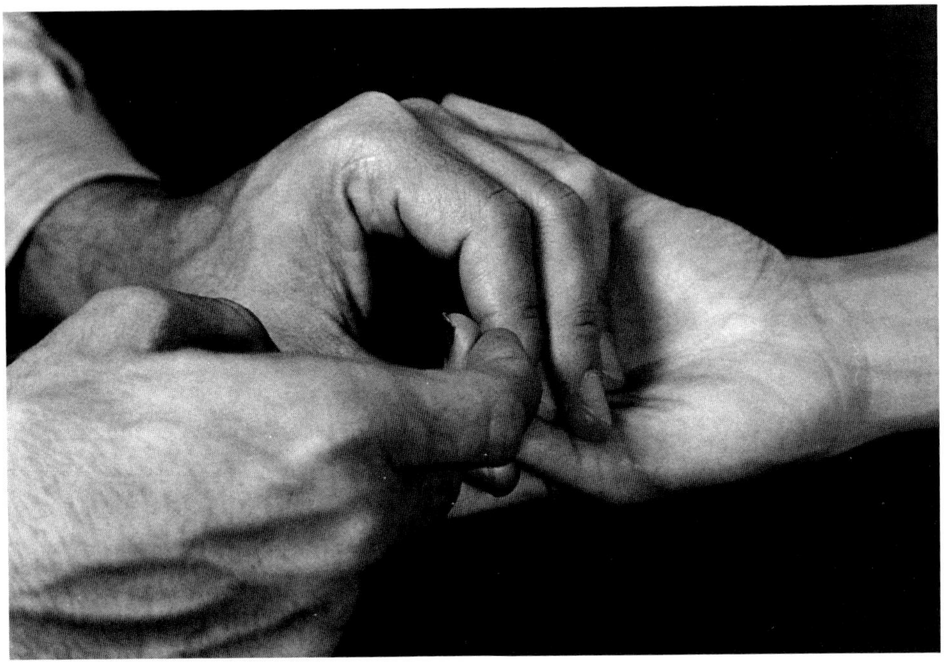

Figure 3-5. Ulnar nerve extrinsic motor function is assessed by having the patient flex the distal interphalangeal joint of the little finger. The examiner then asks the patient to keep the digit in this position and assesses resisted flexion of this distal interphalangeal joint.

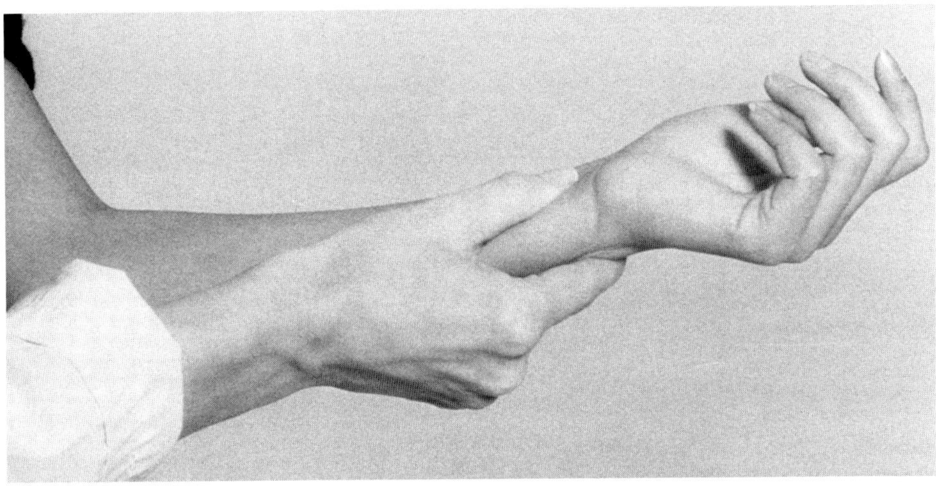

Figure 3-6. Carpal tunnel symptoms can be provoked or aggravated by direct pressure over the median nerve just proximal to the carpal tunnel. Within several seconds, the patient with entrapment of the median nerve in the carpal tunnel will describe paresthesia in the median nerve distribution.

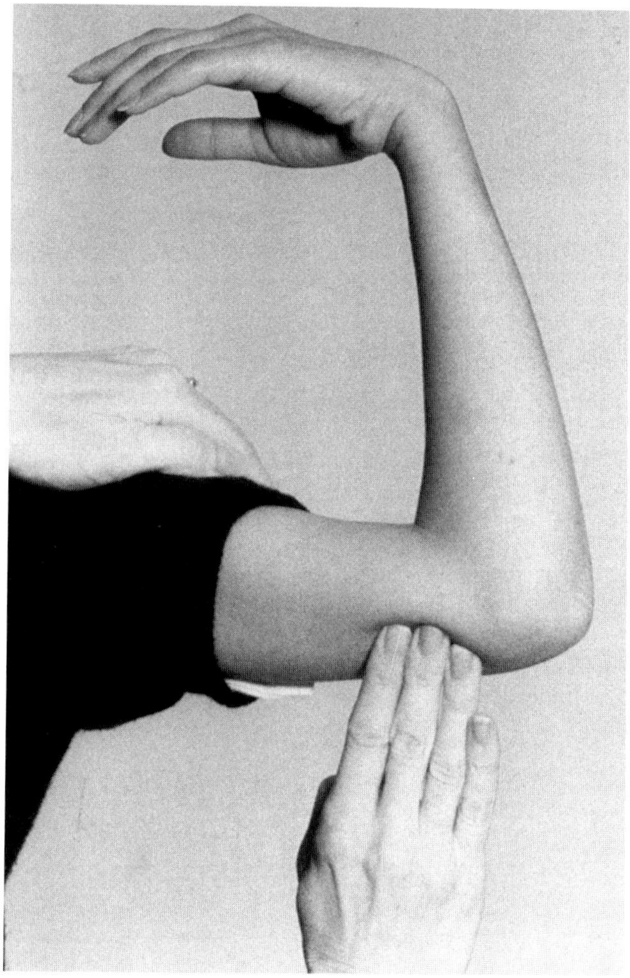

We contrast weakness with wasting. In order for a muscle to undergo wasting, which is the physical appearance of decrease in muscle bulk due to loss of innervation, there has to be a decrease in the number of nerve fibers supplying that muscle. Loss of motor nerve fibers implies degeneration within the nerve fibers. In advanced nerve compression, the nerve undergoes Wallerian degeneration. With degeneration comes loss of neural input to the muscle and actual wasting of the muscle occurs. This degree of wasting can be graded and a rough measure of the degree of wasting or atrophy noted in the patient's record. The implication here is that in early nerve dysfunction due to compression there is weakness in the muscle and with Wallerian degeneration (loss of fibers) there is loss of muscle, or wasting. We can quantitatively measure loss of muscle strength and we can note the degree of muscle wasting (mild, moderate, severe).

What is the analogy in the sensory system? In the sensory system, nerve compression causes changes in threshold, that is, the stimulus intensity required to elicit the normal response to that stimulus is altered. Very early in the course of nerve compression, it appears that an overreaction or a hypersensitive response is present.[4,6,7] Later in the course of nerve compression,

Figure 3-7. Symptoms of ulnar nerve compression in the cubital tunnel can be provoked by elbow flexion and pressure over the ulnar nerve just proximal to the cubital tunnel.

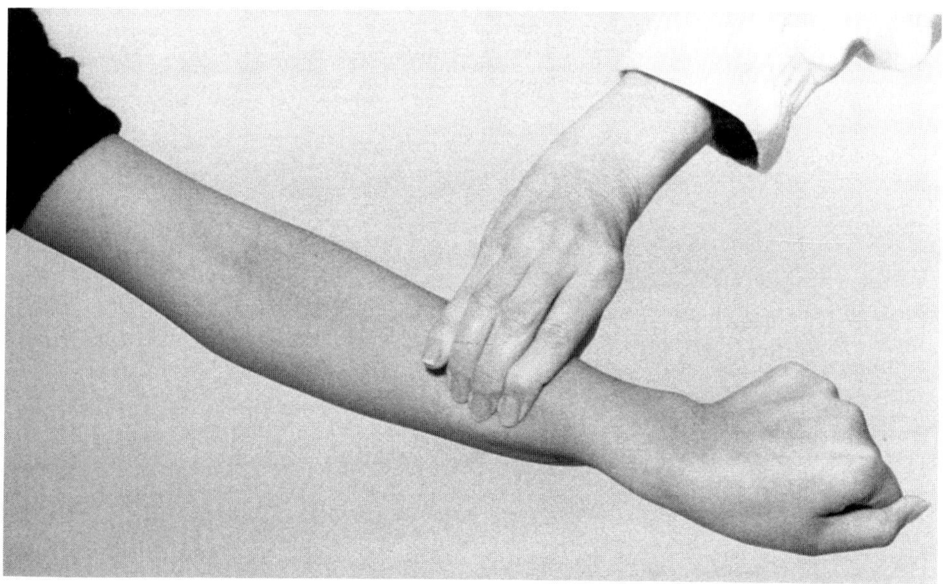

Figure 3-8. Radial sensory nerve entrapment can be provoked by pressure over the radial sensory nerve (just dorsal to the musculotendinous junction of the brachioradialis muscle) and forearm pronation with wrist ulnar flexion.

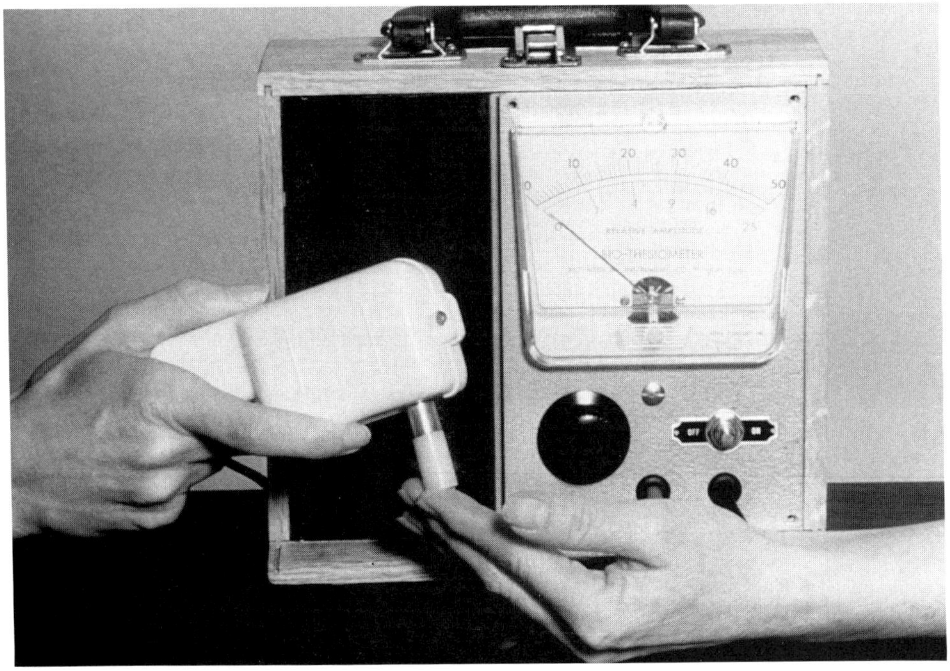

Figure 3-9. A vibrometer can be used to quantitate the cutaneous vibratory threshold of the quickly adapting fiber receptor system. The instrument demonstrated here has a constant frequency but variable amplitude.

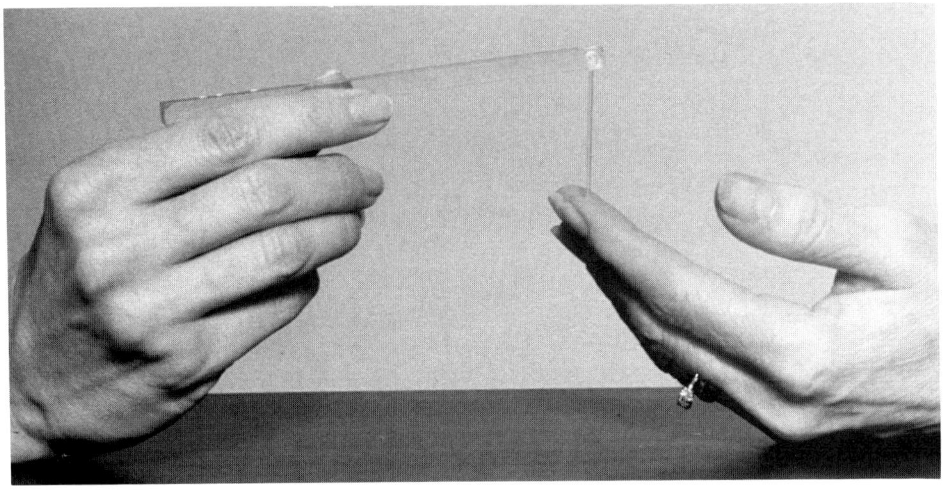

Figure 3-10. Semmes-Weinstein monofilaments can be used to quantitate the cutaneous pressure threshold of the slowly adapting fiber receptor system.

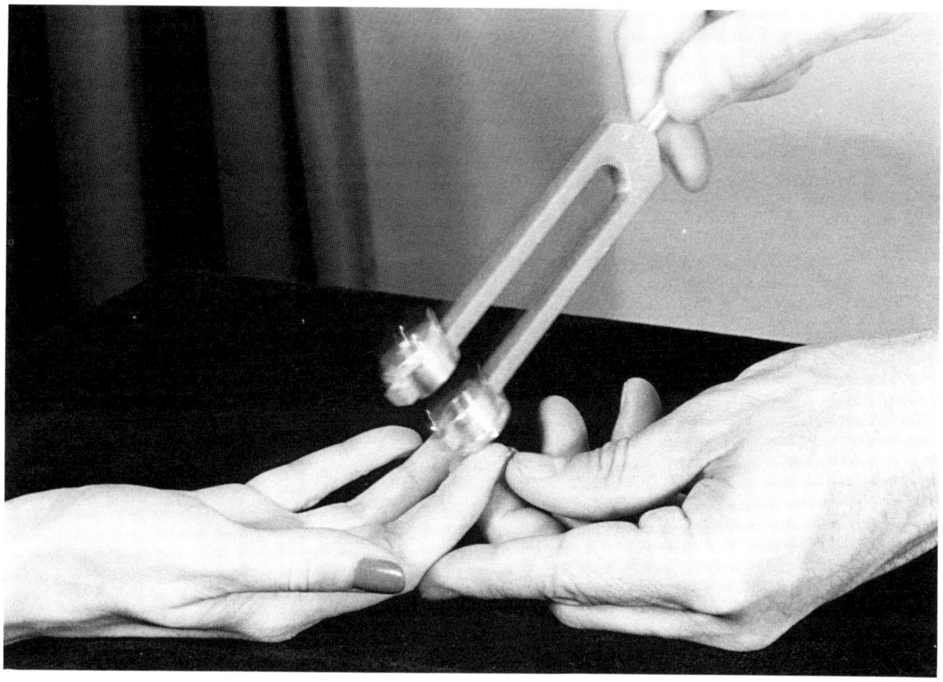

Figure 3-11. The 256 cps tuning fork is an excellent inexpensive tool to assess qualitative vibratory perception. Note the "wrong end" of the tuning fork is used, because the amplitude at this end of the tuning fork is greater than that at the single prong end of the tuning fork. At both ends, the vibration is 256 cps, but the amplitude varies greatly from one end of the tuning fork to the other. The goal is to use a stimulus intensity sufficiently high enough that if the patient does not perceive the stimulus, it is due to a nerve problem, not just a subthreshold stimulus.

it appears that the threshold is raised, so that a greater stimulus intensity is required to elicit the same response as before the injury.[4,6,7] This can be quantitated by cutaneous vibratory threshold (vibrometer) (Fig. 3-9) or cutaneous pressure threshold (Semmes-Weinstein monofilament testing) (Fig. 3-10) or qualitatively by the tuning fork approach[6,7] (Fig. 3-11). A practical example of this is that early in the course of nerve compression, the tuning fork applied to the area affected is perceived as being more sensitive than normal. The patient will often respond to this test by involuntary withdrawing of the finger or altering facial expression. For example, early in median nerve compression at the wrist, the patient's response is that they are feeling more sensitivity in this finger (index) than in another finger (little). Later in the course of nerve compression, they will say the tuning fork is not perceived as well, or it is not as loud, or it is not as strong as that perceived in a sensory area not involved by the nerve compression.

With further compression, and loss of nerve fibers due to Wallerian degeneration, the sensory system will have a diminished number of nerve fibers innervating the territory. This decreased innervation density can be measured by two-point discrimination testing: the static two-point discrimination test for the slowly adapting fiber receptor system or the moving two-point discrimination test[13] (Figs. 3-12, 3-13) for the quickly adapting fiber receptor system can be utilized. An instrument to do this, which has been found to have good interobserver reliability, is the Disk-Criminator.™ [14,15]

The correlations for the motor and sensory system are as follows (Table 3-1). Weakness in the motor system is analogous to altered thresholds in the sensory system. Atrophy or wasting in the motor system is equivalent to abnormal two-point discrimination in the sensory system. Based on these examinations, nerve compression can be staged into early, moderate, or severe, permitting correlation of clinical signs and symptoms with diagnostic testing, such as the vibrometer (Tables 3-2, 3-3) and electrodiagnostic techniques (Table 3-4). Staging for individual nerves is discussed in detail later.

If the nerve is totally divided, the physical examination is compatible with no function in any activity for which that nerve was previously responsible, whether motor or sensory. Physical findings therefore are those simply based on consideration of what nerve may be injured, making a mental list of what functions that nerve previously carried out, examining the patient and finding that there is no function present in the mo-

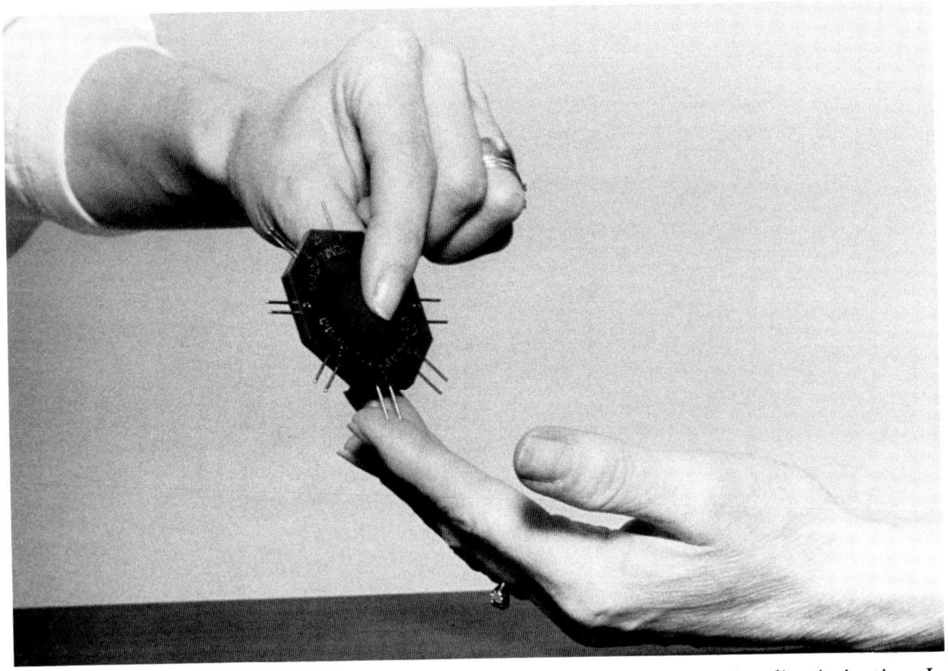

Figure 3-12. The Disk-Criminator™ is used to evaluate static two-point discrimination. In this instance, the autonomous zone of the median nerve is being tested (pulp of index finger).

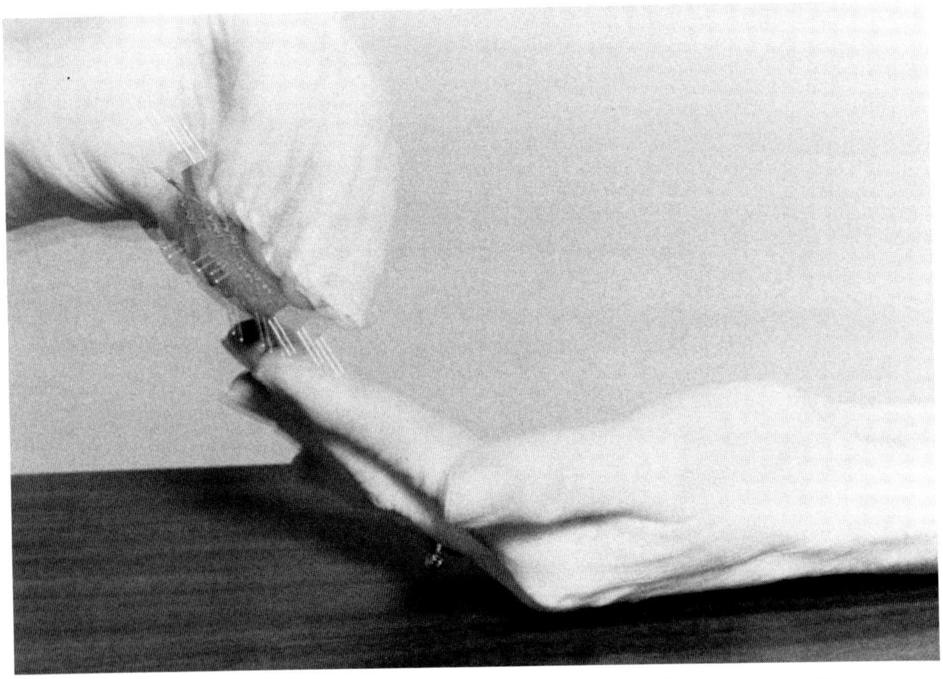

Figure 3-13. The moving two-point discrimination test is evaluated in a similar way but in this instance the Disk-Criminator™ is moved along the distal portion of the thumb pulp in a proximal to distal direction, evaluating the innervation density of the quickly adapting fiber receptor system.

tor or sensory aspects governed by that nerve (Tables 3-5, 3-6, Figs. 3-1 through 3-5). In the instance of partial nerve division, a similar approach is taken and a mental list made of those functions of the nerve that are still functioning and those that are not (Tables 3-7, 3-8).

Table 3-1. Correlation of Motor and Sensory System Findings

	Motor System	*Sensory System*
Moderate nerve compression	Weakness	Abnormal stimulus perception*
Severe nerve compression	Wasting	Abnormal two-point discrimination

*Such as diminished perception of tuning fork vibratory stimulus.

Table 3-2. Vibratory Threshold in Carpal Tunnel Syndrome*

			Vibratory Perception 256 Hz (%)		*Two-Point Discrimination (%)*	
Carpal Tunnel Clinical Stage	*Number of Hands*	*Vibratory Threshold Abnormal (%)*	*Increase*	*Decrease*	*Static (≥6 mm)*	*Moving (≥4 mm)*
Early	7	0	42	0	0	0
Moderate	14	35	21	70	0	0
Severe	13	85	0	100	48	84
Total	34					

*Reprinted with permission from Dellon.[7]

Table 3-3. Vibratory Threshold in Cubital Tunnel Syndrome*

		Vibratory Perception 256 Hz (%)		*Two-Point Discrimination (%)*	
Cubital Tunnel Clinical Stage	*Number of Hands*	*Increase*	*Decrease*	*Static (≥6 mm)*	*Moving (≥4 mm)*
Early	2	100	0	0	0
Moderate	3	0	33	0	0
Severe	5	0	100	80	100
Total	10				

*Reprinted with permission from Dellon.[7]

Table 3-4. Correlation of Clinical and Electrical Sensorimotor Evaluation in the Carpal Tunnel Syndrome*

	Staging of Compression (%)		
Abnormal	*Early*	*Moderate*	*Severe*
Electrical			
Motor	10	50	62
Sensory	80	86	78
Total	80	86	80
Clinical			
Phalen sign	40	64	68
Tinel's test	50	57	64
Vibratory perception	10	50	78
Static two-point discrimination	0	0	32
Moving two-point discrimination	0	0	42
Total	10	50	82
Electrical and clinial studies	80	100	94
Electrical and clinical studies in agreement	30	36	70

*Reprinted with permission from Spindler and Dellon.[23]

Table 3-5. Critical Historical Points in Diagnosis of Nerve Injury[16]

Suggestive of median nerve compression at wrist
- Nocturnal occurrence of numbness in thumb, index, and long fingers
- Worsening of the symptoms with wrist flexion (or extension)

Suggestive of ulnar nerve compression at elbow
- Dropping things, loss of control of fingers, cramping in fingers, numbness in the ring and little fingers, worsening of symptoms when elbow is flexed (talking on telephone, working at desk)

Suggestive of thoracic outlet
- Symptoms predominately in shoulder, upper arm, side of neck, and medial aspect of upper extemity
- Possibly associated with headache
- Symptoms brought on or worsened by working with arms elevated at shoulders

Suggestive of cervical disk disease
- Pain with neck movements
- Pain with coughing or sneezing
- Relief of pain with two-poster brace or cervical collar

Suggestive of vascular compression
- Venous: hand swells, veins stay distended
- Arterial: coldness in hands, color becomes pale when hands are elevated

Table 3-6. Critical Physical Examination Points in Diagnosis of Nerve Injury

1. Muscles to test for unambiguous diagnosis of motor nerve injury
   A. Radial nerve: extrinsic
      1. Wrist extension
      2. Extension of fingers at metacarpophalangeal joints
      3. Extension of thumb
   B. Median nerve: intrinsic
      1. Thumb-palmar abduction
   C. Median nerve: extrinsic
      1. All flexor sublimi
      2. Flexor profundus to index
      3. Flexor pollicis longus
      4. Flexor carpi radialis
   D. Ulnar nerve: intrinsic
      1. First dorsal interossei
      2. Hypothenar muscles
   E. Ulnar nerve: extrinsic
      1. Flexor profundus to little finger
      2. Flexor carpi ulnaris
2. Areas to test for unambiguous diagnosis of sensory nerve injury
   A. Radial nerve: dorsal radial aspect of hand toward the first web
   B. Median nerve: pulp of thumb and index finger
   C. Ulnar nerve: pulp of the little finger
   D. Palmar cutaneous branch of median nerve: proximal palm near thenar eminence
   E. Dorsal cutaneous branch of ulnar nerve: dorsal ulnar surface of hand
   F. Digital nerve: not the tip of the finger (overlap), but the proximal third of the distal phalanx and distal third of middle phalanx, adjacent to the distal skin crease

Table 3-7. Preliminary "Checklist" to Assess Upper Extremity Nerve Function

	Radial	*Median*	*Ulnar*
Sensory (autonomous zone)	Dorsal first web space	Pulp thumb, index finger	Pulp little finger
Motor			
Intrinsic	—	Abductor pollicus brevis	First dorsal interosseous
Extrinsic	Wrist extension	Profundus index finger	Profundus little finger

Electrodiagnosis

The value of electrodiagnosis in the diagnosis and management of peripheral nerve injuries is controversial.[16,17] To the inexperienced diagnostician, who is perhaps not confident in the evaluation of the sensory and motor functions, electrodiagnostic studies are used, unfortunately, as a crutch. To the third party insurance payers, electrodiagnostic studies are all too often used as the "litmus test," or the test of truth, as to whether a problem does or does not exist. To the psychiatrist, the normal electrodiagnostic study often is the reason a patient is referred for evaluation, a patient who may be considered as being "crazy," or having "Workmen's Compensation neurosis" or "an inadequate personality," since the referring physician is unable to find medical support for the patient's symptoms. To the person experienced in the management of peripheral nerve injuries, the appropriate use of electrodiagnostic testing is based on understanding its neurophysiologic basis, its drawbacks, areas in which it cannot give the information desired, a thorough understanding of its potential pitfalls, and of the specific problems with respect to individual nerves and their anatomic anomalies. In this section, the indications and potential pitfalls of electrodiagnosis will be outlined. Further specific details on performance of the individual tests are available in current textbooks[18–20] and as chapters in current hand surgery books.[21–24]

Indications

Before performing electrical testing, we should make a determination by careful history and clinical evaluation of the patient. Electromyography and other electrodiagnostic studies are dynamic evaluations of living tissue and it is imperative that the tests, areas tested and the procedures used be thoughtfully studied and adjustments made in response to the clinical situation.[22]

Table 3-8. Preliminary Checklist to Assess Lower Extremity Nerve Function

	Sciatic				
	Peroneal		*Posterior Tibial*		
	Deep	*Superficial*	*Medial Plantar*	*Lateral Plantar*	*Femoral*
Motor					
Knee		Flexion			Extension
Ankle	Ankle dorsiflexion	Foot eversion	Ankle and toe plantar flexion		—
Toe	Great toe extension	Extensor digitorum brevis	Abductor hallicus brevis	Other intrinsic functions	—
Sensory	Dorsum foot first web only	Dorsum foot except first web	Great toe	Small toe	Anterior thigh and medial calf

The primary indication for referring a patient for electrodiagnostic studies should be inability of the person managing the peripheral nerve injury to arrive at a diagnosis with respect to the patient's presenting problems or to rule out suspected secondary or underlying systemic diseases.

In the following sections of this chapter, our clinical evaluation of the specific nerves will be outlined and the physical findings and historical points that are critical in arriving at a diagnosis will be clearly defined. In the absence of such clear definition, that is, when our standard clinical evaluation fails to lead us to a diagnosis of a patient's presenting problem, then it is appropriate for the physician managing peripheral nerve problems to refer a patient for electrodiagnostic studies. The diagnostic point to be evaluated and the other possibilities to be ruled out must be clearly written on the referral sheet with a copy of the clinical evaluation forwarded to the person who will be doing the electrodiagnostic studies, which serves as a basis for doing the test in the most appropriate manner and for knowing whether one nerve or two nerves need to be examined in one hand, whether a bilateral examination needs to be made, or whether nerves in the lower extremities need to be sampled in addition to those in the upper extremities.

When a patient we are evaluating appears to have multiple peripheral nerve entrapments, it is also appropriate to refer the patient for evaluation to rule out the possibility of systemic conditions, such as diabetic neuropathy or alcoholic neuropathy. The electrodiagnostic techniques are excellent in evaluating the presence of a peripheral neuropathy versus a myopathy. The electrodiagnostic studies are extremely helpful in evaluating the presence of a cervical radiculopathy as a source of the patient's symptoms or in addition to a localized peripheral nerve lesion.

Electrodiagnostic studies are extremely helpful in evaluating the possible recovery of a nerve after an injury, such as a brachial plexus stretch injury or a crush injury, where the electrical parameters may be able to identify, before the clinical evaluation, the recovery of function to the neuromuscular system, thereby guiding the person managing the peripheral nerve injury as to the timing of surgical intervention in this injury.

Electrodiagnostic studies can be valuable in staging a peripheral nerve compression if the studies demonstrate denervation potential or absence of sensory or motor conduction. In these instances, the electrical findings are equivalent to the clinical classification of severe nerve compression and are consistent with an indication for surgical decompression. The electrodiagnostic studies can provide objective measurements by which results of treatment can be compared during serial measurements and therefore may form the appropriate basis for clinical research studies or the management of a particular patient's problem when obtaining objective information is difficult.

Pitfalls

There are many potential problems with electrodiagnostic studies. The most common situation is the patient with significant symptoms in whom the electrodiagnostic testing is intrepreted as being a "normal" study. What is the correct inference of this electrodiagnostic report for the patient, for the managing physician, for the insurance company? It is because of the potential ramifications of the meaning of a "normal interpretation" of an electrodiagnostic study that the physician managing a patient with peripheral nerve injury should be selective in referring patients for these studies. In the worst situation, there is a patient with an injury that occurred at work, in whom the physician believes there is a nerve entrapment based on his clinical evaluation. The physician refers the patient for electrodiagnostic studies and this "normal" interpretation is the result. The Workmen's Compensation carrier may decide to disallow benefits for surgery, since there is "nothing wrong" with the patient and the patient is simply "avoiding returning to work." A more appropriate electrodiagnostic report would say, "Although no specific site of localized nerve entrapment is demonstrated, this study does not exclude the possibility of peripheral nerve entrapment and clinical correlation is advised."

A recent report stresses that patients with normal electrodiagnostic studies but an abnormal clinical evaluation do well with surgery for carpal tunnel release.[25] A series of patients had very detailed electrodiagnostic studies at the request of their rheumatologist. The results of those tests were correlated with a detailed neurosensory evaluation for the carpal tunnel syndrome.[23] The study demonstrated that in the early course of peripheral nerve compression, with mild degree of compression, electrodiagnostic studies were positive for localized nerve entrapment in 80% of the patients, and were also positive on 80% of the patients with clinically staged severe nerve compression. Thus, although the electrodiagnostic studies for median nerve compression at the wrist, for which the electrodiagnostic criteria are the most sensitive and specific, can identify the compression successfully in the early case, electrical studies fail to pick up severe nerve compression in 20% of those patients who had either persistent sensory discomfort, abnormal two-point discrimination, or muscle wasting. There were 20% false-negative results in mild, 14% false-negatives in moderate, and 20% false-negatives in severe degrees of median nerve compression at the wrist even with very sensitive electrodiagnostic testing techniques. The electrical and clinical evaluations disagreed with each other 70% of the time in early carpal tunnel syndrome, 64% in moderate, and 30% in severe nerve compression (Table 3-4).

What is the responsibility of the physician, then, in peripheral nerve entrapment if the electrodiagnostic studies are interpreted as showing median nerve compression at the wrist but there are no denervation potentials on electromyography (EMG) and there is sensory and motor conduction, although delayed, in the median nerve terminal branches? Would such a report be an indication for surgery? As just discussed, patients with mild and moderate degrees of clinical nerve compression for the median nerve at the wrist are found to have abnormal electrodiagnostic studies. It is observed clinically, however, that many patients with this degree of nerve compression may respond to nonoperative management (see Chapter 6). There is at present no study reported in the literature in which a series of patients with abnormal electrodiagnostic studies are followed prospectively for a long period of time and then followed by clinical or electrodiagnostic studies, or both, to determine what percentage of the patients are improved by nonoperative management. Therefore it is our opinion that a normal electrodiagnostic study is not a contraindication to surgery if the clinical evaluation is appropriate. An abnormal electrodiagnostic study is not an absolute indication for surgery unless it is consistent with denervation of muscle and degeneration in the sensory system or as long as the clinical evaluation suggests that there may be room for improvement by nonoperative management techniques.

The pathophysiologic basis for the common situation of symptomatic patients and normal electrodiagnostic studies has been clearly delineated by the recent experimental models of peripheral nerve compression[1,2,5] and by recent reports correlating human material with their preoperative electrodiagnostic testing.[26,27] In summary, these studies demonstrate that in chronic nerve compression there can exist an uneven distribution of disease within the multiple fascicles of the peripheral nerve. This mixed fascicular disease may result in motor wasting out of proportion to the sensory findings in median nerve compression at the wrist if there is more severe compression of the motor fascicle. Conversely, there may be sensory findings that are severe, with abnormal two-point discrimination yet no thenar muscle wasting. More specifically, the middle finger may be significantly disturbing to the patient, whereas his other fingers may not be. For the median nerve in the forearm, there may be varying patterns of loss in median nerve function, for example with weakness in the flexor pollicis longus, but intact function in the thenar muscles and no sensory changes. This has been referred to as an "incomplete anterior interosseous nerve syndrome,"[28] whereas what this really represents is chronic compression of the median nerve. More specifically, because of the band compressing the nerve, there is more decreased function in one of the fascicles, that to the flexor pollicis longus, than there is in the other fascicles. The propensity for a peripheral nerve to manifest signs of compression is related to the arrangement of the fascicles within the peripheral nerve and the location of the force (e.g., a fibrotic band, or fibrotic muscle origin), compressing the nerve.[29]

The electrodiagnostic testing procedures are such that the recording electrode picks up electrical activity in the fastest conducting fibers and does not reveal the occurrence of problems in one or two severely impaired fascicles. Thus, sensory and motor latencies and conduction velocities can be interpreted as within the normal range and there still can be several fascicles involved sufficiently to give the patient significant symptoms. In a similar concept, the EMG needle samples only 6 to 30 muscle fibers about the needle tip. There may be muscle fibers undergoing denervation in other areas of the muscle belly that have not been tested by this single needle insertion technique. This is a sampling error problem. For the clinician faced with a patient with marked symptoms and an electrodiagnostic study computer printout showing many statistical parameters, the discrepancy between the normal report and the abnormal clinical situation should be resolved in favor of the clinical evaluation. Despite the impressive appearance of the computerized printouts for the electrodiagnostic studies, these tests have very significant limitations including the sampling problem just described.

Another potential problem in electrodiagnostic testing is the temperature of the patient at the time of the testing procedure. The ideal situation is when serial tests on the patient are done in a temperature-controlled room by the same testor. The variations in conduction velocity can vary as much as 3 m/s per degree centigrade. Often, the patient comes into the room, is apprehensive, has peripheral vasoconstriction, the hand has become cool, and the electrodiagnostic results may differ based on this factor alone. Frequently, the electrodiagnostic tests are done, in recognition of this fact, after placing the patient's hands in warm towels. How much should the hand be warmed? How is the test standardized? If the patient's initial examination is done in the middle of August, the surgery done in September, and the follow-up examination done in December, the testing temperatures between summer and winter may be significantly different. The patient's degree of body sweating may be significantly different. The patient's set of apprehension may be significantly different. The measurements can vary enough due to these factors to obscure any true changes that have occurred or exist with respect to the normal values for the testing procedure being done. The entire problem of comparisons is even worse when two different persons do the electrodiagnostic testing.

Anatomic variation can present a problem in identifying the underlying localized peripheral nerve entrapment. Radial sensory nerve entrapment in the forearm is a good example.[30] It has been demonstrated that 75% of patients have a significant overlap between the lateral antebrachial cutaneous nerve and the radial sensory nerve.[31] In this situation, the electrodiagnostic recordings done by surface stimulation and surface electrodes may demonstrate normal findings when, in fact, the test was truly recorded from the terminal branch of the musculocutaneous nerve (the lateral antebrachial cutaneous nerve) and not from the underlying radial sensory nerve. Techniques for measuring these two nerves separately in the forearm and comparing the difference in their latencies as the basis for evaluating radial sensory nerve entrapment have been reported.

Yet another potential problem in interpretation of electrodiagnostic studies is related to ulnar nerve entrapment at the elbow. In the initial diagnostic testing, there is a problem in that the types of electrical testing done to identify median nerve compression at the wrist, latency testing, is not accurate when done at the elbow. The reason is that if there is localized compression at the elbow and the nerve is stimulated proximal to the site of compression and the recording picked up at the wrist, the small region of slowing and its effect in terms of a conduction delay are diluted when added into the overall length of time it takes for the electrical impulse to travel from the elbow to the wrist. This is not the situation with median nerve compression at the wrist because the site of localized entrapment is close to the terminal pickup point for the recording electrode. Thus, conduction velocity must be relied on. The conduction velocity must be done segmentally to compare slowing across the elbow with that above and below. It must be recognized by the physician managing the peripheral nerve injury that there is normally about 10 m/s slowing from above to across the elbow to below. Most laboratories will take a cutoff of 50 m/s as being the lower limit of normal for conduction velocity across the elbow. Thus, if someone has just one arm done and the conduction velocity across the elbow is 60, this may be interpreted as being normal. However, if both arms were done and the conduction velocity across the elbow in question was more than a 10 m/s decrease from above to below or more than 10 m/s different from that in the opposite elbow, then an interpretation of ulnar nerve compression at the elbow could be made. Amplitude measurements for the ulnar nerve across the elbow can vary significantly, based on the degree of soft tissue present between the skin and the underlying nerve, and therefore, in general, amplitude measurements are unreliable. The EMG evaluation for ulnar nerve compression at the elbow can be confounded further by anatomic anomalies, such as the Martin-Gruber anastomosis and by the sampling errors already referred to.

Many of the patients on whom we operate for ulnar nerve compression at the elbow, and who have had electrodiagnostic studies performed before being referred to us, have what has been interpreted to be "normal" electrodiagnostic studies. It is our experience therefore that electrodiagnostic studies for ulnar nerve compression at the elbow have at least a 50% false-negative incidence.

In the postoperative period, attempting to evaluate ulnar nerve status is extremely hazardous. The problems with this have recently been investigated.[33] In summary, the ulnar nerve's conduction velocity is determined by the geometry that relates the distance of the skin that is measured to the location of the ulnar nerve, and these measurements change with respect to elbow position, whether it is flexed or extended (Fig. 3-14; Table 3-9). If the skin distance is measured behind (posterior to) the elbow, this distance is longer when the elbow is flexed than when the elbow is extended for the same two skin markings. This is reversed if the skin distance is taken anterior to the elbow. When the ulnar nerve is behind the elbow, it is stretched and under a greater length when the elbow is flexed than when the elbow is extended. Normal ulnar nerve conduction velocities are faster in any given patient with the elbow flexed than when it is extended. Is the converse true when the ulnar nerve has been transposed? In general, there has been no accepted standard for the position in which to do the electrodiagnostic studies after ulnar nerve transposition, and reports are often accompanied by the caveat "interpretation of this report must be guarded because the ulnar nerve has been transposed to a new location." How should the result postoperatively be measured electrodiagnostically so that it may be compared with the one preoperatively? During electrodiagnostic testing, should the elbow be flexed preoperatively and extended postoperatively? Guidelines for these testing techniques are outlined by Dellon et al.[33] The physician managing peripheral nerve injuries should go over this with the person doing the electrodiagnostic studies so that there will be an appropriate basis for comparison of the results after nerve transposition. The physician managing peripheral nerve injuries will be aware that a patient referred to him after ulnar nerve transposition can have electrodiagnostic studies obtained and interpreted in light of these measurement problems.

The interpretation of the reports of electrodiagnostic studies in patients with a peripheral neuropathy are difficult. The peripheral neuropathy by the

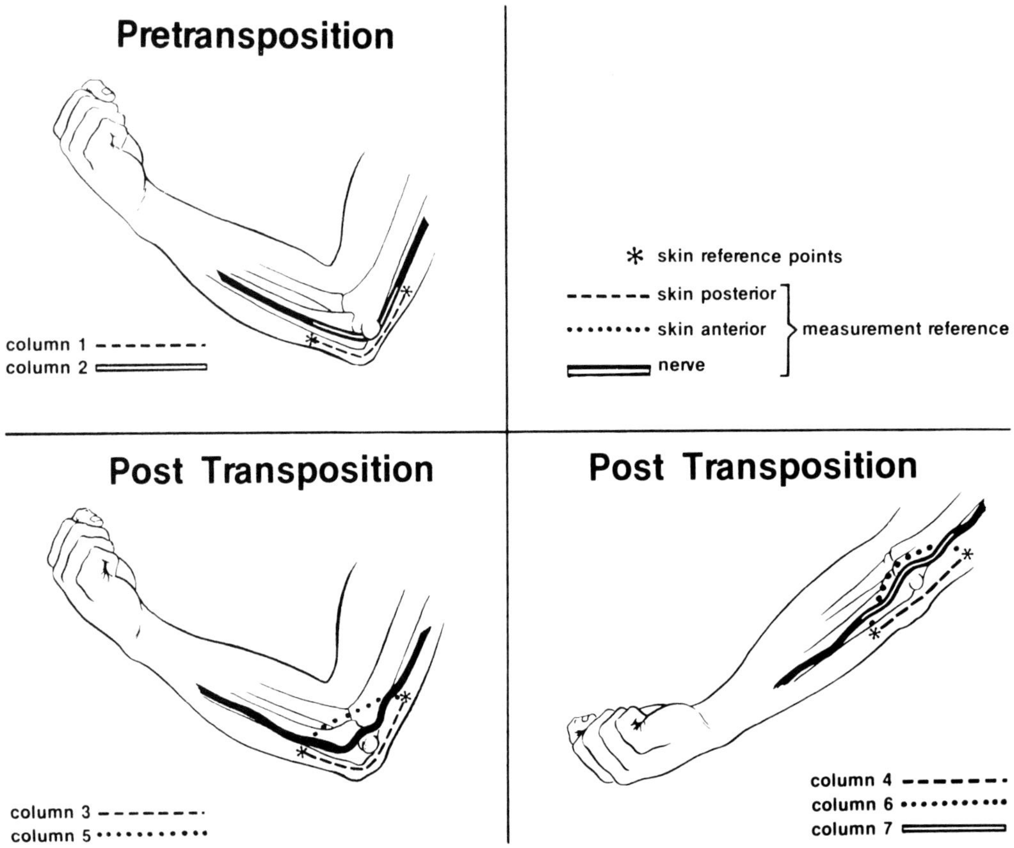

Figure 3-14. Examples of combinations of skin distance markings and elbow position related to performing electrodiagnostic testing in the patient after anterior transposition of the ulnar nerve (see also Table 3-9).

nature of its pathophysiologic characteristics will have some basic neural dysfunction. This is often interpreted as a diffuse conduction velocity slowing with or without amplitude changes in multiple peripheral nerves. This underlying pathologic process makes it difficult to interpret a superimposed peripheral nerve compression. Thus, a patient clinically suspected of having nerve compression associated with a systemic condition, such as diabetes, may have electrodiagnostic studies that are interpreted as showing a "diffuse peripheral neuropathy without localized signs of nerve entrapment." However, an alternate explanation is that the degree of impairment of nerve function by the neuropathy, itself, is such that the electrical testing is not sensitive enough to demonstrate a superimposed compression neuropathy. Therefore in the clinical situation in which the compression is suspected, the physician may still undertake to decompress the peripheral nerve. The problem can be looked at from a different perspective in diabetic neuropathy, since part of the problem may be related to decreased axoplasm flow due to the basic pathophysiologic process itself. Normal anatomic areas of narrowing, such as the spinal neural foramina, the constriction between the clavicle and the first rib, the cubital tunnel, the radial sensory site for peripheral nerve entrapment, the narrowed tunnels at the wrist, the tarsal tunnels, the common peroneal site crossing the fibular head, all may comprise multiple constraints on axoplasmic flow that in and of themselves may create a situation that mathematically can be modeled to be equivalent to a distal axonopathy. Thus, it is possible that a given peripheral nerve compressed at the level of the spine, the thoracic outlet, the cubital tunnel, and Guyon's canal may, in fact, appear from the electrodiagnostic testing at any given point along this course of serial constraints to axoplasmic flow to be a peripheral neuropathy. Certainly, if the report demonstrates a superimposed entrapment on an underlying peripheral neuropathy, the physician managing the peripheral nerve entrapment can feel secure that the situation exists.

Faced with a report indicating a diffuse peripheral neuropathy without site of nerve entrapment, the physician must trust his clinical assessment and realize that the extremity with ulnar nerve compression at the elbow, radial sensory nerve in the forearm, and median nerve compression at the wrist can appear clinically to have a "glove" distribution, such as is seen in the diffuse sensory neuropathy of diabetes. In each instance, however, the physician will be able to "provoke," repro-

Table 3-9. Intraoperative Ulnar Nerve Conduction Velocities (m/sec)*

	Pretransposition		*Posttransposition*				
Patient Number	*1 Skin, Posterior;† Elbow Flexed*	*2 Nerve;† Elbow Flexed*	*3 Skin, Posterior;† Elbow Flexed*	*4 Skin, Posterior;† Elbow Extended*	*5 Skin, Anterior;† Elbow Flexed*	*6 Skin, Anterior;† Elbow Extended*	*7 Nerve;† Elbow Extended*
1	33	35	42	33	44	45	31
2	35	38	48	36	42	55	38
3	44	42	50	44	42	51	42
4	50	57	64	50	57	78	57
5	48	60	60	48	60	65	60
6	49	48	75	59	58	59	52
7	50	39	49	48	41	52	40
8	54	39	54	45	41	47	40

*Reprinted with permission from Dellon et al.[33]

†Distance along which conduction velocities were measured.

Table 3-10. Provocative Tests for Nerve Entrapment

Nerve	*Entrapment Site*	*Provocative Test*
Median	Carpal tunnel	Presure proximal to carpal tunnel Phalen's test Reverse Phalen's (hyperextension of wrist)
Median	Proximal forearm	Pressure over proximal forearm Resisted pronation Resisted sublimus flexion
Ulnar	Guyon's canal	Pressure proximal to Guyon's canal
Ulnar	Cubital tunnel	Pressure proximal to cubital tunnel Elbow flexion
Radial (posterior interosseous)	Arcade of Fröhse	Pressure over supinator Resisted supination
Radial (sensory)	Forearm	Pressure over junction of brachioradialis and extensor carpi radialis tendon Forearm pronation
Posterior tibial	Tarsal tunnel	Pressure at flexor retinaculum
Peroneal	Fibular head	Pressure at fibular head

duce, or aggravate symptoms with specific local provocative tests if superimposed nerve entrapment exists (Table 3-10). The most universally useful and sensitive provocative test in our experience is direct pressure over the nerve just proximal to the entrapment site. The entrapped nerve is exquisitely sensitive to direct pressure. This maneuver will reproduce symptoms within several seconds. A similar maneuver is performed for the contralateral extremity as a control. SURGERY CANNOT CHANGE THE BASIC NATURE OF DIABETIC NEUROPATHY. SURGERY CAN ENSURE THAT THE NERVE IS NOT FURTHER COMPROMISED BY SUPERIMPOSED NERVE ENTRAPMENT.

Clinical Evaluation

Clinical evaluation of the nerve-injured patient begins with observing the injured part of the body. For acute injury, the location of the laceration and the nature of the wounding agent will provide information regarding both the type of injury and the nerve or nerves involved (Table 3-2). The clinical evaluation for nerve compression is similar to that for incomplete or complete nerve division in that the individual muscles that are innervated by the potentially compressed nerve must be considered, but the examination is done in order to allow classification of the degree of nerve compression into mild, moderate, or severe. These evaluation techniques will be discussed for each nerve.

Nerve Compression

Tinel's sign reflects an attempt by an injured nerve to regenerate. Thus, it will be present only if the injury is significant enough to cause nerve degeneration and if the nerve is capable of a regenerative attempt. Thus, Tinel's sign[34,35] will be variably present throughout the natural history of nerve compression. Early in nerve compression, Tinel's sign is negative. In the middle course of nerve compression, when sufficient nerve injury and degeneration have occurred to result in some neural regeneration, Tinel's sign becomes positive. Late in the course of nerve compression, when degeneration has taken its course and no regeneration is occurring, Tinel's sign can be negative again.

The provocative tests, such as wrist flexion to produce signs of median nerve compression at the wrist (Phalen's sign) or elbow flexion to produce signs of ulnar nerve compression at the elbow or forearm pronation to elicit signs of radial sensory nerve compression in the forearm (Dellon-Mackinnon sign),[30] will be positive very early and in the midcourse of nerve compression (Figs. 3-6, 3-7, 3-8). Once the patient has persistent sensory changes due to compression of this particular nerve, the provocative test may be only slightly worse or even be negative because symptoms are already constantly present.

Two-point discrimination is normal early in the course of nerve compression and does not become abnormal, as already discussed, until late in the course of nerve compression. The classic static Weber two-point discrimination test is done (Fig. 3-12), as well as the Dellon moving two-point discrimination test (Fig. 3-13).[6] Nerve compression has not been demonstrated to affect the quickly adapting fibers in preference to the slowly adapting fibers, or vice versa. Therefore neither the moving nor static two-point discrimination test becomes abnormal earlier than the other in the course of nerve compression. We prefer to do the moving two-point discrimination test if just one of these tests is to be done in the sensory testing because of the narrower range of normal values for this test (2 or 3 mm is normal and 4 mm is considered abnormal). This permits a greater degree of confidence in determining when this test has become abnormal.

The tests for threshold (cutaneous pressure threshold [Semmes-Weinstein nylon monofilament] or cutaneous vibratory threshold [vibrometer]) change early in the course of nerve compression. We do not routinely use the quantitative threshold tests, such as Semmes-Weinstein monofilaments or the vibrometer[7] (Figs. 3-9, 3-10). However, these tests are an integral part of all clinical research studies. They are also helpful in evaluating difficult clinical problems when bilateral or multiple nerves are involved. Evaluation of these tests are helpful in following quantitative changes during the early course of nerve recovery. We will often use qualitative vibratory testing with the tuning fork and find that this is a rapid, sensitive, and specific test for this purpose in the clinical situation[7] (Table 3-11).

Staging Nerve Compression

The staging system for nerve compression may be summarized as follows.[7,23] In mild nerve compression, the patient has symptoms that may be related to the motor or sensory system of that nerve, Tinel's sign will be negative, and the only physical examination findings that may be abnormal are a hypersensitive response to the tuning fork stimulation, decreased vibratory thresholds, and a positive provocative test. The symptoms are not persistent, there is no muscle wasting, there is no abnormal moving or static two-point discrimination, and the patient will generally complain of abnormal sensibility and weakness. The more specific symptoms will be described for the particular nerves in subsequent sections. With a moderate degree of nerve compression, the patient's symptoms still are not persistent but are more troublesome throughout the day and usually toward the end of the working day. Tinel's sign may be positive. The provocative tests are still positive. The tuning fork perception now has become decreased and vibratory thresholds increased. The two-point discrimination is still normal. There is no muscle wasting. In the severe category, the patient has one or more of the following three symptoms or signs: persistent sensory changes, muscle wasting, or abnormal two-point discrimination. The concept, then, for nerve compression is a dynamic situation in which the symptoms can be provoked by manipulation of the extremity in the region of the entrapment site and a clinical continuum in which the signs and symptoms vary according to the degree of ischemia, demyelination, and degeneration occurring in the involved nerves. Staging the degree of nerve compression in this manner allows us to alter treatment based on the degree of severity in nerve compression rather than treating all patients with a nerve compression by the same technique without consideration as to its natural history (Tables 3-2, 3-3, 3-4).

Median Nerve at the Wrist

The most commonly compressed peripheral nerve is the median nerve at the wrist as it goes through the carpal tunnel. With the exception of the clinical diagnosis, this subject is thoroughly discussed in Chapter 6. *For the mild degree of median nerve compression at the wrist,* the patient's complaints will be numbness and tingling or, more rarely, pain, or, rarest, coldness in the fingers. The most commonly involved finger and that involved most severely is usually the middle finger with all the hand being the next most common complaint and the thumb, index, middle fingers being the next most common, and the index or thumb alone being the least common complaint. The condition awakens the patient at night, is worse with activities, and is helped when the hand is elevated or rested. The symptoms come and go and there are generally many times throughout the day when the patient's hand feels quite normal. Occasionally, the patient will say that it feels as if there is a tight band around the wrist. Occasionally, he will complain of the joints aching in the fingers, with these symptoms being related to involvement of the joint afferent fibers. The complaints of coldness in the hand may be related to the presence of a significantly contributing persistent median artery, which is also being compressed. Older patients sometimes perceive the changes in their hands as being due to "circulation

Table 3-11. Sensory Tests and Neurophysiologic Correlations

	Pressure (Constant Touch)		*Movement (Moving Touch)*	
Sensory task	Precision sensory grip		Tactilegnosis (object identification)	
Sensory test	Pressure perception	S2PD*	vibration perception	M2PD*
Testing instrument	Semmes-Weinstein monofilaments	Disk-Criminator™	Tuning fork Vibrometer	Disk-Criminator™
Neurophysiologic correlate	Threshold	Innervation density	Threshold	Innervation density
Nerve fiber system	Slowly adapting		Quickly adapting	

*M2PD: moving two-point discrimination; S2PD: static two-point discrimination.

problems" when, in fact, they are due to sensory changes. Phalen's sign is positive (flexion of the wrist with symptoms being elicited within 30 to 40 seconds). Pressure on the nerve, specifically a median nerve compression test as described by McMurtry,[36] will be positive (Fig. 3-6). The tourniquet test, as described by Gilliatt and Wilson,[37] will be positive. In this test, the tourniquet is inflated at the upper arm and within 1 or 2 minutes the patient complains of significant discomfort in the distribution of the median nerve at the wrist. In the absence of median nerve compression at the wrist, the patient's first symptoms usually are in the course of the ulnar nerve distribution and do not begin to occur until approximately 5 minutes of compression with the tourniquet, with pressure increased above systolic. The tuning fork perception in the thumb and index finger in comparison with the little finger of the same hand and in comparison with the contralateral hand will be more sensitive than normal or it will be normal. Two-point discrimination will be normal with no muscle wasting (Tables 3-2, 3-4).

In moderate degree of nerve compression in the carpal tunnel syndrome, the patient will have symptoms as described in the mild degree. The physical examination will now include a positive Tinel's sign over the median nerve at the wrist and tuning fork perception will be diminished. Threshold testing, if done by a Semmes-Weinstein monofilament or vibrometer, will be abnormal and increased. The remainder of the history and physical examination is as described for the mild degree (Tables 3-2, 3-4).

In the severe degree of nerve compression for the carpal tunnel syndrome, the patient may now have a negative Tinel's sign at the wrist, a negative Phalen's sign, but the nerve should still be tender to deep pressure. By history, sensory symptoms are persistent, that is, the patient is aware all day long that there is something wrong with either the thumb, index, middle, or all the fingers. There may be muscle wasting, depending on whether the motor branch is involved to the same degree as the sensory branches. There will be abnormal two-point discrimination because the compression has progressed to the degree that there are degenerative changes in the sensory fibers (Tables 3-2, 3-4).

With *complete median nerve laceration* at the wrist, there will be, shortly after the injury, no muscle wasting, but no function in the abductor pollicis brevis or in the opponens pollicis. The short flexor to the thumb, which is innervated at least 40% by the ulnar nerve,[37] is an unreliable test for median nerve injury. There will be no vibratory perception, or very diminished vibratory perception, in the volar surface of the thumb or index finger. There will be no perception of hot or cold or pinprick. There will be no two-point discrimination. There should be a markedly positive Tinel's sign over the site of injury, which may be too painful to evaluate. Later in the course after median nerve complete division, there will be, in addition to the findings mentioned, wasting of the thenar muscles and narrowing or carroting of the tips of the fingers due to subcutaneous atrophy from loss of neurotrophism and degeneration of the sensory corpuscles. The anesthetic fingers assume a "silk glove" appearance, becoming smooth and shiny.

Ulnar Nerve Compression at the Wrist

The site at which the ulnar nerve is compressed at the wrist, in Guyon's canal, does not contain sensory fibers to the dorsum of the hand and does not contain motor fibers to the profundus to the little finger and does not contain motor fibers to wrist flexion. Abnormalities in dorsal ulnar sensation to the hand, in weakness of grip strength, in weakness of the profundus tendon in the little or ring finger, and in weakness in wrist flexion therefore are not due to ulnar nerve compression at the wrist but must be due to an injury at a higher location. All the following symptoms of ulnar nerve compression at the wrist, however, can also be caused by ulnar nerve compression in the forearm. Localizing signs for ulnar nerve compression at the wrist is tenderness of the ulnar nerve in the region between the pisiform bone and the hook of the hamate and tenderness to palpation over the ulnar nerve in this region. Direct pressure over the ulnar nerve just proximal to Guyon's canal will reproduce the patient's symptoms.

In mild ulnar nerve compression at the wrist, the patient will complain of numbness or tingling, less often pain, and occasionally coldness of the ulnar half of the hand and palm. These symptoms are not persistent, may be aggravated with use of the hand, and do not, in general, cause the patient to be awakened at night. Physical examination may show a positive Tinel's sign over the ulnar nerve. Direct pressure over the ulnar nerve just proximal to Guyon's canal will usually reproduce symptoms. Variations in ulnar nerve innervation of the intrinsics have been well-described.[38] At this stage, there is usually no weakness in pinch strength.

In the moderate degree of ulnar nerve compression at the wrist, the tuning fork perception will be diminished. There is usually measurable weakness in pinch strength if the motor branch of the ulnar nerve is being compressed significantly. The weakness in the pinch muscles, the first dorsal interosseous, and the adductor pollicis is generally out of proportion or worse than the hypothenar muscles, since the branch to the hypothenar muscles arises slightly more proximal to the deep motor nerve and is subjected to only one area of potential compression, which is between the pisiform and the hamate bones. The deep motor is potentially subjected to this compression site and a second site more distally by the leading edge of the flexor digiti quinti muscle. Vibratory perception is decreased in this stage. Tinel's sign is positive. Cutaneous vibratory threshold testing and cutaneous pressure threshold testing will be abnormal.

In the severe degree of compression, there will be weakness and wasting in the various ulnar nerve innervated muscles. These include the hypothenar muscles, which means that, as the patient attempts to abduct and flex the little finger at the metacarpophalangeal joint, there is weakness. The usual wrinkling in the skin over the hypothenar eminence will become lost. Paradoxically, the little finger may remain in an abducted position. This is due to weakness of the fourth palmar interosseous muscle so that little finger strength, abduction strength, is lost and it cannot be kept close to the ring finger. Additionally, in approximately two-thirds of the patients who have the extensor digiti minimi insert partially into a tubercle on the proximal phalanx, there will be an unopposed abduction force imposed by this extrinsic extensor tendon. Thus, even with weakness in the hypothenar muscles, the little finger can be in an abducted position with ulnar nerve compression (Wartenburg's sign).[39] With almost complete loss of strength in the first dorsal interosseous and the adductor, pinch strength can only come through the extrinsic median flexor system, the flexor pollicis longus. In this situation, attempted pinch, which usually occurs with the interphalangeal joint in a neutral position, will occur with the interphalangeal joint of the thumb flexed (Froment's sign)[40] and the metacarpophalangeal joint extended (Jeanne's sign). The intrinsics flex the metacarpophalangeal joint of the little and ring fingers. Although this flexion still can occur through the ulnar innervated profundus, it does not occur until after these extrinsic flexors have exerted their effect on the interphalangeal joints. Thus, the normal sequence of digital balance (flexion of the metacarpophalangeal joints before or at the same time as flexion of the interphalangeal joints) is upset. In this severe degree of ulnar nerve compression, two-point discrimination will be lost in the little finger. Testing in the middle and ring fingers is unreliable because the median nerve can innervate these. Classically, the ulnar half of the ring finger should have diminished two-point discrimination also. At this stage, the patient's symptoms will be persistent in character.

Immediately after *complete division of the ulnar nerve at the wrist,* the findings on the sensory examination will be complete loss of sensation to the palmar aspect of the little finger and the ulnar half of the ring finger, with preservation of sensation over the dorsal aspect of the hand and complete loss of function in the ulnar innervated intrinsic muscles of the hand, but without wasting. Later in the course after ulnar nerve division at the wrist, muscle wasting will be present in these ulnar innervated intrinsic muscles. Those patients with thin, supple fingers and lax finger joints may demonstrate "clawing" of the ulnar two digits almost immediately. By comparison, those with "thick" heavy fingers may never demonstrate any significant claw deformity.

One note of caution in the clinical evaluation for ulnar nerve problems at the wrist is that when a thrombosis of the ulnar artery occurs, the inflammation that may attend this can cause symptoms in the distribution of the ulnar sensory and motor fibers. Thus, in the evaluation of ulnar nerve problems at the wrist, the test for vascular patency of the ulnar artery (Allen's test) should be carried out.

The clinical evaluation of ulnar nerve disease at the wrist can localize a compressive lesion, such as due to a ganglion in Guyon's canal, according to the following sequence. With a compressive site at the level of the hamate, only the deep motor branch may be involved, with just the palmar and dorsal interossei and the adductor pollicis involved. With compression between the pisiform and the hamate, in addition to the findings just described, there will be sensory changes in the little finger and ring finger. With a compressive site just at the level of the pisiform, there will be additional changes in the hypothenar musculature.

Median Nerve Compression in the Forearm

The median nerve can become entrapped from just proximal to the elbow down to the junction of the proximal third with the distal two-thirds of the forearm. The signs and symptoms for entrapment in this area largely run together except for a few instances in which separate types of syndromes have been described. Classically, the sensory distribution of the median nerve proximal to the wrist is the same as it is at the level of the wrist, and the sensory distribution therefore for a median nerve injury in this forearm region is the same as that at the wrist. The median nerve in the forearm region, however, has a much greater distribution of neural fibers to muscles innervating the radial wrist flexor, the palmaris longus, the flexor sublimis, the pronator teres, the flexor pollicus longus, and the profundus to the index and part of the profundus to the middle finger. With a mild degree of nerve compression, the patient's symptoms generally are an aching in the proximal forearm, especially with use of the hand and arm. This is frequently in a situation in which the arm must be used for repetitive pronation and supination movements and repetitive grasping. There is frequently a sensation that the thumb, index and middle fingers do not quite have normal sensation, but this is not a prominent complaint. The hand does not usually awaken the patient at night from sleep. Patients may complain that they have trouble with writing and that their hands feel somewhat weak. Their hands may be clumsy and they may drop things. The symptoms are usually vague, with the exception of aching in the forearm. The physical examination *in the mild stage* will show only aching deep in the forearm with pressure over the course of the median nerve. Some of this aching may be reproduced with forced resistance to flexion of the middle finger at proximal interphalangeal flexion. With this forced contraction of the sublimis muscle belly, fingers are held extended for the index, ring, and little fingers and the middle finger is flexed by the patient against the examiner's resistance. Another provocative sign is for the patient to hold the forearm in pronation, while the examiner attempts to supinate it. This may reproduce an aching in the forearm. Sensory testing is generally normal.

In the *moderate stage of median nerve compression in the forearm,* the sensory symptoms are generally the same, the provocative tests as just described are now positive. There is frequently not a Tinel's sign present because the median nerve is deeply situated beneath muscle bellies. There is no muscle wasting, but weakness in individual muscles, such as the flexor pollicis longus, and the profundus to the index finger may be elicited. In this regard, weakness in the pronator quadratus may be determined by comparing its strength in one hand with that in the other hand, with the pronator teres strength greatly reduced by the technique of elbow flexion. The patient's arm is held flexed at the elbow and then his hand is placed palm upward (supinated). The patient then attempts to pronate the hand against resistance from the examiner, who attempts to keep it supinated.

In the *severe degree of median nerve compression in the forearm,* there will be actual inability to flex the tip of the thumb and inability to flex the tip of the index finger. The middle finger profundus may or may not be involved, depending on cross-innervation from the ulnar nerve. There will be weakness in the pronator quadratus to testing. The patient cannot form a circle with the index and thumb (Fig. 3-15). Muscle wasting cannot be observed in the pronator quadratus and the flexor pollicus longus because the affected muscles are situated quite deeply. There may be observable wasting in muscle bellies of the flexor carpi radialis and the pronator teres. In the severe degree, careful sensory testing of the thumb, index and middle fingers may show changes in the affected hand in comparison with the opposite hand, although, depending on the degree of compression and the site of compression at the median nerve, there may still be no sensory changes elicited. The classic nerve entrapments described for the nerve in this area are the pronator syndrome and the anterior interosseous nerve syndrome. These are discussed in greater detail specifically in Chapter 7.

Ulnar Nerve Compression at the Elbow

The patient's usual complaints for ulnar nerve compression in the elbow are numbness or tingling in the little finger, occasionally pain in the distribution of the ulnar nerve or coldness in the hand, rarely are there complaints about the dorsal aspect of the hand. The patient will often complain of aching in the region of the elbow, and commonly weakness in the hand. If specifically asked, the patient will admit to clumsiness in the hand, dropping objects, inability to use the hand quite as he wishes without specifically being able to express exactly in what way the use of the hand is not normal. A frequent complaint is problems in writing. There may be problems in fine motor coordination. Problems playing a musical instrument, such as the violin, piano, or guitar, or problems with typing are noted by some patients. The patient will frequently notice that when the elbow is flexed, such as when they are driving a car or are talking on the telephone, numbness is experienced in the little and ring fingers. In particular, symptoms such

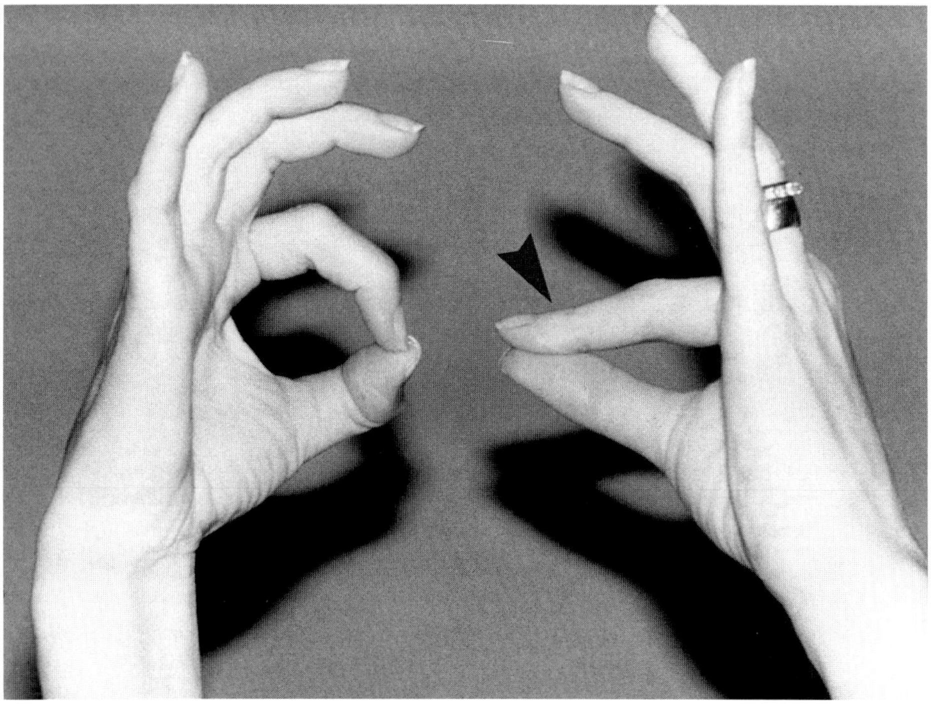

Figure 3-15. With an injury to the median nerve or anterior interosseous nerve in the proximal forearm, the patient is unable to flex the interphalangeal joint of the thumb or the distal interphalangeal joint of the index finger. When attempting to make a "circle" with the thumb and index finger, a "birds-eye" appearance is noted (arrow).

as dropping objects, clumsiness, and weakness are not associated with median nerve compression at the wrist and the mentioning of these symptoms in the patient's history should alert the examiner to consider ulnar nerve compression at the elbow. Dropping objects occurs in median nerve only in severe cases in which sensory loss is such that the object cannot be perceived as being present in the fingers. In the vast majority of the cases, these complaints of dropping things and weakness relate to ulnar nerve compression at the elbow.

In mild degree of ulnar nerve compression at the elbow, the patient will have intermittent symptoms of a sensory nature as just described in the little and ring fingers and on physical examination will have a positive Tinel's sign at the elbow. They will have a positive elbow flexion test and there will be tenderness of the ulnar nerve when pressed, usually between the two heads of the flexor carpi ulnaris. Pressure over the ulnar nerve just proximal to the cubital tunnel will usually provoke symptoms (Fig. 3-7). With light moving touch, there will be a sensory difference between the dorsal ulnar aspect of the hand and the radial dorsal side of the same hand and the dorsal ulnar aspect of the contralateral hand. At this stage, weakness on manual muscle testing of the flexor profundus is variable. The little finger is held extended at the metacarpophalangeal and proximal interphalangeal joints by the examiner's hand and the patient is asked to flex the little finger at its tip and the examiner resists this. Even in the woman who is doing household activities, that is, who is not doing heavy manual work, the profundus to the little finger is extremely strong and little finger distal interphalangeal joint flexion should not be easily overcome by the examiner or weaker when compared with the opposite side. Vibratory perception in the little finger may be hypersensitive. The pinch strength for lateral key pinch and grip strength with the grip meter in the fourth position are thoroughly tested in each hand and at this stage may be normal or slightly weaker than in the opposite hand. If the dominant hand has the same strength as the contralateral nondominant hand, then there is slight weakness present in the dominant hand (Table 3-3).

In *moderate degree of ulnar nerve compression at the elbow,* there will be a positive Tinel's sign at the elbow, a positive elbow flexion test, vibratory perception with the tuning fork will be diminished, and usually there will be an obvious discrepancy in pinch and grip strength between the hand with the nerve compression and the opposite hand. There will be no muscle wasting, two-point discrimination will still be normal, and the symptoms will be intermittent (Table 3-3).

In *severe ulnar nerve compression at the elbow,* there will be one or more of the following: persistent sensory discomfort, abnormal two-point discrimination, or muscle wasting. The wasting is most often observed in the first dorsal interosseous region but, as described for ulnar nerve compression at the wrist, a positive Froment's sign or a positive Wartenberg's sign may be present. There will be wasting of the dorsal interosseous muscles noticed as a depression between the metacarpals in these areas. A pinch strength of 5 lb means essentially no ulnar nerve innervated muscles are being used for pinch, since the flexor pollicis longus alone can generate 5 to 7 lb of pinch strength. (With the ulnar nerve divided at the elbow, the patient will still have the ability to develop 5 to 7 lb of pinch based on the median innervated muscles.) Thus, when the pinch strength is in the 7 to 10 lb range, there is actually extreme weakness of pinch due to ulnar nerve problems. When measuring lateral key pinch, the examiner will note how many pounds of pinch can be generated with the interphalangeal joint of the thumb extended. (In this instance, the patient is using just ulnar innervated muscles.) He will then note the number of additional pounds that can be generated when the interphalangeal joint is flexed (Froment's sign). (In this instance, the patient is using the median nerve innervated flexor pollicis longus.) Flexor carpi ulnaris muscle wasting may be apparent on physical examination but the flexor profundus muscle mass wasting cannot easily be observed (Table 3-3).

Care must be given to a patient's complaint of weakness. We have observed three patients in whom the biceps brachi has ruptured and been repaired. The patient's weakness had erroneously been attributed to the biceps problem, whereas we found a coexisting ulnar nerve compression. This cubital tunnel syndrome in these patients was most likely due to the swelling from the biceps rupture or from the same initial injury itself or the elbow flexed position required in the postoperative period after biceps reconstruction.

An additional source of confusion is the patient with trigger finger release in the ring, middle, or little finger who still has trouble flexing his fingers. Attention here is usually directed toward the triggering problem in the palm, whereas, in fact, it may be flexor profundus weakness due to ulnar nerve compression at the elbow. We have seen four patients with this presentation.

With *ulnar nerve complete division,* initially there is complete anesthesia in the little finger and over the dorsal aspect of the hand when the ulnar nerve lesion is located at the elbow. There can be complete lack of function in the hypothenar muscles and first dorsal interosseous; these are the easiest intrinsic muscles to test unambiguously. There will be complete lack of ability to flex the profundus tendon to the little finger and it is the inability to contract normally the profundus to the little finger and sensory loss over the dorsal ulnar aspect of the hand that localizes the lesion to the proximal forearm or elbow instead of at the wrist. Additional information on ulnar nerve problems at the elbow may be found in Chapter 9.

Radial Sensory Nerve in the Forearm

Compression of the radial sensory nerve in the forearm generally occurs between the distal third and proximal two-thirds of the forearm and, as a result of this, there is no motor involvement. There is a sensory change over the dorsal radial aspect of the hand, but because of overlap between the radial sensory nerve and the lateral antebrachial cutaneous nerve,[28] the textbook territory innervated by the radial sensory nerve may not be involved. The patient's main complaints with radial sensory nerve entrapment in the forearm are abnormal sensation over the dorsal radial aspect of the hand, but they may complain only that their thumb and index finger do not feel normal. Such a complaint may be mistaken for carpal tunnel syndrome. Patients frequently complain that they have pain when they grip or pinch. It is important to realize, as is discussed for radial sensory nerve entrapment in Chapter 10, that with gripping and pinching, the radial sensory nerve is pulled and this pulls against the point of compression causing pain in these actions. This symptom must be evaluated, however, in the context of being sure there are no problems in the trapezial joint or the first dorsal extensor compartment. The patient may complain that his symptoms are worsened with activities, particularly if he has a job requiring repetitive pronation and supination or repetitive grasping movements. There is no nighttime increase in disturbance with this entrapment.

In *mild degree of radial sensory nerve entrapment in the forearm,* there are intermittent symptoms. The perception of vibratory stimuli is hypersensitive. There will be slightly abnormal moving touch perception when this hand is tested compared with the dorsal ulnar aspect of the same hand or the radial sensory aspect of the contralateral hand. There will be a positive Tinel's sign over the radial sensory nerve at the juncture of the tendons of the brachioradialis with the extensor carpi radialis longus. The provocative test with the forearm pronated and the wrist flexed and ulnar deviated will be positive (Fig. 3-8). Finklestein's sign will also be

Table 3-12. Comparison Between de Quervain's and Wartenburg's Syndromes

	deQuervain's Syndrome	*Wartenburg's Syndrome*
Pain dorsoradial wrist	+	+
Positive Finklestein sign	+	+
Pain with resisted thumb extension or abduction	+	−
Tenderness over first extensor compartment	+	−
Tinel's sign present (junction of BR* and ECRL* tendon)	−	+
Exacerbation of symptoms with forearm pronation or pressure over BR and ECRL junction	−	+
Abnormal sensibility testing radial sensory distribution	−	+

*BR: brachioradialis; ECRL: extensor carpi radialis longus.

positive. This syndrome is frequently misdiagnosed as de Quervain's extensor tenosynovitis (Table 3-12).

In *moderate degree of radial sensory nerve entrapment in the forearm,* vibratory perception is decreased. The rest of the examination is the same.

In *severe degree of radial sensory nerve compression in the forearm,* there is abnormal two-point discrimination compared with the contralateral region, and the sensory symptoms are persistent.

When the *radial sensory nerve is divided* in this location, there may, in fact, not be a complete area of anesthesia due to the overlap of the lateral antebrachial cutaneous nerve and occasionally due to an extension of the dorsal cutaneous branch of the ulnar nerve, or the posterior cutaneous nerve of the forearm. The autonomous zone to search for total anesthesia, if it occurs, may be limited to the dorsal radial aspect of the second metacarpal or in the web between the thumb and index finger. On occasion, the converse may be true, with the entire dorsal aspect of the hand numb. Very occasionally, the radial sensory nerve may extend its territory to the volar aspect of the thumb.[41]

Radial Nerve Entrapment at the Elbow

The radial nerve may be entrapped in the region of the elbow and the proximal third of the forearm. The symptom complex related to sites of entrapment here include disturbances in the motor innervation to the brachioradialis, the radial wrist extensors, the thumb extensors, and the finger extensors. Depending on the degree of entrapment and the location of the bands causing the entrapment, these muscles may be completely or incompletely paralyzed. The classic descriptions of entrapments in these areas include the radial tunnel syndrome and the posterior interosseous nerve syndrome. These are more specifically discussed in Chapter 11. The patient generally does not complain of sensory symptoms with entrapment at this proximal level because the nerve contains generally more motor fibers than sensory fibers. The most frequent symptom is aching in the dorsal radial muscle mass and may be easily confused with lateral humeral epicondylitis, or tennis elbow. With use of the hand, aching in this forearm region can be severe, especially when work or sports activities involve repetitive pronation and supination and wrist dorsiflexion and elbow flexion.

In *mild radial nerve compression in this region,* the sensory symptoms are intermittent and the radial nerve may be tender on direct pressure. Tinel's sign is usually not present. There is no tenderness over the lateral humeral epicondyle and weakness on specific muscle testing may be present.

In *moderate degrees of radial nerve compression* in the elbow and forearm region, weakness of the radial wrist extensors may be demonstrated, but more specifically with resisted radial wrist extension, aching may be transmitted to the proximal muscle mass arising from the lateral humeral epicondyle. Specifically, when the entrapment is in the so-called radial tunnel region, resisted middle finger extension produces this symptom. With injury to just the posterior interosseous nerve, both the brachioradialis and the extensor carpi radialis longus are intact. Since the extensor carpi radialis inserts into the base of the second metacarpal, wrist extension with radial deviation will be demonstrated. When the location is somewhat more distal, (the supinator region beneath the arcade of Fröhse), resisted supination causes aching in this area.

In the *severe degree of radial nerve entrapment* in the forearm and elbow region, there will be actual paralysis of involved muscles, which must be distinguished from extensor tendon ruptures. This distinction can be made by looking for the tenodesis effect: When the wrist is flexed or extended, the fingers extend or flex respectively at the metacarpophalangeal joint based on intact tendons. With loss of tendons due to rupture, this tenodesis effect is lost and the fingers remain in the flexed position at the metacarpophalangeal joint regardless of wrist position. Except in the wrist extensor muscle mass, muscle wasting is difficult to detect. The brachioradialis and extensor carpi radialis longus are generally intact regardless of the site of compression unless the radial nerve is injured in the midhumeral region, such as when there is a spiral fracture of the humerus.

With *complete loss of radial nerve function* due to laceration in the elbow and forearm region, there is loss of sensation over the dorsal radial aspect of the hand, with complete inability to extend the fingers and thumb. The wrist is radially deviated because of proximal intact innervation to the extensor carpi radialis longus.

References

1. Mackinnon SE, Dellon AL, Hudson AR, Hunter D: Chronic nerve compression—experimental model in the rat. Ann Plast Surg 13:112–120, 1984.
2. Mackinnon SE, O'Brien JP, Dellon AL, McLean AR, Hudson AR, Hunter DA: A model of chronic nerve compression in the rat model. Ann Plast Surg, 19:430–435, 1987.
3. Seiler WA: Dysesthesia. Unpublished data, 1987.
4. Dellon AL, Schneider R, Burke R: Effect of acute compartmental changes upon response to vibratory stimuli. Plast Reconstr Surg 72:208–216, 1983.
5. Mackinnon SE, Dellon AL, Hudson AR, Hunter DA: A primate model for chronic nerve compression. J Reconstr Microsurg 1:185–194, 1985.
6. Dellon AL: Clinical use of vibratory stimulation to evaluate peripheral nerve injury in compression neuropathy. Plast Reconstr Surg 65:466–476, 1980.
7. Dellon AL: The vibrometer. Plast Reconstr Surg 71:427–431, 1983.
8. Szabo RM, Gelberman RH, Williamson RV, Dellon AL, Yaru NC, Dimick MP: Vibratory sensory testing in acute peripheral nerve compression. J Hand Surg [Am]9:104–108, 1984.
9. Phillips JE, Mackinnon SE, Dellon AL, Beatty SE, O'Brien J: Vibratory sensory testing in acute compartment syndrome. Clinical and experimental study. Plast Reconstr Surg, 79:796–801, 1987.
10. Kendall HO, Kendall FP: *Muscles: Testing and Function.* Williams & Wilkins, Baltimroe, 1949.
11. Mathiowetz V, Weber K, Volland G, et al: Reliability and validity of grip and pinch strength evaluations. J Hand Surg [Am] 9:222–226, 1984.
12. Apfel E: The effect of thumb interphalangeal joint position on strength of key pinch. J Hand Surg [Am] 11:47–51, 1986.
13. Dellon AL: The moving two-point discrimination test; clinical evaluation of the quickly-adapting fiber receptor system. J Hand Surg 3:474–481, 1978.
14. Mackinnon SE, Dellon AL: Two-point discrimination testor. J Hand Surg [Am] 10:906–907, 1985.
15. Dellon AL, Mackinnon SE, Crosby PM: Reliability of two-point discrimination measurements. J Hand Surg 12A: 693–696, 1987.
16. Dellon AL, Hendler N, Hopkins JET, Karas AC, Campbell JN: Team management of patients with diffuse upper extremity complaints. Md Med J 35:849–852, 1986.
17. Dellon AL: Peripheral nerve injuries. In Gardner B, Shaftan GW eds: Surgical Emergencies JB Lippincott, Philadelphia, 1986, pp 533–537.
18. Kimura J: Electrodiagnosis in diseases of nerve and muscle. FA Davis, Philadelphia, 1983.
19. Lenman JAR, Ritchie AE: Clinical electromyograph. Pitman Publishing, London, 1983.
20. Robertson KB: Electrodiagnosis in neurological rehabilitation. In Umphred DA, ed: Neurological Rehabilitation. CV Mosby, St. Louis, 1985.
21. Delagi EF: Electrodiagnosis in peripheral lesions. In Omer GE Jr, Spinner M, eds: Management of Peripheral Nerve Problems. WB Saunders, Philadelphia, 1980.
22. Erdman WJ II: Electromyography and electrical testing in hand rehabilitation. In Hunter DA, Schneider R, Mackinnon SE: Rehabilitation of Hands. CV Mosby, St. Louis, 1984.
23. Spindler HA, Dellon AL: Nerve conduction studies and sensibility testing in carpal tunnel syndrome. J Hand Surg 7:260–263, 1982.
24. Nelson PM: Implications of the electromyographic examination for hand therapy. In Hunter DA, Schneider R, Mackinnon SE, eds: Rehabilitation of the Hands. CV Mosby, St. Louis, 1984.
25. Louis DS, Hankin FM: Symptomatic relief following carpal tunnel decompression with normal electroneuromyographic studies. Orthopedics 10:434–436, 1987.
26. Mackinnon SE, Dellon AL, Hudson AR, Hunter DA: Chronic human nerve compression: A histologic assessment. Neuropathol Appl Neurobiol 12:547–565, 1987.
27. Dellon AL, Mackinnon SE: Correlation of human ulnar nerve entrapment. J Neurol Sci, 1987.
28. Hill NA, Howard FM, Huffer BR: The incomplete anterior interosseous nerve syndrome. J Hand Surg [Am] 10:4–16, 1985.
29. Dellon AL, Mackinnon SE: Musculoaponeurotic variations along the course of the median nerve in the forearm. J Hand Surg [Br] 12B:359–363, 1986.
30. Dellon AL, Mackinnon SE: Radial sensory nerve entrapment in the forearm. J Hand Surg [Am] 11:199–205, 1986.
31. Mackinnon SE, Dellon AL: Overlap of lateral antebrachial cutaneous nerve and superficial sensory branch of the radial nerve. J Hand Surg [Am] 10:522–526, 1985.
32. Spindler H, Dellon AL: Electrodiagnosis of radial sensory nerve entrapment. Unpublished data, 1986.
33. Dellon AL, Mackinnon SE, Schlegel R: Validity of electrodiagnostic studies following anterior transposition of the ulnar nerve. J Hand Surg 12A:700–703, 1987.
34. Tinel J: "The tingling sign in peripheral nerve lesions." Translation by Emanuel B. Kaplan. In Spinner M, ed: *Injuries to the Major Branches of Peripheral Nerves of the Forearm,* 2nd ed., WB Saunders, Philadelphia, 1978, pp 8–13.
35. Dellon AL: Tinel or not Tinel. J Hand Surg [Br] 9:216, 1984.
36. Paley D, McMurty RY: Median nerve compression test in carpal tunnel syndrome diagnosis. Ortho Rev 15:41–45, 1985.
37. Gilliatt RW, Wilson TG: A pneumatic tourniquet test in the carpal tunnel syndrome. Lancet 2:595–597, 1953.
38. Rowntree T: Anomalous innervation of the hand muscles. J Bone Joint Surg 31B:505–510, 1949.
39. Wartenberg R: A sign of ulnar palsy. JAMA 112:1688–1689, 1939.
40. Froment MJ: La paralysie de l'adducteur du ponce et le signe de la prehension. Rev Neurol (Paris) 28:1236–1240, 1915.
41. Dellon AL, Mackinnon SE: Radial sensory nerve entrapment. Arch Neurol 43:833–837, 1986.

Nerve Repair and Nerve Grafting

4

The surgeon, when presented with a peripheral nerve injury for repair, must have a clear understanding of both the anatomy of the peripheral nerve and the neurobiology of nerve degeneration and regeneration. This understanding will significantly influence both the timing and the technique of nerve repair.

Historical Review

The first documentation of repair of a divided nerve is attributed to the Italian Ferrara in 1608,[1] but it really was not until the mid 1800s that any interest was directed toward nerve repair and various repair techniques were introduced. Before this time, it was generally accepted that either no surgery or amputation was indicated after major nerve severance. In 1934, Loyal Davis and David Cleveland published one of the most comprehensive reviews of the history of nerve repairs as an introduction to their own experimental work investigating nerve regeneration across nerve grafts.[2]

The early techniques of nerve repair included many that now appear totally inappropriate. Letievant,[3] in 1872, first described turning back a flap of nerve created from the distal portion of the nerve in a proximal direction, suturing this to a similar flap that was turned down in a distal direction from the proximal end of the nerve. In this fashion, all proximal regenerating nerve fibers were effectively excluded from any of the repair sites. Mackenzie[4] reported good success with use of this technique. It was not until Stookey[5] reviewed their cases and demonstrated no regeneration that the use of these nerve flaps was brought into disrepute. Markoe,[6] in 1885, described a technique whereby the divided ends of the nerve were cut tangentially in order to increase the surface area for nerve contact. In the same year, Rawa[7] described a side-to-side suture in which both the proximal and distal cut nerve stumps were excluded from the nerve repair as the sides of the nerve rather than the ends of the nerve[7] were brought together. Several techniques of suture transfixion similar to those presently used to repair tendons were described.[8–11] Suturing techniques that brought the same suture through the skin and nerve were also noted. In 1886, Assaky[12] described a suture "à distence." He suggested using a scaffolding of sutures between the cut ends of the nerve in hopes that the axons would regenerate along this scaffold. Letievant[3] also described simply inserting the distal stump of the divided nerve between the intact nerve fascicles of the proximal portion of the divided nerve in what was called a nerve implantation technique.

Galen (130-200 AD) was the first to distinguish the difference between nerves and tendons.[13] He did not describe any attempts to repair nerve but did suggest that in the case of partial nerve injury the nerve could be completely cut to prevent what he described as "convulsions." Paulus Aegineta[14] used a combination of agglutination and sutures to repair nerves as early as the 7th century. In the 13th century, Roger of Parma[15] used egg albumin to repair nerves in a similar fashion. Guy de Chauliac[16] in the 14th century reported "I have seen and heard it said that in several cases, cut nerves and tendons have been restored by suture and other remedies that afterward one could not believe that they had been cut." This reference referred to nerve repair in young patients.

A review of the historical descriptions of the management of the nerve gap reveals techniques that were even more creative than those used to perform primary nerve repair. "There are many times when the ends of the divided nerves cannot be approximated easily and several procedures have been advocated in order to obtain end-to-end union. Flexion or extension of neighboring joints, gradual liberation of the nerve trunk from its normal bed, gradual stretching, transposition of the nerve from its normal bed to a shorter anatomical course or a combination of these procedures may bridge gaps as large as 7-8 cm."[2] In reviewing techniques of management of large defects in nerve trunks, Davis and Cleveland[2] described six different techniques (nerve implants,[3,17] nerve flaps,[3] suture à distence,[12] tubulization,[18] nerve crossing,[19] nerve grafts[2]). Presenting their own experimental work, they supported the use of nerve grafts for the management of nerve gaps. Nerve stretching was described first by Assaky[12] in 1886 and then investigated as a method of potential repair by Hoen and Brackett in 1956.[21]

Various types of tubular structures have been suggested as conduits to bridge nerve gaps that could not be managed appropriately with end-to-end suture technique. These have included rubber tubes,[22] rolled Cargile gauze,[23] fat and fascial sheaths,[24] hardened and fresh blood vessels,[25–27] parchment tubes,[28] metal tubes,[29] collagen tubes,[30,31] tantalum,[32] Millipore elastic,[33] polygalactin,[34,35] and polyorthoester.[36] Probably the first description of this tubulization technique was that of Gluck[18] in 1880, who used the central canal of a decalcified bone to serve as the pathway between the separated ends of the divided nerve. In 1810, Philipeaux and Vulpian[37] described the first experiments of nerve grafting. A segment of lingual nerve was used to bridge a defect in the hypoglossal nerve.[37] In 1878, Albert[38] described the first clinical use of a nerve graft. A 3 cm gap in the median nerve was reconstructed using a xenograft. Clinical outcome of this nerve graft was not reported. The first successful nerve graft report is that of Mayo-Robson,[20] who repaired 2.5 cm of the median nerve with a nerve allograft. In 1906, Sherren[39] reviewed 16 cases of nerve grafts and demonstrated some improvement in six of these cases with definite improvement in one. These were all cases of xenografts. In the early history of nerve grafting techniques, there was considerable enthusiasm for use of nerve grafts from cadavers or animals. Emphasis was also directed toward various methods of preserving or storing these grafts. Huber[23] suggested that xenografts were not as successful as autografts or allografts. Scepticism existed regarding the value of nerve grafts even until the early 1970s. Although successful reports of regeneration across nerve autografts were reported in the early 1900s, Stopford[40] and Platt[41] reported failure of functional recovery in 30 cases and concluded that nerve grafting had a small role to play in the management of nerve injury. Stookey[5] suggested that scar tissue at the distal suture line of the nerve graft was the barrier to nerve regeneration. Reviewing 375 cases, Delangeniere[42] noted that the success of nerve transplants diminished with the increased length of the graft. By comparison, Bunnell,[43] in 1928, stated that he had found evidence of regeneration across autogenous nerve grafts that was just as rapid as that after a simple end-to-end suture repair. It is interesting to note that the first facial nerve graft was carried out by Bunnell in 1927.[44]

The two major world wars provided both the clinical material and the major stimulus for experimental studies directed toward nerve repair, but the clinical results of nerve injuries treated at that time were discouraging.[45] In fact, it was not until the introduction of microsurgical technique that the results after the early nerve grafting improved. The extensive history of poor results after nerve grafts tended to blend results of xenografts, allografts, and autografts together. These poor results influenced many present surgeons not to use nerve grafts in their clinical practices. The pioneering and courageous work of Hanno Millesi has brought credibility to nerve grafting technique.[46,47] Millesi is careful to emphasize the importance of microsurgical technique, including instrumentation, sutures, and magnification. He has emphasized the inappropriateness of tension at the site of the nerve repair and has been an advocate for nerve grafts whenever any tension exists.[48] As with almost any surgical technique, nerve grafting can be as easily carried out using poor technique as the appropriate microneurosurgical technique. Some of the poorer results presently realized with nerve grafting probably result from inappropriate tension at the site of the nerve graft. Thus, the problems of using a nerve graft are compounded by using a nerve graft with tension at the two ends of the graft.

Fibrin clot technique was introduced by Young and Medawar[49] in 1940 and popularized by Seddon and Medawar.[50] More recently, Bonard and Narakas[51] have reported success using fibrin glue for nerve repairs. Current concern with transmission of infectious viruses may make this technique relatively unpopular.

Since its first clinical application in 1885, the use of nerve allografts has remained somewhat controversial. Considerable experimental work has been carried out using these allografts. Jacoby et al[52] reported excellent regeneration in a clinical series of nerve allografts. Unfortunately when Kuhlendahl et al[53] reviewed this series of allografts carried out by Jacoby et al, they found no evidence of regeneration across these allografts. This study reported by Kuhlendahl et al placed the use of nerve allografts into clinical disrepute.[53] With the advent of microneurosurgical technique coupled with a greater understanding of the immunology of transplantation, it would appear that allografts may soon find an appropriate clinical role in very extensive nerve injuries when adequate autogenous nerve graft material is not available.

Nerve Repair

As reviewed in Chapter 1, Wallerian degeneration will occur in the distal portion of the nerve after nerve division. This will be characterized by degeneration of both the axon and myelin and a proliferation of columns of Schwann cells that will support subsequent regenerative efforts from the proximal nerve. In the nerve proximal to the lesion, traumatic degeneration will occur. This looks histologically the same as Wallerian degeneration. The proximal extent of the traumatic degeneration will vary directly with the extent of the nerve injury. Significant longitudinal damage will occur after avulsion or crushing injuries. Much lesser longitudinal injury will occur after a sharp laceration. Severe injury can cause actual neuronal death. After this period of degeneration, the proximal nerve will attempt to regenerate. Myelinated and unmyelinated fibers from the proximal stump will sprout into regenerating units or regenerating "clusters," which are composed of a number of fibers that have "sprouted" from a single fiber. This regenerating unit, which is surrounded by perineurium, represents the minimal functional unit for regeneration. The aim of a good nerve repair will be to direct these regenerating fibers successfully into the environment of the distal nerve with minimal loss of regenerating units at the suture line. These extraepineurial sprouts will contribute to a painful suture line neuroma and will represent loss of potential nerve function. As discussed in Chapter 1, it is not clear how many of these regenerating fibers will become functional. It is not known what minimal reinnervation is required in order to restore functional muscle power or cutaneous sensibility. This will probably vary between the motor and sensory systems and between various sensory receptors. With denervation in the motor system, acetylcholine receptors appear throughout the muscle fiber and new neuromuscular junctions may be formed. In the sensory system, on the other hand, the receptors degenerate but are capable of becoming reinnervated with successful nerve regeneration. The potential for successful reinnervation of sensory receptors may vary from receptor to receptor based on the "ease" of reinnervation hypothesis.[54] A single fiber innervates several Merkel cells and several axons may enter a single Meissner corpusle; thus, statistically, it will be easier to reinnervate a Meissner corpusle, which mediates moving touch, than a Merkel cell complex, which mediates static touch.

An effective nerve repair will be dependent on sensory, motor, and autonomic axons making appropriate connections with their distal end organs. The results of nerve repair will be influenced by the level and timing of the repair, the nature and the extent of the injury, the fascicular anatomy and realignment of the injured nerve, the surgical technique, and patient factors. Although the eventual outcome is influenced by many parameters, there are several basic principles of nerve repair that are common to all nerve injuries. We are, thus, able to generate a sequence of eight basic principles or axioms that form the basis of our present management of the nerve-injured patient:

1. Quantitative pre- and postoperative clinical assessment is required for both the motor and sensory system. An assessment of muscle wasting and strength (such as pinch and grip measurements) can be provided for the motor evaluation. A measurement of threshold (vibration or pressure stimulus) and innervation density (both static and moving two-point discrimination) as well as pain and temperature perception (protective sensation) will assess the sensory system.
2. Microsurgical technique, including magnification, microsurgical instruments, and sutures, should be utilized.
3. A nerve repair must be tension free.
4. When a tension-free repair is not possible, an interposition or interfascicular nerve graft should be used.
5. Postural positioning of the extremity to facilitate an end-to-end repair is discouraged. Both the nerve repair and a nerve graft should be carried out with the extremity in a neutral position with no tension on the repair site.
6. When the clinical and surgical condition permits a primary nerve repair, it should be done.

7. When the internal neural topography of the peripheral nerve permits, a group fascicular repair may be done. When the function of the fascicles is primarily mixed sensory and motor without well-defined groups of fascicles, an epineurial repair should be done.
8. A course of postoperative motor and sensory reeducation[54] will maximize the potential surgical result (Chapter 18).

Epineurial Versus Fascicular Repair

There have been both clinical[55–60] and experimental[61–68] studies directed toward the identification of the superiority of one or the other of these two suture techniques (Fig. 4-1). There has been no real conclusive experimental or clinical evidence to suggest that one technique is better than another. Of these, the best were experimental studies, in which retrograde horseradish peroxidase transport studies noted improved specificity of muscle reinnervation after fascicular repair of the rat sciatic nerve when compared with an epineurial repair.[69–71] Normal nerve cell distribution of peroneal and posterior tibial muscles in the spinal cord was compared with that distribution after these two suture techniques. Better organization was noted after the fascicular repair. Experimental studies comparing epineurial to fascicular repairs in primates have demonstrated no advantages in either of the two surgical techniques.[72,73]

Although there have been clinical studies advocating one technique or another, there has been no consensus as to the superiority of either method of repair. As well, there has been no randomized study comparing one technique with the other in which adequate pre- and postoperative clinical and electrophysiologic testing parameters were used. The potential benefits of fascicular alignment are probably not experienced clinically because of the increased surgical manipulation required in order to execute a fascicular repair and the potential for mismatching of fascicles. If it was theoretically possible to align the fascicles completely appropriately and with minimum surgical trauma, it is likely that fascicular repair would produce better clinical results than an epineurial repair. Realistically, it is quite possible that fascicular repairs unintentionally result in alignment of mismatched fascicles resulting in guaranteed loss of nerve function. Although the epineurial repair is not as exact, it may allow for neurotropic effects to exert their influence on the direction of nerve fiber growth (Chapter 1). This is probably why the less exact technique of epineurial repair clinically will produce the same results as fascicular repair, the theoretical benefits of the fascicular repair being lost by the practicality of the technical aspects of the execution of this technique (Fig. 4-2).

It is our recommendation that aspects of both techniques be used in nerve repair. The technique used will depend on the nature of the injury, location of the injury in the extremity, the timing of the nerve repair,

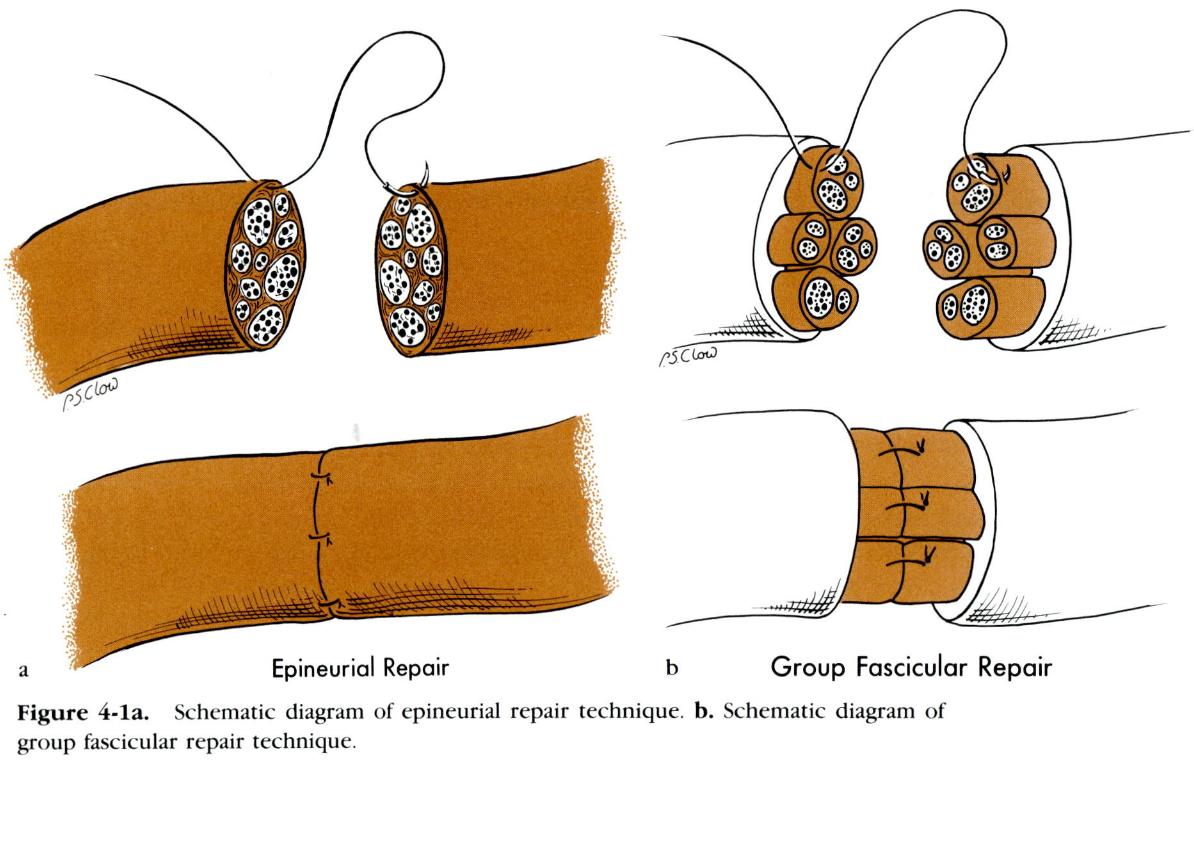

Figure 4-1a. Schematic diagram of epineurial repair technique. **b.** Schematic diagram of group fascicular repair technique.

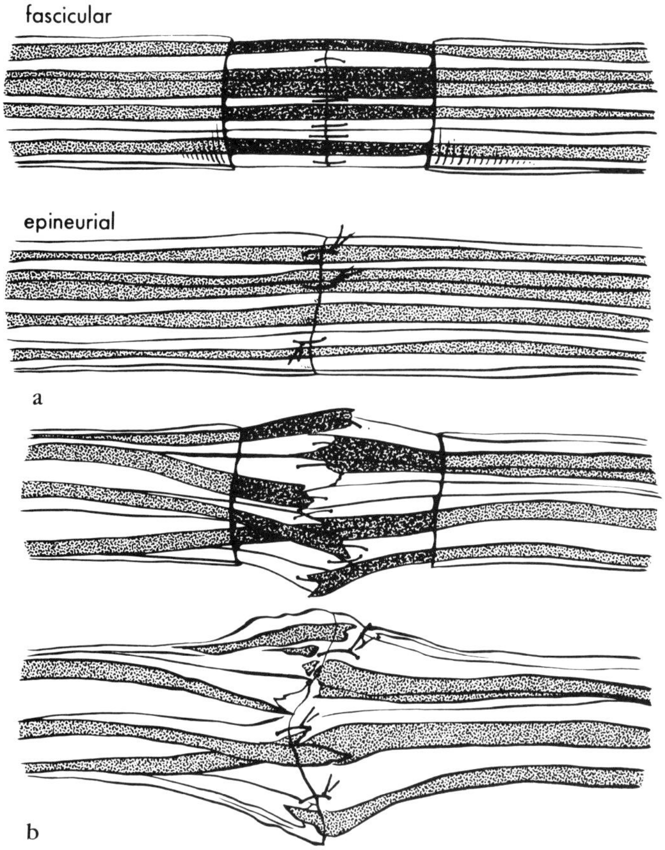

Figure 4-2a. When carrying out a fascicular repair, the surgeon will try to align motor (stippled) and sensory (white) fascicles. When carrying out an epineurial repair, the sutures are placed in the epineurium and surface landmarks, such as blood vessels, are used as anatomic markers to assist in aligning the appropriate fascicles. **b.** Clinical results would suggest that the ideal motor and sensory alignment illustrated in **a** is not realized in the clinical results. In reality, a more disorganized matching of motor and sensory fascicles is experienced at the repair level. Fascicular repair, above, epineurial repair, below.

and the fascicular arrangement of the nerve to be repaired. The goal of the nerve repair will be to align appropriate fascicles with minimal surgical trauma to the nerve.

The nature of the injury will influence repair technique. With acute injuries, when the injuring agent results in a sharp, clean laceration, epineurial repair is usually all that is required. Anatomic vascular markings on the epineurium can be easily matched, and this will help to align fascicles if appropriate magnification is used. If the surgeon has identified a particular fascicle in the proximal and distal stumps as having a specific function, then a fascicular repair of this fascicle is carried out (such as the dorsal cutaneous branch of the ulnar nerve in the forearm, deep motor branch of the ulnar nerve in Guyon's canal, recurrent motor branch of the median nerve at the wrist). Detailed microsurgical technique is critical (Fig. 4-3). A minimum number of fine microsutures will then be used to carry out the remainder of the repair in an epineurial fashion. These sutures can be placed in the external or internal epineurium, thus the neural tissue itself is avoided. The use of fine suture material (9-0, 10-0) ensures that the sutures are used to help align the nerve only and not to take tension off the neurorrhaphy. Millesi[75] has recently emphasized that the "advantages of the microsurgical nerve repair can be exploited only if performed under favourable conditions and without tension. A nerve graft with 2 suture lines but no tension can give better results than a nerve repair with one suture line and tension."

The location of the injury in the extremity will also influence the type of repair that is performed. In the proximal portion of the extremity, the fascicular arrangement is often mono- or oligofascicular in nature. In these instances, an epineurial repair is appropriate. In the distal portion of the extremity, the nerve fascicles are polyfascicular and fascicles often align themselves in a group fascicular pattern. Examining the proximal and distal ends of the divided nerve with the microscope, the surgeon can align these groups. In these instances, it is appropriate for the surgeon to carry out a group fascicular repair using a minimum number of microsutures to ensure that matching fascicular groups are appropriately oriented. Even very distal digital nerve injuries deserve to be explored and treated with microsurgical repair. This is done as much to prevent the development of painful neuroma as to restore sensibility (Fig. 4-4) (Chapter 17).

Intraoperatively, we will assess the effect of movement of adjacent joints on the nerve repair. For example, after a median nerve repair at the wrist if wrist and metacarpophalangeal movement is blocked, movement of the interphalangeal joints will not compromise the nerve repair at all. We routinely immobilize the extremity for 3 weeks after a nerve repair, although we encourage guarded finger flexion in the hopes of achieving some gliding of the tendons past the nerve in its tissue bed. Certainly, if significant scarring occurs at the repair site, it may compromise the potential for recovery.

Nerve Grafts

When an end-to-end nerve repair cannot be carried out with the assurance that there is no tension on the nerve repair, a nerve graft is necessary. Even a minimum amount of tension on the nerve repair will jeopardize the ultimate functional result.[76–78] The effect of tension on the intraneural blood supply is easily demonstrated in the operating room by observing the circulation to the peripheral nerve under the operating microscope.

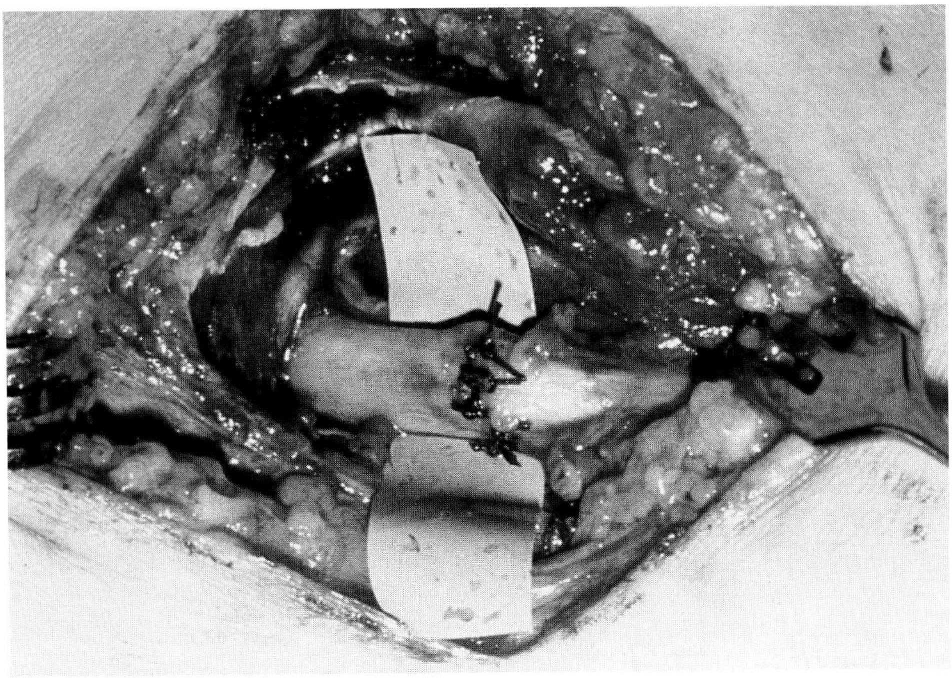

a

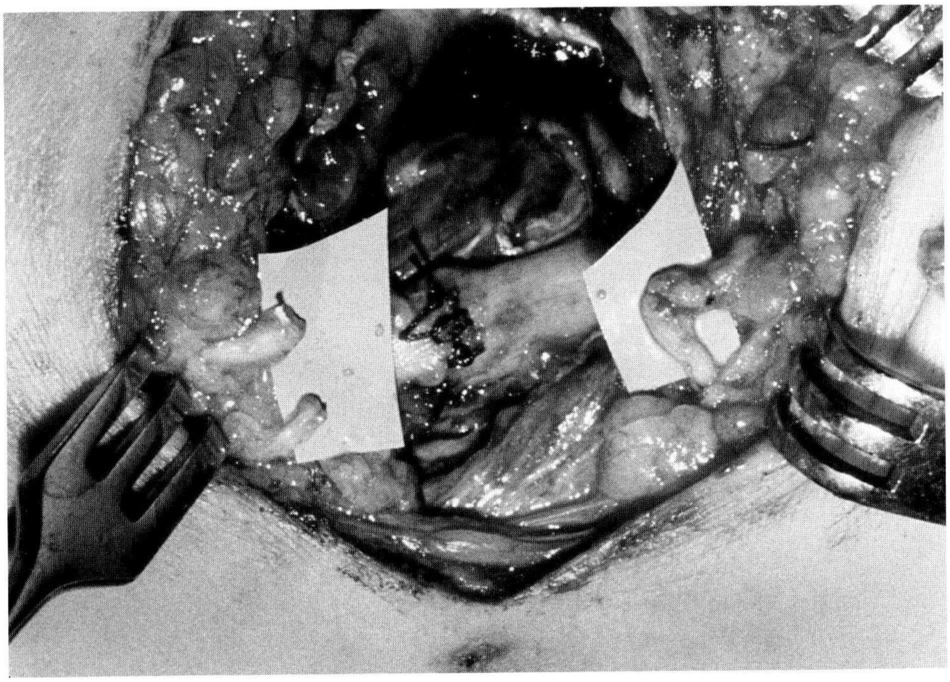

b

Figure 4-3a. This patient was referred for assessment of an ulnar nerve injury. Close-up of surgical exploration of ulnar nerve repair in the proximal forearm. **b.** Not only was the ulnar nerve repair inappropriate (3-0 black silk sutures), but the divided branches of the medial antebrachial cutaneous nerve had been unrecognized and untreated. This nerve injury to the medial antebrachial cutaneous nerve would compound a poor ulnar nerve repair with potential pain from neuroma formation. The proximal ends of the medial antebrachial cutaneous nerve were transposed proximally. The ulnar nerve was transposed anterior to the medial epicondyle, the original repair resected and an epineurial microsurgical repair carried out.

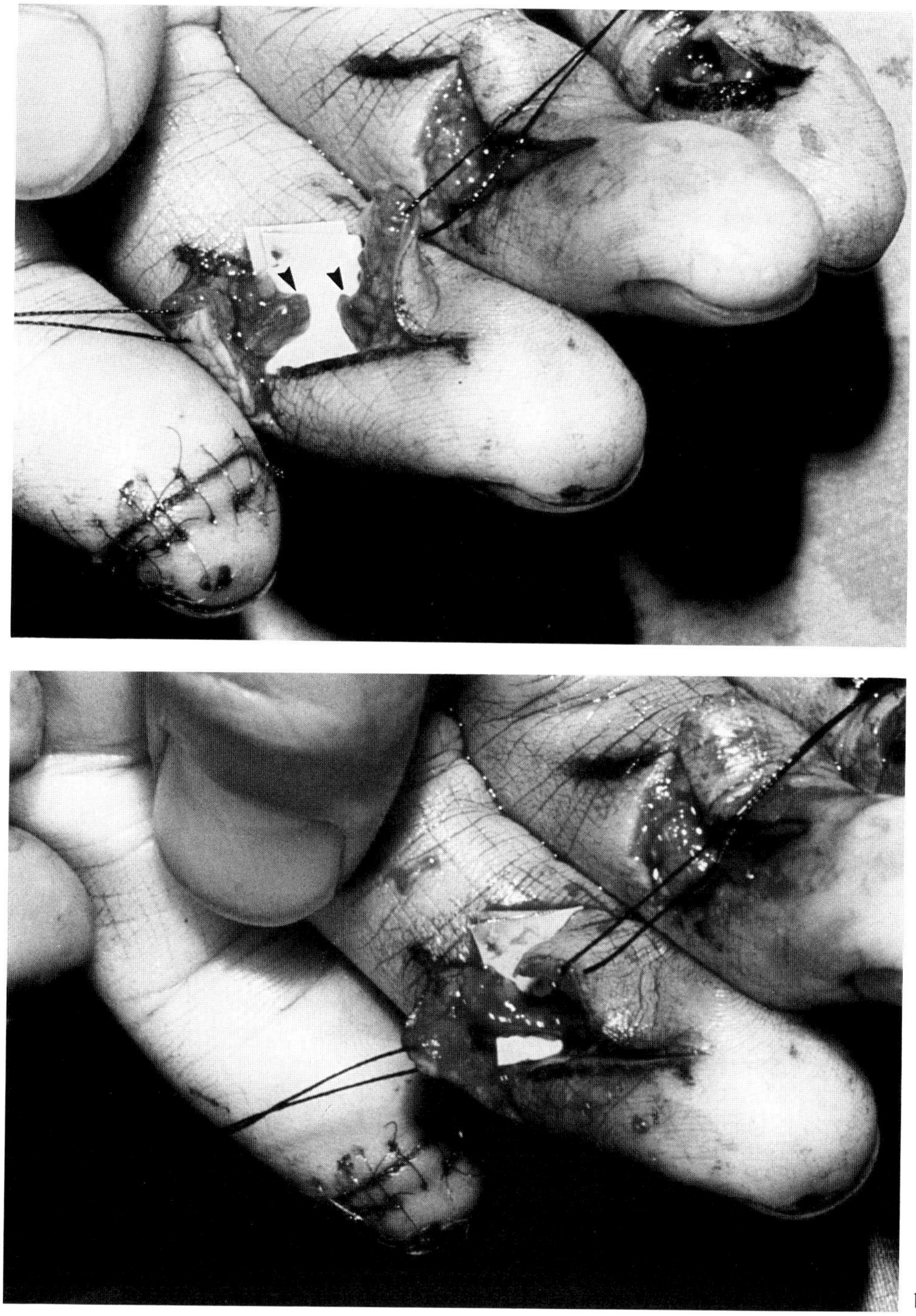

a

b

Figure 4-4a. Multiple injuries to the digits divided the digital nerves at a very distal level (arrow). **b.** A microscopic epineurial repair was possible in all digits.

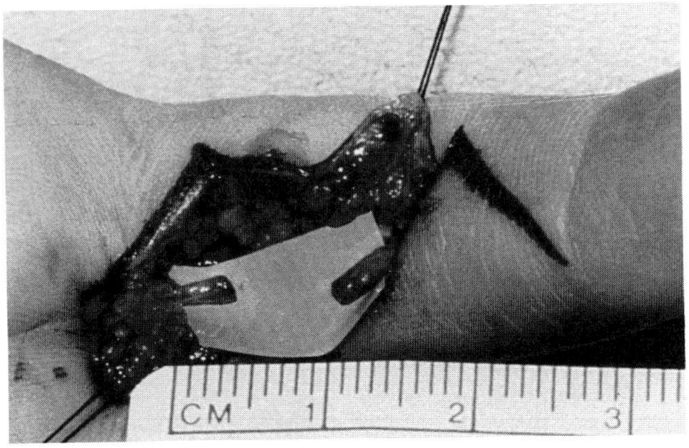

a

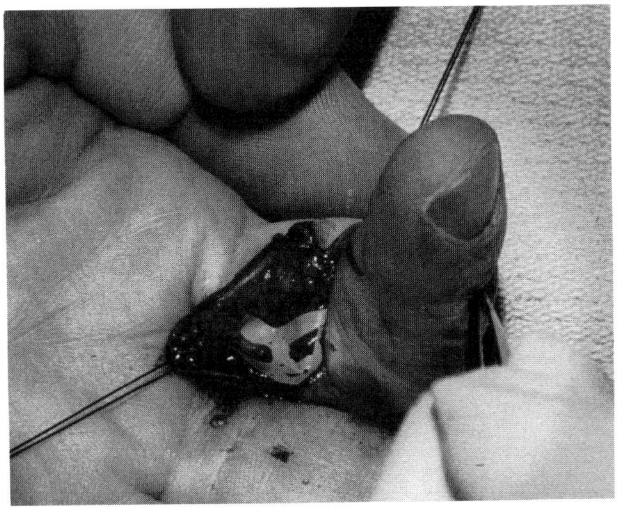

b

Figure 4-5a. In the digit, even a very short nerve gap cannot be managed with an end-to-end epineurial repair. **b.** With almost 90° of flexion at proximal interphalangeal joint, the ends of the nerves are still not easily approximated.

A pair of jeweller's forceps is placed under the nerve and the nerve is then elevated out of its tissue bed. It takes very little tension on the nerve to blanch the nerve completely and arrest blood flow into the nerve. Certainly, repairing a peripheral nerve with the extremity in a flexed position in order to coapt the two nerve ends is inappropriate, especially when one considers that the nerve must glide in its tissue bed as the extremity moves not only to a neutral position but into full extension.

There continues to be disagreement as to the critical length of nerve gap that will necessitate a nerve graft. We tolerate no tension on our nerve repair and move to nerve grafts even with very short nerve gaps. Certainly, the morbidity associated with harvesting a nerve to reconstruct a very short nerve gap is magnified for both the patient and the surgeon in a short gap situation. With the introduction of nerve tubes to accommodate this short gap situation (Chapter 20), these problems may be eliminated. In the digit, a 1 cm gap in a digital nerve, cannot be overcome even with the proximal interphalangeal joint in full flexion and, indeed, it should not be overcome with flexion of the joints (Fig. 4-5). In the forearm, such a short 1 cm gap can more easily be overcome with mobilization of the nerve proximally and distally. For the ulnar nerve, an anterior transposition will provide the surgeon with 5 cm of "extra" nerve tissue.

Technique of Nerve Grafting

The surgical technique of nerve grafting is similar in many ways to that of a primary nerve repair. The surgeon must prepare the proximal and distal ends of the nerve either by evaluating and excising the nonfunctioning portion of the neuroma in-continuity (Fig. 4-6, 4-7) or by excising a proximal neuroma and distal glioma (Fig. 4-8). The surgeon must use the same microsurgical techniques in order to effect a tension-free repair. The proximal and distal repair sites of the grafts must be completely tension free (Fig. 4-9). The surgeon will move the limb through a range of movement to ensure that there is no tension on the graft site repairs as the extremity is moved. It is, thus, not necessary to immobilize a graft for more than 2 weeks because there is never any tension on the repair sites. Longer periods of immobilization will produce unnecessary scarring along the length of the graft and tethering of the nerve graft in the tissue bed (Table 4-1).

Table 4-1. Mechanical Factors Affecting Longitudinal Gliding

	Normal Nerve	*Post-Traumatic*
Elasticity	Normal	Reduced by fibrosis
Gliding properties	Intact	Reduced by fibrosis
Tensile forces	Equally distributed	Increased at site of repair or trauma

In carrying out a nerve graft, it is important to try to achieve as accurately as possible the appropriate sensory and motor match of the individual fascicles of the grafts at proximal and distal repair sites. Techniques of fascicular identification are discussed later. In proximal extremity grafts, frequently the fascicles at the proximal stump will be mixed motor and sensory and, thus, the fascicular alignment of the grafts cannot be specific. At the distal nerve stump, the alignment can usually be quite specific. Using anatomic clues, the surgeon can be certain that the distal alignment at least is exact. An

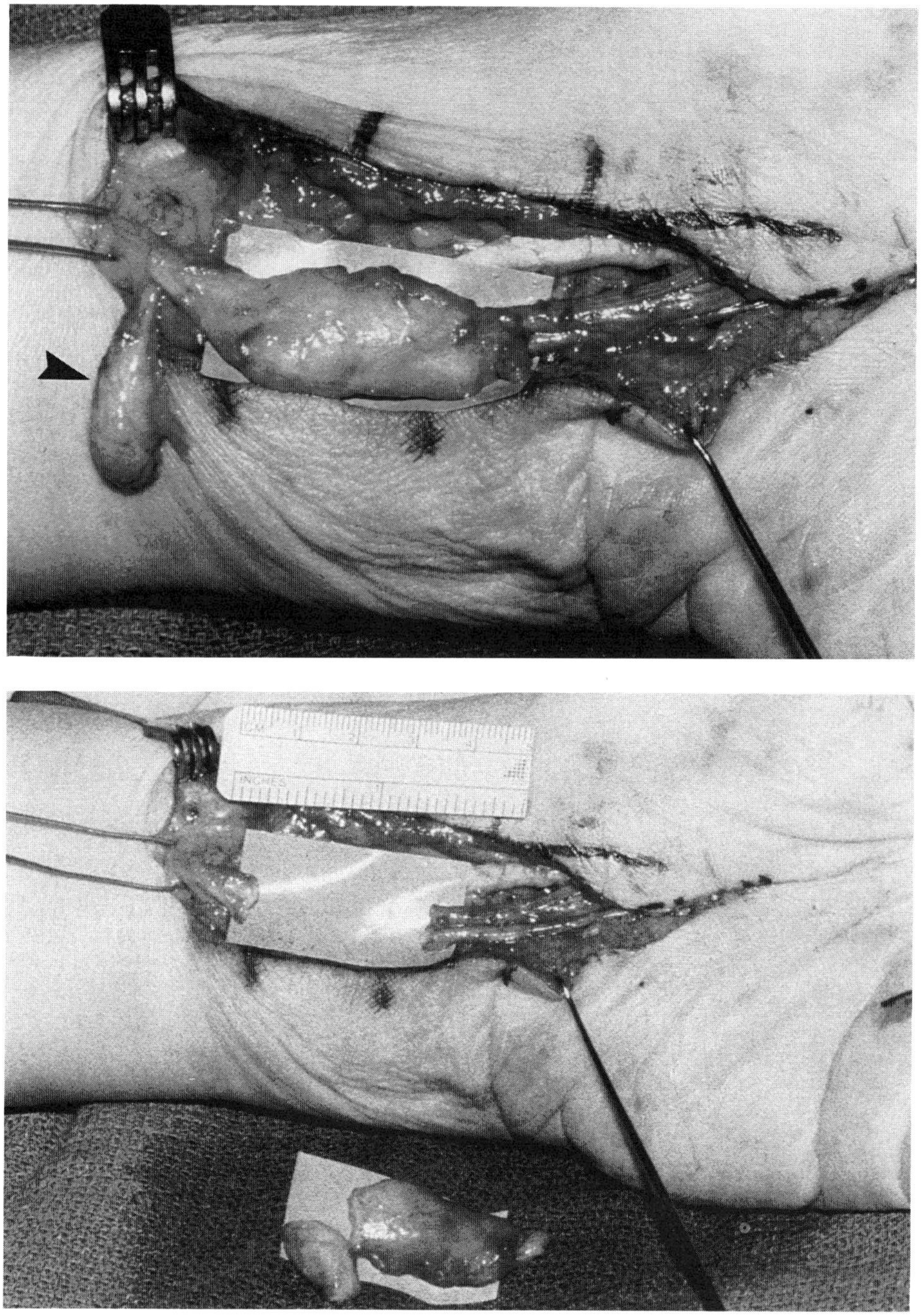

a

b

Figure 4-6a. Several years before exploring this left median nerve, an unsuccessful primary repair had been carried out. The patient clinically had no sensation in the median nerve distribution and had a neuroma of the palmar cutaneous branch of the median nerve. At exploration, a large neuroma in-continuity (fourth degree injury) of the median nerve is noted. A neuroma of the palmar cutaneous branch of the median nerve is also seen (arrow). **b.** The neuroma in-continuity is excised. (*Figure continues.*)

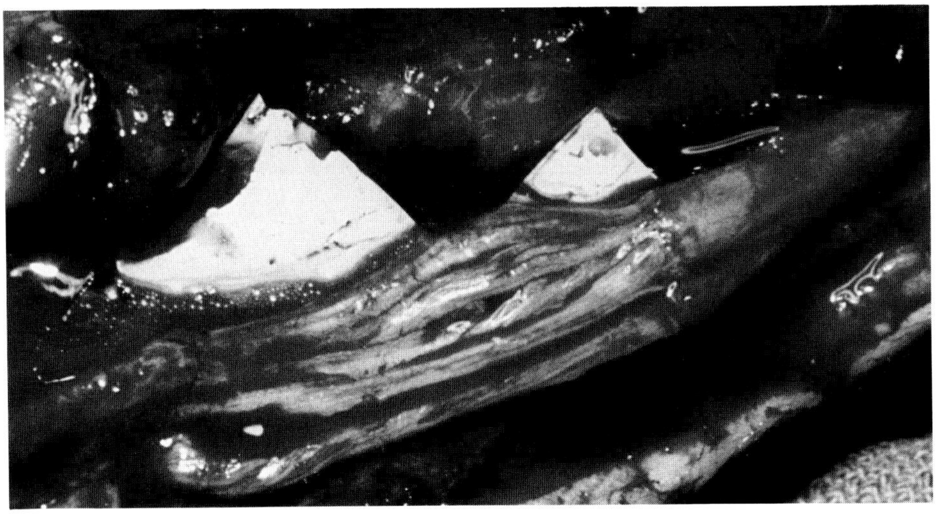

c

Figure 4-6 (*continued*) **c.** Interfascicular nerve grafting is carried out using the sural nerve.

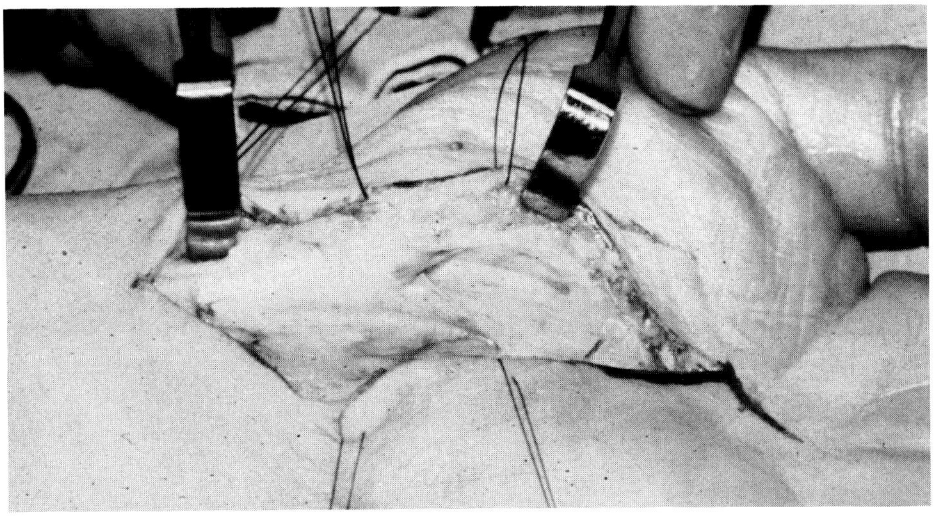

a

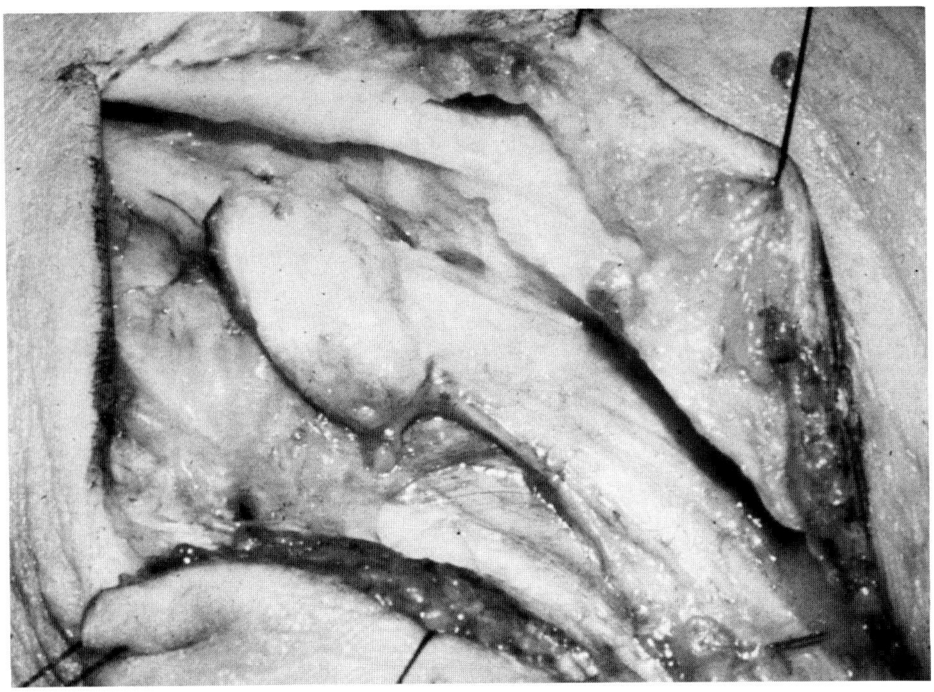

b

Figure 4-7. (*Figure continues.*)

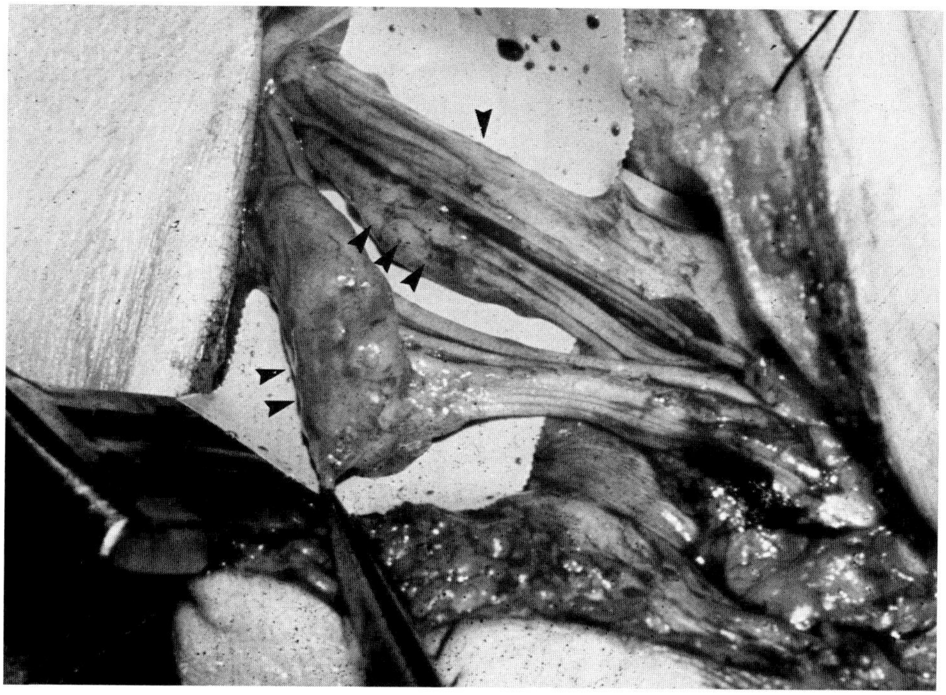

c

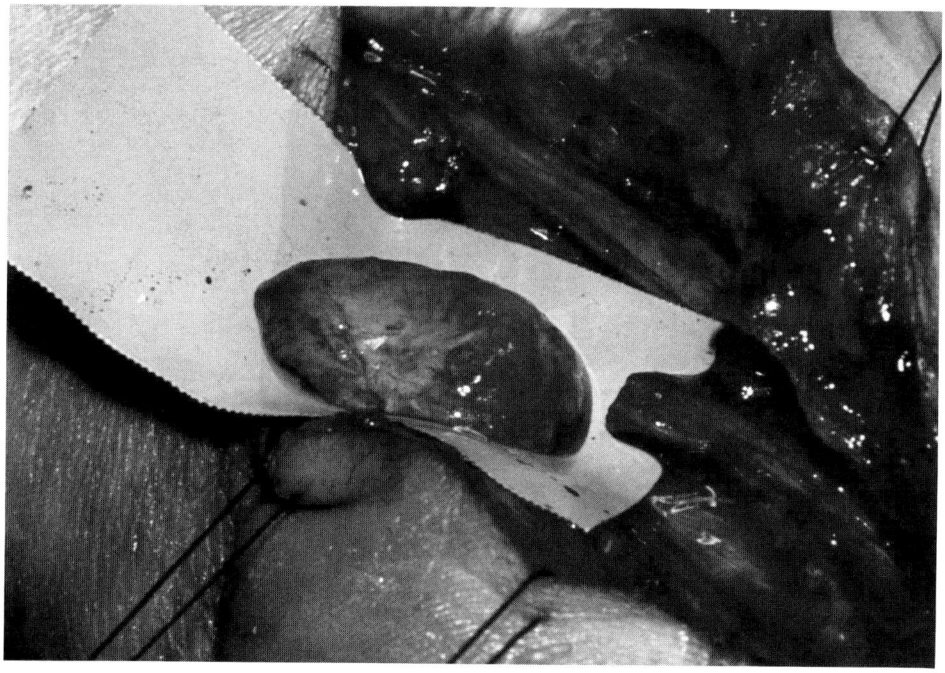

d

Figure 4-7a. After a partial median nerve injury, this patient had no sensation in the thumb, normal sensation in the index finger, diminished but adequate sensation in the long finger (moving two-point discrimination 7 mm) hand toward right. **b.** A neuroma in-continuity of the median nerve was noted (sixth degree injury) **c.** Using microsurgical technique, an internal neurolysis is carried out. A fourth degree injury involved the fascicles to the thumb (double arrow). The fascicles to the index finger were normal (single arrow). The fascicles to the long finger were not normal and corresponded with diminished sensibility (triple arrow). **d.** A neuroma in-continuity involving the fascicles to the thumb was resected. (*Figure continues.*)

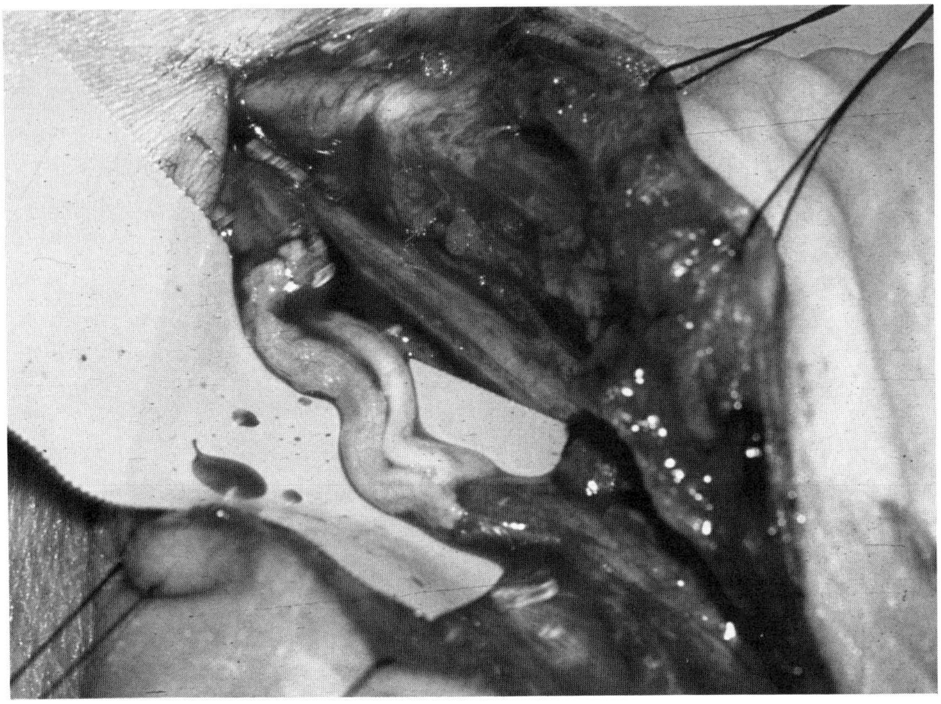

e

Figure 4-7 (*continued*) **e.** The anterior branch of the medial antebrachial cutaneous nerve was used as the donor nerve graft for this portion of the median nerve. The remainder of the median nerve was neurolysed.

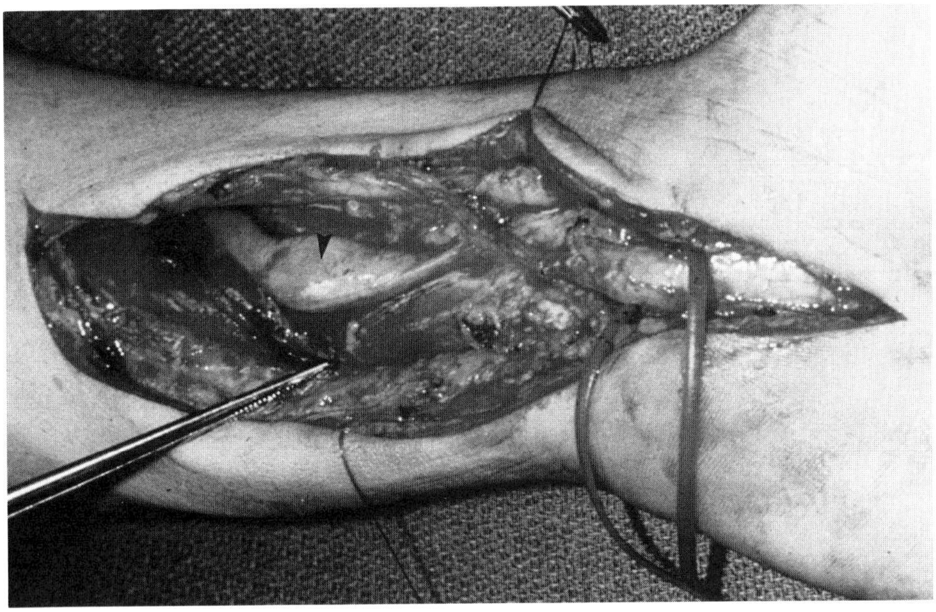

a

Figure 4-8a. This patient had divided his median nerve. The distal portion of the median nerve had been repaired to the proximal portion of the flexor carpi radialis tendon. The proximal neuroma of the median nerve is apparent (arrow). The distal portion of the median nerve, which had been sutured to the flexor carpi radialis tendon, is noted (vessel loop, hand toward right). (*Figure continues.*)

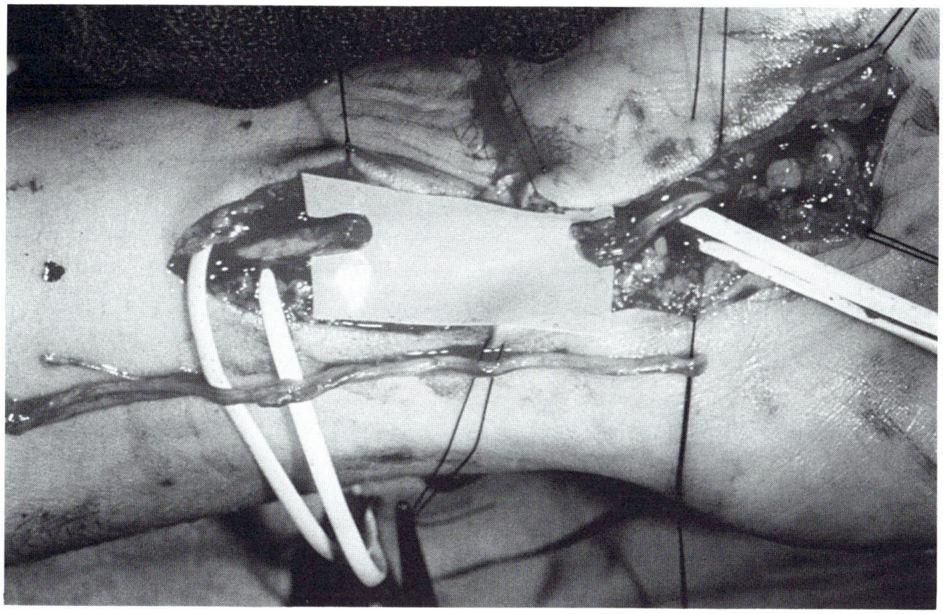

b

Figure 4-8 (*continued*) **b.** The sural nerve will be used to repair the defect.

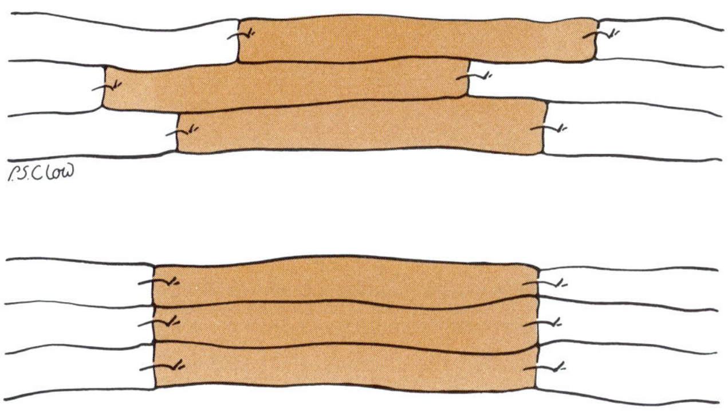

a

Nerve Graft Techniques

Figure 4-9a. We have modified slightly our nerve grafting technique. In situations in which the proximal and distal groups of fascicles have been resected back to good normal tissue and the suture lines for each of the nerve grafts are slightly staggered (above), we have found that when the difference in the distance between fascicles is minimal it is better to increase slightly the length of the nerve gap so that the repairs are all carried out at the same level. We favor this technique (below) because regenerating nerve fibers will have the opportunity to be "captured" by adjacent nerve grafts. In the other technique (above) any regenerating units lost at the nerve repair site will not have the opportunity of being "captured" by the other adjacent nerve grafts. **b.** Hanno Millesi has successfully popularized the use of interfascicular nerve grafting technique for the management of nerve injuries that would, otherwise, be unrepairable or repaired with a neurorrhaphy under tension.

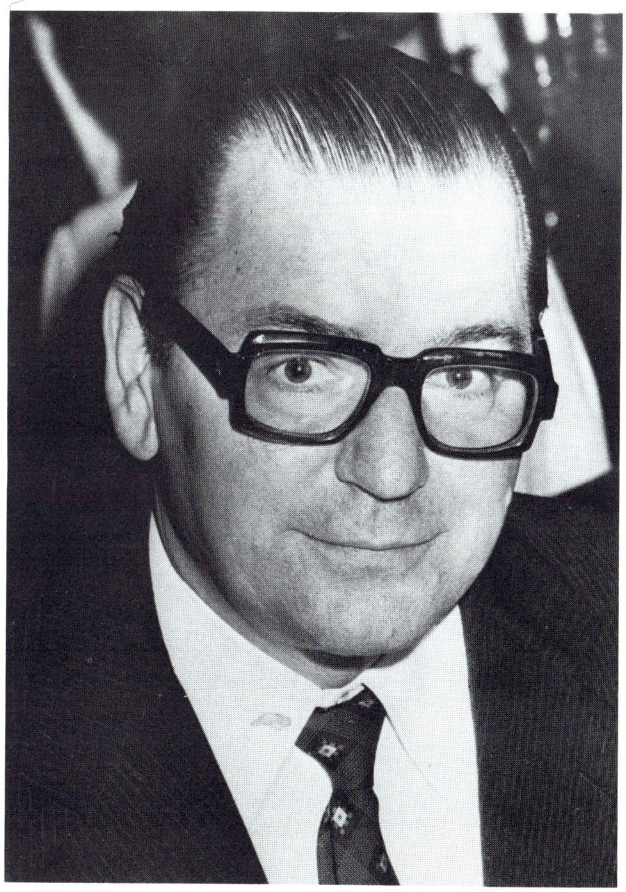

b

excellent example of this technique is seen with peroneal and radial nerve injuries. In the former situations, the injury occurs usually at the knee and, although the distal topography can be determined, the proximal injury usually extends to the level where the fascicles are mixed (motor and sensory). The proximal end of the nerve graft will be aligned with a mixed pattern of both motor and sensory fibers. At the distal end, the nerve has divided into motor and sensory fascicles and the surgeon can choose to reinnervate only motor fascicles. In such a situation, the surgeon has determined that reinnervation of the sensory fascicles is not critical. The surgeon will choose to direct all innervation into the restoration of critical motor function (anterior tibialis function). Likewise, in the radial nerve injuries, the proximal level of the graft is frequently at a point where the fascicles are mixed motor and sensory. Distally, however, the sensory fibers of the superficial radial nerve can be completely excluded from the graft so that all regenerating fibers are directed into the distal motor fascicles and none of the fascicles of the distal graft are aligned with the sensory fascicles (Figs. 4-10, 4-11).

Millesi[79] has emphasized the important difference between a nerve gap and a nerve defect. A nerve defect refers to the amount of actual nerve tissue that is lost and a nerve gap refers simply to the distance between the two nerve ends. Thus, if a nerve is sharply divided, the defect will be 0 while the gap can range from zero to many centimeters if the surgeon moves two ends of the nerves apart. If a 3 cm portion of nerve is excised from a nerve, then the defect will be 3 cm and the gap will range from 3 cm to a larger gap distance if the surgeon pulls the two ends of the nerve apart. Both the gap distance and the defect distance may significantly influence the eventual outcome of the nerve repair. A nerve defect will adversely affect eventual outcome in that actual substance of nerve has been lost and thus the topography of the proximal and distal ends of the nerve stumps will vary, making fascicular alignment very difficult.

Although it has been suggested that longer nerve grafts will be associated with poorer functional results, it is probably not the length of the graft per se that affects the poorer result but rather the fact that longer grafts are usually associated with other factors that are responsible for poorer functional results. Longer nerve grafts are used in reconstruction of long nerve defects which are associated with proximal nerve injuries (increasing the distance and time to reinnervation of motor end plates), and more severe nerve injuries (avulsion traction versus sharp cut), both factors are associated with a greater loss of neurons centrally. It is likely that it is these other prognostic factors that are associated with the longer grafts that are responsible for the "feeling" that long nerve grafts will result in poorer results.

Donor Nerve Grafts

The donor nerves available for nerve grafting are typically the sural nerve, the lateral antebrachial cutaneous nerve, and the anterior division of the medial antebrachial cutaneous nerve. The sural nerve will provide a 30 to 40 cm length of nerve graft material. The patient is left with an area of numbness on the lateral aspect of the foot that diminishes with time. A longitudinal incision extending from the lateral aspect of the ankle to the popliteal fossa will ensure that all sural communicating branches are identified,[80] that no damage is done to the donor nerve, and that the maximum amount of nerve graft material is obtained (Fig. 4-12). When there is a significant lateral sural component from this common peroneal to the sural nerve, additional nerve graft material may also be obtained. The scar is certainly

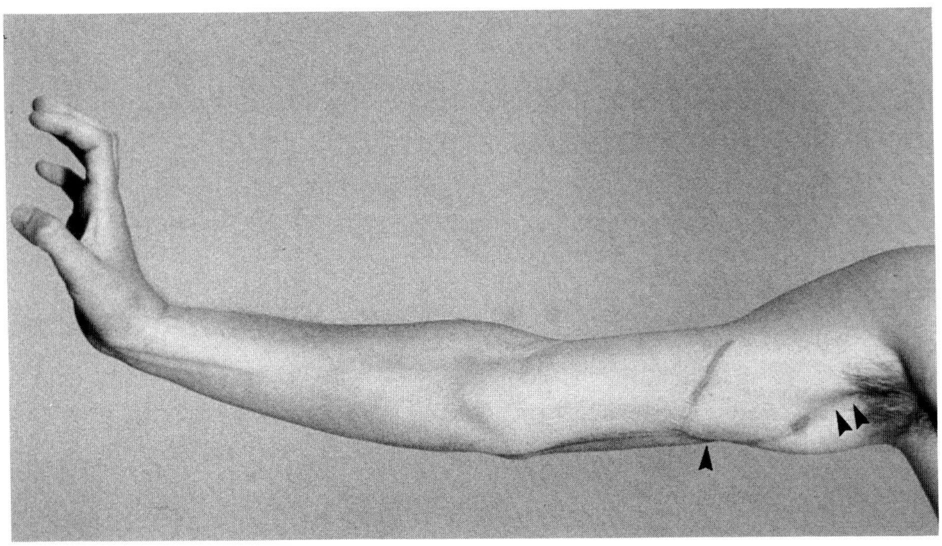

a

Figure 4-10a. (*Figure continues.*)

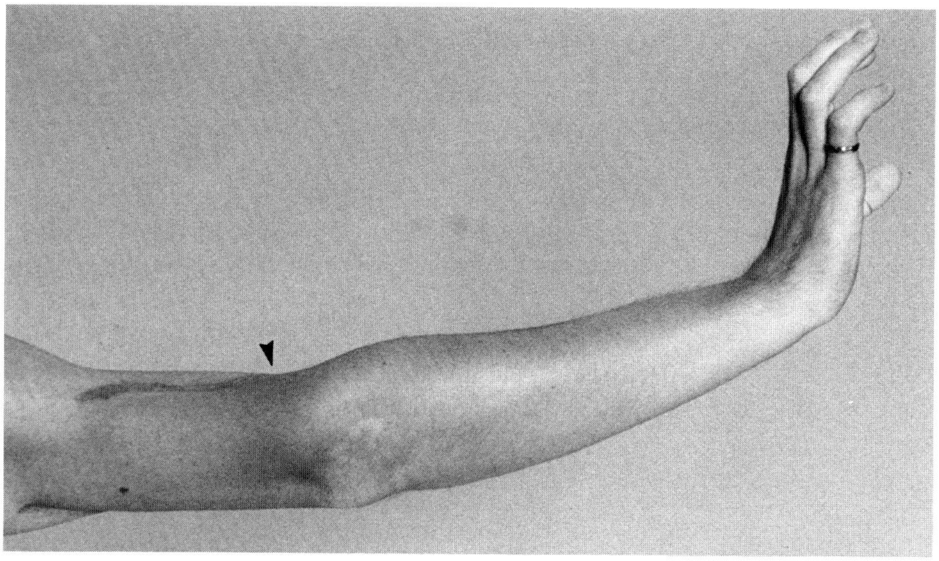

b

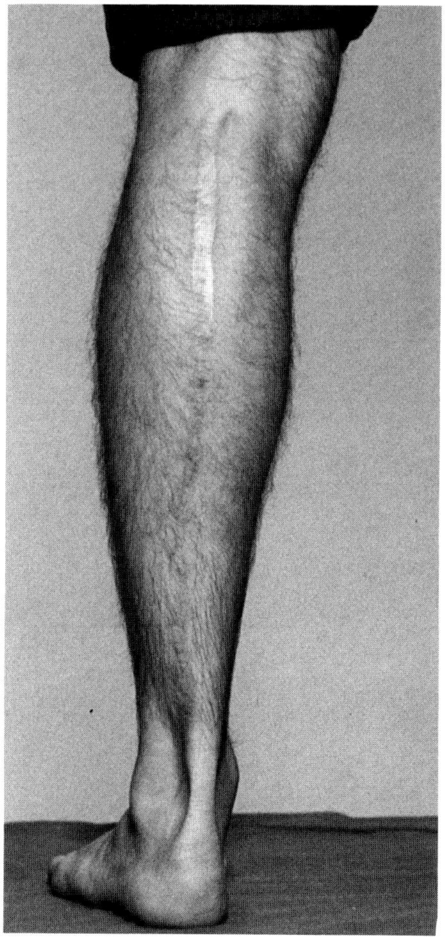

c

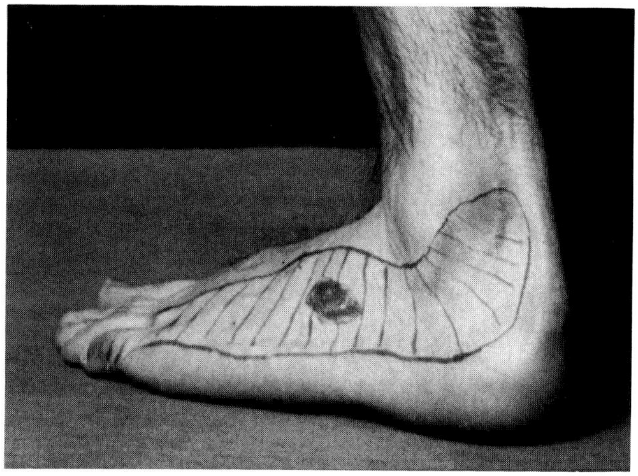

d

Figure 4-10a. This young man fell through a glass window and divided the radial nerve in the mid arm (arrow). Three months after this injury, the patient was referred and the radial nerve was exposed high in the axilla (double arrow). **b.** The radial nerve was also exposed in the antecubital fossa between the brachioradialis and brachialis muscles (arrow). A 14 cm nerve graft was used to reconstruct the defect. Sixteen months after this procedure, the patient demonstrates good wrist extension with limitation of extension of the thumb and digits. **c.** The scar from harvesting the sural nerve graft is apparent. **d.** The patient has marked out the residual area of diminished sensation on the lateral aspect of his foot and a small area of complete anesthesia.

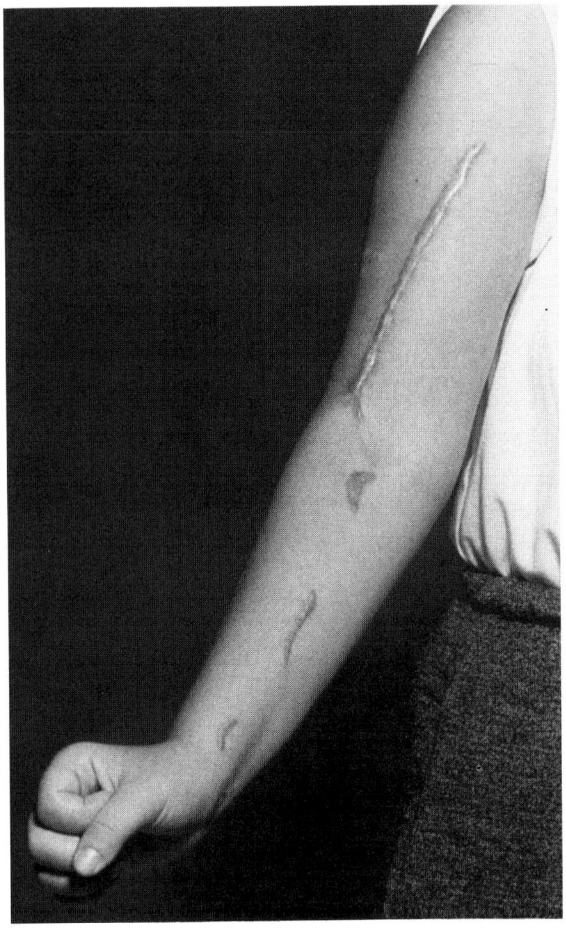

a

Figure 4-11a. Using the same surgical technique, this radial nerve injury was reconstructed using an 18 cm nerve graft. A previous surgeon had noted the radial nerve to be caught under an internal fixation. He tried to repair the long defect in the radial nerve defect and harvested one of the patient's sural nerves but was unable to complete the nerve graft. When we explored the radial nerve, the nerve defect was repaired with the second sural nerve and as well the radial sensory nerve from the injured arm. Ten months after this procedure, the patient has return of wrist extension but no extension of the digits. The scars are still immature and hypertrophic this early after the nerve graft procedure. **b.** The standard exposure for radial nerve grafting will involve an incision in the proximal arm to identify the proximal radial nerve. A second incision is made between the brachioradialis and the brachialis muscles to identify the radial nerve at this level. The nerve graft is placed along the shortest course either anterior or posterior to the humerus. At the distal repair site the radial sensory fascicle is excluded.

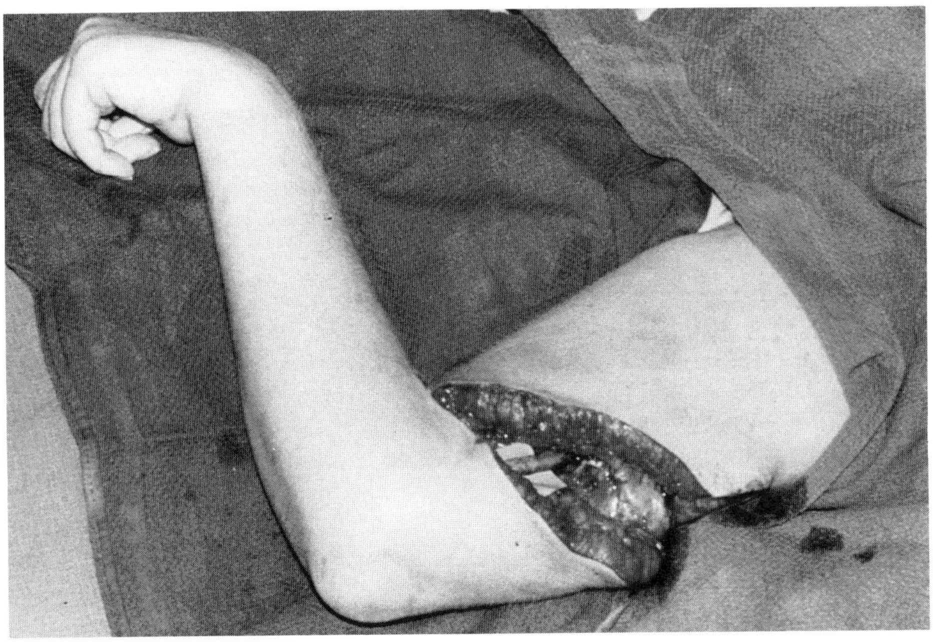

b

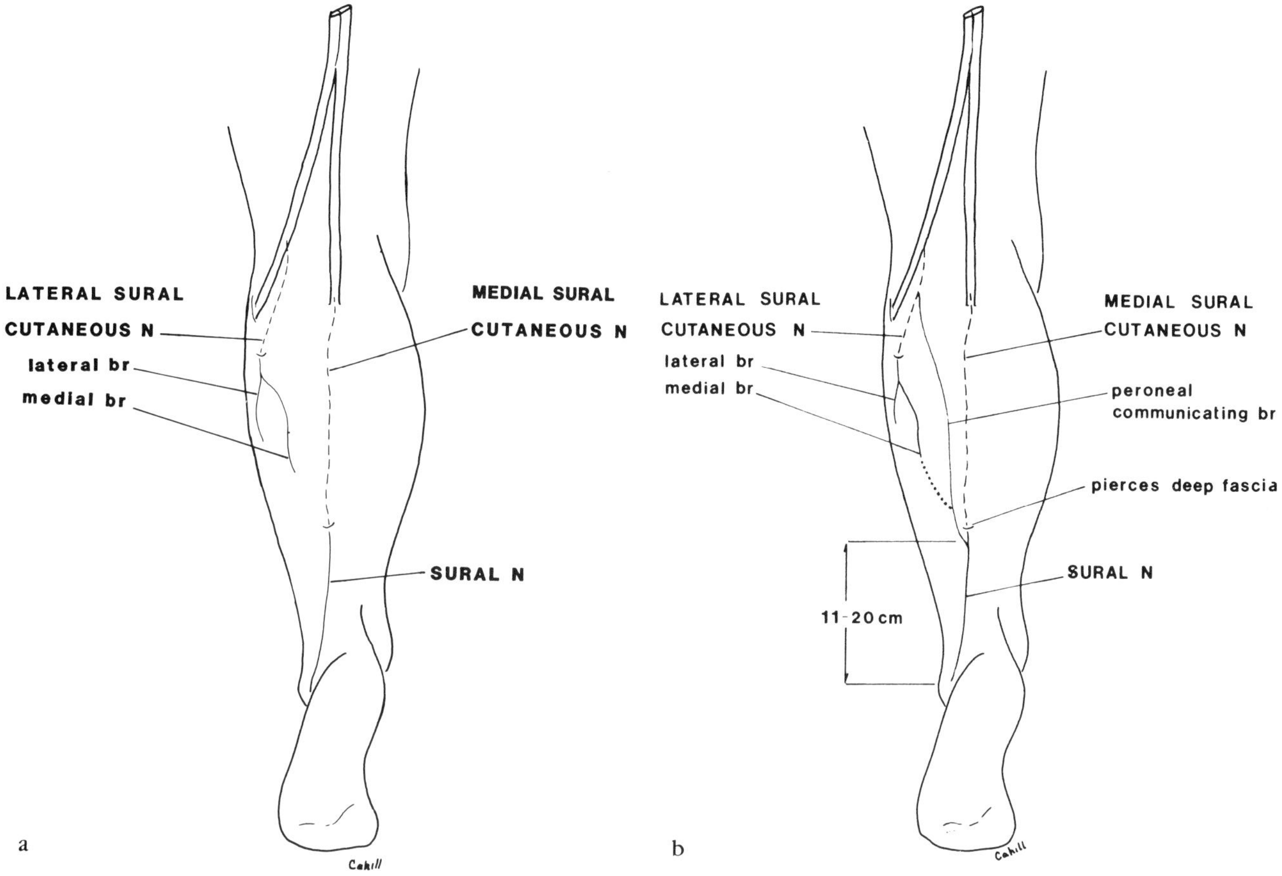

a b

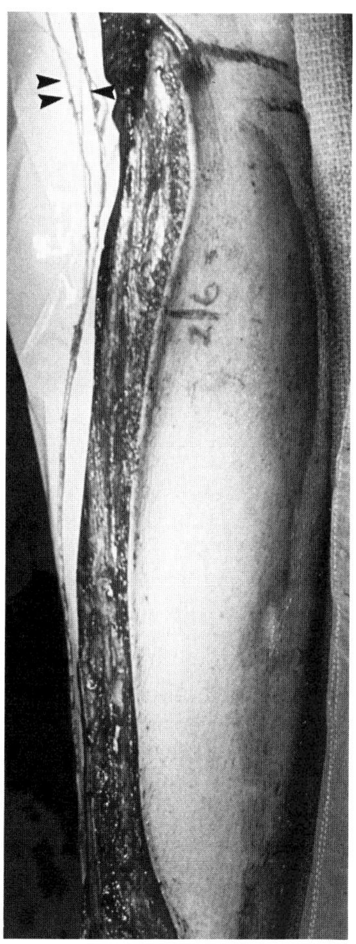

c

Figure 4-12a. In 20% of cadaver dissections, the sural nerve is simply a continuation of the medial sural cutaneous nerve. **b.** In 80% of cadaver specimens, the sural nerve was formed by the union of the medial sural cutaneous nerve with the peroneal communicating branch at a point 11 to 20 cm proximal to the lateral malleolus. (a and b reproduced with permission from Ortiguela et al.[80]) **c.** The posterior aspect of the left leg with the sural nerve graft harvested through a longitudinal incision. The branching point of the sural nerve is noted 26 cm proximal to the lateral malleolus. These two branches represent the medial sural cutaneous nerve (arrow) and the peroneal communicating branch (double arrow). Foot toward bottom, popliteal fossa toward top of photo.

much more unsightly than the multiple transverse "stepladder" type of incision, but the benefits of the longitudinal incision outweigh the cosmetic problems associated with the scar. If a stepladder type of incision is to be used, multiple incisions may be needed across the back of the calf in order to remove communicating branches separately without injuring the main sural nerve.

The lateral antebrachial cutaneous nerve lies adjacent to the cephalic vein in the forearm and can be easily identified (Fig. 4-13). The surgeon will mentally mark out the forearm longitudinally into thirds. The lateral antebrachial cutaneous nerve, which is the cutaneous continuation of the musculocutaneous nerve, lies at the junction between the lateral and middle third of the forearm. At this level, there are often two branches. The nerve is adjacent to the cephalic vein, which is easily palpable but often not visible through the skin. It is most expedient to identify the cephalic vein first and then look for the nerve on either side of this vein. This is an excellent donor nerve for digital nerve grafts and 5 to 8 cm of good nerve graft material can be obtained. The scar on the forearm is somewhat unsightly.

Using the anterior branch of the medial antebrachial cutaneous nerve allows the surgeon to place the scar in the medial aspect of the arm in a much less visible location than that used to harvest the lateral antebrachial cutaneous nerve. The medial antebrachial cutaneous nerve lies adjacent to the bacilic vein (Fig. 4-14). The anterior and posterior branches are identified at this level. Utilizing just the anterior branch of the medial antebrachial cutaneous provides a minimal donor deficit because the sensory loss is along the volar aspect of the forearm. If necessary, the two branches of the medial antebrachial cutaneous nerve may be harvested for a nerve graft and in this instance two nerve grafts of up to 20 cm can be obtained. The extensive loss of sensation on the medial aspect of the arm and elbow will decrease over 2 to 3 years.[81]

We have infrequently used the terminal sensory branch of the posterior interosseous nerve, which is identified in the fourth extensor compartment at the wrist. It is useful for relatively short nerve grafts in the digits.[82] Enough of this small diameter nerve must be harvested so that it can be divided into two lengths and used as two interposition fascicular grafts to match the size of the digital nerve. Only 2 to 5 cm of graft material can be obtained from this site. There is no sensory loss, however, because this nerve provides innervation to the wrist joint and not to the skin.

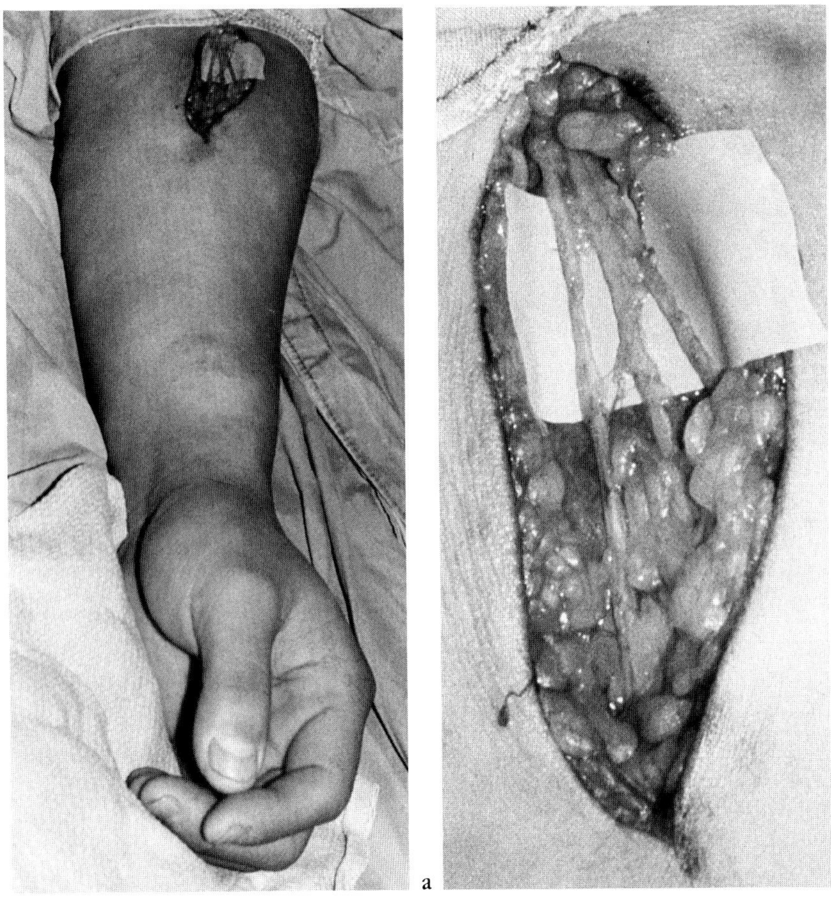

a b

Figure 4-13a. The lateral antebrachial cutaneous nerve can be identified adjacent to the cephalic vein in the proximal forearm. It lies at the medial border of the brachioradialis muscle. The forearm is marked into thirds. This nerve is easily identified at the junction between the lateral and middle thirds. **b.** The branches of the lateral antebrachial cutaneous nerve are noted behind the visibility background. Usually, only two branches are noted at this level, not three as seen here.

The posterior cutaneous nerve of the forearm can be identified at the junction between the brachioradialis muscle and the extensor carpi radialis longus and provides 2 to 5 cm of nerve graft material.[83] The posterior cutaneous nerve of the leg and the lateral femoral cutaneous nerve of the thigh can also, in the rare instance, be used for nerve graft material.

For proximal radial nerve injuries that require nerve grafting, we will frequently use the radial sensory nerve as a donor nerve since it is appropriate to identify this nerve in the distal portion of the radial nerve in order to exclude it from the nerve graft. This maneuver is carried out so that any regenerating nerve fibers will be directed into distal motor nerves rather than being lost to cutaneous reinnervation in the process of reinnervating the functionally unimportant territory of the radial sensory nerve.

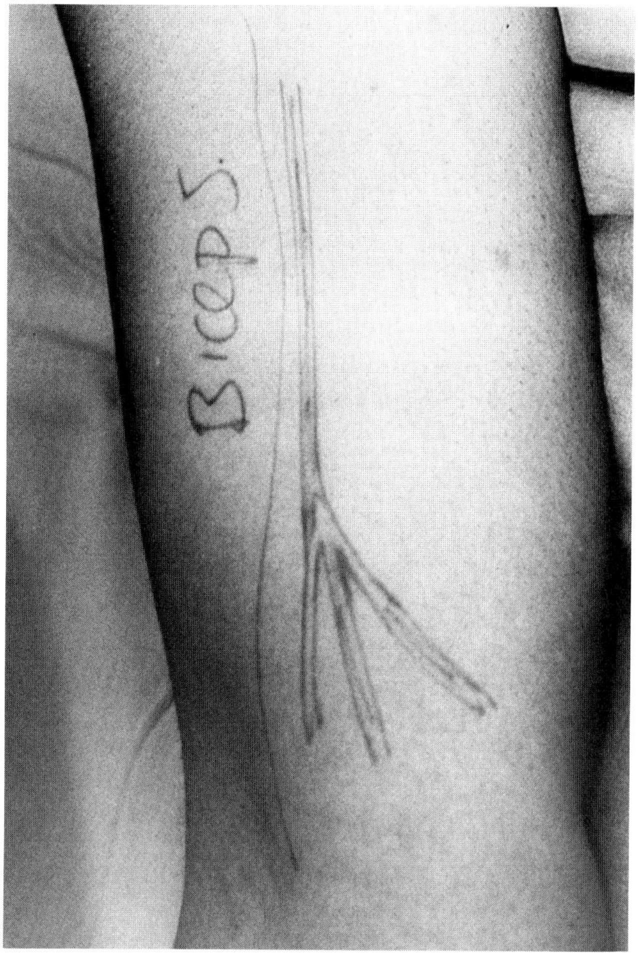

a

Figure 4-14a The medial antebrachial cutaneous nerve can be used as a donor nerve. The nerve is just medial to the biceps muscle and lies adjacent to the bacilic vein (hand toward bottom, axilla toward top). **b.** The vessel loop is around the median nerve, which is just deep to the medial antebrachial cutaneous nerve. The two branches of the medial antebrachial cutaneous nerve are noted (arrows). The anterior branch will be used for the donor nerve because the posterior branch gives important sensibility to the posterior aspect of the elbow and forearm.

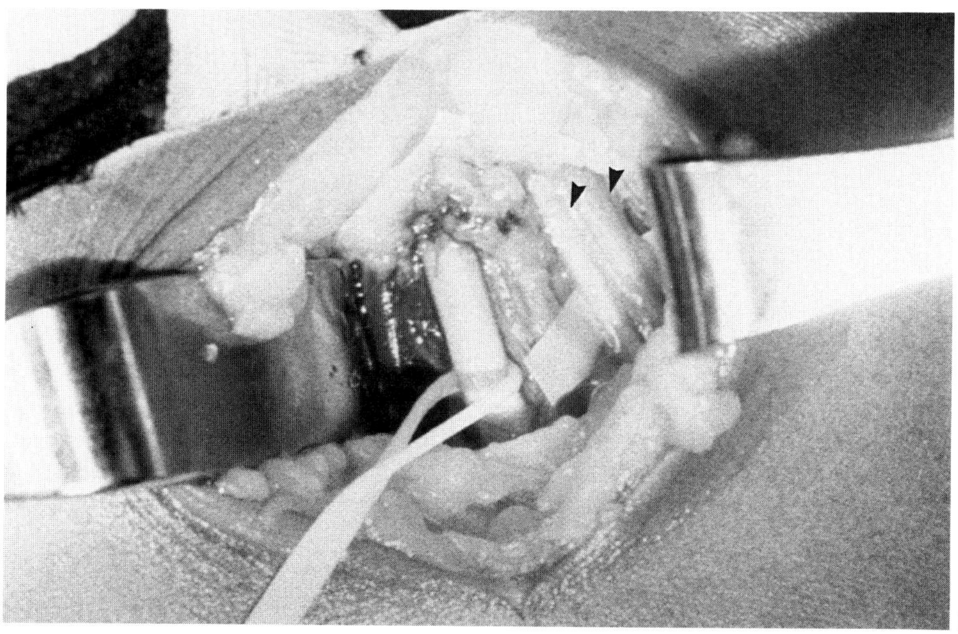

b

Timing of Nerve Repair

The timing of the nerve repair is critical in determining the eventual functional outcome.

Open Nerve Injuries

If there is any suspicion of nerve injury, all open wounds should be explored. If a clean division of the nerve is found, then a microneurosurgical repair is carried out. Likely the same functional results can be realized if the nerve is repaired within the first few days of injury and certainly more damage will be done if an early repair is carried out without the appropriate surgical skill or microsurgical instrumentation and magnification (Fig. 4-15).

Some experimental support for a delay type of repair has been provided by experimental studies investigating conditioning lesions. An increase in the rate of axonal growth was demonstrated by McQuarrie et al[84–86] and Bisby and Keen.[87] A conditioning or priming lesion was presented to the nerve 2 weeks before a second lesion. This resulted in a 23% increase in outgrowth of the sensory axons of the sciatic nerve and gave experimental support for the concept of a delayed repair. Forman et al[88] noted a similar acceleration of axonal growth after only a 2-day interval between the two nerve lesions. This effect is most likely due to increased synthesis in the cell body as a response to nerve injury (Chapter 1). Each time the surgeon trims back the proximal nerve, he is in effect carrying out a conditioning lesion. Richardson et al[89,90] recently noted that a regenerative response after nerve transection was not altered by injury to the proximal stump (crush and colchicine injection) or by nerve growth factor. It is certainly not apparent that such conditioning lesions have any clinical role to play in the management of these injuries.

If the exploration of the open wound reveals an injury to the nerve over a long distance with perhaps some actual loss of nerve tissue, it is best to repair the nerve at a later date when the longitudinal extent of the nerve injury can be ascertained. It may take 3 to 4 weeks for the extent of the nerve damage to be defined.[91] If at the time of the initial surgery the proximal and distal ends of the nerve can be brought together, approximation of nerve ends will prevent retraction. This will, thus, diminish the length of the nerve graft required at the second operation.

Primary nerve grafting is rarely, if ever, indicated because it is impossible to know the proximal or distal extent of the injury pattern at the time of initial injury. Not only does the nerve graft require the use of a valuable potential donor nerve, but more importantly it commits the patient to a waiting period to assess the results of this nerve graft. Valuable time will be lost that will jeopardize the patient's final result if the surgeon has inappropriately estimated the degree of nerve damage at the time of the primary nerve graft.

The secondary nerve graft or repair will be carried out when the wound has healed and some of the edema

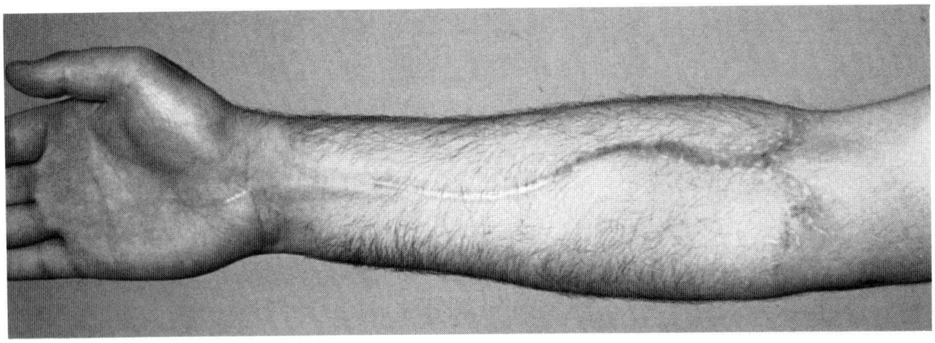

a

Figure 4-15a. This young arm lacerated the volar aspect of the right arm, transecting the radial and median nerves and the brachial artery. The arm was revascularized and the radial and median nerves were repaired using epineurial technique. **b.** Fifteen months after this repair, he has light touch perception in the median nerve distribution but no reinnervation of the intrinsic muscles. His moving and static two-point discrimination in the median nerve distribution was 5 and 6 mm. He was started on a course of sensory re-education when light touch returned to the distribution of the median nerve 6 months after the nerve repair. **c.** The patient demonstrates good anterior interosseous nerve function. **d.** The patient also had good superficialis function with some mismatching of fibers between the fibers to the superficialis muscles and the flexor pollicis longus muscle. Note that the patient flexes the thumb when demonstrating superficialis function and profundus function (**c**). (*Figure continues.*)

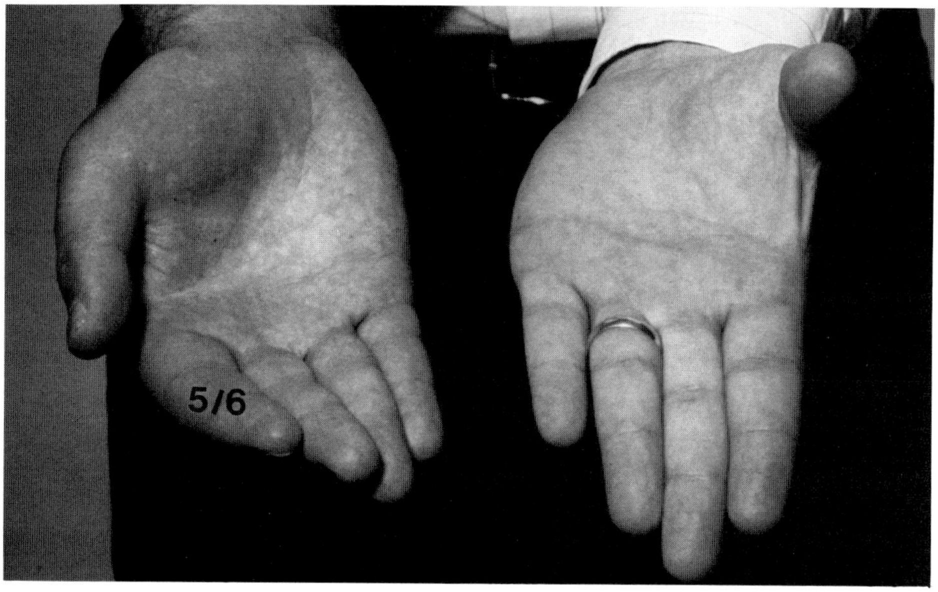

b

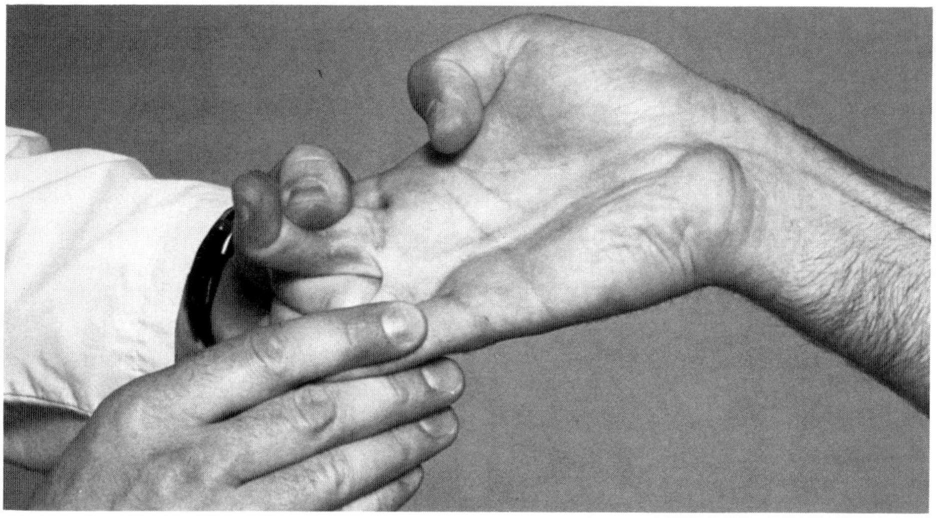
c

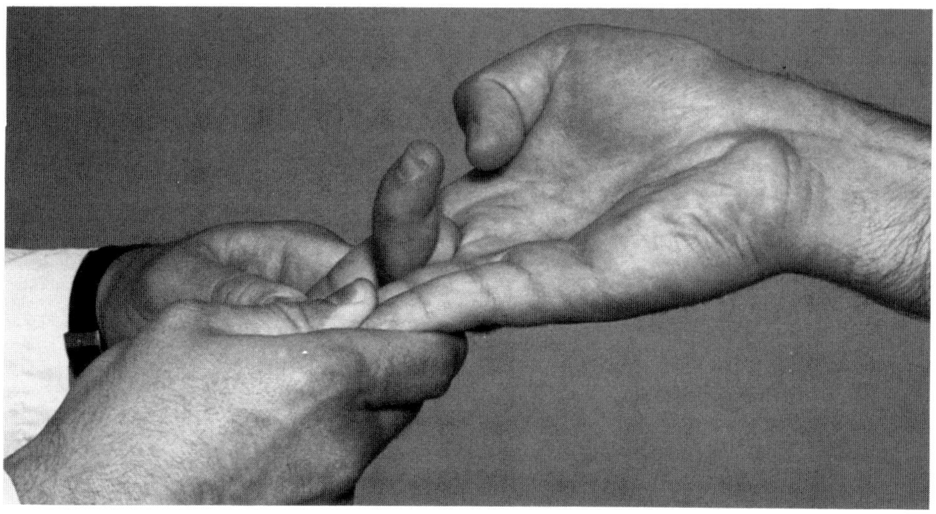
d

and scarring has settled. The secondary repair is usually carried out at about 2 months, and nerve grafts are usually necessary. In proximal injuries that are not clean-cut (such as a chain saw injury to the brachial plexus) we would recommend early (3 weeks) delayed repair with grafts. At this time, the longitudinal extent of the injury will be defined and the wound will not yet have a prohibitive amount of scar tissue. Of course, the wound should be primarily explored in order to line up the plexus elements and oppose these structures appropriately with scaffolding type sutures. Thus, the timing of nerve repair is dictated by the nature of the nerve injury and not by emperical rules about "golden" time periods for repair. If a nerve has been cleanly divided, it should be repaired as soon as the surgeon with the expertise and instrumentation to repair it is available. If the proximal and distal extent of the injury cannot be accurately assessed at the time of the injury, then the nerve can be approximated in a nondefinitive repair and a secondary repair or graft carried out at a later stage. Approximation of the damaged nerve ends may mean that an end-to-end repair or at least a shorter nerve graft is required at the time of the secondary repair.

Closed Nerve Injuries

Timing for the management of closed nerve injuries varies from that of an open nerve injury. In the closed nerve injury with a nerve deficit, there is no indication for primary surgery. The patient is examined carefully over a 3-month period. If by 3 months there is some clinical evidence of recovery or electrical evidence to suggest complete recovery, then the patient's course is followed expectantly realizing that, depending on the level of the injury, it may take several more months for eventual complete return of function. If at 3 months the patient has not demonstrated any evidence of clinical or electrical return of function, then the nerve is explored. Intraoperative evaluation of the nerve injury will include nerve recordings across the area of injury. If a nerve action potential is recorded, then only a neurolysis is performed. If, on the other hand, no electrical activity is recorded, the injured area is excised and grafted. It is our empirical belief that with proximal muscle groups, the maximum time tolerated between the time of the nerve injury and the reestablishment of neuromuscular connection is between 1 year and 18 months. The smaller intrinsic muscles in the hand have to be reinnervated even sooner than that in order to reestablish motor function. The time limits on sensory return vary from those for motor; return of sensation can be restored many years after injury to the nerve.

In dealing with closed nerve injuries, the patient is treated expectantly unless the nerve is located at a specific anatomic site that is known to be susceptible to nerve entrapment. In these instances, the nerve should be decompressed so that the nerve recovery progresses without the superimposed effects of nerve compression. It is generally accepted that a patient who presents with acute carpal tunnel syndrome, with sensory and motor loss after a traumatic injury to the hand or forearm, should be considered for urgent decompression. Unfortunately, other nerves involved in identical clinical situations in known areas of anatomic nerve entrapment are not treated in the same fashion. The patient who demonstrates complete peroneal nerve palsy after a crush injury to the lower extremity is demonstrating the same pathologic condition as the patient who presents with an acute carpal tunnel after a crush injury to the upper extremity. In both instances, the nerve should be decompressed at the site of the anatomic point of nerve compression. When the nerve deficit is not localized to a known anatomic area of nerve compression, it is treated conservatively with frequent clinical examination and electrodiagnostic follow-up.

Identification of Fascicular Function

Critical in determining eventual functional outcome after either nerve repair or nerve grafting is the appropriate identification of sensory and motor fascicles. Unfortunately, the task of matching these fascicles in the proximal and distal nerve stumps remains a tremendous challenge. Currently, there are three techniques available for fascicular identification: anatomic, electrophysiologic, and histochemical.

Intraneural Anatomic Identification

Several investigators[92–95] have recently expanded on Sunderland's classic anatomic work,[96] which identified the fascicular pattern of various peripheral nerves in the extremities. Fascicular maps can be utilized in order to help with the identification of various fascicles at the time of surgery. Equally important is the actual anatomic identification of divisions that can be identified by extending the dissection proximal and distal to the area of injury (Chapter 1) (Fig. 4-16).

Histochemical Differentiation Between Motor and Sensory Nerve Fibers

Histochemical enzyme staining has been used to separate motor from sensory fibers. Acetylcholinesterase and choline acetyltransferase (choline acetylase) have been used to identify motor fibers. Carbonic anhydrase has been used to identify sensory fibers. This technique is most useful for evaluation of the proximal stump be-

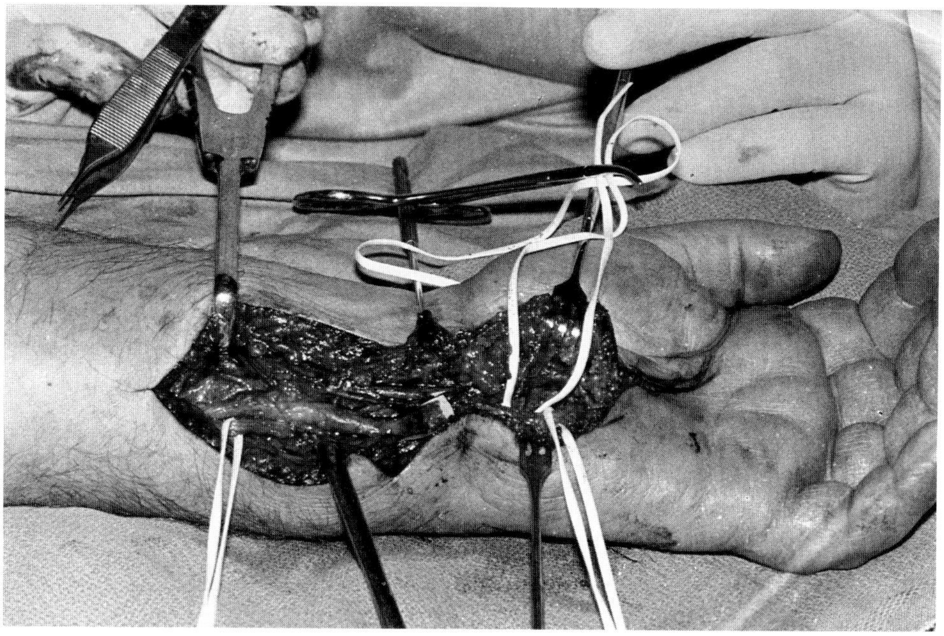

a

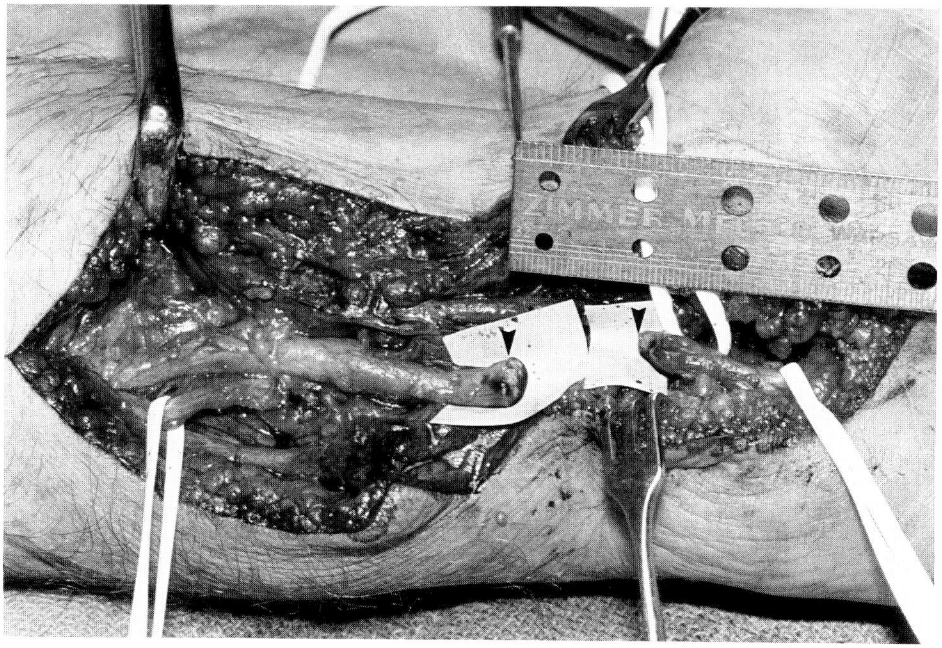

b

Figure 4-16a. This patient with an ulnar nerve injury 5 years before referral complained of numbness in the ulnar nerve distribution and neuromatous type pain. The operation was designed to restore continuity between the proximal and the distal sensory fibers. A vessel loop is placed around the dorsocutaneous branch proximally and the distal branches of the ulnar nerve. **b.** The proximal and distal portions of the ulnar nerve are identified (arrows). **c.** Motor and sensory portions of the distal ulnar nerve can be identified by carrying out a distal dissection will be excluded from the nerve graft so that proximal nerve fibers will all be directed into the sensory component of the ulnar nerve (arrow), (motor fascicles, double arrows). Evaluation of the proximal nerve is done using awake nerve stimulation. In keeping with known fascicular maps, the sensory component was noted to be on the radial side of the ulnar nerve (arrow) and the silent motor component is on the ulnar side (double arrow). The nerve graft will direct proximal sensory fascicles to distal sensory fascicles to maximize sensory regeneration. (*Figure continues.*)

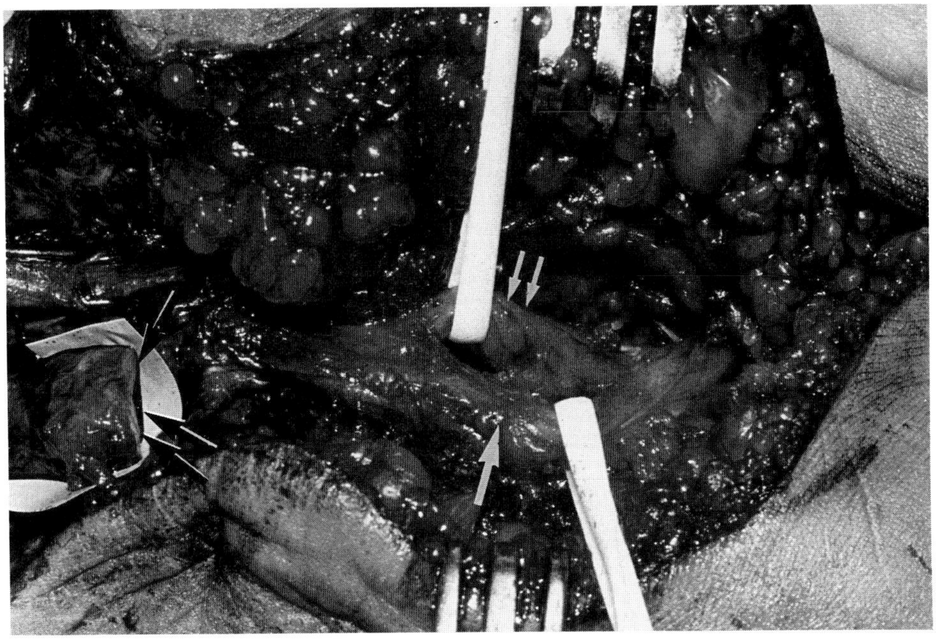

c

Figure 4-16 *(continued)* **c.**

cause this enzyme activity will be present indefinitely in the proximal stump. Enzyme staining response will persist in the distal stump up to 5 days after nerve transection. Carbonic anhydrase staining of Schwann cell activity in the distal nerve may persist much longer. The clinical implication of this technique is currently being investigated.

The activity of the enzyme acetylcholinesterase is markedly higher in ventral (motor) roots than in dorsal (sensory) spinal roots.[97] This has been demonstrated by biochemical and histochemical techniques. Although acetylcholinesterase staining of the nerve stump biopsies will distinguish the highly reactive motor fibers from the less reactive sensory fibers, a critical incubation period of 20 to 26 hours is required.[98] Similar histochemical patterns have been identified in sensory and motor peripheral nerve fascicles with much shorter processing periods (50 minutes).[99] Choline acetyltransferase has been identified in both spinal roots and peripheral nerve tissue.[100,101] The incubation period required for processing tissue specimens has decreased from 24 hours to 1 hour. Recent reports have suggested its clinical use in the identification of sensory and motor fascicles. Riley has shown that carbonic anhydrase histochemistry distinguishes sensory fibers and that the tissue processing can be completed in 1 hour.[102]

Electrical Identification

In 1968, Hakstian reported the use of electrical fascicular identification in humans as an aid to clinical nerve repair.[103] This technique has been used sporadically since then as an intraoperative adjunct to nerve repair.[104,105] The technique of intraoperative awake identification of fascicular function has recently been reviewed.[106] Under appropriate anesthesia, the nerve is explored and the nerve ends prepared for electrical evaluation. The patient is then awakened and the fascicles of the proximal stump are stimulated electrically in order to identify sensory and motor (sensory silent) fascicles. Stimulation of the sensory fascicles will elicit pain or sensation in a precise cutaneous region. Stimulation of the motor fascicles will elicit a slight aching sensation in a deeper less well-defined location corresponding to the approximate location of the muscle.

The benefits of electrical mapping is limited to the proximal nerve stump. Electrical stimulation of the motor fascicles of the distal nerve stump will elicit a motor contraction only in the initial few days after complete transection of the nerve. Success of this technique is dependent on surgeon experience, patient compliance, and anesthesia cooperation.

Neuroma In-Continuity

Seddon and Sunderland have classified nerve injury (Chapter 2). The nerve injury that combines several types of the injury patterns described by Seddon and Sunderland presents the most challenging problem for the surgeon. It is this mixed injury or sixth degree injury that constitutes the surgical dilemma of the true neuroma in-continuity. The type of injury affecting each fascicle will determine the ultimate prognosis and re-

Table 4-2. Relationship of Injury to Recovery

Degree of Injury	Tinel Sign Present/Progresses Distally	Recovery Pattern	Rate of Recovery	Surgical Procedure
I Neurapraxia	−/−	Complete	Fast, days to 12 weeks	None
II Axonotmesis	+/+	Complete	Slow, (1 inch/month)	None
III	+/+	Great variation*	Slow, (1 inch/month)	None or neurolysis
IV	+/−	None	No recovery	Nerve repair or graft
V Neurotmesis	+/−	None	No recovery	Nerve repair or graft
VI	Varies with each fascicle, depending on the combination of injury patterns as noted above			

*Recovery is at least as good as a nerve repair but can vary from excellent to poor, depending on the degree of endoneurial scarring and the amount of sensory or motor axonal misdirection that occurs within the injured fascicle.

covery of the nerve fibers within that fascicle (Table 4-2). The fascicle that sustains a neurapraxia should show complete recovery of normal nerve function within several weeks of the injury. Because the axon has not been injured, no actual axonal degeneration occurs. A Tinel sign indicating an attempt at regeneration will not be present. The return of nerve function will not follow the classic 1 inch per month pattern. As soon as the local conduction block corrects itself or the region of demyelination is repaired, return of function should occur quite quickly and rather dramatically.

If the fascicle has sustained a Sunderland second degree injury, or axonotmesis, axonal degeneration will occur. A Tinel sign will be present and regeneration will occur at the classic rate of 1 inch per month. An advancing Tinel sign will be present. Because the injury is restricted to the axon, the regeneration will be exact and no misdirection of nerve fibers will occur. Thus, the recovery will be complete and normal, as that after a neurapraxia, but the rate of recovery will be much slower and will follow a pattern of serial anatomic recovery corresponding to the advancing level of nerve regeneration.

A Sunderland third degree injury, which has no counterpart in Seddon's classification, describes an injury in which there is some degree of injury to the endoneurium as well as the axons. The perineurium, however, is intact. Nerve regeneration will then occur within the confines of the perineurium. A Tinel sign will be present and recovery will be associated with an advancing Tinel sign. In a Sunderland third degree injury, the identical injury can produce a degree of recovery that is extremely variable, depending on the particular fascicle involved and the level of the injury in the extremity. This third degree injury, more than any of the other injuries, will demonstrate a wider variability of recovery patterns. Depending on the fascicle involved, the identical injury may result in excellent or poor recovery. If the third degree injury involves a fascicle that has mixed, motor and sensory, fibers, then misdirection of these sensory and motor fibers can result in a less than normal pattern of recovery. If, on the other hand, the fascicle that has the third degree injury is a pure fascicle containing nerve fibers that are destined for one particular muscle or one particular cutaneous territory, then even though there may by some mismatching of regenerating nerve fibers and some loss of nerve fibers in the endoneurial scar tissue, the recovery that occurs will at least be appropriate from a sensory and motor point of view. Misdirection of regenerating nerve fibers is possible because of injury to the basal lamina, and less than complete regeneration of the nerve fibers is also possible because of the varying amount of scarring that can be present in the endoneurium. The recovery then with a third degree injury can be very variable. The same type of injury in a proximal fascicle will likely give a poorer result because of the potential mismatching of sensory and motor fibers than a similar injury in a pure fascicle located more distally in the extremity. The prognosis for this type of injury is, however, quite good and certainly very comparable to a primary nerve repair because in the Sunderland third degree injury the perineurium at least is intact.

A fourth degree Sunderland injury will demonstrate no return of function because, essentially, the nerve fibers are in-continuity only with scar tissue. A Sunderland fifth degree injury or a Seddon neurotmesis involves complete division of the nerve and, of course, without surgical repair the prognosis is equally poor.

Thus, it becomes apparent that the surgeon must, with a detailed clinical examination supported by electrodiagnostic testing, assess the nerve injury, recognizing that first, second, and third degree injuries will offer spontaneous recovery, which is superior to that which is provided with surgical repair or grafting techniques. It is the fourth and fifth degree injuries that will require surgical reconstruction.

The surgeon will clinically examine the function of the peripheral nerve involved in order to determine the degree of injury in each of the fascicles or groups of fascicles. Through this clinical examination, he will be making a mental picture of the injury pattern within the nerve.

The technique of internal neurolysis will be critical in evaluating the neuroma in-continuity. Intraoperatively, using microneurosurgical technique, the surgeon explores the nerve beginning with the normal nerve proximal and distal to the area of injury. The surgeon will attempt to separate the fourth and fifth degree injury pattern from those fascicles that have sustained a lesser degree of injury. These former fascicles will require nerve grafting. The latter fascicles will be neurolysed only. Detailed physical examination combined with microsurgical exploration of the nerve will facilitate this surgical decision. Occasionally, intraoperative nerve conduction studies will be required.[108,113] The role of these studies is largely twofold. If a distal nerve injury must be surgically evaluated before enough time has elapsed to allow the ultimate recovery to become apparent, then intraoperative evaluation of group fascicular function is necessary. With proximal nerve lesions (such as brachial plexus), surgical exploration is indicated if there is no evidence of recovery within the first 3 months of the injury. Thus, it is never possible with such a proximal injury to "wait out" the recovery period. If the injury is a fourth and fifth degree injury, an opportunity to recover motor function may be lost unless early (3 to 4 months postinjury) exploration is carried out.

Vascularized Nerve Grafts

The role of vascularized nerve grafts in clinical practice has yet to be established. The theoretical benefits of this technique remain hypothetical. Potential clinical indications include reconstruction of large nerve gaps, proximal injuries, reconstruction in compromised recipient beds, and reconstruction using large caliber donor nerve grafts. Recent advances in transplant immunology suggest that the use of a nerve allograft for extensive and complex reconstructive cases may soon be a clinical reality. In these instances, the problem of donor nerve expendability would no longer exist and vascularized large caliber nerves and those with complex configuration, such as the brachial plexus, could be transferred as vascularized grafts. At the present time, there are neither experimental nor clinical studies to justify the use of a vascularized nerve graft in preference to a conventional nerve graft.

The first vascularized clinical nerve graft was carried out in 1976.[115] The sensory branch of the radial nerve, vascularized with the radial artery, was used to reconstruct a median nerve injury. Recovery of function in this single case was considered to be faster and superior to that observed with conventional grafting techniques. Fachinelli et al[116] reported the clinical use of sural nerve grafts in 1981 (Fig. 4-17). Bonney et al[117] have recently reported their results using vascularized

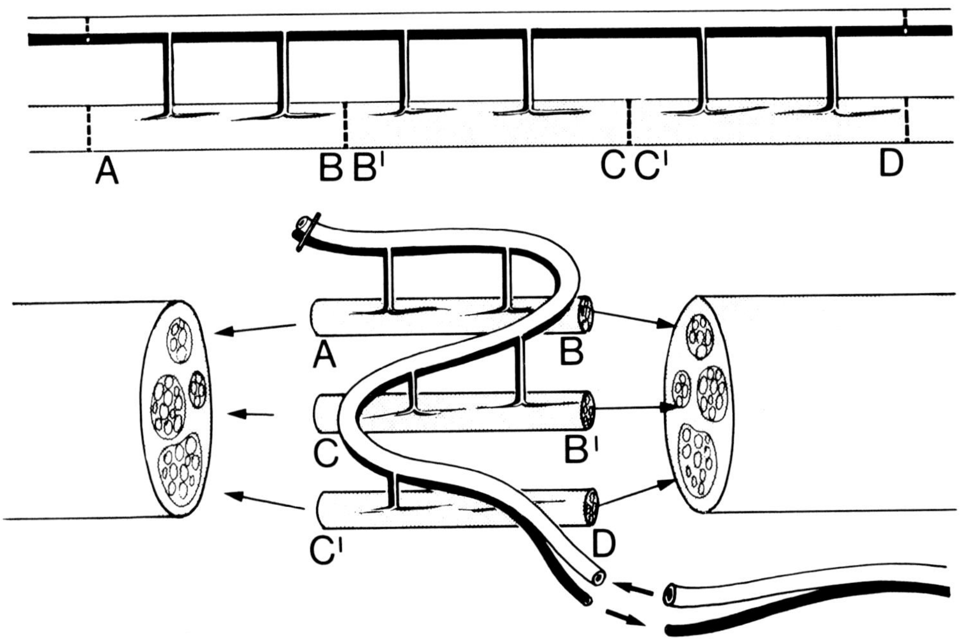

Figure 4-17. This diagram demonstrates Fachinelli's method by which a nerve with a dominant blood supply is divided in segments for multiple fascicular grafts maintained on the same vascular pedicle. (Reproduced with permission from Breidenbach and Terzis.[120])

ulnar nerve grafts in 12 patients with brachial plexus injuries. It 'was their impression that "recovery was superior to that of the use of conventional nerve grafts." Direct comparison of the two techniques, however, was not made. Minderis[118] has had experience with 26 clinical cases of vascularized nerve grafts and is equally pleased with the results using this technique. However, direct comparison between vascularized and conventional nonvascularized nerve grafts was not made.[118]

A single case report comparing regeneration across a vascularized and nonvascularized nerve graft in the same patient demonstrated improved histologic regeneration across the vascularized nerve graft. Functional recovery was also better in the cutaneous territory of the vascularized nerve graft compared with the nonvascularized nerve graft.[119]

Breidenbach and Terzis[120] have investigated potential donor nerve grafts from 241 cadaver dissections. Thirteen potential donor nerves were defined. They described a classification of nerve–blood supply based on the number of extrinsic vascular pedicles (Fig. 4-18, 4-19). They identified six nerves with reliable dominant vascular pedicles that could serve as potential donor nerves for vascularized nerve grafts. Of interest, the results of clinical fluorescence injection studies done on the ulnar and saphenous nerves contradicted dye injection studies in that a much greater length of nerve segment fluoresced than was predicted by cadaver injection studies. This study emphasized the problems of extrapolating cadaver injection studies to the in vivo clinical situation, as well as the importance of the intrinsic blood supply of the nerve. The researchers classified blood supply of nerves in three groups: group 1 had no dominant pedicle, group 2, had one dominant pedicle, and group 3 had multiple dominant pedicles. Logically, group 2 with one dominant pedicle is the ideal arrangement for a vascularized nerve graft. They concluded that the saphenous nerve would provide the most suitable donor vascularized nerve graft because of its length, expendability, and vascular pedicle arrangement.

Kunzel et al[121] has described the clinical use of the ulnar nerve as a vascularized nerve graft. Several experimental studies have compared the vascularized to the nonvascularized nerve graft. The experimental studies, however, are contradictory.[122–125] In particular, an animal model that closely simulates the clinical situation for which vascularized nerve grafts are indicated has yet to be defined. No vascularized nerve grafts of significant caliber or length have been transferred as microvascular free grafts into a soft tissue bed for which the hemodynamics of compromised blood flow have been controlled. A model of a vascularized sciatic nerve graft transferred on a microvascular pedicle as a free nerve graft has recently been described[126] and has potential as an experimental model if the hemodynamics of a compromised bed can be determined.

Results of Nerve Repair and Grafting

It is a challenging task for the reconstructive surgeon to document carefully the degree of recovery noted after nerve repair and grafting. An appreciation of the anticipated results will be important in determining the best reconstructive procedure for the patient. The surgeon will use this information to advise the patient of his potential for functional recovery.

Early Results

Physicians not actively treating peripheral nerve injuries are, for the most part, of the opinion that the results of peripheral nerve surgery are generally poor. This perception stems largely from the published results of experience dealing with nerve injuries during World War II. Three thousand four hundred and fifteen definitive operations were performed on 3656 nerve injuries.[45] The results of the Woodhall and Beebe study demonstrated, with a 5-year follow-up, that radial nerve motor recovery occurred 21% of the time. Median nerve motor recovery occurred 50% of the time, and functional sensation returned in 17% of the cases. Ulnar nerve motor recovery occurred 12% of the time, with sensory recovery in 31%. In these 3415 operations, nerve grafting was performed only 30 times. The results of these nerve grafts were routinely poor. The generally poor results from this extremely large series with long follow-up has definitely colored our perception of the anticipated results after peripheral nerve surgery. It must be emphasized, however, that the majority of these military injuries involved extensive wounds with severe injury to the nerve. Despite this, nerve grafting technique was used in only 30 of the more than 3000 procedures. When a nerve graft was used, the grafts were trunk grafts and in none of the cases was microscopic technique utilized. Seddon's report of the same war experience[180] was compared with the American experience[45] with very similar results. Certainly, the majority of these injuries would now be treated quite differently with microscopic interfascicular nerve grafting techniques. However, there have been no studies of the same magnitude with the same follow-up published since that time, and, thus, these studies continue to command tremendous historical respect.

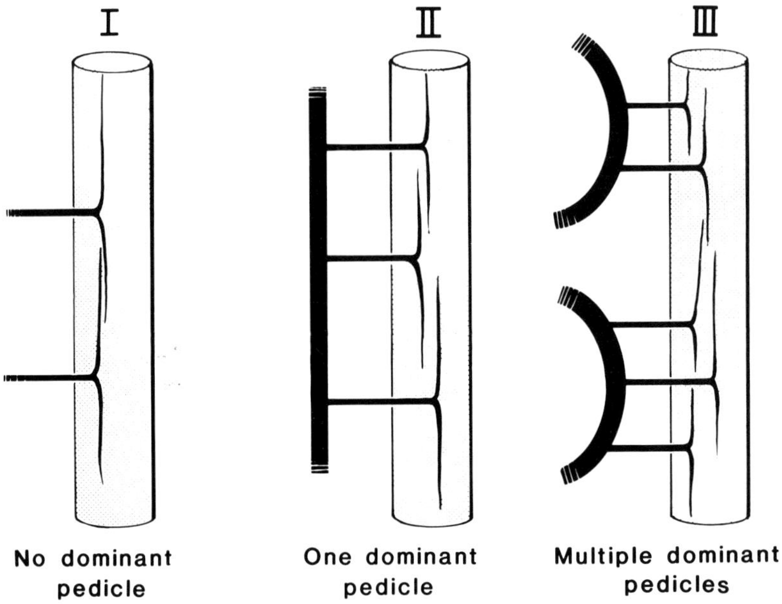

Figure 4-18. Classification of the blood supply to nerves. (Reproduced with permission from Breidenbach and Terzis.[120])

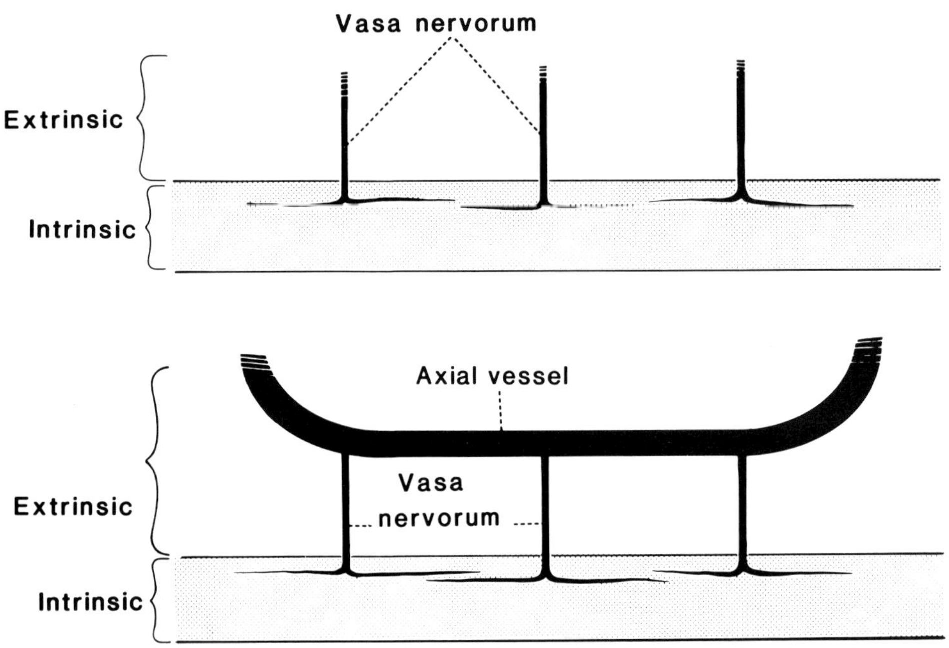

Figure 4-19. The blood supply to the peripheral nerves includes the extrinsic and intrinsic supply. This refers to the location of the blood vessels with respect to the epineurium. Note the two types of extrinsic vessels. Above, the extrinsic vessels arise from fascial, musculocutaneous, and periosteal vessels. Below, the extrinsic vessels arise from axial vessels. (Reproduced with permission from Breidenbach and Terzis.[120])

A review of the results after nerve repair and grafting emphasize four broad factors that will influence the end results of the surgical techniques: *patient, injury, surgical technique, and postoperative rehabilitation. Patient factors,* especially age and patient compliance, are important in determining the eventual functional outcome. The age factor may relate to the potential for central adaptation to the peripheral nerve injury. Certainly, several recent experimental studies have demonstrated that after division or repair of the peripheral nerve, there is reorganization of the central cortex.[127–129] After nerve regeneration and especially with re-education[54] and rehabilitation, these cortical changes return more to normal. The excellent results seen after nerve repair or grafting in young children probably relates to their ability to adapt centrally to the altered profiles seen after nerve repair. This is directed by their constant curious investigations of their environment. The sensory stimuli from this natural re-education process causes central reorganization. Systemic patient factors, such as diabetes or alcoholism, may also influence the results of nerve regeneration (see Chapter 14).

Factors relating to the injury itself are probably the most significant in determining the eventual outcome. More proximal injuries tend to be more severe with greater longitudinal extension of the injury pattern. The more proximal the injury, the more likely there is to be associated death of the cell body.[130] Of course, the more proximal injuries, being farther away from the motor end plates and sensory receptors, are less likely to achieve good functional recovery, especially in the motor system where successful reinnervation of the muscle fibers is time dependent. Finally, in the proximal portions of the extremity, the fascicles tend to contain mixed motor and sensory fibers. Thus, the potential for mismatching of these fibers within a given fascicle is far greater at this proximal level.

In the distal portion of the extremity, the fascicles tend to be organized more discretely into sensory and motor fascicles. The injuries tend to include a large portion that are sharp injuries with less longitudinal damage to the nerve. Finally, the distance between the level of the injury and the distal receptors is much less.

Surgical technique is absolutely critical in determining functional outcome. Microneurosurgical technique with no tension at the suture line is imperative for a good result.

Unfortunately, we still see evidence of very poor quality nerve repairs (Fig. 4-3). Millesi has emphasized that it is equally as possible to carry out a bad nerve graft as it is to carry out a bad nerve repair. Tension at the proximal and distal ends of the nerve graft must be avoided.

Postoperative rehabilitation is critical in determining the final functional result. A recent review of the sensory recovery in transplanted digits and toes demonstrated that the best sensory recovery was noted in those centers where sensory re-education was utilized[131] (Chapter 18). This is equally important in the rehabilitation of motor function, especially in recovery of facial nerve function (Chapter 15).

Although the four factors just discussed will influence the eventual results of the surgical procedure, methods of reporting end results and evaluation techniques currently utilized to quantitate motor and sensory recovery are extremely variable and make it difficult to compare results from center to center.

The majority of studies have reported results according to the modification by Zachary and Holmes[132] of Highet and Sander's scheme[133] (Tables 4-3, 4-4). Although this system does not define good or bad results, it permits interpretation of "a useful median nerve recovery as M3 and S2+, useful ulnar nerve recovery as M2+ and S2+."[134] This grading system, unfortunately, lends itself to considerable variations in what is considered a useful and functional result. McEwan[135] considered "useful" ulnar nerve function as M2+ and "useful" median nerve function as M3. Sakellarides[136] considered M3, S2+, and S3 as "good" and M4 and S3+ as "excellent" for the median nerve. For the ulnar nerve, he regarded M2+, M3, S2+, and S3 as a "good" result and M4 and S3+ as an "excellent" result. Nicholson and Seddon[137] reported M4 and S3+ as useful recovery. In 1980, Posch and delaCruz-Saddul,[138] reviewing 231 peripheral nerve injuries, considered M3 and S2+ as a good result for both median and ulnar nerves and M4 and S3+ as an excellent result. A major flaw in the classification of sensory recovery according to this scheme is the failure to separate painful from painless sensations and a failure to quantitate sensory recovery with measurement of two-point discrimination. A recent report correlated functional recovery with measurements of sensibility and determined measurement of moving two-point discrimination was the best predictor of hand function.[139] Tactilegnosis, or object identification, correlated with the measurement of *moving* two-point discrimination. Measurement of *static* two-point discrimination added some predictive value for hand function because it correlated with how quickly the subjects could identify objects. This would relate to the subject's ability to detect pressure in the hand over a period of time. Recently, the clinical assessment committee for the American Society for Surgery of the Hand has recommended that moving and static two-point discrimination be measured when evaluating nerve function as well as pinch and grip measurements when indicated. This committee also suggested that measurement of pressure thresholds with Semmes-Weinstein monofilaments also be utilized.[140] This would make future reporting of end-stage nerve results more standardized and comparable between different centers.

In order to assess studies of functional recovery,

Table 4-3. Classification of Sensory Recovery

Grade	*Recovery of Sensibility*
S0	No recovery of sensibility in the autonomous zone of the nerve
S1	Recovery of deep cutaneous pain sensibility with the autonomous zone of the nerve
S1+	Recovery of superficial pain sensibility
S2	Recovery of superficial pain and some touch sensibility
S2+	As in S2, but with overresponse
S3	Recovery of pain and touch sensibility with disappearance of overresponse†
S3+	As in S3, but localization of the stimulus is good and there is imperfect recovery of two-point discrimination†
S4	Complete recovery†

†These classifications were modified to include classic two-point discrimination ranges as follows: S3 has two-point discrimination greater than 15 mm, S3+ includes 7 to 15 mm range, S4 includes 2 to 6 mm range.

Table 4-4. Classification of Motor Recovery

Grade	*Motor Recovery*
M0	No contraction
M1	Return of perceptible contraction in the proximal muscles
M2	Return of perceptible contraction in both proximal and distal muscles
M3	Return of function in both proximal and distal muscles to such a degree that all important muscles are sufficiently powerful to act against gravity
M4	All muscles act against strong resistance and some independent movements are possible
M5	Full recovery in all muscles

it is necessary to use the modified Highet scheme. Moberg has suggested that S3+ indicates that some two-point discrimination has returned.[141,142] Thus, we have assigned patients with two-point discrimination of 7 to 15 mm to the S3+ group. Moberg has stated that S4 implies complete recovery and has stated that normal static two-point discrimination is 6 mm; thus, we have assigned a patient with a two-point discrimination of 6 mm to the S4 group. Using these gradings, patients with two-point discrimination greater than 15 mm are assigned in the S3 group. Studies published since the end of the World War II with sufficient information to facilitate interpretation of data have been included in the Tables 4-5 to 4-10.

Low Median Nerve Repair

Of the 864 patients reported with low median nerve repairs, secondary to war injuries, only one patient recovered to S4 level and less than 20% to S3+ level. Approximately 40% recovered to M4 level.[143–146] It is interesting to note that after the Vietnam war, many decades later, the results were no better.[147] In the 465 reported civilian adult low median nerve repairs, the results were not significantly better.[135–138,143–155] Only two patients recovered to S4 level and 33% to S3+ level. Less than 5% recovered to M5 and 40% to M4 (Table 4-5). In a recent review of 150 median and ulnar nerve injuries, Merle et al[155] assessed the effects of the

Table 4-5. Results of Median Nerve Repair—Low

							Motor Recovery (%)				*Sensory Recovery (%)*				
Reference, Date	*Type of Trauma*	*Repair Timing*	*No. Cases*	*Age (yr)*	*% Children*	*Follow-up (yr)*	*M2*	*M3*	*M4*	*M5*	*S2*	*S2+*	*S3*	*S3+*	*S4*
Kirklin et al[143] 1949	War	All	235	Adults	0	2	67				27		73		
Zachary[144] 1954	War	Secondary	290	Adults	0	5	31	14	18	0	47	15	30	9	0.2
Yahr, Beebe; Oester, Davis[146] 1956	War	Secondary	244	Adults	0	4	11	23	29	31	17	28	14	18	
Nicholson, Seddon[137] 1957	Civilian	Secondary	52		16	5	21	27	39	0	21	15	40	25	0
Larson, Posch[148] 1958	Civilian	Primary	54		16	1–7	35	0	65	0					
Larson, Posch[148] 1958	Civilian	Secondary	24		16	1–7	50	0	50	0	3	0	26	71	0
Stromberg et al[149] 1961	Civilian	All	46			2–24									9
McEwan[135] 1962	Civilian	All	27	<14	100	Long	0	0	27	65	4	0	4	7	86
McEwan[135] 1962	Civilian	All	16	>14	0	Long	13	20	27	13	17	0	17	61	0
Sakellarides[136] 1962	Civilian	Primary	38	3–81	26	2–31	13	37	11	0	15	33	13	5	0
Sakellarides[136] 1962	Civilian	Secondary	20	3–81	26	2–31	25	35	25	0	20	29	32	4	0
Flynn, Flynn[150] 1962	Civilian	Primary	40			1–12	25	38	15	7	50	0	7	10	3
Onne[151] 1962	Civilian	Primary	15	<14	100	4–11	20	13	40	27	0	0	0	27	73
Onne[151] 1962	Civilian	Primary	17	>14	0	4–11	30	23	18	29	22	18	18	41	0
Nielsen, Torup[152] 1964	Civilian	All	10	5–58	33	1–3	30		70			30		70	
Boswick et al[153] 1965	Civilian	All	26		35	1					0		88	8	4
Seddon[154] 1972	Civilian	Secondary	110			5	5	47		44	4	5	47	44	0
Omer[147] 1974	War	Secondary	95	Adults	0	1		61	39	0		61		39	0
Posch, delaCruz-Saddul[138] 1980	Civilian	Primary	14		6	2–11	0	43	57	0	7	7	29	57	0

Table 4-6. Results of Median Nerve Repair—High

Reference, Date	Type of Trauma	Repair Timing	No. Cases	Age	Follow-up (yr)	Motor Recovery (%) M2	M3	M4	M5	Sensory Recovery (%) S2	S2+	S3	S3+	S4
Kirklin et al[143] 1949	War	All		Adult	<2					37		47		
Zachary[144] 1954	War	Secondary	95	Adult	5	42	13	6	0	47	23	25	6	0
Yahr, Beebe;[145] Oester, Davis[146] 1956	War	Secondary	124	Adult	>4	17	25	30	13					
Nicholson, Seddon[137] 1957	Civilian	Secondary	6	Adult	5	33	0	50	0	50	0	34	16	0
Larsen, Posch[148] 1958	Civilian	Primary	14		1–7	0	14	36	0		8	50	42	0
Sakellarides[136] 1962	Civilian	All	7	Adult	2–31	42	14	0	0	42	0	14	0	0
Seddon[154] 1972	Civilian	Secondary	100		>5	6	61	30		3	6	61	30	
Omer[147] 1974	War	Secondary	48	Adult	>1	7	3	27	0	7	3	27	0	0
Posch, delaCruz-Saddul[138] 1980	Civilian	Primary	12	Adult	2–11	16	60	8	0	8	8	60	17	0

Table 4-7. Results of Ulnar Nerve Repair—Low

Reference, Date	Type of Trauma	Repair Timing	No. Cases	Age	% Children	Follow-up (yr)	Motor Recovery (%) M2	M3	M4	M5	Sensory Recovery (%) S2	S2+	S3	S3+	S4
Kirklin et al[143] 1949	War	All	158	Adults	0	<2					0	31	69	0	0
Zachary[144] 1954	War	Secondary	384	Adults	0	>5	72	14	5	0	54	15	28	3	0
Yahr, Beebe;[145] Oester, Davis[146] 1956	War	Secondary	441	Adults	0	>4	5	34	38	16	16	24	19	13	0
Nicholson, Seddon[137] 1957	Civilian	Secondary	60		16	>5	32	32	35	0	18	14	47	21	0
Larson, Posch[148] 1958	Civilian	All	62		16	1–7	63	0	37	0	4	0	33	63	0
Stromberg et al[149] 1961	Civilian	All	32			2–24									3
McEwan[135] 1962	Civilian	All	23	<14	100	Long	4	25	67	4	0	0	5	23	72
McEwan[135] 1962	Civilian	All	23	>14	0	Long	32	36	23	0	8	0	24	48	12
Sakellarides[136] 1962	Civilian	Primary	39	3–81	26	2–31	30	6	0	0	25	15	23	5	0
Sakellarides[136] 1962	Civilian	Secondary	29	3–81	26	2–31	20	7	3	0	30	13	27	13	0
Flynn, Flynn[150] 1962	Civilian	Primary	40			1–12	57	15	18	0	50	0	13	7	0
Onne[151] 1962	Civilian	Primary	10	<14	100	5–10	8	30	30	32	0	0	10	30	60
Onne[151] 1962	Civilian	Primary	7	>14	0	5–10					0	0	57	43	0
Nielsen, Torup[152] 1964	Civilian	All	16	5–58	33	1–3	30	70			38		62		
Boswick et al[153] 1965	Civilian	All	19		35	1					4		76	20	0
Seddon[154] 1972	Civilian	Secondary	119			>5	10	43		45	2	10	43	45	0
Omer[147] 1974	War	Secondary	95	Adults	0	>1	61		39	0	61		39		0
Posch, delaCruz-Saddul[138] 1980	Civilian	Primary	20		6	2–11	55	30	10	0	50	0	10	30	0

Table 4-8. Results of Ulnar Nerve Repair—High

Reference, Date	Type of Trauma	Repair Timing	No. Cases	Age	Follow-up (yr)	Motor Recovery (%) M2	M3	M4	M5	Sensory Recovery (%) S2	S2+	S3	S3+	S4
Zachary[144] 1954	War	Secondary	105	Adult	5	23	5	1	0	53	24	23	0	0
Yahr, Beebe[145] 1956	War	Secondary	240	Adult	>4	9	38	32	10					
Nicholson, Seddon[137] 1957	Civilian	Secondary	9	Adult	3	33	22	22	0	33	11	44	11	0
Larsen, Posch[148] 1958	Civilian	Primary	18		1–7	0	0	0	0	0	16	44	44	0
Sakellarides[136] 1962	Civilian	All	18	Adult	2–31	56	11	0	0	40	22	11	0	0
Seddon[154] 1972	Civilian	Secondary	140		>5	13	61		22	4	13	61	22	0
Omer[147] 1974	War	Secondary	48	Adult	>1	73		27	0	73		27	0	0
Posch, delaCruz-Saddul[138] 1980	Civilian	Primary	11	Adult	2–11	54	18	9	0	27	9	27	0	0

Table 4-9. Combined Results of Median and Ulnar Nerve Repairs

		Sensory Recovery (%)		*Motor Recovery (%)*	
Nerve	*Type of Trauma*	*S3+*	*S4*	*M4*	*M5*
Median low	War	20	<1	40	0
	Civilian	33	<1	40	5
Median high	War	3	0	20	5
	Civilian	17	0	30	0
Ulnar low	War	15	0	40	0
	Civilian	34	<1	32	0
Ulnar high	War	0	0	23	6
	Civilian	20	0	17	0

level of the injury on the functional outcome. Good to excellent results were experienced in 53.5% of the low nerve injuries (wrist) and 36.8% of the injuries in the forearm. This study included primary, delayed, and nerve grafts of both median and ulnar nerves but summarized all results together. They concluded:

1. There were neither excellent nor very good results when the nerve repair was delayed.
2. Primary neurorrhaphy gave 50% useful results.
3. Secondary neurorrhaphy gave 50% fair results and interfascicular grafting gave a poor result in 57% of cases.
4. The percentage of failures found after nerve repair performed on an emergency basis was higher than the percentage of failures observed after secondary repair.[155]

High Median Nerve Repair

Results after high median nerve repairs were significantly poorer than those after low median nerve repairs (Table 4-6). None of the patients with war injuries recovered S4 function. Only 3% recovered S3+ function and only 20% recovered M4 motor function.[143–147] In the civilian injuries, again no patients recovered S4 function, although 17% recovered S3+ function. No patients recovered M5 motor function and 38% recovered M4 motor function.[136–138,148,154,155]

Ulnar Nerve Repair

The results of ulnar nerve repair were generally less, especially with respect to sensory[135–138,143–155] recovery than for median nerve repair (Table 4-7, 4-8, 4-9).

Digital Nerve Repair

The results for sensory recovery after digital nerve repair are generally good,[138,148,151,156–167] although two recent studies demonstrated that the results can be quite variable.[136,161] Young et al[161] compared patients treated with a fascicular or epineurial digital nerve repair. They found no difference between the two types of repair and noted that 90% of the patients obtained S3+ or S4 recovery. By comparison, Posch and dela-Cruz-Saddul[138] reported, in 1980, that 20% of patients with digital nerve repair had only a S2 recovery (Table 4-10). Berger et al. recently reported 91% S3+ or S4 results with digital nerve repair.[191]

Reviewing all the articles written on the results of digital nerve repairs, we find that 60% of patients having a digital nerve repair will recover two-point discrimination.[138,148,151,156–167] The more favorable results of digital nerve repair noted in the last decade probably relate to improved technique and the addition of sensory re-education to some center's postoperative management.

Digital Nerve Graft

The results after digital nerve grafting are noted in (Table 4-11). There have been very few reports on the results of digital nerve grafts.[162–169] Seddon reported in 1947[162] the results of 15 digital nerve grafts. Eighteen percent had recovery of two-point discrimination (S3+, S4). In 1955, however, Brooks[163] reported 17 digital nerve grafts with none of the patients recovering two-point discrimination. In contrast, McFarlane and Moyer[164] in 1976 reported the results of 13 digital nerve grafts and noted that 46% had recovery of two-point discrimination. In 1984, Beazley[167] reported the results of 12 digital nerve grafts, with 58% recovering two-point discrimination. Rose et al[168] presented the results of vascularized digital nerve grafts and noted that 93% recovered two-point discrimination. Our own results in 33 patients with digital nerve grafts demonstrated that 31 patients (94%) recovered two-point discrimination.[170] Before these two reports,[168,170] the average results for digital nerve grafting demonstrated that only 30% of patients recovered two-point discrimination. This is compared with the average recovery for digital nerve repair in which we find that at least 60% of patients after digital nerve repair recovered two-point discrimination. The improved results in these two studies[168,170] may relate to the potential added benefits of vascularizing the nerve graft[168] or adding an intense course of sensory re-education[170] to the postoperative management.

Ulnar Nerve Grafting

The results of ulnar nerve grafting are noted in Table 4-12. Millesi's series[173,174] provides the largest number of patients published to date. Haase et al[171] have also

Table 4-10. Results of Digital Nerve Repair

Reference, Date	*Type of Trauma*	*Repair Timing*	*No Cases*	*Age (yr)*	*% Children*	*Follow-up (yr)*	*Nerve Block*	*Sensory Recovery (%)* S2	*S2+*	*S3*	*S3+*	*S4*
Bunnell[156] 1927	Civilian	All	105				No					
Larsen, Posch[148] 1958	Civilian	All	142		16	1–7	No	7	0	29	64	0
Weckesser[157] 1961	Civilian	Primary	12	7–55	8		No	0	0	16	42	25
Weckesser[157] 1961	Civilian	Secondary	12	7–48	8		No	0	16	16	21	63
Onne[151] 1962	Civilian	Primary	8	<14	100	4–15	Yes	0	0	0	0	100
Onne[151] 1962	Civilian	Primary	14	>14	0	4–15	Yes	28	0	29	43	0
Honner et al[158] 1970	Civilian	Primary	24	<19	100	2–6	Yes	12	0	20	20	48
Honner et al[158] 1970	Civilian	Primary	50	>19	0	2–6	Yes	28	0	28	28	16
Buncke[159] 1972	Civilian	All	18	6–51	5		No	0	0	22	28	50
Poppin et al[160] 1979	Civilian	Primary	62	6–67	22	5–15	Yes	0	10	16	55	19
Posch, delaCruz-Saddul[138] 1980	Civilian	Primary	71		6	2–11	No	20	0	32	48	0
Young et al[161] 1981	Civilian	Primary	27	3–67		2–4	No	0	0	10	57	33
Berger et al[191] 1988	Civilian	Primary	129			2	No	← 9 →			← 91 →	

Table 4-11. Results of Digital Nerve Graft

Reference, Date	*Type of Trauma*	*Gap Grafted (cm)*	*No. Cases*	*Age*	*Follow-up (yr)*	*Nerve Block*	*Sensory Recovery (%)* S2	*S2+*	*S3*	*S3+*	*S4*
Seddon[162] 1947	War	3–8	15	Adults	2–4	No	46	12	24	6	12
Brooks[163] 1955	Civilian	>2	17		>5	No	18	0	47	0	0
McFarlane, Moyer[164] 1976	Civilian	1.5–3.5	17	20–59	0.75–2	No	0	15	39	46	0
Young et al[165] 1980	Civilian	>2	27	15–57	0.5–5	Yes	0	0	60	25	15
Yamano et al[190] 1982	Replant	2–5	5	28–56	2	No	0	0	0	100	0
Wilgis, Maxwell[169] 1979	Civilian	1–2.5	11	17–54	.9–2	Yes	0	0	0	33	67
Beazley et al[167] 1984	Civilian	1–5	12	0.5–71	2–6	No	42			58	
Rose, Kowalski[166] 1985	Civilian	5–8	5	Adults	3–7	No	0	20	0	20	60
Rose et al[168] 1987	Civilian	4.5	13	19–55	1	No	0	0	7	55	38
Mackinnon[170] 1988	Civilian	1–5	31	18–62	4	No	6	0	0	40	54
Berger et al[191] 1988	Civilian	1–6			3–7	No		←	85	→	

published a relatively large series of ulnar nerve grafts. Reviewing all the results published to date that have documented any sensory testing end results,[163,167,171–174,176,177] we see as a whole 28% of patients recovered two-point discrimination (S3+ and S4 level; 25 of 88 patients). Similarly, reviewing all the articles that report published data on motor recovery, we see that 54% of patients (49 of 90) recovered to the M4 or M5 level (Table 4-12).

Median Nerve Grafts

The results of median nerve grafts are given in Table 4-13. Taken as a whole, 2% of the nerve graft patients recovered to S4; 24%, to S3+; 20%, to M5; 13%, to M4.

Radial Nerve Repair and Graft

Sakellarides[136] reviewed the results of 13 patients with high and low radial nerve injuries. He noted that with high radial nerve injuries only one of the six patients recovered motor function to the M3 level. With low radial nerve injury, two of seven patients recovered to M4 or M5. These results were not an improvement on the combined American and British war experience.[45,180] In 1974, reviewing 917 nerve injuries, Omer[147] described the results of 190 radial nerve injuries. Spontaneous recovery occurred in 139 (73%) cases (Table 4-14).

Young et al[179] have recently described Hudson's results with surgery of the posterior interosseous nerve (Table 4-15). The results after surgery, including repair, neurolysis, and interfascicular nerve grafting were excellent (90%).

Lower Extremity Nerve Surgery

There have been very few reports detailing the incidence of nerve injuries in the lower extremity or the results after surgical treatment of these problems.[181–187] In 1980, Kline[183] reported his experience with lower extremity nerve lesions. Chen and Yu[182] reported the results of 27 cases of replanted limb surgery. In their study, there were eight instances of grade I function (34.8%), 11 of grade II function (47.8%), and four of

Table 4-12. Results of Ulnar Nerve Graft

Reference, Date	Type of Trauma	Gap Grafted (cm)	No. Cases	Age (yr)	% Children	Follow-up (yr)	Motor Recovery (%) M2	M3	M4	M5	Sensory Recovery (%) S2	S2+	S3	S3+	S4
Bunnell, Boyes[175] 1939	Civilian	3–15	32			1–15									0
Millesi et al[173,174] 1972, 1976	Civilian	2–20	39	11–69	23	5–11	8	31	18	31	0	15	65	15	5
Walton, Finseth[176] 1977	Civilian	2–6	2	16–50		1.5–2.5	0	50	0	0	50	0	50	0	0
Tallas et al[177] 1978	Civilian	3–7	10			1.5–3.5	20	50	30	0	20	20	40	20	0
Young et al[165] 1980	Civilian	>2	5	15–57		1–5				20		0	0	60	0
		40													
Hoase et al[171] 1980	Civilian	1.5–7	26	9–73		2.5–5	7	45	48	0	30	5	15	50	
Yamano[172] 1982	Civilian	5–9	2	6.5	100	2.5–5	0	0	100	0			?		
Beazley et al[167] 1984	Civilian	2–7	6	.5–71		2–6	average M2		0			average S1		0	

Table 4-13. Results of Median Nerve Graft

Reference, Date	Type of Trauma	Gap Grafted (cm)	No. Cases	Age (yr)	% Children	Follow-up (yr)	Motor Recovery (%) M2	M3	M4	M5	Sensory Recovery (%) S2	S2+	S3	S3+	S4
Bunnell, Boyes[175] 1939	Civilian	3–15	32			1–15									3
Seddon[162] 1947	War	5–15	11	Adult		2–3	0	36	18	0	10	18	45	18	0
Brooks[163] 1955	Civilian	>7	33			>5	0	69	0	0	21	0	69	0	0
Millesi et al[173,174] 1972, 1976	Civilian	2–20	38	8–62	3	5–11	7	21	14	46	3	0	60	34	3
Walton, Finseth[176] 1977	Civilian	5–10	8	17–38	0	1.5–2.5	12	0	50	0	13	0	12	63	12
Tallas et al[177] 1978	Civilian	4–15	6			1.5–2.5		33	16	33				33	
Young et al[165] 1980	Civilian	>2	8	15–57	0	1–5		0	0	0	0	37	38	25	0
Beazley et al[167] 1984	Civilian	4–6	5	.5–71	2–6		average M2+		0			average S2		0	

Table 4-14. Results of Radial Nerve Repair

Reference, Date	Type of Trauma	No. Cases	% Motor Recovery, M4 to M5
Seddon[180] 1954	War	114	37
Woodall, Beebe[45] 1956	War	197	21
Sakellarides[136] 1962	Civilian	13	14
Brown[178] 1970	War	5	Some return 40%

Table 4-15. Posterior Interosseous Nerve Palsy, Surgical Results*

	Excellent/Good	Fair/Poor	Failure
External neurolysis	20	1	2
Internal neurolysis	1		
Tendon Transfer	4		
Group Fascicular Graft	11	1	—
Total	36	2	2

*Reprinted with permission from Young et al.[179]

grade III function (17.4%). There were no instances of grade IV function. These investigators graded function as follows:

Grade I: Normal gait, good sensation

Grade II: Slight limp, good sensation

Grade III: Patient can walk with an elevated shoe, fair sensation

Grade IV: No sensation, patient cannot walk without crutches

The most complete summary of the results after surgery for lower extremity nerve lesions was recently published by Millesi[181] (Table 17-18). Millesi's proposed grading system for functional recovery after lower extremity nerve injuries is recommended (Table 4-19).

Our own experience with lower extremity nerve grafting has been good.[188] We have returned pain-free sensation with good localization to the sole of the foot in nine of nine patients with posterior tibial nerve grafts, five of the nine have recovered to S3+ level. We have found grafting the superficial peroneal nerve to be largely unsuccessful because the patients frequently report unpleasant sensitivity on the dorsum of the ankle or lower leg over the site of the nerve graft. These injuries are usually better managed with proximal transposition of the superficial peroneal nerve into the deep tissue of the lower leg. This nerve and its response to nerve grafting is similar to that seen with nerve grafts of the radial sensory nerve.[189] Regeneration will occur across the graft but because of the movement of the ankle and the tissue bed of skin and tendons, the grafting procedure is frequently also associated with unacceptable pain.

Table 4-16. Functional Results after Peroneal Nerve Lesions with Severe Loss of Nerve Substance (21 Patients)*†

Result	*NG Only (1st Series)*	*NG Only (2nd Series)*	*Same Patients (2nd Series) After TPTT‡*	*NG‡ + Simultaneous TPTT (3rd Series)*
Good				
With good nerve regeneration			5	5
Satisfactory				
With partial nerve regeneration			1	4
Fair				
With partial nerve regeneration				
Without nerve regeneration			1	
Poor				
With partial nerve regeneration	5	5		
Without nerve regeneration		2		
Total	5	7	—	9 (= 21)

*Reprinted with permission from Millesi.[181]

†All were treated by secondary nerve grafts at more than 4 months after injury.

‡NG = nerve graft; TPTT = tibialis posterior tendon transfer.

Table 4-17. Functional Result in 39 Patients with a Post-Traumatic Sciatic Nerve Lesion*

			According to Site of Lesion and Type of Operation				
			Foramen Infrapiriforme	*Gluteal Area*	*Thigh*		
Level	*Results*	*All Cases*	*NL + NG†*	*NL (Injection Lesion)*	*NG*	*NG + NL*	*NL*
3	Good	28	9	5	7	2	5
3 (T + P)	Tibial and peroneal nerves	6	2	1	2	1	—
3 (T)	Tibial nerve only	22	7	4	5	1	5
2	Satisfactory	6	1	1	3	1	—
1	Poor	5	—	—	4	—	1
0	Nil	—	—	—	—	—	—
Total		39	10	6	14	3	6

*Reprinted with permission from Millesi.[181]

†NG = nerve graft; NL = neurolysis.

Table 4-18. Functional Results after Clean Transection of the Peroneal Nerve (10 Patients)*

		Nerve Graft		
Result	*Neurorrhaphy*	*Within 4 Months*	*After 4 Months*	*More Than 4 Months After Injury + Simultaneous TPTT†*
Good				
With good nerve regeneration		3		3
Satisfactory				
With partial nerve regeneration				
Fair				
With partial nerve regeneration				
Without nerve regeneration				
Poor				
With partial nerve regeneration	1‡		2‖	
Without nerve regeneration	1§			

*Reprinted with permission from Millesi et al.[181]

†TPTT: Tibialis posterior tendon transfer.

‡Improved to fair result after neurolysis.

§Improved to fair result after TPTT.

‖One patient improved to a fair result and the other to a good result after secondary TPTT.

Table 4-19. Evaluation of Functional Recovery after Sciatic Nerve Lesions*

Level	*Result*
3	Good result Good vasomotor function Protective sensibility Active plantar flexion Active dorsal flexion—two possibilities must be distinguished 3 (T+ P†): Dorsal flexion due to useful recovery of the muscles innervated by the common peroneal nerve 3 (T†): Dorsal flexion due to functioning tibialis posterior tendon transfer; in this case there must be useful recovery not only in the gastrocnemius and soleus but in the other muscles innervated by the tibial nerve as well
2	Satisfactory result Good vasomotor function Protective sensibility Active plantar flexion due to reinnervation of the gastrocnemius (M3 or better) An orthopedic device is required
1	Poor result Good vasomotor function Protective sensibility No useful motor recovery An orthopedic device is required
0	Nil No nerve regeneration

*Reprinted with permission from Millesi.[181]

†T + P = tibial and peroneal nerves; T = tibial nerve only.

References

1. Ferrara G: Nuova Selva di Cirurgia Divisia in tre Parti Venice. S Combi. 1608.
2. Davis L, Cleveland DA: Experimental studies in nerve transplants. Ann Surg 99:271–283, 1934.
3. Letievant JJE: Traite des sections nerveuses. JB Baillie-reetfils, Paris, 1872.
4. Mackenzie JAJ: Resection of the sciatic nerve, neuroplasty, end results. Surg Gynecol Obstet 9:30–44, 1909.
5. Stookey B: The futility of bridging nerve defects by means of nerve flaps. Surg Gynecol Obstet 29:287–311, 1919.
6. Markoe TM: Secondary nerve suture. Ann Surg 2:181, 1885.
7. Rawa AL: Ueber die Nervennaht. Wien Med Wchnschr 35:358, 1885.
8. Snyder CC, Webster H, Pickens JE, et al: Intraneural neurorrhaphy. A preliminary clinical and histological evaluation. Ann Surg 167: 691, 1968.
9. Spitzy H: Bemerkung zur Ueberbruckung von Nervendefekten. Munch Med Wochenschr 64:372, 1917.
10. Hirschel G: Erfahrungen uber Schussverletzungen der Nerven. Munch Med Wochenschr 62:159, 1915.
11. Heinemann O: Ueber Schlussverletzungen der peripheren Nerven. Arch Klin Chir 108:107, 1916.
12. Assaky G: Du la suture des nerfs a distence. Arch Gen Med 17:529–553, 1886.
13. Brock AJ: Greek Medicine. JM Dent & Sons, New York, 1929.
14. Paulus Aegineta. The seven books translated by F. Adams, 2 vol, London 1844-1847, Sydenham Society.
15. Roger of Parma, quoted by Henderson HE: Gilbertus Anglicus Medicine of the 13th century, Medical Library Association, Cleveland, 1918.

16. Guy de Chauliac on wounds and fractures (translated by W.A. Brennan), W.A. Brennan, Chicago, 1923.
17. Hoffmann F: Einige Falle von Nervenlahmung und Nervennaht. Mitt Chir Klin 118:24, 1884.
18. Gluck T: Ueber Neuroplastik auf dem Wege der Transplantation. Arch Klin Chir 25:606–616, 1880.
19. Flourens P: Experiences sur la reunion ou cicatrisation des plaies de la moelle epiniere et des nerfs. Ann Sci Nat 13:113–122, 1828.
20. Mayo-Robson AW: Nerve grafting as a means of restoring function in limbs paralysed by gunshot or other injuries. Br Med J 1:117, 1917.
21. Hoen TI, Brachett CE: Peripheral nerve lengthening. 1. Experimental. J Neurosurg 13:43, 1956.
22. Garriety RW: The use of plastic and rubber tubing in the management of irreparable nerve injuries. Surg Forum 6:517, 1955.
23. Huber GC: A study of the operative treatment for loss of nerve substance in peripheral nerves. J Morphol 11: 629, 1895.
24. Kirk EG, Lewis D: Fascial tubulization in the repair of nerve defects. JAMA, 65:486–492, 1915.
25. Weiss P: Nerve reunion with sleeves of frozen dried artery in rabbits, cats and monkeys. Proc Soc Exp Biol Med 54:274, 1943.
26. Moyer EK, Kimmel DL: The repair of severed motor and sensory spinal nerve roots by the arterial sleeve method of anastomosis. J Comp Neurol 88:285, 1984.
27. Hirasawa Y, Marmor L: The protective effect of radiation combined with sheathing methods on experimental nerve heterografts. Silastic, autogenous veins and heterogenous arteries. J Neurol 27:401, 1967.
28. Verne J, Iselin M: Reflexions sur deux picels de reparation nerveuse sur l'homme prelevees dix semaines et six mois l'operation. Presse Med 49:789, 1941.
29. Payr E: Beitrage zur Technik der Blutgefass und Nervennaht nebst Mittheilungen ubre die Verevendung eines resorbibaren Metalles in der Chirurgie. Arch Klin Chir 62:67, 1900.
30. Braun R: Comparative studies of neurorrhaphy and sutureless peripheral nerve repair. Surg, Gynecol Obstet 120:15, 1966.
31. Madison R, DaSilva CF, Dikkes P, Sidman RL, Chiu TH: Increased rate of peripheral nerve regeneration using bioresorbable nerve guides and laminin-containing gel. Exp Neurol 88:767–772, 1985.
32. Weiss P: Suturless reunion of severed nerves with cuffs of tantalum. J Neurosurg 1:219, 1944.
33. Campbell JB, Bassett CA, Girado JM, et al: Application of monomolecular filter tubes in bridging gaps in peripheral nerves and for prevention of neuroma formation. A preliminary report. J Neurosurg 13:635, 1956.
34. Molander H, Olsson Y, Engkvist O, et al: Regeneration of peripheral nerve through a polyglactin tube. Muscle Nerve 5:54–57, 1982.
35. Seckel BR, Ryan SE, Gagne RG, et al: Target specific nerve regeneration through a nerve guide in the rat. Plast Reconstr Surg 78:793–798, 1986.
36. Bora FW, Brown MJ, Summer AJ: Prosthetic nerve grafts. The use of a resorbable tube as an alternative to autogenous nerve grafting. Presented at the 41st Annual Meeting of the American Society for Surgery of the Hand, New Orleans, September, 1986.
37. Philipeaux JM, Vulpian A: Note sur sa essais de greffe d'un troncon de nerf lingual entre les deux vouts de thypoglose. Arch Physiol Norm Pathol 3:618, 1817.
38. Albert E: Einige Operationen an Nerven. Wien Med 26:1285, 1878.
39. Sherren J: Some points in the surgery of peripheral nerves. Edinburgh Med J 20:297–332, 1906.
40. Stopford JSB: The treatment of large defects in peripheral nerve injuries. Lancet 2:1296–1327, 1920.
41. Platt H: On the results of bridging gaps in injured nerve trunks by autogenous fascial tubulization and autogenous nerve grafts. Br J Surg 7:384–389, 1919.
42. Delageniere H: A contribution to the study of the surgical repair of peripheral nerves based on 375 cases. Surg Gynecol Obstet 39:543–553, 1924.
43. Bunnell S: Repair of nerves and tendons of the hand. J Bone Joint Surg 10:1–16, 1928.
44. Bunnell S: Suture of facial nerve within temporal bone with report of first successful case. Surg Gynecol Obstet 45:7, 1927.
45. Woodall B, Beebe WG: In Peripheral Nerve Regeneration, A follow-up study of 3,656 World War II injuries. VA Medical Monograph, US Government Printing Office, Washington, D.C., 1956.
46. Millesi H: Microsurgery of peripheral nerves. Hand 5:157–160, 1973.
47. Millesi H: Indication, technique and results of nerve grafting. Handchirurgie [Suppl] 2:1–24, 1977.
48. Millesi H, Berger A, Meissl G: Experimentelle Untersuchungen zur Heilung durchtrennter peripherer Nerven. Chir Plast 1:174, 1972.
49. Young JZ, Medawar PB: Fibrin suture of peripheral nerves. Lancet 2:126, 1940.
50. Seddon HJ, Medawar PB: Fibrin suture of human nerves. Lancet 2:87, 1942.
51. Bonnard C, Narakas A: Comparison in clinical results of neurosynthesis when using microsutures of fibrin glue. Presented at the 3rd Annual Meeting, American Society for Reconstructive Microsurgery, San Antonio, Texas, September, 1987.
52. Jacoby W, Fahlbusch R, Mackert B, et al: Transplantation lyophilisierter Homoioplasticher Nerven sur Uberbrukung peripherer Nervendefekte beim Menschen. Fortschr Med 88:183, 1970.
53. Kuhlendahl H, Mumenthaler M, Penzholz H, et al: The treatment of peripheral nerve injuries with homologous nerve grafts. Acta Neurochir (Wien) 26:339, 1972.
54. Dellon AL: Evaluation of Sensibility in Re-education of Sensation of the Hand. Williams & Wilkins, Baltimore, 1981.
55. Donoso RS, Ballantyne JP, Hansen S: Regeneration of sutured human peripheral nerves. An electrophysiological study. J Neurol Neurosurg Psychiatry 42:97–106, 1979.

56. Edsage S: Peripheral nerve suture. A technique for improved intraneural topography. Acta Chir Scand (Suppl) 331:1–104, 1964.
57. Hakstian RW: Perineurial neurorrhaphy. Orthop Clin North Am 4:945–956, 1973.
58. Kutz JE, Shealy G, Lubbers L: Interfascicular nerve repair. Orthop Clin North Am 12:277–286, 1981.
59. Lilla JA, Phelps DB, Boswick JA: Microsurgical repair of peripheral nerve injuries in the upper extremity. Ann Plast Surg 2:24–31, 1979.
60. Snyder CC: Epineurial repair. Orthop Clin North Am 12:267–276, 1981.
61. Bora FW: Peripheral nerve repair in cats. The fascicular stitch. J Bone Joint Surg 49A:659–666, 1967.
62. Bora FW, Pleasure DE, Didizian NA: A study of nerve regeneration and neuroma formation after nerve suture by various techniques. J Hand Surg 1:138–143, 1976.
63. Chabaud HE, Rodkey WG, McCarroll HR, et al: Epineurial and perineurial fascicular nerve repairs. A critical comparison. J Hand Surg 1:131–137, 1976.
64. Kline DG, Hudson AR, Bratton BR: Experimental study of fascicular nerve repair with and without epineurial closure. J Neurosurg 54:513–520, 1981.
65. Levinthal R, Brown WJ, Rand RW: Comparison of fascicular, interfascicular and epineural suture techniques in the repair of simple nerve lacerations. J Neurosurg 47:744–750, 1977.
66. Orgel MG, Terzis JK: Epineurial versus perineural repair. An ultrastructural and electrophysiological study of nerve regeneration. Plast Reconstr Surg 60:80–91, 1977.
67. Wise AJ: A comparative analysis of macro and microsurgical neurorrhaphy techniques. Am J Surg 117:566–572, 1969.
68. Yamamoto K: A comparative analysis of the process of nerve regeneration following funicular and epineurial suture for peripheral nerve repair. Arch Jpn Chir 43:276–301, 1974.
69. Brushart TM, Mesulam MM: Alteration in connections between muscle and anterior horn motoneurons after peripheral nerve repair. Science 208:603–605, 1980.
70. Brushart TM, Tarlov E, Mesulam MM: A comparison of motor neuron pool organization after epineurial and perineurial repair of the rat sciatic nerve. Orthop Trans 4:19–20, 1980.
71. Brushart TM, Henry EW, Mesulam M: Reorganization of muscle afferent projections accompanies peripheral nerve regeneration. Neuroscience 6:2053–2061, 1981.
72. Chabaud HE, Rodkey WG, McCarrol HR: Peripheral nerve injuries. Studies in higher nonhuman primates. J Hand Surg 5:201–206, 1980.
73. Grabb WC, Bement SL, Kaepke GH, et al: Comparison of methods of peripheral nerve suturing in monkeys. Plast Reconstr Surg 46:31–38, 1970.
75. Millesi H: Founders lecture: Microsurgery of Peripheral Nerves: A Surgical Technique or a Biological Approach. American Society for Surgery of the Hand. San Antonio, Texas, 1987.
76. Terzis JK, Faibisoff BA, Williams B: The nerve gap: Suture under tension versus graft. Plast Reconstr Surg 56:166, 1975.
77. Miyamoto Y, Tsuge K: Effects of tension on interneural microcirculation in end to end neurorrhaphy. In Gorio A, Millesi H, Mingrino S, eds: Posttraumatic Peripheral Nerve Regeneration. Raven Press, New York, 1981, p 81.
78. Millesi H, Meissl G: Consequences of tension at the suture site. In Gorio A, Millesi H, Mingrino S, eds: Posttraumatic Peripheral Nerve Regeneration. Raven Press, New York, 1981, p 277.
79. Millesi H: The nerve gap. Theory and clinical practice. Hand Clin 2:651–664, 1987.
80. Ortiguela ME, Wood MD, Cahill DR: Anatomy of the sural nerve complex. J Hand Surg [Am] 12:1119–1123, 1987.
81. Louie G, Mackinnon SE, Dellon AL, Patterson GA, Hunter DA: Medial antebrachial cutaneous—lateral femoral cutaneous neurotization in restoration of sensation to pressure bearing areas in a paraplegic. Ann Plast Surg 19:572–576, 1987.
82. Dellon AL: Partial dorsal wrist denervation: Resection of posterior interosseous nerve. J Hand Surg [Am] 10:527–533, 1985.
83. Hall H, Mackinnon SE, Gilbert R: Approach to the posterior interosseous nerve. Plast Reconstr Surg 74:435–437, 1984.
84. McQuarrie IG, Grafstein B: Axon outgrowth enhanced by a previous nerve injury. Arch Neurol 29:53–55, 1973.
85. McQuarrie IG, Grafstein B, Gershon MD: Axonal regeneration in rat sciatic nerve. Effect of a conditioning lesion and of dcb-AMP. Brain Res 132:443–453, 1977.
86. McQuarrie IG: Acceleration of axonal regeneration in rat somatic motor neurons by using a conditioning lesion. In Gorio A, Millesi H, Mingrino S, eds: Posttraumatic Nerve Regeneration. Raven Press, New York 1981, pp 49–58.
87. Bisby MA, Keen P: The effect of a conditioning lesion on the regeneration rate of peripheral nerve axons containing substance P. Brain Res 336:201–206, 1985.
88. Forman DS, Wood DK, Desilva S: The rate of regeneration of sensory axons in transected rat sciatic nerve repaired with epineurial sutures. J Neurol Sci 44:55–59, 1979.
89. Richardson PM, Issa VMK: Peripheral injury enhances central regeneration of primary sensory neurones. Nature 309:791–793, 1984.
90. Richardson PM, Verge VMK: The induction of a regenerative propensity in sensory neurons following peripheral axonal injury. J Neurocytol 15:585–594, 1986.
91. Zachary LS, Dellon AL, Seiler WA: Relationship of intraneural damage in the rat sciatic nerve to the method of injury. Microsurgery 8:182–185, 1987.
92. Chow JA, Sunderland S, Van Beek AL: Surgical significance of the motor fascicular group of the ulnar nerve in the forearm. J Hand Surg [Am] 9:605, 1985.
93. Jabaley ME, Wallace WH, Heckler FR: Internal topography of major nerves in the forearm and hand. A current view. J Hand Surg 5:119, 1980.
94. Williams HB, Jabaley ME: The importance of interneural anatomy of the peripheral nerves to nerve repair in the forearm and hand. Hand Clin 2:689–707, 1986.
95. Shizhen Z, Xiangluo T, Muzhil I: The microsurgical anatomy of peripheral nerves. In Shizhen Z, Yongjian H,

Wencyun Y, eds: Microsurgical Anatomy. MTP Press, Lancaster, England; 1985, pp 299–350.
96. Sunderland S: The intraneural topography of the radial, median and ulnar nerves. Brain 68:243, 1945.
97. Adams CWM, Grant RT, Davis OB: Cholinesterases in peripheral nervous system. 1. mixed, motor and sensory trunks. Brain Res 5:366–367, 1967.
98. Gruber H, Zenker W: Acetylcholinesterase: Histochemical differentiation between motor and sensory nerve fibres. Brain Res 51:207—214, 1973.
99. Yunshao H, Shizhen Z. Further exploration of acetylcholinesterase: Histochemical identification of motor and sensory fascicles in human peripheral nerve and its applicability during operation. Plast Reconstr Surg 82:125, 1988.
100. Engel J, Ganel A, Melamed R, et al: Choline acetyltransferase for differentiation between human, motor and sensory nerve fibres. Ann Plast Surg 4:367–380, 1979.
101. Ganel A, Engel J, Raymond S: Intraoperative identification of peripheral nerve fascicle: Use of a new rapid biochemical assay technique. Orthop Rev 15:85–88, 1986.
102. Riley DA, Lang DH: Carbonic anhydrase activity of human peripheral nerves. A possible histochemical aid to nerve repair. J Hand Surg [Am] 9:112–124, 1984.
103. Hakstian RW: Funicular orientation by direct stimulation: An aid to peripheral nerve repair. J Bone Joint Surg 50:1178–1186, 1968.
104. Nakatsuchi Y, Matsui T, Honda Y: Funicular orientation by electrical stimulation and internal neurolysis in peripheral nerve suture. Hand 12:65–73, 1980.
105. Vanderput J, Tanner JC, Huypens L: Electrical physiological orientation of the cut ends in primary peripheral nerve repair. Plast Reconstr Surg 44:378–382, 1969.
106. Gaul JS: Electrical fascicle identification as an adjunct to nerve repair. Hand Clin 2:709–722, 1986.
107. Seddon HH: Three types of nerve injury. Brain 66:237, 1943.
108. Sunderland S: A classification of peripheral nerve injuries producing a loss of function. Brain 74:491, 1951.
109. Van Beek AL: Electrodiagnostic evaluation of peripheral nerve injuries. Hand Clin 2:747–760, 1986.
110. Terzis JK, Dykes BW: Electrophysiological recordings in peripheral nerve surgery. A review. J Hand Surg 1:52–66, 1976.
111. Kline DG, Hackett ER, May PF: Evaluation of nerve injuries by evoked potentials and electromyography, J Neurosurg 31:136–138, 1969.
112. Kline DG, Hackett ER: The value of electrophysiologic tests for peripheral nerve neuromas. J Surg Oncol 2:299–310, 1970.
113. Williams HB, Terzis JK: Single fascicular recordings an intraoperative diagnostic tool for the management of peripheral nerve lesions. Plast Reconstr Surg 57:562–569, 1976.
114. Kline DG, Nulsen FE: The neuroma incontinuity. Its preoperative and operative management. Surg Clin North Am 52:1189–1209, 1972.
115. Taylor EG, Ham FJ: The free vascularized nerve graft. Plast Reconstr Surg 57:413, 1976.
116. Fachinelli A, Masquelet A, Restrepo J, Gilbert A: A vascularized sural nerve. Int J Microsurg 3:157, 1981.
117. Bonney G, Birch R, Jamieson AM, Eames RA: Experience with vascularized nerve grafts. In Terzis JK, ed: Microreconstruction of Nerve Injuries. WB Saunders, Philadelphia, 1986, pp 403–414.
118. Minderis M: Experience in vascularized sural nerve transplantation. Personal communication, Vilnius, Lithuania, December, 1987.
119. Mackinnon SE, Hunter D, Kelly L: A histological and functional comparison of regeneration across a vascularized and conventional nerve graft. A case report. J Microsurg 9:226—233, 1988.
120. Breidenbach WC, Terzis JK: The blood supply of vascularized nerve grafts. J Reconstr Microsurg 3:43–56, 1986.
121. Kunzel KH, Fischer C, Ander H: The ulnar nerve of the vascularized transplant. J Reconstr Microsurg 2:175, 1986.
122. Settergren CR, Wood MB: Comparison of blood flow in free vascularized versus nonvascularized nerve grafts. J Reconstr Microsurg 1:95, 1984.
123. Lind R, Wood MB: Comparison of the patterns of early revascularization of conventional versus vascularized nerve grafts in the canine. J Reconstr Microsurg 2:229, 1986.
124. Seckel BR, Ryan SE, Simons JE, et al: Vascularized versus nonvascularized nerve grafts. An experimental structural comparison. Plast Reconstr Surg 78:211, 1986.
125. Gu Y, Zheng Y, Li H, Zu Y: Arterialized venous free sural nerve grafting. J Plast Surg 15:332, 1985.
126. Bain J, Mackinnon SE, Hudson AR, Hunter DA: A comparison of regeneration across a vascularized and nonvascularized nerve graft—an experimental study in the rat. 1988. In preparation.
127. Merzenich MM: Alteration in cortical map following preferential digital stimulation in the adult monkey. (Abstr.) Neuroscience 10:34, 1984.
128. Merzenich MM, Nelson RJ, Stryker MP, et al: Somatosensory cortical map changes following digital amputation in adult monkey. J Comp Neurol 224:591–605, 1984.
129. Jenkins WM, Merzenich MM: Reorganization of neocortical representations after brain surgery. Brain Res 71:249–266, 1987.
130. Kristensson K: Retrograde signalling of nerve cell body response to trauma. In Regeneration. Gorio A, Millesi H, Mingrino S, eds: Posttraumatic Peripheral Nerve. Raven Press, New York, 1981, pp 115–128.
131. Dellon AL: Sensory recovery in replanted digits and transplanted toes. A review. J Reconstr Microsurg 2:123—129, 1986.
132. Zachery RB, Holmes W: Primary suture of nerves. Surg Gynecol Obstet 82:632–651, 1946.
133. Highet WB, Sanders FK: The effects of stretching nerves after suture. Br J Surg 30:355, 1943.
134. Sanders FK: Histopathology of nerve grafts. In Seddon HJ, ed: Peripheral Nerve Injuries. Her Majesty's Printing Office, London, 1954, pp 134–155.
135. McEwan LE: Median and ulnar nerve injuries. Aust NZ J Surg 32:89–104, 1962.

136. Sakellarides H: A follow-up study of 173 peripheral nerve injuries of the upper extremity of civilians. J Bone Joint Surg 44A:140–148, 1962.
137. Nicholson OR, Seddon HJ: Nerve repair in civil practise. Br Med J 2:1065–1071, 1957.
138. Posch JL, delaCruz-Saddul F: Nerve repair in trauma surgery. A 10 year study of 231 peripheral injuries. Orthop Rev 9:35–45, 1980.
139. Dellon AL, Kallman CM: Evaluation of functional sensation in the hand. J Hand Surg 8:865–870, 1983.
140. Clinical Assessment Committee, American Society for Surgery of the Hand, Dean Louis, Chairman.
141. Moberg E: Objective methods for determining the functional value of sensibility in the skin. J Bone Joint Surg 40B:454–476, 1958.
142. Moberg E: Criticism in study of methods for examining sensibility in the hand. Neurology (Minneap) 12:8–19, 1962.
143. Kirklin JW, Murphy F, Berkson J: Suture of peripheral nerves. Factors affecting prognosis. Surg Gynecol Obstet 88:719–730, 1949.
144. Zachary RB: Results of nerve sutures. In Seddon HJ, ed: Peripheral Nerve Injuries. Her Majesty's Stationery Office, London, pp 334–388, 1954.
145. Yahr MD, Beebe GW: Recovery of motor function. In Seddon HJ, ed: Peripheral Nerve Regeneration. U.S. Government Printing Office, Washington, DC, 1956, pp 71–202.
146. Oester VT, Davis L: Recovery of sensory functions. In Woodhall B, Beebe GW, eds: Peripheral Nerve Regeneration. U.S. Government Printing Office, Washington, DC, 1956, pp 241–310.
147. Omer G: Injuries to nerves of the upper extremities. J Bone Joint Surg 56A:1615–1624, 1974.
148. Larsen RD, Posch JL: Nerve injuries in the upper extremity. Arch Surg 77:469–482, 1958.
149. Stromberg WB, McFarlane RM, Bell LL: Injury of the median and ulnar nerves. J Bone Joint Surg 43A:717–730, 1961.
150. Flynn JE, Flynn WF: Median and ulnar nerve injuries. Ann Surg 156:1002–1009, 1962.
151. Onne L: Recovery of sensibility in sudomotor activity in the hand after nerve suture. Acta Chir Scand (Suppl) 300:1–70, 1962.
152. Nielsen JB, Torup D: Nerve injuries in the upper extremities. Dan Med Bull 11:92–95, 1964.
153. Boswick JA, Schneewind J, Stromberg W: Evaluation of peripheral nerve repairs above the elbow. Arch Surg 90:50–51, 1965.
154. Seddon HJ: Surgical disorders of the peripheral nerves. Williams & Wilkins, Baltimore, 1972.
155. Merle M, Amend P, Cour C, Foucher G, Michon S: Microsurgical repair of peripheral nerve lesions: A study of 150 injuries of the median and ulnar nerves. Peripheral Nerve Repair Regeneration 2:17–26, 1986.
156. Bunnell S: Surgery of the nerves of the hand. Surg Gynecol Obstet 44:145–152, 1927.
157. Weckesser EC: The repair of nerves in the palm and the fingers. Clin Orthop 19:200–207, 1961.
158. Honner R, Fragiadakis FG, Lamb DW: An investigation of factors affecting the results of digital nerve division. Hand 2:21–31, 1970.
159. Buncke HJ: Digital nerve repairs, Surg Clin North Am 52:1267–1285, 1972.
160. Poppin NK, McCarroll HR Jr, Doyle JR, et al: Recovery of sensibility of the sutured digital nerves. J Hand Surg 4:212–226, 1979.
161. Young L, Wray RC, Weeks PM: A randomized prospective comparison of fascicular and epineural digital nerve repairs. Plast Reconstr Surg 68:89–92, 1981.
162. Seddon HJ: The use of autogenous grafts for repair of large gaps in peripheral nerves. Br J Surg 35:151–167, 1947.
163. Brooks D: The place of nerve grafting in orthopedic surgery. J Bone Joint Surg 37A:299–326, 1955.
164. McFarlane RM, Moyer JR: Digital nerve grafts with the lateral antebrachial cutaneous nerve. J Hand Surg 1:169–173, 1976.
165. Young VL, Wray CR, Weeks PM: The results of nerve grafting in the wrist and hand. Ann Plast Surg 5:212–215, 1980.
166. Rose EH, Kowalski TA: Vascularized nerve grafts in the dorsum of the foot. J Hand Surg [Am] 10:514–521, 1985.
167. Beazley RW, Milek MA, Reiss BH: Results of nerve grafting in severe soft tissue injuries. Clin Orthop 188:208–212, 1984.
168. Rose EH, Kowalski TA, Norris MS: The reversed venous arterialized nerve graft in digital nerve reconstruction across scarred beds. Plast Reconstr Surg 1988. In press.
169. Wilgis EFS, Maxwell GP: Distal digital nerve grafts: Clinical and anatomical studies. J Hand Surg 4:439–443, 1979.
170. Mackinnon SE: Sensibility recovery across digital nerve grafts. 1988. In preparation.
171. Hoase J, Bjerre P, Simesen K: Median and ulnar nerve transections treated with microsurgical interfascicular cable grafting with autogenous sural nerve. J Neurosurg 53:73–84, 1980.
172. Yamano Y: Electrophysiological study of nerve grafting. J Hand Surg 7:588–592, 1982.
173. Millesi H, Meissl G, Berger A: The interfascicular nerve grafting of the median and ulnar nerves. J Bone Joint Surg 54A:727–750, 1972.
174. Millesi H, Meissl G, Berger A: Further experience with interfascicular grafting of the median, ulnar and radial nerves. J Bone Joint Surg 58A:29–118, 1976.
175. Bunnell S, Boyes JH: Nerve grafts. Am J Surg 44:64–75, 1939.
176. Walton R, Finseth F: Nerve grafting in the repair of complicated peripheral nerve trauma. J Trauma 17:793–796, 1977.
177. Tallas R, Staniforth P, Fisher TR: Neurophysiological studies of autogenous nerve grafts. J Neurol Neurosurg Psychiatry 41:677–683, 1978.
178. Brown PW: The time factor in surgery of upper extremity peripheral nerve injury. Clin Orthop 68:14, 1970.
179. Young MC, Richards RR, Hudson AR: The results of surgical treatment of posterior interosseous nerve palsy. J Bone Joint Surg 1988. In press.

180. Seddon HJ: Peripheral nerve injuries. Medical Research Council, Special Report Series 282, Her Majesty's Stationery Office, London, 1954.
181. Millesi H: Lower extremity nerve lesions. In Terzis JK, ed: Microreconstruction of Nerve Injuries, WB Saunders Philadelphia, 1987, pp 239–251.
182. Chen ZW, Yu HL: Lower limb replantation. In Urbaniak JR, ed: Microsurgery for Major Limb Reconstruction, CV Mosby, St. Louis, 1987, pp 67–73.
183. Kline DG: Operative experience with major lower extremity nerve lesions including the lumbosacral plexus and the sciatic nerve. In Omer G, Spinner M, eds.: Management of Peripheral Nerve Problems. WB Saunders, Philadelphia, 1980, pp 607–625.
184. Clawson DK, Seddon HJ: The results of repair of the sciatic nerve. J Bone Joint Surg 42B:205, 1960.
185. Clawson DK, Seddon HJ: The late consequences of sciatic nerve injury. J Bone Joint Surg 42B:213, 1960.
186. MacCarty CS: Two stage autograft for repair of extensive damage to the sciatic nerve. J Neurosurg 8:319, 1951.
187. White J: The results of traction injuries to the common peroneal nerve. J Bone Joint Surg 40B:346, 1968.
188. Mackinnon SE, Dellon AL: Nerve grafting in the lower extremity. 1990. In preparation.
189. Mackinnon SE, Dellon AL: Pain after radial sensory nerve grafting. J Hand Surg [Br] 11:334–341, 1986.
190. Yamano Y, Namba Y, Hino Y, et al: Digital nerve grafts in replanted digits. Hand 4:255–262, 1982.
191. Mailander P, Berger A, Schaller E, Ruhek. Results of primary nerve repair in the upper extremity. Miscrosurg 10:147—150, 1989.

Internal Neurolysis

5

The endoneurolysis consists in separating the fascicles of the nerve from ... the endoneurial cicatrix. The separating of the bundles of a normal nerve is easy over a short distance, but for a longer distance is not possible without injuring an inner plexus.... To separate a fascicle within the nerve from the cicatrix, it is necessary first to separate the nerve fibers above the cicatrix. One splits the neurilemma and fixes it with a fine clamp. One isolates with a small scalpel the individual fascicles which can be seen within the nerve. After a large fascicle is free in one place, one introduces a small hook and it becomes easy to follow this fascicle in the direction of the cicatrix and to free it. In a similar manner, one proceeds distally within the nerve. If the endoneurial growth is not too rough, one can free individual fascicles and remove the cicatrix. The tighter the cicatrix, the more laborious is the work and the more imperfect is the success. One can make this task easier in wetting the nerve with saline.... The neurolysis is therefore quite appropriate in traumatic neuralgia (pressure from cicatrix and callus) and in inflammatory perineuritis, and in the case of neuritis following gunshot wounds.

Lehmann, 1936[1]

Historical Review

Perhaps no subject within the field of peripheral nerve surgery remains as controversial as internal neurolysis. The causes for the controversy are: (1) conflicting results from the few studies that have attempted to investigate internal neurolysis; (2) various hypotheses regarding the pathophysiologic characteristics of nerve compression; (3) lack of an experimental model of nerve compression with which to test these hypotheses; and (4) anecdotal accounts of dangers of internal neurolysis. Babcock in 1907[2] and again in 1927[3] discussed his concept that it would be valuable to open the thickened nerve sheath in a compressed nerve to permit the escape of fluid, thereby reducing the internal pressure within the nerve. His technique included splitting the nerve sheath and separation of the bundles. He termed his procedure "hersage" to emphasize his technique of "combing" the nerve fascicles. The first clear description of an internal neurolysis that approaches the concepts that will be employed in this chapter is that by Lehmann in his chapter in the text, *Allgemeine Thera-*

pie, published in German in 1936. It is clear from Lehmann's description of his surgical technique that in the degree of nerve pathologic alterations that were severe and that would require an internal neurolysis, there was intraneural fibrosis. His technique emphasized meticulous intraneural neurolysis. His writing simply was a description of a technique without reference to its clinical effectiveness. The concept of internal neurolysis implies there is scarring within the nerve that requires release. The first description of which we are aware that this pathologic condition does occur was in a case report described by John B. Murphy in 1916[4] in which he reported what we would now term an "anterior subcutaneous ulnar nerve transposition." That patient had developed a post-traumatic ulnar "neuritis" and Murphy states "the nerve having been removed from the source of irritation, the connective tissue which is formed within it was allowed to remain." Thus, although expressing the concept that, in the pathophysiologic changes of nerve trauma, intraneural fibrosis will occur, Murphy, at the same time, initiated the controversy as to whether or not that fibrosis can resolve without an operative procedure within the nerve. The next brief mention of the occurrence of intraneural fibrosis with severe nerve compression is made by Stopford in 1926[5] in describing progressive changes that occur with increasing severity of nerve compression. No histologic substantiation of this was offered nor suggestion for treatment made. The first histologic investigations to suggest that severe nerve compression results in intraneural fibrosis were the observations by Marie and Foix,[6] described in 1913, on a postmortem median nerve specimen. This report contained no photomicrographs for histologic documentation.[6] The first published histologic confirmation of intraneural fibrosis was in the postmortem evaluation of a median nerve from the carpal tunnel reported by Thomas and Fuller in 1963.[7] Beginning in 1961, Raymond M. Curtis, one of the founding members of The American Society for Surgery of the Hand, began to use internal neurolysis in the treatment of severe carpal tunnel syndrome. His observation had been that a significant number of patients failed to get excellent results by simple decompression of the median nerve. He used a modification of the technique described by Babcock. His indications for doing an internal neurolysis as an adjunct to the treatment of carpal tunnel syndrome were for patients with: (1) constant sensory loss; (2) abnormal (static) two-point discrimination; (3) thenar atrophy; or (4) failure to improve after previous division of the transverse carpal ligament. It is clear from his writing that abnormal two-point discrimination was an indication for internal neurolysis, although he did not define the degree to which this test needed to be abnormal. His report of the internal neurolysis of 101 hands in 83 patients represents the first large clinical series with careful preoperative testing of the patients. The results of his treatment indicated that 72% of the patients who had abnormal motor signs and symptoms before surgery had a return to normal of thenar muscle function, with an additional 23% demonstrating improvement in function. Only two patients were unimproved after this surgery. Of the 95 patients in his series who had abnormal sensory signs and symptoms before the internal neurolysis, 89 had a return to normal or near-normal sensation, with just 5% of the cases remaining with less than normal two-point discrimination. One patient had a complication of a "disabling shoulder-hand syndrome." The published photomicrographs and his description of the operative technique indicated that the epineurium was opened and the degree of intraneural dissection varied according to the pathologic findings, with the dissection, however, not going completely through to the posterior aspect of the nerve. Preserving the posterior epineurium was an attempt to preserve "whatever vascular supply" came through this "mesoneurium." The dissection was continued until there was clear identification of the different fascicles and the intraneural fibrosis was excised from within the nerve.[8]

The publication of the report by Curtis and Eversmann[8] in 1973 represents the transition in the history of internal neurolysis to attempted clinical and experimental investigations with this technique. Because of the concerns that this degree of intraneural dissection would create more scarring and result in worsening of the clinical situation, there was a great reluctance by surgeons to accept this technique. The first basic investigation of the response of a peripheral nerve to an internal neurolysis came from the laboratory of Gören Lundborg in 1976. Lundborg, in the introduction to his work, states: "Internal neurolysis per se implies a significant trauma to the nerve which may induce microvascular damage and formation of new intraneural scar tissue. Such a procedure, therefore, appears justified only when the preoperative intraneural fibrosis is more severe than the scarring which might be induced by the surgical procedure."[9] The results of that study indicated "an experimental internal neurolysis per se may induce fibrosis in all layers of the nerve and may cause some nerve fiber damage. However the barrier function of the perineurium and the endoneurial vessels seems to be generally well preserved." It must be emphasized that this research work utilized an internal neurolysis on a normal rabbit tibial nerve. This work from Lundborg's laboratory proceeded with the evaluation of intraneural blood flow.[10] This study demonstrated the intrinsic vascularization of human peripheral nerves and the discussion of the anatomic demonstration of the intraneural blood flow pattern emphasized "that intraneural dissection produces considerable trauma to the nerve and an inflammatory reaction in extrafascicular layers." However, it must be emphasized that this latter research article did not include any additional new experimental work on intraneural dissection. The only other basic experimental study currently available for evaluation is that from Alan Hudson's group. This report in 1981 carried out internal neurolysis in normal rat sciatic nerves. This study was similar to that carried out by Lundborg in terms of the comprehensive evaluation of neurophysiologic and morphologic effects on the nerve. Hudson and colleagues concluded: "The results of this study indicate that under the circumstances of this experiment, it is possible to perform internal neurolysis without producing any significant long lasting morphological or physiological alterations in a peripheral nerve. The tissues must be handled very gently in order to avoid damage to the larger myelinated fibers at the periphery of the fascicle. The crucial maneuver, however, is that of preservation of the perineurium. With experience, the use of magnification and modern microsurgical technique, this can be accomplished relatively easily."[11] Thus, the only two experimental studies on internal neurolysis were conducted in normal nerves and came to opposite conclusions. It is not surprising therefore that in a guest editorial in 1981, George Phalen, the "father of the carpal tunnel syndrome," stated "with the advent of microsurgery, some hand surgeons are advocating internal neurolysis of the median nerve as a routine part of every operation for carpal tunnel syndrome. Such advice courts disaster. Although the immediate result may be good, the later inevitable interfascicular scarring can produce irreparable damage to the median nerve."[12]

The next stage had to await the development of satisfactory models for chronic nerve compression. This subject was reviewed in an earlier chapter. The presently available models for chronic nerve compression in the rat sciatic nerve[13] and the primate median nerve[14] have been successful in producing a model that allows the evaluation of the intraneural changes. These changes demonstrate progressive inter- and extrafascicular epineurial fibrosis and perineurial thickening. These studies suggested that such interfascicular epineurial fibrosis can serve as the appropriate plane for an intraneural dissection in these chronically compressed nerves (Fig. 5-1). Utilizing this experimental model for chronic nerve compression, the most recent study has demonstrated that after 6 months of median nerve compression at the wrist, when either decompression of the median nerve alone is carried out versus decompression plus microsurgical internal neurolysis of the median nerve, there is no significant neurophysiologic or morphometric difference between the nerves in the two treatment groups at 6 months after the operative procedure.[15] In particular, the internal neurolysis procedure did not produce scarring within the nerve (Fig. 5-2).

The most recent work involving models using chronic peripheral nerve compression have documented that a histologic basis exists for an intraneural dissection, that this basis is the interfascicular epineurial fibrosis, and that, if this dissection is done without disruption of the perineurium and after 6 months of postoperative healing, the procedure of internal neurolysis has not produced a worsening of scarring in or about the nerve.

Clinical acceptance of internal neurolysis has been confounded by the absence of well-defined staging systems for chronic nerve compression. This problem becomes apparent from recent writings about the carpal tunnel syndrome. For example, one report suggests 93% "satisfactory results" may be obtained at 6 months after surgery, without any "complications," by simple division of the transverse carpal ligament.[16] These results are in marked contrast to other reports that suggest a much higher failure rate, but they may be better understood by considering the patients selected for this outpatient local anesthesia procedure, that is, by clinical staging. These patients were symptomatic from median nerve compression but had no thenar muscle atrophy present. They were in an "early stage" and were not patients who "might require internal neurolysis."[16] Another report attempted to treat patients with carpal tunnel on a prospective basis, randomizing them between simple decompression of the nerve alone and decompression plus cortisone injection and external neurolysis.[17] This report concluded that there was no difference in the results obtained by either of these treatment methods. The report had very comparable distribution of patients, 11 in each group, but within each group the patients ranged from those who had sensory symptoms alone to those who had thenar atrophy, that is, the groups were not homogenous by clinical staging.[17]

A similar attempt to define on a prospective basis the value of steroid injection and splinting in the carpal tunnel syndrome was made in 50 patients. The average period of follow-up was 15 months. The group of patients studied comprised the full spectrum of those who had symptoms only, an "early stage," to those with abnormal two-point discrimination and thenar atrophy, a "severe stage." The conclusion of that study was that "hands with severe symptoms of more than one year duration and findings of atrophy, weakness and distal motor latencies of more than six milliseconds, or absent sensory responses had the poorest response to injections and experienced a high rate of relapse."[18] These most recent studies by good investigators suggest variations in response, depending on the degree of severity of the clinical problem.

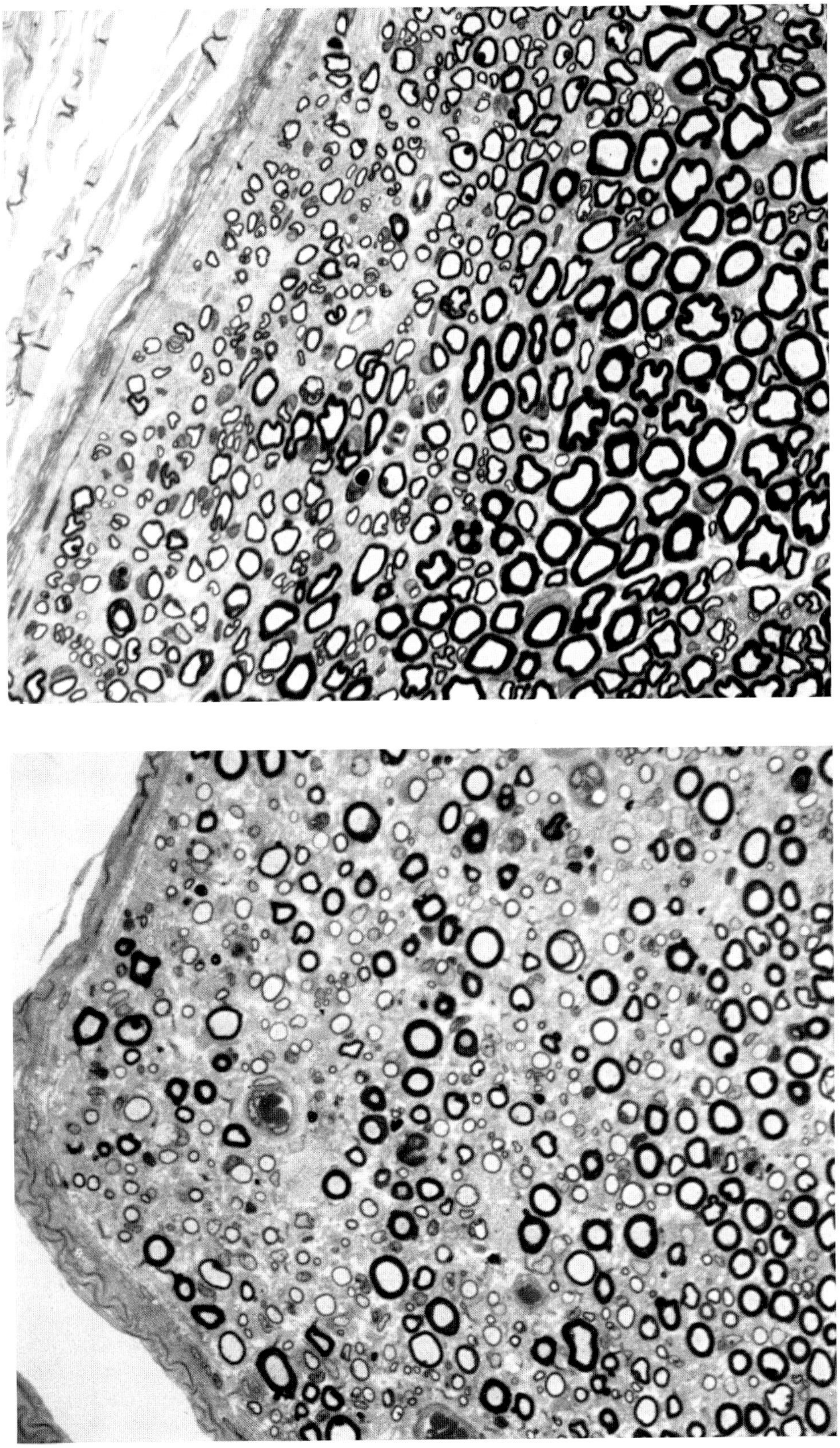

a

b

Figure 5-1. Morphometric changes in rat sciatic nerve with increasing duration of a mild degree of compression. Note increased thickness of the perineurium and of extrafascicular epineurium. After 4 months (a) and 6 months (b) of compression. (Toluidine blue ×345.) (Reproduced with permission from Mackinnon et al.[13]) (*Figure continues.*)

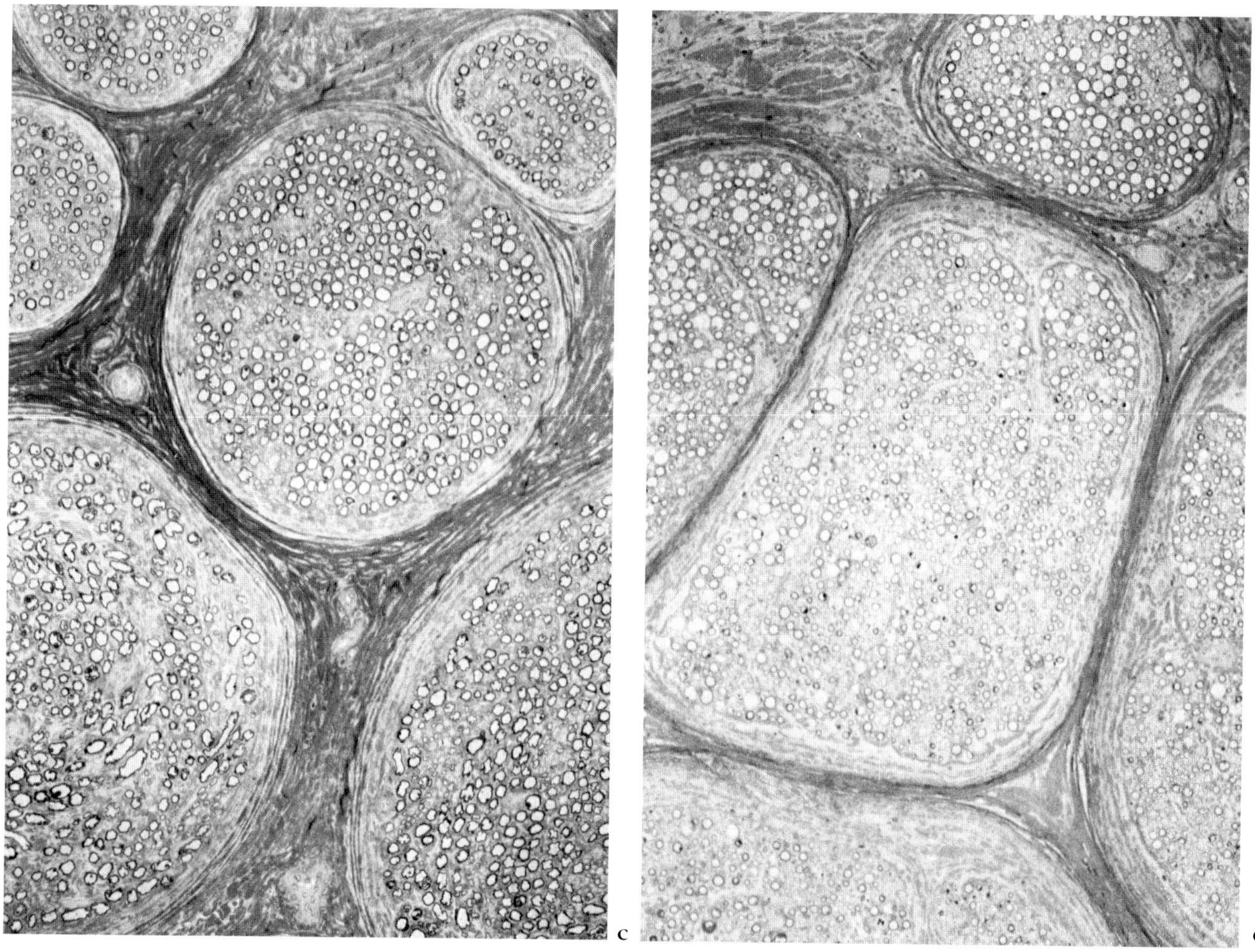

c d

Figure 5-1. *(continued)* In the monkey, note that the area of interfascicular epineurial fibrosis and thickening (c) is the plane for intraneural dissection. With severe chronic compression (d), loss of intrafascicular volume due to demyelination and axonal degeneration result in attenuation of this interfascicular plane, increasing the need for gentleness during the internal neurolysis. (Toluidine blue, ×137.) (Reproduced with permission from Mackinnon et al. [14]).

Once the pathophysiologic changes of a disease process are understood, the condition may be clinically staged and treatment varied according to the degree of severity. These most recent studies suggest that we are approaching this basis in our understanding of nerve compression syndromes. Nevertheless, an acceptable staging system has not been universally accepted. This will become essential if new forms of treatment or even old forms of treatment are to receive appropriate study. For example, the recent work with the effects of pyridoxine and carpal tunnel syndrome[19] represents a perfect example of a new therapeutic approach that will require careful staging of the patients entered into the study if the results are to be appropriately understood. Clinical staging will eliminate the confusion that has led multiple surgical procedures for the same disease currently championed by different training centers or "authorities."

This is the exact situation that exists today with multiple forms of treatment for ulnar nerve entrapment at the elbow. Thus, there is still controversy as to whether simple decompression of the ulnar nerve is suitable or whether the nerve should be transposed anteriorly and then located either subcutaneously, intramuscularly, or submuscularly. Most of the articles addressing this question have not attempted to stage the degree of severity of the nerve compression. The first article to attempt to stage ulnar nerve compression at

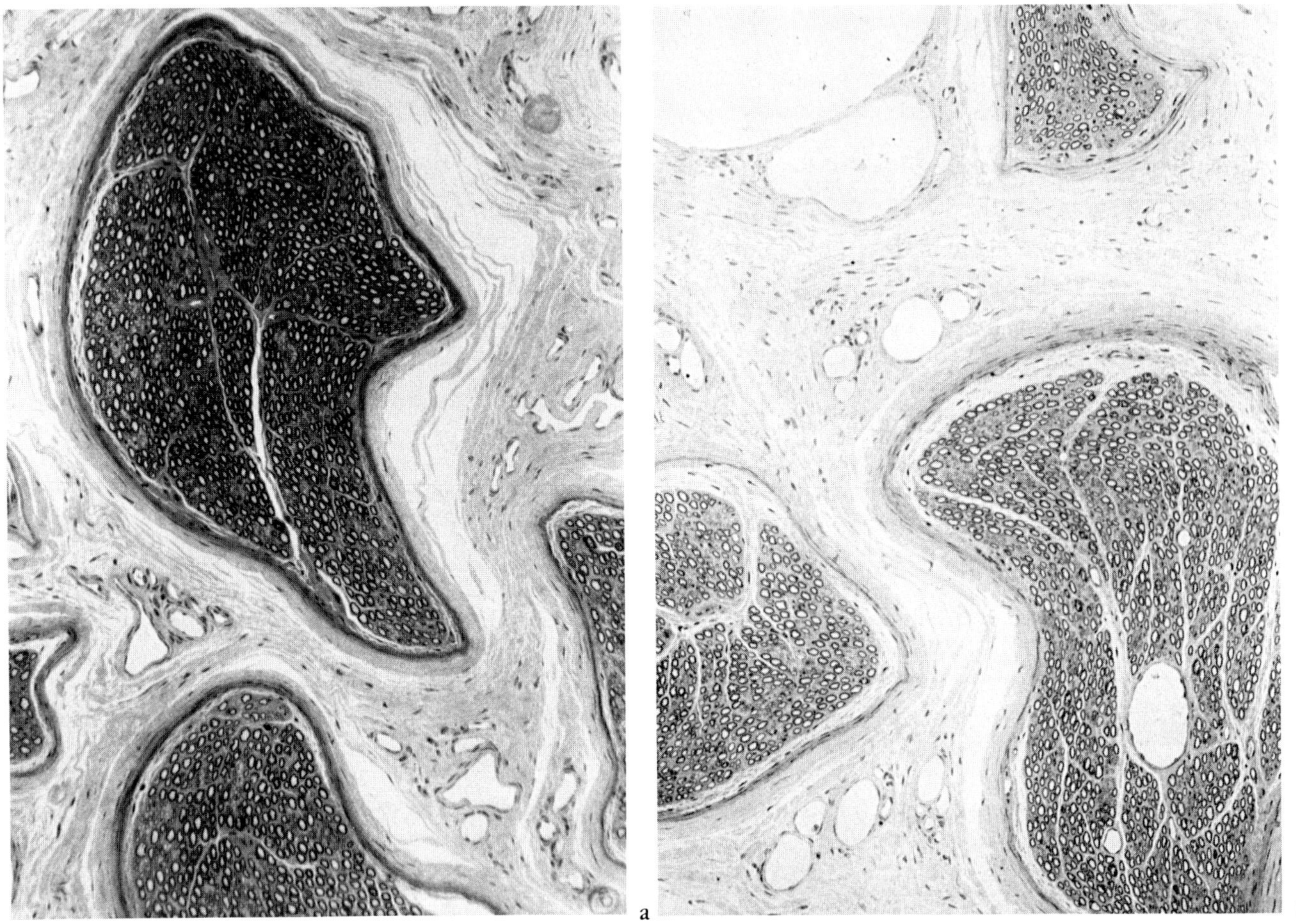

Figure 5-2. No difference in degree of interfascicular scarring was noted 6 months after treatment of chronic median nerve entrapment at the wrist in a monkey group treated by surgical decompression alone (a) versus decompression plus internal neurolysis (b). (Toluidine blue transverse section, ×137.) (Reproduced with permission from Mackinnon et al.[14]).

the elbow is that by McGowan,[20] and this staging system only included changes in motor function. Recently, it has become appreciated that attempts to determine the result of ulnar nerve treatment must be related to the preoperative situation of both the patient's sensory and motor ulnar nerve status.[21]

An attempt to stage peripheral nerve compression that is related to potential surgical choices has been proposed.[22,23] This system would define an early stage in nerve compression that would manifest itself by clinical symptoms due to either the motor or sensory system in terms of paresthesias, pain, weakness, or lack of coordinated muscle function. At this stage, there are few positive clinical signs. However, provocative tests, such as Phalen's sign or the elbow flexion test, are positive. The most commonly positive clinical test would be an increased response to vibratory testing. This group of patients would be treated by nonoperative measures. The intermediate stage in nerve compression would be patients who have progressed to the point where clinical signs include further motor weakness, diminished perception of vibratory stimulus, and abnormal cutaneous vibratory or pressure thresholds. This group of patients, if not previously treated, would enter a nonoperative regimen of treatment or if they were patients who had progressed to this stage and no longer wished to continue with the nonoperative approach would become surgical candidates for simple decompression alone or cortisone injection into the carpal tunnel alone. The severe or advanced group would be those who have persistent sensory changes and either muscle atrophy or abnormal two-point discrimination. Either of these three situations suggests the presence of intraneural fibrosis and the presence of muscle atrophy or abnormal two-point discrimination suggests actual axonal loss. These situations imply a pathophysiologic situation that may not be reversible by simple decompression alone.

Review of the Literature

The subject of internal neurolysis is complicated by the lack of standardization of terminology used to describe operations on nerves. Thus, a review of the literature on neurolysis indicates a wide variety of operations performed on a wide variety of nerves. However, the majority of these reports do not deal with internal neurolysis. Although only in an anecdotal fashion, the first mention of internal neurolysis in ulnar nerve surgery was by Adson[24] in 1918. Adson describes an anterior transposition in which the nerve was placed into an intramuscular groove and a fascical sling was created to hold it in place. However, he clearly adds that "if judging from the neurologic findings the patient has complete or three-fourths paralysis of the ulnar nerve, complete resection of the diseased portion of the nerve with anastamosis of the severed ends are advised, but if the paralysis is less than half, instead of resection, we advise the longitudinal splitting of the epineurium and perineurium in several places about the nerve in order to liberate the columns of nerve fibers from the contracting scars".[24] As is apparent from the previous discussions of the normal anatomy (Chapter 1), "splitting of the perineurium" is not considered today as part of an internal neurolysis, as Adson had suggested. In 1975, there is a mention by Lluch,[25] in his case report, that "an endoneurolysis revealed intact funicular continuity with moderate proximal pseudoneuroma formation." In an article that attempted to discuss the results of cubital tunnel decompression alone versus anterior subcutaneous transposition alone, it was specifically mentioned that "an epineurotomy was not done but an epineurotomy with an internal neurolysis was done if intraneural fibrosis was noted." However, it is unclear from their patient list or statistics what percent of the patients in their series were considered to have intraneural fibrosis present.[21] For example, one of the earliest descriptions of the use of neurolysis is that given by Platt[26] in 1928 in his description for an intramuscular transposition of the ulnar nerve: "where there is incongruity between the nerve and its bed, an ideal neurolysis is available, the operation of anterior transposition in which the nerve is displaced to the front of the elbow and implanted in a new bed". The extensive article on ulnar nerve compression at the elbow by Wadsworth[27] in 1977 described "neurolysis" of the ulnar nerve, and again it is clear that what is meant is movement of the nerve from its bed and an anterior transposition, although in one place within the text he indicates that "neurolysis, together with intraneural injection of saline and perineural injection of hydrocortisone, produced minimal improvement in (patients with advanced) palsy." There is no statistical analysis or a number of patients mentioned that had had an external neurolysis versus those who had had additional work done inside the nerve, as his latter phrase suggests.[27] The same use of the term "neurolysis" with respect to ulnar nerve surgery continues into the 1980s.[28] The term neurolysis as it is most commonly utilized is synonymous with an external neurolysis. In each case in which the ulnar nerve is transposed anteriorly, it must be separated from any scarring along the course of the postcondylar groove and therefore an external neurolysis of the ulnar nerve also becomes synonymous with any form of anterior transposition of the ulnar nerve. Indeed, it is difficult to do an anterior transposition of the ulnar nerve without doing an external neurolysis of the ulnar nerve. The only specific distinction made in the writings about ulnar nerve surgery at the elbow with respect to forms of neurolysis is that by Leffert.[29] In his series of 15 patients operated on for recurrent or persistent ulnar nerve entrapment at the elbow, he specifically makes the point that "in all cases where there was significant scarring or opacity of the epineurium, an external neurolysis and epineurectomy was carried out. In no case was an internal neurolysis done." As will be discussed later, an epineurectomy may be considered as the first part of an internal neurolysis. Nevertheless, it may be stated that at the present time there is no series of ulnar nerve patients in the literature for whom internal neurolysis has either been reported or suggested as the appropriate treatment.

An area in which there remains controversy but in which the distinction between external and internal neurolysis is clearly made in the literature relates to drug injection injuries. Among the earliest writings are those regarding injection injury of the sciatic nerve. In 1950, Matson[30] reported on two patients with drug injection injuries. In the first case operated on in 1948, an external neurolysis of the sciatic nerve was clearly done, based on the operative description given: "Thorough neurolysis of the involved area was carried out. There was no neuroma formation or evidence of division of any part of the nerve." This patient recovered partially. His second patient was a 2-year-old girl with drug injection injury to the sciatic nerve, which was operated on in August of 1948. Matson noticed that "after the nerve had been mobilized from the surrounding reaction (scar tissue), it was apparent that the same type of fibrosis was present within the neurilemmal sheath itself. The sheath was therefore split longitudinally and the peroneal and tibial components of the nerves separated. The sheaths around these separate bundles also appeared fibrotic and they, in turn, were split longitudinally together with the sheath of the nerves of the short head of the biceps femoris. All areas of constriction were divided in such a manner as to preserve the integrity of the axons." This child by 13 months after surgery had no measurable muscle atrophy and no demonstrable weakness. The child carried out all activities requiring the use of the leg in a normal manner. Matson's conclusion was that "if there is not progressive evidence of improvement in paralysis incident to a faulty intramuscular injection, exploration of the involved nerve, accompanied by a thorough neurolysis, should be performed without further delay."[30] This report suggests the meaning of the term, "neurolysis," as we will use it, which is that the intraneural dissection is carried out until a good fascicular pattern is present. We use this as an operational definition.

The classic description by French[31] clearly describes the pathologic condition found in 16 cases of injection injury to the sciatic nerve in children. The observations made in that study attempted to discriminate between two categories of patients, those with and those without perineural adhesions. French indicated that there were three objections to early "neurolysis." One-third of the patients recovered completely after drug injection injuries in periods ranging from 24 hours to 13 months. However, in the early stages they could not determine those patients who would not require "neurolysis" from those who might potentially benefit from it. He noted that in experimental animals, much of the neurologic sequelae of drug injection injuries was attributed to axonal degeneration and "intraneural scarring as well as to extraneural scar formation. Neurolysis affects only the removal of extraneural scar tissue." It was also his opinion that the ischemic nerve does not necessarily undergo axonal degeneration unless it is manipulated. Thus, French believed that intraneural dissection might hasten axonal degeneration due to manipulation of the nerve and that intraneural neurolysis would not be able to remove the intraneural scarring caused by the drug injection injury.[31] Thus, the report by French, who was in the Department of Pediatrics and Division of Neurology, and not a neurosurgeon as Matson was, came to a different conclusion about the treatment of the sciatic nerve injuries and suggested limitations on the ability of intraneural neurolysis to effect removal of scar tissue. However, French's final conclusion was that in cases in which palpable granulomas existed along the course of the sciatic nerve after injury the nerve should be explored and a neurolysis, an external neurolysis, carried out.

With further understanding of drug injection injury mechanisms, it became clear that the histopathologic findings could include not just intraneural fibrosis but actually the formation of a neuroma in-continuity. Thus, subsequent writing has suggested that: "At operation the surgeon has three options: neurolysis, resection and suture, or a combination of neurolysis with intent to reoperate and resect if no recovery occurs in a stated period of time."[32] These investigators suggested that once the nerve was exposed, it should be inspected under magnification, such as an operating microscope, and that "this affords much greater opportunity to inspect the damage and is helpful in the dissection in the rare instances when internal neurolysis is done. Stimulating and recording equipment capable of measuring evoked responses in the nerve is also required."[32] In contrast to these investigators, internal neurolysis in the treatment of peripheral nerve injuries has been enthusiastically supported by Brown.[33] Brown's belief with respect to drug injection injuries is that there may be a "high price to pay" for waiting for the nerve to undergo spontaneous recovery. This price being paid in terms of changes in muscle, motor end plate, joints, and in the skin, changes that can become irreversible. Brown's writing has artist drawings that clearly show a stepwise approach to internal neurolysis beginning with saline injection into the subepineurial layer and then a stepwise lysis of internal fibrosis until individual fascicles are clearly seen. "Dissection is carried down between the nerve bundles and the scarred epineural. The perineurial expansions are further opened to give as much freedom as possible to nerve bundles." Postoperatively, he emphasizes that "gentle motion of the extremity is started at once and is gradually increased in order to avoid, insofar as possible, adherence of the nerves to underlying tissues." He states that "the old concept of neurolysis, i.e., merely freeing a nerve from the surrounding scar, was inadequate to release the axons and nerve bundles from the intrinsic scar which follows trauma." Although Brown does not indicate any specific numbers of patients he has treated, his conclusion is that "neurolysis is indicated when no motor or sensory recovery is evident within four to six weeks after injury. The technique of internal neurolysis requires gentle handling of nerve tissues with the aid of magnification methods and special instruments. The results in 35 years of experience with these problems has been most rewarding. Hospital stay is brief, the risks are slight and we have never seen a patient worsened by the procedure."

Subsequent experimental studies with local anesthetic agents[34] and steroids[35] have continued to delineate the pathologic characteristics of nerve injection injuries. When the injuries are produced, intraneural fibrosis does occur and the lesions should be considered as a neuroma in-continuity. It becomes clear then that the present approach to surgery for nerve injection injuries may require intraneural dissection, and the appropriate guidelines for this will require intraoperative electrodiagnostic recording techniques that have been clearly outlined by Kline and colleagues[36,37] and Terzis and colleagues.[38,39] Among the few other reports that discuss neurolysis is the extensive series of 917 war injuries to nerves of the upper extremities described by

Omer in 1974.[40] Among those patients, "neurolysis" was performed in 59 cases in which the injured nerve was found in-continuity but bound in fibrous scar. Neurolysis was successful in 60% of the cases that were adequately followed. It is clear from this description that the term "neurolysis" as used is an external neurolysis and a description of the value of internal neurolysis in these patients was not discussed. Similarly, the most recent article, entitled "Axillary Nerve Injuries—21 Cases Treated by Nerve Graft and Neurolysis,"[41] is primarily a description of external neurolysis carried out within the brachial plexus. "If the nerve appears only compressed by scar tissue once the mobilization is complete is sufficient to effect an accurate microsurgical neurolysis." However, a more extensive description of the use of neurolysis in brachial plexus is suggested by Clodius et al[42] in their description of the treatment of irradiation plexitis of the brachial plexus. Another nerve that has been operated on and the term "neurolysis" used has been the facial nerve.[43–45] These have been carried out in patients with hemifacial spasm and the techniques again are more consistent with an external neurolysis. The only peripheral nerve for which literature exists with regard to the use of internal neurolysis is the median nerve at the wrist.

Following the description by Curtis and Eversmann in 1973[8] with their indications for internal neurolysis and the excellent results with just one complication in 101 hands, their technique was taken up first in the German-speaking countries. Samii[46] reported internal neurolyses done in 51 patients for carpal tunnel syndrome in whom there was muscle atrophy and loss of sensibility. He indicated "in almost all instances, it was possible to nearly repair the sensory and the motor function. The previously existing atrophy of the thenar muscles could not be found anymore in almost all instances."[46] Gassmann et al,[47] whose study was published in 1977, utilized Curtis' criteria for doing the internal neurolysis and reported on a series of 72 patients. Forty-two of these were treated by simple decompression, 19 were treated by decompression and an external neurolysis. Eleven patients were treated by an internal neurolysis. Their results were carefully analyzed according to preoperative problems. They found that decompression alone or decompression and external neurolysis did not cause reversal of muscle atrophy in any of the seven patients in whom it was done. However, internal neurolysis caused reversal of muscle atrophy in six of the seven patients in whom it was done. They had no postoperative complications related to the internal neurolysis per se. In addition to their internal neurolysis technique, they resected the palmaris longus tendon to prevent its pressure across the median nerve and they also released the ulnar nerve in Guyon's canal "prophylactically." They examined the excised epineurial tissues and found them to contain significant fibrosis. It was their belief that leaving this tissue would result in an abnormal compressive force about the fascicles and that resection of this pathologically changed tissue was indicated. "The pathologically changed and augmented interfascicular connective tissue is resected with a microsurgical technique so that the fascicles which are very thin and rolled out because of the massive compression lie loosely and next to each other. Where patients had abnormal nerve conduction studies beforehand, all of these were improved postoperatively."[47] They concluded that "our results after epineurial and interfascicular neurolysis are so far encouraging and seem to justify this extensive intervention in carpal tunnel syndrome where there is long-lasting loss of sensitivity and/or thenar atrophy."[47]

In another series of patients reported by Eversmann and Ritsick[48] in which before and after carpal tunnel release nerve conduction studies were measured intraoperatively, there were seven patients who had an internal neurolysis according to the criteria and methods reported by Curtis and Eversmann. Of interest in the intraoperative recordings was that in these severe cases, release of the transverse carpal alone did not result in improvement in the intraoperative nerve conduction recordings. Five of the seven patients had values of the intraoperative nerve conduction recordings improve within 15 minutes after the internal neurolysis.

Another article reporting different surgical techniques in a different series of patients included three patients in whom an internal neurolysis was done.[49] Their indication for this was that at surgery the sheath appeared thickened. However, it could not be ascertained by their analysis how this particular group of patients did with respect to other patients in the series. They did have one case of "Sudeck's syndrome" result in their total series of 95 patients, and this was in one of the three cases in whom the internal neurolysis was done. In a series of patients reported by Hoehn,[50] internal neurolysis was used in all patients, irrespective of their presenting symptoms, and the nerve conduction studies were compared before and after in 23 hands. Twenty-one of the 23 had improvement in the nerve conduction study after surgery. There were no postoperative complications. In another series of patients in whom Curtis' indications were utilized, namely, "constant sensory loss and/or palsy or thenar atrophy," and for whom there was a postoperative follow-up of at least 6 months, there was restored or improved sensory or motor function in more than 90% of the 50 patients operated on with internal neurolysis.[51] No complications from the technique were reported. A recent report, again utilizing Curtis' indications for surgery and Curtis' technique, with internal neurolysis being done through only the volar 50% of the nerve, reported 76%

of 36 hands recovering sensation or muscle strength.[52] No complications from the procedure were recorded. The conclusion was that "internal neurolysis, if done by a surgeon educated in microsurgery, is recommended as a safe and effective procedure in patients with severe carpal tunnel syndrome."

One of the most enthusiastic supporters of internal neurolysis has been Hanno Millesi, Professor of Plastic Surgery in Vienna. His first publication[53] on internal neurolysis in 1975 shortly followed that of Curtis and Eversmann. His approach, which is very similar technically to the one we use, was presented at the Combined Austrian and Swiss Plastic Surgery Meeting in 1981 at Innsbruck, at a plastic surgery symposium in Anaheim, California in 1981, in 1982 at a course on microsurgery in Oklahoma City, in 1983 at a similar course in Toronto, and appears carefully worked in a recent book chapter.[54] Millesi's concept of intraneural fibrosis and the need for intraneural neurolysis is identical to our own. His technique differs only in that he deflates the pneumatic tourniquet and observes the changes in the nerve before proceeding with internal neurolysis. If the compressed nerve expands sufficiently after tourniquet deflation, then he does not proceed.

Surgical Technique

The operative technique used for internal neurolysis of a nerve is based on the concept that injury to the nerve produces fibrosis within the connective tissue components of the nerve. For the epineurium, this means a thickening in the extrafascicular as well as the interfascicular epineurium (Fig. 5-1). The perineurium is thickened. There may also be endoneurial fibrosis. With the concept that the perineurium provides and maintains a special internal milieu for the individual nerve fibers within the fascicle, the operative technique may not breach or injure the perineurium. Therefore the operative technique becomes one of removing the extrafascicular epineurial fibrosis and separating the fascicles from the interfascicular epineurial fibrosis. Since the degree of intraneural fibrosis varies depending on the extent of the nerve injury, it follows that the extent to which an intraneural neurolysis is required will vary correspondingly. Therefore it follows that the definition of how much of an intraneural resection is done in an internal neurolysis is an operational definition, which is to say that the intraneural neurolysis is continued until there is a good fascicular pattern present and ideally the perineurial markings on each fascicle are apparent (Figs. 5-1 through 5-7).

The operation is begun for any given nerve by surgically approaching the nerve through the ideal surgical exposure. (You are referred to the appropriate chapters for each individual nerve with respect to the surgical approach to the nerve itself.) After the nerve has been identified and appropriately freed from corresponding external compressive forces, that is, flexor tenosynovitis in the transverse carpal ligament in the carpal tunnel or the roof of the cubital tunnel and scarring in the postcondylar groove for the ulnar nerve at the elbow, the nerve is ready for the internal neurolysis.

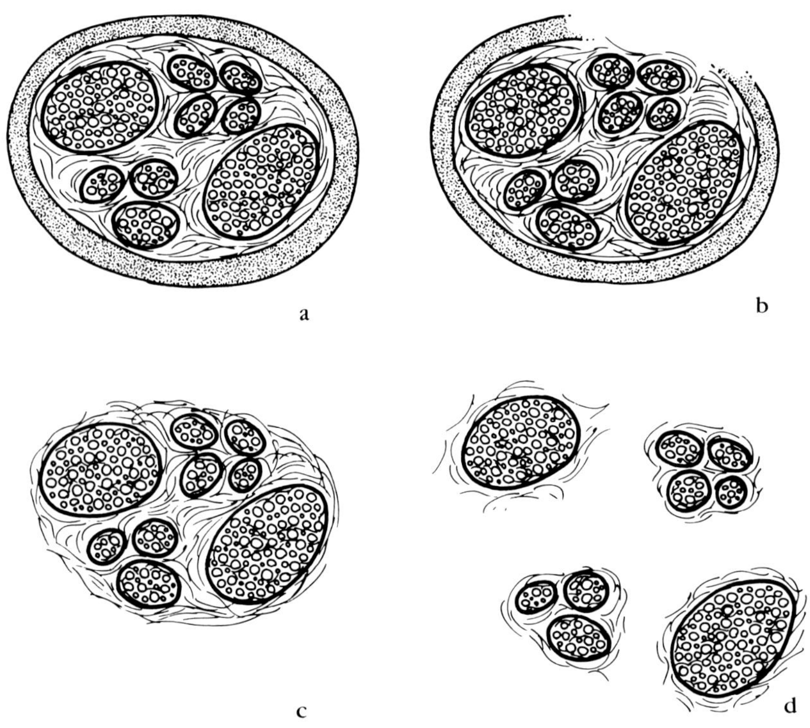

Figure 5-3. Schematic illustration of operative technique for internal neurolysis. The compressed nerve is illustrated in **a**. An epineurotomy is noted in **b**. **c.** The epineurium has been removed (external neurolysis). **d.** An internal neurolysis has been carried out.

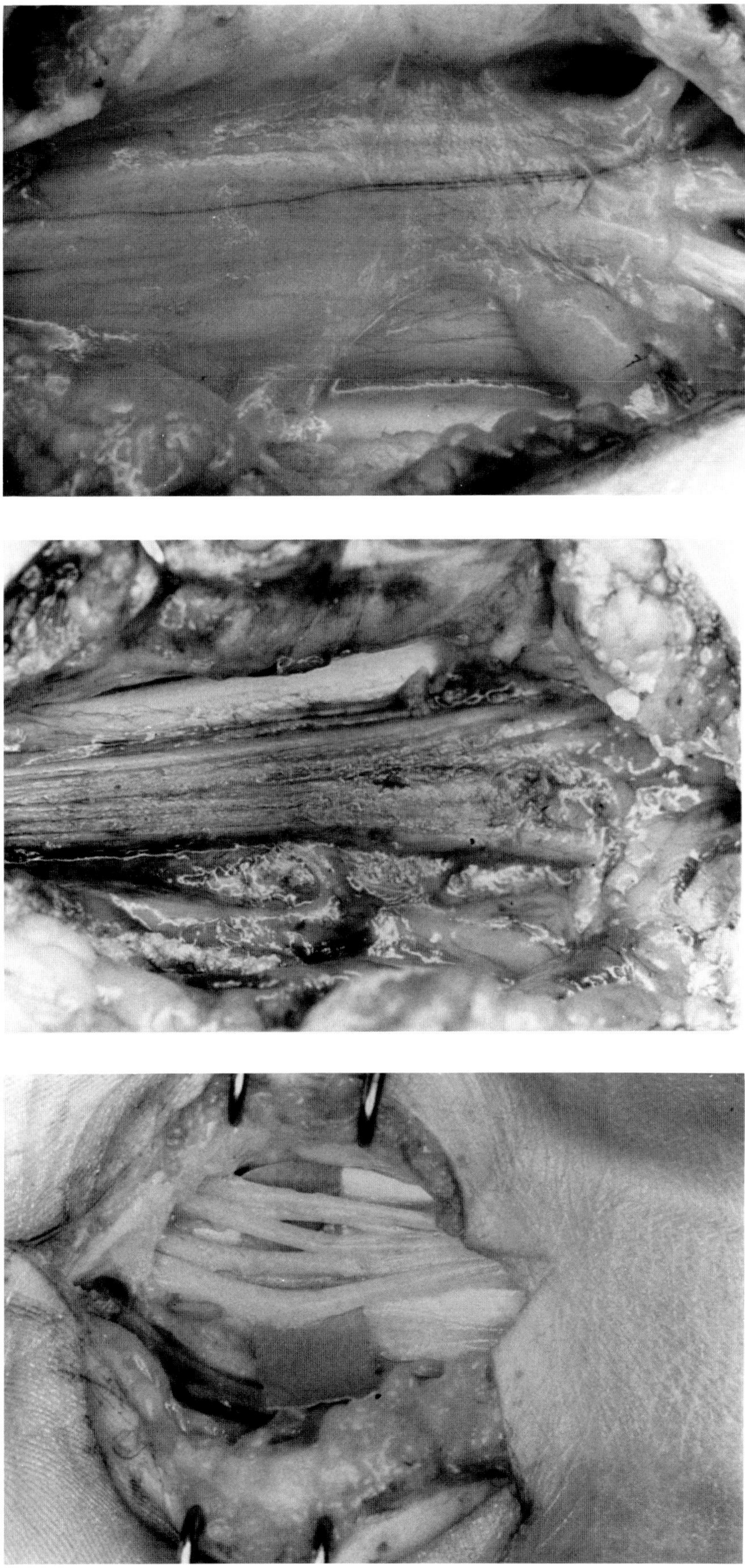

a

b

c

Figure 5-4. Median nerve internal neurolysis as an example of the "operational definition," that the intraneural neurolysis is continued until there is a good fascicular pattern with perineurial markings (**a**). No intraneural fibrosis and no intraneural dissection required. Moderate degree of intraneural fibrosis requiring a degree of neurolysis is shown in **b**. **c.** Severe intraneural fibrosis requiring extensive intraneural dissection.

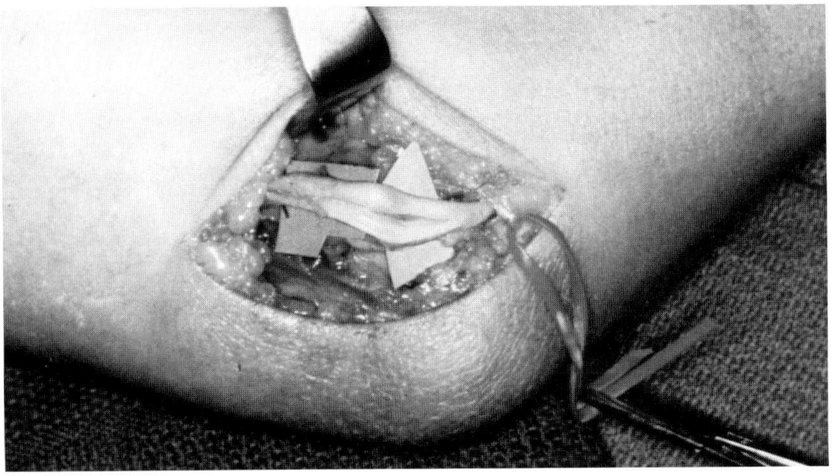

a

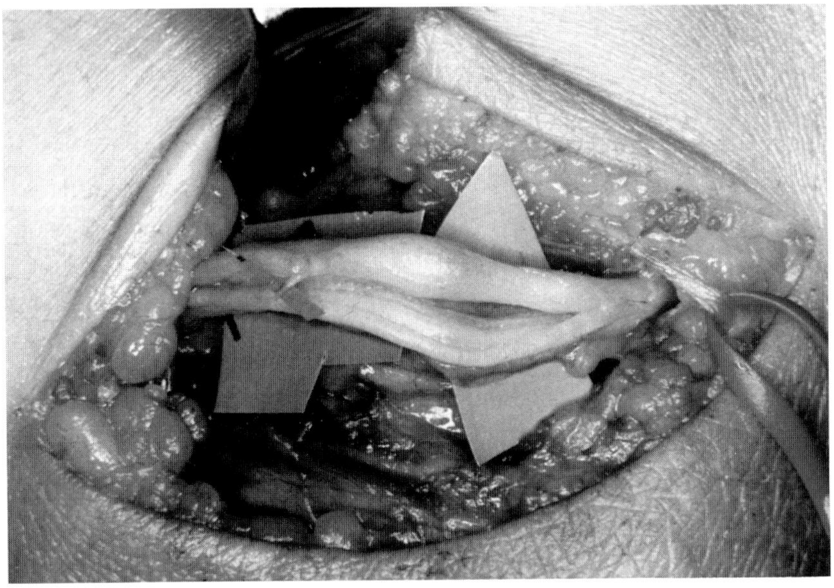

b

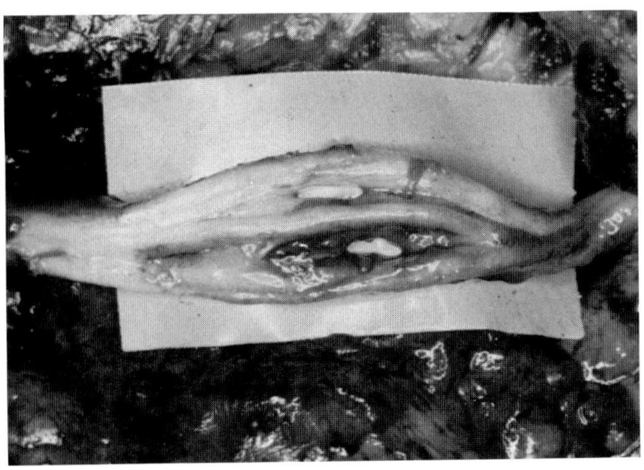

c

Figure 5-5. Plexus formation must be distinguished from intraneural fibrosis. This problem most commonly occurs for the ulnar nerve at the elbow (**a**). Orientation view of ulnar nerve hand toward the right. Examples of intraneural fibrosis and intraneural neurolysis in the ulnar nerve at the elbow with varying degrees of plexus formation (**b-d**). (See also Figures 6-2c, 6-6c, 6-7d, and 17-52)

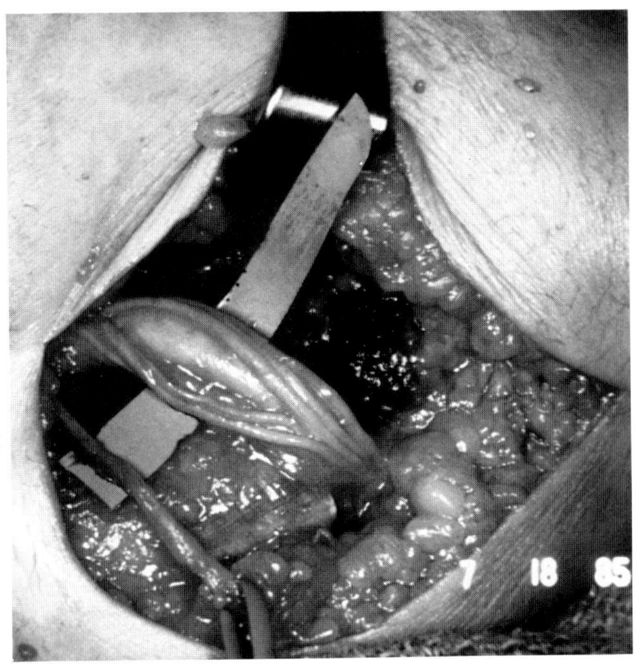

d

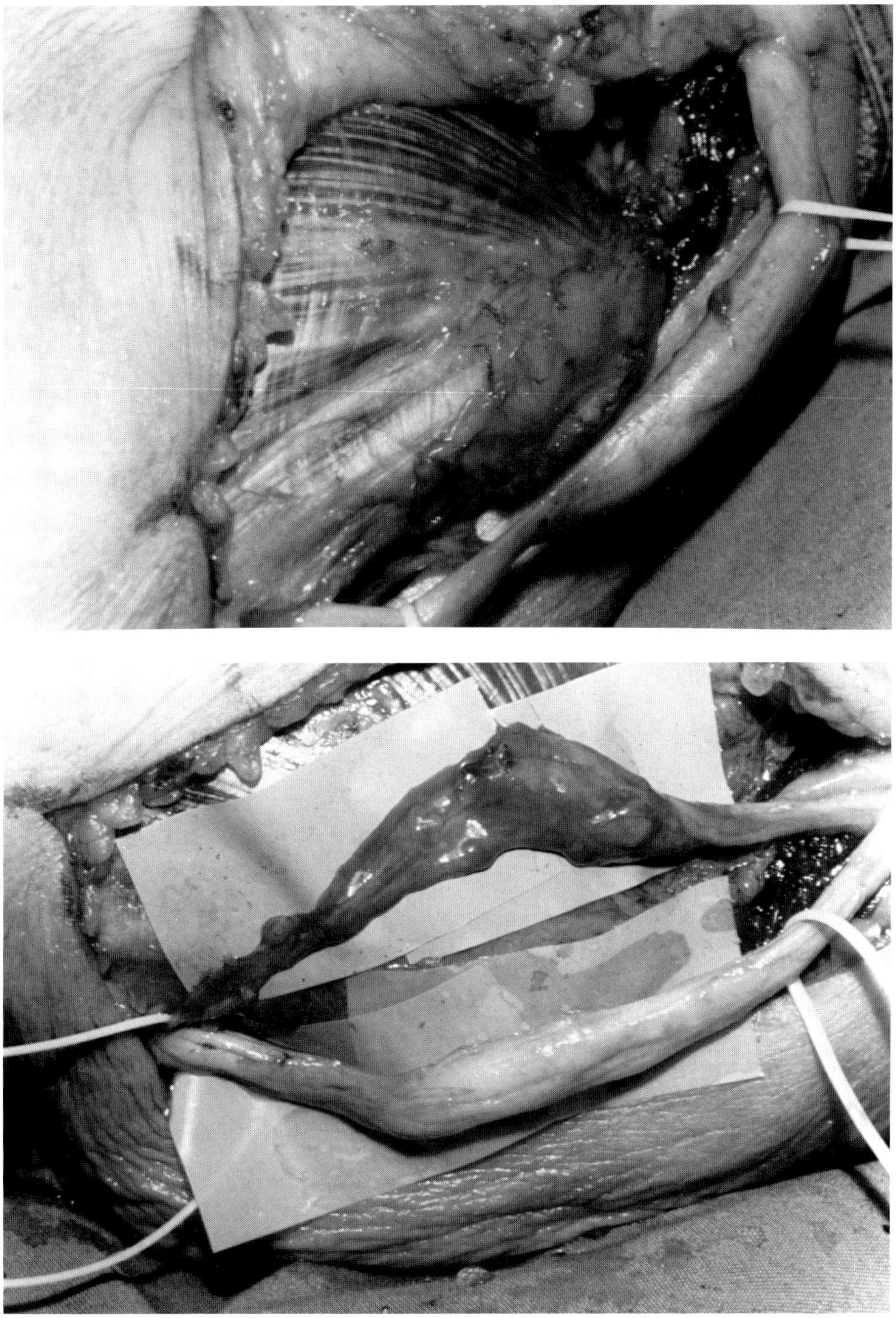

a

b

Figure 5-6. Internal neurolysis of the right ulnar nerve at elbow is not possible due to extensive plexus formation and large pseudoneuroma formation hand toward left (**a**). Just the epineurium, on the above background material, could be resected safely (**b**).

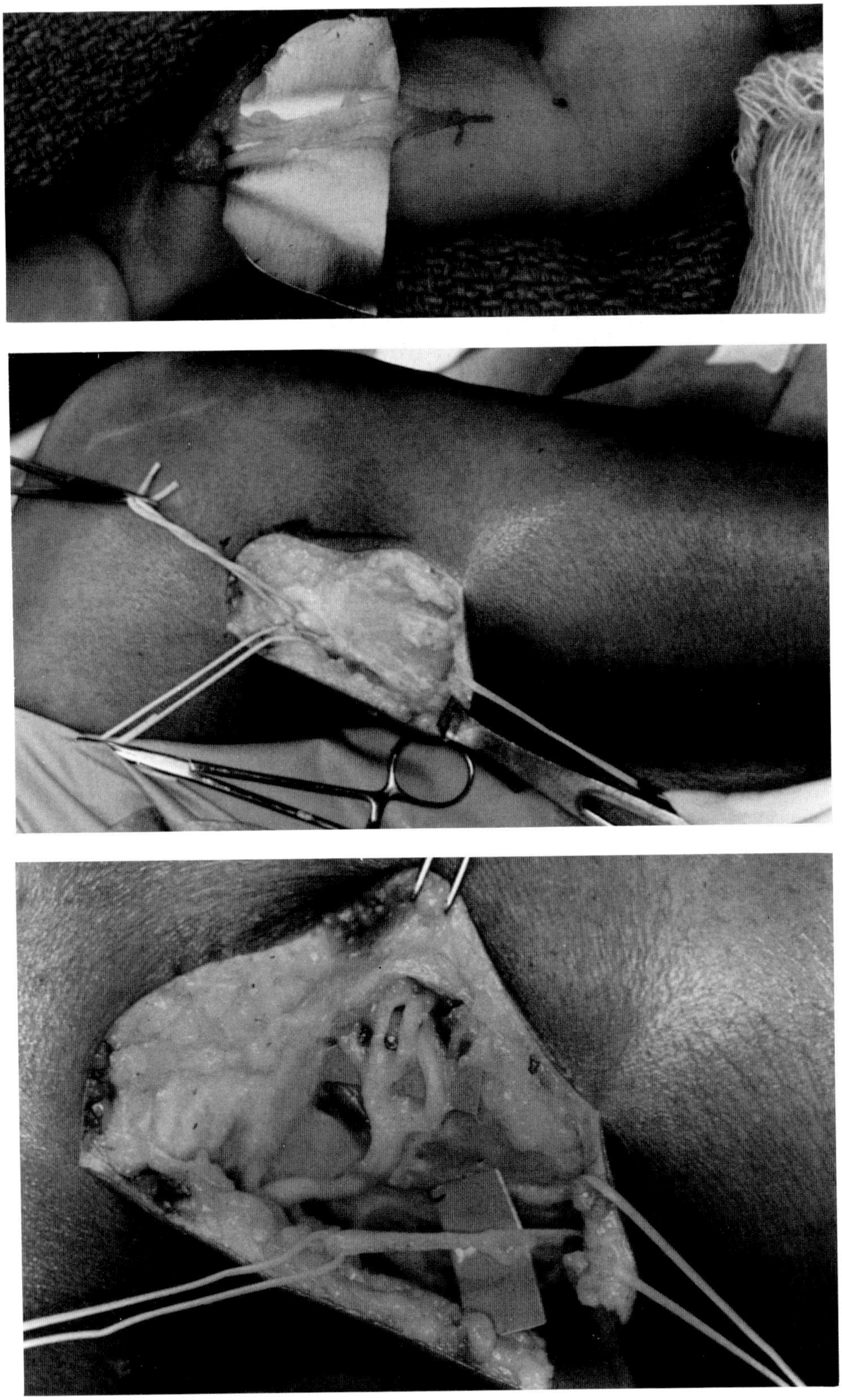

a

b

c

Figure 5-7. Legend on page 145.

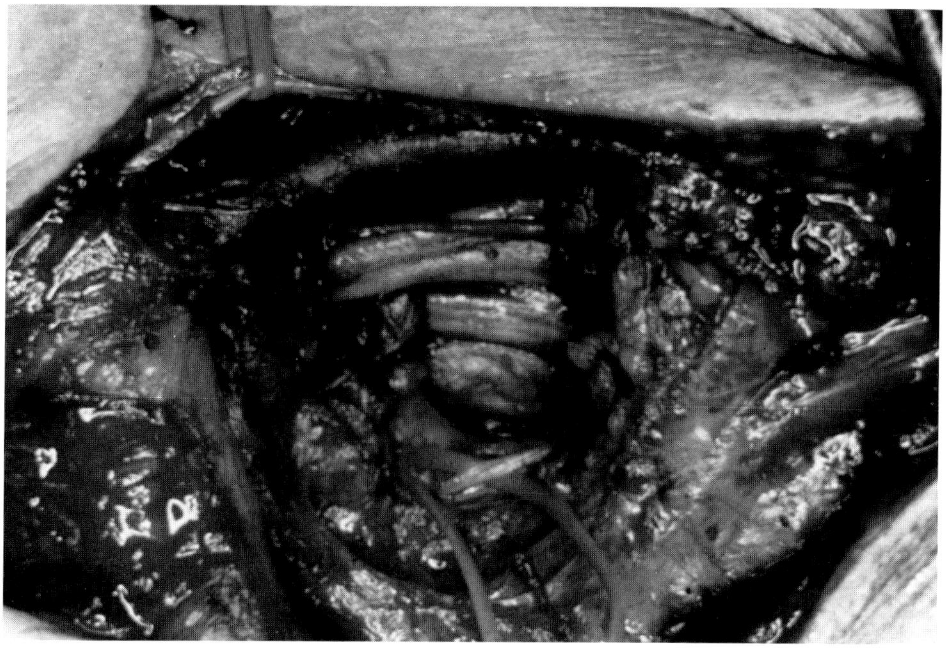

d

Figure 5-7. Examples of internal neurolysis for chronic nerve compression of the digital nerve (**a**), common peroneal nerve (right peroneal nerve foot toward the right) (**b** and **c**) brachial plexus (**d**). The phrenic nerve is retracted with the vessel loop on the left, the supraclavicular nerves with the vessel loop to the right. All three trunks of plexus are seen well with fascicles visualized. (For posterior tibial nerve, see Figures 12-9b and 12-11c and for radial nerve see Figure 11-8.)

Microsurgical instruments and technique are utilized always for an internal neurolysis. At least 3.5 power magnification is utilized and once the surgeon is appropriately familiar and skilled in the technique of intraneural neurolysis, loupes of 3.5 power magnification may be suitable for the procedure. The intraneural neurolysis is always done under tourniquet control so that the intraneural topography may be adequately visualized. The dissecting instrument may be either a scalpel or sharp pointed microscissors. We prefer the latter instrument. Although saline injection beneath the epineurium has been recommended by some, we believe that this distorts the intraneural topography so that we do not use it. Furthermore, we have not found it necessary once sufficient skill is obtained with the intraneural dissection technique. The extrafascicular epineurium is incised and this incision is continued down until the first fascicle is apparent. It may be appropriate at this point to place two traction sutures of 6-0 silk or other fine suture material into the epineurium on either side of this slit to aid in dissection and stabilize the nerve (Fig. 5-4). With additional experience in the dissection technique, this, too, has been found not to be absolutely required. Then the points of the fine-tipped scissors are inserted beneath the next layer of intraneural fibrosis, which would be between the two most superficial fascicles. The tip of the fine-pointed scissors is now visible beneath the overlying thin film of fibrosis and the scissors are gently slid down between the fibers. Great care is taken to visualize and be aware of plexus formation. The interchange of nerve fibers between adjacent fascicles makes up these plexi. Distinguishing between a plexus formation and fibrosis between two fascicles may sometimes be difficult and extreme care must be taken. This situation occurs almost never within the median nerve in the carpal tunnel and almost never in the radial-sensory nerve in the forearm but is extremely common in the ulnar nerve at the elbow (Figs. 5-5, 5-6). In the latter region, the intraneural fibrosis when present appears as fine parallel whitish fibers being almost transverse between fascicles, whereas the nerves forming the plexus formation leave at an acute angle from one fascicle and journey over a period of several millimeters into the adjacent fascicle. In all instances, if the tip of the fine-pointed scissors is kept just superficial to a thin film of transverse fibers, the surgeon may be assured that intraneural fibrosis is being lysed and that a plexus is not being interrupted. Once the intraneural fibrosis between two fascicles has begun to be opened, the fine-pointed scissors is placed between the fascicles and the prongs of the scissor are spread apart, gently separating the fibers from each other. This gives a new opening beneath the next more distal region of fibrosis and the scissors are inserted here and the procedure repeated. The epineurium that is extrafascicular that was opened at the earliest portion of the procedure is dissected from the surface of the fascicles, first to one side and then to the other side. Once it has been dissected, it may be used as a traction mechanism, as the dissection is then carried down between fascicles, first in the central portion of the nerve and then proceeding to each edge or periphery of the nerve. If the intraneural fibrosis proceeds all the way through to the posterior aspect of a nerve, then the intraneural dissection continues all the way through to the posterior aspect of the nerve (Fig. 5-4). On each fascicle longitudinal vessels in the perineurium are visible and these are not injured. Segmental blood supply into the extrafascicular epineurium does not occur generally within the carpal tunnel unless a persistent median artery is present. In the region of the ulnar nerve at the elbow, segmental vessels enter proximal to the cubital tunnel and just distal to the cubital tunnel, and these may be preserved occasionally during the anterior transposition procedure.

In general, the length of the intraneural neurolysis corresponds to the segment of nerve that has been compressed. In cases in which blunt trauma has occurred, such as with a fall or a wrist fracture or after contusions to the elbow, the extent of intraneural fibrosis within the nerve exceeds that usually due to the constricting band imposed by the normal anatomic structures. In these cases, the length of intraneural neurolysis must be correspondingly longer.

At the completion of the dissection, the extrafascicular epineurium is resected and submitted to the pathologist. In the region of the median nerve at the wrist and the radial sensory nerve in the forearm, this generally imposes no additional risk. For the ulnar nerve at the elbow, branches to the flexor carpi ulnaris frequently arise from the ulnar nerve proximal to the cubital tunnel and may lie relatively loosely in the epineurium instead of being tightly apposed to the main ulnar nerve fascicles. Thus, care must be taken in resecting the extrafascicular epineurium in the ulnar nerve at the elbow that critical fascicles to the ulnar wrist flexor are not excised with the specimen.

After the intraneural neurolysis, the wound is irrigated with saline and the nerve placed into the most optimal bed available. In the carpal tunnel, the nerve remains in the radial side of the carpal tunnel with the transected edge of the transverse carpal ligament remaining on the most ulnar side of the carpal tunnel adjacent to the hamate, so that the scarred edge of the ligament does not adhere to the surface of the median nerve. For the ulnar nerve at the elbow, the preferred site is for the nerve that has had an internal neurolysis to lie in the intermuscular plane between the brachialis muscle and the overlying reconstructed flexor pronator muscle mass, a submuscular transposition. As far as possible, the nerve should lie in a well-vascularized bed and not lie subjacent to a skin incision. Thus, for the radial sensory nerve in the forearm, the incision is deliberately placed several centimeters to the volar aspect of the proposed course of the radial sensory nerve.

Steroids are not routinely placed about the nerve after neurolysis.[55]

Postoperative Care

The region that was operated on is splinted for 7 to 8 days until time of suture removal. After that time, the nerve is allowed movement within its bed by action of the appropriate muscles and underlying joint. It is no longer supported by splints. This early movement is believed to be essential in order to prevent the nerve from becoming adherent to its bed. Various surgeons over time have commented, for example, that placing a nerve within an incised muscle, such as intramuscular or submuscular placement of the ulnar nerve at the elbow, in and of itself, is a cause for scarring to occur between the nerve and the structure in which it is placed. A recent experimental study in the primate in which the ulnar nerve was placed in one extremity in a submuscular position and in the other extremity in an intermuscular position at the elbow has demonstrated that there is no difference 6 months after the operative procedure either in the interface between the epineurium of the ulnar nerve and the adjacent or subjacent muscle, in the degree of intraneural fibrosis in the nerve, or in the axon to myelin ratios of the fibers within the ulnar nerve.[56] In that experimental study, the primate elbows were splinted in 90° of flexion for 3 weeks, after which they were permitted unrestricted use of their elbows. In our patients after submuscular transposition, the plaster splint is removed after 8 days and the elbow is prevented from extension past 90° by continued wearing of a splint for an additional week. During this second week, flexion within the sling is permitted. Postoperatively, beginning in about 10 days, the patient is instructed in vigorous massage of the wound to be practiced with a suitable hand cream for 5 minutes two or three times a day. This is continued until the scar is softened and the skin is freely mobile over the underlying tissues.

After an intraneural neurolysis there is frequently a period, beginning at about 1 to 2 weeks and extending up to 3 months after surgery, of hypersensitivity in the region innervated by the internally neurolyzed nerve. This is explained to the patient beforehand. The patient is told that they may feel heat or cold or sensitivity or burning pain in the region that was previously numb as "the new life" returns to that area. It is explained to them that after a prolonged period of sitting, they are aware that their foot goes to sleep and when they begin to stand up there is occasionally a period of intense discomfort in their foot as the circulation returns to the nerve and sensibility returns to the foot. The aspect of reinnervation of their hand is explained to them in this manner. It is not believed that this represents causalgia. Most patients simply say that their hand is extremely sensitive. During this time, patients who previously had had a diminished perception of vibratory stimuli will now have an increased perception of vibratory stimuli. Previously reduced cutaneous vibratory or pressure thresholds will be returning toward normal. Patients may require additional support in terms of medication and in this regard hydroxyzine instead of narcotics has been helpful. The patient may even require a period with the therapist for desensitization during this time.

We have experienced two cases of postoperative reflex sympathetic dystrophy after an internal neurolysis for carpal tunnel syndrome in 600 cases of internal neurolysis of the median nerve, and no cases of reflex sympathetic dystrophy in 250 cases of internal neurolysis in the ulnar nerve at the elbow. We have had no cases of reflex sympathetic dystrophy in 30 cases of internal neurolysis in the radial-sensory nerve in the forearm.[57]

Results of Internal Neurolysis

In the experimental model of severe nerve compression for the rat sciatic nerve, internal neurolysis gave statistically significantly better results when judged morphometrically and electrophysiologically than did simple decompression of the nerve.[55] The reader is referred to the appropriate chapter on the particular nerve for the clinical results of internal neurolysis. Figure 5-7 gives clinical examples of internal neurolysis for the brachial plexus, digital nerve, common peroneal nerve, and posterior tibial nerve.

References

1. Lehmann W: In Foester O, et al, eds: *Allgemeine Therapie.* Springer-Verlag, Berlin, 1936, pp 165, 205.
2. Babcock WW: Nerve disassociation; a new method for the surgical release of certain painful or paralytic afflictions of nerve trunks. Ann Surg 46:686–693, 1907.
3. Babcock WW: A standard technique for operations on peripheral nerves, with a special reference to the closure of large gaps. Surg Gynecol Obstet 45:364–378, 1927.
4. Murphy JB: Cicatrical fixation of ulnar nerve from ancient cubitus valgus—release and transference to new site. Clin John B. Murphy 661–670, 1916.
5. Stopford JB: Compression of peripheral nerves. Br Med J 1:1027–1028, 1926.
6. Marie P, Foix C: Atrophie isolee de l'eminence thenar d'origine neuritique, Role du ligament annulaiare anterieus du carpedans la pathoogenie de la lesion. Rev Neurol (Paris) 26:647–648, 1913.
7. Thomas PK, Fuller PM: Nerve fiber size in the carpal tunnel syndrome. J Neurol Neurosurg Psychiatry 26:520–527, 1963.
8. Curtis RM, Eversmann WW Jr: Internal neurolysis as an adjunct to the treatment of the carpal tunnel syndrome. J Bone Joint Surg 55A:733–740, 1973.
9. Rydevik B, Lundborg G, Nordborg C: Intraneural tissue reactions induced by internal neurolysis. Scand J Plast Reconstr Surg 10:3–8, 1976.
10. Lundborg G: Intrinsic vascularization of human peripheral nerves: Structural and functional aspects. J Hand Surg 4:34–41, 1979.
11. Gentili F, Hudson AR, Kline DG, Hunter D: Morphological and physiological alterations following internal neurolysis of normal rat sciatic nerve. In Gorio A, et al, eds: Post-Traumatic Peripheral Nerve Regeneration: Experimental Basis and Clinical Implications. Raven Press, New York, 1981, pp 183–210.
12. Phalen GS: The birth of a syndrome, or carpal tunnel revisited. J Hand Surg 6:109–110, 1981.
13. Mackinnon SE, Dellon AL, Hudson AR, Hunter D: Chronic nerve compression—an experimental model in the rat. Ann Plast Surg 13:112–120, 1984.
14. Mackinnon SE, Dellon AL, Hudson AR, Hunter D: A primate model for chronic nerve compression. J Reconstr Microsurg 1:185–194, 1985.
15. Mackinnon SE, Dellon AL: Evaluation of microsurgical internal neurolysis in a primate median nerve model of chronic nerve compression: Internal neurolysis versus decompression. J Hand Surg 13A:345–351, 1988.
16. Lichtman DM, Florio RL, Mack GR: Carpal tunnel release under local anesthesia: Evaluation of the outpatient procedure. J Hand Surg 4:545–46, 1979.
17. Freshwater MF, Arons MS: The effects of various adjuncts on the surgical treatment of carpal tunnel syndrome secondary to chronic tenosynovitis. Plast Reconstr Surg 61:93–96, 1978.
18. Gelberman RH, Aronson D, Weisman MF: Carpal tunnel syndrome: Results of a prospective trial of steroid injection and splinting. J Bone Joint Surg 62A:1181–1184, 1980.
19. Byers CM, Delisa JA, Frankel DL, Kraft GH: Pyridoxine metabolism in carpal tunnel syndrome with and without peripheral neuropathy. Arch Phys Med Rehabil 65:712–716, 1984.
20. McGowan AJ: Results of transposition of the ulnar nerve for traumatic ulnar neuritis. J Bone Joint Surg 32B:293–301, 1950.
21. Foster RJ, Edshage S: Factors related to the outcome of surgically managed compressive ulnar neuropathy at the elbow level. J Hand Surg 6:181–192, 1981.

22. Spindler HA, Dellon AL: Nerve conduction studies and sensibility testing in carpal tunnel syndrome. J Hand Surg 7:260–263, 1982.
23. Dellon AL: The vibrometer. Plast Reconstr Surg 71:427–431, 1983.
24. Adson AW: Surgical treatment of progressive ulnar paralysis. Minn Med 1:455–460, 1918.
25. Lluch AL: Ulnar nerve entrapment after anterior transposition at the elbow. NY State J Med 75:75–76, 1975.
26. Platt PT: The operative treatment of traumatic ulnar neuritis at the elbow. Surg Gynecol Obstet 47:822–825, 1928.
27. Wadworth PG: The external compression syndrome of the ulnar nerve at the cubital tunnel. Clin Orthop 124:189–204, 1977.
28. Fromison AI: Treatment of compression neuropathy of the ulnar nerve at the elbow by epicondylectomy and neurolysis. J Hand Surg 5:391–395, 1980.
29. Leffert RD: Anterior submuscular transposition of the ulnar nerve by the Learmonth technique. J Hand Surg 7:147–155, 1982.
30. Matson DD: Early neurolysis in treatment of injury to the peripheral nerves due to faulty injection of antibiotics. N Engl J Med 242:973–975, 1950.
31. French JH: Post-injection sciatic nerve palsies in infants and children. J Pediatr 58:195–204, 1961.
32. Clark K, Williams PE Jr, Willis W, McGavran WL III: Injection injury of the sciatic nerve. Clin Neurosurg 8:17:111–125, 1970.
33. Brown HA: Internal neurolysis in the treatment of peripheral nerve injuries. Clin Neurosurg 17:99–107, 1970.
34. Gentili F, Hudson AR, Hunter D, et al: Nerve injection injury with local anesthetic agents: A light and electron microscopic, fluorescent microscopic and horseradish peroxidase study. Neurosurgery 6:263–272, 1980.
35. Mackinnon SE, Hudson AR, Gentili F, et al: Peripheral nerve injection study with steroid agents. Plast Reconstr Surg 69:482–490, 1982.
36. Kline DG, Hackett ER: Value of electrophysiologic tests for peripheral nerve neuromas. J Surg Oncol 2:299–310, 1970.
37. Kline DG, Nulsen FP: The neuroma-in-continuity: Its preoperative and operative management. Surg Clin North Am 52:1189–1209, 1972.
38. Terzis JK, Dykes RW, Hahstian RW: Electrophysiologic recordings in peripheral nerve surgery—a review. J Hand Surg 1:52–66, 1976.
39. Williams HB, Terzis JK: Single fascicular recordings—an intraoperative diagnostic tool for the management of peripheral nerve lesions. Plast Reconstr Surg 57:562–569, 1976.
40. Omer GE Jr: Injuries to nerves of the upper extremity. J Bone Joint Surg 56A:1615–1624, 1974.
41. Petrucci FS, Morelli A, Raimondi PL: Axillary nerve injuries—21 cases treated by nerve graft and neurolysis. J Hand Surg 7:271–278, 1982.
42. Clodius L, Uhlshmid G, Hess K: Irradiation plexitis of the brachial plexus. Clin Plast Surg 11:161–165, 1984.
43. Woltman HW, Williams HL, Lambert EH: An attempt to relieve hemifacial spasm by neurolysis of the facial nerve: A report of two cases of hemifacial spasm with reflections on the nature of the spasm, the contracture and mass movement. Proc Staff Meet Mayo Clin 26:236–240,1951.
44. Auger RG, Piepgras DG, Laws ER, Miller RH: Microvascular decompression of the facial nerve for hemifacial spasm. Clinical and electrophysiological observations. Neurology (NY) 31:346–350, 1981.
45. Iwakuma T, Matsumoto A, Nakamura N: Hemifacial spasm: Comparison of three different operative procedures in 110 patients. J Neurosurg 57:753–756, 1982.
46. Samii M: Intraneurale Neurolyse des Nervus medianus beim Karpaltunnel Syndrom. Handchirurgie 8:117–119, 1976.
47. Gassman N, Stegmuller G, Stanisic M: Das karpaltunnel Syndrom. Indikation, Technik und Resultate nach epineuraler und inter aszikularer Neurolyse. Handchirurgie 9:137–142, 1977.
48. Eversmann WW Jr, Ritsick JA: Intraoperative changes in motor nerve conduction latency in carpal tunnel syndrome. J Hand Surg 3:77–81, 1978.
49. Fissette J, Onkelinx A: Treatment of carpal tunnel syndrome. Comparative study with and without epineurolysis. Hand 11:206–210, 1979.
50. Hoehn JG: Neurolysis in the treatment of carpal tunnel syndrome. A preliminary report. Orthop Rev 9:103–107, 1980.
51. Althaus B, Maillard GF: Spatrsultate nach chirurgis cher behandlung fon fifty karpaltunnel syndromen unter anwendung der mikrochirurgis chen endoneurolyse. Helv Chir Acta 48:89–93, 1981.
52. Rhoades CE, Mowery CA, Gelberman RH: Results of internal neurolysis of the median nerve for severe carpal tunnel syndrome. J Hand Surg 67A:253–256, 1985.
53. Millesi H: Unfallschaden peripherer Nerven. In Zenker R, Deucher F, Schink W, eds: Chirurgie der Gegenwart, vol. 4—Unfallchirurgie. Munchen, Urban & Schwarzenberg, 1975, pp 1–75.
54. Millesi H: Microsurgery of peripheral nerves: Neurolyses, nerve grafts, brachialplexus injures. In Bunke HJ, and Furnas DW, eds: Symposium on Clinical Frontiers in Reconstructive Microsurgery. St Louis, CV Mosby, 1984, pp 353–373.
55. Mackinnon SE, O'Brien J, Dellon AL, MacLean AR, Hudson AR, Hunter DA: An assessment of the effects of different treatment strategies, including internal neurolysis on a chronically compressed rat sciatic nerve model of chronic entrapment. Plast Reconstr Surg 81:251–256, 1988.
56. Dellon AL, Mackinnon SE, Hudson AR, Hunter DA: Effect of submuscular versus intramuscular placement of the ulnar nerve: An experimental model in the primate. J Hand Surg 11B:117–119, 1986.
57. Dellon AL, Mackinnon SE: Radial-sensory nerve entrapment in the forearm. J Hand Surg 11A:199–205, 1986.

Carpal Tunnel Syndrome

6

Historical Review of Controversies

The carpal tunnel syndrome was the first peripheral nerve entrapment syndrome described,[1] and remains the most frequently recognized. This syndrome has been well-described in both personal reminiscences and clinical series by Phalen and colleagues,[2–4] in a textbook devoted to peripheral nerve entrapment by Spinner,[5] and in an encyclopedic chapter by Eversmann in Green's textbook on hand surgery.[6] Although a comprehensive historical review of the syndrome is not the purpose of this chapter, it is relevant to review the origins of some of the controversies that still surround treatment of this common problem. It is also important to emphasize that even in 1988, standard preoperative evaluation for the diagnosis of this syndrome, standard operative treatment for this syndrome, and a standard for judging successful postoperative results do not exist. It is our belief that the underlying reason for continued controversy of such a common human condition lies in the previous lack of an experimental model for chronic nerve compression, and the lack of good pre- and postoperative evaluation of sensibility, which would allow investigation of the controversies just described.

The description in 1893 by Schultz[7] of numbness and tingling in the fingertips and his introduction of the term "acroparesthesia" led to the grouping of patients with symptoms of numbness and tingling in their fingertips among those patients with systemic diseases that may cause similar problems. Recognition by Wilson[8] in 1913 that the presence of a cervical rib could cause acroparesthesia may well have led to the emphasis for the next 30 years of proximal causes for this problem (by Halsted in 1916,[9] Sargent in 1921,[10] Adson and Coffey in 1927,[11] and Walshe et al in 1944[12]). Despite the fact that surgical approaches to the cervical rib, first rib, scalene muscles, and subclavian artery frequently failed to relieve the patient of symptoms and despite the fact that the patient's symptoms often occurred in the absence of muscle wasting, the attribution of these symptoms of acroparesthesias to a distal cause frequently was not made.

Although the earliest description by Paget was in a patient who had post-traumatic median neuritis from "excessive callus formation after a Colles' fracture," the concept of surgical decompression of a compressed median nerve did not appear to have occurred to anyone until the 1940s. Zachary in 1945[13] and Cannon and Love in 1946[14] are generally attributed with the early operative treatment of carpal tunnel syndrome. However, careful review of the early literature demonstrates that James R. Learmonth, a surgeon at the Mayo Clinic, may have performed the first median nerve decompression on July 30, 1933,[15] and another in 1941.[16] The reason for the obscurity of this latter reference to Learmonth's operation is that he is attributed as the surgeon by Woltman, a neurologist, who was reporting a single case of median nerve entrapment in a patient with acromegaly in the neurology literature. Woltman had for diagnostic signs in that patient blistering of the tips of the thumb, index and middle fingers, and atrophy of the thenar muscles. With that degree of physical findings, the surgeon at the Mayo Clinic thought that he was warranted to explore the median nerve in the carpal tunnel and, in fact, did divide the deep transverse carpal ligament. Learmonth later developed a right-angled scissors for division of this ligament through a proximal incision.

With the realization that the symptoms of acroparesthesia could be due to compression of a peripheral nerve, the emphasis switched and an increasing number of publications reported the success rate of this procedure for carpal tunnel "release." The belief that proximal causes for compression in and around the region of the brachial plexus could be the source of distal symptoms became seriously doubted. Case after case was reported in which patients with previous surgical procedures at the more proximal levels had failed to improve until they had distal median nerve decompression. Recently, 1000 cases of carpal tunnel syndrome were reviewed on this point, concluding that the diagnosis of "thoracic outlet syndrome" was "elusive" at best.[17]

Today, we continue to live with the legacy of this historical controversy. Although the earliest cases of carpal tunnel syndrome required obvious physical findings of sensory and motor impairment, today, if a patient complains of numbness and tingling in the thumb, index or middle finger, which may worsen throughout the day and which awakens him at night, then even in the absence of obvious physical signs of sensory or motor impairment and even in the presence of normal electrodiagnostic studies, this patient may become a candidate for surgery. In contrast, patients who have compression of the brachial plexus, but who have more vague distal symptoms, are today frequently treated with more distal procedures before any proximal operation. Indeed, there are many surgeons trained today who still doubt that the so-called thoracic outlet is a legitimate diagnosis. Our current approach to diffuse upper extremity, neck, and shoulder discomfort has been reported recently[18] and is reviewed in detail in the Chapter on "Brachial Plexus Injuries."

The relationship of proximal and distal sources of compression to the patient's symptoms raises the possibility of the simultaneous presence of two sources of nerve compression. This possibility was first published as a hypothesis in *Lancet* in 1972 by Upton and McComas.[19] Preliminary experimental observations that appeared to demonstrate the double crush syndrome[20] have since been confirmed.[21] Although these aspects of the carpal tunnel syndrome as discussed in greater detail in Chapter 14 on "Multiple Crush Syndrome," it is noted here that the double crush concept provides a basis for the observations that some patients are relieved by either proximal or distal decompression, whereas others require both decompressions to be relieved.

The history of the surgical treatment of the carpal tunnel syndrome is generally one of decompression of the entrapped median nerve. This assumes that the source of the compression can be identified and that it lies outside the nerve itself. From the earliest descriptions of the surgical release of the transverse carpal ligament in the 1940s, there would appear to be little change in the basic therapeutic approach to this problem. Perhaps the reason for this apparent unanimity in the approach to the surgical treatment lies in what is generally regarded to be the high success rate for the treatment of this syndrome achieved with this procedure. Most surgeons probably would indicate that their success rate lies in the 90% range. Early publications, for example, by Kendall,[22] give this impression. Kendall indicated that his review of 327 patients who were treated under his care between the years 1948 and 1958 resulted in 70% success rate by nonoperative management and, in those patients resistant to conservative care, who numbered 116, the operative procedure was successful in all except two patients whose "relief of sensory symptoms remained incomplete." This type of reporting, however, is difficult to support when one carefully reviews the patients' reported physical findings. For example, Kendall's series contained "severe weakness and wasting in 21% of the patients thenar muscles." There is no mention in his results section of the recovery of these thenar muscles. Kendall's sensory examination consisted of preoperative testing with pinprick. It was noted that impaired pinprick was common over the volar surface of the index and middle fingers. Present concepts of peripheral nerve compression suggest that the large myelinated fibers are more susceptible to ischemia and compression than are the more thinly myelinated fibers responsible for the perception of pain.[23] Thus, it might be expected that if patients had impaired perception of pain, their sensory problems would be in the more advanced group. Preoperative evaluation of innervation density in touch fibers by static or moving two-point discrimination was not reported. There was no mention postoperatively of improved perception of pinprick. Another example of this type of reporting is a description relating the "new" carpal tunnel syndrome to the presence of systemic disease (rheumatoid arthritis, gout, myeloma).[24] Each of the three patients in this report, after decompression of the median nerve at the wrist, recovered "promptly with complete relief of symptoms." Review of each case, however, indicates no mention of improvement of their thenar muscle wasting.

The historical perspective of the success of surgical decompression must be viewed with the present concepts of peripheral nerve compression. These suggest that the duration of chronic nerve compression induces structural changes in the nerve, which may eventuate in loss of function of sensory or motor fibers with attendant abnormal physical findings of abnormal two-point discrimination and muscle wasting.[25,26] Superimposed on these physical findings would be increased symptoms with increased use of the hand, increased flexor synovitis, increased flexion or extension of the wrist, since each of these temporarily produce an increased degree of neural ischemia. Without doubt, this increased neural ischemia results in increased symptoms. The simple operative decompression of the median nerve by release of the deep transverse carpal ligament causes an immediate change in acute ischemic changes in the nerve and response of the hand to use and nighttime wrist position. Thus, it is possible that a surgeon may report that his patients' "symptoms" are relieved, yet in the absence of reporting the postoperative degree of thenar wasting or weakness still present and in the absence of doing a preoperative evaluation of innervation density of the touch corpuscles (static or moving two-point discrimination test), he is unable to make a correct interpretation as to whether decompression alone, in fact, allows the complete recovery of the motor and sensory system. Interestingly, the most recent reports of results in the carpal tunnel syndrome, when careful preoperative assessment has been made and the patient treated with simple decompression, have demonstrated improvement in only 75% of the patients.[27,28] This leaves approximately 25% of the patients with carpal tunnel syndrome who may benefit further, perhaps by alteration in the operative technique.

Theoretically, operative decompression may be extended to within the nerve, where interfascicular fibrosis exists. In the few reported cases of entrapment of the median nerve that have been examined microscopically, it was clear that severe entrapment can result in morphometric changes.[29–35] These observations have also been demonstrated recently from the experimental models of chronic nerve entrapment.[36,37] These studies demonstrate that part of the histopathologic changes of chronic nerve compression is the development of intraneural fibrosis in the form of increased intrafascicular epineurium. It is possible that this serves as a source of increased pressure within the nerve that is not relieved by simple decompression of the nerve in the traditional surgical approach. If this were to be the case, there would be room for further improvement in the more difficult or advanced case. The concept of this type of internal decompression, or internal neurolysis of the median nerve, is an adjunct to the historical surgical treatment of carpal tunnel syndrome as described by Curtis and Eversmann.[38]

The controversy surrounding the intraneural neurolysis of a compressed peripheral nerve began with this description of improved results in previously failed carpal tunnel release patients by Curtis and Eversmann.[38] They described an internal neurolysis technique that was indicated in patients who have muscle wasting, abnormal two-point discrimination, or persisent sensory discomfort, and for recurrent carpal tunnel syndrome patients. The first three categories imply that a careful preoperative assessment of the sensory and motor function has been recorded and the patient's degree of nerve compression, in effect, has been staged. This implies that a different degree of treatment should be given to those with the worst degrees of entrapment neuropathy. This represented a truly innovative approach to the treatment of this disease. It became immediately apparent that the degree of dissection within the nerve may cause increased scarring.

In the laboratory, Lundborg investigated this problem.[39] His model, however, consisted of internal neurolysis in a normal rabbit tibial nerve. He found that there was "some" increased fibrosis produced within the nerve after this procedure. Lundborg's results seemed to justify the approach of most surgeons, which was not to attempt to operate within the nerve. As a response to this criticism of his described procedure, Curtis began to place cortisone intraoperatively about the median nerve to minimize this theoretical increase of fibrosis.[40] However, a recent surgical investigation of internal neurolysis in a normal nerve, this time the rat sciatic nerve model, demonstrated that after a brief period of alteration in the blood–nerve barrier, there was no increase of fibrosis present in the nerve 6 months later.[36] Our own most recent work demonstrates that an internal neurolysis done on the monkey on a median nerve compressed for 6 months causes no increased intraneural scarring when compared with a simple decompression of that monkey's contralateral median nerve after a similar period of compression.[37]

A recent report from Gelberman's group suggests that a Curtis-Eversmann type internal neurolysis can be done safely in patients.[41] Our own clinical observations also indicate that a carefully done intraneural neurolysis is possible by a surgeon trained in microsurgical technique. It remains for more detailed work on a large series of clinical patients who have been treated according to a staging of their disease (nerve compression) before there will be sufficient scientific support to suggest any alteration of the current widespread surgical approach to carpal tunnel surgery.

Anatomic Considerations in the Patient with Carpal Tunnel Syndrome

The carpal tunnel may be thought of as an inverted table with the carpal bones forming the table top and the hook portion of the hamate, the pisiform, the tubercle of the trapezium, and the distal pole of the scaphoid forming the table legs. Variation in carpal canal size has recently been implicated as a predisposing factor to carpal tunnel syndrome.[42] Across the top of these four legs is stretched the deep transverse carpal ligament. One view of the carpal tunnel then would be from proximal to distal beneath the deep transverse carpal ligament. Thus, the surgeon should have in mind what constitutes the distal end of the tunnel. The carpal tunnel ends when the fat surrounding the superficial palmar arch is reached. In the operative procedure, all fibrous bands are searched for and divided distally. The beginning of the carpal tunnel, or its proximal entrance, is not well-defined anatomically. Indeed, the antebrachial fascia blends distally with the thick transverse carpal ligament. The region of transition from the thinner antebrachial fascia to the thick, deep transverse carpal ligament may be termed the "superficial carpal ligament" or the "superficial volar ligament." This region is imporant in that it presents a relationship between the superficial transverse carpal ligament and the volar lip of the radius. In serial transverse sections from the distal forearm toward the metacarpal, this area represents a narrowed segment. This area is particularly likely to be vulnerable in cases of fracture of the distal radius where callus formation or changes in the angulation of the distal radius may further narrow this already narrowed entrance into the carpal tunnel. The occurrence of carpal tunnel syndrome after fractures of the distal radius is well-documented.[43–49] Accordingly, as part of the carpal tunnel release procedure, this proximal entrance to the carpal tunnel, the distal antebrachial fascia, must also be released (Fig. 6-1a). Also in this region, exploration of the volar wrist ligaments is required to evaluate the presence of other pathologic changes related to increased carpal tunnel pressure, such as a volar wrist ganglion (Fig. 6-1b).

The literature continues to expand in descriptions of anomalies of hand and forearm muscles.[50–55] These include extra muscle bellies and tendon slips, going in and above the transverse carpal ligament. The presence of these must be appreciated, noted, and, when necessary, divided.

The variations in the takeoff of the motor branch of the median nerve have been carefully documented.[56,57] Since the motor branch usually comes from the radial side of the median nerve, all attempts to release the deep transverse carpal ligament should be done on the most ulnar side of the carpal tunnel adjacent to the hamate. There may even be a separate fibrous tunnel where the motor branch enters into the thenar muscles.[58] In patients with thenar atrophy, this fibrous, compressive tunnel should be looked for and, if present, released. It has been our personal observation that the motor branch is most often more centrally located in the median nerve, in those patients in whom there is thenar atrophy. In this position, in contrast to its more usual radial position, the motor fascicle is under more direct pressure from the transverse carpal ligament (Fig. 6-2). This observation may also be the anatomic basis for the electrodiagnostic recordings of patients with severe motor findings but sensory sparing.[59]

The variations of the median artery should be known.[60,61] This artery may be present in up to 10% of reported anatomic studies. It may be of significance when it contributes to the superficial palmar arch in the presence of incomplete normal arches between the radial-ulnar arteries. Accordingly, unless you have determined that there is adequacy of flow through the radial and ulnar artery, division or excision of the median artery is to be discouraged. When the median artery represents a significant contribution to the blood flow dynamics of the hand, a potential variation in the presentation of the patient's symptoms may be complaints of coldness in the fingers related to compression of this artery.[62] The median nerve, in our experience, is generally split into two separate nerves when there is a persistent median artery; there is a higher division of the median nerve in the presence of a persistent median artery (Fig. 6-1d). This has been previously reported.[63,64] The median nerve also may have a high division in the absence of a persistent median artery.[65,66]

Blood supply to the median nerve must be recognized as being principally longitudinal and within the nerve itself, having segmental contributions occurring from the ulnar artery proximal to the carpal tunnel and from the superficial palmar arch distal to the carpal tunnel. Thus, the investing sheath of flexor synovium with the epineurium about the median nerve is not signifi-

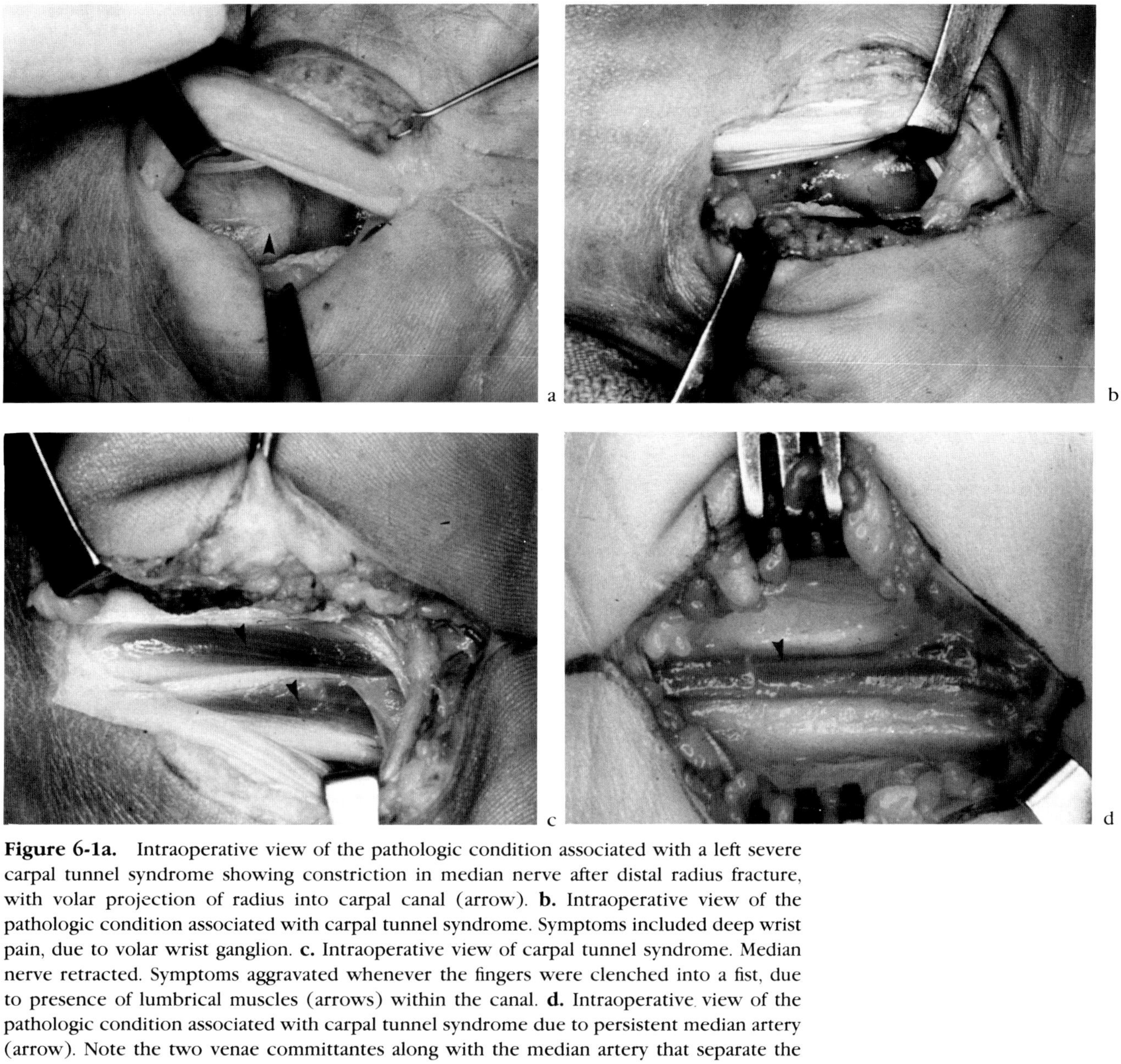

Figure 6-1a. Intraoperative view of the pathologic condition associated with a left severe carpal tunnel syndrome showing constriction in median nerve after distal radius fracture, with volar projection of radius into carpal canal (arrow). **b.** Intraoperative view of the pathologic condition associated with carpal tunnel syndrome. Symptoms included deep wrist pain, due to volar wrist ganglion. **c.** Intraoperative view of carpal tunnel syndrome. Median nerve retracted. Symptoms aggravated whenever the fingers were clenched into a fist, due to presence of lumbrical muscles (arrows) within the canal. **d.** Intraoperative view of the pathologic condition associated with carpal tunnel syndrome due to persistent median artery (arrow). Note the two venae committantes along with the median artery that separate the median nerve into two separate fascicles before its entrance into the carpal canal.

cant as a mesoneurium or source of blood supply. This allows the surgeon to carry out an epineurectomy of the median nerve completely without concern for disruption of any significant segmental blood supply within the carpal tunnel.[62,67] The postoperative feeling of warmth expressed by patients may be related to the "sympathectomy" effect achieved because the epineurectomy causes a denervation of the sympathetic fibers found in the median nerve at this level.[68]

The relationship of the incision for carpal tunnel release and the palmar cutaneous branch of the median nerve is now well-appreciated.[69] The palmar cutaneous branch will be found running deep to and parallel with the tendons of the palmaris longus and flexor carpi radialis. Accordingly, transverse incisions and incisions that lie in the thenar crease are likely to injure the innervation of this region and leave a postoperative painful scar (Fig. 6-3). An incision in the radial axis of the ring finger (Fig. 6-2) is likely to split the territory between the palmar cutaneous branch of the median nerve and the palmar cutaneous branch of the ulnar nerve, resulting in the least likelihood of a painful scar.

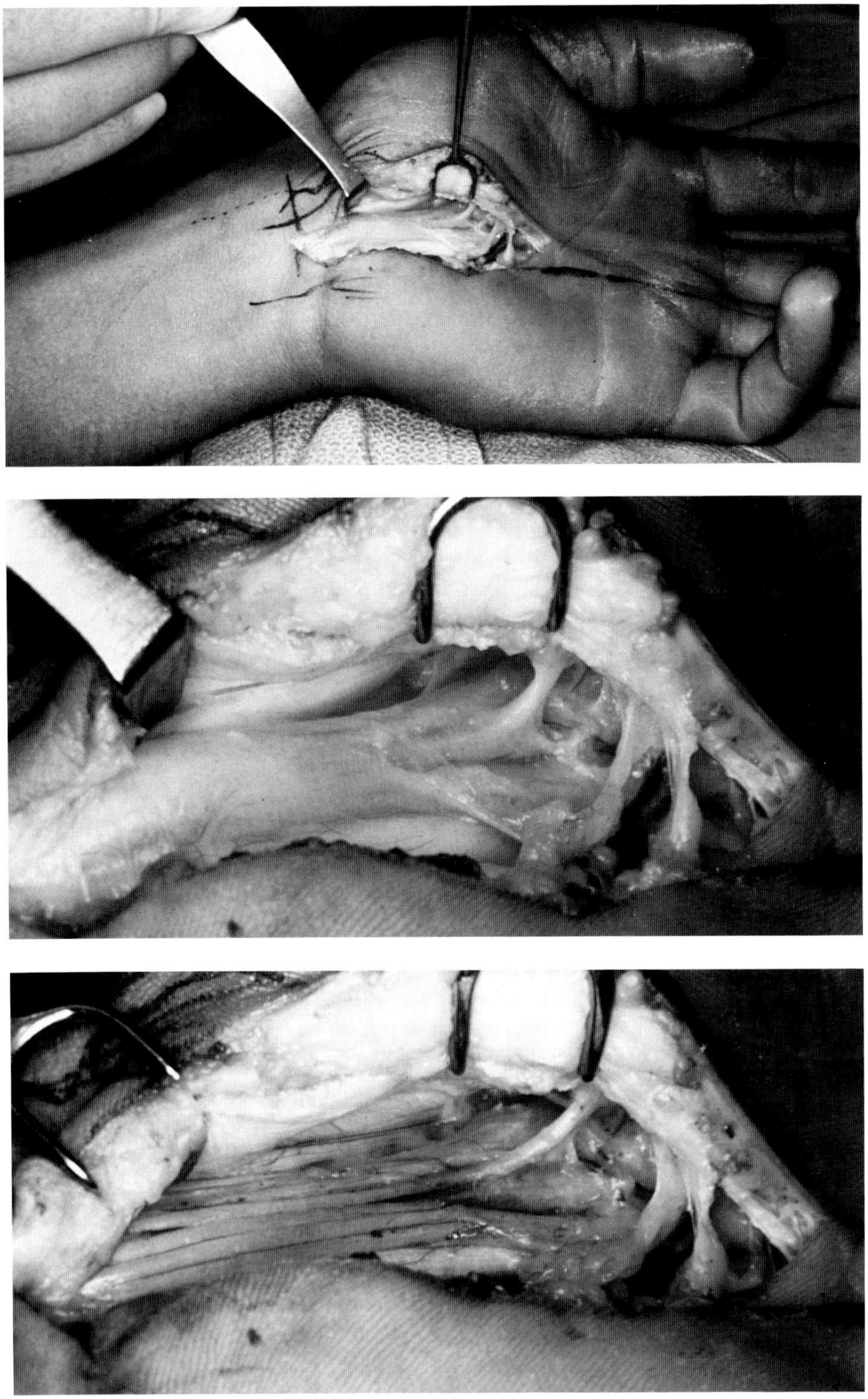

a

b

c

Figure 6-2. Relationship of palmar cutaneous branch of median nerve to carpal tunnel surgery. The marking (a) is the longitudinal axis of the ring finger, to the radial side of which lies the territory of the palmar cutaneous branch. Note moderate compression (b) of the median nerve, with intraneural fibrosis. **c.** After internal neurolysis, note also that the motor branch arises topographically from the center of the median nerve. Thenar muscle atrophy was present in this case.

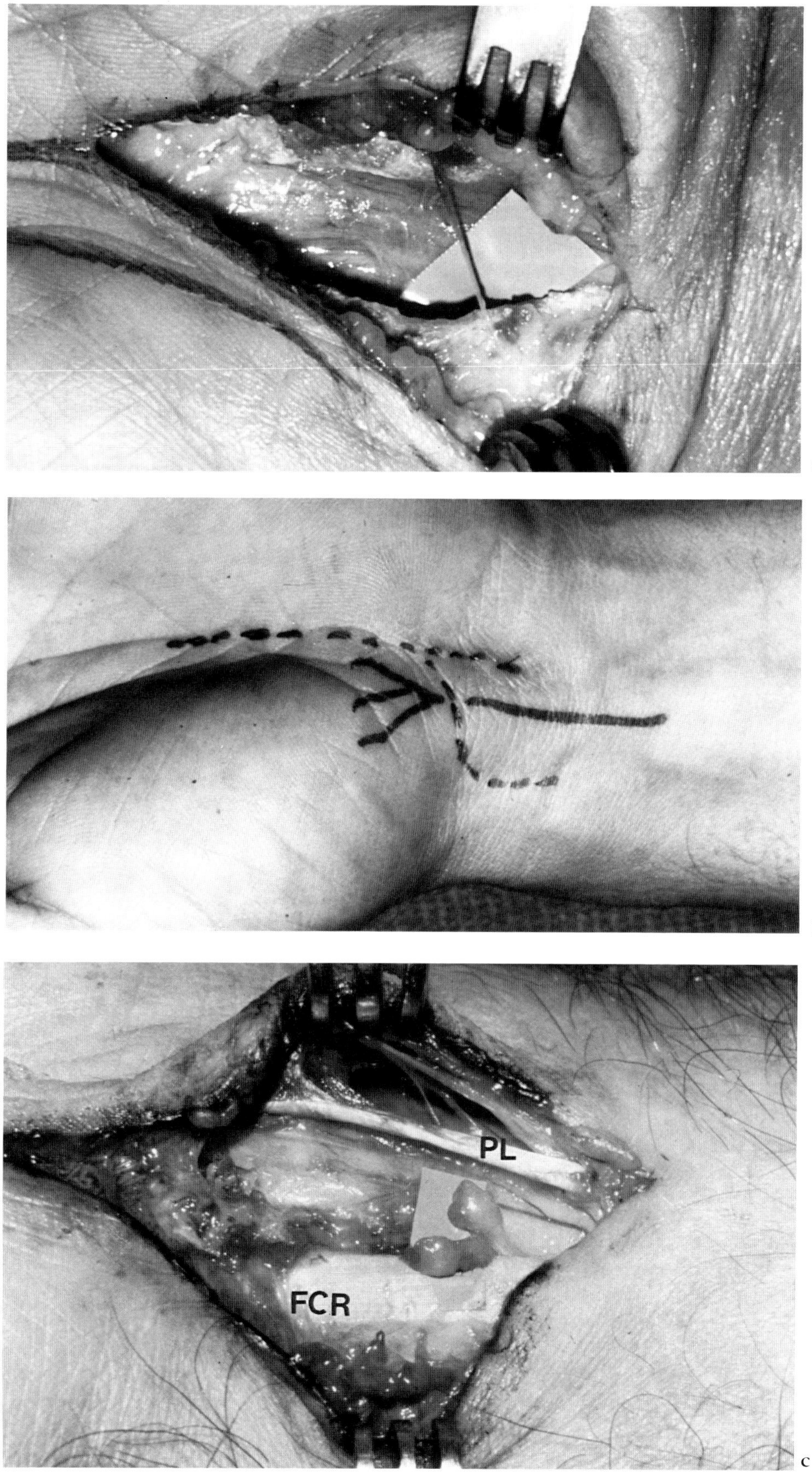

a

b

c

Figure 6-3. Relationship of palmar cutaneous branch of median nerve to carpal tunnel surgery. **a.** Branch of the palmar cutaneous is only ocassionally observed during the dissection into the carpal tunnel through the thenar crease, and this branch is preserved. **b.** Second patient in whom previous carpal tunnel surgery through the thenar crease has divided the palmar cutaneous nerve. **c.** Third patient in which previous surgery resulted in division of the same nerve, identified proximally first, resulting in neuroma formation (digits toward the left). FCR, flexor carpi radialis, PL, palmaris longus.

Diagnosis: Staging Degree of Compression

Throughout the history of medicine, as knowledge about a disease has been gained, treatment of that disease has shifted from a more empiric to a more scientific basis. In particular, it has become clear that a given disease progresses naturally through stages, usually worsening in degree, and treatment will then vary in accordance with the degree of the disease. As understanding of peripheral compression neuropathy increases, treatment of this disease should also alter accordingly. Furthermore, reports of results of treatment of this disease should now reflect appropriate preoperative testing to permit preoperative staging of the nerve compression. A basis for this approach for the carpal tunnel syndrome has been reported.[70,71]

A patient may be categorized as having a minimal degree of carpal tunnel syndrome if they have: (1) symptoms that are intermittent; (2) physical examination that demonstrates only positive provocative tests, such as Phalen's sign or Tinel's sign; and (3) the nonprovocative finding of hypersensitive response to the 256 Hz cps vibratory stimulus. Patients with this minimal degree are placed on a regimen of day and night splinting and 100 mg of vitamin B_6 per day (see the last section of this chapter for further discussion of pyridoxine). They are seen in 3 months and the physical examination repeated. If they are the same or improving, they are continued on this regimen and seen again in an additional 3 months. If they are improving, they are taken off daytime splinting and continued on night splinting. Vitamin B_6 is discontinued. They are seen again in 3 months and if they continue to improve, they go to alternate night splinting. Along with this, their lifestyle, in terms of hobbies and extracurricular activities and their work duties are carefully evaluated and appropriate restrictions may be given. If any of the symptoms are not improved or are worsening, or if the findings on physical examination become more severe, and the patient does not desire further splinting, this patient becomes a candidate for surgery at this time. If surgery is medically contraindicated, cortisone injection into the carpal tunnel can be expected to give them 3 months' relief of symptoms. The most recent investigation suggests that dexamethasone is the safest of the steroid preparations with respect to nerve injection injuries.[72]

Moderate degree of carpal tunnel syndrome patients on physical examination have: (1) vibratory perception that is decreased in the median nerve distribution; (2) positive provocative signs, such as the Phalen's and Tinel's; and (3) weakness of thenar muscles but no wasting. These patients frequently have previously been treated conservatively, but if not they are placed on the same type of regimen as described with minimal degree of carpal tunnel syndrome and managed in a similar fashion.

The severe degree of carpal tunnel syndrome is characterized by: (1) sensory symptoms that are persistent in nature; (2) abnormal static two-point discrimination (greater than 6 mm); or abnormal moving two-point discrimination (4 mm or greater); and (3) muscle wasting. The patient in the severe category has the histopathologic development of intraneural fibrosis and becomes a candidate for surgery without a trial of splinting, unless his medical condition contraindicates surgery, in which case he becomes a candidate for a cortisone injection. The surgery we recommend for this degree of compression is carpal tunnel decompression plus internal neurolysis of the median nerve (see Figs. 6-3c, 6-6d, 6-7c).

If electromyography demonstrates denervation potentials in the thenar muscles, the patient also is considered to be severe in degree. For any other findings in the electrodiagnostic studies, the patient may still go into either the minimal or moderate category, with the exception that if the orthodromic or antidromic sensory potentials are not recordable, the patient would be placed in the severe category. We have observed usually that when the sensory potentials cannot be recorded, there is also abnormal two-point discrimination, and thus the patient would have been staged as severe even without the electrodiagnostic studies.

Surgical Technique

With the patient in the supine position, with satisfactory anesthesia, and with a tourniquet placed about the upper extremity over a soft roll, the hand is prepared with povidone-iodine and draped in the appropriate manner. The hand is elevated and exsanguinated with an elastic bandage and the tourniquet inflated. An incision is made 6 mm to the ulnar side of the thenar crease and paralleling the crease with a zig-zag extension across the wrist. The incision is deepened into the subcutaneous tissue and hemostasis obtained throughout with the bipolar coagulator. The palmar fascia is split longitudinally. If crossing branches of the palmar cutaneous branch of the median nerve or the ulnar nerve should, in fact, be found across the incision, every attempt is made to preserve them. The superficial transverse carpal ligament (thickened distal antebranchial fasia) is identified and opened adjacent to the hamate. The median nerve is identified. Then the deep transverse carpal ligament is divided adjacent to the hamate going distally until the fat surrounding the superficial palmar arch is

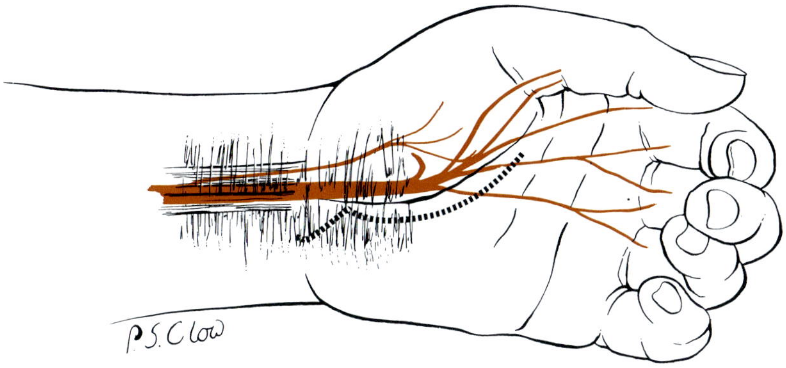

Figure 6-4. Illustration of operative technique for surgical decompression of the carpal tunnel.

reached. Proximally, with the skin elevated, the distal portion of the antebrachial fascia is divided under direct vision. The deep transverse carpal ligament is taken with a double hook and reflected to the radial side. The median nerve may be adherent to the underside of the deep transverse carpal ligament and is gently and bluntly dissected from it, being aware that within this region may be motor branches entering through the deep transverse carpal ligament. The observations are now made of the condition of the median nerve and the degree of flexor tenosynovitis present. The carpal tunnel is explored and any pathologic conditions or congenital anomalies noted (Fig. 6-4).

It is our procedure to take a portion of flexor tenosynovium, even in the absence of extensive flexor tenosynovitis, for examination by a pathologist, since the carpal tunnel syndrome may be a presenting symptom of a systemic condition. If the synovium is thickened and densely white, it may be more consistent with chronic buildup of synovium from repetitive trauma or a residua of post-traumatic synovitis. If the synovium is well-vascularized and purplish or juicy yellowish-orange, this may be an ongoing arthritic process. If the patient preoperatively has been suspected of having a chronic systemic illness, a thin segment from the palmar edge of the deep transverse carpal ligament may be resected and sent to the pathology department to stain for the presence of amyloid. The synovium, itself, may also be tested for the presence of amyloid material. If specific immunologic tests are requested, to identify types of autoimmune disease, the synovium should be submitted in saline instead of formalin (Fig. 6-5).

It is then part of our procedure to utilize the microsurgical instruments, and at least 3.5 loupe magnification, to open the epineurium and inspect the condition of the fascicles. If the fascicles appear soft with obvious bands of Fontana (perineurial markings), and there is no evidence of intraneural fibrosis, then the procedure is terminated. The wound is closed with interrupted and continuous sutures of 5-0 nylon.

The dressing is nonadherent gauze fluff, soft roll, a volar plaster splint, kling, and stockinette. Then an elastic bandage is applied and the tourniquet is let down. The elastic bandage remains in place for the first postoperative hour.

A microsurgical intraneural neurolysis would be done if preoperatively the patient had one of the indications of intraneural fibrosis (persistent sensory discomfort, abnormal two-point discrimination, or muscle wasting), and if after doing the epineurotomy there appeared to be intraneural fibrosis (Fig. 6-5). For a fuller description of the technique for internal neurolysis, you are referred to Chapter 5.

If preoperatively there were indications that ulnar nerve compression at the level of the wrist also is present, then, following the procedures already described, the ulnar nerve is released in Guyon's canal. For a description of this technique, you are referred to Chapter 8.

If the patient had extensive flexor tenosynovitis present, then a radical flexor tenosynovectomy is carried out from the distal forearm to the superficial palmar arch before skin closure (Fig. 6-5).

It should be noted that in our technique the deep transverse carpal ligament is not resutured. The location of the division of the deep transverse carpal ligament, at its most ulnar edge, allows the ligament to provide an interface between the median nerve and the overlying skin.

Postoperative Management

The volar plaster splint is removed with the sutures 8 to 10 days postoperatively and the patient allowed to begin unrestricted use of the hand and wrist at that time. The patient is allowed unrestricted opening and closing of the fingers in the early postoperative period. This combination of procedures allows the median nerve to regain normal excursion without adhering to the tendons, or the overlying deep transverse carpal ligament,

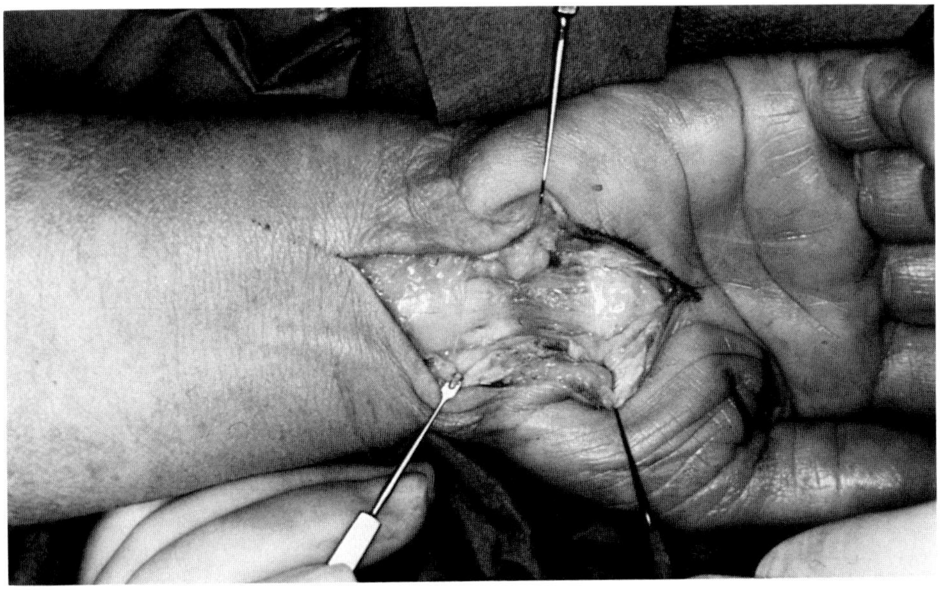

a

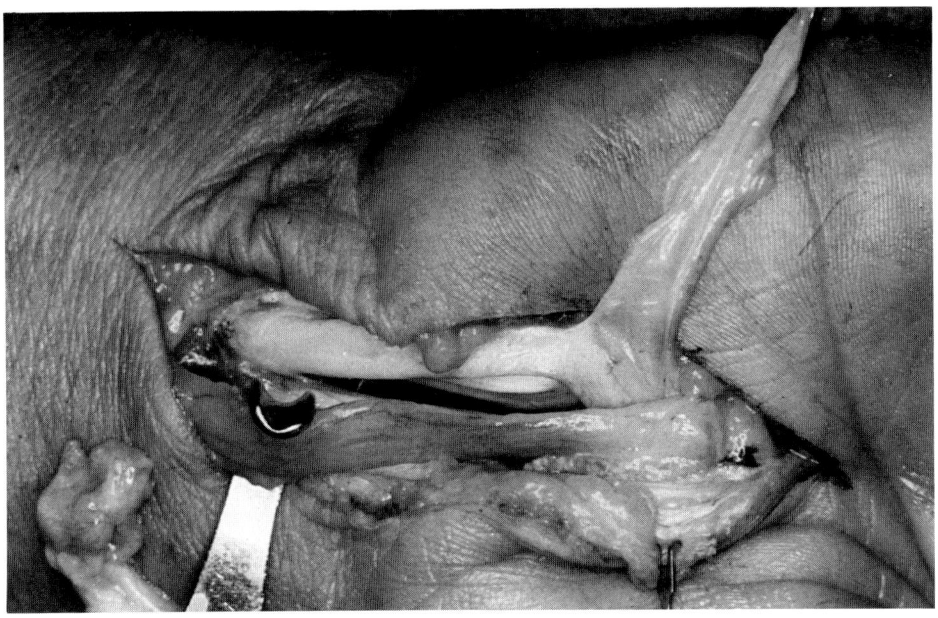

b

Figure 6-5. Flexor synovectomy done in conjunction with carpal tunnel decompression. Note flexor synovitis, here due to rheumatoid arthritis **(a)**, covering flexor tendons, with severe compression of median nerve. Note discoloration of median nerve **(a, b)**, indicative of advanced neural pathologic processes. The glossy appearance of the fascicles is suggestive of Wallerian degeneration, and an extensive intraneural dissection may be increasingly hazardous to these delicate fascicles. The flexor synovium is excised **(b)**.

and allows the fascicles in the median nerve after any intraneural neurolysis to move with respect to each other in their surrounding tissues. Postoperative therapy is begun by the patient with massage of the scar with skin cream beginning the second week after surgery, for approximately 5 minutes several times a day.

The patient is seen the third week after surgery and checked again. At this time, if the scar has areas of tenderness or residual swelling, the patient is encouraged to continue the massage. The patient is checked again at approximately 8 weeks after the surgery. If the scar has any areas of thickened redness or discrete areas of pain, the patient is begun on a topical cortisone cream and massage. The patient is seen thereafter at 3 months, 6 months, and 1 year. The baseline sensory and motor testing done at the initial examination are repeated at 6-month and 1-year follow-up visits.

Surgical Complications of Carpal Tunnel Release

The incidence of complications (12 to 15%) after carpal tunnel release for treatment of carpal tunnel syndrome is a subject infrequently reported.[73,74] The most common "complication" should probably be considered as a treatment failure. Although often reported to occur as infrequently as 7%,[75] this complication alone exceeds 20% in clinical series where careful preoperative measurements of sensibility are contrasted with postoperative measurements.[27,28] The next most common complication is a painful scar.[73,74] This includes pain due to palmar branches of digital nerves, as well as the palmar branch of the median nerve. Painful scars were most often seen after use of the transverse incision at the wrist (Figs. 6-6, 6-7), still frequent with incisions placed directly in the thenar crease, and are the least common utilizing the incision recommended by Taleisnik,[69] and described in the operative technique section of this chapter. Other complications are well-known, although much less frequent, such as injury to the superficial palmar arch, bow-stringing of the flexor tendons, and reflex sympathetic dystrophy. Rare complications continue to appear as case reports, such as division of the motor branch[75] and division of the communicating ramus between the median and ulnar nerve.[76]

The complications in one of our own series of 500 carpal tunnel syndrome procedures from 1978 through 1985 include: painful scar requiring surgery (1), painful scar requiring cortisone injection (4), reflex sympathetic dystrophy requiring stellate ganglion block (1), reflex sympathetic dystrophy requiring prednisone and hydroxyzine orally and physical therapy (2), recurrence requiring repeat surgery (2 in patients with rheumatoid arthritis with recurrent flexor tenosynovitis), division of thenar motor branch requiring primary repair (1), division of superficial palmar arch (1), infection requiring oral (1, in a diabetic with wound dehiscence) antibiotics or local wound care (2, one in a diabetic and one who used a cane in the operated hand). We have had no complications with injury to the palmar cutaneous branch, division of communicating ramus median-to-ulnar, flexor tendon bow-stringing, damage to the median nerve itself requiring surgery, bleeding requiring drainage or reoperation, infection requiring intravenous antibiotics, and wound dehiscence requiring reoperation. These 14 complications, or about 5% incidence, occurred using the staging system and treatment schema and operative technique described.

A postoperative problem that is receiving recognition now is aching discomfort or pain about the wrist after release of the transverse carpal ligament. Theoretically, this ligament acts as the volar ligament to maintain the carpal arch whose volar projections are the tubercle of the navicula and trapezium radially and the pisiform and hamate ulnarly. With this ligament released, it is hypothesized that there will be a carpal shift.[77] Of historic interest, treatment of carpal tunnel syndrome was once suggested to include resection of this ligament.[78] On the other extreme, some today advocate a partial reconstruction of this ligament routinely with carpal tunnel surgery.[79] It is possible, however, that these vague aching discomforts are related to a different problem, such as small cutaneous nerve branches divided by the incision, or a second, associated injury, such as a volar wrist sprain, with traction injury to the terminal branches of the anterior interosseous nerve. Injury to the terminal branches of the anterior interosseous nerve has been found in association with a carpal tunnel syndrome.[80] This nerve also is involved with the pain related to a ganglion of the volar carpal ligament, and the undiscovered presence of such a cyst may be the source of this residual deep aching pain.[80] The recent report of 10.4% widening of the carpal arch, associated with weakening of grip strength postoperatively,[77] is retrospective and required "adjustment" for the dominant hand. Its conclusions await affirmation by a prospective study.

The treatment of complications after carpal tunnel release follows from accurate diagnosis. If the patient has persistent symptoms, either the carpal tunnel was not completely released or intraneural fibrosis is present in the median nerve. Treatment is reexploration with complete release. The release, especially if there was an associated Colles' fracture, should come well proximally. An internal neurolysis should also be done.

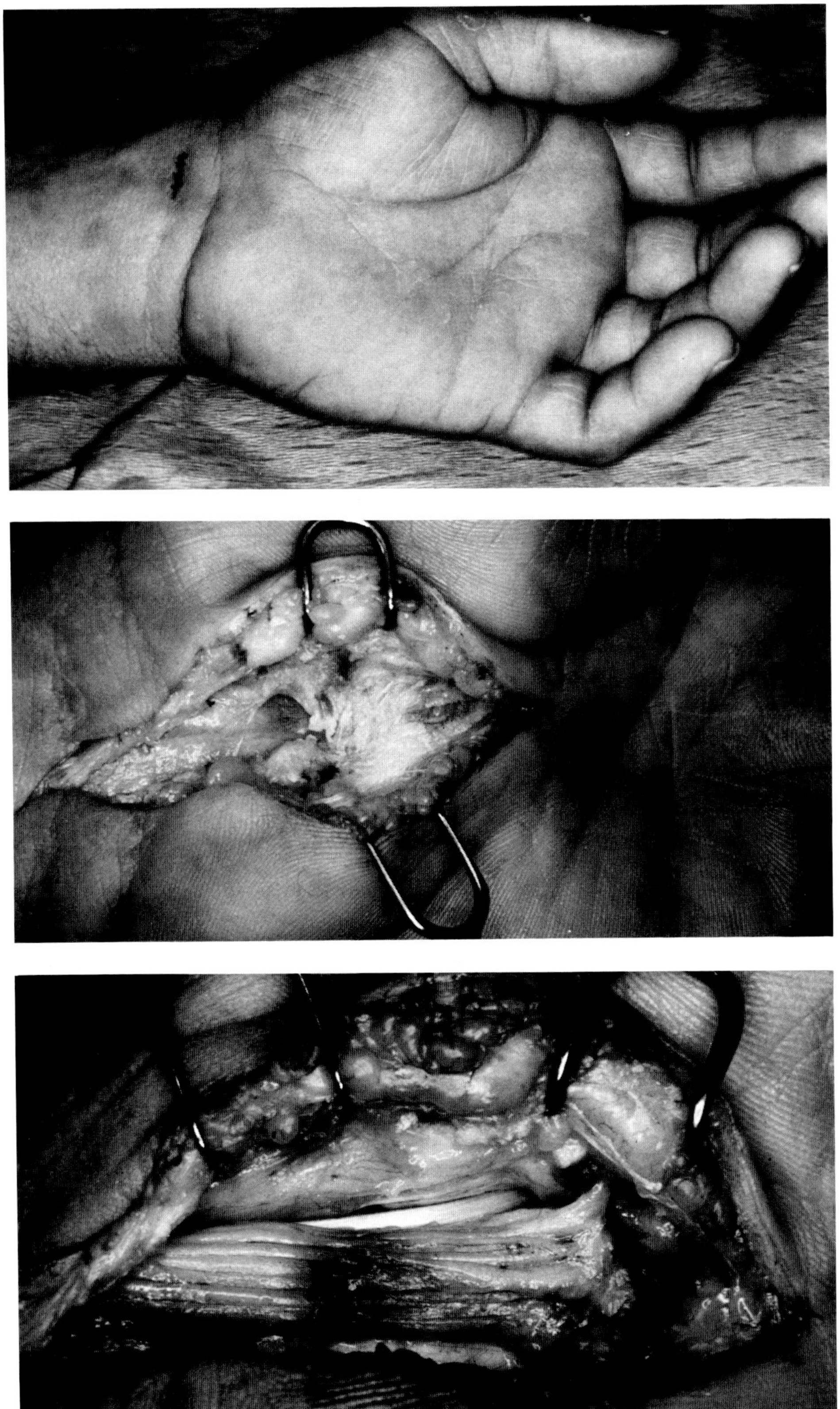

a

b

c

Figure 6-6. Example of problems associated with transverse incision for carpal tunnel decompression **(a)**. This patient had persistent symptoms of carpal tunnel syndrome requiring reexploration. The deep transverse carpal ligament had not been divided completely initially **(b)**. The severe compression of the median nerve is apparent after the tunnel is finally released. **c.** The appearance of the median nerve after internal neurolysis.

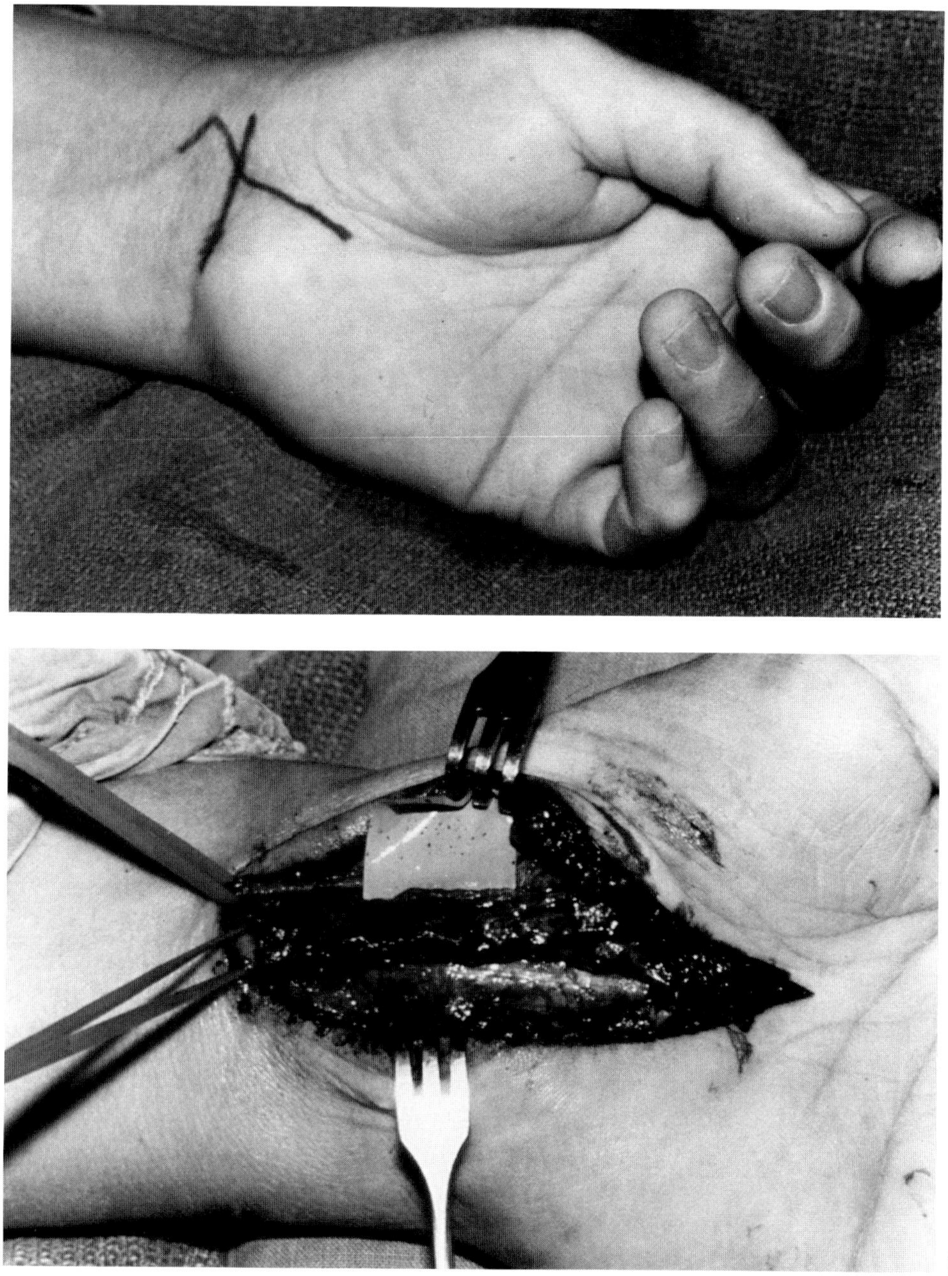

a

b

Figure 6-7. Example of problems associated with a transverse incision for carpal tunnel decompression. For persistent carpal tunnel syndrome symptoms and pain after the initial "release" through a transverse approach, a reexploration through a thenar crease incision was done. Note the previous two surgical incisions. **a.** Postoperatively, incapacitating pain was the predominant feature of the complaints. At a third operative exploration **(b)** an in-continuity neuroma of the median nerve was found. (*Figure continues.*)

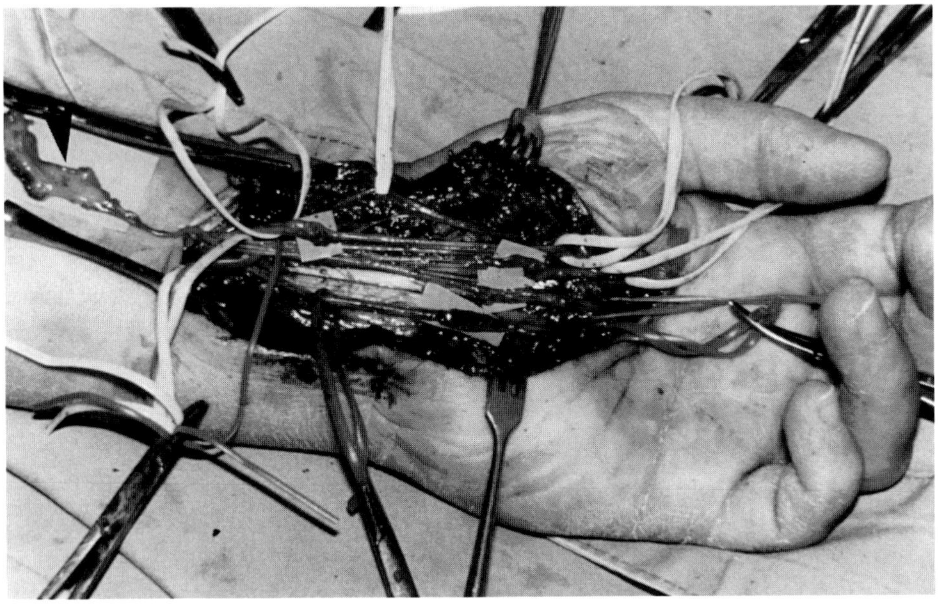

c

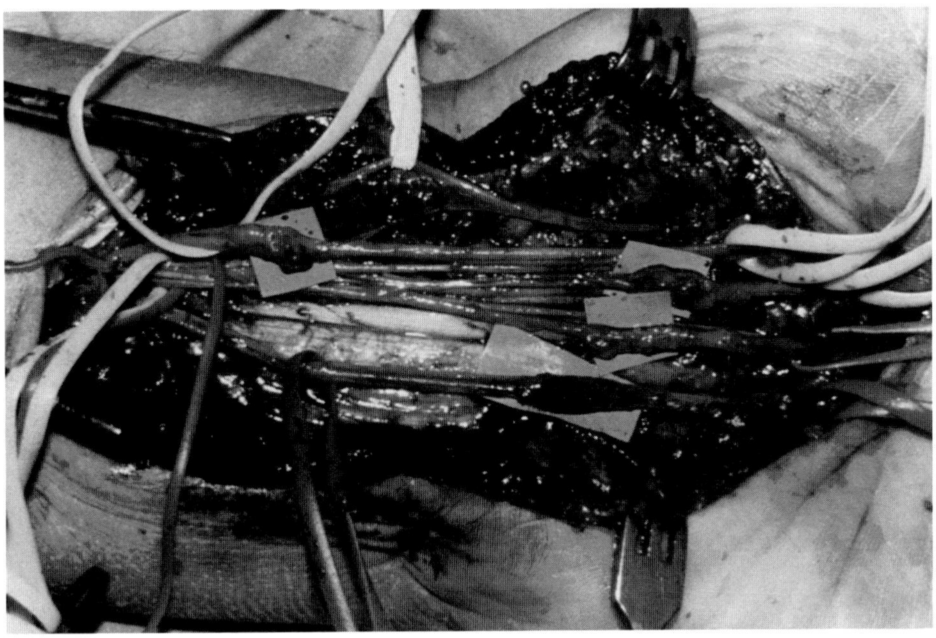

d

Figure 6-7. *(continued)* After intraneural neurolysis (c), identified were an "end-bulb" neuroma of the palmar cutaneous branch of the median nerve (single arrow), and four in-continuity neuromas on separate fascicles of the median nerve (on distal background) (close-up, d). Each of these small neuromas was excised, an interposition nerve graft placed, and the area covered with an abductor digiti minimi muscle flap.

Treatment of a painful incision is treated first by massage, with topical application of a cortisone cream and a program of desensitization. If a discrete spot remains as the source of pain, a steroid is injected into the scar. As already indicated, recent observations on drug injection suggest that a dexamethasone preparation would be the safest for this purpose.[72] If after 6 months of this treatment the pain is limiting use of the hand, the incision can be reopened, the skin elevated, the scar excised, and the wound closed again. A definite neuroma of the palmar cutaneous branch of the median nerve usually occurs at the wrist level or more proximally and is not the source of the painful scar just described. Before a planned resection of such a neuroma, diagnostic nerve block is done (see Chapter 17, "Painful Sequelae of Peripheral Nerve Injury").

A treatment of the complication of direct injury to the median nerve during carpal tunnel release, whether it be division of the motor branch, a communicating branch, or the main trunk of the nerve, should be primary repair of the injured nerve. If the surgeon does not become aware of the injury until the postoperative period, secondary repair or nerve grafting is required.

The painful sequelae of carpal tunnel surgery are further discussed in Chapter 17.

Results of Carpal Tunnel Surgery

The initial anecdotal or isolated case reports of carpal tunnel release have been followed with reports of series of patients operated on for carpal tunnel syndrome (Tables 6-1, 6-2, 6-3). These series, however, were usually not staged in terms of degree of severity, contained patient descriptions that did not permit separate analysis of results based on degree of sensory or motor impairment, and offered a variety of surgical approaches. Often an excellent result meant just relief of night pain and return to work, since residual sensory disturbances and muscle wasting, in fact, impaired hand function very little.

One surgical approach claiming excellent results was the short transverse incision and transverse carpal ligament division with the "retinaculotome." Paine[81] used this approach, which required "no more than five minutes" of operating time, obtaining "in all except two cases immediate relief of their painful burning and tingling." Patrick,[82] similarly, using a "cartilage" knife, noted that "the whole operation, including injection of local anesthetic and the insertion of two stitches, can be completed without haste in under three minutes," with the results that "all were immediately relieved of their pain."

There is an increasing trend to recognize that more severe degrees of compression should be treated differently. All of the patients reported by Cannon and Love[14] had severe fibrosis of the median nerve noted at surgery and all received an "internal neurolysis," type unspecified. The Mayo Clinic review[83] noted that a few "internal neurolyses" were done, depending on the findings, yet in their subsequent report on patients with recurrent carpal tunnel syndrome,[84] an internal neurolysis was not reportedly done. In the report from Stockholm,[85] a "selective" internal neurolysis was done, since the motor branch was "dissected out" separately in cases with thenar atrophy. The type of internal neurolysis reported by Curtis and Eversmann[38] and utilized by Gelberman's group[41] is a "50% volar" intraneural neurolysis because Curtis believed preservation of the posterior epineurium was critical for median nerve blood supply. The internal neurolysis we advocate has an "operative definition," meaning the intraneural neurolysis is continued until there is no further intraneural fibrosis, even if a 100% epineurectomy is done, emerging on the posterior aspect of the median nerve.

Table 6-1. Results of Treatment of Carpal Tunnel Syndrome by Splinting

				Results					
Reference	*No. Patients Followed*	*Staging**	*Splinting*	*Symptomatic Relief Complete*	*Atrophy Corrected*	*Weakness Corrected*	*Sensory "Loss" Corrected*	*2 PD† Corrected*	*Recurrence (n)*
Kendall,[22] 1960	173	Minimal-moderate	100%	70%		N/A†	N/A	ND†	
	125					50%	N/A	ND	
		Minimal-moderate, 70%	100%	100%	—	N/A	—	—	
		Severe, 30%	100%	95%	0%	50%	N/A	ND	1
Longloh, Linscheid[84] 1972	33	Severe, 100% (all recurrent)		51%	0%	84%	84%	ND	

*Patients staged as described in this chapter.

†N/A: data not available; ND: examination not done; 2 PD: two-point discrimination.

Table 6-2. Results of Treatment of Carpal Tunnel Syndrome by Decompression

				Results					
Reference	*No. Patients Followed*	*Staging**	*Just Decompression*	*Symptomatic Relief Complete*	*Atrophy Corrected*	*Weakness Corrected*	*Sensory "Loss" Corrected*	*2PD† Corrected*	*Recurrence (n)*
Paine[81] 1963	133	N/A†	100%	99%	0%	25%‡	50%‡	ND†	1
Patrick[82] 1965	32	N/A	100%	100%	N/A	N/A	N/A	N/A	2
Phalen[3] 1966		Minimal-moderate, 44%	100%	N/A	—	N/A	78%	ND	2
	212	Severe, 56%	100%	N/A	68%	83%	78%	ND	
Cruez et al[83] 1966	313	N/A	95%	46%	ND	N/A	81%	ND	0
Reitz, Önne[85] 1967	65	Minimal-moderate, 40%	100%	100%	—			—	
		Severe, 60%	50%	92%	75%			ND	
Semple, Cargill[100] 1969	150	N/A	100%	75%	N/A	N/A	N/A	ND	
Posch, Marcotte[101] 1976	681	N/A	100%	91%	N/A	N/A	N/A	ND	
Eversmann, Retsick[102] 1978	51	Moderate, 86%	100%			§			
Graham[27] 1983	214	Minimal-moderate, 44%	100%	75%	N/A	N/A	N/A	ND	
Gelberman et al[86] 1987	33	Severe, 100%	100%	62%	65%	90%		85%	31%
Kulick et al[28] 1986	100	Minimal-moderate, 80%	100%	85%‡		70%	N/A	ND	6
		Severe, 20%	100%¶	35%‡	5%		N/A	ND	

*Patients staged as described in this chapter.

†N/A: Data not available; ND: Examination not done; 2PD: two-point discrimination.

‡Estimated.

§Ninety-one percent of these patients had improvement in motor conduction latencies, only parameter tested.

¶Epineurotomy added

Table 6-3. Results of Treatment of Carpal Tunnel Syndrome by Decompression Plus Internal Neurolysis

				Results					
Reference	*No. Patients Followed*	*Staging**	*Decompression† Internal Neurolysis*	*Symptomatic Relief Complete*	*Atrophy Corrected*	*Weakness Corrected*	*Sensory "Loss" Corrected*	*2PD† Corrected*	*Recurrence (n)*
Cannon, Love[14] 1946	7	Severe, 100%	100%	86%	40%	N/A†	N/A	ND†	
Cruez et al[83] 1966	313	N/A	5%	46%	ND	N/A	81%	ND	0
Reitz, Önne[85] 1967	65	Severe, 60%	50%	92%	75%			ND	
Curtis, Eversmann[38] 1973	96	Severe, 100%	100%		70%			94%	
Eversmann, Retsick[102] 1978	51	Severe, 14%	100%			§			
Graham[27] 1983	214	Severe, 56%	100%	58%	N/A	N/A	N/A	ND	
Rhoades et al[41] 1985	36	Severe, 100%	100%	33%	56%	70%	60%	76%	67%

*Patients staged as described in this chapter.

†N/A: data not available; ND: examination not done; 2PD: two-point discrimination.

‡Estimated.

§ Eighty-six percent of these had improvement in motor conduction latencies, the only parameter tested.

The study with the most complete pre- and postoperative assessment of patients is that by Gelberman's group.[41,86] From their tables, each degree of preoperative loss of two-point discrimination or thenar strength can be related to the postoperative outcome (see Tables 6-2 and 6-3).

In summary, from this review, the chances of obtaining excellent symptomatic improvement in patients with carpal tunnel syndrome with minimal to moderate degree of severity by simple decompression of the tunnel is 80 to 100%, whereas for patients with severe degree of compression, simple decompression offers a range from 51 to 95% for excellent symptomatic relief. Simple decompression has been reported to correct muscle atrophy in from 0 to 68% of cases. Treatment of the severe degree of compression by some form of internal neurolysis has been reported to correct muscle atrophy in 50 to 75% of patients, and abnormal two-point discrimination in 76% of patients.

The controversy over including an internal neurolysis as an adjunct to treatment of the severe degree of compression in carpal tunnel syndrome continues.[86] In his own group Gelberman's recommendation has varied, at first pro[41] and then con[86]. Statistically he could show no improvement when internal neurolysis was added to the treatment of a comparable group of patients. However, by reference to Table 6-2 and 6-3, it is clear that his results for simple decompression are the best, while for internal neurolysis the worst reported in the literature. Furthermore, their two groups were not treated cotemporaneously. The question must be raised, "What have they done to give such poor results from internal neurolysis?" From the discussions and studies reviewed in Chapter 5, it is clear that the neurolysed nerve must be mobilized to prevent recurrent scar formation. Gelberman's technique however immobilizes the neurolyzed median nerve for three weeks with the wrist in 20° of dorsiflexion. We feel this postoperative difference, plus their not carrying the neurolysis through to the posterior aspect of the median nerve when necessary (in the severely constricted nerve) contribute to the difference in results their group observed and that which we found in our patients.

Steroid Injection into the Carpal Tunnel

There is a long history of the use of intratunnel injection of a steroid compound to reduce, theoretically, the flexor tenosynovitis presumed to be responsible for the increased pressure on the median nerve. Ever since Kopell[87] reported improvement in symptoms, without recurrence, in one patient, there has been a steady stream of reports on this subject. Phalen[3] in 1966 recommended it as a diagnostic as well as therapeutic modality, finding 62% of 270 patients were improved, with only 28% of those improved having recurrence. Phalen still recommends this approach.[4] However, other studies,[89–91] while finding 75 to 90% of their (combined) 303 patients improved after injection, found 89 to 94% of their patients having recurrent symptoms.

Green[90] has analyzed his series of 222 carpal tunnel injections further. Just 20% of his patients had no recurrence of symptoms, but only 82 of those with recurrent symptoms were severe enough to have surgery. Of those having surgery, 94% had a "good" result from surgery. In contrast, just 82% of those who did not have a good response from steroid injection had a good response to surgery. Thus, Green suggests that a patient's response to steroid injection has prognostic value. A chi-square analysis of this suggestion (77 of 82 versus 14 of 17) reveals there is no statistically significant difference in these values. Another variable that Green isolated is that patients whom we would stage as severe, with thenar atrophy, are not included in his injection group. Thus, his 90% improvement occurs in patients we would stage as minimal or moderate degree of severity.

In summary, the literature supports the view that steroid injection into the carpal tunnel can temporarily improve symptoms in at least 80% of patients whose nerve compression is not severe in degree, and that in about 10% of these patients, their symptomatic relief may be permanent. Our personal approach is that the injection is not required to make a diagnosis, and that we use it only as a temporizing procedure, for example, severe symptoms or recent onset or increasing severity until surgical release can be scheduled, or in whom surgery may be contraindicated medically or refused by the patient.

Vitamin B_6

Pyridoxine (vitamin B_6) has received increasing publicity in the lay as well as the scientific press for the treatment or adjunctive treatment of the carpal tunnel syndrome. The basic question, if formulated as follows, is simple to answer: Can a vitamin B_6 deficiency result in the carpal tunnel syndrome? If the answer is "yes," then surely correcting the deficiency with vitamin B_6 should be effective and should be done. At the present time, medical diagnostic laboratories are not set up to run a vitamin B_6 assay, as they are, for example, vitamin B_{12} or folate.

Vitamin B_6 is a cofactor for transamination reactions. Just as the SGOT can be determined for liver function, there is an assay for red blood transamination (EGOT) reactions that can be used to determine vitamin B_6 levels.[92,93] At present, only Folkers Laboratory in Austin, Texas, is making the test available.

Folkers, a Ph.D. biochemist, is largely responsible for the investigations into this relationship.[94,95] He has demonstrated a deficiency of pyridoxine in patients with carpal tunnel syndrome. His patient population has included patients with systemic complaints, as well as those with just isolated peripheral entrapment neuropathies. His patients have had symptomatic relief and "cures" after treatment with pyridoxine, 200 mg/day, for 3 to 6 months. Serial (EGOT) measurements have shown return to normal levels in these patients.

Investigation of this problem, without EGOT determinations, has been reported by Amadio[96] in 19 patients with just isolated distal median nerve entrapment symptoms. Just two of these patients, and these had a "minimal" degree of symptoms, improved on pyridoxine alone. Most recently, Arem et al[97] reported a series of ten patients who, in a double-blinded study, had their pretreatment blood evaluated by Folkers for EGOT determinations. Five patients received 500 mg/day of pyridoxine and five received placebos. The group of patients who received pyridoxine did benefit from their vitamin B_6 therapy and had electrodiagnostic confirmation of this, whereas those who did not receive vitamin B_6 did not improve.

It has been our personal practice in the past to prescribe pyridoxine, 100 mg/day, to all patients receiving nonoperative management. (Vitamin B_6 toxicity has been reported[98] but not at levels less than 500 mg/day, and usually at levels of 1000 mg/day.) It should be possible for a medical diagnostic laboratory to do the EGOT assay, and allow us to prescribe vitamin B_6 only to those whose test results justify it.

Electrodiagnostic Testing

The general agreement in the surgical literature has been to operate on carpal tunnel syndrome if electrodiagnostic testing suggests median nerve entrapment. Our approach, as already suggested, has been to relate these electrodiagnostic results to a clinical staging system in the following way: abnormal electromyography with denervation potentials is considered severe in degree and an indication for surgery. Abnormal sensory testing, only to the extent of "no recordable sensory potentials" is considered severe in degree and an indication for surgery, since this suggests degeneration in the sensory system.

There is no good correlation between detailed clinical sensibility evaluation and electrodiagnostic studies.[70] In 74 patients with carpal tunnel syndrome diagnosed and staged clinically, it was found that nerve conduction studies were positive in 80% of minimal and in 80% of severe cases. Surgery is only recommended for the severe cases. At present, there is no reported investigation to document the natural history of patients with clinically minimal or moderate degree of nerve compression at the wrist who have positive nerve conduction studies, and who are not operated on.

There is a report[99] now of 33 of 220 carpal patients with tunnel syndrome who had normal nerve conduction studies. These patients were operated on. They would be staged as "minimal" by our criteria for degree of severity. At surgery, few pathologic changes were noted in the median nerve. Excellent results were obtained in 96% of these patients.

Our present recommendation is that electrodiagnostic testing be done only when we suspect systemic disease, multiple levels of nerve entrapments, need documentation of the nerve's condition for medicolegal reasons, or the patient presents some other diagnostic dilemma. These tests are not recommended routinely.

References

1. Paget J: Lectures on Surgical Pathology, 2nd ed. Lindsay and Blakiston, Philadelphia, 1854, p. 42.
2. Phalen GS, Gardner WJ, LaLonda AA: Neuropathy of median nerve due to compression beneath transverse carpal ligament. J Bone Joint Surg 32A:109–112, 1950.
3. Phalen GS: The carpal tunnel syndrome. Seventeen years experience in diagnosis and treatment of 654 hands. J Bone Joint Surg 48A:211–228, 1966.
4. Phalen GS: The birth of a syndrome, or carpal tunnel revisited. J Hand Surg 6:109–111, 1981.
5. Spinner M: Injuries to the Major Branches of Peripheral Nerves of the Forearm, 2nd ed., WB Saunders, Philadelphia, 1978.
6. Eversmann WW Jr: Entrapment and compression neuropathies. In Green DP, (ed): Operative Hand Surgery, 2nd ed, Churchill Livingston, Inc., New York, pp 1423–1478, 1988.
7. Schultz F: Dtsch Z Nervenheilk, 3:300, 1893.
8. Wilson SAK: Proc Soc Med (clinical section), 6:133–141, 1913.
9. Halsted WS: As to the cause of the dilatation of the subclavian artery observed in some cases of cervical rib: A clinical and experimental study Trans. Am Surg Assoc 34:272–288, 1916.
10. Sargent P: Lesions of the brachial plexus associated with rudimentary ribs. Brain 44:95–124, 1921.
11. Adson AW, Coffey JR: Cervical rib—a method of anterior approach for relief of symptoms by division of the scalenus anterior. Ann Surg 85:839–844, 1927.
12. Walsche FMR, Jackson H, Wyburn-Mason R: On some pressure effects not associated with cervical and with

rudimentary and "normal" first ribs, and the factors entering into their causation. Brain 67:141–177, 1944.
13. Zachary RB: Thenar palsy due to compression of the median nerve in the carpal tunnel. Surg Gynecol Obstet 81:213, 1945.
14. Cannon BW, Love JG: Tardy median nerve palsy: median neuritis amenable to surgery. Surgery 20:210–216, 1946.
15. Learmonth JR: Technique for transplanting the ulnar nerve. Surg Gyn Obst 75:792–793, 1942.
16. Woltman HW: Neuritis associated with acromegaly. Arch Neurol Psychiatry 45:680–682, 1941.
17. Carroll RE, Hurst LC: The relationship of thoracic outlet syndrome and carpal tunnel syndrome. Clin Orthop 164: 149–153, 1982.
18. Dellon AL, Hendler N, Hopkins JET, Karas A: Team management of patient with diffuse upper extremity complaints. Md State Med J 35:849–852, 1986.
19. Upton ARM, McComas AJ: The double crush syndrome in nerve entrapment syndromes. Lancet 2:359–362, 1972.
20. Seiler WA, Schlegel R, Mackinnon SE, Dellon AL: The double crush syndrome: Development of a model. Surg Forum 34:596–598, 1983.
21. Dellon AL, Mackinnon SE: The double crush syndrome: basic scientific and clinical applications of nerve regeneration. In Nyhus LM, ed: Surgery Annual. Appleton, Lange, Norwalk, Connecticut, 1988, pp 81–83.
22. Kendall D: Aetiology, diagnosis and treatment of paraesthesiae in the hands. Br Med J 2:1633–1640, 1960.
23. Dellon AL: Evaluation of Sensibility and Re-education of Sensation in the Hand. Williams & Wilkins, Baltimore, 1981.
24. Grossman LA, Kaplan HJ, Ownby FD, Grossman M: Carpal tunnel syndrome—initial manifestation of systems disease. JAMA 176:259–261, 1961.
25. Mackinnon SE, Dellon AL, Hudson AR, Hunter DA: Chronic nerve compression—an experimental model in the rat. Ann Plast Surg 13:112–120, 1984.
26. Mackinnon SE, Dellon AL, Hudson AR, Hunter DA: A primate model for chronic nerve compression. J Reconstr Microsurg 1:185–194, 1985.
27. Graham RA: Carpal tunnel syndrome: A statistical analysis of 214 cases. Orthopedics 6:1283–1287, 1985.
28. Kulick MI, Gordillo G, Javidi T, Kilgore ES, Newmeyer WL III: Long-term analysis of patients having surgical treatment for carpal tunnel syndrome. J Hand Surg [Am] 11:59–66, 1986.
29. Marie P, Foix C: Atrophie isolee de l'eminence thenar d'origine nevritique. Role du ligament annulaiare anterieus du carpe dans la pathoogenie de la lesion. Rev Neurol (Paris) 26:647–648, 1913.
30. Thomas PK, Fullerton PM: Nerve fiber size in the carpal tunnel syndrome. J Neurol Neurosurg Psychiatry 26:520–527, 1963.
31. Neary D, Eames RA: The pathology of ulnar nerve compression in man. Neuropathol Appl Neurobiol 1:69–88, 1975.
32. Mackinnon SE, Dellon AL, Daneshvar A: Histopathology of the tarsal tunnel syndrome: Examination of a human posterior tibial nerve. Contemp Orthop 9:43–48, 1984.
33. Jefferson D, Eames RA: Subclinical entrapment of the lateral femoral cutaneous nerve: An autopsy study. Muscle Nerve 2:145–154, 1979.
34. Neary D, Ochoa J, Gilliatt RW: Subclinical entrapment neuropathy in man. J Neurol Sci 24:283–298, 1975.
35. Mackinnon SE, Dellon AL, Hudson AR, Hunter DA: Histopathology of compression of the superficial radial nerve in the forearm. J Hand Surg [Am] 11:199–205, 1986.
36. Gentili F, Hudson AR, Kline DG, Hunter D: Morphological and physiological alterations following internal neurolysis of normal rat sciatic nerve. In Gorio A, et al, ed: Post-traumatic Peripheral Nerve Regeneration: Experimental Basis and Clinical Implications. Raven Press, New York, 1981, pp 183–210.
37. Mackinnon SE, Dellon AL: Effect of intraneural neurolysis upon chronic median nerve entrapment in the primate. J Hand Surg 13A:345–351, 1988.
38. Curtis RM, Eversmann WW Jr: Internal neurolysis as an adjunct to the treatment of the carpal tunnel syndrome. J Bone Joint Surg 55A:733–740, 1973.
39. Rydevik B, Lundborg G, Nordborg C: Intraneural tissue reactions induced by internal neurolysis. Scand J Plast Reconstr Surg 10:3–8, 1976.
40. Curtis RM: Personal communication, 1978.
41. Rhoades CE, Mowery CA, Gelberman RH: Results of internal neurolysis of the median nerve for severe carpal tunnel syndrome. J Bone Joint Surg 67A:253–256, 1985.
42. Bleecker ML, Bohlman M, Moreland R, Tipton A: Carpal tunnel syndrome: Role of carpal canal size. Neurology (Cleve) 35:1599–1604, 1985.
43. Abbott LC, Saunders JB: Injuries of the median nerve in fractures of the lower end of radius. Surg Gynecol Obstet 57:507, 1933.
44. Frykman G: Fracture of the distal radius including sequelae—shoulder-hand syndrome, disturbance of the distal radioulnar joint and impairment of nerve function. A clinical and experimental study. Acta Orthop Scand [Suppl] 108:1, 1967.
45. Lynch AC, Lipscomb PR: The carpal tunnel syndrome and Colles' fracture. JAMA 185:363, 1963.
46. Sponsel KH, Palm ET: Carpal tunnel syndrome following Colles' fracture. Surg Gynecol Obstet 121:1252, 1965.
47. Lidstrum A: Fractures of distal end of radius. A clinical and statistical study of end result. Acta Orthop Scand [Suppl] 41:1, 1959.
48. Chapman DR, Bennett JB, Bryan WJ, Tullos HS: Complications of distal radial fractures: Pins and plaster treatment. J Hand Surg 7:509–512, 1982.
49. Stewart HD, Innes AR, Burke FP: The hand complications of Colles' fractures. J Hand Surg [Br] 10:103–106, 1985.
50. Backhouse KM, Church-Davidson D: Anomalous palmaris longus muscle producing carpal tunnel-like compression. Hand 7:22–24, 1975.
51. Ametewee K, Harris A, Samuel M: Acute carpal tunnel syndrome produced by anomalous flexor digitorum superficialis indicis muscle. J Hand Surg [Br] 10:83–84, 1985.
52. Jabaley M: Personal observations on the role of the

lumbrical muscles in carpal tunnel syndrome. J Hand Surg 3:82–84, 1978.
53. Brones MF, Wilgis EFS: Anatomical variations of the palmaris longus, causing carpal tunnel syndrome. Plast Reconstr Surg 62:798–800, 1978.
54. Fatah MF: Palmaris profundus of Frohse and Frankel in association with carpal tunnel syndrome. J Hand Surg [Br] 9:142–144, 1984.
55. Lahey MD, Aulicino PL: Anomalous muscles associated with compression neuropathies. Orthop Rev 40:19–28, 1986.
56. Lanz V: Anatomic variations of the median nerve in the carpal tunnel. J Hand Surg 2:44–53, 1977.
57. Bennett JB, Crouch CC: Compression syndrome of the recurrent branch of the median curve. J Hand Surg 7:407–409, 1982.
58. Johnson RK, Shrewbury MM: Anatomical curse of the thenar branch of the median curve—usually in a separate tunnel through the transverse carpal ligament. J Bone Joint Surg 52A:269–273, 1970.
59. Jhee WH, Oryshkevich RS, Wilcox R: Severe carpal tunnel syndrome with sparing of sensory fibers. Orthop Rev 15:93–96, 1986.
60. Barfred T, Hojlund AP, Bertheussen K: Median artery in carpal tunnel syndrome. J Hand Surg [Am] 10:864–867, 1985.
61. Rayan GM: Persistent median artery and compression neuropathy. Orthop Rev 40:89–92, 1986.
62. Pecket P, Gloobe H, Nathan H: Variations in the arteries of the median nerve. Clin Orthop 97:144–147, 1973.
63. Eicken O, Carstam N, Eddland A: Anomalous distal branching of the median nerve. Scand J Plast Reconstr Surg 5:149–152, 1971.
64. Nathes A, Chacha PB, Lim P: Acute carpal tunnel syndrome secondary to thrombosis of a persistent median artery. Ann Acad Med Singapore 9:118–121, 1980.
65. Moneim MS: Unusually high division of the median nerve. J Hand Surg 7:13–14, 1982.
66. Kitayamo Y, Tsukasass S, Kurokawa M: High division of the median nerve: Unusual anatomical variations. Ann Plast Surg 14:74–76, 1985.
67. Blunt MJ: The vascular anatomy of the median nerve in the forearm and hand. J Anat 93:15–22, 1959.
68. Morgan RF, Reisman NR, Wilgis EFS: Anatomic localizaton of sympathetic nerves in the hand. J Hand Surg 8:283–288, 1983.
69. Taleisnik J: The palmar cutaneous branch of the median nerve and the approach to the carpal tunnel: An anatomic study. J Bone Joint Surg 55:1212–1217, 1973.
70. Spindler HA, Dellon AL: Nerve conduction studies and sensibility testing in carpal tunnel syndrome. J Hand Surg 7:260–263, 1982.
71. Dellon AL: The vibrometer. Plast Reconstr Surg 71:427–431, 1983.
72. Mackinnon SE, Hudson AR, Gentili F, Hunter DA: Peripheral nerve injection study with steroid agents. Plast Reconstr Surg 69:482–490, 1982.
73. Das SK, Brown GH: In search of complications in carpal tunnel decompression. Hand 8:243–249, 1976.
74. MacDonald RI, Lichtman DM, Hanlon JJ, Wilson JN: Complications of surgical release for carpal tunnel syndrome. J Hand Surg 3:70–76, 1978.
75. Lilly CJ, Magnell TD: Severance of the thenar branch of the median nerve as a complication of carpal tunnel release. J Hand Surg [Am] 10:399–402, 1985.
76. May J, Rosen H: Division of the sensory ramus communicans between the ulnar and median nerve: A complication following carpal tunnel release. J Bone Joint Surg 63:836–838, 1981.
77. Gartsman GM, Kovach JC, Crouch CC, Noble PC, Bennett JB: Carpal arch alteration after carpal tunnel release. J Hand Surg [Am] 11:372–374, 1986.
78. Simeone FA: Acute and delayed traumatic peripheral entrapment neuropathies. Surg Clin North Am 51:1329–1336, 1972.
79. Wilgis EFS: Personal communication, 1986.
80. Dellon AL, Mackinnon SE, Daneshvar A: Terminal branch of the anterior interosseous nerve as a source of wrist pain. J Hand Surg [Br] 9:316–322, 1984.
81. Paine KWE: The carpal tunnel syndrome. Can J Surg 6:446–449, 1963.
82. Patrick J: Carpal tunnel syndrome. Br Med J, 1:1377–1378, 1965.
83. Creuz KA, Thoms JE, Lambert EH, Love JG, Lipscomb PR: Long-term results of operation for carpal tunnel syndrome. Mayo Clin Proc 41:232–241, 1966.
84. Langloh ND, Linscheid RL: Recurrent and unrelieved carpal-tunnel syndrome. Clin Orthop 83:41–47, 1972.
85. Rietz KA, Önne L: Analysis of sixty-five operated cases of carpal tunnel syndrome. Acta Chir Scand 133:443–447, 1967.
86. Gelberman RH, Pfeffer GB, Galbraith RT, Szabo RM, Rydevik B, Dimik M: Results of treatment of severe carpal tunnel syndrome without internal neurolysis of the median nerve. J Bone Joint Surg 69A:896–903, 1987.
87. Kopell HP: Carpal tunnel compression median neuropathy treated nonsurgically. NY State J Med 58:744–745, 1958.
88. Crow RS: Treatment of the carpal tunnel syndrome. Br Med J 1:1611–1615, 1960.
89. Gelberman RH, Aronson D, Weisman MH: Carpal tunnel syndrome. Results of a prospective trial of steroid injection and splinting. J Bone Joint Surg 62A:1181–1184, 1980.
90. Green DP: Diagnostic and therapeutic value of carpal tunnel injection. J Hand Surg [Am] 9:850–854, 1984.
91. Schuchmann JA, Melvin JL, Duran RJ, Coleman CR: Evaluation of local steroid injection for carpal tunnel syndrome. Arch Phys Med Rehabil 52:253–255, 1971.
92. Kishi H, Kishi T, William RH, Folkers K: Human deficiencies of vitamin B_6. I. Studies on parameters of the assay of the glutamic oxaloacetic transaminase by the CAS principle. Res Commun Chem Pathol Pharmacol 12:557–569, 1975.
93. Solomon LR, Hillman RS: Regulation of vitamin B_6 metabolism in human red cells. Am J Clin Nutr 32:1824–1831, 1979.
94. Ellis JM, Folkers K, Levy M, Shizukuishi S, Lewandowski

J, Nishii S, Schubert HA, Ulrich R: Response of vitamin B-6 deficiency and the carpal tunnel syndrome to pyridoxine. Proc Natl Acad Sci USA 79:7494–7498, 1982.

95. Ellis J, Folkers K, Levy M, Takemura K, Shizukuishi S, Ulrich R, Harrison P : Therapy with vitamin B_6 with and without surgery for treatment of patients having the idiopathic carpal tunnel syndrome. Res Commun Chem Pathol Pharmacol 33:331–344, 1981.

96. Amadio PC: Pyridoxine as an adjunct in the treatment of carpal tunnel syndrome. J Hand Surg [Am] 10:237–241, 1985.

97. Arem A, Halvarson G, Vadhanavikit S, Kolkers K: Effects of vitamin B_6 in carpal tunnel syndrome. Presented at the Plastic Surgery Research Council meeting, May, 1985.

98. Schaumburg H, Kaplan J, Windebank A, Vick N, Rasmus S, Pleasure D, Brown MJ: Sensory neuropathy from pyridoxine abuse: A new megavitamin syndrome. N Engl J Med 309:445–448, 1983.

99. Grundberg AB: Carpal tunnel decompression in spite of normal electromyography. J Hand Surg 8:348–349, 1983.

100. Semple JC, Cargill AO: Carpal tunnel syndrome: Results of surgical decompression. Lancet 1:918–919, 1969.

101. Posch JL, Marcotte DR: Carpal tunnel syndrome: An analysis of 1201 cases. Orthop Rev 5:25–35, 1976.

102. Eversmann WW Jr, Retsick JA: Intraoperative changes in motor nerve conduction latency in carpal tunnel syndrome. J Hand Surg 3:77–81, 1978.

103. Reisman NR, Dellon AL: The abductor digiti minimi muscle flap: A salvage technique for palmar wrist pain. Plast Reconstr Surg 72:859–863, 1983.

7

Median Nerve Entrapment in the Proximal Forearm and Brachium

Historical Review

Injury to the median nerve proximal to the wrist constitutes a challenging variety of problems, primarily in determining the site of injury to the median nerve. These problems have been considered by previous investigators, with encyclopedic descriptions of these contributing problems, diagnostic approaches, and treatment results.[1–5] The purpose of the present chapter is to place these considerations into perspective to permit a practical approach for the surgical management of this peripheral nerve injury. In general, the problems with the median nerve that are encountered in the brachium, or upper arm, are frequently associated with vascular problems. This is due to the close relationship of the median nerve, from its origin from the medial and lateral cords of the brachial plexus, to the axillary and then the brachial artery. In contrast, problems with the median nerve at the elbow and proximal forearm are more likely due to compression of the median nerve by various anatomic structures. This may be associated with a single act of trauma or, increasingly in our daily experience, with repetitive traumatic disorders (workmen's compensation). The diagnosis depends on a thorough understanding of the anatomy of the median nerve and the various muscle and fibrous arch anomalies that can occur along its length. Various nerve anomalies, such as the Martin-Gruber anastomosis, must be appreciated. The surgical approach to this region must take into account, the concept of the multiple crush syndrome (Chapter 14). Inherent in the concept of the multiple crush syndrome will be the surgical requirement of release of all potential compressive sites along the course of the nerve. A detailed understanding of these potential compressive sites will be extremely important in determining the diagnosis of the problem.

Surgical Anatomy

Brachium

The median nerve is formed in the axilla and generally located anterior to the axillary artery. The median nerve is formed by a branch of the lateral cord and the medial cord of the brachial plexus and thus contains contributions from C5, C6, C7, C8, and T1 through the an-

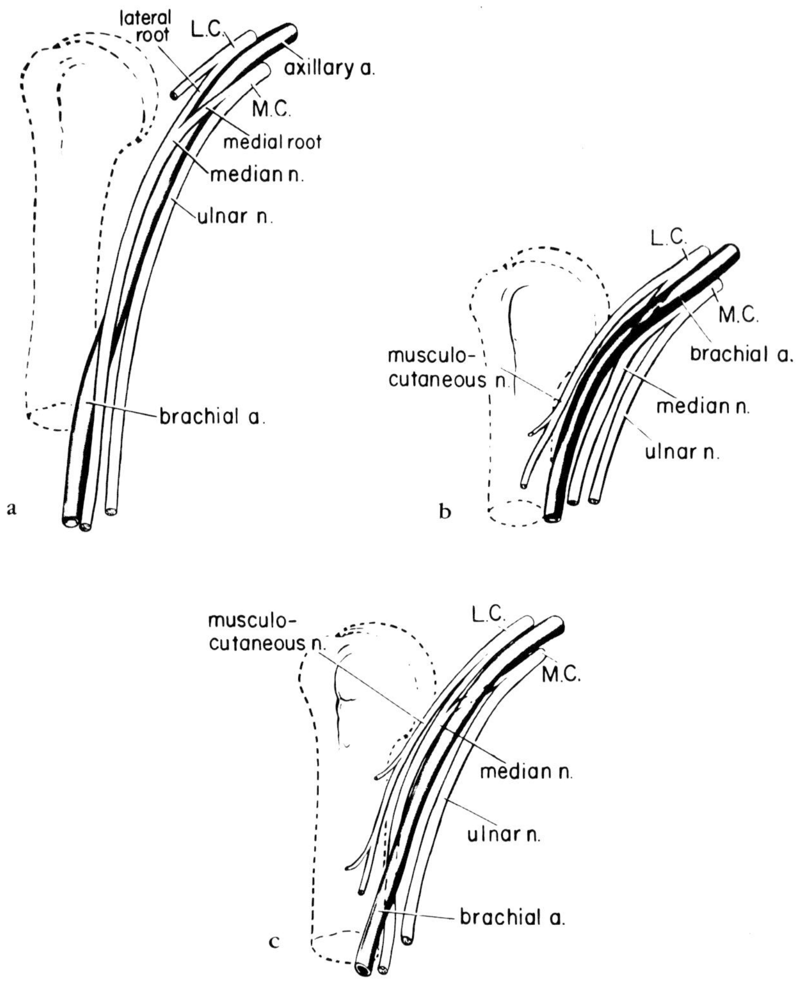

Figure 7-1. Variations in origin of the median neve with respect to the axillary artery. **(a)** The usual pattern with the nerve anterior to the artery. The lateral **(b)** and the medial **(c)** and contribution to the median nerve pass posterior to the artery. L.C.: lateral cord; M.C.: medial cord. (Reproduced with permission from Kaplan and Spinner.[6])

terior divisions of the upper, middle, and lower trunks of the brachial plexus. The medial cord contribution is constant in size. Occasionally, the lateral cord contribution will be smaller and may be either double or triple in terms of branches that join the medial cord component. Furthermore, either the medial or lateral cord component may pass posterior to the axillary artery (Fig. 7-1). The contribution from the lateral cord may be "deferred," ultimately joining the median nerve as a branch from the musculocutaneous in the upper portion of the upper arm, rather than in the axilla. The medial and lateral cord contributions themselves may not join together in the axilla but may await a juncture until the proximal third of the upper arm.[6] When the lateral cord contribution to the median nerve is small, it is increasingly likely that there is a contribution from the musculocutaneous to the median nerve in the proximal portion of the arm. This arrangement has been noted to occur in 24% of cadaver dissections[7,8] (Fig. 7-2). The median nerve, once formed, crosses the medial intermuscular septum and will ultimately continue across the elbow into the forearm on top of the brachialis muscle in the central portion of the arm approximately half way from medial to lateral. The medial relationship of the median nerve to the brachial artery and then the biceps tendon provides a useful anatomic arrangement that facilitates surgical exploration (TAN: tendon, artery, nerve, from lateral to medial at the elbow). However, in one significant variation, described by Struthers in 1848,[9] a bony process, arising on the medial aspect of the distal humerus and termed a "supracondylar spur," was noted by Struthers in his cadaver dissections. Struthers, an anatomy professor, after noting the presence of this supracondylar spur in approximately 3% of his cadaver dissections, made further observations on this anomaly. He found that he could palpate the bony spur through the skin. He also noted a ligament going from the end of the supracondylar process toward the medial humeral epicondyle and through this passed the median nerve accompanied by an artery. In our clinical experience we have not noticed one example of Struthers' supracondylar process or Struthers' ligament. The anatomic dissections done on 104 extremities in 64 cadavers,[10] just one arm was

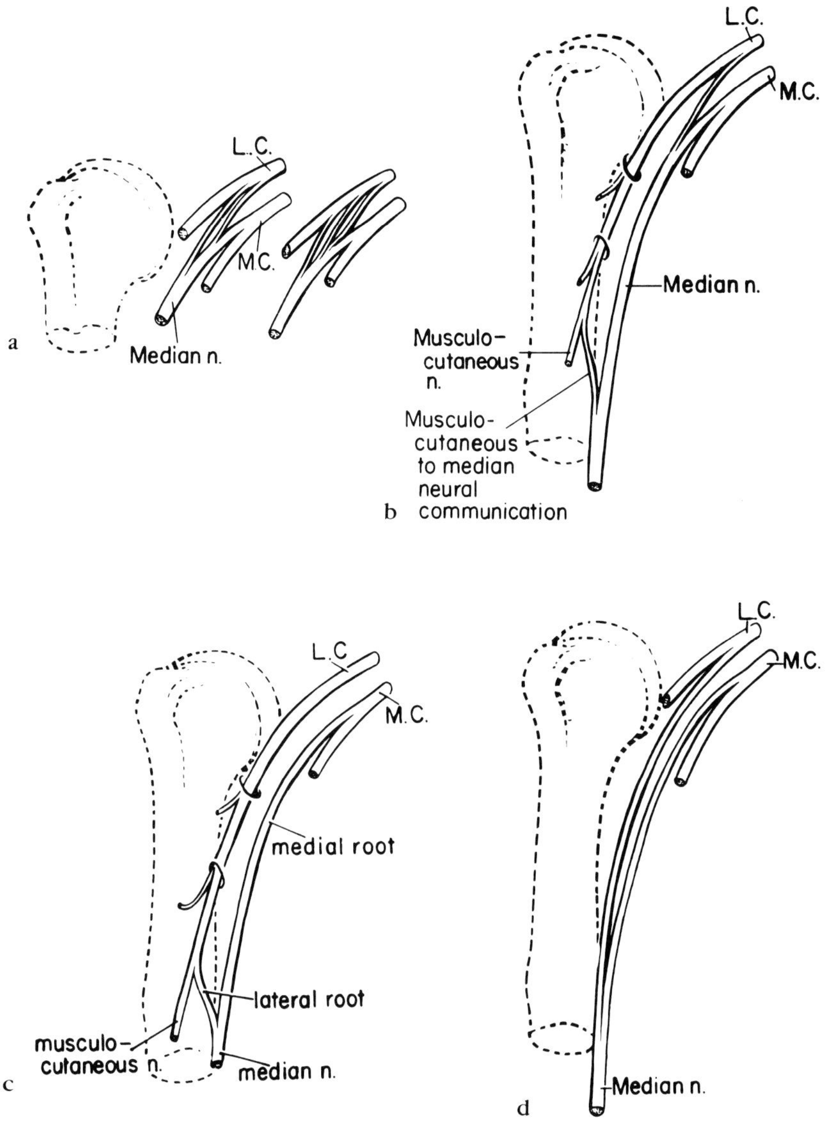

Figure 7-2. Variations in lateral cord contribution to the median nerve. These may be multiple branches **(a)**. There may be a contribution from the musculocutaneous, as well as the lateral cord (L.C.). There may be no lateral cord contribution, but rather a significant contribution from the musculocutaneous **(c)**. The medial (M.C.) and lateral cord may join to form the median nerve in the proximal third of the branchium instead of the axilla **(d)**. (Reproduced with permission from Kaplan and Spinner[6])

found to have a rudimentary supracondylar process. Struthers observed that the supracondylar process was a remnant from the evolutionary process of the formation of the distal humerus based on three separate observations in cats.[11] Today, at least three generations past Struthers anatomic observations, we have found the incidence of the supracondylar process decreasing and therefore the occurrence of median nerve problems from this cause will probably continue to decrease in importance. We may make the conjecture that the supracondylar process through evolution is disappearing.

When there was a high division of the brachial artery into the radial and ulnar artery, the ulnar artery accompanied the median nerve (Fig. 7-3). Symptoms from this problem thus can be vascular as well as neurologic, but they infrequently occur in the absence of trauma. Many reports have noted problems related to this anatomic variation in the setting of trauma.[12–18] In such instances, surgical exploration with resection of the bony spur and the ligament has been successful in relieving symptoms. (This potential site of entrapment, the ligament of Struthers, is the only entrapment site described by Struthers. Struthers, himself, did not describe the so-called "arcade of Struthers" which supposedly entraps the ulnar nerve [see Chapter 9].[10])

The relationship of the median nerve to arterial venous structures in the upper arm is the basis for additional sources of nerve injury. A common one, and one being seen with increasing frequency, is nerve compression due to bleeding from diagnostic and therapeutic procedures. For example, drawing blood from the brachial artery in the antecubital fossa can lead to

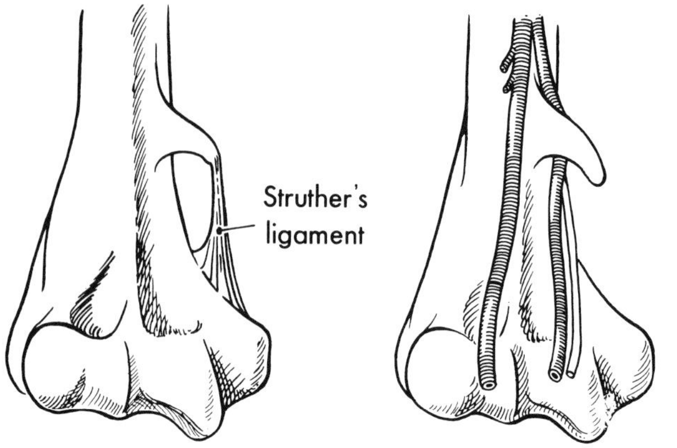

Figure 7-3. Struthers supracondylar bone process and ligament, (left), and associated median nerve and artery (may be either brachial artery or, as is the case here, when there is a high division of the brachial artery, the ulnar artery) passing beneath the ligament, (right). (Reproduced with permission from Stewart.[5]).

extravasaton of blood, especially in patients receiving anticoagulants. Bleeding in this location causes compression of the median nerve beneath the overlying unyielding lacertus fibrosis.[19] Cases of this type have been described and the appropriate treatment is surgical intervention with release of the lacertus fibrosis and evacuation of the hematoma. Similar problems have been reported in patients with bleeding disorders[20] and for axillary arteriotomies.[21] A related problem is diagnostic procedures, such as arteriography. Catheter insertion into axillary arteries or veins can lead to bleeding, causing nerve compression in the brachial sheath.[22,23] Again in this instance, surgical exploration with release of the sheath and evacuation of the hematoma is the indicated treatment. Diagnosis in these situations is based on the clinical observation of sensory symptoms in the distribution of the median nerve, followed by an associated muscle weakness, swelling in the forearm, elbow, or axillary site where the iatrogenic intervention occurred. In the awake cooperative patient, vibratory testing is carried out in the distribution of the median nerve.[24] It has been demonstrated that abnormal perception of the 256 cps vibratory tuning fork correlates with an intracompartmental tissue pressure of 40 to 45 mmHg. This would be an appropriate pressure for a surgical intervention (for additional discussion of vibratory testing and nerve injuries, see Chapter 3).

At the extremes of the brachium are the axilla and the antecubital fossa. Compression of the median nerve by virtue of compression by anatomic structures in the axilla is best considered under brachial plexus problems where compression beneath the pectoralis minor is discussed (Chapter 14).

Continuing with problems associated with arteries and median nerve compression in the brachium, Omer and Spinner[3] have reported on six patients who had either partial or complete median nerve paralysis caused by anomalous vascular perforations (an artery or vein perforating the median nerve) or vascular arches that compressed or tethered the median nerve in the axilla. In particular, a well-documented case had perforation of the median nerve high in the axilla by the posterior humeral circumflex artery. Preoperative diagnosis was made by means of an arteriogram.[25] Spinner has emphasized that either a brachial arteriogram or venogram may be required with the arm either at the side first and then with the arm elevated in order to distinguish whether an artery or vein is contributing to the proximal compressive site. The diagnosis is made when the normal artery or venous pattern disappears with elevation of the arm. The patient with the posterior circumflex humeral artery perforation of the median nerve presented with a sudden onset of pain in the shoulder, loss of ability to flex the terminal phalanx of the thumb, and tenderness along the medial aspect of the arm below the coracoid process. Surgical approach in this case required ligation of the perforating vessels with a good postoperative relief of symptoms and progressive improvement in function of the thumb with full recovery by 4 months.

Bony injury in the brachium is rarely associated with median nerve problems. For example, in a series of 73 anterior shoulder dislocations and fractures of the surgical neck of the humerus, only one of the 73 patients had a median nerve problem, whereas 22 patients had axillary nerve injury.[26] The majority of nerve problems associated with fractures in the brachium are due to direct crush injury or high velocity missile secondary effects on the nerve. These do not require direct surgical approach to the nerve.[27,28] Approximately 85% of the lesions have spontaneous recovery within 4 months. Parenthetically, failure to recover after four months would lead us to suggest earlier exploration especially in an area of known anatomic nerve compression to ensure that there is no superimposed component of compressive neuropathy that is providing an additive effect to the existing degree of nerve injury [see Chapter 3]. Complete nerve lesions associated with gunshot wounds above the elbow or stretch injuries from dislocated joints and fractures adjacent to joints should be explored by 3 to 4 months. Fifty percent of these are found to have a neuroma in-continuity (for discussion of approach to this problem, see Chapters 4, 5, and 17). With regard to the distal end of the brachium, the anatomic structures are best considered with respect to the proximal forearm (see next section).

Proximal Forearm and Elbow

The median curve crosses the elbow superficial to the brachialis muscle. This muscle in general protects the median nerve from underlying bony problems. Nevertheless, a large brachialis muscle has been reported to contribute to median nerve compression, against the overlying bicipital aponeurosis and lacertus fibrosis.[13,29] Additional anomalous ligaments have also been reported to compress the median nerve in this area.[30] We have identified an origin of the superficial head of the pronator teres arising 2 cm proximal to the medial humeral epicondyle in 20% of cadaver dissections.[10] It has been postulated that in this situation, the pronator teres superficial head now is in position to compress the median nerve directly against the underlying trochlear process of the humerus with elbow extension and with forearm pronation (Figs. 7-4, 7-5). Struthers, in 1854, continuing his observations on the supracondylar process, noted that there was a "high origin to the pronator teres, which may at first form a separate muscle, this appears to be frequently, if not generally present in cases of supracondyloid process."

Bony ligamentous injuries about the elbow can be responsible for median nerve injury. In particular, supracondylar fractures have been reported to cause injury to either the entire median nerve or to a particular distribution of the median nerve, such as the anterior interosseous nerve.[31–36] Posterior dislocation at the elbow has been reported to cause similar injuries to the median nerve.[37–39] As well, the nerve has been found

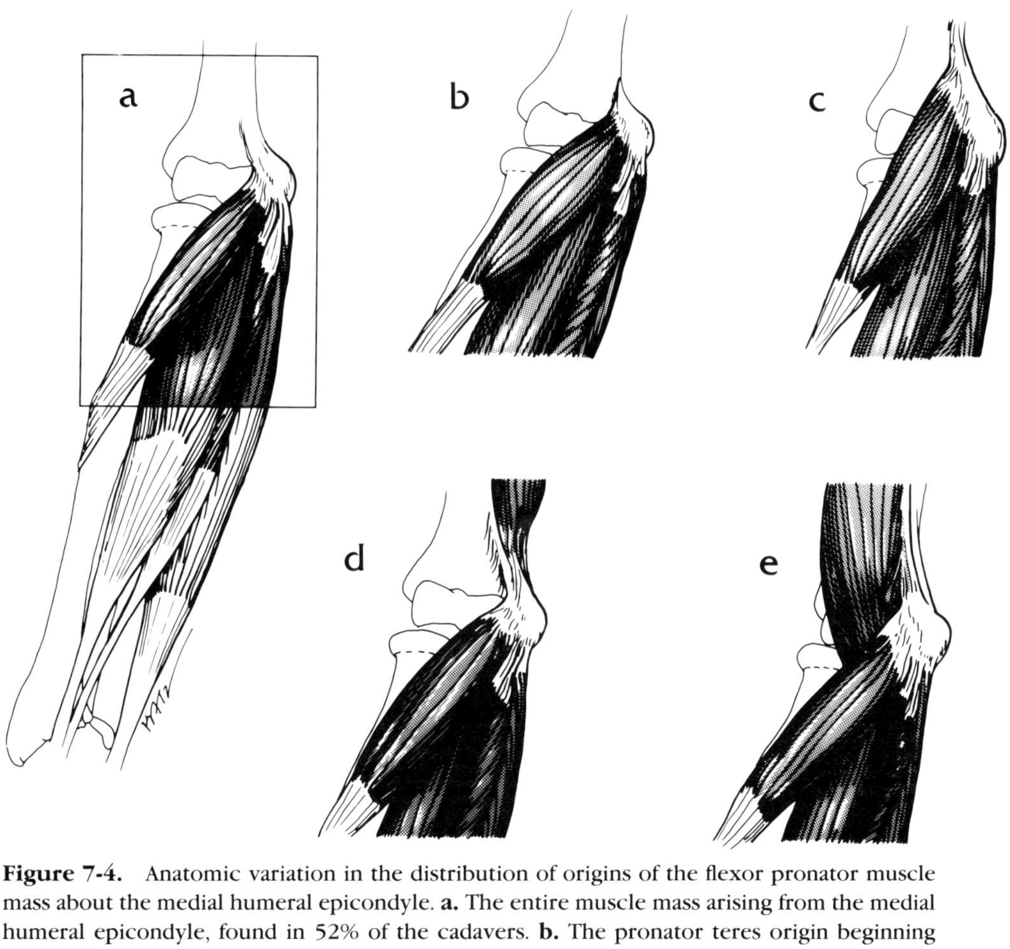

Figure 7-4. Anatomic variation in the distribution of origins of the flexor pronator muscle mass about the medial humeral epicondyle. **a.** The entire muscle mass arising from the medial humeral epicondyle, found in 52% of the cadavers. **b.** The pronator teres origin beginning up to 2 cm proximal to the epicondyle, found in 31% of the cadavers. **c.** A high origin of the pronator teres, 2 cm or more proximal to the epicondyle, found in 17% of the cadavers. Among those with the high origin of the pronator teres was one fibrous origin coming from the medial head of the triceps tendon joining with fibers from the medial intermuscular septum (**d**), and one muscular coming from brachialis muscle fibers and the median intermuscular septum in one cadaver (**e**). (Reproduced with permission from Dellon.[10])

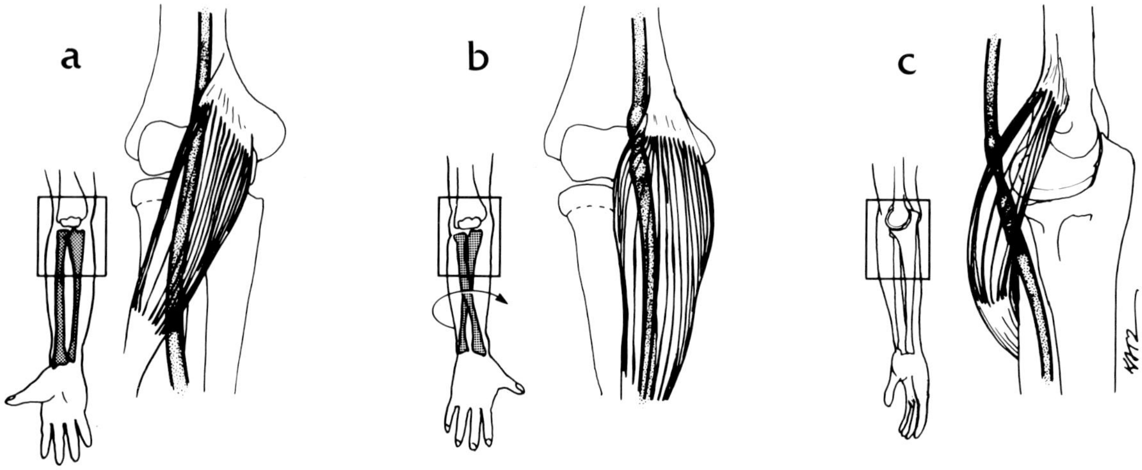

Figure 7-5. Relationship of median nerve to high origin of flexor pronator muscle mass. **a.** With origin below axis of elbow flexion, the median nerve is not compressed by the pronator teres. With a high origin, pronation of the forearm may cause compression of the median nerve beneath the edge of the pronator (b), and extension of the elbow may cause compression of the median nerve against the trochlear process of the humerus (c). (Reproduced with permission from Dellon.[10])

to be entrapped between an untreated fracture of the distal humerus.[40] Injuries to the nerves due to this fracture dislocation problem frequently occur in children. This often makes the diagnosis a further challenge. Use of vibratory testing in these pediatric cases is especially useful[41] (Chapter 3).

Awareness of the potential nerve injury is the most critical factor in making the correct diagnosis. Correction of the fracture and dislocation by the appropriate orthopedic maneuvers is mandatory. Careful follow-up of the extremity for the period of time any edema is present is the recommended course of action. Frequent physical examination looking for any sensory deficits in the median nerve, inappropriate or increasing pain, and an inability to flex the interphalangeal joint of the thumb and index finger are the best guidelines. As already described, one of the best ways to carry out the sensory testing in children is with vibratory stimuli. This is especially useful in children who may view other forms of sensory testing as either painful or frightening. When the child perceives the tuning fork, he either smiles or gently moves his head away or, in fact, may laugh.

A wide range of clinical presentations of these median nerve injuries has caused speculation as to the mechanism of nerve injury. It is interesting to speculate on the reason for anterior interosseous nerve injuries in the presence of normal sensation. Millesi's theory, which we support, is that an entire median nerve may be compressed by various arches, but the anterior interosseous nerve receives an additional "crush" effect in that it is relatively tethered at its "takeoff" from the median nerve proper. Although the median nerve proper can thus glide longitudinally in the forearm, the anterior interosseous nerve is subjected to a traction injury at the relatively immobile branching point. Anatomic factors that also account for this finding of preferential injury to the nerve are the facts that the anterior interosseous nerve fibers lay in the posterior aspect of the median nerve and therefore are most likely to come in direct contact with the bony surface of the humerus in the trauma. This has also been suggested as the reason for index and middle finger sensory changes, as supposedly these nerve fibers are in the posterior aspect of the nerve. In fact, however, a review of anatomy books[42] suggests that the anterior interosseous nerve is not always depicted by the illustrator as being posterior and, in fact, most reported cases with intraoperative photographic documentation of anterior interosseous nerve compression (see next section) suggests that the anterior interosseous nerve arises on the radial side of the median nerve. Based on our own series of 43 extremities in 31 cadavers, we found the anterior interosseous nerve to arise on the radial side of the median nerve in 19 of the 31 cadavers.[42]

As will be discussed later, there are a series of fibrous arches that occur across the median nerve just distal to the antecubital fossa, caused by the muscular origins of the deep and superficial heads of the pronator teres and the flexor digitorum superficialis (Fig. 7-6). It has been postulated[42] that symptoms of anterior interosseous nerve syndrome are related to whether the anterior interosseous nerve arises on the radial side of the median nerve and its relationship with a fibrous arch. This hypothesis may be extended further to the situation with fractures and ligamentous injuries about the elbow in terms of the wide variation in the clinical pic-

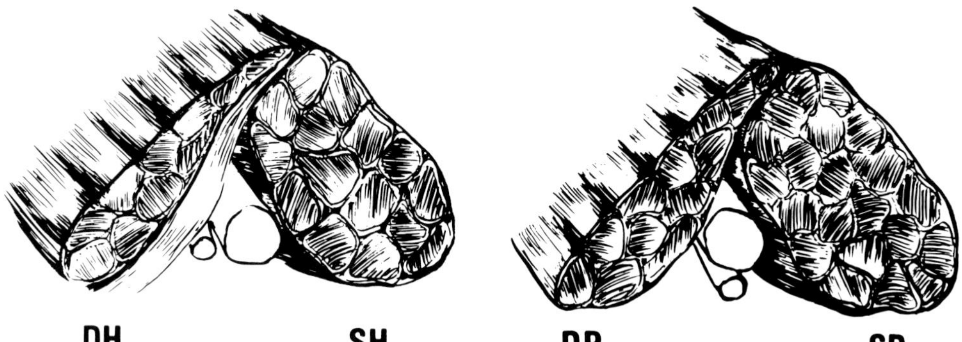

Figure 7-6. Schematic diagram of "at risk" concept for nerve compression related to a presence of a fibrous band or edge to a muscle crossing the nerve (left) and location of branch to be compressed with respect to the fibrous arch and the main nerve trunk (right). Thus, in the example at the left the fibrous edge of the deep head of the pronator teres (DH) and the radial origin of the anterior interosseous nerve from the median nerve make this anatomic arrangement "at risk" in contrast to the one on the right.[42] SH.SP, superficial head of pronator teres; DH.DP, deep head of pronator teres where DH has fibrous bind on deep surface head of pronator teres.

ture that is presented. When the fibers of the anterior interosseous nerve are posterior to the median nerve or if they arise radial and are in a relationship to a distal fibrous arch, then these nerve fibers will either be more likely to be injured directly by bone in the first instance or be tethered distally if a dislocation occurs in the latter instance. Thus, the anatomic arrangement present at the time of the injury most likely determines the spectrum of signs and symptoms that will occur. These anatomic factors must be borne in mind during the physical examination and during any surgical exploration undertaken to decompress the nerves (see further discussion later).

The significant anatomic variations with respect to the median nerve itself relate to a high origin of a sensory branch to the web space between the middle and ring fingers and the contribution from the median nerve to the ulnar nerve described as the Martin-Gruber anastomosis. Winkelman and Spinner[43] in 1973 described a branch arising from the median nerve approximately 4 cm distal to the anterior interosseous nerve that went through an opening in the flexor sublimis muscle and then ran distally along the surface of the anterior sublimis muscle lying just beneath the antebrachial fascia until it entered the carpal tunnel. Spinner[2] additionally quotes Sunderland, who noted that Gruber in 1870 reported four specimens similar to the one described by Winkelman and Spinner. Additionally, Spinner[2] quotes Hartman in an article in French in 1888 with a similar anatomic specimen. The surgical significance of this clearly is that if unusual sensation occurs in the web space between the middle and ring fingers or if sensation is lost after a relatively superficial injury in the forearm or deeper proximal forearm, exploration for this anatomic variation should be considered and searched for possible nerve repair. At the wrist level, there is what is frequently termed a "high division of the median nerve." This is described in Chapter 6 and is different from the anatomic variation just described. Martin[44] in 1763 and Gruber[45] in 1870 described a branch from the median nerve to the ulnar nerve that carried motor fibers. This branch can arise either directly from the median nerve or as a branch from the anterior interosseous nerve. Clearly, this nerve anomaly is not a true anastomosis. Nerve fibers are primarily carried to the first dorsal interosseous and the palmar and dorsal interossei to the second and third web spaces, as well as occasionally to the hypothenar muscles and also occasionally to the adductor pollicis muscle. The surgical significance of this is that an ulnar nerve lesion at the elbow could be present and yet all the intrinsic muscles of the hand still function. A lesion of the median nerve at the elbow or more proximally when the Martin-Gruber anastomosis is present would therefore also result in the loss of all intrinsic muscle functions of the hand, although the ulnar nerve would be without a lesion.[46] Sunderland[47] has reviewed the anatomic studies that have looked toward the incidence of this anastomosis that was reported by Gruber to be present in 20% of dissections. Sunderland quotes Thompson in 1893 as having demonstrated 15% incidence. Thane in 1895 and Piersol in 1907 as demonstrating a 20 to 25% instance, Hirosawa in 1931 as demonstrating a 10.5% incidence. The most recent clinical and experimental study has been done by Mannerfelt,[48] who identified this neural anomaly as being present in 15%. From the comparative anatomy standpoint, we have identified the Martin-Gruber anastomosis as being present in 100% of baboons, rhesus monkeys, and cynomolgus monkeys.[49] In these animals, the anastomosis was noted in the very proximal portion of the forearm. This has clear relevance with respect to anatomic models for neural regeneration of the median or ulnar nerve. Dèpending on the experimental design, the Martin-Gruber anastomosis will require division at the outset in these studies or its presence be accounted for in evaluation of the results.

Anatomic Studies

The anatomic arrangement of the muscles with the median nerve has a relationship to and plays a signifciant role in nerve compression distal to the elbow. There are variations in the pronator teres, in the flexor digitorum sublimis, and in the flexor pollicis longus contributing to possible sites of nerve entrapment. The relationship of the median nerve to the pronator teres and flexor digitorum sublimis is best understood in terms of the nerve's relationship to a passageway beneath an arch. There may be either no arch, one arch, or two arches present across the median nerve. This relationship was best described from a series of cadaver dissections[42] and the results of that study are depicted schematically in Figure 7-7. The pronator teres muscle's superficial head, arising from the medial humeral epicondyle, was present in all specimens. The fascial covering of the flexor pronator muscle mass is continuous proximally with the lacertus fibrosis and thereby forms a continuous sheath with the fascia in the upper arm. The median nerve crosses beneath this fibrous sheath and beneath the superficial head of the pronator teres in all instances. The pronator teres was missing a deep head in 6% of the specimens and in this situation there was no true arch formed across the median nerve. In the remaining 94% of the specimens, the deep head of the pronator teres, which has a variable origin from either the coranoid process of the ulna or from the interossous membrane or from both, joins the superficial head of the pronator teres, forming the first arch. Eleven of the 31 specimens had a fibrous arch beneath the superficial head and 15 and 31 specimens had a distinct fibrous arch on the ulnar side of the deep head of the pronator teres. The flexor digitorum superficialis may have from one to three heads. The relationship between the presence of these origins of the sublimis muscle with respect to the presence of arches and the pronator teres is depicted schematically in Figure 7-7. In all instances, there was a head arising from the medial

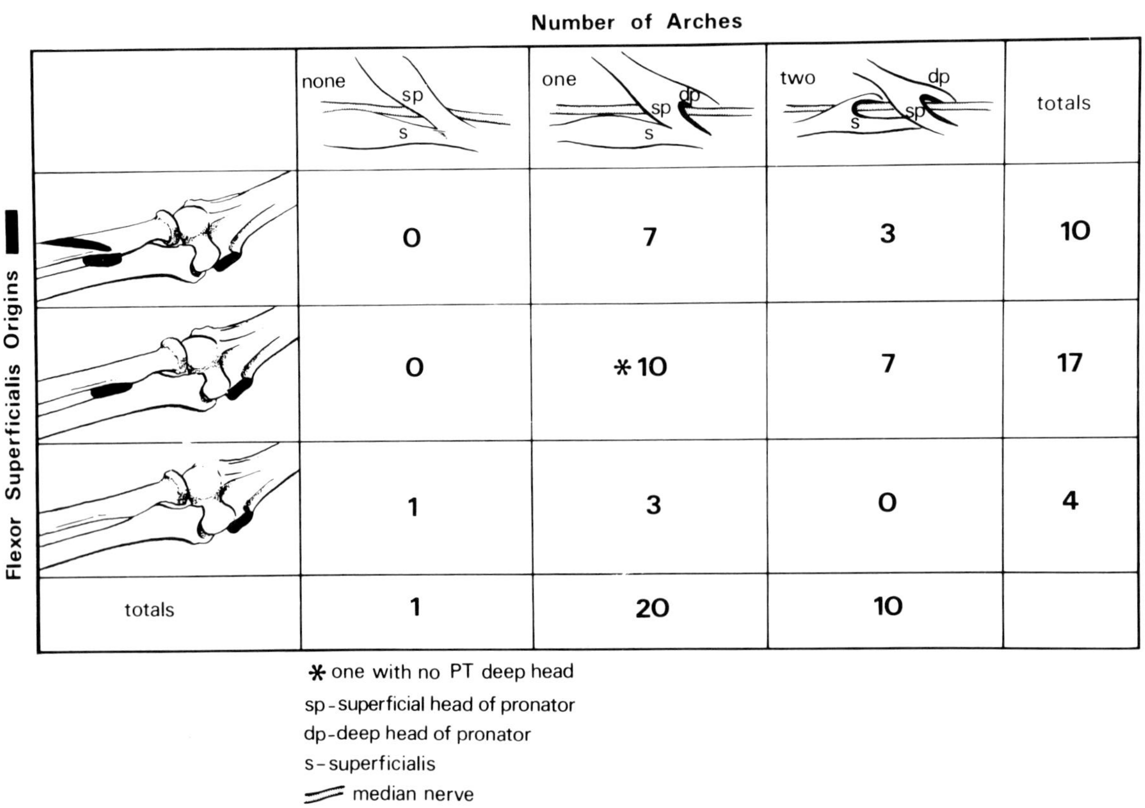

Number of Arches

Flexor Superficialis Origins	none	one	two	totals
(row 1)	0	7	3	10
(row 2)	0	*10	7	17
(row 3)	1	3	0	4
totals	1	20	10	

Figure 7-7. Relationship of a number of arches crossing the median and flexor superficialis origin. (Reproduced with permission from Dellon and Mackinnon.[42])

humeral epicondyle. In 4 of the 31 specimens, this was the only head present. In 17 of the 31 specimens, there was a deep or second origin that arose from the interosseous membrane. This deep origin was in a direct distal line with the deep head's origin of the pronator teres. In 10 of the 31 specimens, the superficialis had a wide third origin from a diagonal area on the volar aspect of the radius. Here, it lay just distal to the pronator teres insertion and just proximal to the origin of the flexor pollicis longus. Eleven of the 31 specimens had a fibrous arch beneath the superficialis muscle junctures of its superficial and deep head. The deep head of the pronator teres and of the superficialis muscle are separated by approximately 1 cm in their origin. When the superficialis muscles do not take additional origin or do not join with the pronator teres, then a second arch is formed (Figs. 7-8, 7-9). In 10 of the 31 cases, there were two distinct arch systems present.

The surgical implication of these arches is that the presence of the fibrous arch places the nerve in relationship to a potentially compressive structure. If the patient's work activity requires a significant amount of pronation of the forearm or flexion of the fingers, the muscle hypertrophy plus the presence of this fibrous arch predisposes the patient to nerve compression. If, in addition, the anterior interosseus nerve, as described in the preceding section, arises on the radial instead of the posterior aspect of the median nerve, then the anterior interosseous nerve is particularly predisposed to compression beneath this fibrous arch (Fig. 7-6).

During the surgical exploration, the arch system must be completely excised. This implies that the surgeon must look to see if a second arch is present. Correcting the presence of a first arch will clearly be insufficient to treat the problem if a second arch is also present. Where the sublimis muscle arises with the deep head of the pronator, there is a cojoined arch, but after release of the first arch, the technique for which will be discussed later, the surgeon must continue to look distally to be sure that a second arch separated in space due to a more distant sublimis deep head origin does not coexist.

The flexor pollicis longus muscle originates from the radius beginning at the juncture of the proximal and distal two-thirds and from the interosseous membrane. The best way to conceptualize the variations that are found is to think of them as variations in the flexor pollicis longus muscle. The most common anomaly is the muscle described by Gantzer in 1818. The most complete anatomic study related to this was done by Mangini[50] in 1960 and his findings were confirmed by our own dissection study.[42] Gantzer's muscle is best understood as an accessory slip of the flexor pollicis longus muscle at its most proximal location. It was present in 45% of our cadaver dissections. It was always found to be innervated by a proximal branch from the anterior interosseous nerve. In all instances, Gantzer's muscle arose deep to the anterior interosseous nerve, and in no instance did it cross superficial to the anterior interosseous nerve. The muscle originates from the medial humeral upper condyle deep to the other muscles. The muscle varied in its length and some were joined by just a short tendon to the tendon of the flexor pollicis longus but in most instances it was joined by a tendinous length of at least 3 cm (Figures 7-8, 14-6). In this location, Gantzer's muscle may compress the anterior interosseous nerve. The surgeon, after releasing the flexor sublimis arch, must look to see if either a large muscle belly of Gantzer's muscle could compress the anterior interosseous nerve from below against an overlying structure or whether there is any variation with respect to the nerve and the tendinous origin of this muscle. Kaplan has noted that fibrosis and secondary contraction of this muscle could produce a flexion contracture of the thumb. Clearly, this would not be part of the presentation of a median nerve injury but is noted as a possible instance in which Gantzer's muscle or its tendon would require resection or division.[51] Two other anomalous muscles, much rarer in occurrence, may arise in relationship to the flexor pollicis longus origin. The palmaris profundus can originate via a tendinous origin near the proximal aspect of the flexor pollicis and then be extended by its muscle belly beneath the flexor carpi radialis to insert by its tendon either into the transverse carpal ligament or go superficial or deep to the transverse carpal ligament.[52] The flexor carpi radialis brevis is similar in that it can arise from the central region of the flexor pollicis longus and, by means of a distal tendon, insert with the flexor carpi radialis.[2] Either of these muscles, by means of its fibrous origin and muscle belly, may compress the median nerve in the more distal portion of the forearm (Fig. 7-10).

Other structures that may be of importance to median nerve compression in this region are the arteries and veins that may cross the median nerve, such as the ulnar collateral vessels.

Diagnosis

The diagnosis of median nerve injury will be apparent from a consideration of the functions of the median nerve. Primarily, any loss of thumb abduction and opposition and loss of sensation over the volar aspect of the thumb, index, and middle fingers and the radial half of the ring finger, loss of flexor pollicis longus function, loss of the flexor profundus to the index and middle fingers, loss of the pronator teres, flexor carpi radialis,

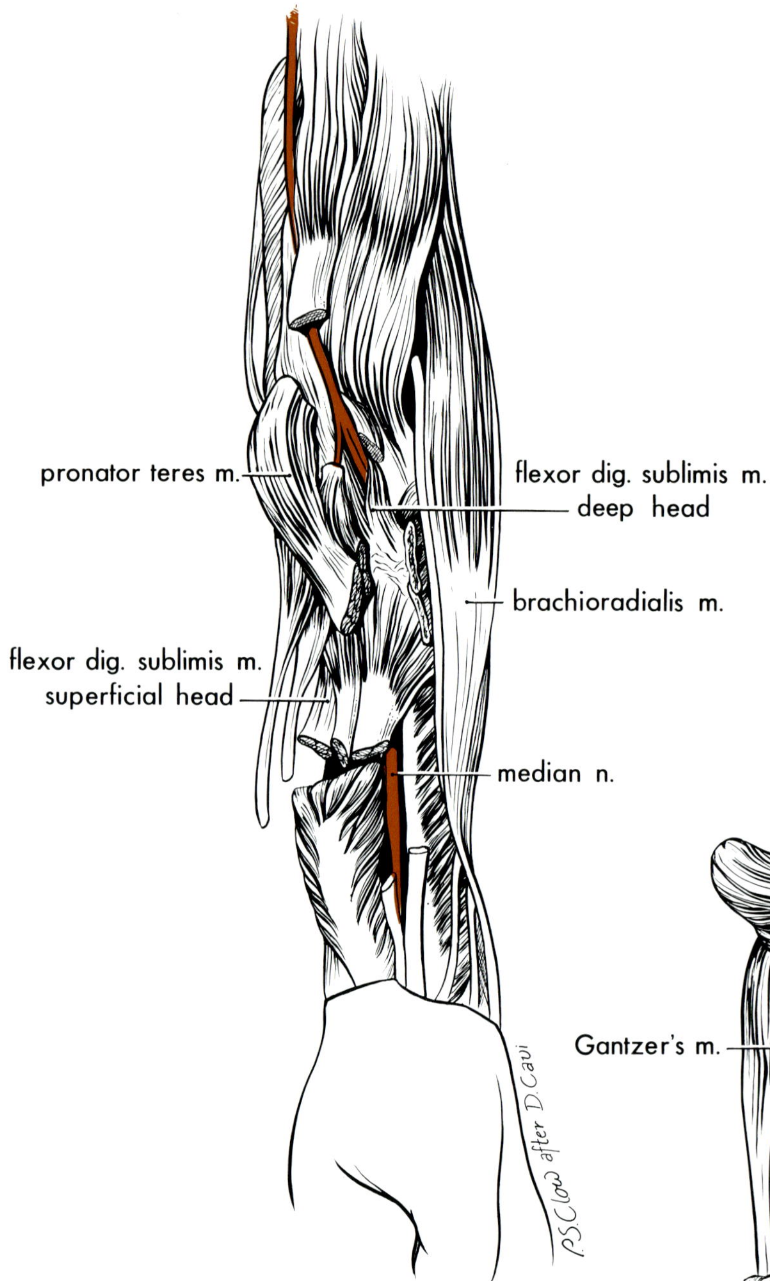

a

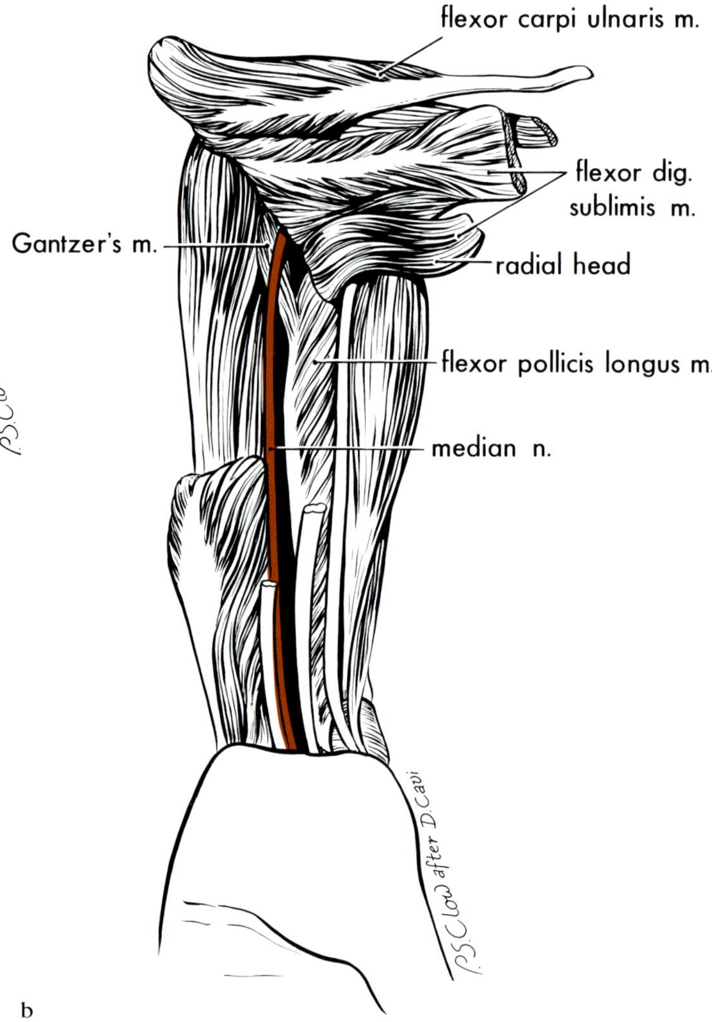

b

Figure 7-8. Illustration of wide origin of flexor sublimis with, in addition to its universally present origin from the medial humeral epicondyle and its usually present (87%) deep head from the ulna or interosseous membrane **(a)**, its radial head present in 32% of the specimens. All three heads divided and reflected proximally **(b)**. Note also Gantzer's muscle and the median nerve. (Reproduced with permission from Dellon and MacKinnon.[42])

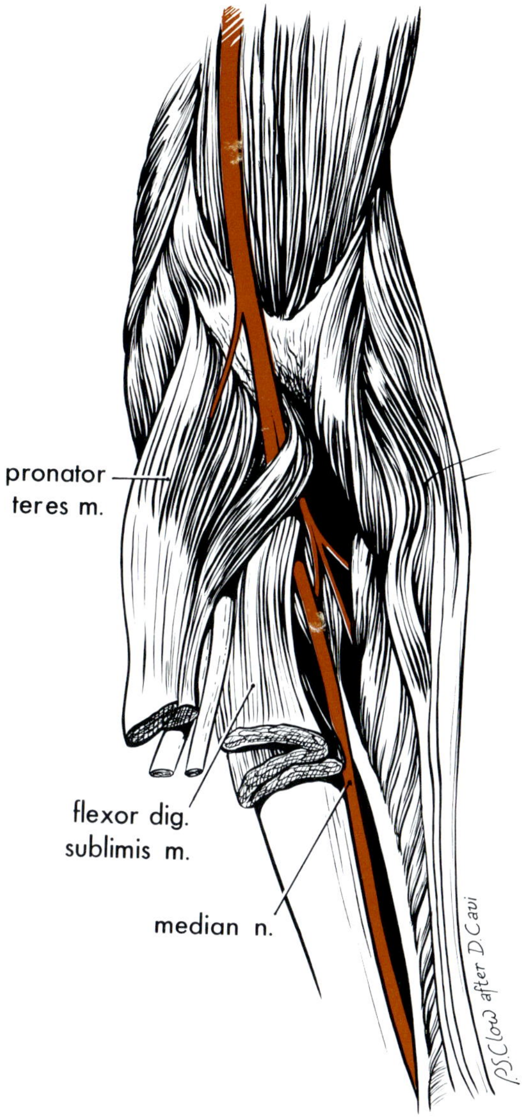

a

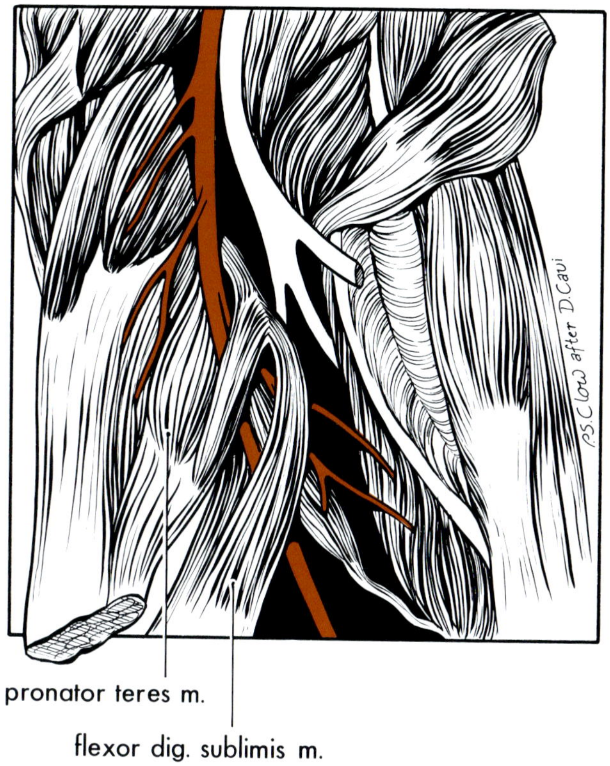

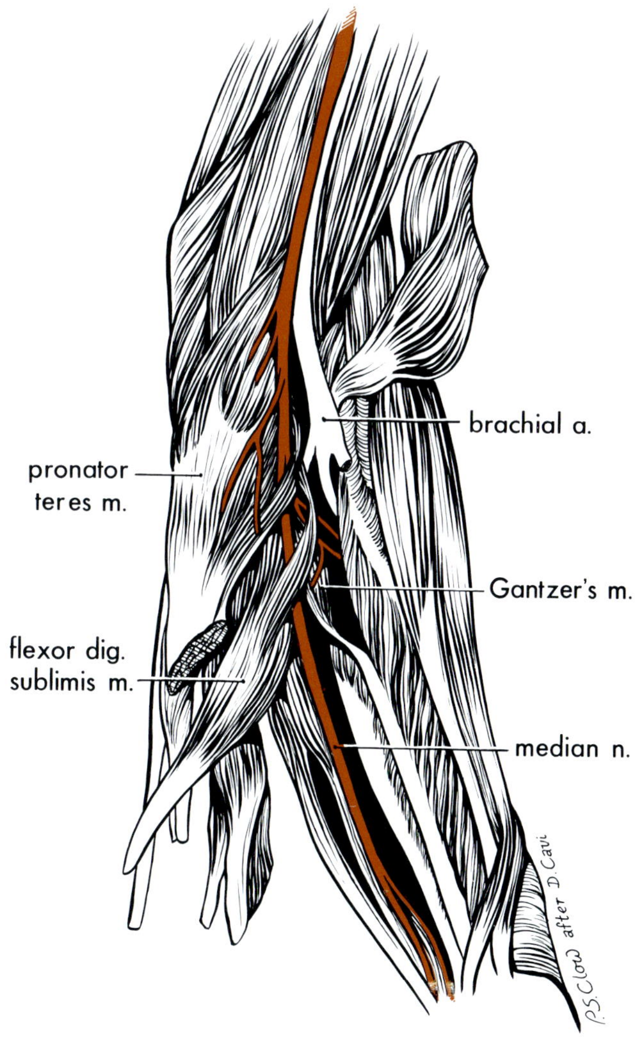

Figure 7-9. Illustration of median nerve being crossed by single arch **(a)**, and double arch **(b)**. The proximal arch is formed by the juncture of the deep and superficial heads of the pronator teres. The second arch is formed by the flexor sublimis where the deep head from the ulna joins the head from the medial humeral epicondyle. (Reproduced with permission from Dellon and MacKinnon.[42])

b

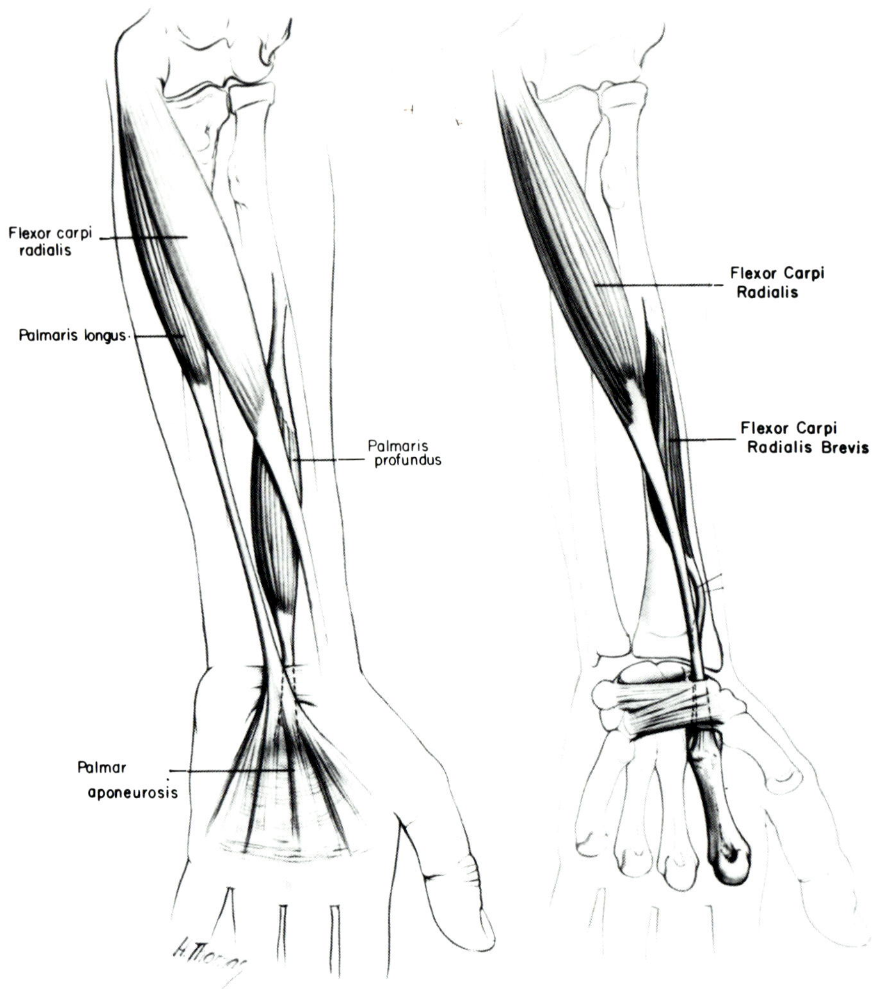

Figure 7-10. Anomalous muscles originating from radius in relationship to the flexor pollicis lognus. These muscles, the palmaris profundus and the flexor carpi radialis brevis, may cause median nerve compression in the mid forearm. (Reproduced with permission from Spinner.[2])

and pronator quadratus. The combination of the sensory and muscle losses that are noted suggests the site of the nerve injury. There are, however, many possible situations in which a mislocalization of the site of injury can occur. When the loss is primarily sensory, with the complaints being numbness and tingling in the thumb, index, and middle fingers and with the symptoms being worsened at night with nighttime awakening, and few other complaints on the part of the patient, attention should be directed to a site at the level of the wrist. The carpal tunnel syndrome is discussed in detail in Chapter 6. The complaint of nighttime awakening is explained by the fact that during sleep the flexor muscles cause wrist flexion, resulting in compression of the median nerve at the wrist. The physical examination reproducing this provocative test (the Phalen's sign) and the presence of a positive pressure provocative test, or a Tinel's sign, at the wrist are the physical findings that again point to median nerve compression at the wrist level as the source of this problem. However, additional proximal sites of nerve compression can exist as discussed in Chapter 14 with the multiple crush syndrome. Thus, a frequent association of median nerve entrapment in the proximal forearm and the carpal tunnel syndrome has been identified when this coexistence has been carefully sought.[53] Unfortunately, frequently a proximal site of compression is not considered until a patient has failed to make an appropriate recovery from a distal median nerve release. Preoperative electrodiagnostic studies may not be helpful, for although they are highly sensitive for detecting median nerve entrapment at the wrist, they are generally not helpful in confirming median nerve entrapment in the proximal forearm, so that even a recent article has suggested that the pronator teres syndrome is "controversial."[5] Clearly, at any site from the axilla to the wrist, an appropriate injury to the median nerve can cause sensory loss in the entire distribution or partial distribution of the nerve, as well as wasting of thenar muscles. Therefore a careful history and careful physical examination are essential in attempting to localize median nerve injury.

When the mechanism of injury is a shoulder dislocation, a midshaft fracture of the humerus, a supracondylar fracture of the humerus, an elbow dislocation, or a gunshot or knife wound, then the location for the median nerve injury is apparent. These are the usual clues the surgeon has when the median nerve injury is in the brachium. When there is no overt history of trauma but the patient complains of symptoms that may be referable to the median nerve, then a meticulous investigation by physical examination and history is required in the proximal forearm and elbow region.

So-Called Pronator Teres Syndrome

The so-called pronator teres syndrome has been well-described by multiple investigators beginning in 1951.[54–59] The patient's only complaints may be aching in the proximal forearm. Usually, this is brought on by some type of work activity. When there is a history of crush injury to the forearm, the concept of median nerve compression of the forearm is not so obscure. In the absence of such a history, the questioner must carefully ask the patients about their hobbies, in particular, activities that require wringing out of cloths or towels or carpenter or machine work where the forearm must constantly go through pronation, supination, and range of motion. A history that reveals a job in which the person must work with the arm forcefully pronated should bring this location of compression to mind. Physical examination may show a positive Tinel's sign over the median nerve in the proximal third of the forearm. Pressure over this same area may produce pain in the forearm and sensory complaints in the hand. If the patient is asked to keep his arm pronated while the examiner attempts to supinate the forearm, the pain should be produced by this provocative test (Fig. 7-11). There may be findings with nerve conduction and electromyographic studies,[57,60] although these are uncommon. There may be complaints by the patient of some numbness and tingling in the fingers when the forearm is aching after work. Weakness to manual muscle testing of the pronator teres, the flexor sublimis, and the thenar intrinsic muscles is occasionally demonstrated. The patient may indicate that the hand becomes weaker with prolonged work activities. However, if this symptom is mentioned by the patient, the ulnar nerve at the elbow

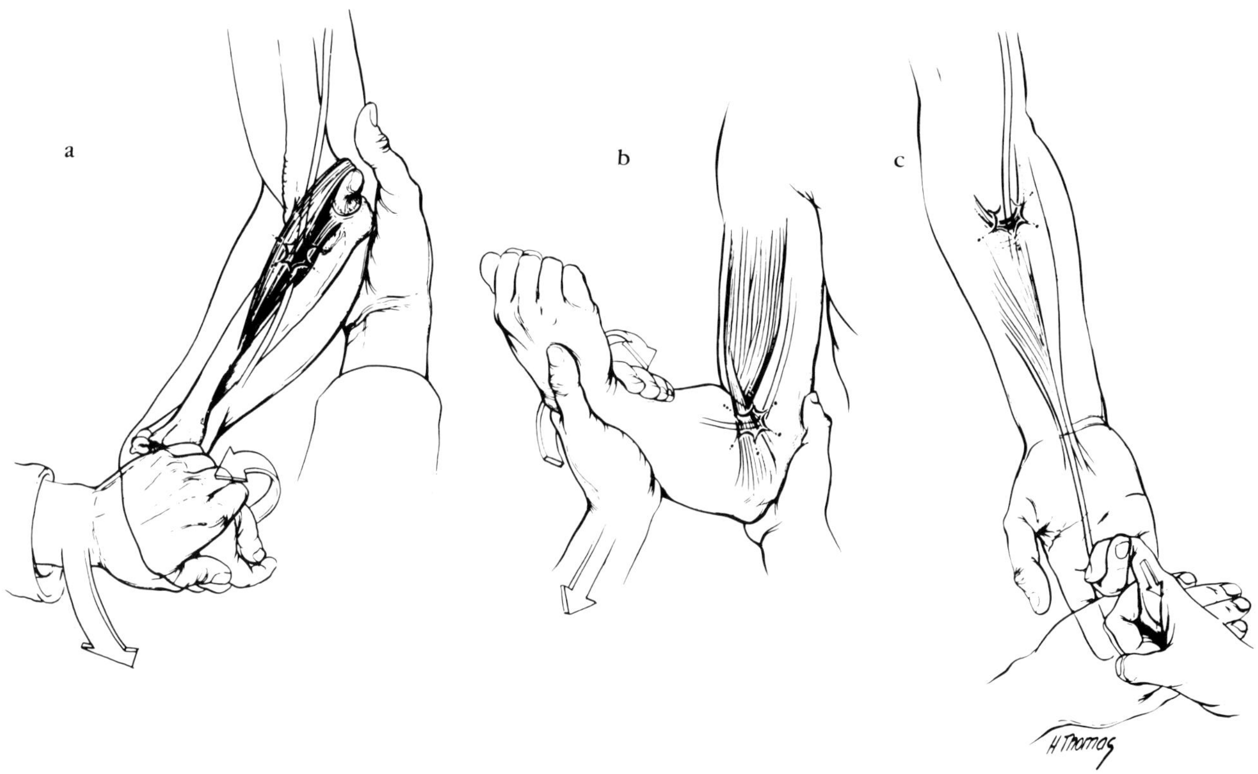

Figure 7-11. Physical examination techniques that provide a provocative test for median nerve entrapment in forearm. Resisted pronation suggests entrapment beneath the pronator **(a)**, resisted forearm flexion and supination suggest entrapment beneath the lacertus fibrosis **(b)**, and resisted middle finger sublimis flexion **(c)** suggests entrapment at the sublimis arch if these resisted movements create pain or aching in the proximal forearm. (Reproduced with permission from Spinner.[2])

should also be examined as a possible coexisting site of nerve entrapment (see Chapter 9). Similar complaints to those of the so-called pure pronator teres syndrome can be due to compression beneath the lacertus fibrosis, and resisted elbow flexion and supination causes tightening in the lacertus fibrosis by means of the biceps brachii contraction.

Anterior Interosseous Nerve Syndrome

Another supposedly "pure" syndrome is that of anterior interosseous nerve compression. This was first described by Kiloh and Nevin.[61] Spinner, however, cites an earlier description by Tinel in 1918 of two cases of anterior interosseous nerve syndrome that Tinel described under the heading of "dissociated paralysis of the median nerve." Subsequently, there has been an extensive reporting in the literature of so-called isolated anterior interosseous nerve compression.[62–69] In its complete form, the anterior interosseous nerve syndrome is manifested by inability to flex the thumb at its interphalangeal joint, the index finger at its distal interphalangeal joint, and variably of the middle finger at its interphalangeal joint (Fig. 7-12). If there is loss of function of the pronator quadratus muscle and the first and second lumbricals, the patients will generally not have complained of loss of lumbrical and pronator function but do note inability to use the thumb and index finger in the normal fashion. The patients have no sensory complaints. There is, however, a sensory component to the anterior interosseous nerve, since its terminal branch innervates the volar wrist capsule.[70] As described in the preceding section, other investigators have described injury to this nerve after supracondylar fractures and elbow dislocations, but these reports are in patients in whom this type of trauma in general had not occurred. The patients present without pain and with a history of what may have occurred to them as either a sudden onset of loss of function or gradual weakness and loss of coordination in the use of their fingers. Physical examination shows the classic inability to pinch the thumb and index finger together to create a round "O," but rather in this attempted pinch function, the distal interphalangeal joints of the thumb and index finger remain straight (Figs. 7-12 through 7-14). Flexing the elbow, thereby removing the pronator teres from most of its function, allows testing of the pronator quadratus. Strength can be compared with the opposite side. Weakness in the flexor digitorum profundus to the middle finger may or may not be demonstrable if the ulnar nerve has a partial innervation of this muscle branch. The absence of middle finger distal interphalangeal joint loss of function should not be considered as weighing against this diagnosis. Sensory testing generally is within normal range. Electrical testing is pri-

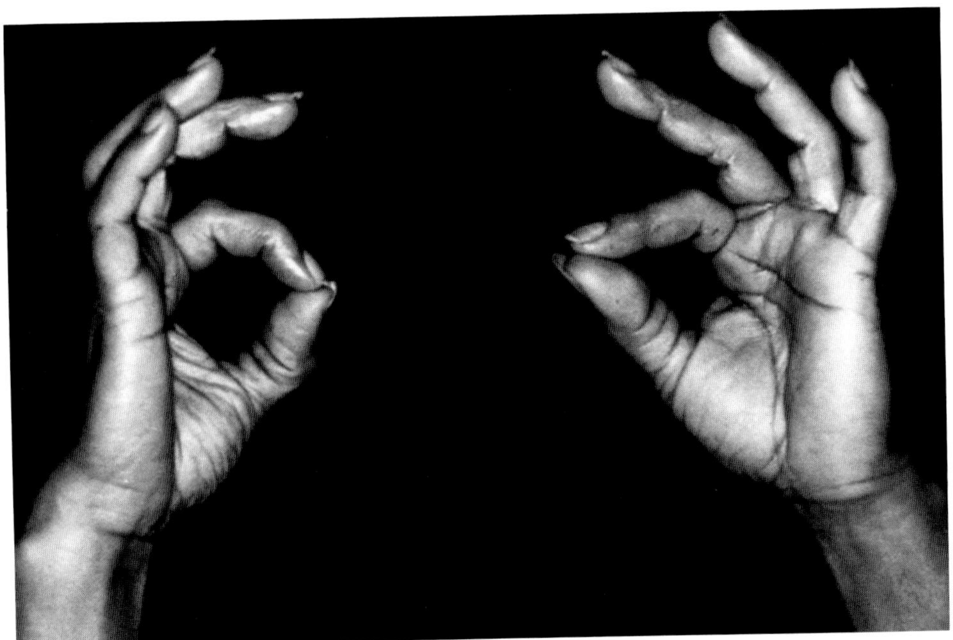

Figure 7-12. Diagnosis of anterior interosseous nerve palsy demonstrated by inability to form a circle between index and thumb because the flexor pollicis longus and the index profundus do not function.

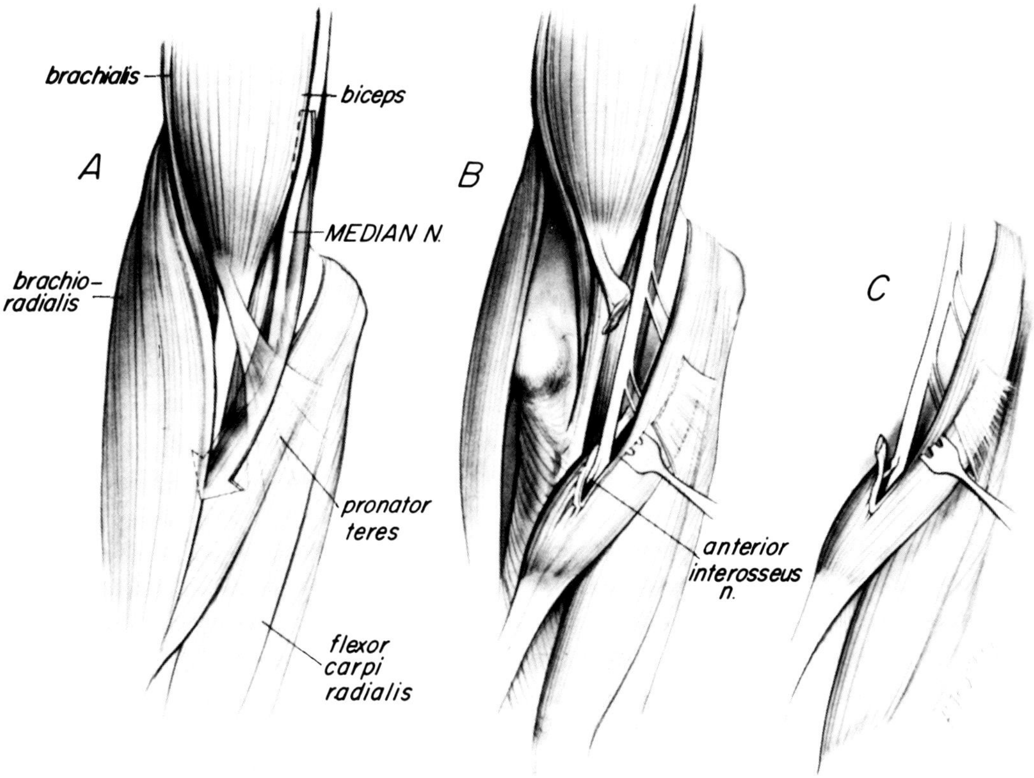

a

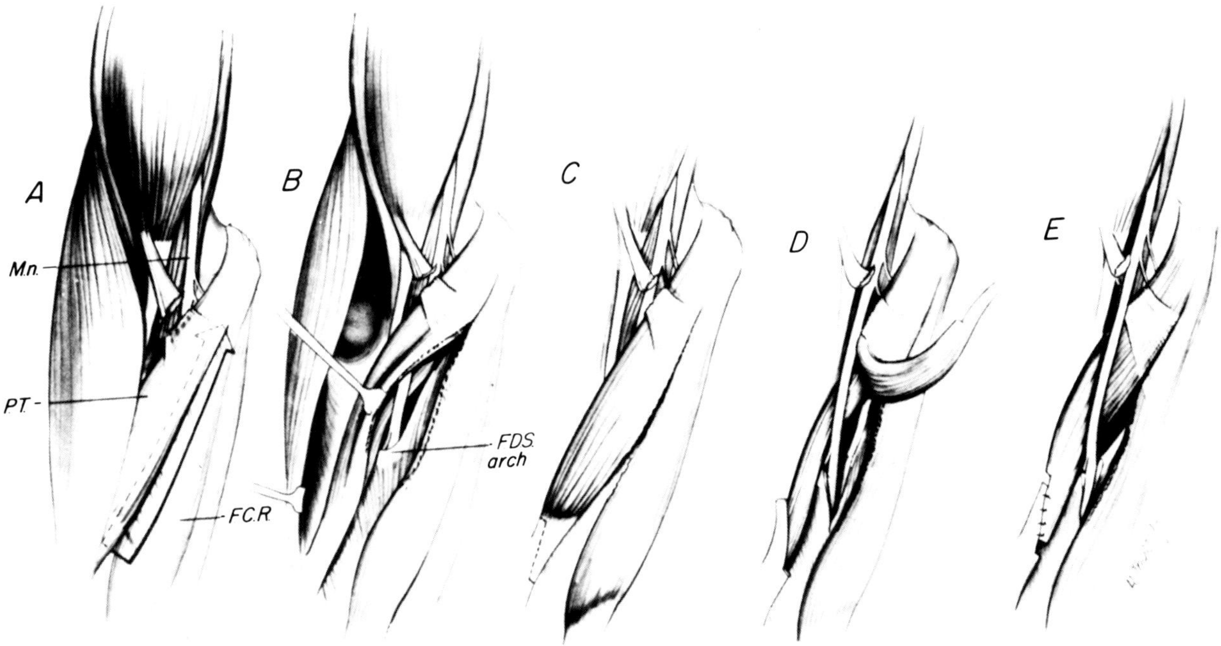

b

Figure 7-13. Exposure of the median nerve in the proximal forearm requires identification of the median nerve proximal to the elbow. This is identified at the medial side of the biceps brachii after going through the fascia in the brachium **(a).** The lacertus fibrosis, which is a blend of the brachial fascia into the fascia overlying the flexor pronator muscle mass, is then released, with care being taken not to damage the biceps tendon insertion **(b).** Through this approach, the most proximal branches of the median nerve into the pronator teres superficial head will be identified on the medial aspect of the median nerve. When there is the anatomic variation of a high origin of the pronator teres superficial head (Fig. 7-4), this will require division in order to reach this stage of the dissection. The deep head of the pronator teres, if present, will then be identified and may be divided from its origin from the coranoid process of the ulna and from the interosseous membrane **(c).** (Reproduced with permission from Spinner.[2])

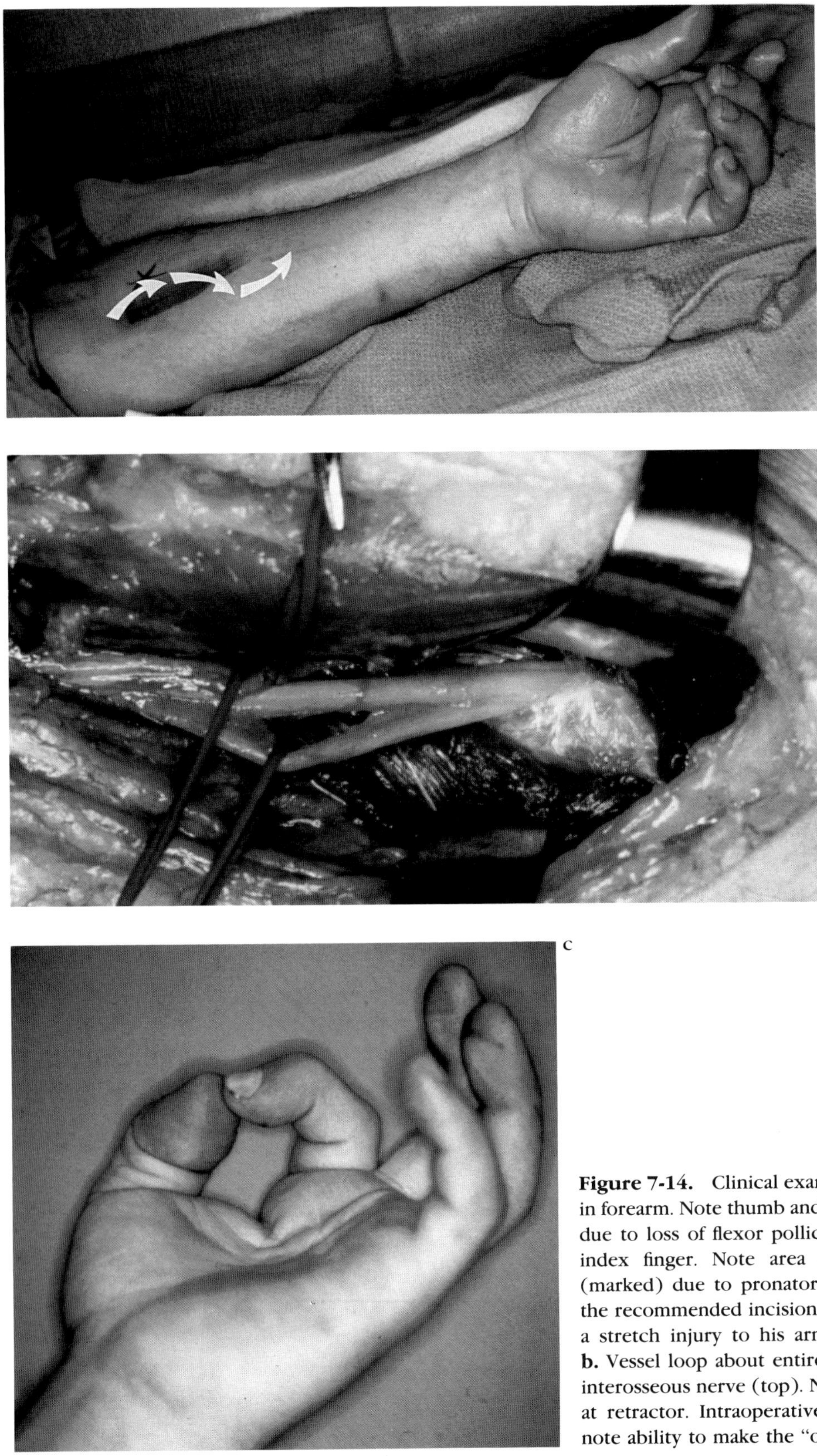

a

b

c

Figure 7-14. Clinical example of median nerve compression in forearm. Note thumb and index are extended at distal joints due to loss of flexor pollicis longus and flexor profundus to index finger. Note area of proximal forearm depression (marked) due to pronator teres wasting. **a.** The location of the recommended incision is marked (arrows). This man had a stretch injury to his arm during an automobile accident. **b.** Vessel loop about entire median nerve (left) and anterior interosseous nerve (top). Note thick white fibrous single arch at retractor. Intraoperative views **(b, c)**. **c.** Postoperatively note ability to make the "o" sign.

marily of value with electromyography, which can demonstrate denervation occurring in the flexor pollicis longus and the profundus to the index finger and the pronator quadratus. The diagnosis then of anterior interosseous nerve syndrome has little confusion about it when present in its complete form or the possible confusion of it with a tendon rupture. Clearly, rupture of the flexor pollicis longus or the profundus to the index finger, such as can occur with rheumatoid arthritis, from flexor synovitis, or from bony spurs in the region of the carpal tunnel,[71–73] can give a similar picture. In this instance, electromyographic findings will be abnormal in the flexor pollicis longus and part of the profundus. Electromyographic testing of the pronator quadratus should be normal, and the normal tenodesis effect at the wrist for the thumb and index finger is lost if the tendon rupture has occurred. The tenodesis effect is still present if the tendons are intact, in which case the cause is an anterior interosseous nerve compression. Deep aching pain in the volar wrist, worsened with wrist extension and which may be worsened with wrist flexion, has been described due to injury to the terminal branch of the anterior interosseous nerve.[70] This is usually due to volar wrist ligamentous sprain or previous fracture of the distal radius with entrapment of the nerve and callus formation or actual disruption of the terminal fibers in the volar wrist ligaments with small neuroma formation. This source of volar wrist pain may be diagnosed with a block of the terminal branch of the anterior interosseous nerve, and pain relief may be obtained by a partial volar wrist denervation procedure.[70,74]

Multiple Crush Syndrome

The multiple crush syndrome (see Chapter 14) is a syndrome in which symptoms are due to multiple sites of compression, each of which by itself may be insufficient to cause symptoms. Median nerve compression in the forearm is a prime example of a multiple crush syndrome. From anatomic considerations already described, it is clear that the median nerve can be compressed in sequence from proximal to distal by the lacertus fibrosis, a high origin of the pronator teres muscle, a fibrous arch between the deep head of the pronator teres and the superficial head, a fibrous arch between the deep origins of the flexor sublimis and the superficial head of the flexor sublimis, crossing branches of the ulnar collateral vessels, Gantzer's muscle, anomalous muscles, such as the palmaris profundus or the flexor carpi radialis brevis. It is also clear from the previous description that, depending on the topographic orientation within the median nerve of its component fascicles, such as the location of the anterior interosseous nerve, different fascicles and therefore different sensory motor functions, will be more likely at risk to be compressed by the series of potential compressive sites just listed. Additionally, in a person susceptible to nerve compression, for example, a person with a peripheral neuropathy such as diabetes, other anatomic regions may contribute to the multiple crush syndrome, including the cervical spine, the thoracic outlet, or the transverse carpal ligament at the wrist. Thus, it should be no surprise that a patient's symptoms and the physical examination may be confused to the point that either an initial surgical procedure fails or that the physical findings are atypical. This, unfortunately, has given rise to description of a series of problems defined as "incomplete syndromes" or variations on the classic presentation. This most particularly has been described for the anterior interosseous nerve syndrome.[67,75,76] It is clear that the correct course of action should be to carry out the history-taking and physical examination and the operative procedure with the consideration that all structures that compress the nerve should be released and that any possible combination of symptoms and signs can occur. For example, resisted middle finger sublimis flexion causes aching in the forearm. There has not been described, as yet, a "sublimis syndrome." This is the likely extension if the alternate course of action is followed. In fact, resisted flexor sublimis function (Fig. 7-11) has been described as being a sign of the pronator syndrome. A positive flexor sublimis resistance test is a provocative sign demonstrating that a fibrous arch exists beneath the sublimis, and the surgeon's attention is therefore directed to continue with release of potential compressive structures, as just outlined.

Additional diagnostic testing is conceivable, such as stress electromyography and nerve conduction studies. Whereas nerve conduction tests might be normal before the induction of work activity, it may become positive after completion of a stressful exercise. However, an awareness of the potential sites of compression and physical diagnosis, as previously described, should permit appropriate diagnosis without the need for these more invasive type of testing procedures. For completeness of the differential diagnosis, it is possible to have signs of median nerve dysfunction related to an acute brachial plexus neuropathy. This type of neuropathy has been described by Parsonage and Turner and by others.[77–80] In this instance, there is diffuse aching in the neck and shoulder generally of more sudden onset and the situation is often painful. Electrodiagnostic studies of the brachial plexus can distinguish the site of this neuropathy. Radiculopathies of C5 or C6 roots may give sensory dysfunction in the distribution of the median nerve, but there is usually pain associated with neck movements and weakness or positive electromyographic changes present in other C5 and C6 innervated muscles, such as the supraspinatus and deltoid. Radiculopathies at C8 or T1 are less common than C5 or C6 but when present may be associated with wasting in the thenar muscles. There is, however, usually a more diffuse wasting in all the intrinsic muscles. There is an associated neck pain and in these situations, electrodiagnostic testing is again valuable, as well as cervical spine films and computed tomography scans with contrast media.

Operative Technique

The operative approach to patients with median nerve injuries in the brachium is usually dictated by the approach required for the bony injury or through the gunshot or knife wound, and no particular surgical technique need be described for this. This section will mainly describe our approach to decompression of the multiple structures that can compress the median nerve in the forearm.

The patient is placed in the supine position with satisfactory anesthesia, which may be general or brachial plexus regional, and a pneumatic tourniquet is placed over the upper extremity over a soft roll and the arm is extended on an arm board. The hand is elevated and exsanguinated with an elastic bandage and the tourniquet inflated. An incision is made that is toward the radial side of the flexor pronator muscle mass. The incision must be planned so that it can extend down to the mid forearm and proximal to the antecubital crease. We recommend a lazy-S type of incision, which does not cross the antecubital crease. Unfortunately, the far more cosmetic transverse incision will not allow adequate release of proximal and distal structures.

The incision is deepened into the subcutaneous tissue and hemostasis obtained throughout with the bipolar coagulator, and the forearm branches of the lateral antebrachial cutaneous nerve must be looked for. These will arise 1.5 to 2 cm distal to the antecubital crease and will accompany the cephalic or accessory cephalic vein. Approximately one-third of the lateral antebrachial cutaneous nerves have a high division with a branch coming toward the medial portion of the forearm. As the incision approaches the medial portion of the forearm, care must be taken not to injure the medial antebrachial cutaneous nerve. This portion is given off the posterior branch and continuing as its anterior branch. These vessels are identified and encircled with a vessel loop.

The fascia of the upper arm is entered medial to the biceps and the lacertus fibrosis is excised. The median nerve and brachial artery are identified. Palpation in this area is carried out in an attempt to identify a supracondylar process of the humerus, and, if one is there, it is resected. If there is a medial displacement of the median nerve with either the brachial artery or the ulnar artery, should there be a high split to the brachial artery, a crossing Struthers ligament is searched for and, if present, it is excised. The resection is then carried distally by reflecting the pronator teres superficial head medially. In those patients with a high origin of the superficial head of the pronator teres, this is taken down directly at its origin from the medial edge of the humerus from the medial intermuscular septum and sometimes with fibers originating from the brachialis muscle. When this head is taken down, branches from the median nerve into the flexor pronator muscle mass are searched for and their integrity preserved. These branches come off the medial aspect of the median nerve. Dissection is then carried distally directly on the median nerve, and crossing veins and further distally crossing ulnar collateral vessels are divided. The next structure will be the deep head of the pronator teres coming up on the lateral side of the median nerve, and its process from either the coranoid of the ulna and then always from the interosseous membrane is divided and the fibrous arch joining it to the superficial head, if present, is resected. This frees the median nerve from the first of the possible fibrous arches. The surgeon's finger then can slide distally on the surface of the nerve and continue to feel if there are any distal structures. The more distal portions can be reached either by elevating the pronator teres and looking beneath and carrying out additional divisions of fibrous bands through this approach or by extending the incision more distally and coming into the plane between the flexor carpi radialis and the pronator teres, reflecting the pronator teres now laterally. Depending on the anatomy, the sublimis muscle will be found either partially to take origin from the pronator teres arch or to have a separate, more distal arch (Fig. 7-15). If a fibrous arch is present, this deep head of the sublimis is also resected and then distally Gantzer's muscle and possible fibrous origins that may be compressing the ulnar nerve from anomalous muscles, such as the palmaris profundus, are looked for and released or resected as needed.

The direct observations of the median nerve may show areas of increased vascularity at the sites of compression or decreased vascularity with narrowing or a swelling in a pseudoneuroma formation proximal to the swelling (Figs. 7-15, 7-16). The nerve may feel firm or fibrotic in areas beneath the swelling, or where multiple areas of compression have contributed to the

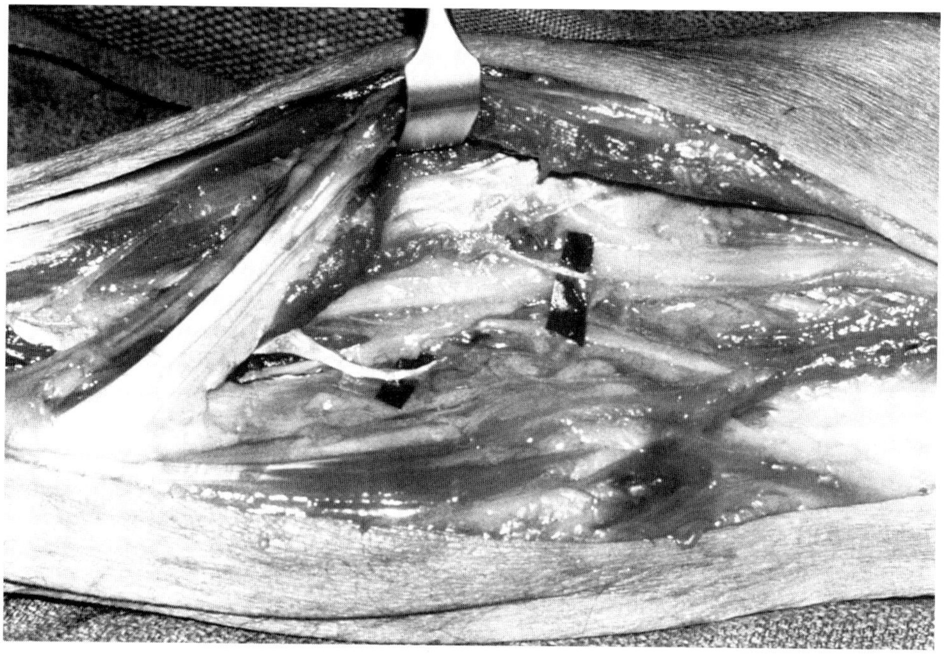

Figure 7-15. Cadaver view of a double arch: Distal toward the left and radial toward the top. These arches are well-separated and each is narrow (dark visibility background markers). Note fibrous proximal arch (already partially divided) from deep head of pronator teres at take off of anterior interosseous nerve. The distal fibrous arch is an origin of flexor sublimis muscle crossing the anterior interosseous nerve directly.

problem, the nerve may not have one single area of narrowing. Microsurgical instruments and technique are used and the epineurium is opened. In patients who have muscle wasting or persistent sensory discomfort, it will be anticipated that there will be intraneural fibrosis. In areas where there are multiple areas of compression, there may not be one single area with significant intraneural fibrosis. The epineurium is opened and the nerve is evaluated in the areas of the compression, and, if intraneural fibrosis is present, an intraneural neurolysis is carried out (see Chaper 5). Occasionally 5 ml of dexamethasone may be placed in the operative site to inhibit scar formation. The wound is closed with interrupted 4-0 absorbable sutures and the skin with subcuticular absorbable sutures. The dressing is nonadherent gauze, fluff, soft roll and a posterior plaster splint allowing the elbow to stay in approximately 60° flexion. This dressing is brought down across the wrist, keeping the wrist in neutral position. It is held in place with kling, paper tape, stockinette, and tensor wrap. The tourniquet is let down and circulation returned and the tips of the fingers evaluated. The tensor wrap is removed 1 hour after the operative procedure. In the early postoperative period, the patient is encouraged to move the fingers and forearm to encourage gliding of the nerve in its new bed.

Median Nerve Exploration in the Forearm with Coexisting Transposition of the Ulnar Nerve

In patients who have a coexisting ulnar nerve entrapment at the elbow, an anterior submuscular transposition of the ulnar nerve may be carried out simultaneously with the median nerve decompression in the forearm. As discussed in Chapter 9, the approach to anterior submuscular transposition has an incision paralleling the ulnar nerve in the postcondylar groove. This incision may have its proximal portion placed, coming distal to the medial humeral epicondyle, then coming proximal and angling back across the antecubital crease to the midportion of the arm and then extending as a Z limb along the pronator teres course distally. The anterior submuscular transposition as carried out by us includes a step-cut lengthening of the flexor pronator muscle mass and fascia, and this results in a partial median nerve decompression in and of itself. When the proximal limb of the step-cut lengthening of the flexor pronator fascia is carried out, it releases the lacertus fibrosis from the thick fibrous origin of the common flexor tendon, and the flexor pronator muscle mass is cut and released distally. It lengthens the flexor sublimis origin from the medial humeral epicondyle. This loos-

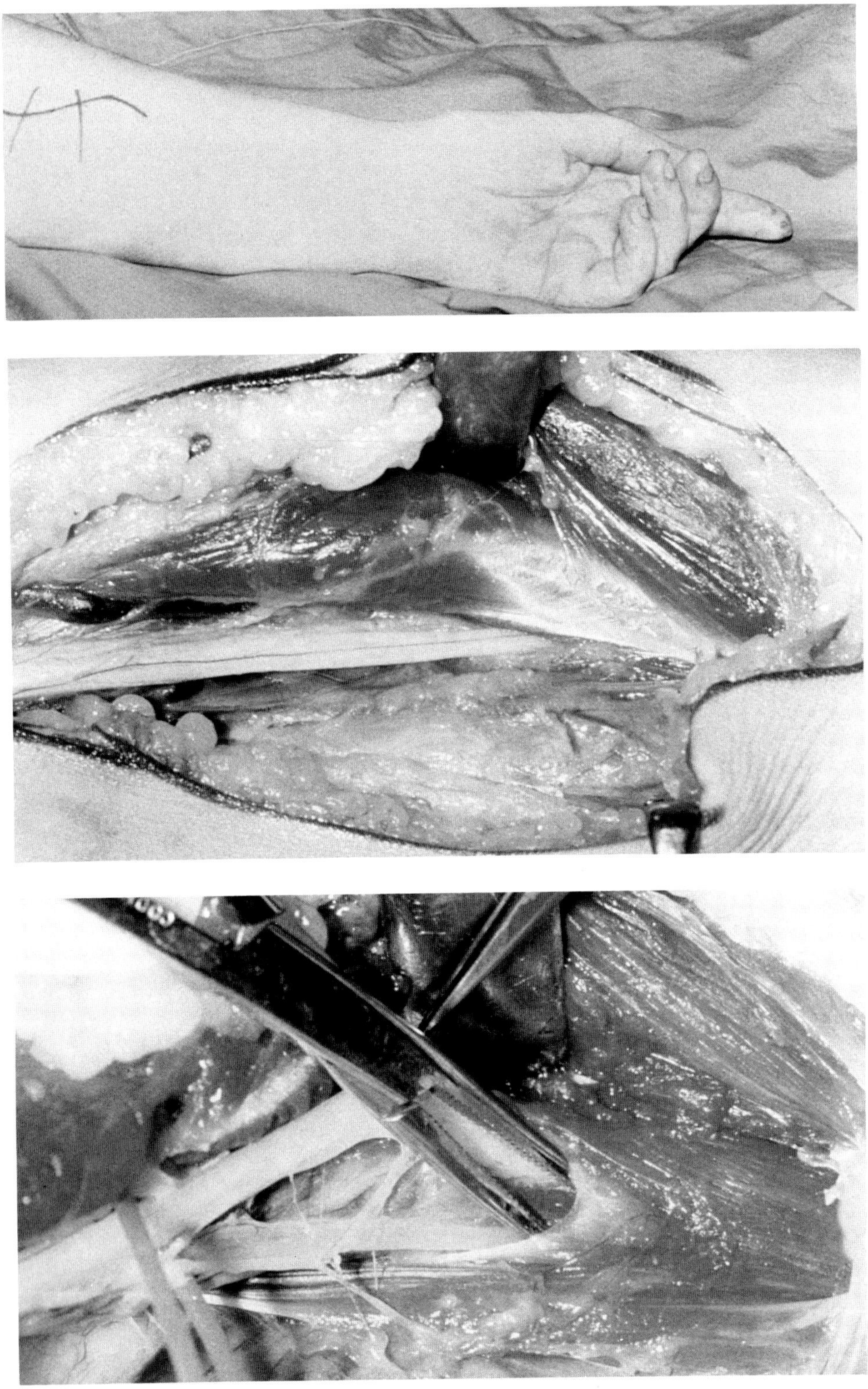

a

b

c

Figure 7-16. Intraoperative view of a patient with a single arch. **a.** Initial view with extended thumb and index finger. **b.** Superficial head of pronator teres. **c.** Clamp beneath fibrous arch over anterior interosseous nerve with vessel loop on median nerve. (*Figure continues.*)

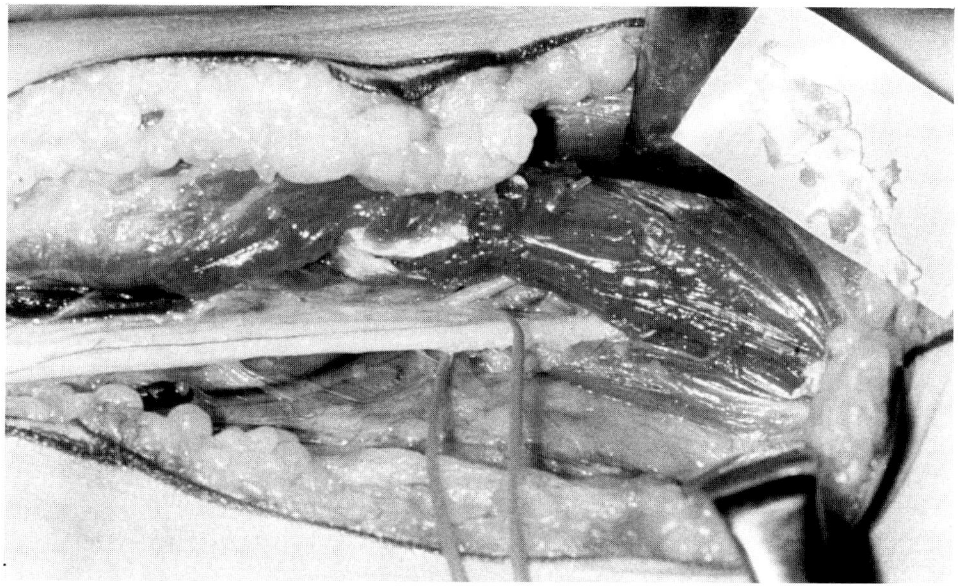

d

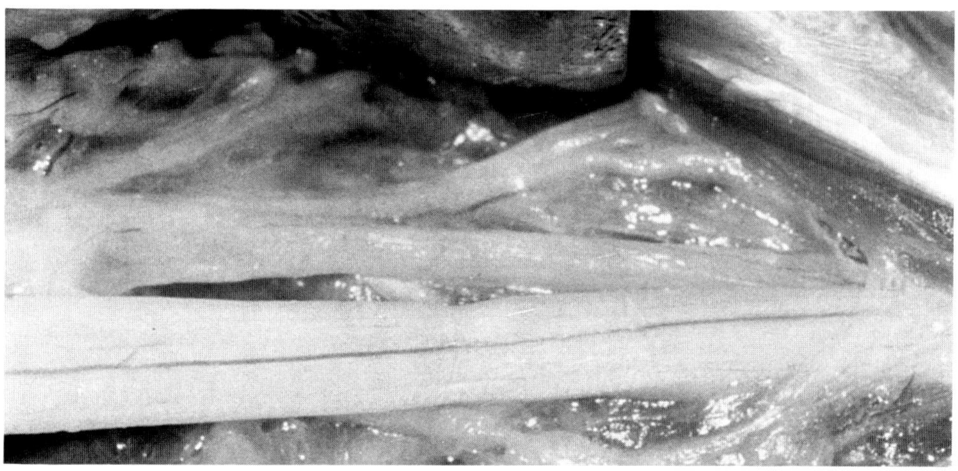

e

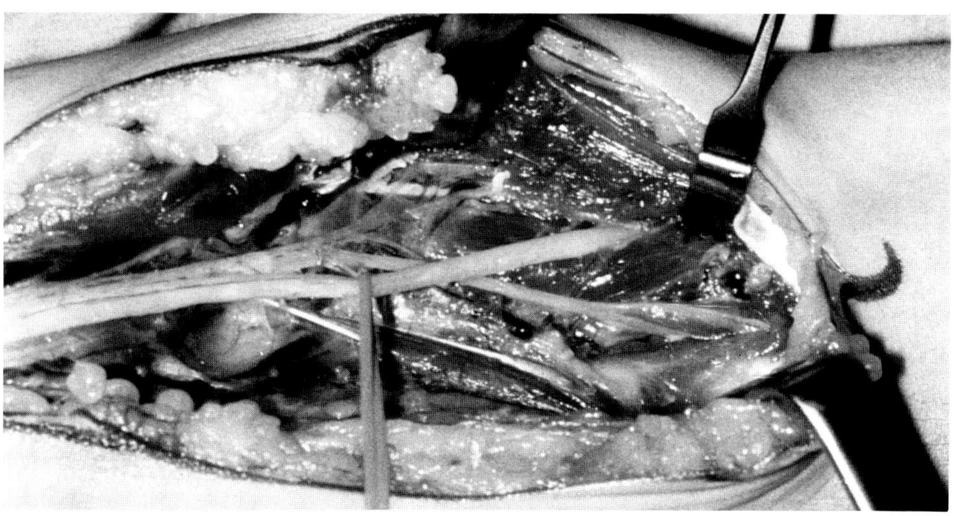

f

Figure 7-16 *(continued)* **d.** Arch and deep head of pronator teres resected on white square. **e.** Close-up of compressed areas on anterior interosseous nerve (note also the color change compared with 'whiter' median nerve). **f.** Total length of released nerve with internal neurolysis.

ens the fibrous arch of the sublimis, if it is present across the median nerve. The step-cut lengthening of the flexor pronator muscle mass lengthens the origin of the superficial head of the pronator teres by approximately 1.5 cm, thereby releasing this structure. Thus, the anterior submuscular transposition as carried out by us decompresses the median nerve in the forearm from the major structures that compress it, namely, the lacertus fibrosis, the pronator teres, and the flexor sublimis. The flexor pronator muscle mass step-cut and elevated the dissection along the median nerve may be carried out as previously described. In this instance, a fibrous arch from the deep head of the sublimis and pronator teres deep head would still be divided. Neither in this approach nor the approach already described would the insertion of the pronator teres be step-cut and placed deep to the median nerve to lengthen it in this fashion.[2] This has not been found to be necessary if the maneuvers described here are used. If the patient is thin, it is possible to decompress the median nerve satisfactorily through the ulnar nerve transposition incision. In all other instances, a separate incision has been required to decompress both nerves adequately.

Postoperative Care

The patient is given a sling and if the operation is done as an outpatient procedure, the patient is given a prescription for oral pain medication. He is not given antibiotics. The patient is admitted to the hospital for one postoperative night. The patient returns on the eighth day after surgery and the dressing is removed and any sutures may be removed. The patient is allowed then immediate wrist and elbow flexion and extension as desired; the only exception being if a concomitant submuscular transposition of the ulnar nerve is carried out, in which case the patient is required to wear the sling an additional week to prevent tearing or overstretching of the repaired flexor pronator muscle mass. Bruising, if present, is treated by application of warm compresses at home. Beginning the third week, the patient is instructed to begin massaging the scar with some type of hand cream, such as Intensive Care Lotion or vitamin E cream or cocoa butter. He is instructed that the massage is more important than the cream, itself, and that the cream reduces the heat of friction. He is to massage it for just 3 to 4 minutes twice a day. As discomfort lessens, the patient is begun on exercises to strengthen the hand and begin exercise tolerance. These exercises primarily consist of squeezing either exercise putty or Play-Doh. He is instructed to do it just until his hand aches or swells and not to push his activities further than this. He is seen at 3 weeks, at 6 to 8 weeks, and at 3 to 4 months after surgery. During this period of time, the expectation is that function should be returning to the paralyzed muscles and that abnormal sensibility will have been returned. The usual return to work date is 8 to 10 weeks after this operative procedure. Generally, if the patient's job activity is such that he has to do assembly line type work or work with a vibrating or pneumatic torque wrench or hammer, he is advised to seek an alternate type of employment within the same company.

Results of Surgery

The technique of nerve repair and nerve grafting is discussed in great detail in Chapter 4. With particular respect to the median nerve in the brachium and proximal forearm, however, it is appropriate to review the available literature at this point. Frustration continues to be the guideword in an attempt to see improved nerve results from our microsurgical approach. This may be reflected in the scarcity of articles that actually give results for median nerve repair and grafting in this region. For example, a recent article on "Microsurgical Repair of Peripheral Nerve Injuries in the Upper Extremity"[81] indicated only that "several patients with median nerve injuries at the distal forearm or wrist level had two-point discrimination of less than one cm. at the fingertips within eight months." Articles on epineurial versus perineurial repair of peripheral nerves continue to appear,[82] discussing the theoretical basis of each without giving clinical results. Entire monographs on symposia on peripheral nerve trauma[83] have no results of repair of peripheral nerve injuries or grafting in this region, with the exception of the chapter written by Millesi.[84] Millesi most recently has summarized his results for grafting of the median nerve and these are presented in Table 7-1, as well as his results with median nerve repair, presented in Table 7-2. Although Millesi uses the term "Repair" in Table 7-2, he indicates in his text that in 28 of the 30 cases, the median nerve was bridged by a nerve graft. Thus, his results in Tables 7-1 and 7-2 represent median nerve grafts, the difference being that in Table 7-2 the median nerve was injured at the same time as the ulnar nerve. In Table 7-1, although there were 39 patients, only 20 were followed for motor function, since there was anomalous innervation of the thenar muscles from the ulnar nerve in 19 of these cases.[84] Although Millesi does not indicate exactly the location of the median nerve defects, the extent of the graft, the majority being greater than 5 cm, suggests that the location of the lesion was proximal to the wrist in the majority of cases, at least with respect to the proximal extent of the nerve, nerve graft juncture site, and these results are therefore included in this Chapter. Sunderland's encyclopedic monograph does

Table 7-1. Results of Median Nerve Repair by Nerve Grafting*

	Mixed Innervation†			*M4-5*			*M3*			*M2*		
	Age (yr)	*Interval (mo)*	*Defect (cm)*	*Age (yr)*	*Interval (mo)*	*Defect (cm)*	*Age (yr)*	*Interval (mo)*	*Defect (cm)*	*Age (yr)*	*Interval (mo)*	*Defect (cm)*
S3+ −4	21	4	5.0	19	6	2.5				23	4	7.0
	20	1	2.0	22	8	8.0						
	25	2	3.5	18	7	7.0						
	40	2	2.0	21	2	6.0						
	27	2	3.5	10	9	5.0						
	49	1	6.5	9	2	5.0						
	44	8	5.0	20	3	5.0						
	7	2	2.0	46	5	3.5						
	13	4	4.0	50	2	2.0						
				10	4	4.0						
S3	21	4	4.5	35	6	2.0	43	8	5.0	41	28	15.0
	21	2	6.0	19	2	4.0	44	36	12.0			
	46	4	2.0	50	2	3.0	48	18	7.0			
	24	4	5.0				25	2	5.0			
	27	2	4.0				6	5	4.0			
	52	12	4.5									
	30	9	10.0									
	23	5	4.0									
	61	3	4.0									
S2	26	11	16.0									

*Reprinted with permission from Millesi.[84]

†These patients had an innervation anomaly in which the thenar muscles were innervated by the ulnar nerve as well as by the median nerve.

Table 7-2. Results of Median and Ulnar (Simultaneous Injury) Nerve Repair by Grafting in 29 Patients*

	M4-5 S3+ −4	*M4-5 S3*	*M3 S3+ −4*	*M3 S3*	*M3 S2*	*M2+ S3*	*M2 S3+ −4*	*M2 S3*	*M2 S2*	*M1 S3*	*M0 S3+ −4*	*M0 S3*	*M0 S2*
Median nerve n_1 = 30													
n	4	3 + 1NS†	2	7			2	3	3	2	2		1NL†
Interval 6	4	1	1	6				1					
(mon) 6–12		2					1		2	2			
12		1NS	1				1	2	1		2		1NL
Ulnar nerve n_1 = 28													
n	2	8	1	5 + 1NS	2	6		1		1		1	
Interval 6	2	5		2	1	3							
(mon) 6–12		2	1	2		2		1		1		1	
12		1		1 + 1NS	1	1							

*Reprinted with permission from Millesi et al.[84]

†NS: nerve sutures; NL neurolysis.

not list the results of median nerve repair or graft in the brachium or proximal forearm.[1] Seddon[85] has given his British experience through 1972 and this is listed in Table 7-3.

The most complete review of median nerve repair and grafting in the brachium and forearm region, listed as "high repair," has been given in Dellon's monograph. Each report from World War II through 1980 was included, subcategorized as to whether the injury was civilian or war type, whether the repair was primary or secondary, whether children were included in the series, the length of follow-up of the series noted, and the results categorized into sensory and motor recovery based on the British system of classification. This classification is listed in Table 7-4. The results of this review of the literature[28,85–101] are listed in Table 7-5.

Table 7-3. Results of Median Nerve Repair: Brachium and Forearm*

	Number of Patients			
	Good	*Fair*	*Poor*	*Bad*
Primary suture				
Brachium	—	1	—	—
Forearm	—	1	2	—
Secondary suture				
axilla	1	2	—	—
Brachium	15	20	4	2
Forearm	14	39	2	1

*Reprinted with permission from Seddon.[85]

The results of release of median nerve entrapment syndrome in the proximal forearm may be obtained from the individual references just cited. The largest series, however, is that by Johnson et al,[102] who com-

Table 7-4. Classification of Sensory and Motor Recovery*

Grade	
Recovery of Sensibility	
S0	No recovery of sensibility in the autonomous zone of the nerve
S1	Recovery of deep cutaneous pain sensibility with the autonomous zone of the nerve
S1+	Recovery of superficial pain sensibility
S2	Recovery of superficial pain and some touch sensibility
S2+	As in S2, but with overresponse
S3	Recovery of pain and touch sensibility with disappearance of over-response
S3+	As in S3, but localization of the stimulus is good and there is imperfect recovery of two-point discrimination
S4	Complete recovery
Motor Recovery	
M0	No contraction
M1	Return of perceptible contraction in the proximal muscles
M2	Return of perceptible contraction in both proximal and distal muscles
M3	Return of function in both proximal and distal muscles to such a degree that all important muscles are sufficiently powerful to act against gravity
M4	All muscles act against strong resistance and some independent movements are possible
M5	Full recovery in all muscles

*Reprinted with permission from Dellon.[86]

Table 7-5. Results of Median Nerve Repair and Grafting for High Lesion*

	Degree of Recovery (%)				
	No.	*M4*	*M5*	*S3+*	*S4*
Repair					
War injury	266	20	5	3	0
Civilian injury	139	30	0	17	0
Graft					
All	104	13	20	24	2

*Reprinted with permission from Dellon.[86]

bined their experience of 71 cases over a 20-year period. Fifty-one of these 71 cases were operated on. The sites of entrapment that they found in order of the highest frequency were the pronator teres, the superficialis arch, and the lacertus fibrosis. Follow-up ranged from 6 months to 19 years, and just 4 of the 51 cases were considered to be failures. All patients who had decompression of the median nerve in the forearm for only sensory complaints had relief the day after operation. Cases that were surgical failures were believed to be due either to a "misdiagnosis or a recurrent scarring around the scar associated with a new injury." They included no pre- or postoperative measurements for pinch and grip strength in the reporting of results nor comments on patients' return to work activities. The report did not include specifically cases of anterior interosseous nerve palsy, but rather was restricted to what was referred to in the diagnosis section as the "pure" pronator syndrome.

References

1. Sunderland S: Median nerve lesions. In Sunderland S, ed: Nerve and Nerve Injuries. Churchill Livingston, Edinburgh, 1978.
2. Spinner M: The median nerve. In Spinner M, ed: Injuries to the Major Branches of Peripheral Nerves of the Forearm, 2nd ed. WB Saunders, Philadelphia, 1978.
3. Omer GE, Spinner M: Management of Peripheral Nerve Problems. WB Saunders, Philadelphia, 1980.
4. Dawson DM, Hallett M, Millender LH: Entrapment Neuropathies. Little, Brown & Co, Boston, 1983.
5. Stewart JD: Focal Peripheral Neuropathies. Elsevier, New York, 1987.
6. Kaplan EB, Spinner M: Normal and anomalous innervation patterns in the upper extremity. In Omer G, Spinner M, eds: Management of Peripheral Nerve Problems. WB Saunders, Philadelphia, 1980.
7. Vallois HV: Recherches sur le trajet et les anastomoses du nerf musculo-cutane au niveau du bras. Arch Anat Histol Embryol 1:183, 1922.
8. Kerr AT: The brachial plexus of nerves in man, variations in its formation and branches. Am J Anat 23:285–395, 1918.
9. Struthers J: On a peculiarity of the humerus and humeral artery. Monthly J Med Sci 28:264–267, 1848.
10. Dellon AL: Musculotendinous variations about the medical humeral epicondyle. J Hand Surg [Br] 11:175–181, 1986.
11. Struthers J: On some points in the abnormal anatomy of the arm. Br For Med Chir Rev 14:170–179, 1854.
12. Solieri S: Nevralgia del nervo mediano del processo sopraepitrocleare. Chir Organi Mov 14:171–180, 1929.
13. Mandruzzato F: Patholgeia e chirurgia del processo sopraepitrocleare del'omero. Chir Organi Mov 24:123–132, 1938.
14. Barnard LB, McCoy SM: The supercondyloid process of the humerus. J Bone Joint Surg 28:845–850, 1946.
15. Kessel L, Wang M: Supercondylar spur of the humerus. J Bone Joint Surg 48B:765–769, 1966.
16. Lehar K, Dujobny M, deCastro SC: Entrapment of median nerve by supercondylar process of the humerus. J Neurosurg 46:252–255, 1977.
17. Suramyi L: Median nerve compression by Struthers' ligament. J Neurol Neurosurg Psychiatry 46:1047–1049, 1983.
18. Gessini L, Jandolo B, Pietrangeli A: Entrapment neuropathies of the median nerve at and above the elbow. Surg Neurol 19:112–116, 1983.
19. Luce EA, Futrell JW, Wilgis EF, Hoopes JE: Compression neuropathy following brachial arterial puncture in anticoagulated patients. J Trauma 16:717–721, 1976.
20. Silverstein A: Neuropathy in hemophilia. JAMA 190:534–535, 1964.

21. Molner W, Paul DJ: Complications of axillary arteriotomies. Radiology 104:269–276, 1972.
22. Stall LA, Van Voorthuisen AE, Van Dijk LM: Neurological complications following arterial catheterization by the axillary approach. Br J Radiol 39:115–116, 1966.
23. Braun RM, Newman J, Thatcher B: Injury to the brachial plexus as a result of diagnostic arteriography. J Hand Surg 3:90–94, 1978.
24. Ebeatty S, Mackinnon SE, Dellon AL, O'Brien J, Phillips JE: Vibratory sensory testing in acute compartment syndrome: A clinical and experimental study. Plast Reconstr Surg 79:796–801, 1987.
25. Spinner M: Cryptogenic infraclavicular brachial plexus neuritus. Bull Hosp Joint Dis 37:98–104, 1976.
26. Blom S, Dahlback LO: Nerve injuries in dislocations of the shoulder joint and fractures of the neck of the humerus. A clinical and electromyographical study. Acta Chir Scand 136:461–466, 1970.
27. Omer GE Jr: The results of untreated traumatic injuries. In Omer GE Jr, Spinner M eds: Management of Peripheral Nerve Problems. WB Saunders, Philadelphia, 1980.
28. Omer GE JR: Injuries to nerves of the upper extremity. J Bone Joint Surg 56A:1615–1624, 1974.
29. Martinelli P, Gabollini AS, Poppi N, et al: Pronator syndrome due to thickened bicipital aponeurosis. J Neurol Neurosurg Psychiatry 45:181–182, 1982.
30. Kelly MJ, Jackson BT: Compression of median nerve at the elbow. Br Med J 2:283–286, 1976.
31. Lipscomb PR, Burleson RJ: Vascular and neural complications in supercondylar fractures of the humerus in children. J Bone Joint Surg 37A:487–492, 1955.
32. Warren JD: Anterior interosseous nerve palsies. A complication of forearm fractures. J Bone Joint Surg 45B:511–513, 1963.
33. Henrickson B: Supracondylar fractures of the humerus in children. Acta Chir Scand [Suppl] 369:1, 1966.
34. El-Sharkawai AH, Fattah HA: Treatment of displaced supracondylar fractures of the humerus in children on full extension and supination. J Bone Joint Surg 47B:273–276, 1965.
35. Spinner M, Schrieber SN: The anterior interosseous nerve paralysis as a complication of supercondylar fractures in children. J Bone Joint Surg 51A:1584–1590, 1969.
36. Jones ET, Louis DS: Median nerve injuries associated with supercondylar fracture of the humerus in children. Clin Orthop 150:181–186, 1980.
37. Rana NA, Kenwright J, Taylor RG, Rushworth G: Complete lesion of the median nerve associated with dislocation of the elbow joint. Acta Orthop Scand 45:365–369, 1974.
38. Matev I: A radiologic sign of entrapment of the median nerve in the elbow joint after posterior dislocation. J Bone Joint Surg 56B:353–355, 1976.
39. Hallett J: Entrapment of the median nerve after dislocation of the elbow: A case report. J Bone Joint Surg 63B: 408–412, 1981.
40. Holmes JC, Skolnick MD, Hall JE: Untreated median nerve entrapment in bone after fracture of the distal end of the humerus: Postmortem findings after 47 years. J Bone Joint Surg 61A:309–310, 1979.
41. Dellon AL: Clinical use of vibratory stimuli to evaluate peripheral nerve injury in compression neuropathy. Plast Reconstr Surg 65:466–476, 1980.
42. Dellon AL, Mackinnon SE: Musculoaponeurotic variations along the course of the median nerve in the proximal forearm. J Hand Surg [Br] 12:359–363, 1987.
43. Winkelman NZ, Spinner M: A variant high sensory branch of the median nerve to the third web space. Bull Hosp Joint Dis 34:161–163, 1973.
44. Martin R: Tal om Nervus allmanna Egenskaper i Mannsikans Krobp. Stockholm, Lars Salvius, 1763.
45. Gruber W: Ueber die Verbindung des Nervus Medianus mit dem Nervus ulnaris am Unterarme des Menschen und der Sangethiete. Arch Neurol Physiol 37:501–522, 1870.
46. Spinner M. Injuries to the Major Branches of Peripheral Nerves in the Forearm, 2nd ed. WB Saunders, Philadelphia, 1978, pp 208–211.
47. Sunderland S: Nerve and Nerve Injuries, 2nd ed. Churchill Livingson, Edinburgh, 1978, p 663.
48. Mannerfelt L: Studies on the hand in ulnar nerve paralysis. A clinical-experimental investigation in normal and anomalous innervation. Acta Orthop Scand [Suppl] 87:1, 1966.
49. Dellon AL, Mackinnon SE, Seiler WA: Models for peripheral nerve research. In Adams RJ, Swindle MM eds: Induced Animal Models of Human Disease. Williams & Wilkins, Baltimore, 1988.
50. Mangini U: Flexor pollicis longus muscle. Its morphology and clinical significance. J Bone Joint Surg 42A:467–470, 1960.
51. Kaplan EB: Correction of a disabling flexion contraction of the thumb. Bull Hosp Joint Dis 3:51–54, 1942.
52. Reimann AF, Daseler EH, Anson BJ, Beaton LE: The palmaris longus muscle and tendon. The study of 1600 extremities. Anat Rec 89:495–505, 1944.
53. Breidenbach W, Tsai T, Manstean C: Ipsilateral pronator teres in carpal tunnel compression of the median nerve. Presented at the Annual Meeting of the American Society for Surgery of the Hand, January, 1985. J Hand Surg [Am] 10:432, 1985.
54. Seyffarth H: Primary myoses in the M. pronator teres as a cause of lesion of the N. medianus (the pronator syndrome). Acta Psychiat Neurol [Suppl] 74:1, 1951.
55. Solnitzky O: Pronator syndrome: Compression neuropathy of the median nerve at the level of the pronator teres muscle. Georgetown Med Bull 13:232–238, 1960.
56. Kopell HP, Thompson WAL: Pronator syndrome. N Engl J Med 259:713–715, 1958.
57. Morris HH, Peters BH: Pronator syndrome: Clinical and electrophysiologic features in seven cases. J Neurol Neurosurg Psychiatry 39:461–464, 1976.
58. Kojima T, Harase M, Ietsune T: Pronator syndrome: Report of six cases. Orthop Surg (Jpn) 19:1147–1148, 1968.
59. Hartz CR, Linscheid RL, Gramser RR, et al: The pronator teres syndrome. Compressive neuropathy of the median nerve. J Bone Joint Surg 63A:885–890, 1981.
60. Buchthal F, Rosenthalk A, Trojaborg W: Electrophysio-

logical findings in entrapment of the median nerve at the wrist and elbow. J Neurol Neurosurg Psychiatry 37:340–360, 1974.
61. Kiloh LG, Nevin S: Isolated neuritis of the anterior interosseous nerve. Br Med J 1:850–851, 1952.
62. Bell GE Jr, Goldner JL: Compression neuropathy of the median nerve. South Med J 49:966–972, 1956.
63. Thomas DF: Kiloh-Nevin syndrome. (Abstr.) J Bone Joint Surg 44B:962, 1962.
64. Fearn CB, D'a Goodfellow JW: Anterior interosseous nerve palsy. J Bone Joint Surg 47B:91–93, 1965.
65. Farber JS, Bryan RS: The anterior interosseous nerve syndrome. J Bone Joint Surg 58:521–523, 1968.
66. Sharrard WIW: Anterior interosseous neuritis. Report of a case. J Bone Joint Surg 50B:804–805, 1968.
67. Spinner M: The anterior interosseous nerve syndrome with special attention to its variations. J Bone Joint Surg 52A:84–94, 1970.
68. Schmidt H, Eiken O: The anterior interosseous nerve syndrome. Scand J Plast Reconstr Surg 5:53–56, 1971.
69. Gardner-Thorpe C: Anterior interosseous nerve palsy: Spontaneous recovery in two patients. J Neurol Neurosurg Psychiatry 37:1146–1150, 1974.
70. Dellon AL, Mackinnon SE, Daneshvar A: Terminal branch of anterior interosseous nerve as source of wrist pain. J Hand Surg [Br] 9:316–322, 1984.
71. Nolebuff EA, Potter TA: Rheumatoid involvement of tendon and tendon sheaths in the hand. Clin Orthop 59:147–159, 1968.
72. Mannerfelt L, Norman O: Attrition ruptures of flexor tendons in rheumatoid arthritis caused by bony spurs in the carpal tunnel. J Bone Joint Surg 51B:270–277, 1969.
73. Wertsch JJ, Senger JR, Matloub HS: Pseudo-anterior interosseous nerve syndrome. Muscle Nerve 8:68–70, 1985.
74. Dellon AL: Interruption of nerve function. In Marsh J, ed: Current Therapy in Plastic and Reconstructive Surgery. BC Decker, Toronto, 1988.
75. Cragg C: Isolated paralysis of the flexor pollicis muscle. An unusual variation of the anterior interosseous nerve syndrome. Case report. Scand J Plast Reconstr Surg 8:250–252, 1974.
76. Hill NA, Howard FM, Huffer BR: The incomplete anterior interosseous nerve syndrome. J Hand Surg [Am] 10:4–16, 1985.
77. Spillane JD: Localized neuritis of the shoulder girdle. Lancet 2:532–534, 1943.
78. Parsonage MJ, Turner JWA: Neuralgic amyotrophy: The shoulder girdle syndrome. Lancet 1:973–978, 1948.
79. Turner JWA, Parsonage MJ: Neuralgic amyotrophy (paralytic brachial neuritis). Lancet 2:209–212, 1957.
80. Tsairis P, Dyck PJ, Molder DW: Natural history of brachial plexus neuropathy. Arch Neurol 27:109–117, 1972.
81. Lilla JA, Phelps B, Boswick JA Jr: Microsurgical repair of peripheral nerve injuries in the upper extremity. Ann Plast Surg 2:24–31, 1979.
82. Orgel MG: Epineurial versus perineurial repair of peripheral nerves. Clin Plast Surg 11:101–104, 1984.
83. Michon J, Moberg E: Traumatic Nerve Lesions of the Upper Limb. Churchill Livingston, London, 1975.
84. Millesi H: Nerve grafting. Clin Plast Surg 11:105–114, 1984.
85. Seddon H: Surgical Disorders of the Peripheral Nerves. William & Wilkins, Baltimore, 1972, p 303.
86. Dellon AL: Evaluation of Sensibility and Re-education of Sensation in the Hand. William & Wilkins, Baltimore, 1981.
87. Kirklin JW, Murphy F, Berkson J: Suture of peripheral nerves: Factors affecting prognosis. Surg Gynecol Obstet 88:719–730, 1949.
88. Zachary RB: Results of nerve suture. In Seddon HJ, ed: Peripheral Nerve Injuries. Her Majesty's Stationery Office, London. pp 34–388.
89. Yahr MD, Beebe GW: Recovery of motor function. In Woodhall B, Beebe GW, eds: Peripheral Nerve Regeneration. U.S. Government Printing Office, Washington, DC, 1956, pp 71–202.
90. Oester VT, Davis L: Recovery of sensory functions. In Woodhall B, Beebe GW, eds: Peripheral Nerve Regeneration. U.S. Government Printing Office, Washington DC, 1956, pp 241–310.
91. Nicholson OR, Seddon HJ: Nerve repair in civil practice. Br Med J 2:1065–1071, 1957.
92. Lansen RD, Posch JL: Nerve injuries in the upper extremity. Arch Surg 77:469–482, 1958.
93. Sakellaridies H: A follow-up study of 173 peripheral nerve injuries in the upper extremity of civilians. J Bone Joint Surg 44A:140–148, 1962.
94. Posch JL, dela Cruz-Saddul F: Nerve repair in trauma surgery: A ten-year study of 231 peripheral injuries. Orthop Rev 9:35–45, 1980.
95. Bunnell S, Boyes JH: Nerve grafts. Am J Surg 44:64–75, 1939.
96. Seddon HJ: The use of autogenous grafts for repair of large gaps in peripheral nerves. Br J Surg 35:151–167, 1947.
97. Brooks D: The place of nerve grafting in orthopedic surgery. J Bone Joint Surg 37A:299–326, 1955.
98. Millesi H, Meisse G, Berger A: The interfascicular nerve-grafting of the median and ulnar nerves. J Bone Joint Surg 54A:727–750, 1972.
99. Millesi H, Meisse G, Berger A: Further experience with interfascicular grafting of the median, ulnar and radial nerves. J Bone Joint Surg 58A:209–218, 1976.
100. Young VL, Wray CR, Weeks PM: The results of nerve grafting in the wrist and hand. Ann Plast Surg 5:212–215, 1980.
101. Tallas R, Staniforth P, Fisher TR: Neurophysiological studies of autogenous nerve grafts. J Neurol Neurosurg Psychiatry 41:677–683, 1978.
102. Johnson RK, Spinner M, Shrewsburg MM: Median nerve entrapment syndrome in the proximal forearm. J Hand Surg 4:48–51, 1979.

Ulnar Nerve Entrapment at the Wrist

8

Historical Review

The subject of ulnar nerve entrapment at the wrist is made interesting by the ability to localize the site of entrapment due to the relationship of the normal anatomy of the distal ulnar nerve and its unique relationship to other anatomic structures about the wrist. The differential diagnosis of this problem is based not only on the wide variety of etiologies, but also on the variety of anatomic anomalies that occur in this nerve and in this region. Furthermore, the close relationship of the ulnar nerve to the median nerve at the wrist presents interesting diagnostic and therapeutic problems. The treatment of ulnar nerve entrapment at the wrist is perhaps the least controversial and most mutually agreed on surgical technique of all the nerve entrapments.

Ulnar nerve entrapment at the wrist is most commonly called ulnar nerve entrapment in Guyon's canal. Jean Casimir Felix Guyon, as a 30-year-old anatomist, became interested in the small protrusion that occurs in the distal forearm adjacent to the hypothenar eminence when pressure is placed on the hypothenar eminence. His anatomy dissections were descriptions of the fibrofatty contents of a triangular-shaped space or "loge." He did note that through this space passed the ulnar artery, accompanying veins, and the ulnar nerve, where it divided into the motor and sensory branches, and he indicated the possibility for nerve entrapment in this location.[1] Indeed, it has been pointed out by Grantham[2] that Guyon did not describe semantically what we call a canal. "A canal should have a bed, a floor and sides and be unroofed. This space (described by Guyon) is constructed more like a scout's lean-to."[2] Guyon became a professor of surgical pathology and was best known for his urinary tract surgery.[3]

It is not clear who first described the space or loge of Guyon as a canal. Perhaps, the first true description of a "tunnel" through which a portion of the ulnar nerve could be entrapped was by McFarlane et al,[4] who described the pisohamate tunnel through which the deep motor branch may become compressed against the overlying fibrous arch, giving origin to the hypothenar muscles. The extent to which the anatomy in this region lends itself to further description and attempt at classification is best exemplified by the recent exhaustive description by Gross and Gelberman,[5] who attempt to divide this region into three separate zones (Figs. 8-1, 8-2). We believe, however, that the description of the patient's symptom complex in terms of the motor and sensory distribution of the complaints and findings, and the relationship of these findings to the anatomic site

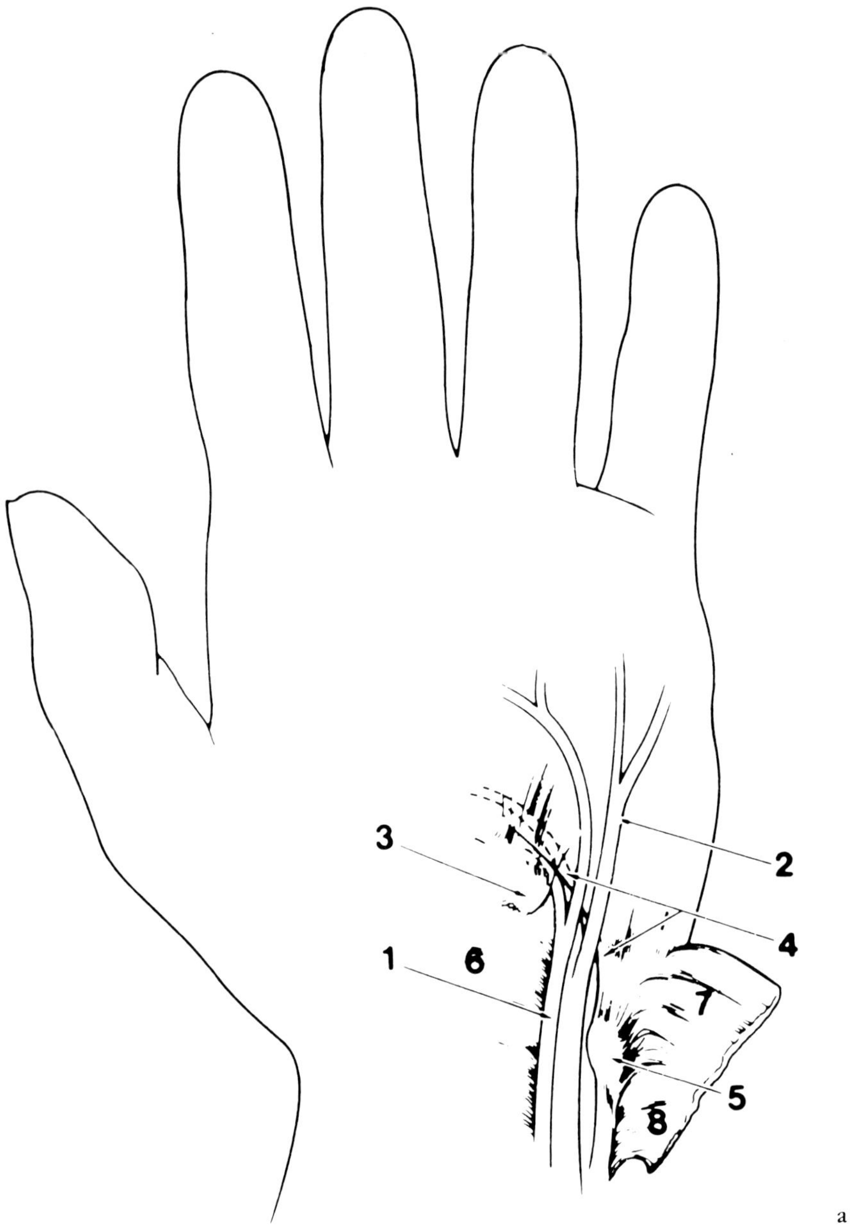

Figure 8-1. Left: The distal ulnar tunnel showing anatomic landmarks. 1. ulnar artery (H); 2. superficial branch of the ulnar nerve (N); 3. hamulus (H); 4. fibrous arch of the hypothenar muscles; 5. pisiform (P); 6. transverse carpal ligament; 7. palmaris brevis; 8. palmar carpal ligament. Right: Location of the three zones: Zone 1 (coarse stippling); zone 2 (lines); zone 3 (fine stippling). (Reproduced with permission from Gross and Gelberman.[5])

along the ulnar nerve, can best be described in relationship to the known anatomic landmarks, such as the pisiform and the hamate. We see no need to introduce new nomenclature or classification to this region and will not incorporate such into this chapter.

The first description of compression of the ulnar nerve at the wrist was probably that by Jay Ramsey Hunt in 1908[6] and subsequent articles written over the next few years.[7–9] He described clearly the entrapment of the ulnar nerve at the wrist with various clinical presentations based on the site of the entrapment, so that this nerve entrapment has been called by some the Ramsey Hunt syndrome. Hunt's description is also one of the earliest reported cases of occupational trauma causing nerve entrapment. The next descriptions of ulnar nerve problems in this region were identified in relationship to vascular problems. The extensive description by Middleton[10] in 1933 not only called attention to this fact but again to the role of occupation in the cause of problems with the ulnar nerve at the wrist level. Subsequently, the relationship between the ulnar artery, which in the distal portion of this region lies superficial to the ulnar nerve terminal sensory fibers and compression of the ulnar nerve, either directly due to aneurysm formation, or secondary to inflammation attendant on thrombosis of the vessel, has been extensively described and documented[11–19,21–28] (Fig. 8-3).

Ulnar nerve compression at the wrist was next

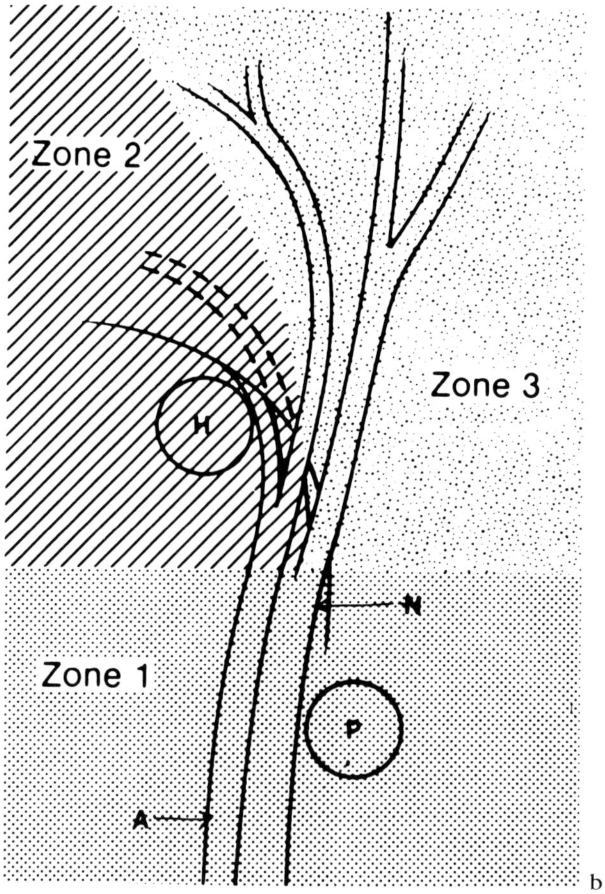

Figure 8-1 (*continued.*)

described as being due to a common tumor, the ganglion, independently by Brooks[29] and Seddon[30] in 1952. Brooks described the ganglion arising at the level of the pisiform, causing altered function in the motor and sensory components of the ulnar nerve, whereas Seddon described the ganglion arising in the pisohamate hiatus causing altered function in just the deep motor branch of the ulnar nerve. Both Brook's and Seddon's observations have been confirmed by subsequent researchers.[31–36] Although the ganglion is the most common tumor of the hand, virtually any tumor may occur along the course of the ulnar nerve at the wrist level, and other tumors causing ulnar nerve compression have been reported, such as lipomas,[4,36–38] giant cell tumor,[39] and rheumatoid synovial cyst.[40]

Trauma can play a role in ulnar nerve compression at the wrist in three classic ways other than the "hypothenar hammer syndrome," which is responsible for impinging the ulnar artery[41,42] or nerve against the hamate. Injuries that fracture the hook of the hamate can cause injury to the ulnar nerve by the force, itself, by displacement of the fractured piece, or by scarring subsequent to the fracture healing.[3,43–47] Fractures through the distal radius[43,48–52] and carpal dislocations,[53,54] indeed, in a bipartite hamulous have been reported to cause ulnar nerve compression at the wrist.[55] The incidence of ulnar nerve compression at the wrist was 2 in 213 cases of Colles' fracture, in comparison with 37 cases of carpal tunnel syndrome in this same group of

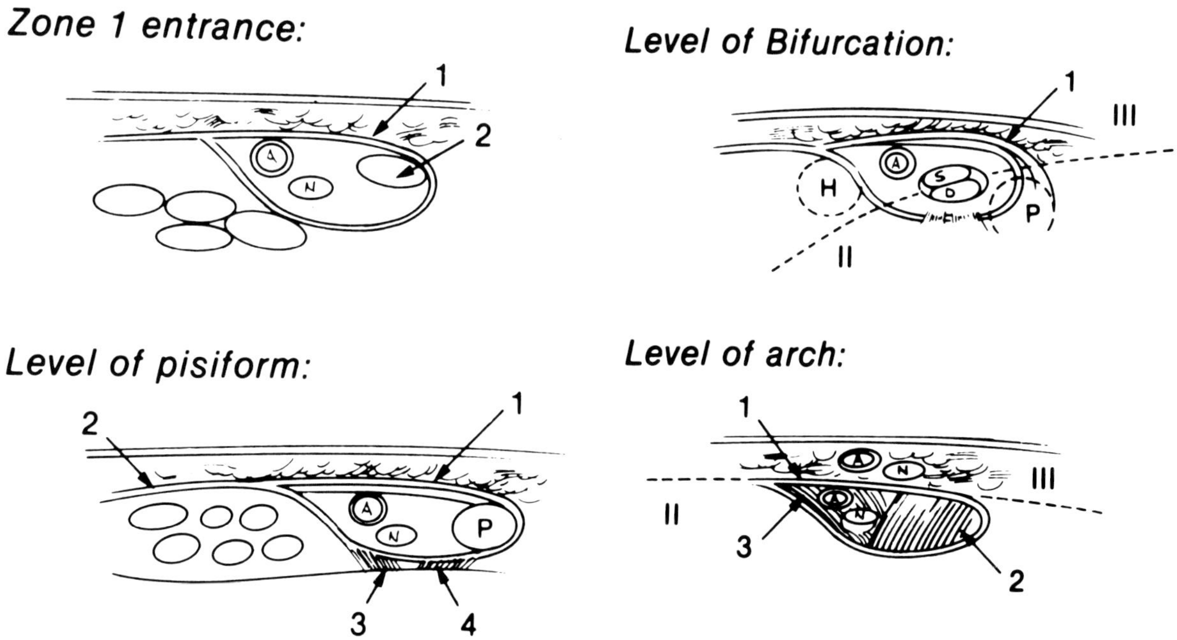

Figure 8-2. Schematic cross-sections of the distal ulnar tunnel. Entrance to zone 1: A. ulnar artery; N. ulnar nerve; 1. palmar carpal ligement; 2. tendon of flexor carpi ulnaris. Level of the pisiform: A. ulnar artery; N. ulnar nerve; P. pisiform, 1. palmaris brevis; 2. transverse carpal ligement; 3. pisohamate ligament; 4. pisometacarpal ligament. (Reproduced with permission from Gross and Gelberman.[5])

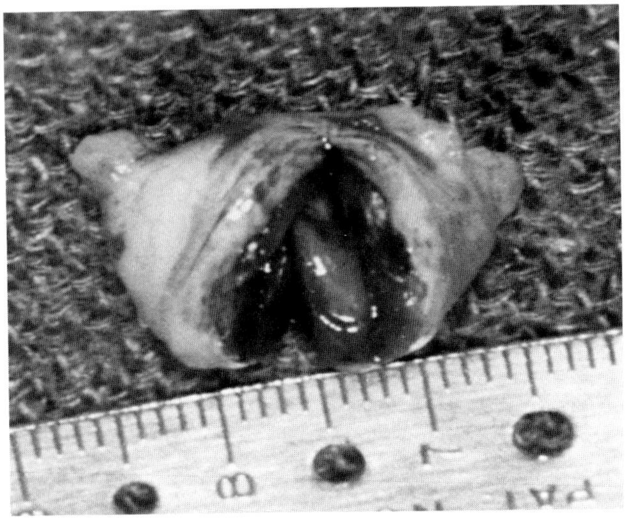

a

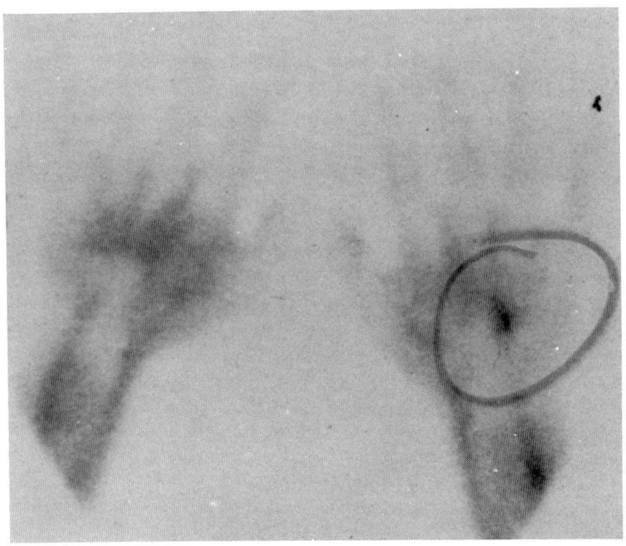

b

Figure 8-3. Ulnar nerve compression at the wrist due to aneurysm of the ulnar artery. Mass in hypothenar area developed slowly after a blow from a lacrosse ball. This was associated with numbness in the little and ring fingers with normal motor function. At surgery, a traumatic aneurysm of the ulnar artery was found, excised, and reconstructed with a vein graft (a). Nucleotide study documenting aneurysm preoperatively (b). (Reproduced with permission from Ho et al.[17])

patients. After these bony injuries, the next main group of injuries occur from the hobby or pastime of bicycle riding. One of the earliest descriptions of nerve entrapment was by Destot[55] who, in 1896, described ulnar nerve paralysis at the elbow from bicycle riding. Other reports of ulnar nerve entrapment due to the hypothenar eminence pressing against the bicycle during long rides have also been reported.[56–58] A source of trauma of increasing frequency that we have observed has been compression of the ulnar nerve at the wrist due to automobile accidents. The typical situation has the driver of the car being hit from the back or side while the driver's hands are both on the wheel. In the ensuing rocking forward and backward that occurs, the hand, in the hypothenar and thenar and palm are directly hit against the steering wheel and are then stretched and with shearing forces moving forward and backward, compression and contusion are directly caused to the median and ulnar nerves in the wrist. The subsequent swelling may not be noticed but over a period of between 1 and 2 years after the accident, this area has undergone chronic compression, usually of both the ulnar and median nerves together at the wrist level, with the patient complaining of numbness in all of the fingers. We have noted a positive Tinel's sign over the ulnar nerve at the wrist in these instances. With confirmatory electrodiagnostic studies and on exploration of the ulnar nerve in this area, generally dense fibrosis is present within the canal with adherence of the artery to the nerves and significant fibrous tissue in and around the normally loose fat.[59] An additional type of trauma is that due to burns. Thermal burns, whether directly from flame[14] or from electrical injuries (Fig. 8-4), can cause ulnar nerve compression at the wrist secondary to edema and subsequent fibrosis in the hand.

Surgical Anatomy

The ulnar nerve in the mid forearm has three main fascicular groups. The most ulnar or medial of the fascicles contains the fibers that will become the dorsal cutaneous sensory branch of the ulnar nerve. Approximately 9 cm proximal to the wrist, the dorsal ulnar branch courses dorsally, leaving just the terminal motor and sensory branches, to transverse the distal third of the forearm toward the wrist. The motor fascicles lie between the fascicles to the dorsal ulnar aspect of the hand and the sensory fascicles to the little and ring fingers. Thus, proximal to the takeoff of the dorsal ulnar branch, they are the fascicles in the middle of the ulnar nerve, whereas once the dorsal ulnar fascicle has separated from the main nerve, the motor fascicles are the ulnarmost fascicles in the ulnar nerve as it approaches the wrist. Passing the pisiform bone, the motor fascicles move deep to the sensory fascicles ultimately to enter the deep tunnel crossing the pisohamate ligament and go beneath the fibrous arch of the hypothenar muscles to cross the hand as the deep motor branch. Thus, the motor fascicles pass from medial or ulnar to the sensory fascicle to the little and ring fingers proximal to the wrist, to deep to these fascicles in the region between the pisiform and the hamate, to radial or lateral to the sensory fascicles in their ultimate destination (Fig. 8-5). This anatomic relationship allows clear identification of

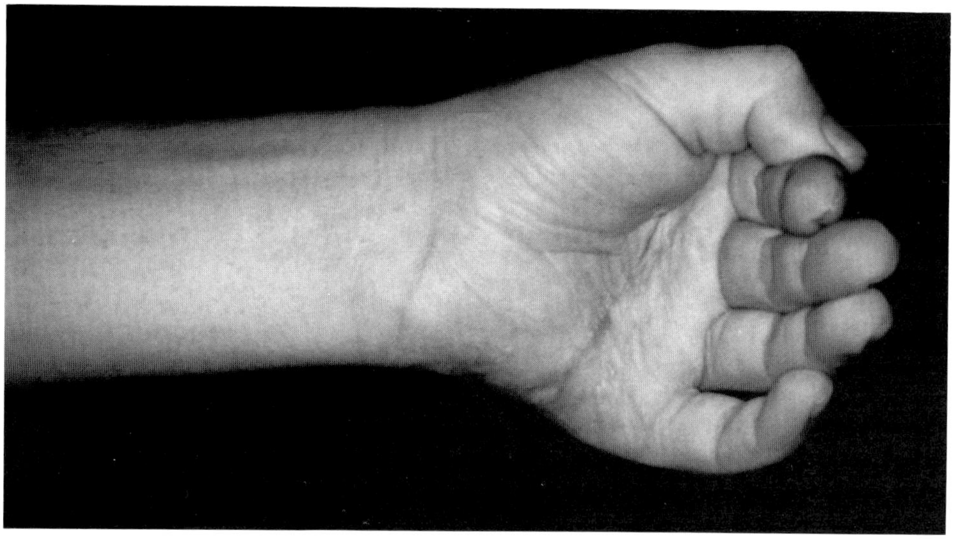

a

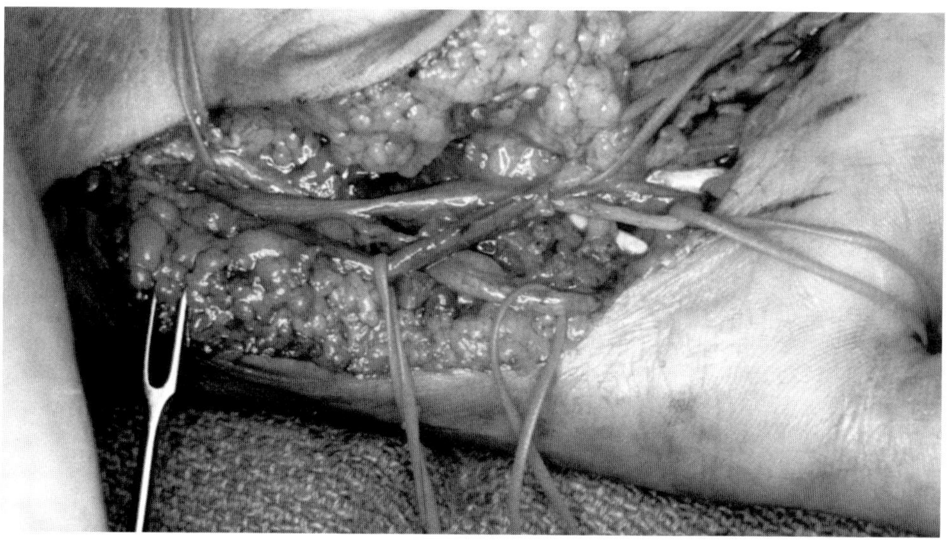

b

Figure 8-4. Ulnar nerve compression at the wrist due to electrical burn. The third degree palmar loss of skin was replaced by grafts, which were subsequently revised as thick scars. The patient had severely diminished sensation in little and ring fingers and no ulnar innervated motor function. At exploration, the ulnar nerve branches were intact but densely scarred (a). After an internal neurolysis, good sensation was recovered, as well as pinch strength (b).

the motor from the sensory fascicle when nerve repair or nerve grafting is required in this region.

During surgical decompression of the ulnar nerve at the wrist level, the deep motor branch is most easily found, therefore, by retracting the ulnar artery and accompanying veins toward the ulnar side or the pisiform. This brings the sensory branch into view. Moving this sensory branch toward the ulnar side, the origin of the hypothenar muscles from the hamate is then identified. At its proximal edge will be the entrance of the deep motor branch into the tunnel between the pisohamate ligament and the flexor digiti minimi. It is actually the leading edge of the flexor digiti minimi that can compress the motor branch. This muscle had a fibrous edge in 40% of cadaver dissections (Fig. 8-5).[61] This fibrous edge should be divided surgically when one is present, since it may produce an area of compression (Fig. 8-6). This fibrous origin of the flexor digiti minimi has been noted to vary from 1 to 6 mm, occasionally presenting an even wider band. The ulnar artery and accompanying veins lie radial or lateral to the ulnar nerve and slightly superficial to it. This relationship is true proximal to the wrist and through the canal. Past the hamate, the vessels move to a more superficial position as the ulnar nerve splits into its motor and sensory fascicles. The vessels lie completely superficial to the terminal sensory fibers in the region past the hamate (Figs. 8-1, 8-2, 8-4).

The ulnar nerve at the wrist crease represents mo-

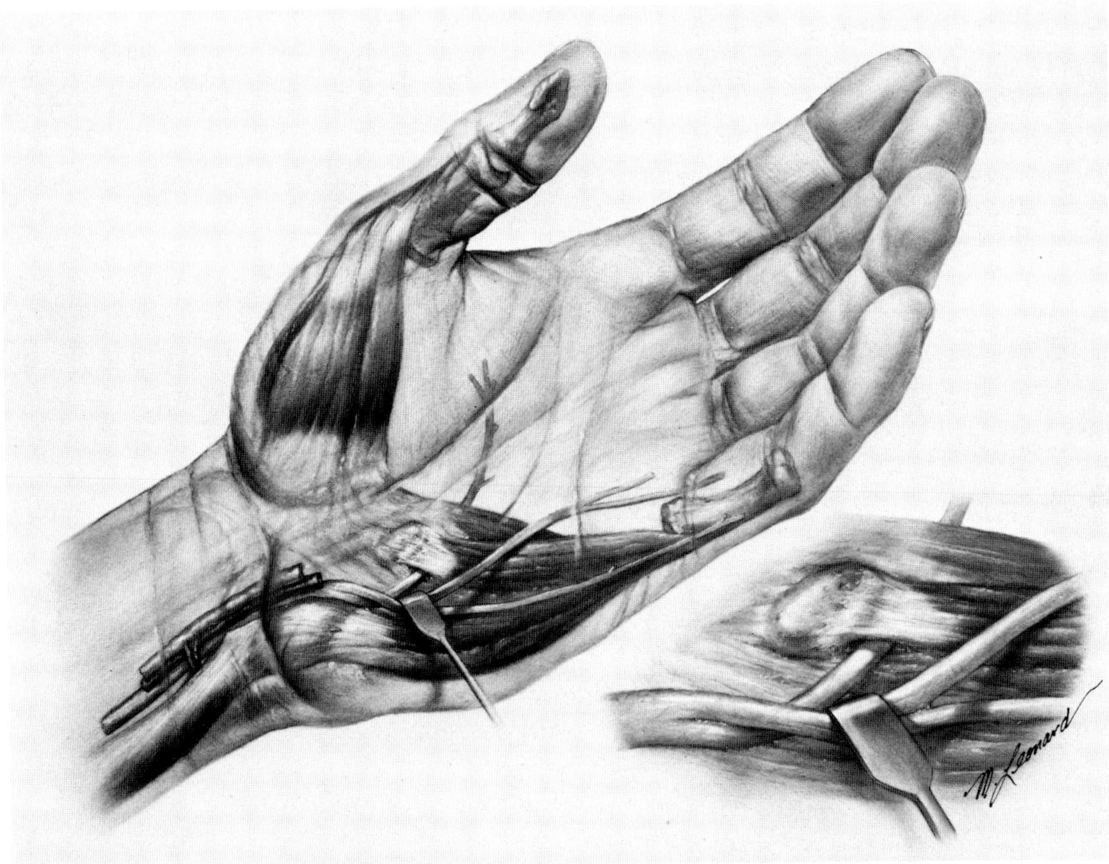

Figure 8-5. Anatomy of the ulnar nerve at the wrist demonstrating change of position of motor fascicles from ulnar (medial) to the sensory fascicles proximal to the wrist, to a position deep to them as they cross the pisohamate ligament, to radial (lateral) to them as the motor branch crosses beneath the arch of the hypothenar muscle origin. This arch is fibrous, in 40% of hands. (Reproduced with permission from Dellon and Mackinnon.[50])

tor and sensory fascicles that are clearly discrete from each other in terms of grouped fascicles, but they lie within a common sheath. Superficial to them at this point is the antebrachial fascia fibers blending with a thin layer of fibers termed the palmar or volar carpal ligament. Deep to the ulnar nerve at this point lies the transverse carpal ligament fibers inserting into the pisiform. The most medial or ulnar portion of the space that the ulnar nerve will enter is formed by the flexor carpi ulnaris. Just distal to this, as the pisiform itself is reached and the flexor carpi ulnaris blends into the pisiform, the floor of this space makes the transition from inserting fibers of the transverse carpal ligament to fibers from flexor carpi ulnaris. The radial or lateral side of this space is now made up completely of the transverse carpal ligament, and the roof to the space, the thin palmar carpal ligament, has, in some instances, been reinforced by the palmaris brevis muscle, which is present only to a variable degree and in some is completely absent (Fig. 8-2). Just distal to the pisiform, the fascicles of the ulnar nerve begin the transition just described, with the motor fascicles moving deep around the hook of the hamate. At this point, the two discrete divisions of the ulnar nerve are discernable. The sensory fibers continue to move superficially and distal to come above or superficial to the hypothenar muscle, the flexor digiti minimi that is arising from the hamate. The motor branch continues deep distal and moving radial to curve around the hamate and go beneath this flexor digiti minimi. At this point, the floor of the space is composed of the opponens digiti minimi, and the most medial or ulnar portion of the space is bounded by the abductor digiti minimi muscle. The artery accompanying the deep motor branch is the ulnar artery's contribution to the deep palmar arch where the ulnar artery's branch accompanying the sensory fascicles has become the superficial palmar arch (Fig. 8-2).

Variations in the anatomy in the region of the ulnar nerve at the level of the wrist may contribute to entrapment of the nerve. The most common variations

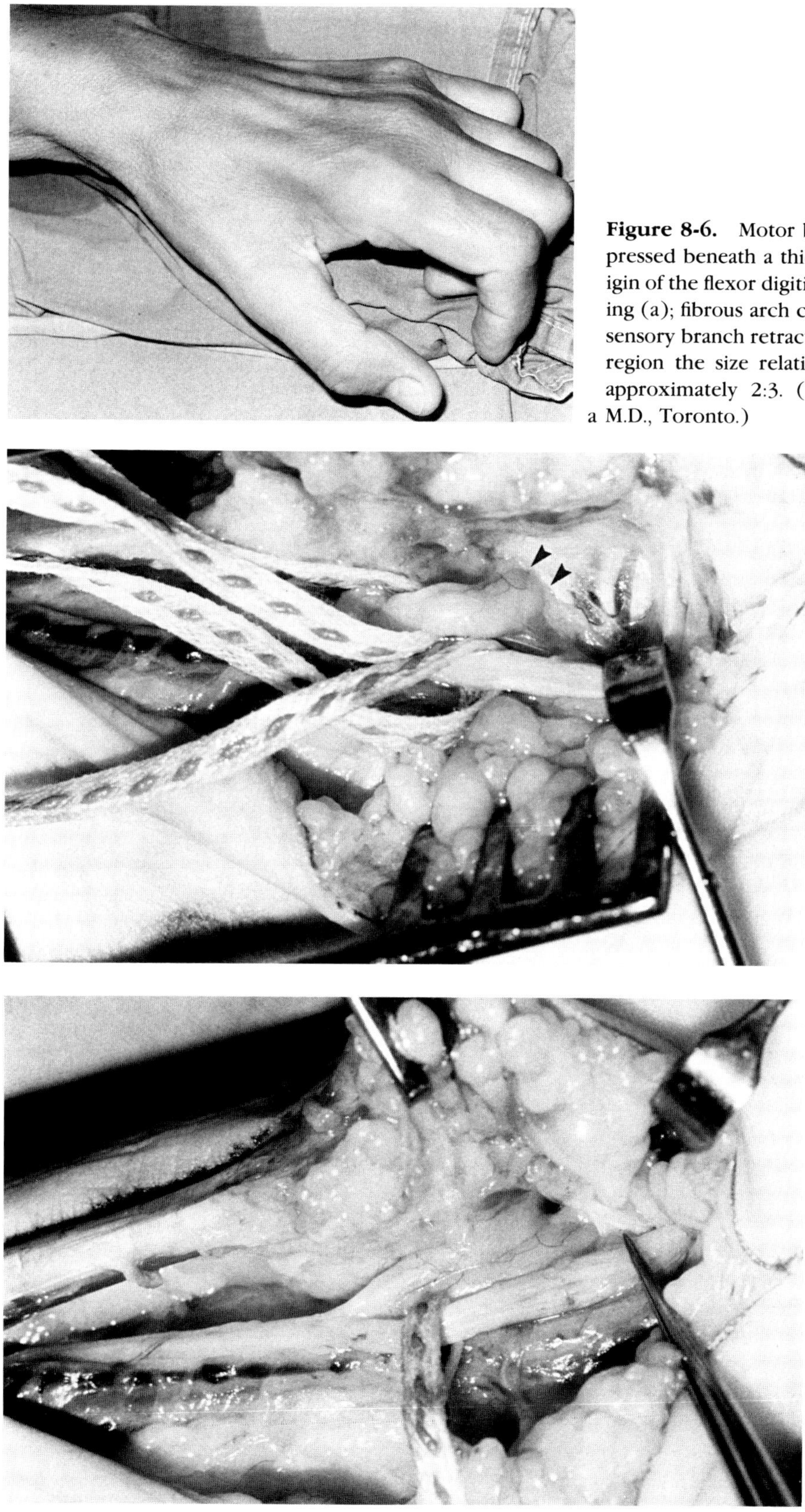

a b c

Figure 8-6. Motor branch of the ulnar nerve may be compressed beneath a thick fibrous arch, representing part of origin of the flexor digiti minimi from the hamate. Intrinsic wasting (a); fibrous arch compressing motor branch (arrow) with sensory branch retracted (b); fibrous arch released (c). In this region the size relationship of the motor:sensory groups is approximately 2:3. (Photograph courtesy of R. Knowlton, M.D., Toronto.)

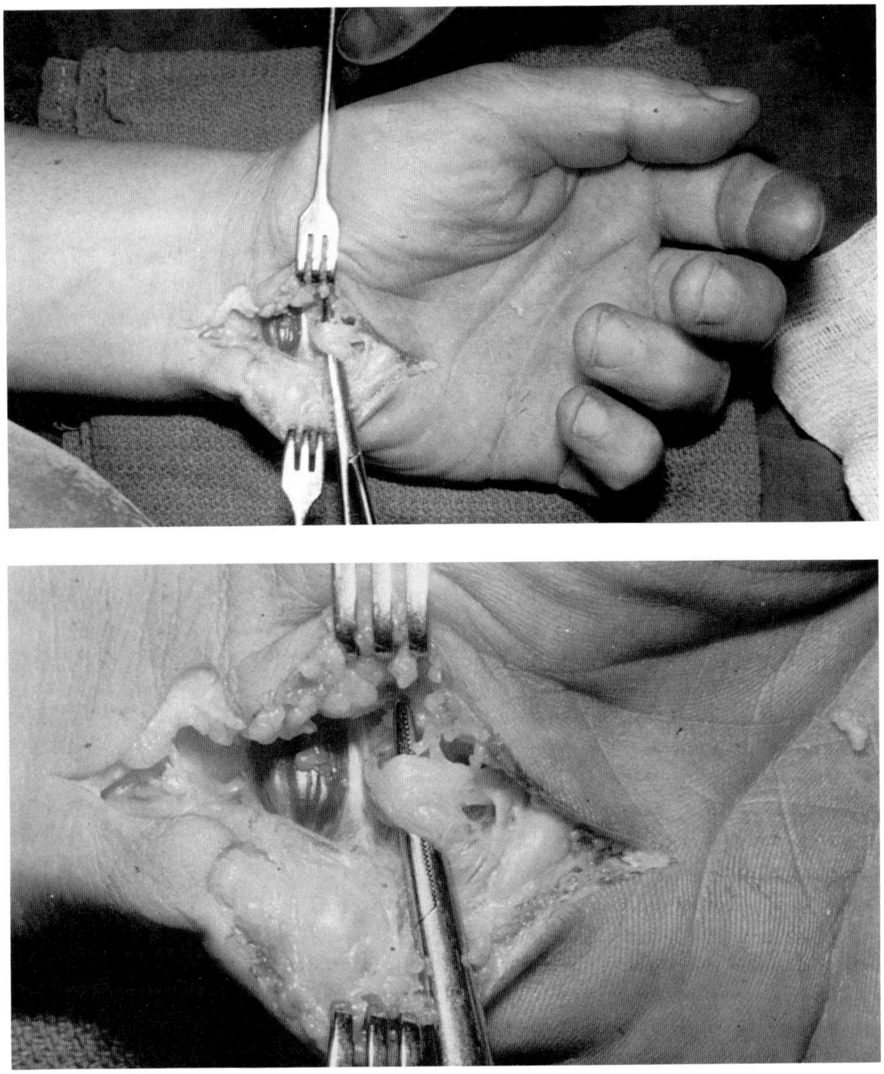

a

b

Figure 8-7. The palmaris brevis muscle can have a fibrous edge **(a)** causing ulnar nerve compression in Guyon's canal with both motor and sensory dysfunction **(b)** (Photograph courtesy of James F. Murray, M. D., Toronto)

are those associated with the palmaris longus. The most common variation is an accessory slip of the palmaris longus tendon that arises proximally and inserts into the pisiform, thus creating an arch through which the undivided ulnar nerve, accompanied by the ulnar artery, passes. There may be a reverse relationship in which the palmaris longus seemingly originates from the flexor retinaculum at the wrist, having a tendinous insertion into the medial humeral epicondyle.[62] An accessory palmaris longus has been noted to cause compression of the ulnar nerve at the wrist.[63] Anomalous muscles have been described in the space of Guyon as having variable relationships to the motor or sensory branch[64–67] and causing nerve compression. Ulnar nerve compression in this region has been reported to be due to a duplication of the palmaris longus,[68] of the abductor digiti minimi,[69,70] and of the entire set of hypothenar muscles,[71] where the palmaris brevis was approximately six times normal size and the entire mass duplicated a tumor of the hand. A fibrous edge to the palmaris brevis may cause compression (Fig. 8-7). Further anomalies in this region causing ulnar nerve compression have been reported.[18,72,73] Additional anomalies no doubt will be reported in the future. The significance of these anatomic abnormalities is to be aware of the normal, recognize the presence of the anomaly when exploring the wrist for ulnar nerve compression, and be prepared to resect the compressive anomalous muscle or tendon as needed.

Variations in the ulnar nerve can occur at the wrist level. For example, the deep motor branch, instead of passing distal to the hamate, may split, with a branch passing proximal and radial to the hamate, that is, through the carpal tunnel, joining its other branch distal to the hamate.[74,75] The deep motor branch near its terminal portion may send a branch to join the motor branch of the median nerve. This so-called anastomosis was described by Riche[76] and Cannieu.[77] Variations in the sensory distribution have been clearly described. The most common is the communication between the ulnar nerve sensory branch and the web space between the ring and little fingers, which may give a branch to the middle finger as well by communicating with the median nerve branch to this third web space.[78] The innervation to the little finger may be partially contributed to by sensory branches that travel with the dorsal cutaneous branch of the ulnar nerve, which, at the level of the pisiform, loop backward to join the sensory branch to the little finger.[79] The sensation to the dorsal ulnar aspect of the hand can occasionally become an unreliable sign in localizing the level of the nerve lesion. When present, this dorsal sensation suggests that the ulnar nerve lesion is located at the wrist, since loss of dorsal ulnar sensation usually means a problem with the dorsal cutaneous branch that arises proximal to the wrist. Learmonth,[80] in 1919, described a variation in which the entire dorsal ulnar aspect of the hand was supplied by the radial nerve. The dorsal ulnar area also can be innervated by the posterior cutaneous nerve of the forearm and by a posterior branch of the lateral antebrachial cutaneous nerve (Fig. 8-8). In these instances, the presence of sensation over the dorsal ulnar aspect of the hand may falsely localize the lesion to the ulnar nerve at the wrist when, in fact, the lesion may be more proximal.

Spinner[81] has clearly described the appearance of the hand based on the interplay of the normal and the anomalous anatomy of the ulnar nerve as it affects the diagnosis of the site of an ulnar nerve lesion (Figs. 8-9 through 8-11). The attitude of the hand depends on the

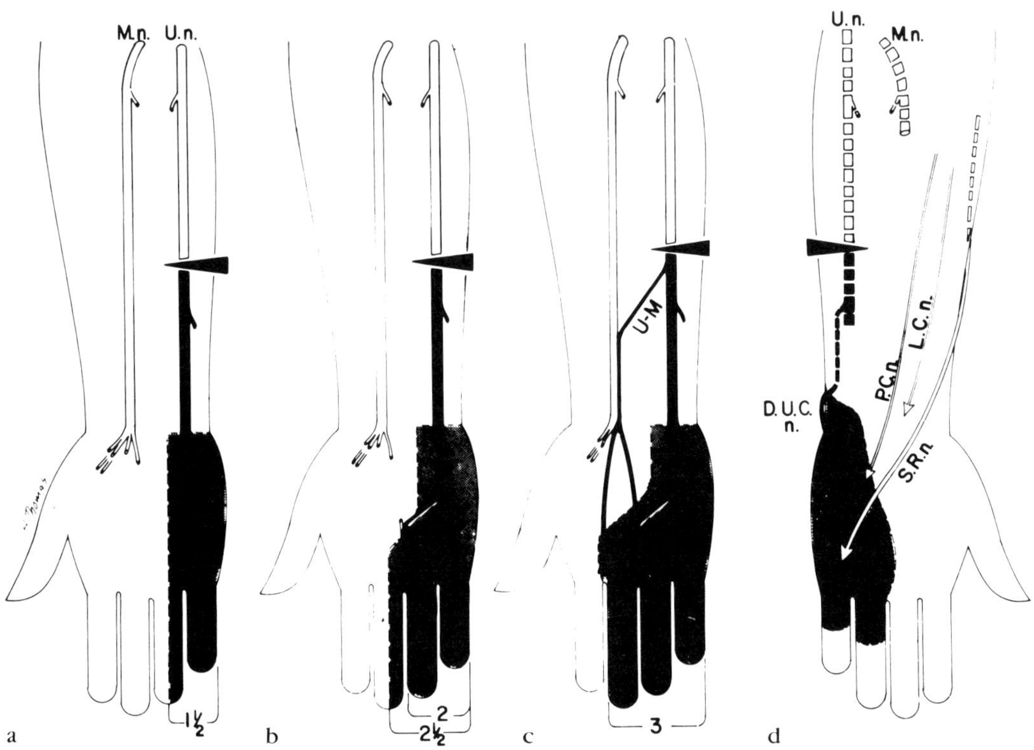

Figure 8-8. The typical sensory distribution of the ulnar nerve (U.n.) to the medial 1½ digits **(a)** can be increased to the adjacent digits by neural communications in the palm **(b)** and in the forearm **(c)**. **d.** The superficial radial nerve (S.R.n.) can supply the dorsal ulnar aspect of the hand, which is usually innervated by the dorsal ulnar cutaneous nerve (D.U.C.n.). The posterior cutaneous nerve of the forearm (P.C.n.) and the lateral cutaneous nerve of the forearm (L.C.n.) can also supply some of the dorsal ulnar aspect of the hand. M.n.: medial nerve. (Reproduced with permission from Spinner.[71])

location of the ulnar nerve lesion. When the intrinsic muscles have lost their nerve supply, flexion at the metacarpophalangeal joint is lost. The ulnar-innervated extrinsic flexors still function so that the interphalangeal joints will be flexed. The radially innervated extensor tendons can still extend the metacarpophalangeal joints. The effect of the unopposed action of these latter two extrinsic tendon units without the "balancing" effect of the intrinsic muscles produces the appearance of a claw deformity. The claw deformity, thus, occurs with a low ulnar nerve lesion (Fig. 8-9). If the median nerve innervates the ring finger lumbrical, only the little finger will be clawed. If dorsal ulnar sensation is present, associated with the claw deformity, the lesion will be between the wrist level and the takeoff of the dorsal cutaneous branch of the ulnar nerve, approximately, the distal third of the forearm to the wrist. If dorsal ulnar sensation is lost, but the fingers remain in a flexed position at the interphalangeal joints, then the lesion is located between the takeoff of the dorsal cutaneous branch and the innervation of the flexor digitorum profundus or somewhere between the distal third and proximal third of the forearm. The claw deformity will be lost if the ulnar nerve lesion is proximal to the innervation of the ulnar nerve to the flexor digitorum profundus, since there will be no flexion at the distal interphalangeal joint. If anomalous innervation of the median nerve to the profundus to the little and ring fingers exists, however, due to innervation within the flexor profundus muscle belly itself, then, even with a high ulnar nerve lesion, clawing may still be present (Fig. 8-10). Since any possible combination may exist,

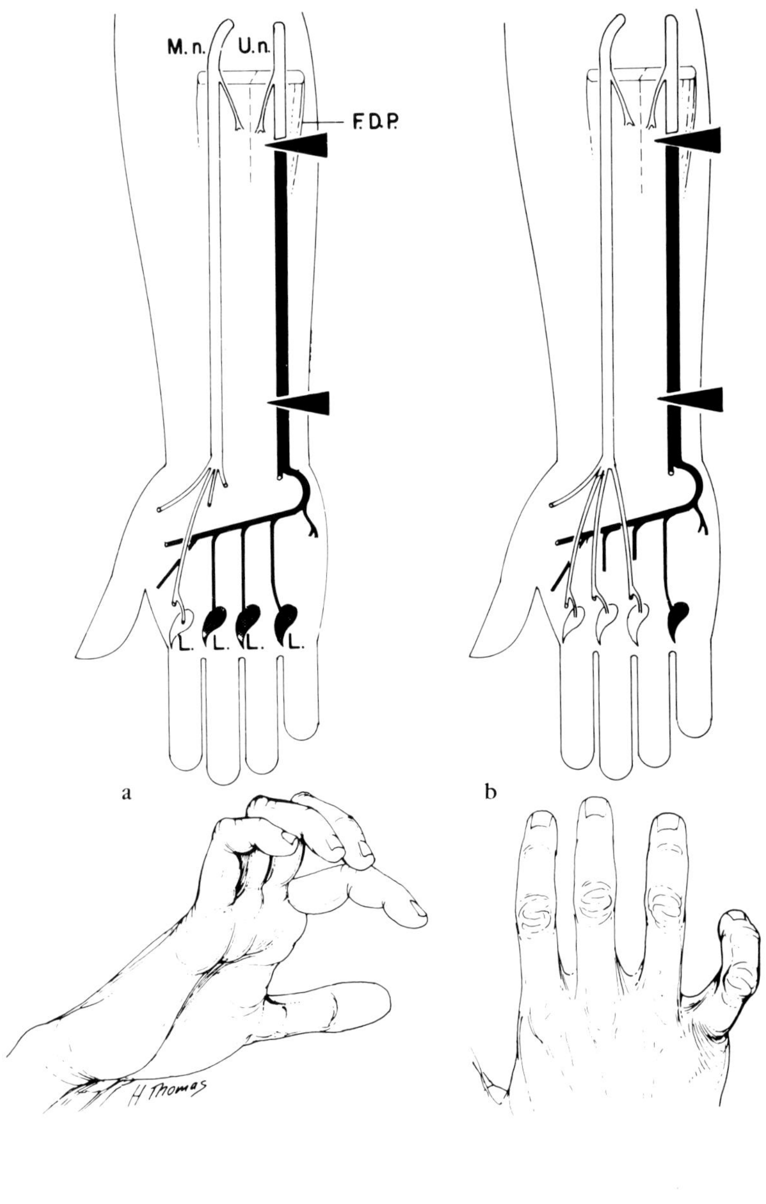

Figure 8-9a. A complete ulnar nerve lesion results in a three-finger clawhand when the lumbrical to the long finger is innervated by the ulnar nerve. **b.** Claw deformity of the little finger only occurs with a complete low ulnar lesion when the ring finger lumbrical is innervated by the median nerve. (Reproduced with permission from Spinner.[71])

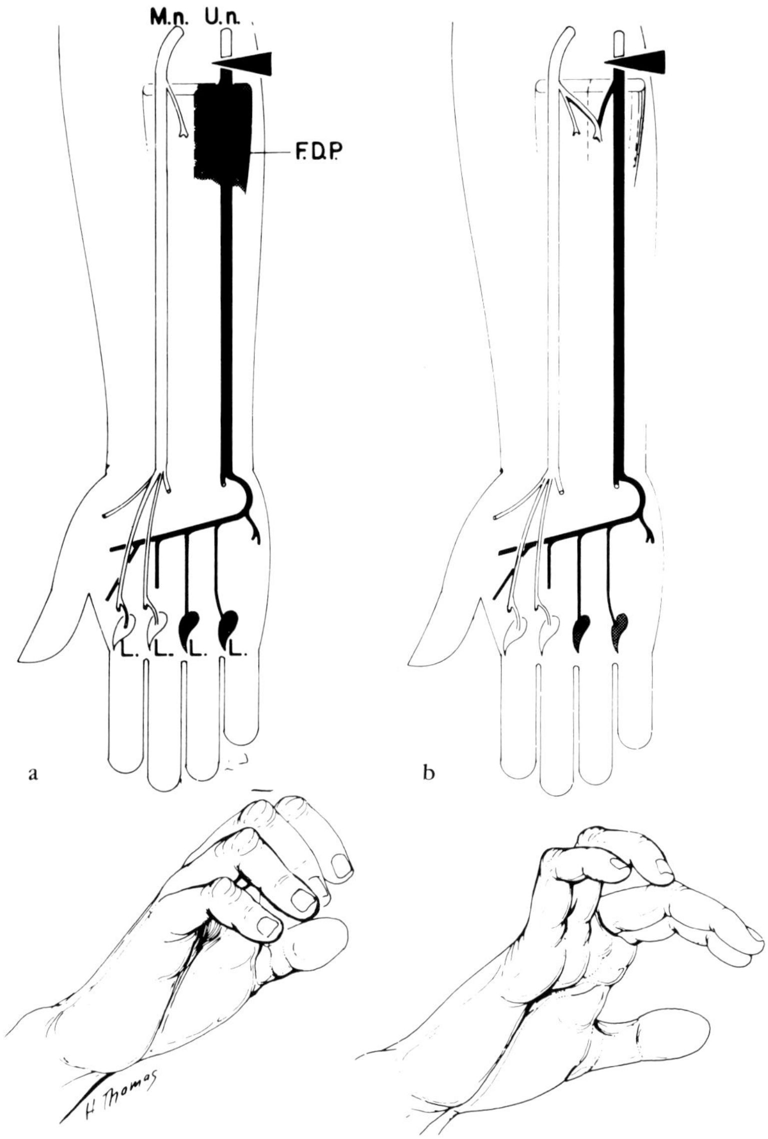

Figure 8-10a. A complete high ulnar nerve lesion is usually observed without digital claw deformity. **b.** However, complete high ulnar nerve lesions produce a clawed hand when the intact median nerve supplies the flexor digitorum profundus to the ring finger and little finger. (Reproduced with permission from Spinner.[71])

compensating anomalies may give further unusual combinations (Fig. 8-11). Therefore in addition to careful sensory examination, detailed electromyographic examination or diagnostic nerve blocks, or both, may be required to understand completely the appearance of the hand or the site of the ulnar nerve injury.

Diagnosis

The diagnosis of ulnar nerve entrapment at the wrist relies on being able to identify sensory loss in the hand and muscle weakness in the hand. The basic approach to each of these subjects is given in Chapter 3. Recalling the normal ulnar innervation of the hand, a detailed motor and sensory examination is performed. Motor evaluation will examine, in particular, the function of the flexor digitorum profundus to the little finger, the function of the hypothenar muscles, the function of the palmar and dorsal interossei, and the first dorsal interosseous muscle. Evaluation of pinch and grip strength will be critical. Sensibility testing in the little finger and dorsum of the hand will evaluate ulnar nerve sensory function. Analysis of the findings of such a motor and sensory examination will determine whether or not an ulnar nerve lesion is present. The location then of the lesion becomes the subject of the differential diagnosis. Table 8-1, taken from Stewart's monograph,[82] assists in determining if the lesion is due to problems in the C8 and T1 roots, the lower trunk of the brachial plexus, or the median cord of the brachial plexus. In essence, the

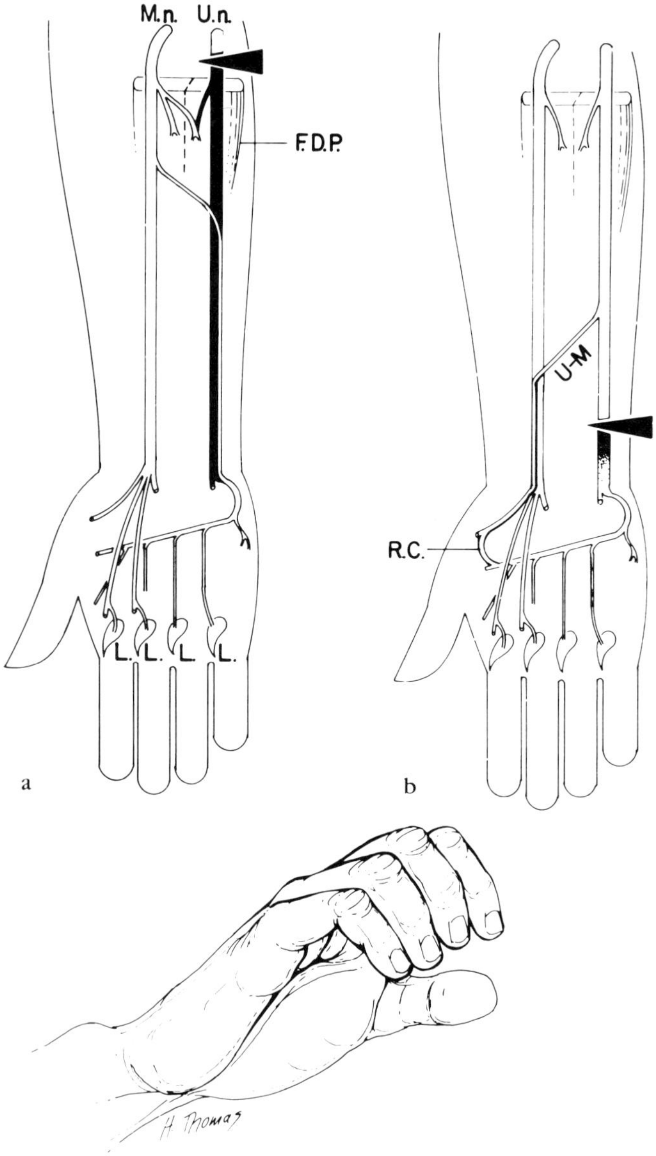

Figure 8-11a. A high ulnar nerve lesion has a normal attitude even though the flexor profundus muscles of the index, long, ring, and little fingers are innervated by the anterior interosseous branch of the median nerve because the intrinsic muscles are also innervated by the anomalous Martin-Gruber communication. **b.** Similarly, a complete low ulnar nerve lesion can also present with a normal-appearing hand when both an ulnar to median nerve (U-M) and a Riche-Cannieu (R.C.) communication are present. (Reproduced with permission from Spinner.[71])

differential diagnosis lies in identifying muscles that have weakness or wasting that are in addition to those traditionally supplied by the ulnar nerve itself. Electromyography may be esential in this endeavor.

Very proximal lesions have been described as the source of intrinsic atrophy, such as a meningioma compressing the spinal cord at the level of the foramen magnum.[83] A classic central nervous system source for intrinsic wasting is the spinal cord syrinx. In addition to muscle wasting of all the intrinsic muscles in the hand, there is a unique sensory loss: pain, heat, and cold sensation is lost but the perception of touch is preserved (Table 8-2; Fig. 8-12). The cataloging of the various sensory and motor losses will, in the absence of anatomic variations such as described in the preceding section, allow localization of the lesion to above-elbow, elbow, distal third of the forearm, and the various levels in the region of the wrist itself, that is, pisiform, deep and superficial within the pisohamate hiatus, and at the level of the hamate. As will be discussed in Chapter 9, the presence or absence of the flexor carpi ulnaris, which is difficult to determine accurately, varies when there is a lesion present at the elbow. With trauma that damages the entire nerve in this segment, such as a posttraumatic ulnar neuropathy at the elbow, the wrist flexor does not function, but with the classic cubital tunnel syndrome, as described by Osborne[84] and by Feindel and Stratford,[85] there is preservation of the wrist flexor. This occurs because the branch to the flexor carpi ulnaris arises proximal to the cubital tunnel, so

Table 8-1. Differential Diagnosis in Ulnar Nerve Problems Due to Proximal Injury Site: Muscle Testing*

C8- and T1-innervated muscles	
Triceps	Radial nerve†
Extensor digitorum	Radial nerve
Extensor carpi ulnaris	Radial nerve
Extensor pollicis longus, brevis	Radial nerve
Flexor carpi ulnaris	Ulnar nerve
Flexor digitorum profundus (digits 4,5)	Ulnar nerve
Flexor digitorum profundus (digits 2,3)	Median nerve
Flexor pollicis longus	Median nerve
Intrinsic muscles of the hand	Ulnar and median nerves
Lower trunk-innervated muscles	
Triceps	Radial nerve†
Extensor digitorum	Radial nerve
Extensor carpi ulnaris	Radial nerve
Flexor carpi ulnaris	Ulnar nerve
Flexor digitorum profundus (digits 4,5)	Ulnar nerve
Flexor digitorum profundus (digits 2,3)	Median nerve
Flexor pollicis longus	Median nerve
Intrinsic muscles of the hand	Ulnar and median nerves
Medial cord-innervated muscles	
Flexor carpi ulnaris	Ulnar nerve
Flexor digitorum profundus (digits 4,5)	Ulnar nerve
Flexor digitorum profundus (digits 2,3)	Median nerve
Flexor pollicis longus	Median nerve
Intrinsic muscles of the hand	Ulnar and median nerves

*Reprinted with permission from Stewart.[82]

†These radial-innervated muscles are largely supplied by C6 and C7, but often have a significant C8 (though not T1) contribution.

that in the passage through the cubital tunnel, the main ulnar nerve, itself, becomes the recipient of the pressure and this fascicle, which has already separated from the ulnar nerve proper, is relatively shielded, its function preserved. Determining the location of the ulnar nerve compression presents a considerable diagnostic problem. Other problems in the differential diagnosis may arise from ulnar nerve dysfunction due to the presence of a hereditary neuropathy. This problem may mimic pressure palsy[86] or neural tumors.[87,88] The presence of such a hereditary neuropathy or a neural tumor will become evident when the surgical exploration is carried out at the site of the entrapment. In the hereditary neuropathies there is usually a hypertrophic type of neuropathy and the nerve may appear much larger than normal. The presence of a neural tumor will be obvious as a space-occupying mass within the site of the compression.

Arthritis can also be a problem in the differential diagnosis. Arthritis between the pisiform and triquetrum,[89,90] so-called pisotriquetrial arthritis, can cause pain and inflammation and calcification in the region of the ulnar nerve at the wrist. Attempts at placing lidocaine and cortisone in an attempt to treat arthritis may also decrease inflammation and swelling about the nerve. In a similar fashion, diagnostic nerve block at the level of the ulnar nerve at the wrist in an attempt to impute the problem to a nerve injury may anesthetize the pisotriquetrial joint covering up this arthritis as the source of the pain, rather than ulnar nerve compression. The two problems may coexist. The pisotriquetrial ar-

Table 8-2. Variations in Signs and Symptoms of Ulnar Nerve Injury Related to Injury Site*

	Sensory		*Motor*				
					Intrinsics†		
Injury Site	*Dorsal hand*	*Little & Ring Finger*	*Wrist Flexor*	*Profundus V*	*ADM FDM ODM*	*IDI and others*	*APB OPB*
Syrinx‡					X	X	X
Above elbow	X	X	X	X	X	X	
Elbow	X	X	±	X	X	X	
Forearm, distal third		X			X	X	
At pisiform		X			X	X	
Pistohamate hiatus,							
Deep					X	X	
Superficial		X					
At hamate						X	

*Normal anatomy assumed.

†ADM: abductor digiti minimi; APB: abductor pollicis brevis; FDM: flexor digiti minimi; IDI: complete ODM: opponens digiti minimi; OPB: opponens pollicis brevis.

‡For differential diagnosis of other proximal injury site, see Table 8-1.

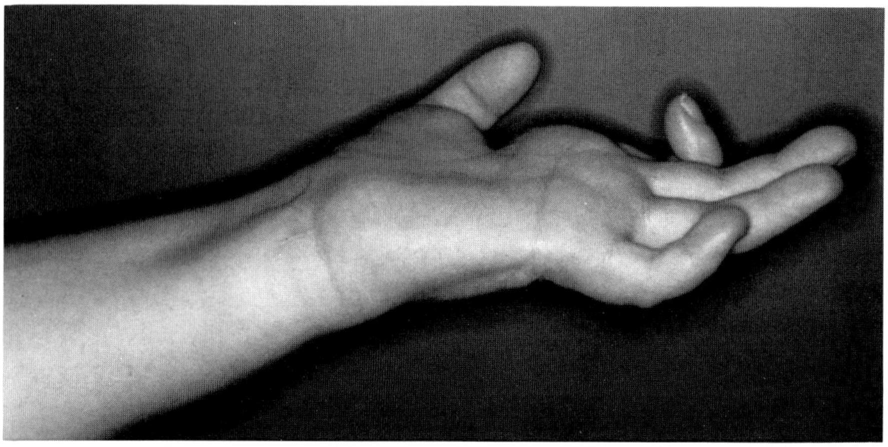

Figure 8-12. Appearance of the hand in a patient with a syrinx of the cervical cord. All intrinsic muscles have wasted. The differential diagnoses include anterior horn cell disease, such as amyotrophic lateral sclerosis (ALS) or poliomyelitis, but with a syrinx there is a unique sensory loss due to compression of the anterior spinothalmic tract: loss of pain, hot and cold perception with preservation of touch perception.

thritis may be determined by wrist extension, which causes pain, resisted wrist flexion, which causes pain, and pressure of the pisiform against the underlying triquetrum, which causes pain, none of which is present with ulnar nerve compression at the wrist level (Fig. 8-13).

Once it has been determined that the problem resulting from ulnar nerve dysfunction is due to ulnar nerve compression at the level of the wrist, further differential diagnosis in terms of what the cause may be relates to what type of anomalous structures or tumors may be producing the distribution of symptoms. To a large extent, this problem has been dealt with in the introductory "Historical" section and in the "Surgical Anatomy" section. The best differential diagnosis of this problem, however, is that given by Gross and Gelberman.[5] Reviewing a total of 142 cases in the English literature, they grouped these according to their zone (1, 2, or 3) classification. Combinations of motor and sensory deficit together occurred virtually exclusively in zone 1, which is before the division of the ulnar nerve into its motor and sensory branches. Motor symptoms alone as the presentation occurred, virtually exclusively, in zone 2, which relates to the deep terminal branch of the ulnar nerve. Pure sensory symptoms, of the 17 cases they found, occurred in 10 of the 17 in zone 3, which is the superficial sensory branch, whereas 7 of the 17 occurred with lesions that compressed the ulnar nerve in zone 1. The leading causes for the compression in these zones are listed in Table 8-3, in which it can be seen that the majority of the problems that resulted in combined motor and sensory loss were due to ganglions arising proximally in the carpus, fractures about the distal radial-ulnar joint, followed by anomalous muscles. The most common cause of the pure motor problems arising in zone 2 were ganglion, followed by carpal fractures, whereas the most common cause of pure sensory deficits occurring in zone 3 were vascular problems in the superficial arch or end of the ulnar artery.[5]

One of the most common diagnostic problems the surgeon must face in this area is whether to decompress the ulnar nerve at the wrist level when median nerve decompression surgery is being carried out for the carpal tunnel syndrome. The usual situation involves the patient with symptoms that are clearly related to carpal tunnel syndrome, such as numbness in the middle and ring fingers or thumb and index finger with nocturnal awakening. The patient may say that his "whole hand" goes to sleep at times or the "whole hand is dead" when he awakens at night. The patient must be carefully questioned as to whether, in fact, he is aware that the little finger truly has sensory abnormalities. If the patient is quite clear that the little finger is involved, it is incumbent on the physician to rule out coexisting ulnar nerve compression at the wrist or, what is more common, ulnar nerve compression at the level of the elbow. In this situation, pinch strength and grip strength loss suggest problems at the level of the elbow. If the ulnar nerve is not tender at the elbow, and if dorsal ulnar sensation in the hand is relatively preserved, then ulnar nerve compression at the wrist must be seriously entertained in the diagnosis. The most common cause of this problem in patients that we have seen is from motor vehicle accidents. The patient is driving, the hands are on the wheel, the automobile is struck from the back,

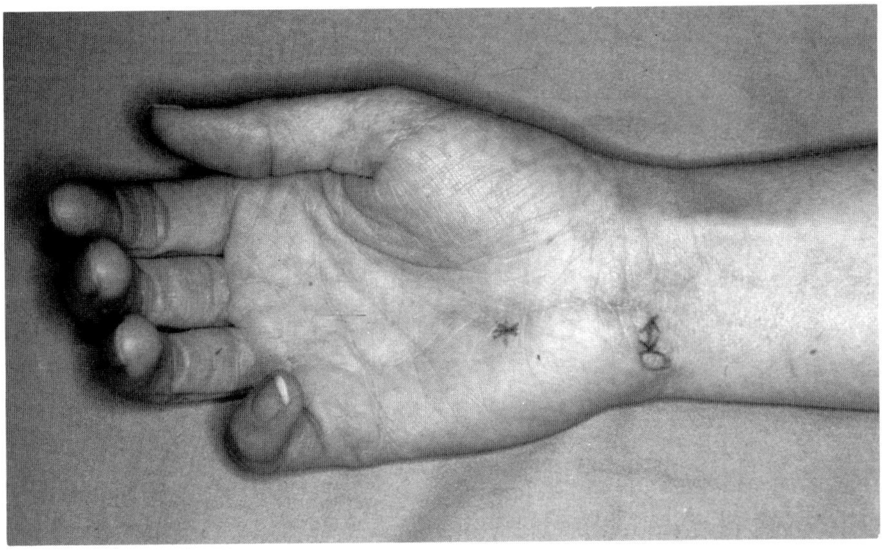

Figure 8-13. Diagnostic pitfall: Pisotriquetrial arthritis. The close proximity of the pisiform (circle) to the ulnar nerve may associate pain of pisotriquetrial arthritis and ulnar nerve compression. Also, as in this patient, pisiform excision can create sufficient scarring that requires subsequent ulnar neurolysis.

as described in the preceding section, giving rise to problems with the ulnar nerve at this level. There is usually a positive Tinel's sign over the ulnar nerve at the level of the pisiform. A positive pressure provocative test can be elicited (pressure just proximal to Guyon's canal produces numbness in the little finger and ulnar aspect of the ring finger). Electrodiagnostic testing may be helpful. It must be recalled, however, that observations have been made of approximately a 30% incidence of abnormal distal ulnar sensory latency when electrodiagnostic studies are done for median nerve compression at the wrist and the ulnar nerve is simultaneously tested.[91] It is possible that there may be some type of crossover or common connection between sensory fibers in the C7 or C8 root level or dorsal root ganglion that direct fibers in both the median nerve and ulnar nerve, so that compression in the carpal tunnel may cause simultaneous symptoms in the little finger. Such mechanisms are amenable to experimental tracing with multiple tracer studies.[92] Many surgeons have practiced decompression of Guyon's canal at the same time as they do a carpal tunnel release[93] (Fig. 8-14). From 1980 through 1985, we did this on a routine basis. Influenced by a report by Gelberman[94] and because a few patients complained of pain occurring in the cutaneous area of the hypothenar eminence related to this release and because it was not clear that adding this release improved results, we presently only decompress the ulnar nerve simultaneously with carpal tunnel release in those patients with abnormal sensation in the little finger. This problem has been studied thoroughly by Gelberman's group.[94] They identified 20 of 59 hands in patients having carpal tunnel syndrome as having concomitant abnormalities in ulnar nerve function. This was demon-

Table 8-3. Common Causes of Compression Neuropathy by Zone and Deficit*

	Zone (Deficit)†					
Cause	*1 (M/S)*	*1 (M)*	*1 (S)*	*2 (M)*	*3 (S)*	*Total*
Ganglia	19	1	1	21		42
Fractures	13			5	1	19
Anomalous muscles	3		1	1	2	7
Thrombosis			1		5	6
Bursitis			4			4
Thickened pisohamate ligament				3		3
Others	4			6	2	12
Total	47 (total Zone 1)			36	10	93

*Reprinted with permission from Gross and Gelberman.[5]

†M/S: both motor and sensory deficits; M = motor deficit only; S = sensory deficit only.

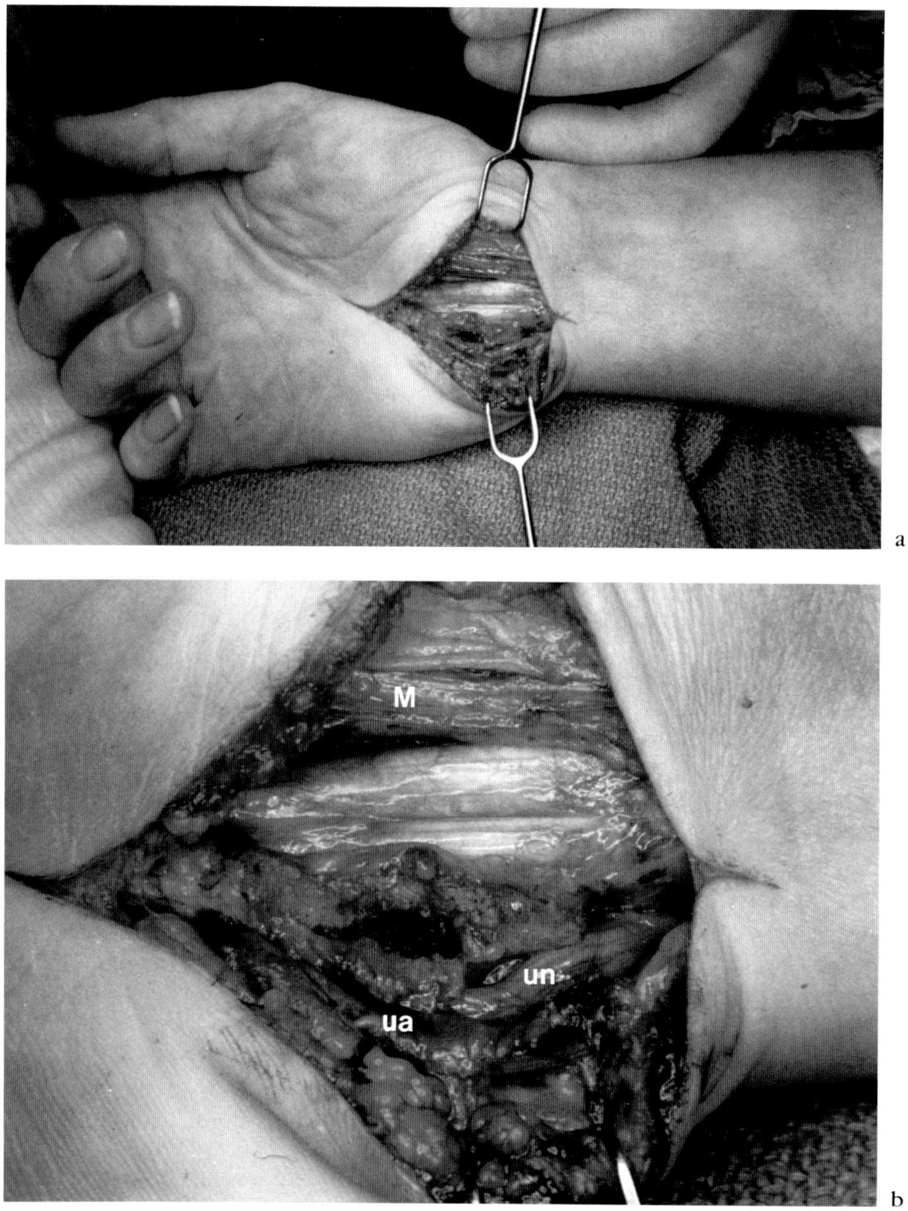

Figure 8-14. Example of decompression of ulnar nerve at the wrist when there is concomitant median nerve compression at the wrist and ulnar nerve compression at the elbow. Since it is possible that a multiple crush problem exists with respect to the ulnar nerve, when the median nerve is released at the wrist **(a)**, the ulnar nerve is simultaneously routinely decompressed also. **b.** The appearance of the decompressed ulnar nerve (un), the ulnar artery (ua) and veins adjacent, and the median nerve (M). Two separate incisions at the wrist are not necessary.

strated by either two-point discrimination, cutaneous pressure threshold testing, or both. Fifty-three percent of this group complained of paresthesia or numbness in the ulnar nerve distribution. One percent of the patients had abnormal electromyographic testing of the ulnar nerve. Patients were treated, however, with just median nerve decompression, and Guyon's canal was not released. After surgery, 89% of the patients had improvement in paresthesias or numbness, or both, in the ulnar nerve distribution, with 94% having improvement in their abnormal cutaneous pressure thresholds and 86% having improvement in their two-point discrimination. The mechanism for patients having ulnar nerve symptoms when their problem is median nerve compression at the wrist remains obscure. Routine decompression of the ulnar nerve at the time of median nerve decompression is not recommended.

Surgical Technique

To approach ulnar nerve entrapment at the wrist, the patient is placed under satisfactory anesthesia, either general or, most commonly, brachial block, in the supine position with a pneumatic tourniquet placed about the upper extremity over a soft roll. After preparing the arm, the hand is elevated and draped appropriately. The hand is elevated, exsanguinated with an elastic bandage, and the tourniquet inflated to an appropriate pressure. The incision as recommended by Taleisnik[95] is utilized and is essentially 6 to 7 mm to the ulnar side of the thenar crease, which is in essence in the radial axis of the ring finger. This incision splits the boundary between the palmar cutaneous branch of the median nerve and the ulnar innervation to the hypothenar area. The incision continues with a zigzag at the wrist and a proximal extension can be made if needed. Going through the subcutaneous tissue, hemostasis is obtained with the bipolar coagulator. In those patients with a palmaris brevis muscle, the origin of this is divided and coagulated. The incision then approaches the palmar carpal ligament. This ligament is generally a formation of interdigitating fibers, some coming from the transverse carpal ligament, some coming from the palmaris longus and inserting toward the pisiform and the fascia of the abductor digiti minimi muscle. The surgical approach can begin either distal or proximal. When the operation is not done in conjunction with a transverse carpal ligament division, then the approach is often easiest starting distally. When the subcutaneous tissue distal to the palmar carpal ligament is identified, the approach is just to the ulnar side of the slip of the palmarar fascia that goes to the little finger. In this region, the superficial palmar arch may be seen, and, utilizing the superficial palmar arch as a guide, the scissors are placed bluntly going proximally along the course of this vessel. By gentle spreading in this fatty tissue and lifting upward, the interdigitating fibers described are identified and divided, taking their course toward the pisiform. No structures from either the ulnar artery or ulnar nerve generally cross this area. Having said that, occasional small nerve twigs in the situation where the palmar cutaneous branch of the ulnar nerve has traveled with the ulnar nerve may be present and if divided, may give rise later to subsequent pain in this hypothenar region. This dissection is continued toward the pisiform, revealing the ulnar artery and accompanying two veins. Coming back toward the pisiform, at this point, almost always, a fascial structure is encountered. It either comes from the palmaris longus toward the pisiform or goes from the pisiform to the transverse carpal ligament, but in either case or if both are present, it represents a remaining structure to be divided that bridges the ulnar nerve in the pisohamate hiatus from the ulnar nerve in the distal forearm. A vein may accompany this structure, and this, indeed, may be a segmental vascular supply to the median nerve from the ulnar artery. If this is present and divided, it is coagulated with the bipolar coagulator. This decompresses the ulnar nerve from the wrist to the superficial palmar arch.

Furthermore, neurolysis of the ulnar nerve may now be undertaken. The ulnar artery and its accompanying veins are retracted radially or toward the ulnar side of the hand. This will take with it the associated sensory branches of the ulnar nerve, which are superficial to the motor terminal branch at this point. Looking on the radial side of this group of structures, the origin of the flexor digiti minimi, the hypothenar muscle originating from the hamate superficially, is identified as already described. Palpation of the hook of the hamate is a maneuver that reliably aides identification of this arch. There may be a fibrous edge to the proximal edge of this arch (Fig. 8-5). When present as a fibrous edge, this edge is divided, the motor fibers gently spread and the motor nerve followed down beneath this arch as it goes through its tunnel distal to the hamate.

Utilizing loope magnification, the sensory branches and the motor branches may now be further identified and, if necessary, the epineurium opened and an internal neurolysis carried out.

During the exploration, as already described, ganglia, if they are present, are identified and excised. Lipomas or other tumors, if present, are identified and excised. A nonunion of a fractured hook of the hamate may be subperiosteally excised and any anomalous muscles or tendinous structures may be excised.

This, then, completes the surgical treatment of ulnar nerve entrapment at the wrist level. If the median nerve is to be released simultaneously, it usually is done first, as described in Chapter 6, and then the ulnar nerve decompressed, although the choice as to which nerve is released first can simply be left to the surgeon as a matter of preference. We will frequently decompress the median nerve at the time of release of the ulnar nerve at the wrist because of the simplicity of this operation, the high frequency of carpal tunnel syndrome, and the potential inducement of carpal tunnel syndrome with postoperative hand swelling. If the surgeon plans to release the carpal tunnel as well as Guyon's canal, a very simple maneuver is to carry out a standard carpal tunnel release: identify the superficial arch and then follow the arch proximally into Guyon's canal. Of course, two separate incisions to decompress these two nerves at the wrist are never required.

The wound is closed with interrupted and continuous sutures of 5-0 nylon. The dressing is a well-padded hard dressing with a soft roll and a volar plaster splint holding the wrist in a neutral position, held in place with kling paper tape stockinette and an Ace wrap. The tourniquet then is let down and circulation observed in the fingers.

Postoperative Care

During the postoperative period, the patient may wear a sling for the first 3 days. He is encouraged to move his fingers. The dressing is removed on the eighth day after surgery and the sutures are removed if this is appropriate with regard to any other medical or wound-healing problems. The patient is instructed to utilize the hand as needed, stopping whenever swelling or aching discomfort occurs in the palm. Usually by approximately 3 to 6 weeks, the scar is somewhat thickened and pink and a cortisone cream is prescribed to be massaged into the wound twice daily.

Complications

The complications from ulnar nerve decompression at the wrist have not been described in the literature. Our experience has been, most commonly, of some tenderness within the hypothenar eminence, some hypertrophy or tenderness of the scar, itself. We have had no other complications after ulnar nerve decompression at the wrist level.

Results

The results of ulnar nerve repair at the wrist level and more proximally have been reviewed[96] (Table 8-4).

Table 8-4. Summary of Results

	No. in Group	*Degree of Recovery (%)*			
		M4	*M5*	*S3+*	*S4*
Ulnar					
Low repair					
War injury	1098	40	0	15	0
Civilian injury*	466	32	0	34	0.7
Children	33	55	12	24	70
High repair					
War injury	393	23	6	0	0
Civilian injury	196	17	0	20	0
Graft					
Civilian injury	56	20	23	14	7

*Group included 49 children.

The results of ulnar nerve decompression at the wrist have not been previously reviewed. From a review of the literatuare,[22–26] it may be determined that of the 43 reported cases, all but two improved. One of these patients had severe wasting, the other was not described as to his preoperative condition. Thirty-seven (86%) had excellent results after decompression of the ulnar nerve in Guyon's canal. Four (9%) had good results.

Discussion

To be inclusive, the dorsal ulnar branch does cross the wrist level and may be entrapped at this point. For example, Stopford[97] described it as being compressed by a wristwatch, much as the radial sensory nerve can be compressed by a wristwatch or handcuff (Chapter 10). In fact, although most series of cases of entrapment of the dorsal ulnar branch have been reported, treatment of this problem has been one of the most difficult for us. We have seen five patients with this problem. The nerve has been injured by a crush-type injury to the dorsal ulnar surface of the hand and, in general, has been associated with tendinitis in the sixth dorsal extensor compartment. Management by nonoperative techniques, such as splinting and cortisone injection, have not been successful. Release of the sixth dorsal extensor compartment and neurolysis of the dorsal branch of the ulnar nerve has given only fair results, with three of the patients requiring wearing of a permanent leather wrist gauntlet in order to enable them to return to work. One of the patients, whose nerves were significantly injured initially, developed a neuroma that required resection and implantation proximally into the muscle belly of the flexor carpi ulnaris.

References

1. Guyon F: Note sur une disposition anatomique propre a la face anterieure de la region du poignet et non encore decrite par le docteur. Bull Soc Anat Paris 6:184–186, 1861.
2. Grantham SA: Ulnar compression in the loge de Guyon. JAMA 197:229–230, 1966.
3. Boyes JH: On The Shoulder of Giants: Notable Names in Hand Surgery. JB Lippincott, Philadelphia, 1976, pp 103–105.
4. McFarlane RM, Mayer JR, Hugill JV: Further observations on the anatomy of the ulnar nerve at the wrist. Hand 8:115, 1976.
5. Gross MS, Gelberman RH: Anatomy of the distal ulnar tunnel. Clin Orthop 196:238–247, 1985.
6. Hunt JR: Occupational neuritis of the deep palmar branch of the ulnar nerve. J Nerv Ment Dis 35:676–689, 1908.

7. Hunt JR: Thenar and hypothenar types of neural atrophy of the hand. Am J Med Sci 141:224, 1911.
8. Hunt JR: Neural atrophy of the muscles of the hand without sensory disturbances. Rev Neurol Psychiatr 12:137, 1914.
9. Hunt JR: Thenar and hypothenar types of neural atrophy of the hand. Br Med J 2:642, 1930.
10. Middleton DS: Occupational aneurysms of palmar arteries. Br J Surg 21:215–218, 1933.
11. Barker NW, Hines ES Jr: Arterial occlusion in the hands and fingers associated with occupational trauma. Proc Staff Meet Mayo Clinic 19:345–349, 1944.
12. Costigan DG, Riley JM, Coy FE: Thrombofibrosis of the ulnar artery in the palm. J Bone Joint Surg 41A:702–704, 1959.
13. Smith JW: True aneurysms of traumatic origin in the palm. Am J Surg 104:7–13. 1962.
14. Kleinert HE, Boliantis GJ: Thrombosis of the palmar arterial arch and its tributaries: Etiology and newer concepts in treatment. Trauma 5:447–457, 1965.
15. Milling MAP, Kinmonth MH: False aneurysm of the ulnar artery. Hand 9:57–59, 1977.
16. Kalisman M, Laborde K, Wolff TW: Ulnar nerve compression secondary to ulnar artery false aneurysm at the Guyon's canal. J Hand Surg 7:137–139, 1982.
17. Ho PK, Dellon AL, Wilgis EFS: True aneurysms of the hand resulting from athletic injury: Report of two cases. Am J Sports Med 13:136–138, 1985.
18. Hayes JR, Mulholland RC, O'Connor BT: Compression of the deep palmar branch of the ulnar nerve. J Bone Joint Surg 51B:469–472, 1969.
19. Jackson JP: Traumatic thrombosis of the ulnar artery in the palm. J Bone Joint Surg 36B:438, 1954.
20. Teece LG: Thrombosis of the ulnar artery. Aust NZ J Surg 19:156–157, 1949.
21. Bakke JL, Wolff HG: Occupational pressure neuritis of the deep palmar branch of the ulnar nerve. Arch Neurol Psychiatry 60:549–555, 1948.
22. Blunder R: Neuritis of the deep branch of the ulnar nerve. (Abstr.) J Bone Joint Surg 40B:354, 1958.
23. Dupont C, Cloutier GE, Prevost Y, Dion MA: Ulnar-tunnel syndrome at the wrist. J Bone Joint Surg 47A:757–761, 1965.
24. Hart UL: Two unusual injuries of the wrist. J Bone Joint Surg 23:948–949, 1941.
25. Kleinert HE, Hayes JE: Ulnar tunnel syndrome. Plast Reconstr Surg 47:21–24, 1971.
26. Lamb D: Ulnar nerve compression lesions at the wrist and hand. Hand 2:17–18, 1970.
27. Nicolle FV, Woolhouse FM: Nerve compression syndromes of the upper limb. J Trauma 5:313–318, 1965.
28. Stern PJ, Vice M: Compression of the deep branch of the ulnar nerve—a case report. J Hand Surg 8:72–74, 1983.
29. Brooks DM: Nerve compression by simple ganglia. J Bone Joint Surg 34B:391–400, 1952.
30. Seddon HJ: Carpal ganglion as a cause of paralysis of the deep branch of the ulnar nerve. J Bone Joint Surg 34B:386–390, 1952.
31. Ebeling P, Gilliatt RW, Thomas DK: A clinical and electrical study of ulnar nerve lesions in the hand. J Neurol Neurosurg Psychiatry 23:1–9, 1960.
32. Vanderpool DW, Chalmers J, Whiston TB: Peripheral compression lesions of the ulnar nerve. J Bone Joint Surg 50B:792–802, 1968.
33. Uriburu IJF, Marchio FJ, Marin JC: Compression syndrome of the deep motor branch of the ulnar nerve. J Bone Joint Surg 58A:145–147, 1976.
34. Mallet BL, Zilkha KJ: Compression of the ulnar nerve at the wrist by the ganglion. Lancet 1:890, 1955.
35. Richmond DA: Carpal ganglion with ulnar nerve compression. J Bone Joint Surg 45B:513, 1963.
36. Tashima Y, Kimata Y: A case of ganglion causing paralysis of intrinsic muscles innervated by the ulnar nerve. J Bone Joint Surg 43B:153, 1961.
37. Zahrawi F: Acute compression ulnar neuropathy at Guyon's canal resulting from lipoma. J Hand Surg 9A:238–240, 1984.
38. White WL, Hauna DC: Troublesome lipomata of the upper extremity. J Bone Joint Surg 44A:1353, 1962.
39. Rengachary SS, Arjunan K: Compression of the ulnar nerve at Guyon's canal by soft tissue giant cell tumor. Neurosurgery 8:400–405, 1981.
40. Dell PC: Compression of the ulnar nerve at the wrist secondary to rheumatoid synovial cyst: Case report and review of literature. J Hand Surg 4:468–473, 1979.
41. Conn J Jr, Bergan JJ, Bell JL: Hypothenar hammer syndrome: post-traumatic digital ischemia. Surgery 68:1122–1128, 1970.
42. Corradi M, Mandrioli R, Rinaldi E, Ugolotti U: La sindrome dell "uncinato. Riv Chir Mano 20:445–449, 1983.
43. Howard FM: Ulnar nerve palsy in wrist fractures. J Bone Joint Surg 43A:1197, 1961.
44. Baird DB, Fredenberg ZB: Delayed ulnar nerve palsy following a fracture of the hamate. J Bone Joint Surg 50A:570, 1968.
45. Shea JD, McClain EJ: Ulnar nerve compression syndromes at and below the wrist. J Bone Joint Surg 51A:1095–1103, 1969.
46. Nisenfield FG, Neviaser RJ: Fracture of the hook of the hamate: A diagnosis easily missed. J Trauma 14:612, 1974.
47. Foucher G, Schuind F, Merle M, Brunelli F: Fractures of the hook of the hamate. J Hand Surg [Br] 10:205–210, 1985.
48. Zoega H: Fracture of the lower end of the radius with ulnar nerve palsy. J Bone Joint Surg 48B:514–516, 1966.
49. Vance RM, Gelberman RH: Acute ulnar neuropathy with fractures at the wrist. J Bone Joint Surg 60A:692--695, 1978.
50. Kornberg M, Aulicino PL, Dupuy TE: Laceration of the ulnar nerve with a closed fracture of the distal radius and ulna. Orthopedics 6:729–731, 1983.
51. McCarroll HR: Nerve injuries associated with wrist trauma. Orthop Clin North Am 15:279–287, 1984.
52. Watson-Jones R: Carpal semilunar dislocations and other wrist dislocations with associated nerve lesions. Proc R Soc Med 22:1071, 1929.
53. Dunn WA: Fractures and dislocations of the carpus. Surg Clin North Am 52:1513, 1972.

54. Greene MH, Hadied AM: Bipartite hamulus with ulnar tunnel syndrome—case report and literature review. J Hand Surg 6:605, 1981.
55. Destot M: Paralysie cebritale par l'usage de la bicyclette. Gaz Anaphitaux 69:1176–1177, 1896.
56. Eckman PB, Pearlstein G, Altorcchi PH: Ulnar neuropathy in bicycle riders. Arch Neurol 32:130–131, 1975.
57. Hoyt CS: Ulnar neuropathy in bicycle riders. Arch Neurol 33:372, 1976.
58. Dellon AL: Unpublished observations, 1987.
59. Stewart HD, Innes AR, Burke FD: The hand complications of Colles' fractures. J Hand Surg [Br] 10:103–106, 1985.
60. Frank DH, Robson MD: Unusual occurrence of chronic nerve compression syndromes at the wrists of thermally injured patients. Orthop Rev 8:180, 1979.
61. Dellon AL, Mackinnon SE: Anatomic investigations of nerves at the wrist: II. Instance of fibrous arch overlying the motor branch of the ulnar nerve. Ann Plast Surg 21:36, 1988.
62. Spinner M, Freundlich BD: An important variation of the palmaris longus. Bull Hosp Joint Dis 28:126–130, 1967.
63. Thomas CG: Clinical manifestations of an accessory palmaris muscle. J Bone Joint Surg 40A:929–930, 1958.
64. Schjelderup H: Aberrant muscle in the hand causing ulnar nerve compression. (Abstr.) J Bone Joint Surg 46B:361, 1964.
65. Swanson AB, Biddulph SL, Boughman FA, DeGroot G: Ulnar nerve compression due to an anomalous muscle in the canal of Guyon. Clin Orthop 83:64, 1972.
66. Gloobe H, Picket P: An anomalous muscle in the canal of Guyon. Anat Anz 133:477, 1973.
67. Turner MS, Caird DM: Anomalous muscles in ulnar nerve compression at the wrist. Hand 9:140–142, 1977.
68. King TS, Orahilly RM: Palmaris accessorius and duplication of the M. palmaris longus. Acta Anat [Suppl] 10:327–331, 1950.
69. Jeffrey AK: Compression of the deep palmar branch of the ulnar nerve by an anomalous muscle. J Bone Joint Surg 53B:718, 1971.
70. Fahrer M, Millroy P J: Ulnar compression neuropathy due to an anomalous abductor digiti minimi: Clinical and anatomic study. J Hand Surg 6:266, 1981.
71. Lipscomb PR: Duplication of hypothenar muscles simulating soft tissue tumor of the hand. J Bone Joint Surg 42A:1058–1060, 1960.
72. Wood J: On some varieties in human myologies. Proc R Soc Lond 13:299–303, 1864.
73. Fennay JB: Deep ulnar nerve paralysis resulting from an anatomical abnormality. J Bone Joint Surg 47A:1381, 1965.
74. Lenz U: Lahmung des Tiefen Hohlhandastes des Nervus Ulnaris, bedingt durch eine Anatomsche Variante. Handchirurgia 6:83–86, 1974.
75. Lass R, Shrewsbury MM: Variation in the path of the deep motor branch of the ulnar nerve at the wrist. J Bone Joint Surg 57A:990–991, 1975.
76. Riche P: Le nerf cubital et les muscles de l'eminence thenar. Bull Mem Soc Anat Paris 5:251–252, 1897.
77. Cannieu JMA: Recherches sur une anastomse. Entra la branche profnude du cubitale et le median. Bull Soc Anat Physiol Bordeaux 18:339–340, 1897.
78. May JW, Rosen H: Division of sensory ramus communicans between the ulnar and median nerves: A complication following carpal tunnel release: Case report. J Bone Joint Surg 63A:836–838, 1981.
79. Kaplan EB: Variation of the ulnar nerve at the wrist. Bull Hosp Joint Dis 24:85–88, 1963.
80. Learmonth JR: A variation in the distribution of the radial branch of the musculospiral nerve. J Anat 53:371–372, 1919.
81. Spinner M: Injuries to the Major Branches of the Peripheral Nerves of the Forearm. WB Saunders, Philadelph'a, 1978, pp 245–252.
82. Stewart JD: Focal Periphera Neuropathies. Elsevier, New York, 1987.
83. Liveson JA, Renschoff J, Goodgold J: Electromyographic studies in the case of foramen magnum meningioma. J Neurol Neurosurg Psychiatry 36:561–564, 1973.
84. Osborne G: Surgical treatment of tardy ulnar neuritis. J Bone Joint Surg 39B:782, 1957.
85. Feindel W, Stratford J: Role of the cubital tunnel in tardy ulnar palsy. J Surg 1:296–298, 1958.
86. Earl CJ, Fullerton PM, Wakefield GS, Shutta HD: Hereditary neuropathy with liability to pressure palsies. Q J Med 33:41–98, 1964.
87. Jenkins SA: Solitary tumors of peripheral nerve trunks. J Bone Joint Surg 34B:401–411, 1952.
88. White NB: Neurilemomas of the extremities. J Bone Joint Surg 49A:1605–1610, 1967.
89. Phalen GS: Calcification adjacent to the pisiform bone. J Bone Joint Surg 34A:579–580, 1952.
90. Jenkins SA: Osteoarthritis of the pisiform-triquetral joint. J Bone Joint Surg 33B:532–534, 1957.
91. Sedal L, McLeod JG, Walsh JC: Ulnar nerve lesions associated with the carpal tunnel syndrome. J Neurol Neurosurg Psychiatry 36:118–123, 1973.
92. Brushart T: Personal communication.
93. Goldner JL, Dellon AL: Personal communication.
94. Silver MA, Gelberman RH, Gellman H, Rhoades CE: Carpal tunnel syndrome: Associated abnormalities in ulnar nerve function and the effect of carpal tunnel release on these abnormalities. J Hand Surg [Am] 10:710–713, 1985.
95. Taleisnik J: The palmar cutaneous branch of the median nerve and the approach to the carpal tunnel. An anatomic study. J Bone Joint Surg 55A:1212–1217, 1973.
96. Dellon AL: Evaluation of Sensibility and Re-education of Sensation in the Hand. Williams & Wilkins, Baltimore, 1981, chapter 11.
97. Stopford JSB: Neuritis produced by a wristlet watch. Lancet 1:993–994, 1922.

9 Ulnar Nerve Entrapment at the Elbow

Historical Review

The careful study of the subject of ulnar nerve-compression at the elbow is both interesting and frustrating. Despite more than 100 years of clinical experience in the diagnosis and treatment of this nerve compression, the present-day student remains without a firm data base for scientific decision analysis in terms of patient treatment. Despite more than 50 separate reports of series of patients treated for ulnar nerve compression at the elbow, there remains only personal bias for choosing one surgical technique over another. The current status of surgical training remains the one in which the student learns the technique most utilized by his teacher. The teachers, themselves, have frequently changed techniques even in the latter stages of their professional careers, based on their last complication or personal dissatisfaction. From the time when surgeons believed that virtually cvcry case of ulnar nerve compression at the elbow should be operated on, because there appeared to be no instances of spontaneous recovery, we see recently the development of a tendency toward surgical nihilism, and the recommended treatment is to place the arm with the entrapped nerve into a splint.[1] From statements such as: "In no case is the operation futile,"[2] we have witnessed reports of ulnar nerve surgery in which 14 of 38 reported cases are reoperations for previous failures,[3] and of a surgeon's personal series of 500 ulnar nerve compressions at the elbow, 200 were for recurrent ulnar nerve problems.[4] Over the last decade, however, basic anatomic and physiologic studies have done much to help us understand the pathophysiologic mechanisms involved with ulnar nerve compression at the elbow. As will be seen later from the information, this provides a basis for evolving a rational plan of operative and nonoperative treatment. The quagmire of surgical end-result reporting is due to the lack of a classification scheme that permits preoperative staging of the ulnar nerve compression, as well as a lack of accurate preoperative and postoperative recordings by the surgeons that would permit critical evaluation of the results of surgery on both motor and sensory ulnar nerve functions. In the review that follows, the disparate elements in the history of treatment for ulnar nerve compression at the elbow are placed in perspective, and the basis is provided to permit science to guide the care of these patients in the future.

What's in a Name?

In 1878, Panas[5] reported on three patients whose presenting problems were related to ulnar compression at the elbow. The causes of his patients' problems included previous fracture at the elbow with late (12½ years) development of ulnar nerve compression, hypertrophic osteoarthritic spurring at the elbow joint, and a bony irregularity in the postcondylar groove. Subsequent reports by Broca and Mouchet[6] in 1899 and Mouchet in 1914 emphasized the role of trauma and, in particular, fractures of the lateral humeral epicondyle. These fractures can heal with angulation at the elbow joint and the development of cubitus valgus. This deformity was viewed as causing stretching and friction of the ulnar nerve, leading to its compression in the postcondylar groove. Because of the role of trauma and because of the variable, often delayed, appearance of the nerve compression with respect to the date of the trauma, the clinical syndrome was called "post-traumatic ulnar neuritis" or "tardy ulnar palsy." In 1926 and 1928, the name for the syndrome was further elucidated and complicated by Platt,[8,9] who correctly reported that, although the lateral humeral epicondyle was fractured, the mechanism of injury concerned a downward and outward stretch of the ulnar nerve and that similar ulnar nerve compression could be caused by supracondylar humeral fractures, as well as fractures through the medial humeral epicondyle. The distinctions were made between the nerve injury appearing immediately at the time of fracture (primary post-traumatic ulnar neuritis) or the appearance of the symptoms within a few weeks after the fracture (secondary post-traumatic ulnar neuritis) or the appearance of the symptoms many years later (tardy ulnar neuritis or tardy ulnar palsy). The early reported series of cases of ulnar nerve compression at the elbow contained a very high percentage of cases in which the cause involved trauma of some type. Yet there was always a small percentage of cases for which no explanation could be determined, and these cases were called "idiopathic ulnar neuritis" or "idiopathic ulnar nerve compression" at the elbow (Table 9-1).

The name for the clinical syndrome reflected, then, the major cause of the problem, that is, trauma. As often happens, what we call something either reflects or determines, or both, the way we think about and treat the subject. With post-traumatic ulnar neuritis and tardy ulnar palsy, the surgical attempts were early directed at freeing the ulnar nerve from scar tissue in the postcondylar groove, altering the angle of the forearm with respect to the humerus, and transposing the ulnar nerve away from the site of trauma. Panas[5] directly explored the ulnar nerve in one of his patients. Unfortunately, this patient died of sepsis. Attempts were made by other surgeons to deepen the postcondylar groove by surgically gouging the medial humeral epicondyle and the olecranon. The first report of anterior transposition of the ulnar nerve has been reported to have been described by Roux of Lausanne in 1897.[8,10] Apparently, this first subcutaneous transposition met without success. Sunderland,[11] who has written one of the best accounts of the history of the operative treatment of ulnar nerve compression at the elbow, has indicated that Broca, in 1903, Savariaud, in 1903, and Mouchet, in 1914, all objected theoretically to the concept of transposing the ulnar nerve to such an exposed external position. They also observed that the ulnar nerve would still be stretched across the elbow when the elbow was in complete extension. Mouchet[7] described a supracondylar osteotomy to correct the cubitus valgus deformity without operating on the ulnar nerve itself. Subsequently, Mouchet[12] was to discard his own osteotomy in favor of anterior transposition of the ulnar nerve. The techniques to deepen the postcondylar groove were reported by Davidson and Horowitz[10] to have been carried out by Broca and Sengennse of Bordeaux, as well

Table 9-1. Changing Spectrum of Etiologies of Ulnar Nerve Compression at the Elbow

Series	*Date*	*Trauma (%)*		*Arthritis, Subluxation, Ganglion, Other (%)*	*Idiopathic (%)*	*Metabolic (%)*	*Occupational (%)*
		Fracture	*Other*				
Mouchet[7]	1914	100					
Adson[14]	1918	67			33		
Sheldon[19]	1921	50	41		9		
Richards[85]	1945	60		32			8
McGowan[25]	1950	47	5	33	15		
Vanderpool et al[31]	1968	13	25	15	45	2	
Paine[79]	1970	18	12	18	43	9	
Harrison and Nurich[91]	1970	13	17	44	26		
Payan[92]	1970	9	27	28	36		
Wilson and Krout[67]	1973	0	26		26		48
Campbell et al[87]	1974	44	23		33		
Hagstrom[95]	1977	4	32		64		
MacNichol[71]	1979	11	5	26	58		
Laha and Panchal[100]	1979	0	27	10	36	9	18

as by Guillemain of Mally. However, these techniques were discarded because it was realized that the nerves did not recover due to recurrent involvement with fibro-osseous scar formation.

Since the name for ulnar nerve entrapment at the elbow was related to trauma, which implied scarring, the early surgeons attempting to treat this problem were among the first to use the technique of neurolysis (Chapter 5). On May 3, 1898, B. Farquhar Curtis presented a patient to the New York Neurological Society. His case presentation was entitled, "Traumatic Ulnar Neuritis—Transplantation of the Nerve."[13] The 28-year-old woman had, in childhood, sustained a fracture of both condyles at the elbow. At surgery, the nerve was found to lay on an exposed surface instead of in the postcondylar groove. The nerve was found to be "thickened for a distance of about an inch and one-half and to be about twice its normal diameter. On incision through the sheath, there seemed to be a general increase of the fibrous tissue of the nerve. The nerve was split and stretched gently, and then removed from its exposed situation to a more protected part, i.e., to the front of the elbow. The result has been surprisingly satisfactory, so she has been able to resume her long hours of writing without discomfort." (The second patient that Curtis reported on at that meeting was a woman in whom he had carried out a secondary repair of the median nerve at the wrist. See Chapter 4.) Adson,[14] from the Mayo Clinic, described in 1918 what is best understood today in terms of a neurolysis. His neurolysis accompanied also an anterior transposition of the ulnar nerve, but his transposition was into an intramuscular location. Adson advised that, "The longitudinal splitting of the epineurium and perineurium in several places about the nerve [be done] in order to liberate the columns of nerve fibers from the contracting scars." Adson noted that, "The nerve in its new position causes very little trouble and the results are most gratifying in that the progressive paralysis ceases, or improves to an appreciable degree, particularly if the nerve has not been injured too severely." The clinicians had noticed that palpation of the ulnar nerve in the postcondylar groove demonstrated nodular thickenings along the course of the ulnar nerve. The early surgical explorations described these thickenings as "neuromas." The surgical approach to such a damaged nerve is predictable: excision. Earle,[15] in 1816, was the first to report operative treatment for ulnar neuritis by excising the injured segment of the ulnar nerve. This was reportedly successful in relieving the patient of severe neuralgia. Similar occurrence was reported by Calder[16] in 1833 for a patient operated on by Schott for severe ulnar neuralgia. In 1908, Sherren[17] excised the neuroma in a post-traumatic ulnar neuritis and sutured the ulnar nerve back together. Sunderland reports that Andrae had done a similar procedure to shorten and tighten a recurrent subluxing ulnar nerve in 1889.[18] Adson,[14] already described, noted that: "The treatment of the thickening of the neuroma depends largely on the amount of paralysis present. If, judging from the neurologic findings, the patient has complete or three-fourths paralysis of the ulnar nerve, complete resection of the diseased portion of the nerve with anastomosis of the severed ends is advised.... After the nerve has been transferred to its new position (intramuscular), the flexor tendon, as well as its tendinous fibers from the common flexor tendon, are sutured back to their normal position, thus making a new groove for the entrance of the ulnar nerve for covering the ulnar nerve and preventing it from going back into the postcondylar groove." The trend against resection was begun by Shelden,[19] in 1921, who cautioned that: "It is not expedient to resect a pseudoneuroma because of the additional damage which may be produced in numerous instances in which the sheath of the nerve has been split over the pseudoneuromas and where constrictions appear in the hope that this relief of tension may provide better nutritional conditions for the nerve fibers."

The latest addition to the nomenclature problem was coined by Feindel and Stratford[20] from Saskatoon. In April 1956, October 1956, and January 1957, these surgeons operated on three patients who had no previous history of trauma and who had motor and sensory findings consistent with ulnar nerve entrapment at the elbow, except for sparing of flexor carpi ulnaris function. They reported their results in 1958. As indicated in Table 9-1 there had always been a group of patients with ulnar nerve compression at the elbow who had no apparent cause for their problems, so-called idiopathic ulnar palsy. Feindel and Stratford noted a thick fibrous band running between the two heads of the flexor carpi ulnaris causing compression on the ulnar nerve as it entered between the two heads of these muscles. Geoffrey Osborne, from Liverpool, in fact, received the first credit for describing this band because the abstract of the paper he presented to the British Society for Surgery of the Hand appeared in print in 1957.[21] Osborne indicated that he had 13 patients with this problem, that they had been treated by release of the band, and the results had been "as satisfactory as in those patients who had been treated by transposition of the nerve." For the syndrome of ulnar nerve compression at the elbow with sparing of the flexor carpi ulnaris and where there is no antecedent trauma, Feindel and Stratford coined the term, "cubital tunnel syndrome." Both Osborne and Feindel and Stratford confused the issue by linking this band to previous nomenclature. Osborne entitled his paper, "Surgical Treatment of Tardy Ulnar Neuritis," whereas Feindel and Stratford entitled their article, "The Role of the Cubital Tunnel in Tardy Ulnar Palsy." However, from the description previously given, it is clear that the term "tardy ulnar palsy" is related to the development of ulnar nerve compression of the elbow after previous trauma, and from the intent of Osborne and of Feindel and Stratford, the syndrome they described is unrelated to trauma. The use of the new terminology, "cubital tunnel syndrome," generated an interest in the surgical approach to the problem of simple decompression of the ulnar nerve without transposition.

The causes for ulnar nerve compression at the elbow can be many and can be multifactorial (Table 9-2). Accordingly, when a specific cause is important in understanding the pathophysiologic features of the syndrome or in dictating the course of treatment, that cause should be described. Terms such as "post-traumatic ulnar neuritis," "tardy ulnar palsy," and "cubital tunnel syndrome," unless immediately followed by a descriptive term to define their meaning, are better left unused. Accordingly, this Chapter is titled "Ulnar Nerve Entrapment at the Elbow."

Table 9-2. Causes of Ulnar Nerve Compression at the Elbow

Trauma
Fractures[5,7–9,19,85]
Lateral humeral epicondyle (Fig. 9-8)
Medial humeral epicondyle (Fig. 9-9)
Supracondylar (Fig. 9-9)
Dislocation of elbow
Direct soft tissue injury (Fig. 9-7)
Arthritis
Osteoarthritis[25,79,85,91] (Fig. 9-11)
Rheumatoid[113–115] (Fig. 9-10)
Congenital
Cubitus valgus (Fig. 9-8)
Subluxing ulnar nerve[25,31,85,116,117] (Fig. 9-1)
Epitrochleoanconeus[31,43] (Fig. 9-3)
Snapping triceps[37–40]
Enlarged medial head of triceps[32,33] (Fig. 9-14)
Deep flexor-pronator aponeurosis[53,54]
Osborne's band[20,21,41,42] (Figs. 9-6, 9-12, 9-13)
Band in floor of cubital tunnel (Fig. 9-12)
External compression
Postanesthetic[94,118–120] (Fig. 9-1)
Chronic bed–ridden patients[121]
Hemorrhage
Metabolic
Diabetes[122–124]
Alcoholism[72]
Toxic, nutritional, etc.
Occupational[67,85,100]
Assembly line, office worker (desk job)
Truck driver
Computer keypuncher, secretarial
Miscellaneous
Torticollis[125]
Leprosy[126]
Biceps rupture[22]

Epidemiology of Ulnar Nerve Compression at the Elbow

The incidence of nerve compression has been observed by those involved in peripheral nerve surgery to be increasing over the last decade. This phenomenon has not been investigated statistically in terms of actual incidence or prevalence. However, a review of 14 of the series of ulnar nerve compressions at the elbow from the literature (Table 9-1) demonstrates a changing pattern in the spectrum of causes. This changing spectrum gives insight into the apparent epidemic of nerve compressions just alluded to. Through the first half of the 20th century, the reported series in general had no less than 50% and often 60 to 90% or more of their patients with the problem due to trauma. As the orthopedic surgeons became more successful in treating complex humeral fractures about the elbow and elbow dislocation, the incidence of complications involving the ulnar nerve in trauma in this region related to fractures has steadily decreased. Thus, in the decade from 1968 to 1979, the series of ulnar nerve compressions at the elbow frequently had just 15 to 30% due to trauma, with many series having less than 10% of the patients with problems related to fractures or fracture dislocations at the elbow. The general percentage of patients in each series with ulnar compression due to the group of problems related to osteoarthritis, rheumatoid arthritis, ulnar nerve subluxation, ganglion, and lipomas remains generally constant, in the range of 15 to 30%. The remaining group of patients, which generally have fallen into the wastebasket category of idiopathic or unknown causes of ulnar nerve compression at the elbow, are becoming increasingly identifiable as being related to either an increased susceptibility to nerve compression due to an underlying disease, such as diabetes or alcoholism, or, more commonly, due to the changing patterns in the activities of daily living of our population, due to the workplace.

The awareness that the ulnar nerve in the postcondylar groove is susceptible to external compression has been well-described in patients whose arms have been positioned in the prone position in the operating room or restrained by straps during operative procedures[120] (Fig. 9-1) and in patients who place continual pressure on their elbows as they attempt to maintain themselves in bed, where they are placed due to chronic debilitating diseases.[23] Increasing members of the work force find themselves confined to desk jobs, where the flexed position of the elbow and the contact between the elbow and the desk creates a similar external compression situation that causes ulnar nerve entrapment at the elbow. In addition, specific jobs cause compression of the

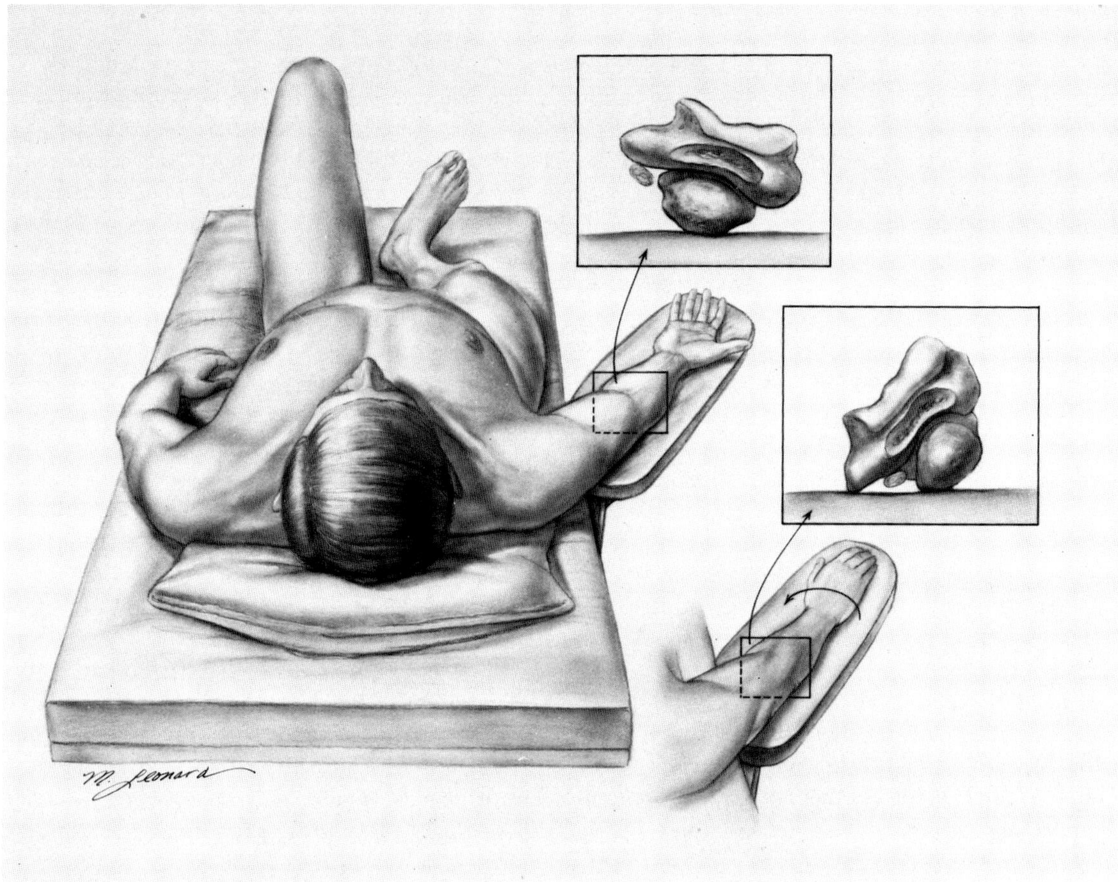

Figure 9-1. Postanesthesia ulnar nerve compression at the elbow is most commonly due to positioning the forearm prone. In this position, the ulnar nerve is most superficial in the cubital tunnel, exposing it to trauma. In contrast, if the forearm is supinated, the olecranon sustains the burden of the compression.

ulnar nerve at the elbow, such as the truck driver whose left arm remains flexed on the window sill, the assembly line worker carrying out frequent flexion-extension, pronation-supination movements, especially when these positions must be carried out with the elbow not only flexed but the arm abducted at the shoulder. The soft tissue trauma that results from falls in the workplace is accounting for an increasing number of patients who present with ulnar nerve compression at the elbow. Additionally, automobile accidents cause a significant number of ulnar nerve compressions at the elbow, primarily by a mechanism in which the driver, with his arms on the steering wheel, has his car struck and goes through rapid forward and backward movements causing stretch and compression injuries to the ulnar nerve at the elbow, in addition to any direct trauma caused by the elbow hitting the car door or other structure.

In Table 9-2 a list of causes of ulnar nerve compression at the elbow is given. It is believed that enough specific causes have been identified, so that the patient with ulnar nerve compression at the elbow who does not have one of these causes identified before surgery will be found at surgery to have one of the anatomic factors listed under "Congenital" in Table 9-2. It is suggested therefore that the old category of idiopathic causes for ulnar nerve compression at the elbow be dropped. At present, our own experience in more than 500 cases of ulnar nerve compression at the elbow has a breakdown of approximately 1% due to fracture, 20% due to direct soft tissue injury, 29% due to osteoarthritis, subluxation, ganglion, congenital anatomic structures, 20% due to underlying metabolic causes that predispose the peripheral nerve to compression, and 30% occupation related.[22] In a practice with more orthopedic trauma the incidence of venor neuropathy due to fracture will be higher.

The change in epidemiologic findings helps to understand from a historical perspective the changing emphasis in the surgical literature. For example, in 1921, Shelden[79] indicated that with respect to post-traumatic ulnar neuritis and tardy ulnar neuritis that follow fractures of the elbow joint, "Deformity of the elbow joint constitutes the essential etiologic factor.... Except for paresthesia and tenderness of the ulnar nerve, the first symptom to appear is atrophy of the small muscles of the hand, particularly in the first interosseous space." It was therefore appropriate for Shelden, seeing ulnar nerve compression at the elbow due to trauma with significant scar formation, to consider anterior transposition (he carried out a subcutaneous transposition) and to recommend this operation, which was designed to "relieve the nerve of the unusual tension induced by the deformed elbow and to protect it against frequent trauma." Since the nature of the ulnar nerve entrapment at the elbow that was being seen was of this character, presenting with atrophy of the intrinsic muscles. When the causative factor is progressive fibrosis, it is understandable that Donald Brooks,[23] writing in an editorial in 1950, said, "It is clear that early transposition of the [ulnar] nerve is desirable; there is no conservative treatment." (This editorial preceded McGowan's classic article, which contained the staging for post-traumatic ulnar compression.) Since the presenting symptoms included paresthesias in virtually all patients but various degrees of muscle weakness and atrophy accompanied most cases, it is not surprising that McGowan's[25] classification of the degree of severity of the nerve compression was based on motor changes (Table 9-3).

Whereas the writers in the first half of the 20th century saw not a single case of ulnar nerve compression at the elbow improve without surgery, and indeed saw only cases worsen if left untreated, by 1974 we find Eisen and Dannen[26] describing the so-called early or mild cubital tunnel syndrome and arriving at an electrophysiologic definition for the early diagnosis of "ulnar nerve palsy"[27] (Table 9-4). Eisen[26] had been seeing patients with numbness and tingling in the little and ring fingers that were intermittent and there was no motor weakness and no muscle atrophy. As already described, the changing epidemiologic features of the cause of the nerve compression probably is the basis for this changing clinical spectrum. With a program of nonoperative management that included avoiding pressure on the elbow and keeping the elbow extended as much as possible, with appropriate alterations in work activities, 90% of the patients with this mild degree of ulnar nerve compression at the elbow had relief of symptoms with a mean follow-up of 22 months.

It is clear, then, that as the cause for ulnar nerve compression has begun to shift, the possibility begins to exist that the pathophysiologic changes associated with the new epidemiologic causes of ulnar nerve compression will be such that there may be a time when it is reversible. In this instance, the physical examination, on which the diagnosis of ulnar nerve entrapment at the elbow can be made, will need to rely on the clinician's ability to distinguish more subtle neurologic changes than gross muscle atrophy. Such physical examination and findings include the increased response to vibratory stimuli at 256 cps[28] and the reproduction or induction of the patient's symptoms by flexing the elbow. This test, which we have called in the past a positive elbow flexion test, has recently been correlated with electrodiagnostic testing by Fine and Wongjirad.[29] As will be described later in the section on treatment of ulnar nerve compression at the elbow, the group of patients staged as having a minimal degree of compression have been observed by us, in more than 50% of the patients followed prospectively for at least 2 years, to have obtained relief of their symptoms.[30]

Table 9-3. Staging of Ulnar Nerve Compression at the Elbow, McGowan's Classification*

Grade 1	Minimal with no detectable motor weakness
Grade 2	Intermediate
Grade 3	Severe with paresis or paralysis of intrinsic muscles

*Reprinted with permission from McGowan.[25]

Table 9-4. Staging of Ulnar Nerve Compression at the Elbow Electrodiagnostic Criteria*

		Ulnar Nerve Compression	
	Normal Population (n=48)	*Mild (n=56)*	*Severe (n=34)*
Motor conduction velocity (m/sec)			
Above elbow	59.2 ± 8.2	52.7 ± 8.5	52.8 ± 9.7
Across elbow	53.2 ± 7.8	47.7 ± 10.1	34.8 ± 8.8
Below elbow	54.6 ± 6.7	52.9 ± 6.5	48.2 ± 9.4
Motor latency (msec)			
Elbow to ADM†	7.9 ± 0.9	9.1 ± 1.2	11.3 ± 2.0
Wrist to ADM	3.0 ± 0.4	3.3 ± 0.5	3.9 ± 0.7
Sensory latency (msec)			
V to wrist	2.3 ± 0.5	2.5 ± 0.4	3.7 ± 1.0

*Reprinted with permission from Eisen.[27]

†ADM: abductor digiti minimi.

Surgical Anatomy

The ulnar nerve is the continuation of the medial cord of the brachial plexus and contains sensory and motor nerve fibers from C8 and T1 nerve roots. Accompanied by the superior ulnar collateral vessels, the ulnar nerve approaches the medial humeral epicondyle in relationship to the medial head of the triceps muscle on its medial side and the humerus on its lateral side. Posteriorly, it is in relationship to the medial head of the triceps and anteriorly it is related to the fascia that goes from the medial head of the triceps to the medial intermuscular septum. The ulnar nerve then passes through a region bounded by the medial humeral epicondyle superiorly and laterally, the postcondylar groove in the olecranon that lies posterior to the ulnar nerve and slightly medial, and a roof or connective tissue that extends from these two bony prominences distally to the two heads of the flexor carpi ulnaris. The ulnar nerve passes between the two heads of the flexor carpi ulnaris and then proceeds distally.

Cubital Tunnel

The cubital tunnel has been variously described. In its shortest extent, it has been limited to a passage just between the two heads of the flexor carpi ulnaris. The anatomy of the region suggests that the cubital tunnel is most appropriately considered as the length along which the ulnar nerve passes from superficial to the forearm flexor pronator muscle group to the location deep to and within the flexor pronator muscle group. Accordingly, the term, "cubital tunnel" is utilized in this chapter to include the fascial covering that is frequently loose and variable in its proximal extent at the level of the medial humeral epicondyle and the olecranon to that distal area that is frequently tight between the two heads of the flexor carpi ulnaris, which may be bounded by a thickening in the fascial covering (Osborne's band). The normal biomechanics of this entire roof of the tunnel will be discussed later. This entire roof in both its loose and its thicker, tighter distal part acts as a single functional unit, which again lends support to considering the entire length of this fascial roof as the length of the cubital tunnel.

The biomechanics of the normal anatomy related to the ulnar nerve at the elbow have been described in a series of four articles.[31–34] In 1968, Vanderpool from Houston, Texas, and Chalmers and Lamb from Edinburgh, and Whiston from Melrose, Scotland, combined to write one of the classic papers in peripheral nerve surgery.[31] In addition to the epidemiologic aspects of ulnar nerve compression, which has already been referred to, and in addition to their presentation of their surgical results of the treatment of ulnar nerve compression at the elbow, which will be discussed later, they made important observations on the relationship of anatomy to ulnar nerve compression at the elbow, which form the basis of our understanding of this nerve compression syndrome.[31] They observed the relationship between forearm positioning in the operating room and the development of postanesthetic ulnar palsy (Fig. 9-1). They evaluated 18 human cadavers and noted that "with flexion of the elbow, the cubital tunnel decreases in volume as the aponeurosis (the roof of the cubital tunnel) becomes stretched." The distance this aponeurosis stretched was increased by 5 mm for each 45° of flexion, with elongation being 40% from full extension to 135° of elbow flexion. They further built on Sunderland's 1945 observations of the intraneural arrangement of the ulnar nerve at the elbow. These observations demonstrated that the motor fibers to the intrinsic muscles of the hand lay most superficial, that is, most anterior and most medial, while the sensory afferents from the hand lay also superficial but more posterior.[35] They observed that the intrinsic muscles to the hand and the sensory afferents from the little and ring fingers were most likely to become compressed by the overlying aponeurosis as it tightened. They noted that Sunderland had depicted the motor branches to the flexor carpi ulnaris and flexor digitorum profundus to lie deepest in the cubital tunnel, that is, most lateral and most posterior. Therefore, pathologic changes arising in the joint, itself, such as synovitis or hypertrophic osteoarthritic bone spurring, would be more likely to cause problems in grip strength and wrist flexion, with possibly these motor signs presenting first rather than numbness in the little and ring fingers or intrinsic muscle problems. Relating the type of clinical presentation for ulnar nerve compression at the elbow to the intraneural topography of the ulnar nerve at the elbow and the anatomy of the cubital tunnel, as Vanderpool et al did,[31] has been incorporated into the writings of most subsequent researchers' considerations of these problems.

Apfelberg and Larson[32] carried out the most complete anatomic evaluation of the mechanism described by Vanderpool et al.[31] In a series of 15 cadaver dissections, they demonstrated that the aponeurosis from the medial humeral epicondyle to the olecranon became stretched because the geometry was such that the distance between these two bony points was the closest when the elbow was in extension and was the farthest apart when the elbow was in flexion. Apfelberg and Larson noted that the ulnar nerve was found to stretch approximately 4.7 mm during elbow flexion and that the ulnar nerve appeared to be larger within the postcondylar groove (an average of 5.4 mm in diame-

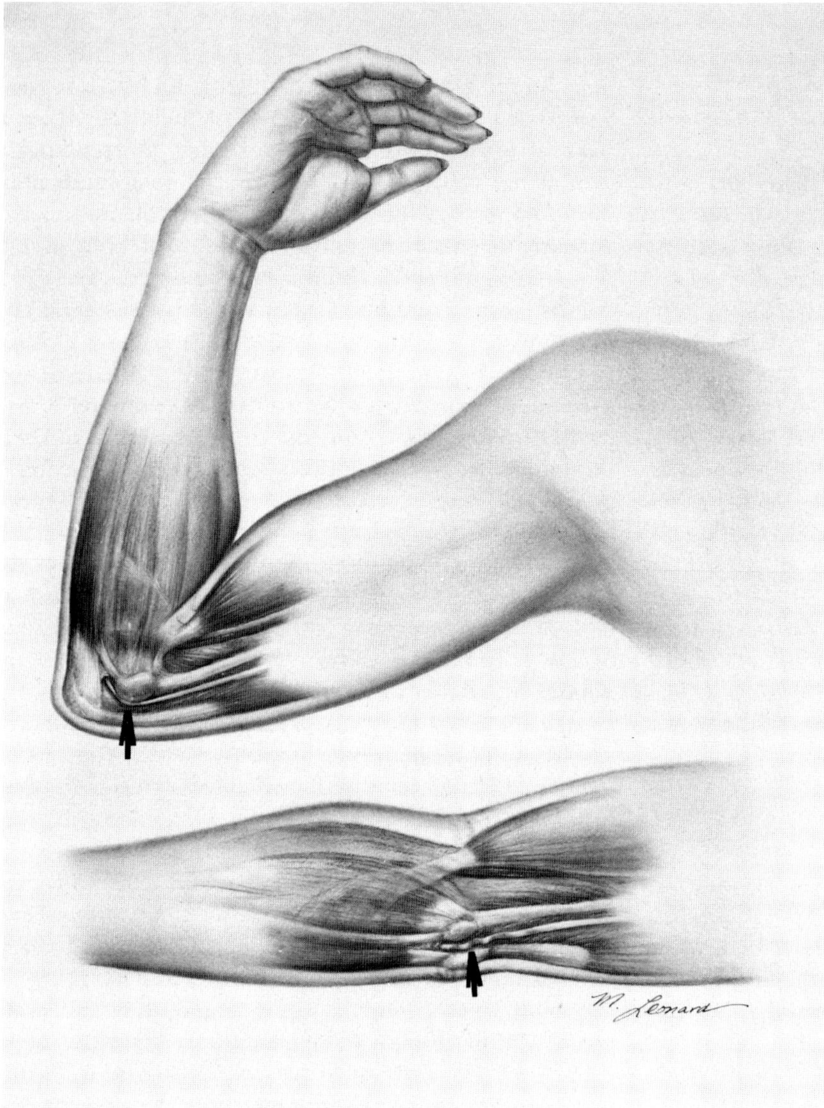

a

Figure 9-2. Illustration of Apfelberg and Larsen's[32] observation that the ulnar nerve increases in length (stretches) an average of 4.7 mm with elbow flexion (a). They demonstrated alteration in volume of cubital tunnel by its acceptance of a 6 mm dilator with the elbow extended (b) and just a 3 mm dilator with the elbow flexed (c). (Modified from Apfelberg and Larsen.[32])

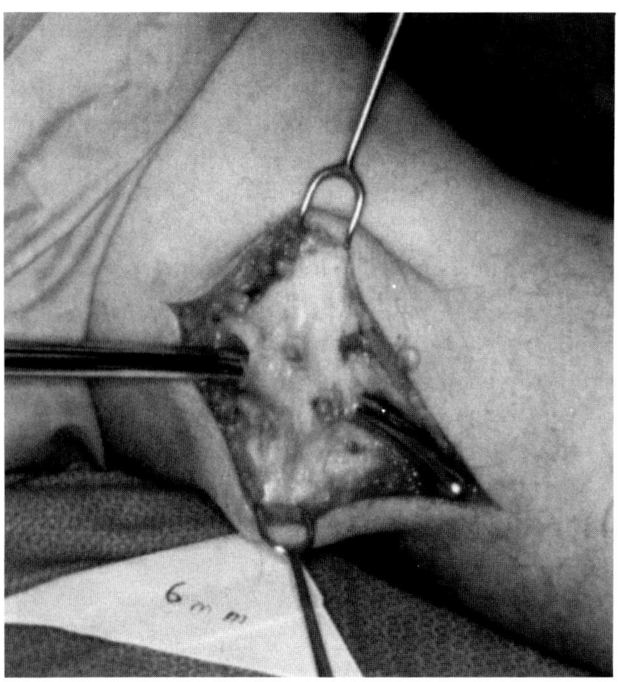

b

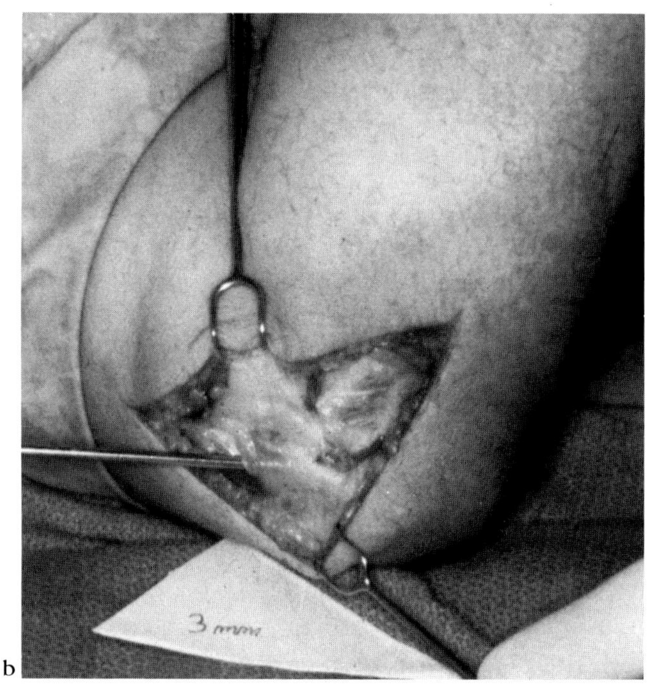

c

ter) than it was proximal (an average of 4.7 mm) or distal (an average of 4.7 mm) below the postcondylar groove (Fig. 9-2a). Chang et al[36] noted in 1963 from an extensive study of cadaver dissections that the ulnar nerve appeared to be enlarged in the postcondylar groove. They found that 47% of their anatomic specimens showed a swelling in the postcondylar groove and that this was proportional to the age, with 60% of these enlargements being found in men older than age 35 years. Chang et al noted that this enlargement was related to an increase in the amount of connective tissue present. They believed that it was a pathophysiologic reaction, rather than a normal variation. Furthermore, the cross-sectional area of the tunnel in this region was round with the elbow in extension, but became narrowed by a rising or bulge in the floor of the tunnel due to a bony process of the olecranon as the elbow came into flexion. Thus, the ulnar collateral ligament of the elbow joint, which is on the medial side of the elbow and which forms the floor of the cubital tunnel, bulges into the tunnel with elbow flexion. These investigators demonstrated this narrowing by the placement of Bake dilators into the cubital tunnel (Fig. 9-2b). A 6 mm dilator could be inserted into the postcondylar groove with the elbow in extension. With the elbow in flexion, a 3 mm dilator was the largest that could be inserted (Fig. 9-2c). Medical grade acrylic was injected into the cubital tunnel with the elbow in flexion and extension and allowed to harden into a mold to demonstrate the shape. In extension, the molds were rounded with an average height of 5.8 mm, and when the elbow was extended, the cross-sectional area flattened, with an average height of 3.2 mm.

Apfelberg and Larson[32] made one further observation related to the medial head of the triceps. They observed that during flexion the bulge of the medial head of the triceps pushed the ulnar nerve anteriorly and slightly medially for an average of 0.73 cm, causing it to become compressed in the angle formed by the medial intermuscular septum and the aponeurosis or roof of the cubital tunnel. The medial head of the triceps has been, as already noted, related to ulnar nerve compression at the elbow in two additional ways. A large medial head to the triceps can bulge completely around the medial humeral epicondyle during elbow flexion. This is associated with a loud snapping sound and compression of the ulnar nerve against the medial humeral epicondyle in the syndrome known as the "snapping triceps tendon."[37–40] Furthermore, the medial head of the triceps has been observed by Dellon[33] in a series of 64 cadaver dissections to have the ulnar nerve located within the triceps muscle, so that portions of the medial head of the triceps can form a roof over the ulnar nerve. In 19 of the 33 cadavers dissected in that study, the medial head of the triceps had an insertion into the floor of the cubital tunnel. In this location, contraction of the medial head of the triceps would contribute to ulnar nerve subluxation. Fourteen of the 18 (78%) cadavers that had ulnar nerve subluxation also had the medial head of the triceps in the floor of the cubital tunnel. This is in contrast to an incidence of the triceps in the floor of the cubital tunnel in just 11% of the overall number of cadavers in the series. This difference was found to be significant at the $p < 0.001$ level.

The only physiologic study of the cubital tunnel was that reported in 1975 by Pechan and Julis.[34] These investigators studied human fresh autopsy material (number of specimens not given). They directly measured the intraneural pressure by placing a needle beneath the epineurium of the ulnar nerve within the cubital tunnel. They found that with the elbow in extension, the mean pressure in the ulnar nerve was 7.2 mmHg. When the arm was kept at the side and the elbow flexed, the pressure increased to 11.1 mmHg. When the wrist was extended, in addition to the elbow being flexed, the pressure increased to 17.9 and when the shoulder was elevated in an anterior direction with the elbow flexed and the wrist extended, the pressure increased to 24 mmHg. When the elbow was flexed, the wrist extended, and the arm brought to a position over the head, the pressure increased to 45.7 mmHg. Division of the aponeurosis (roof of the cubital tunnel) caused reduction of this pressure increase (Table 9-5). These anatomic findings taken together demonstrate unequivocally that, with elbow flexion, the ulnar nerve is subjected to increased pressure. This pressure is further increased when the elbow flexion is accompanied by wrist extension, which tightens the origin of the flexor carpi ulnaris at the point at which the ulnar nerve goes from superficial to deep and the pressure is again increased with shoulder abduction and increases with increasing degrees of elevation of the arm. These further increases in ulnar nerve compression within the cubital tunnel, as the shoulder is abducted, presumably result

Table 9-5. Ulnar Intraneural Pressure in the Cubital Tunnel Related to Elbow Position*

	Intraneural Ulnar Pressure (mmHg)	
Position	*Mean*	*Range*
Elbow at side		
Elbow extended	7.2	2.7–13.8
Elbow flexed	11.1	6.3–16.4
Elbow flexed plus wrist extended	17.9	8.2–28.5
Shoulder elevated: anterior		
Elbow flexed plus wrist extended	24.0	13.8–32.2
Shoulder elevated: overhead		
Elbow flexed plus wrist extended	45.7	28.5–72.6

*Reprinted with permission from Pechan and Julis.[34]

from traction of the ulnar nerve, which is fixed at the elbow against the proximal point of fixation in the brachial plexus.

The roof to the cubital tunnel, which we previously described as being of varying thickness and laxity, depending on the position of the elbow, was noted by Osborne[21] in 1957 to have a thickened most distal part between the two heads of the flexor carpi ulnaris, which can be responsible for ulnar nerve compression in that precise region. This thickened region, which has been subsequently called Osborne's band, was identified also by Feindel and Stratford[20] and subsequent writers[41,42] as the site, if not the mechanism, of compression in patients presenting with so-called cubital tunnel syndrome (Figs. 9-12c, 9-20b). As may be understood from the immediate preceding description, whether or not there is a thickened area within this aponeurosis, the entire aponeurosis tightens with elbow flexion and can cause compression of the ulnar nerve. The incidence of this thickening, or Osborne's band, in normal cadavers was examined.[33] The presence of such a band occurred in 49 of the 64 cadavers (77%). In 23% there was no fibrous thickening between the two heads of the flexor carpi ulnaris. The findings were bilateral. Therefore it appears that the presence of this thickened band, when in existence, may aggravate the normal physiologic mechanism of increased pressure that occurs with elbow flexion.

The roof of the cubital tunnel may be formed by an anomalous muscle. This muscle, which is termed the epitrochleoanconeus (Fig. 9-3), has been best described in a review by Hirasawa.[43] He has noted the incidence to be from 1 to 30% of cadavers containing this muscle. In a recent series of cadaver dissections, it was noted to be present in 4 of 33 (12%) cadavers in which the specimen was suitable to allow investigation of this muscle. The muscle was present to an equal extent on both sides of the specimen when it was present.[33] A particular pattern was noted in these cadaver dissections. This pattern was that in the seven cadavers with an epitrochleoanconeus muscle, just two had an Osborne's band present in comparison with Osborne's band being present in 47 of the 57 cadavers that did not have an epitrochleoanconeus muscle. Six of the seven cadavers with an epitrochleoanconeus muscle had a large medial head to the triceps with the ulnar nerve in the triceps muscle. This prominent medial head to the triceps was present in just 10 of the 57 cadavers that did not have an epitrochleoanconeus muscle. This relationship was significant at the $p < 0.001$ level. Our observations in baboons and monkeys had demonstrated that the ulnar nerve appears almost always to be completely located within the triceps muscle, with the medial head of the triceps entering into the floor of the cubital tunnel and an epitrochleoanconeus muscle being present. In the rhesus and cynomolgus monkey, the ulnar nerve was more superficial than it was in the baboon but was still usually covered by a thin sheet of the medial triceps head, the fibers blending almost directly into the medial intermuscular septum. The subhuman primates did not have a well-developed Osborne's band. It was thus speculated[33] that in the course of evolution the comparative anatomy has changed from having an ulnar nerve being completely covered by triceps, with the triceps, in fact, entering into the floor of the cubital tunnel and the triceps fibers and fascia seeming to blend with an epitrochleoanconeus muscle. This muscle was innervated by the ulnar nerve. This system restrains the nerve in and about the region of the medial humeral epicondyle. With evolution, it appears that the medial head of the triceps has regressed, leaving a thinner layer of fascia to go from the medial head of the triceps to the medial intermuscular septum, with the ulnar nerve in man lying below this thin film of fascia. With evolution, the epitrochleoanconeus muscle may have resolved to the point at which its remnant is represented by the fibrous aponeurosis that now forms the roof of the cubital tunnel. As man has become increasingly required to work with his elbow flexed, the series of constraints, loosened through evolution, has permitted ulnar nerve subluxation.

"Arcade of Struthers"

The relationship of the ulnar nerve proximal to the medial humeral epicondyle has been variously described as the "arcade of Struthers".[44–47] In cadaver dissections, Spinner and associates[47] have reported an incidence varying from 20 to 70% of a thick fascial structure from the medial head of the triceps to the medial intermuscular septum located approximately 8 cm proximal to the medial humeral epicondyle, which can be a source of ulnar nerve compression. They have credited this structure to Struthers. Very careful reading of Struthers' writings from 1848 and 1854[48,49] indicates his clear description of the supracondylar bony process and ligament that bear his name and are related to median nerve compression. Struthers does clearly describe the fascia just mentioned but nowhere uses the term "arcade." This so-called arcade described and depicted by Spinner (Fig. 9-4) can best be understood by realizing that it was recognized by Spinner in patients with recurrent ulnar nerve symptoms after ulnar nerve transposition. In our personal series of more than 500 ulnar nerve explorations,[22] a discrete arcade of Struthers has never been identified. However, in patients who have previously had an anterior transposition and who have failed to improve, the surgical reexploration clearly shows an

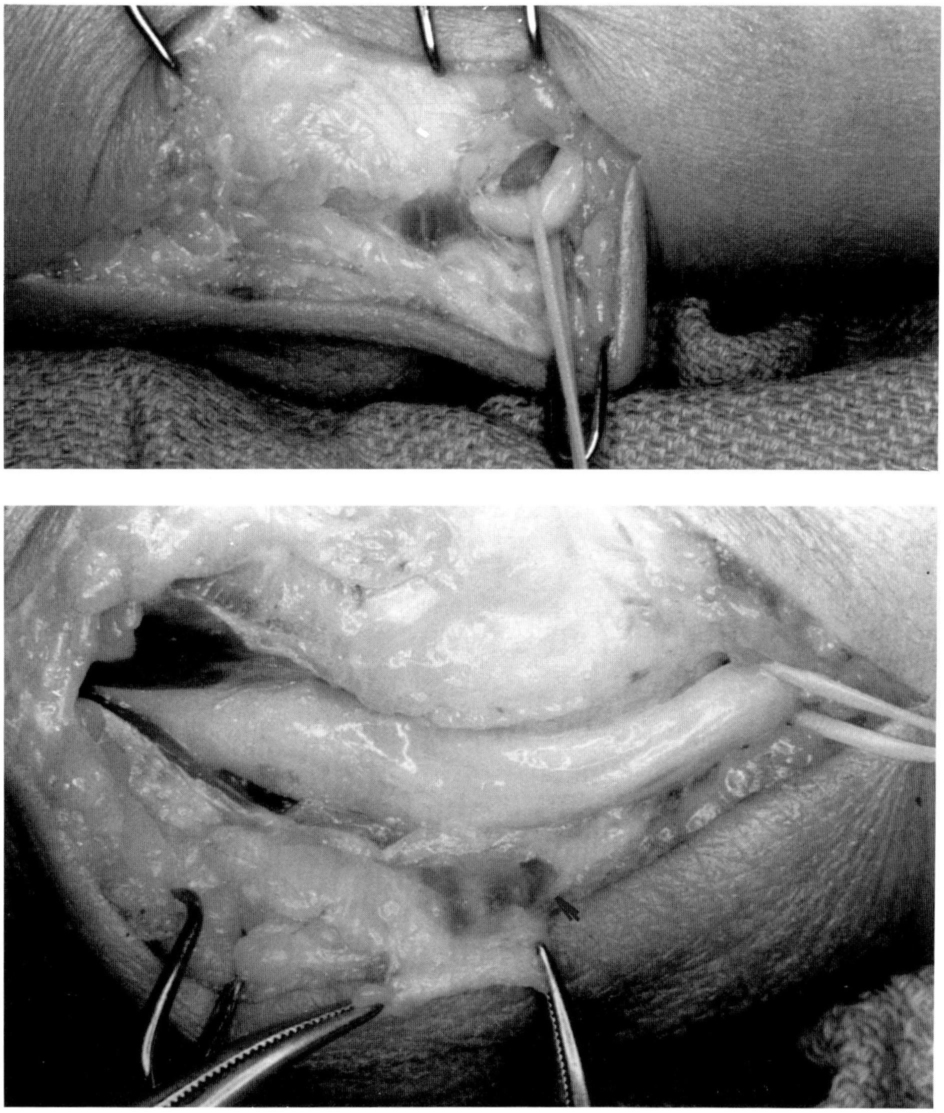

a

b

Figure 9-3. Epitrochleoanconeus muscle remains in situ **(a)** and after internal neurolysis **(b)**. Note multiple fascicles, little plexus formation, no pseudoneuroma. Note (arrow) innervation to muscle from ulnar nerve.

ulnar nerve being tethered proximally and usually about 8 cm proximal to the medial humeral epicondyle by the fascia already described, which runs from the medial head of the triceps to the medial intermuscular septum. At any surgical procedure, the surgeon may convince himself of the ability to create such an arcade simply by incising this fascia for only a length of 4 to 5 cm. Then, when the ulnar nerve is transposed anteriorly, it appears that there indeed exists an arcade compressing the ulnar nerve. Simply releasing the fascia to a higher level immediately makes this anatomic arcade disappear.[33] It is thus recommended (see later) that in the surgical procedure this fascia is split well proximal to the medial humeral epicondyle, although the incision, itself, need not extend that far proximally.

Pseudoneuroma

The intraneural topography of the ulnar nerve at the elbow has been described by Sunderland[35] and has been represented as being comprised of several fascicles. Sunderland's intent during this dissection was to relate the location of the fascicle along the length of the ulnar nerve with the type of function its fibers were carrying. One of the observations made by Sunderland was that there are connections between nerves, so-called plexus formation (Chapter 1). With regard to the subject of intraneural neurolysis, or internal neurolysis (Chapter 5, Figs. 5-5, 5-6), it is noted that for the median nerve at the wrist, there is very little plexus formation. Sun-

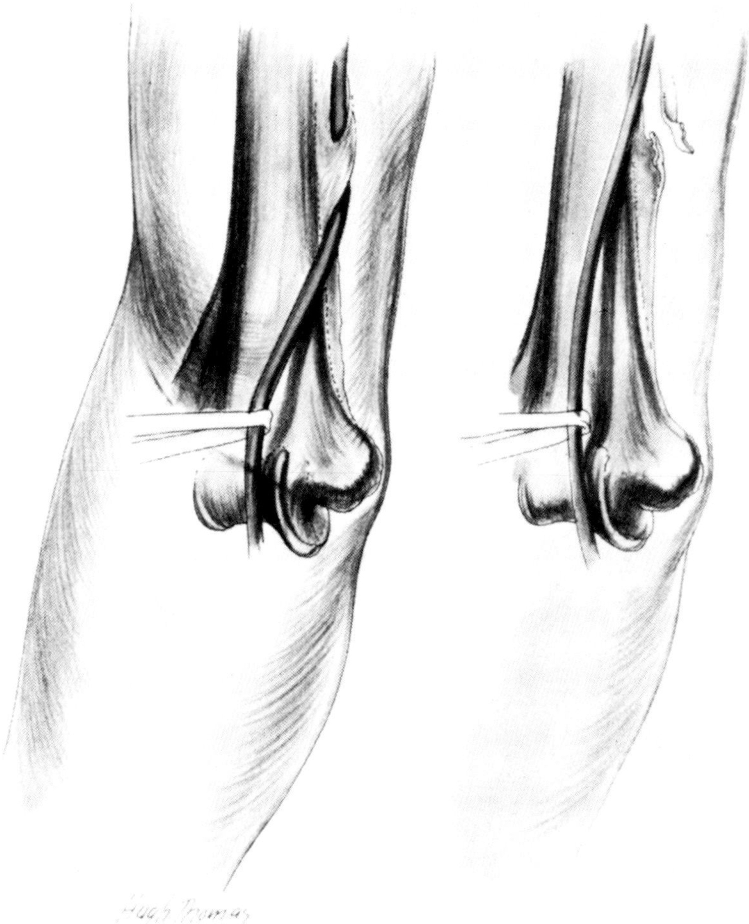

Figure 9-4. The postulated "arcade of Struthers."[47] This may be formed by insufficient proximal release of the fascia from the medial head of the triceps to the medial intermuscular septum (see text). (Drawing reproduced with permission from Spinner.[47])

derland did not specifically address the degree to which plexus formation was present at the level of the elbow. The observations made by the earliest investigators of ulnar nerve compression at the elbow concerned the presence of so-called pseudoneuroma formation. It has been our observation[22] that there is a relationship between the presence of pseudoneuroma formation and plexus formation. It has been noted that there is a subpopulation of ulnar nerves that are comprised of six to ten individual fascicles with little or no plexus formation present in the region of the cubital tunnel. The hypothesis would be that the absence of plexus formation permits movement of these fascicles with respect to each other, therefore minimizing the effect of shear and stress forces, thereby reducing the degree of intraneural fibrosis that would contribute to the pseudoneuroma formation. In contrast, there is a subpopulation of ulnar nerves that are comprised of one to four large fascicles with extensive plexus formation between them. The hypothesis would be that these fascicles have little ability to adjust their positions with respect to each other, thereby not having the ability to reduce shearing forces and friction. Thus, the group with increased plexus formation and few fascicles would be more likely to have intraneural fibrosis and pseudoneuroma formation. This hypothesis has been found to be correct in our personal series of ulnar nerve explorations at the elbow in that there is a positive correlation between the presence of pseudoneuroma and the degree of interfascicular plexus formation in the cubital tunnel (Figs. 5-5, 5-6, 9-5a, b, 9-12a).

Medial Antebrachial Cutaneous Nerve

The cutaneous nerve innervating the region into which the incision for ulnar nerve decompression is to be placed is of importance. The medial antebrachial cutaneous nerve is one of the terminal branches of the medial cord of the brachial plexus. Its course is anterior and lateral to the medial humeral epicondyle. In the region of the antecubital crease or slightly proximal to

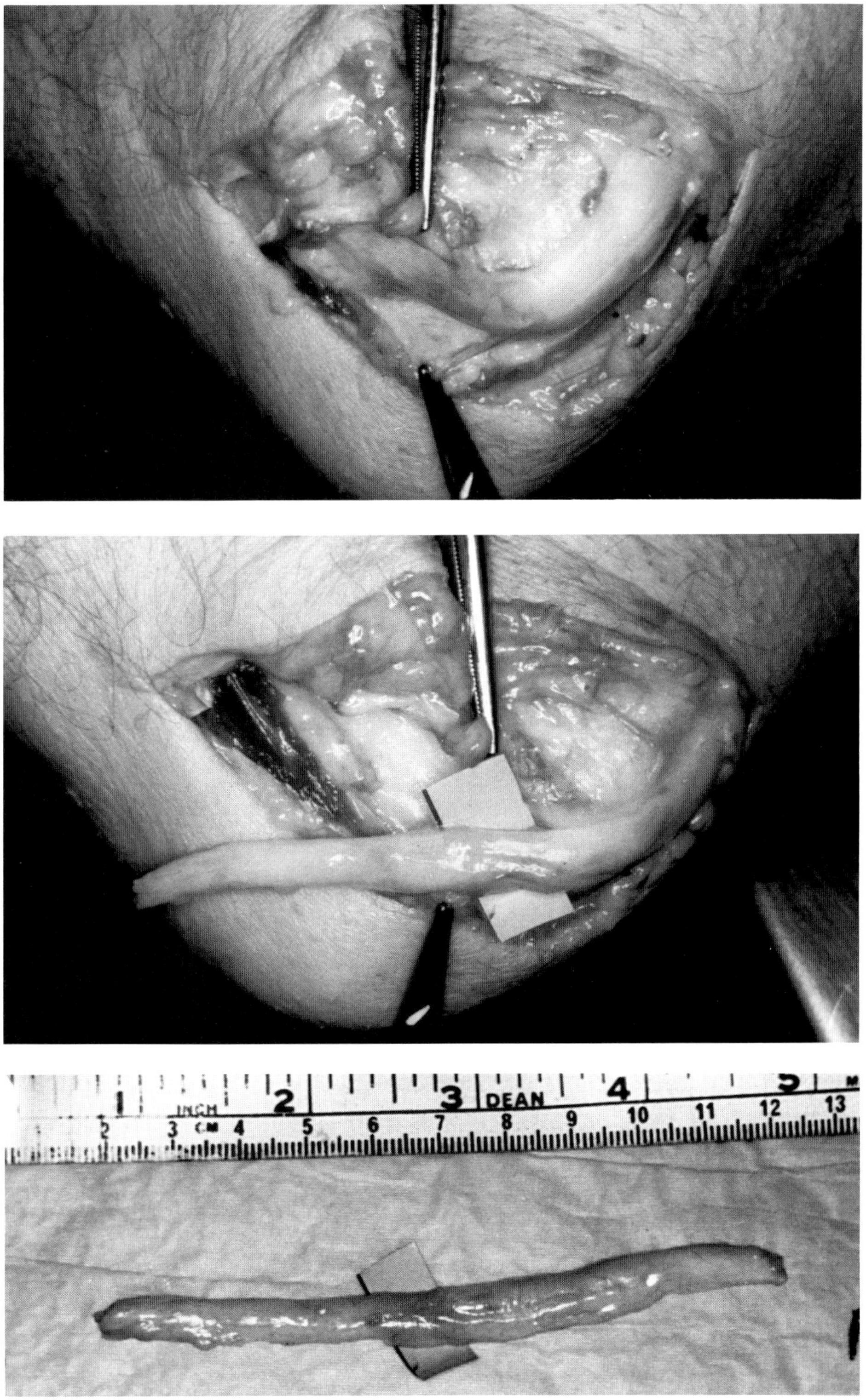

a

b

c

Figure 9-5. Histopathologic findings of human ulnar nerve compression continued.[58] Autopsy findings for right ulnar nerve at elbow. **a.** Clamp grasps divided Osborne's band at entrapment site of ulnar nerve; **b.** distal transection of ulnar nerve, the narrowed area that was compressed beneath Osborne's band is apparent (note small proximal pseudoneuroma); **c.** excised right ulnar nerve demonstrating proximal, central and distal sites available for morphometric analysis; **d.** excised left ulnar nerve, sectioned, for histologic study. Morphometric analysis was done from these histopathologic findings of the left ulnar nerve, stained with toluidine blue, transverse sections. **e.** Proximal to Osborne's band, there is "loss" of large myelinated fiber population (×588). (*Figure continues.*)

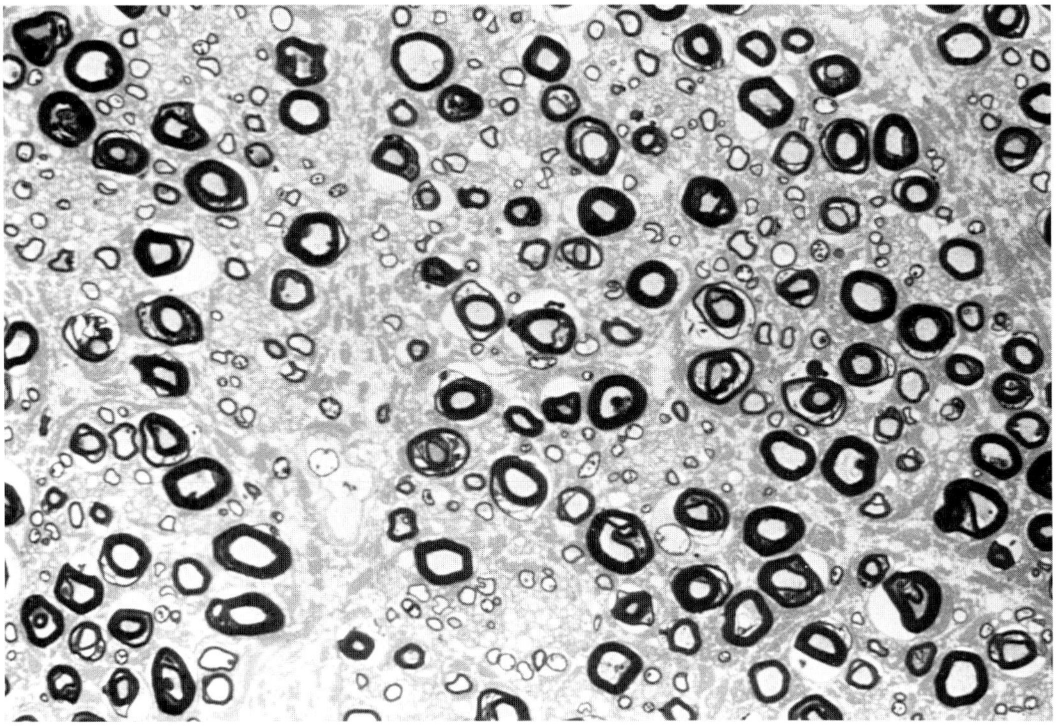

d

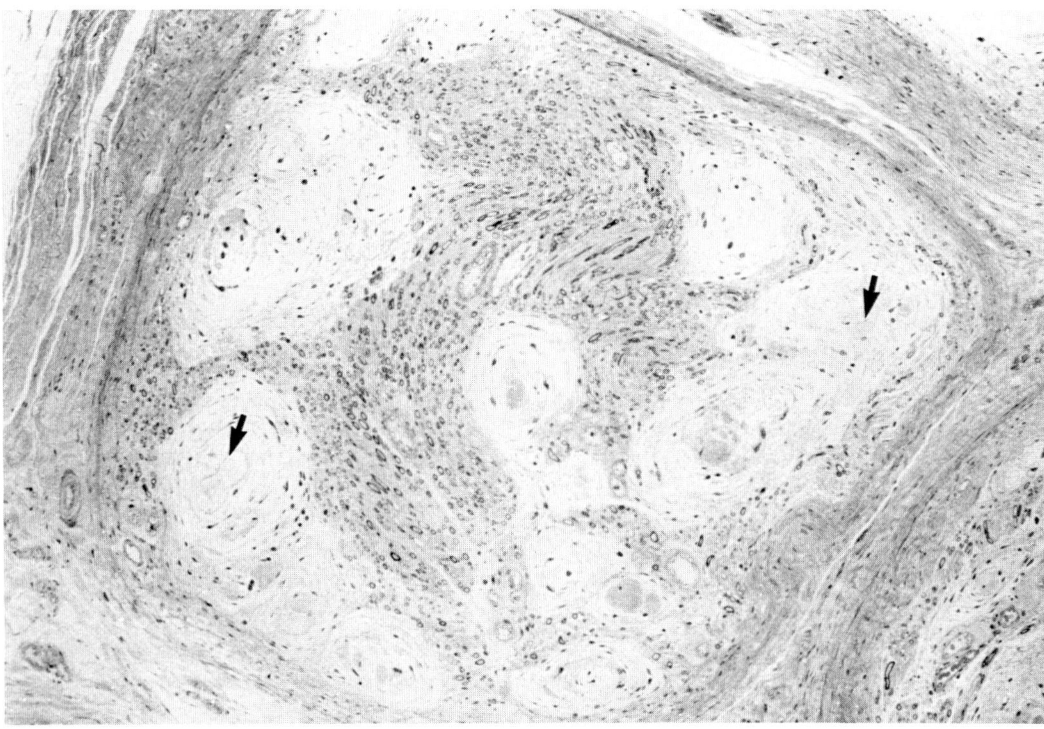

e

Figure 9-5 *(continued).* At the site of compression, there are Renaut bodies (arrows) × 147) associated with marked perineurial thickening and **(f)** severe myelin thinning (× 588). Distal to the band **(g)**, some remyelination has occurred, but there is still profound loss of neural tissues. (× 588.)

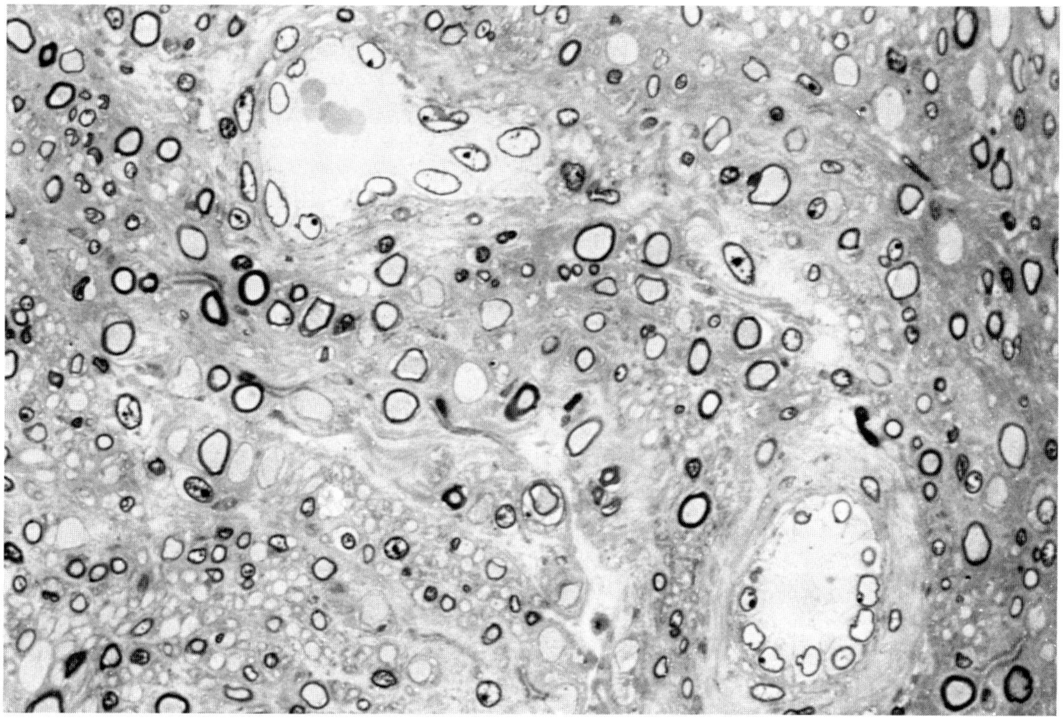

f

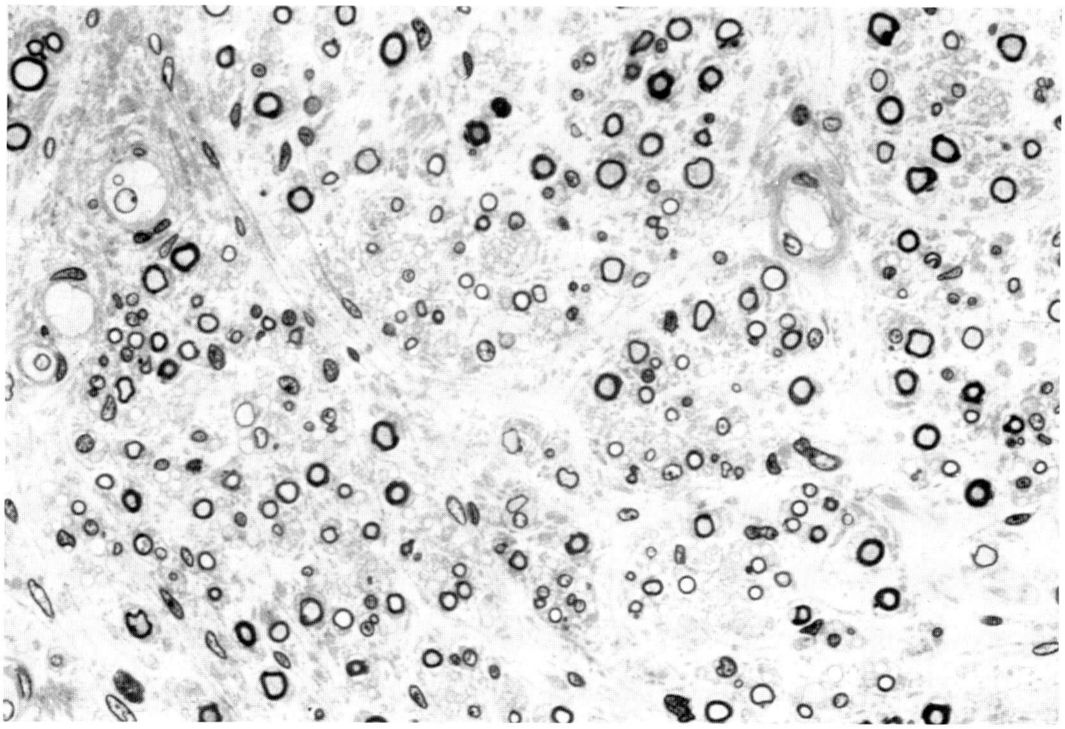

g

Figure 9-5 *(continued).*

it, it splits into an anterior and posterior branch. The posterior branch may have one or more smaller branches that cross the region of the medial humeral epicondyle on the postcondylar groove to innervate the posteromedial aspect of the olecranon. The anterior branch of the medial antebrachial cutaneous nerve continues down the forearm to innervate the medial volar third of the forearm. Another cutaneous branch of the medial cord of the plexus, the medial branchial cutaneous nerve, may extend into the surgical incision area by coming directly posterior to the medial humeral epicondyle and entering the most posterior aspect of the incision. When the incision is overlying the course of the ulnar nerve in the postcondylar groove (Figs. 9-18, through 9-20), the likelihood of injuring one of these branches is very real. As will be discussed later in "Postoperative Complications" section, the most common complication of ulnar nerve transposition is an injury to a branch of this nerve causing either a painful scar, an area of decreased sensitivity inferior to the scar, or, in the worst cases, a painful neuroma that requires subsequent neuroma resection[50] (Figs. 9-21, 9-24).

Intramuscular Placement

The intramuscular placement of an anteriorly transposed ulnar nerve has been largely condemned,[2,3,47,51] primarily because of scarring found in patients who have had intramuscular placement and subsequently have had the operative procedure fail. The scarring has been variously attributed, however. The most common reason given is the extent of exposed muscle fibers and fibrous bands to which the ulnar nerve becomes adherent in the postoperative period. This hypothesis was directly tested in an experimental study[52] in baboons, and intramuscular placement was done on one side and a submuscular placement done on the contralateral side. Each of the five baboons had no splints applied in the postoperative period. Three months after surgery, a block of tissue was excised that included the flexor pronator muscle mass and the ulnar nerve. These muscle blocks were examined and there was no difference between the ulnar nerves in any of the morphometric measurements. There was a gliding tissue plane of loose mesoneural tissue between the muscle nerve interface in all specimens. This study demonstrated that the mere location of the ulnar nerve next to divided muscle and fibrous tissue did not, in and of itself, create scarring if the nerve was allowed to glide in the postoperative period. There was no sign of nerve compression as demonstrated by mean nerve fiber diameter or change in the axon to myelin ratio between either of these intramuscular or submuscular specimen groups. Our dissections about the medial humeral epicondyle[33] demonstrated that what is commonly called the common flexor tendon, in fact, represents a thick fibrous origin from the medial humeral epicondyle that largely gives rise to the flexor digitorum sublimis head from the humerus. This fibrous band is 3 to 5 mm in width and may rise a height of 1 cm in length above the ulna. Thus, when an intramuscular placement is carried out, the ulnar nerve is usually placed on top of this fibrous band. Then, any type of tunnel reconstruction to maintain the nerve in the intramuscular position must compress the ulnar nerve against the underlying fibrous structure. This prevents the ulnar nerve from sliding and this tethering mechanism and site of compression becomes the reason that intramuscular placement of the ulnar nerve frequently fails (see "Results" section later) Figs. 9-25, 9-26). It may be inferred that those reports of intramuscular placement where there is success either do not create a roof over the newly located ulnar nerve or have carried out a deep intramuscular placement, in which case the surgeon must have divided these thick fibrous structures. This common flexor tendon has been described in a more distal location[53,54] to be a potential source of ulnar nerve compression distal to the cubital tunnel. Such fibrous structures distally may be identified when the flexor pronator muscle mass is divided to allow the submuscular positioning, especially if the common flexor tendon is divided as described in the operative section later. These distal bands should not provide a more distal site of compression.

Ruptured Biceps and Ulnar Nerve Compression

The anatomy of the biceps tendon may contribute to ulnar nerve compression. With rupture of the biceps, which has been well-described,[23] there are several possible mechanisms by which ulnar nerve compression can occur. Three patients with ulnar nerve compression after biceps rupture have been noted.[22] The patient with biceps rupture has weakness of elbow flexion. The patients noted were referred because of weakness in the upper arm after biceps rupture. However, this was weakness in grip, determined by careful evaluation. The mechanisms for ulnar nerve compression after biceps rupture can include the trauma itself initially, bleeding after the biceps rupture, which causes compression of the ulnar nerve at the elbow due to the secondary swelling, and placement of the elbow in flexion during the 6 to 12 weeks during which the tendon healing occurs after repair of the biceps rupture.

"Trigger Finger" and Ulnar Nerve Compression

The innervation of the flexor profundus muscle by the ulnar nerve must be remembered during the evaluation of possible weakness and inability to flex the little and ring fingers. It has been noted in our series of ulnar nerve compressions at the elbow that there were four patients who presented with weakness and inability to flex the ring or little finger due to "recurrent trigger finger" problems. Each of these patients had been operated on at least twice and one had three operations for trigger finger problems. At the time of presentation, each patient was unable to flex the little or ring finger completely. Careful evaluation revealed weakness in the profundus to the little and ring fingers without problems with the tendon related to the first annular ligament. In each instance, anterior submuscular transposition with neurolysis of the flexor profundus motor branch restored ability to flex the involved finger.

Histopathology

The pathophysiologic characteristics of nerve compression is discussed in general in Chapter 2. In particular, the ulnar nerve has been examined from a postmortem specimen of a patient who was known preoperatively to have had ulnar nerve compression.[55] There has been an additional report of the incidence of ulnar nerve compression in postmortem material from patients who were known not to have signs or symptoms of ulnar nerve compression before their death.[56] The latter report by Neary et al in 1975 is instructive in that their 12 patients were found to have a high incidence of histopathologic changes in the median and ulnar nerves. In particular, 5 of the 12 cases had either bulbus swellings in the myelin or intercalated segments of demyelination. Thus, approximately 40% of routine postmortem specimens, from patients in the age range of 40 to 70 years, demonstrated histopathologic evidence of ulnar nerve compression at the elbow. This is appropriately called subclinical ulnar nerve compression at the elbow. These nerves, in addition, demonstrated the presence of Renaut bodies. The Renaut body (as described in Chapter 2) is identifiable in areas where a nerve is compressed and subjected to shearing or tension and traction forces.[57] The experimental models of chronic nerve compression, in which the nerves are not subjected to such shearing forces, have not been found to contain Renaut bodies. Thus, the presence of Renaut bodies in subclinical ulnar nerve entrapment is in support of the pathophysiologic findings of ulnar nerve compression at the elbow already described: increased pressure on the ulnar nerve in the cubital tunnel with elbow flexion, tethering of the ulnar nerve beneath the thickened distal end of the roof of the cubital tunnel (Osborne's band), stretching of the ulnar nerve with flexion, and the frequent compounding of these effects by a subluxing ulnar nerve. The ulnar nerves in the subclinical group demonstrated a slight shift to the left in the myelinated fiber histogram (smaller diameter mean fibers in the area beneath the cubital tunnel) than was present proximal or distal. There appeared histologically to be a loss of the large myelinated fibers (large fiber dropout); however, these large fibers were present in the distal segment consistent with loss only of myelin and no Wallerian degeneration in the area of compression. Contrast the previous report from Neary and Eames[55] in 1975 of the patient with more severe ulnar nerve compression who had a more significant shift of fiber histogram in the ulnar nerve toward the left and had the mean fiber population shifted to the left in the distal segment, with accompanying Wallerian degeneration in some of the more distal fascicles. The patient reported by Neary and Eames had had the preoperative diagnosis of ulnar nerve compression but the patient had not been extensively evaluated.

Recently, we have had the opportunity to examine bilateral ulnar nerves from a patient with severe ulnar nerve compression.[58] One side had already had an anterior transposition of the ulnar nerve. The patient's electrodiagnostic studies had been carried out preoperatively, as well as an extensive clinical evaluation. The intraoperative appearance of the nerve previously operated on and that of the previously unoperated ulnar nerve are demonstrated in Figure 9-5. The histologic evaluation of the previously unoperated severely compressed ulnar nerve at the right elbow is demonstrated in Figure 9-5 d–g.

Preoperatively, the patient complained of persistent numbness and tingling in the little and ring fingers of each hand and over the dorsal aspect of each hand. He also complained of profound weakness in pinch and grip strength. He indicated that he was unable to utilize his hands to carry out movements easily. Seven years previously, he had had an anterior transposition of the left ulnar nerve at the elbow. This operation had not been successful in alleviating the problems in his hand. After the surgery, muscle wasting in each hand persisted. The preoperative examination demonstrated a 16 cm scar in the left elbow region. There was a bilateral, markedly positive Tinel's sign at each ulnar nerve. The right was located in the postcondylar groove. The left was located anterior to the medial humeral epicondyle, where the patient's nerve had been placed

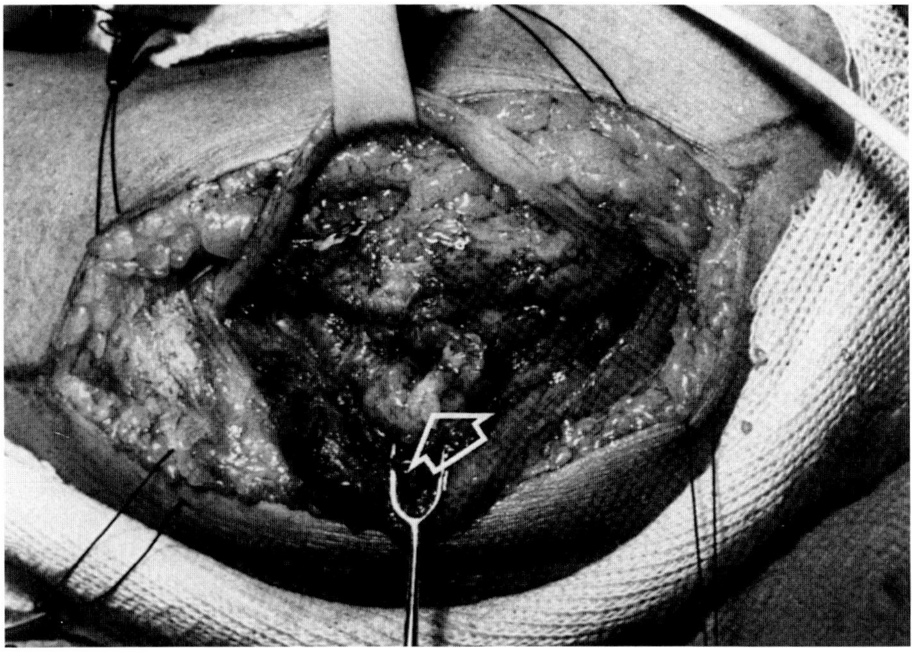

Figure 9-6. Diagnosis of ulnar nerve compression at the elbow: rheumatoid synovitis (arrow).

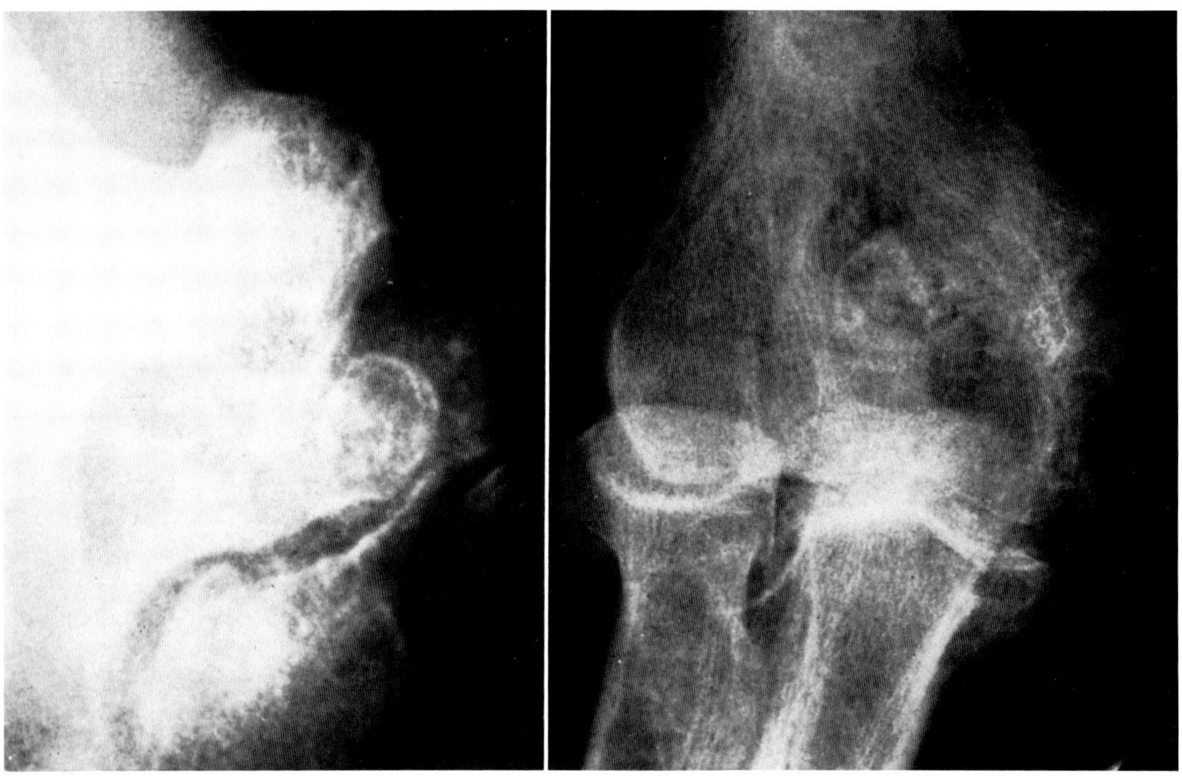

Figure 9-7. Diagnosis of ulnar nerve compression at the elbow: osteoarthritic bone spur.

in a subcutaneous position. Additionally on the left, there was pain in the scar with an area of distal diminished sensibility of the posteromedial aspect of the forearm. (For this complication of injured medial antebrachial cutaneous nerve,[50] see the later section on "Postoperative complications.") There was severe wasting of the first dorsal interosseous and a bilateral positive Froment's and Wartenberg's sign. Pinch strength in the right dominant hand was 10 pounds and 6 pounds in the left. Grip strength was 40 pounds in the right and 15 pounds in the left. There was barely a perceptible first dorsal interosseous function with attempted pinch. There was weakness to manual muscle testing of the flexor profundus to the little finger in each hand. There was decreased ability to cross the index and long fingers of each hand. There was abnormal vibratory perception that was decreased to the 256 cps vibratory stimuli in the little finger of each hand in comparison with the index finger of each hand. Moving two-point discrimination was 3 mm in the index finger of each hand, 6 mm in the right little finger, and 8 mm in the left little finger. Static two-point discrimination was 4 mm in each index finger, 6 mm in the right little finger, and 7 mm in the left little finger. There was markedly diminished moving-touch perception over the dorsal ulnar aspect of the left hand and just slightly reduced over the dorsal ulnar aspect of the right hand. There was normal strength in the wrist flexors.

At surgery, the left ulnar nerve was found to have been placed in a subcutaneous position with flexor pronator fascial structures having been sutured back over the nerve to maintain the position. The medial intermuscular septum was still in place and there was a neuroma of the medial antebrachial cutaneous nerve. A neuroma resection and an internal neurolysis of the ulnar nerve were carried out, and the medial intermuscular septum was resected. The flexor pronator muscle mass was elevated and the nerve placed in a submuscular location. The day after surgery, the patient sustained a fall, fracturing his hip. In the ensuing week after a hip-pinning procedure, the patient developed a pulmonary embolism and died. At autopsy, permission was obtained to take the bilateral ulnar nerves for morphometric assessment.

The right ulnar nerve was characterized by the severe fibrosis inside the nerve (Fig. 9-5a-c). Sunderland[11] has described the mechanism whereby some initial injury causes swelling within the ulnar nerve, and then subsequent chronic tension and friction between the ulnar nerve and its overlying fibrous aponeurosis and its bony confines cause persistent irritation, subsequent inflammation, leading ultimately to intraneural fibrosis. The histopathologic findings of the chronic ulnar nerve compression[55] and the subclinical ulnar nerve compression[56] reported by Neary and coworkers are demonstrated on the photomicrographs as interfascicular fibrosis. This was also confirmed by ourselves[58] (Fig. 9-5d-f). The implication for treatment, discussed later, is that in addition to the treatment of the external compression, surgical treatment should be directed at this intraneural fibrosis by doing a microsurgical internal neurolysis.

Diagnosis

The diagnosis of ulnar nerve compression at the elbow frequently can be suspected, if not made, at the initial interview with the patient if specific questions are asked. The patient's most common symptoms are numbness and tingling in the little and ring fingers. There may be complaints of pain. The pain is usually not in the little and ring fingers, but is frequently described as being at the elbow or along the medial aspect of the hand or forearm. Shooting pains may be described into the little and ring fingers. There are commonly complaints of weakness in the hand, of clumsiness, which may be described by the patient in terms of difficulty with writing or in carrying out fine manipulations. A common complaint of musicians is inability to play their instruments for prolonged periods of time or with the same dexterity that they previously had. Particularly, this is common in guitarists, those who play other stringed instruments, such as the violin, and in piano players, but similar complaints may be present in typists or in the dental hygienist who notes that she cannot manipulate the instruments as well. Another common complaint is of dropping things or being unable to open jars. These complaints are rarely, if ever, associated with median nerve problems unless there is severe loss of function in the muscles innervated by the anterior interosseous nerve or severe sensory loss in the median nerve. In particular, there is a pertinent negative question in the history: ulnar nerve compression in the elbow only occasionally awakens the patient from sleep. The patient is frequently aware that the symptoms are worsened with use of their hands, particularly when they have to do activities that cause the elbow to be flexed. Patients will say, for example, that their hands go numb when holding a steering wheel, when holding a hairdryer, or, most commonly, when holding a telephone for a prolonged period of time. Thus, activities requiring elbow flexion are implicated in the patient's symptoms.

During the history-taking, if ulnar nerve compression is suspected, a good technique is to ask the patient simply to flex their elbows while you are asking them questions and to let you know if "anything happens." In less than a minute, they frequently will describe numb-

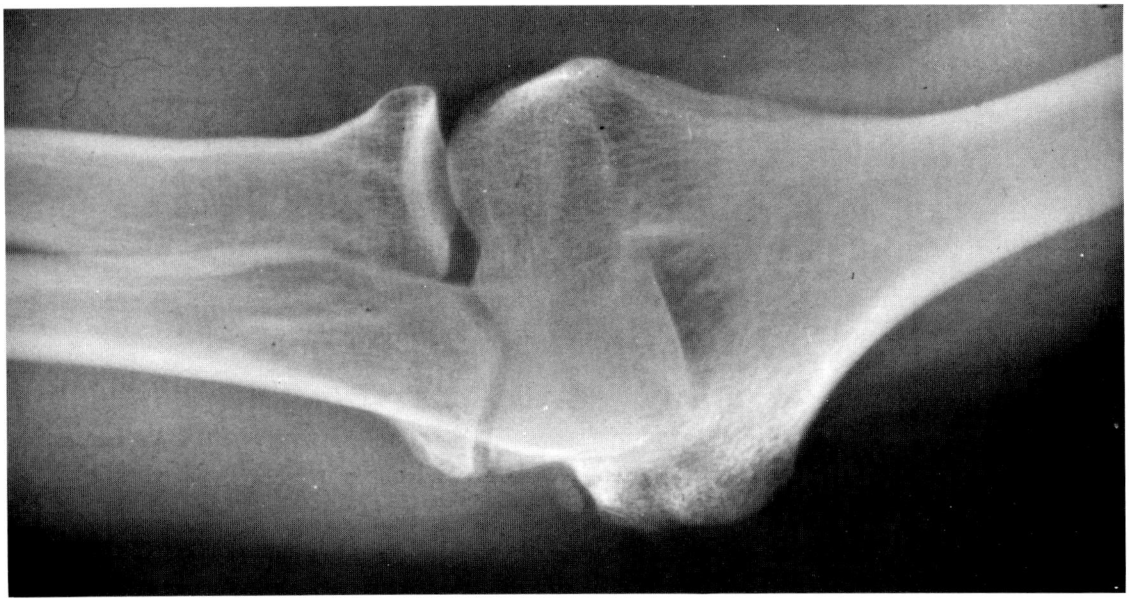

Figure 9-8. Diagnosis of ulnar nerve compression at elbow: childhood fracture with subsequent cubitus valgas.

ness or tingling in their little and ring fingers, or their whole hand is becoming cold. This provocative test, which we have always termed the elbow flexion test and which we have found to be quite reliable, has recently been presented and published as an abstract, correlating this finding with electrodiagnostic studies.[29] In particular, this "ulnar flexion maneuver" was found in 11 of 12 patients who had positive results to correlate with electrophysiologic criteria that is diagnostic of ulnar nerve compression at the elbow. Pressure over the ulnar nerve just proximal to the cubital tunnel with elbow flexion will hasten these symptoms.

Other important historical questions are: is there a history of trauma, such as a fracture (Figs. 9-8, 9-9) or fall, are work functions repetitive, for the disorder might be involved with occupations such as computer programming, assembly line work, desk job with external compression on the elbow. It is also important to rule out underlying medical problems that may make the patient more susceptible to nerve compression, such as diabetes, alcoholism, thyroid problems, or arthritic conditions associated with vasculitis, such as rheumatoid synovitis (Fig. 9-6) or arthritic conditions associated with hypertrophic bone spurs, such as osteoarthritis (Fig. 9-7). The following pertinent questions must be answered to rule out the possibility of the symptoms coming from a C8 or T1 radiculopathy or from compression of the lower trunks of the brachial plexus: Is there pain when the head is turned or extended? Is there aching in the neck and shoulders and worsening of the symptoms in the little and ring fingers when the arm is held elevated at the shoulder? The patients will occasionally complain of cramping in the small muscles of the hand and of the little and ring fingers pulling in toward the palm. (See Table 8-1).

The physical examination of the patient with signs of ulnar nerve compression at the elbow must produce evidence that the sensory and motor dysfunction of the ulnar nerve is occurring proximal to the wrist and distal to the brachial plexus, that sensory function in the little finger and half of the ring finger is diminished, and that there is ulnar-innervated muscle dysfunction only. The findings that there are abnormal perceptions of sensation over the dorsal ulnar aspect of the hand a Tinel's sign at the elbow (Figs. 9-10, 9-11) and that there is weakness in the ulnar wrist flexor (Fig. 9-12) and that there is weakness in the flexor digitorum profundus to the little finger all point to a location proximal to the wrist. This is because the dorsal ulnar branch of the ulnar nerve divides from the ulnar nerve approximately 9 cm proximal to the pisiform, the innervation to the flexor digitorum profundus to the ulnar nerve arises just proximal to the elbow and innervates the flexor muscles

Figure 9-9. Diagnosis of ulnar nerve entrapment: Complex elbow fracture treated open and no direct injury to ulnar nerve noted. Elbow flexion contracture developed and treatment with splint was instituted. Progressive ulnar nerve dysfunction **(a)** resulted in clawing **(b)**, Froment's sign **(c)**, note just 2 kg of pinch using flexor pollicis longus, and decreased vibratory perception **(d)**.

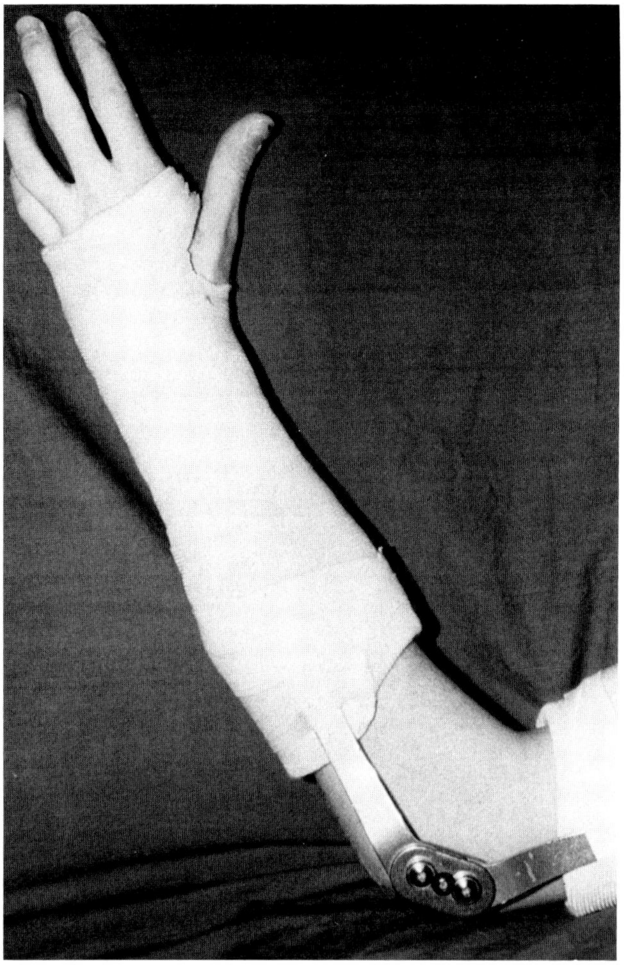

a

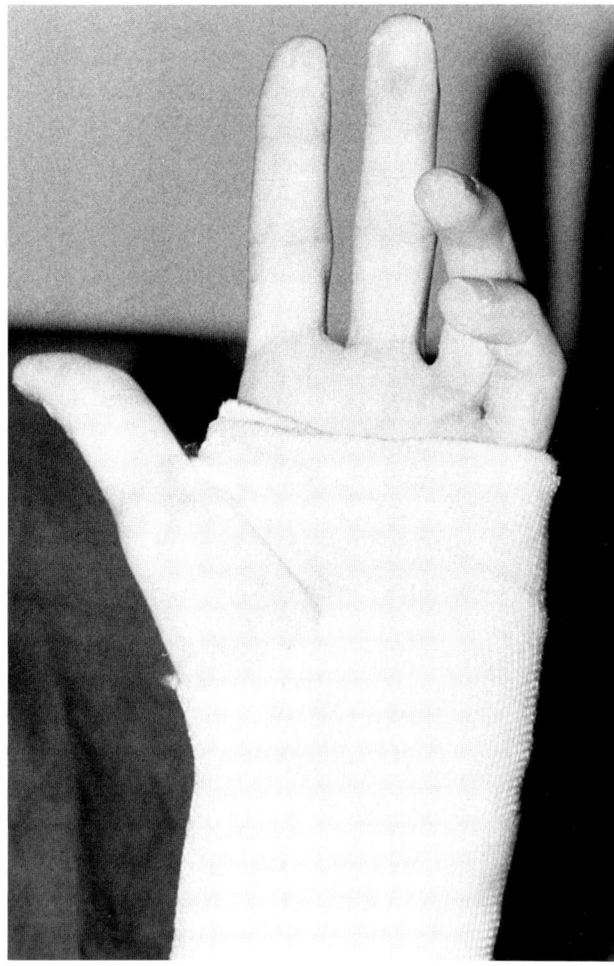

b

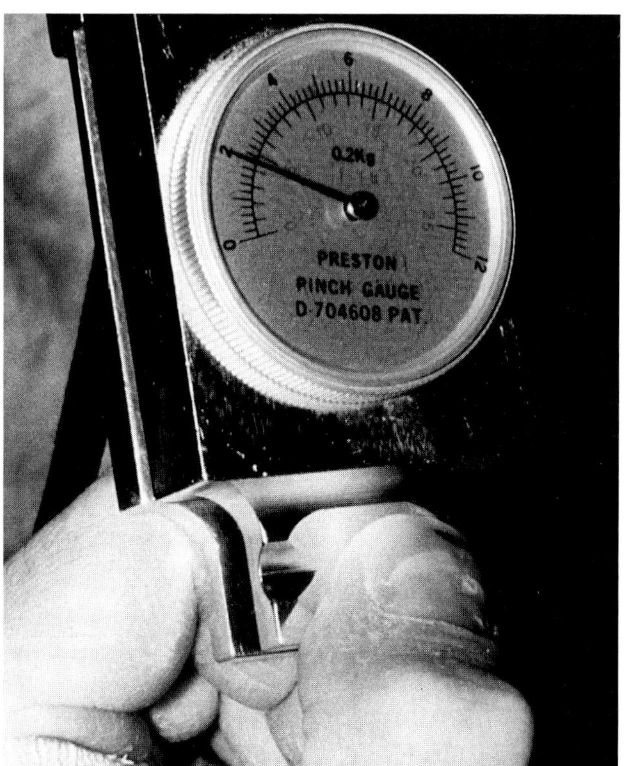

c

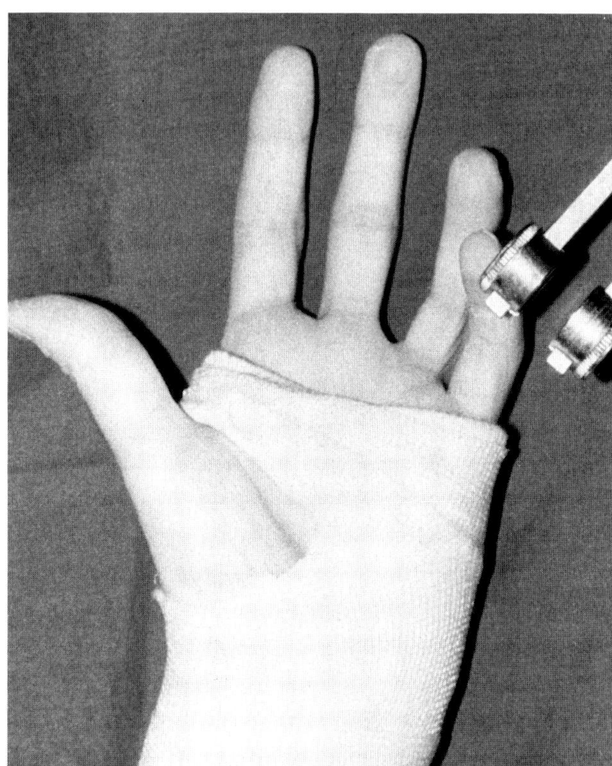

d

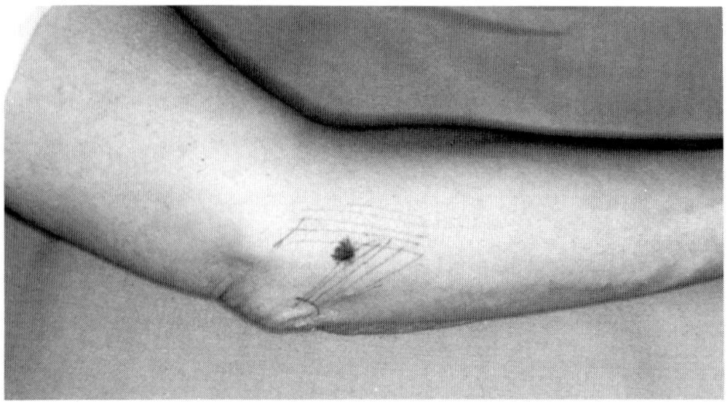
a

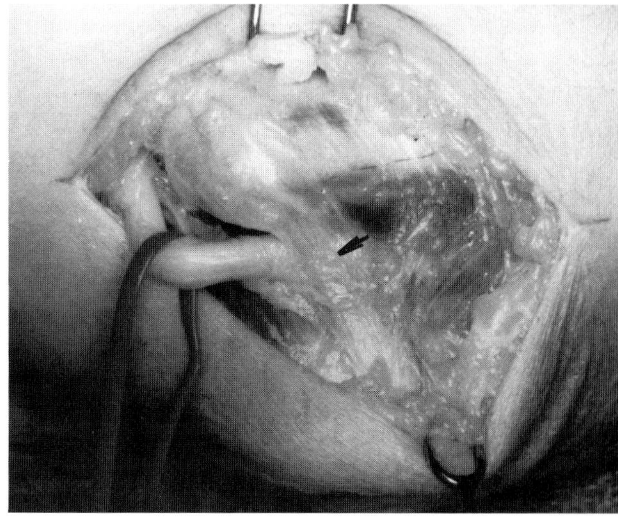
b

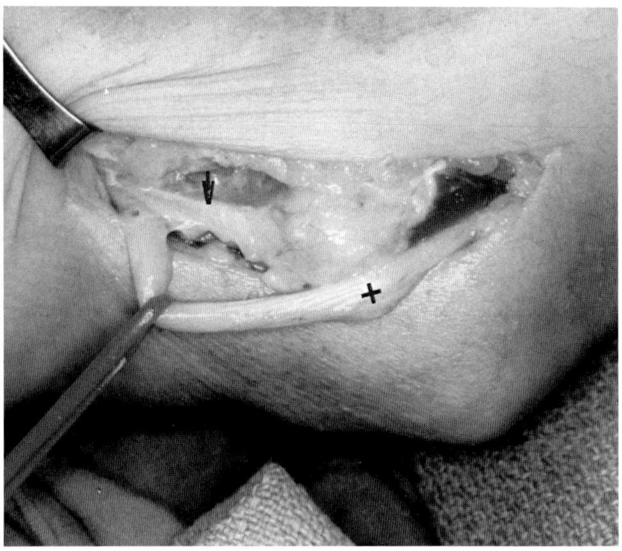
c

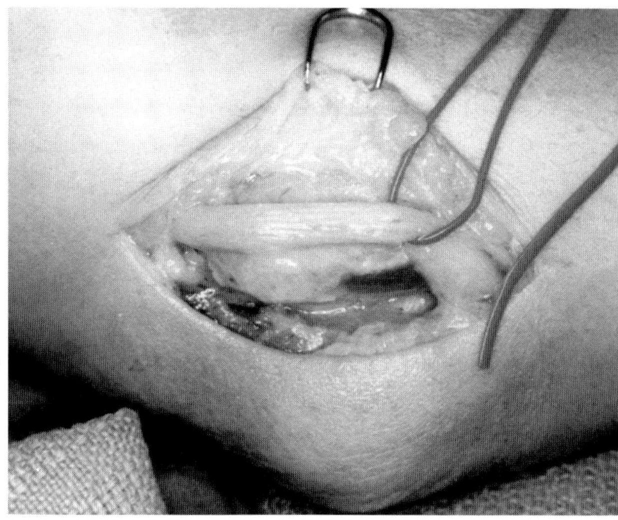
d

Figure 9-10. Diagnosis of ulnar nerve entrapment at elbow. **a.** A positive Tinel's sign at or proximal to Osborne's band. **b.** This correlates intraoperatively with Osborne's band (arrow) and (c) a mild pseudoneuroma (+). Note medial intermuscular septum (arrow). **d.** After internal neurolysis.

proximal third of the forearm, and the flexor carpi ulnaris branch comes off most proximal to the elbow and innervates the flexor carpi ulnaris just distal to the elbow. A localization proximal to the elbow, which does not mean that there is not a coexisting entrapment at the elbow, would be suggested by a positive Roos' sign (see Chapter 14), which is duplication of the patient's symptoms when the arm is elevated at the shoulder. This sign, combined with tenderness over the brachial plexus beneath the anterior scalene muscles, localizes to the plexus, itself. A more proximal site, that of a C8 or T1 radiculopathy, would include a demonstration of pain with neck movement and an abnormal triceps tendon reflex. With an even more central lesion, such as a syrinx, there would be wasting of the median-innervated intrinsic muscles, such as the opponens and abductor pollicis brevis, and there would be a dissociated sensory loss, so that touch sensation is present but pain, heat, and cold perception are absent. Wasting of all the intrinsic muscles in the presence of normal sensation might also suggest a motor neuron problem, such as amyotrophic lateral sclerosis.

Localization of ulnar nerve entrapment to the elbow on physical examination may also be determined by the presence of a positive Tinel's sign directly over the ulnar nerve in the postcondylar groove. This may be either directly at Osborne's band or at any site more proximal, including proximal to the medial humeral epicondyle, depending on the cause of the nerve compression in this region (Figs. 9-10 through 9-13). When the ulnar nerve compression is related to subluxation of the ulnar nerve, then the positive Tinel's sign in the site of most sensitivity is usually proximal to the medial humeral epicondyle. When the site of compression is again at the medial humeral epicondyle associated with a loud snapping sound, such as is made by a snapping of the medial head of the triceps over the medial humeral epicondyle, Tinel's sign[35–38] is also just proximal to the

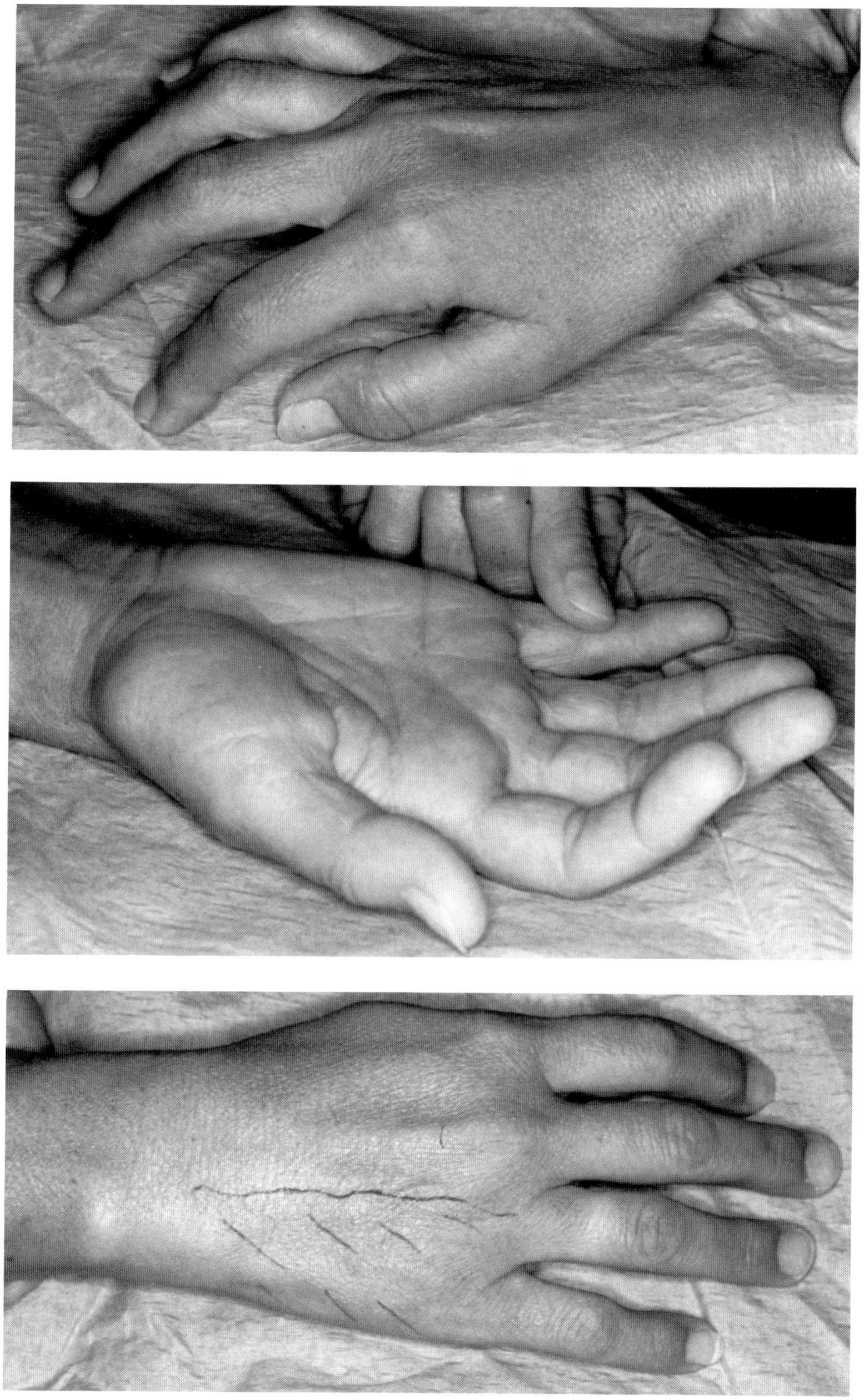

a

b

c

Figure 9-11. Diagnosis of ulnar nerve entrapment at the elbow. Previous injury: On physical examination, with a severe degree of compression, there is clawing of the little and ring fingers and wasting of the interossei muscles **(a)**, lack of profundus function to little finger **(b)** altered sensation over dorsal ulnar aspect of the hand **(c)** (*Figure continues.*)

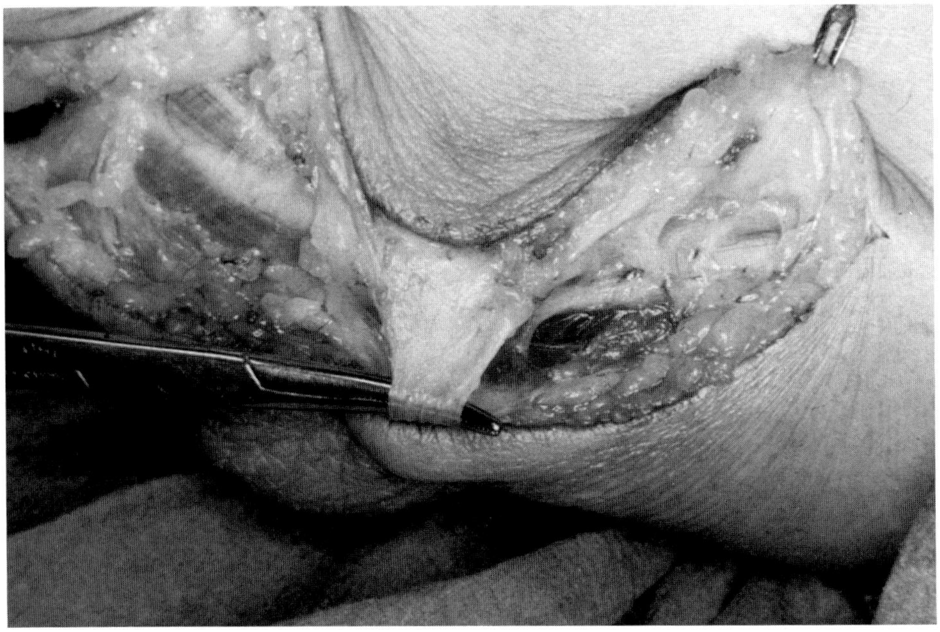

d

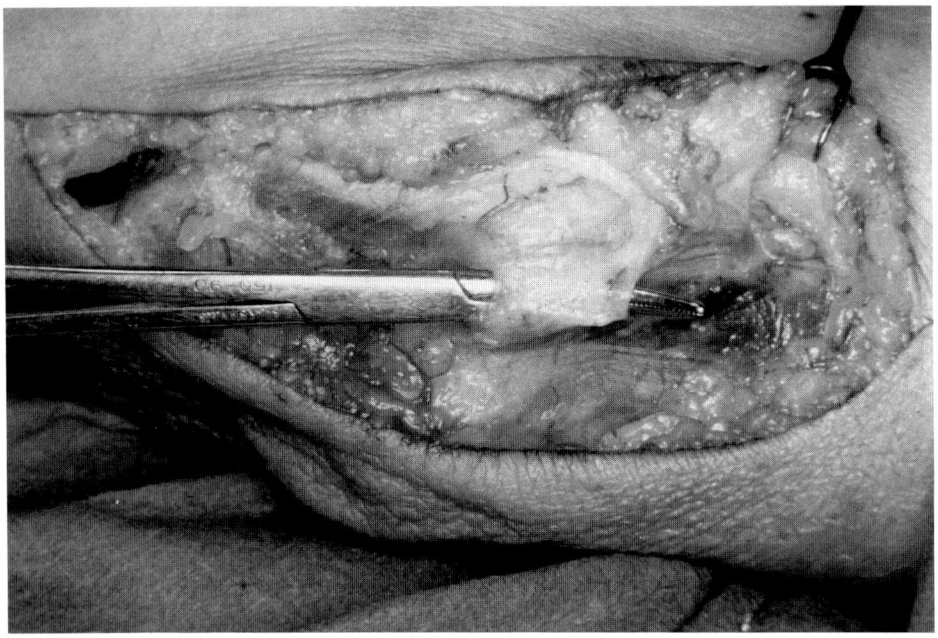

e

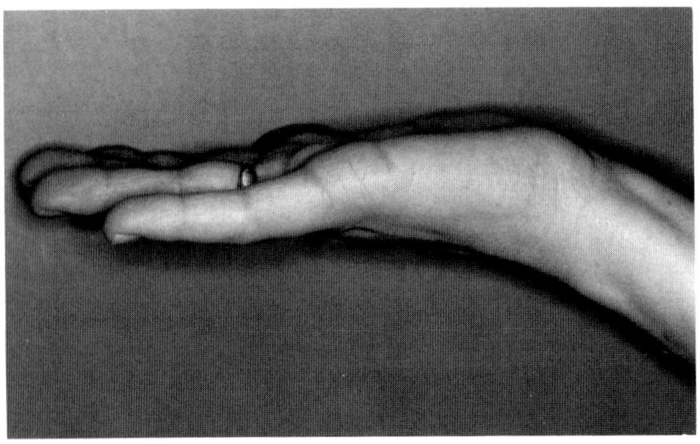

f

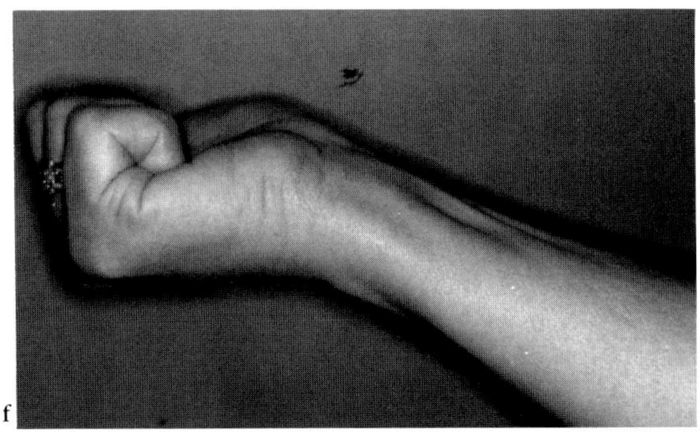

g

Figure 9-11 *(continued).* Subcutaneous fibrosis **(d)**, thickened roof of cubital tunnel due to blunt trauma **(e)**. Postoperatively there is no clawing **(f)** and good flexor profundus function **(g)**.

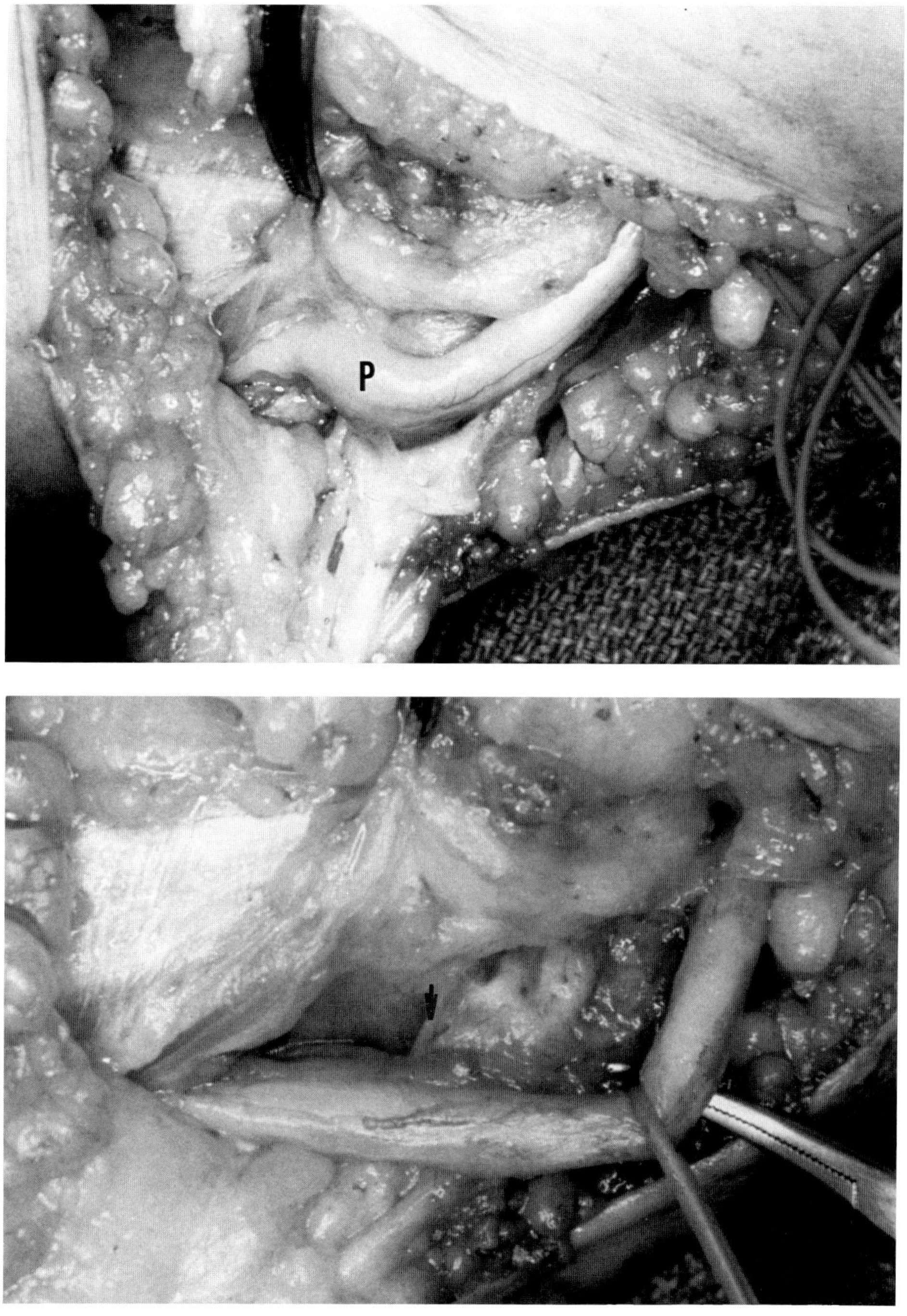

a

b

Figure 9-12. Diagnosis of ulnar nerve entrapment. This patient has had two previous ulnar nerve releases: the first a simple decompression; the second, an anterior subcutaneous transposition. Intraoperatively, there was compression still distally at Osborne's band site (clamp) and a pseudoneuroma (P) was present **(a)**. **b.** In the floor of the cubital tunnel was a band (arrow) running transversely across the postcondylar groove, where it could compress the deepest fascicles (which, according to Sunderland,[35] contain the fibers to the flexor carpi ulnaris (FCU) and flexor digitorum profundus (FDP) IV and V; (*Figure continues.*)

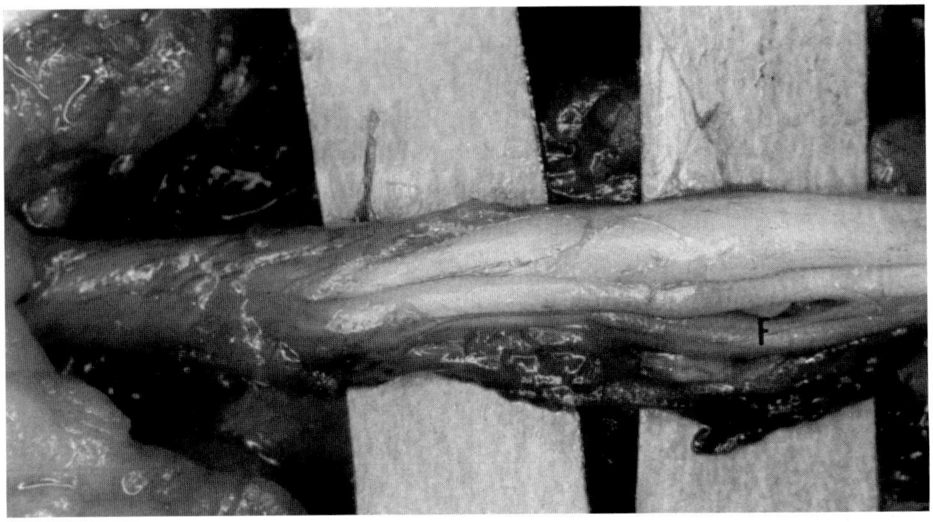

c

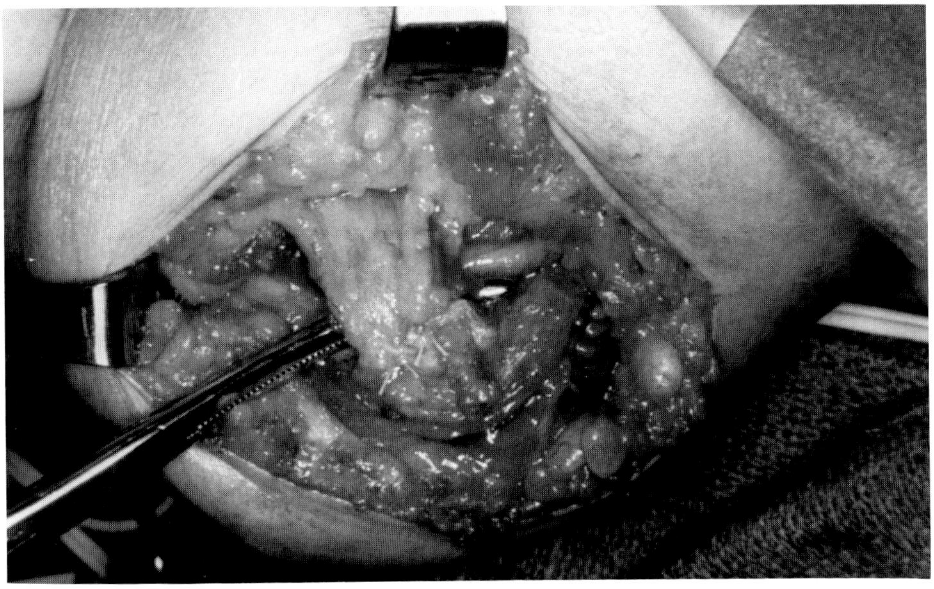

d

Figure 9-12 *(continued).* After neurolysis and after submuscular transposition (**c** and **d**). (F, fibers to FCU.)

medial humeral epicondyle. The examiner can determine an enlarged medial head of the triceps inserting into the postcondylar groove (Fig. 9-14),[32,33] contributing to ulnar nerve compression, by placing a finger in the postcondylar groove and having the patient attempt to extend the elbow. The large bulge in the medial head of the triceps may be palpated in this area, along with a pushing up of the ulnar nerve toward the medial humeral epicondyle. In this instance, the positive Tinel's sign is also just proximal to the medial humeral epicondyle. Palpation along the ulnar nerve in the postcondylar groove may demonstrate a swelling. This swelling may be the pseudoneuroma that has developed directly as a result of friction and intraneural fibrosis (Figs. 9-3, 9-10, 9-12) or may be due to the presence of a tumor, such as a ganglion, or a neural tumor, such as a schwannoma. The presence of such a mass in this region clearly helps to localize the problem to this area. A positive Tinel's sign may be noted in patients who previously had some type of anterior transposition. When this Tinel's sign is located proximal to the medial humeral epicondyle and along the course of the medial intermuscular septum, it generally means that the medial intermuscular septum (Fig. 9-10) was either not excised or was incompletely excised and that the ulnar nerve as it crosses this structure has found a new site of entrapment (see also section "Postoperative Complications"). In a patient who has had an ulnar nerve transposed, there may be a Tinel's sign distal to the medial humeral epicondyle. Here the ulnar nerve is usually compressed against the periosteal origin of the flexor carpi ulnaris (Figs. 9-19, 9-20). See also "Surgical Technique".

The patient may have ulnar nerve compression at

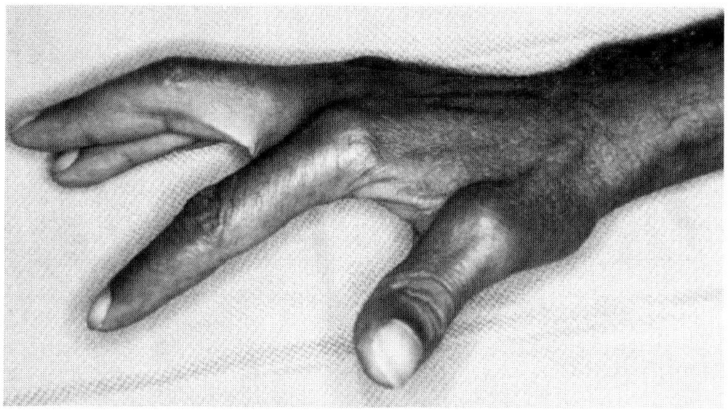

a

Figure 9-13. Diagnosis of ulnar nerve compression at the elbow. Severe first dorsal interosseous wasting **(a)**, due to presence of an Osborne's band **(b)**.

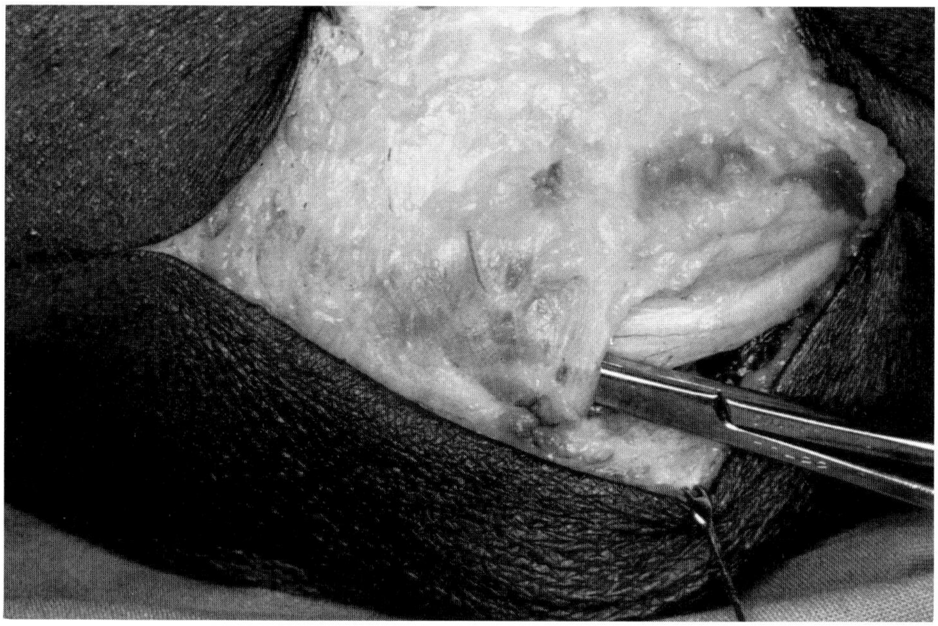

b

the elbow in the absence of a Tinel's sign. Early in the course of nerve compression and there are no neural structures that are regenerating, or when it is extremely late in the course of ulnar nerve compression and none of the degenerated structures are capable of regenerating, then Tinel's sign will be absent[59] (Tables 9-6, 9-7). The physical examination for determining sensory and motor dysfunction is given in detail in Chapter 3. Vibratory testing becomes abnormal first (Fig. 9-9). Vibratory perception is first increased in early ulnar nerve compression and then decreased with more advanced ulnar nerve compression[28,60] (Table 9-8). The moving and static two-point discrimination do not become abnormal until the more severe degree of ulnar nerve compression[61] (Table 9-9), at which point there is often wasting of the intrinsic muscles (Figs. 9-10 through 9-13).

Provocative tests for ulnar nerve dysfunction at the elbow include the elbow flexion test,[29] direct compression over the ulnar nerve at the elbow, following which numbness and tingling will be either increased or brought on, and the placement of a tourniquet about the upper arm, after which, over a very short period of time, numbness and tingling will be brought on in the distribution of the ulnar nerve. In this latter provocative test, the time at which this occurs should be compared with that in a contralateral asymptomatic extremity.

The Froment sign[62] and the Wartenberg sign[63] are indicative of ulnar nerve compression but are not helpful in localizing the site of the compression.

The diagnosis of ulnar nerve compression at the elbow provides the basis for a clinical staging classification. The information obtained in order to make the diagnosis of ulnar nerve compression at the elbow provides the information necessary to categorize the patient's degree of compression into either mild, moderate, or severe. An attempt to do this has been made in the past primarily by McGowan[25] (Table 9-3). McGowan's classification was listed as grades I, II, and III and these were termed "minimal, intermediate, and severe." This staging classification made no mention of

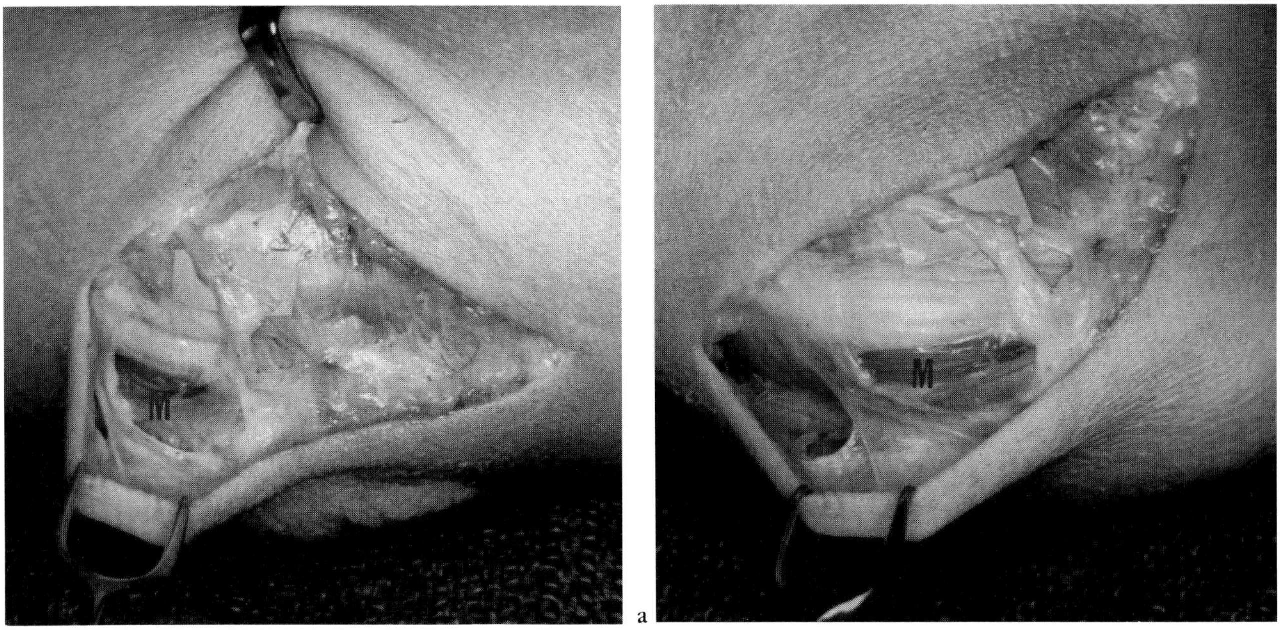

a b

Figure 9-14. Diagnosis of ulnar nerve compression at the elbow. The medial antebrachial cutaneous nerve, preserved at background. **a.** Medial head of triceps (M) is large and inserts into floor of the cubital tunnel. Note change that occurs in relationships of muscle, ulnar nerve, and medial humeral epicondyle as elbow moves from extension **(a)** to flexion **(b)**. With flexion, there is ulnar nerve subluxation **(b)**.

sensory changes and the degree of sensory impairment from ulnar nerve compression at the elbow did not make a difference in her staging system. Dawson et al[51] have modified McGowan's classification to include a sensory descriptor (Table 9-9). However, this classification is inadequate because it considers persistent symptoms as a moderate degree of compression, whereas it would better be placed into the severe category, as determined from the pathophysiologic findings of nerve compression (see before and Chapter 2). Persistent symptoms imply the presence of intraneural fibrosis, which implies the need for internal neurolysis (see Chapter 5 and the "Nonoperative Treatment" and "Results" sections later). Furthermore, Dawson et al continued to use the terminology of McGowan, which confused the word "paresis" with "paralysis." These investigators also do not clearly distinguish between weakness and atrophy. Most writers have not distinguished between atrophy, weakness, and wasting. The term "paralysis," means a loss of power of voluntary movement in a muscle. This may be due either to injury or disease of the muscle, itself, or of its nerve supply (also has a sensory meaning). Paralysis in the sensory system means anesthesia, a loss of sensation in a part. Paresis means "partial or incomplete paralysis." Atrophy means a wasting of tissues and implies degeneration.[64] Weakness does not imply atrophy and is not synonymous with atrophy or wasting. A muscle can be weak without atrophy being present. Weakness is therefore not synonymous with paralysis. Weakness would be more synonymous with paresis. Because the grading system for ulnar nerve compression should include sensory and motor components and because the intraneural topography may permit an uneven distribution of pressure to sensory or motor fibers, separate clear definitions of minimal or mild, moderate, and severe must be included in the classification system. Because the term "paralysis" can be applied to either motor or sensory component of the nervous system, it should not be included in the staging definitions. Terms that clearly relate to either motor or sensory function should be utilized. The staging system recommended is given in Table 9-10. This is similar to one proposed by Osborne,[65] and later modified by him[66] (Table 9-11).

The conceptual basis for the staging of ulnar nerve compression at the elbow, given in Table 9-10, is that with a mild degree of nerve compression, the patient has symptoms. The only findings present on physical examination may be those induced by provocative tests, such as the elbow flexion pressure test or tapping over the ulnar nerve in the postcondylar groove. In terms of treatment (see "Nonoperative Treatment" section

Table 9-6. Human Ulnar Nerve Compression at the Elbow, Clinical Correlation, Nerve Conduction Study*

	Latency (ms)				
Nerve	*Onset*	*Peak*	*Distance (mm)*	*Velocity* (ms^{-1})	*Amplitude* (μv)
Right ulnar					
Digit 5 to wrist	2.9	3.6	146	48	6
Wrist to ADM†	3.3				5,000
Below elbow to ADM	8.1		265	55	5,000
Above elbow to ADM	10.3		110	50	2,500
Across elbow				(70)	
Left ulnar					
Digit 5 to wrist	NR†				
Wrist to ADM	2.7				5,000
Below elbow to ADM	8.1		275	51	4,500
Above elbow to ADM	12.8		125	27	3,500
Across elbow (derived velocity)				(32)	
Left median					
Digit 2 to wrist	3.5	4.1	162	46	6
Wrist to APB†	4.5				10,000
Elbow to APB	9.5		272	54	10,000
F wave	33.8				
Right median					
Digit 2 to wrist	2.9	3.5	145	48	11
Wrist to APB	3.7				10,000
Elbow to APB					10,000

*Reprinted with permission from Dellon and Mackinnon.[58]

†ADM: adductor digiti minimi; APB: abductor pollicis brevis; NR: no reaction.

Table 9-7. Human Ulnar Nerve Compression at Elbow, Morphometric Evaluation*

	Mean Fiber Diameter (± SD)	*Neural Tissue (%)*	*Myelin (%)*	*Axon/Myelin Ratio*
Right ulnar nerve				
Proximal	6.6 ± 2.38	31	66	0.5
Cubital tunnel	5.0 ± 2.37	29	49	1.0
Distal	6.6 ± 2.87	34	63	0.6
Left ulnar nerve				
Proximal	6.9 ± 3.1	34	64	0.5
Cubital tunnel	5.2 ± 1.69	15	36	1.7
Distal	4.1 ± 1.28	10	52	0.5

*Reprinted with permission from Dellon and Mackinnon.[58]

Table 9-8. Physical Diagnosis in Ulnar Nerve Compression at the Elbow: Sensory Changes Related to Stage of Severity*

	Vibratory Threshold (%)					*Innervation Density (%)*	
		Qualitative (Tuning Fork)				*Two-Point Discrimination*	
		30 Hz		*256 Hz*			
Clinical Stage	*Quantitative (Vibrometer % Abnormal)*	*Increased*	*Decreased*	*Increased*	*Decreased*	*(≥ 6 mm) Static*	*(≥ 4 mm) Moving*
Mild	50	100	0	100	0	0	0
Moderate	33	0	33	0	33	0	0
Severe	100	0	80	0	100	80	100

*Reprinted with permission from Dellon.[60]

Table 9-9. Staging of Ulnar Nerve Compression at the Elbow: Dawson et al's Classification*

Group I	Recent and mild symptoms of intermittent paresthesias and hypoesthesia
Group II	Persistent symptoms and varying degrees of weakness and intrinsic atrophy
Group III	Marked intrinsic muscle atrophy, weakness and deformity

*Reprinted with permission from Dawson et al.[51]

Table 9-10. Proposed Staging of Ulnar Nerve Compression at the Elbow

Stage	Category	Findings
Mild	Sensory	Paresthesias come and go
		Vibratory perception increased
	Motor	Subjective weakness, clumsiness, or loss of coordination
	Tests	Elbow flexion test or Tinel's sign or both are positive
Moderate	Sensory	Paresthesias come and go
		Vibratory perception normal or decreased
	Motor	Measurable weakness in the pinch or grip strength
	Tests	Elbow flexion test or Tinel's sign or both are positive
		Finger crossing may be abnormal
Severe	Sensory	Paresthesias are persistent
		Vibratory perception decreased
		Abnormal two-point discrimination
	Motor	Measurable weakness in pinch and grip plus muscle atrophy
	Test	Positive elbow flexion test or positive Tinel's sign or both may be present
		Finger crossing usually abnormal

later), this group has the best potential to be improved by nonoperative means. The mild group primarily has changes related to altered motor and sensory thresholds. In contrast, in the severe group, the ulnar nerve compression has progressed to the point where there is degeneration in the motor and sensory nerves, which leads to loss of nerve fibers. In the motor system, this induces atrophy. In the sensory system, it induces loss of innervation density. Thus, the physical examination reflects on the motor system weakness plus atrophy and in the sensory system changes in vibratory and pressure thresholds plus loss of innervation density abnormal static and moving two-point discrimination (Table 9-8). In the moderate degree of staging, there has not been a significant degree of Wallerian degeneration. There are more advanced changes in threshold. For the motor system, this translates into measurable weakness in pinch and grip strength. In the sensory system, it translates into diminished thresholds that may be detected with von Frey hairs or with cutaneous pressure threshold testing, such as the Semmes-Weinstein monofilaments, or by use of the vibrometer[60] for quantitative testing or the tuning fork for a qualitative testing technique.[28] Electrodiagnostic testing is described in the next section. Electrodiagnostic testing does not directly relate to this clinical staging category. However, if with nerve conduction there is no obtainable sensory conduction, or with electromyography there are denervation potentials present, then the electrical testing has demonstrated evidence of denervation, and conceptually patients with these findings on the electrodiagnostic testing would be categorized in the severe group. Table 9-4 presents an attempt at staging of ulnar nerve compression into mild and severe but does not categorize severity based on nerve fiber degeneration.[27] (This is discussed further in the next section.)

Table 9-11. Grades of Ulnar Neuritis as Described by Osborne[65,66]

	Sensory	*Motor*
1. Subjective features only	Tingling, numbness Discomfort in hypothenar muscles	Clumsiness and weakness of fingers Loss of dexterity
2. Early objective signs	Hypoesthesia and paresthesia to touch or pressure. Sensation to light touch and pinprick diminished TPD abnormal	Slight intrinsic wasting and "objective" weakness of intrinsics Little finger stands away from ring. Early clawing
3. Established clinical pattern of ulnar neuritis	Well-marked sensory deficit in ulnar distribution. Sweating diminished, skin dry	Obvious intrinsic wasting and weakness Clawing of ring and little fingers
4. Advanced ulnar palsy Compare ulnar nerve division	Total sensory anesthesia and loss of sweating	Paralysis of all intrinsics, weakness of long flexors

Electrodiagnostic Testing

The use of electrodiagnostic techniques for making a diagnosis of ulnar nerve compression at the elbow can be very helpful. In the previous section it was indicated that with a careful history and physical examination, the clinician may arrive at a diagnosis of ulnar nerve compression at the elbow without doing electrodiagnostic testing. Electrodiagnostic testing may be specifically recommended when difficult diagnostic problems occur. This is commonly seen in the setting of multiple sites of nerve compression, such as the patient who complains of neck pain, shoulder and anterior chest discomfort, numbness in the little and ring fingers, where the localization to cervical spine, thoracic outlet, wrist, or elbow may be difficult to determine. Furthermore, some patients are truly difficult to examine. Some are examined in the setting of a work-related injury or of a car accident where litigation is involved. Some patients have had previous surgery. Some patients have difficulty communicating their symptoms. All of these are excellent indications for preoperative electrodiagnostic testing.

There are ample reports in the literature in which results of electrodiagnostic testing do not correlate or correlate only imprecisely with the patient's symptoms. For example, Wilson and Krout[67] found that after surgery nerve conduction studies did not correlate with the clinical improvements in their patients and could not distinguish between the patient who had a good or bad result from surgery. One of the most important pathophysiologic reasons for lack of correlation is that the demyelination that accompanies nerve compression (see previous section on "Histopathology" and Chapter 2) causes delays in motor and sensory nerve conduction, but this may be unrelated to the clinical situation. Myelin thinning and nerve conduction delay do not correlate with muscle atrophy and loss of sensory receptors. Thus, there may be early electrical changes in patients who do not have significant nerve compression. Conversely, with early nerve compression, there is an associated neural ischemia that immediately translates into symptoms for the patient and yet at this stage there may be no electrical changes. These types of correlation have been carefully made for the carpal tunnel syndrome[68] in which 20% of patients with mild carpal tunnel syndrome had normal electrodiagnostic studies and 20% of patients with clinically severe carpal tunnel syndrome still had normal electrodiagnostic studies.

There should be no need for routine preoperative electrodiagnostic testing. Clark[69] has written that "in evaluating a case for signs of cubital tunnel syndrome ... clinical signs are more reliable than electrical studies." Even a study designed to define the electrical abnormalities in this syndrome found 80% of "mild" and 47% of "severe" cubital tunnel syndrome patients to have normal electrical values for motor conduction velocity across the elbow.[27] The most common electrical abnormality in that study, the motor latency from elbow to abductor digiti minimi, was still found to be normal in 37% of the "mild" and 9% of the "severe" clinical cases. Foster and Edshage,[70] in a study of 110 patients over a 10-year period indicated "electromyography was not performed on any patient in this study." Similarly, MacNichol,[71] in a review of 100 patients treated surgically for ulnar nerve compression at the elbow over a 10-year period, noted that "nerve conduction studies were seldom available." Of Lugnegard et al's[72] 33 patients, 20 did not have preoperative electrical testing. Of Chan et al's[73] 235 patients, 45 did not have preoperative electrical testing. Although there are studies in which all of those patients who had preoperative electrical studies had positive studies,[74–77] only Craven and Green[78] have indicated that "a normal (electrodiagnostic) value is a contraindication to surgery." Yet there are studies reported in which patients with preoperative "normal values" have been operated on. Of Paine's[79] 63 patients, 35 had preoperative electrical studies and 11 of these 35 were *normal.* Of Eaton et al's[80] 16 patients, ten had preoperative testing and two of the ten were normal. Of Culver's[81] 46 patients, just 15 had preoperative testing and 6 of these 15 were normal. It is clear from this discussion that there is a wide spectrum of the use of preoperative electrical testing. It is also clear that *there is no reason to deny surgery to a patient with a normal preoperative electrical study, or to require all patients to have such a study if the history and physical examination of the patient are themselves consistent with ulnar nerve compression at the elbow.* (See Fig. 9-15 and discussion on electrodiagnostic testing after anterior transposition of the ulnar nerve in the "Results" section of Chapter 9. See also Chapter 3.)

Nonoperative Treatment

Once a diagnosis of ulnar nerve compression at the elbow has been made based on the patient's history and physical examination, and supplemented by electrodiagnostic testing if necessary, the treatment decision is initially based on the degree of severity of the nerve compression. For a patient with a mild degree of nerve compression, the initial treatment is nonoperative. Since, as described previously, the pathophysiologic mechanism involves increased pressure on the ulnar nerve in the cubital tunnel with degrees of elbow flex-

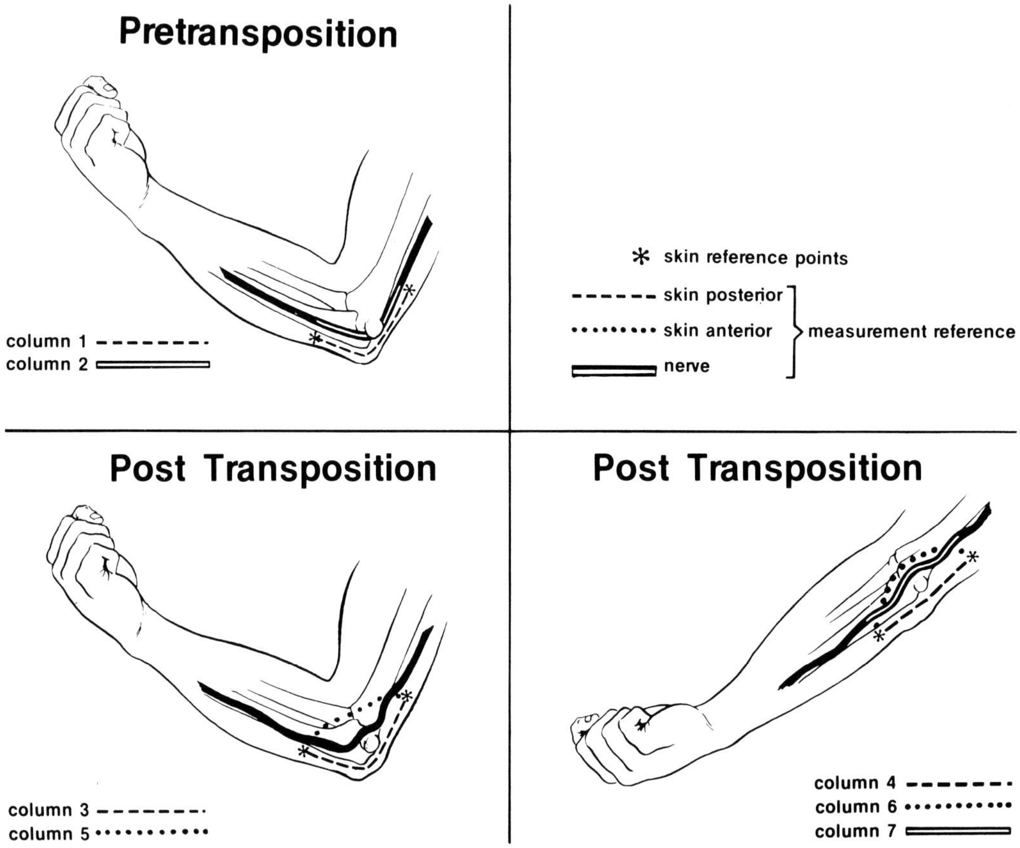

Figure 9-15. Electrodiagnostic testing pitfalls with respect to the ulnar nerve at the elbow. Examples of combination of skin distance marking and elbow positions used in Table 9-21. Left side has elbow flexed, right side with elbow extended. Top is pretransposition; bottom is post-transposition. For the same patient, same nerve, varying the skin site marking from anterior to posterior or the elbow position from flexed to extended can cause changes in the conduction velocity across the elbow to vary up to 10 m/s. (Reproduced with permission from Dellon et al.[112])

ion and shoulder abduction, aggravated by shear, friction, and tension forces with repetitive elbow flexion, the nonoperative treatment is based on maintaining the elbow in a nonflexed position (Fig. 9-2). It is recognized that a patient may not successfully get through a day without severe inconvenience if the elbow is prevented from flexing at all. Thus, placing the patient in a cast or a nonremovable splint is not recommended. Removable elbow splints that prevent the patient from assuming a fully flexed position at the elbow can be used. We have found that the standard hockey elbow pads are frequently satisfactory. The patient is instructed to sleep with the arm at his side, and, to facilitate this, he may wrap a rolled-up towel about his arm. He may set the alarm clock to awaken him at 1 or 2 o'clock in the morning and readjust his position until this habit is learned. He is instructed not to sleep with his arm curled about him. When he is working at a desk, he is instructed to place a padded pillow beneath his elbow and sit with his chair farther from the desk so that his forearm rests on the desk. If the patients have an occupation requiring work at a typewriter or computer console where the elbow and wrist are flexed, they are instructed to alter the angle of the computer console and the height of the desk chair to bring the wrist into a neutral position and the elbow in only 30° of flexion. If they do a significant amount of reading, they are instructed to get a reading stand. This may be placed on the bed to straddle their legs and then the arm only needs to be raised to turn the page, not to hold the book. They are instructed not to leave their elbow flexed on the window sill of a car. They are instructed when relaxing to sit with the arm placed in the lap and the forearm supinated and the elbow in 30° of flexion. They are instructed not to cross their arms or to lean their head on their hand. They are instructed to minimize the use of the telephone in this hand and if their occupation requires considerable telephone use, they are instructed to get a headset or a speakerphone. Work routines or schedules, musical practice schedules, and other activities must be altered to accommodate to these new requirements until the patient's symptoms are improved. Such treatment is continued for 3 months and then the patient is reevaluated. If there is no worsening of the clinical status, that is, if the patient has not moved into the moderate degree of nerve compression, then they may continue in this nonoperative treatment mode for an additional 3 months and then be reevaluated. If they have worsened, then a surgical approach should be considered. If the patient presents with a moderate degree of nerve compression or has moved from a minimal to a moderate degree, there is still the possibility that they may be improved with nonoperative techniques and the treatment routine outlined above is utilized for a 3-month period and the patient then is reevaluated. If the patient in the moderate degree has such severity of symptoms that he refuses or tires of the nonoperative technique and cannot sustain the alterations in daily and work activities, then a surgical approach may be considered. If the patient presents with a severe degree of nerve compression, then the possibility for improvement with nonoperative technique does not exist or is vanishingly small. The patient with a severe degree of nerve compression is a surgical candidate unless surgery is refused.

Surgical Technique

Once the diagnosis of ulnar nerve compression at the elbow has been made (see previous section), decision analysis may be utilized to select from the treatment options. Although various algorithms have been suggested for treatment methods[51,109] (Fig. 9-16) if surgery is selected, then the surgical technique that we recommend is the anterior submuscular transposition. James Learmonth, writing from Edinburgh, described the technique in 1942[82] (Fig. 9-17). His article, which is just two pages in length, contains 11 figures. They are artist drawings. He reported no patients. He gave no statements as to the success he had with this operation. His rationale for doing a submuscular placement was that he believed he "placed the nerve in an intermuscular interval where nerves normally run." The technique Learmonth illustrated clearly shows *excision* of the medial intermuscular septum and placement of the ulnar nerve to lie on the brachialis muscle. It shows the flexor pronator muscle mass cut obliquely and sutured back to itself in place. Adson's[14] 1928 diagram shows the medial intermuscular septum left intact and Platt's[9] 1928 diagram clearly shows this septum *incised.* Shelden's[19] 1921 article had no diagram to illustrate his transposition technique and his text did not mention

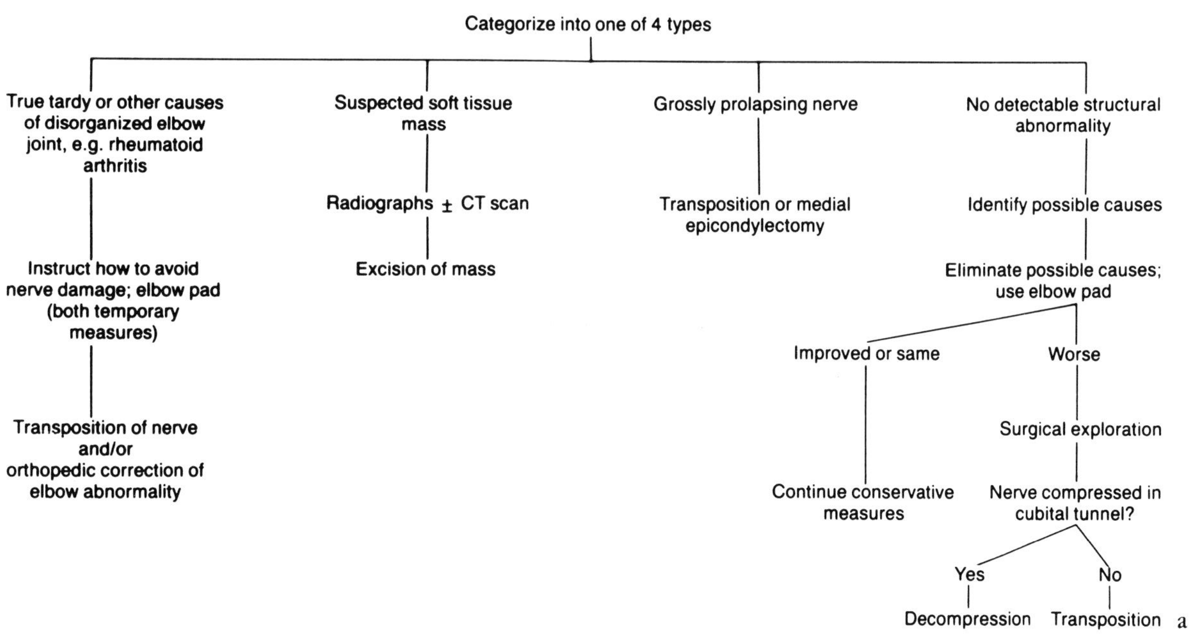

Figure 9-16. Treatment decisions for ulnar nerve compression at the elbow: algorithm for patient management based upon patient symptoms **(a)**[51] or based on cause of compression **(b)**.[109]

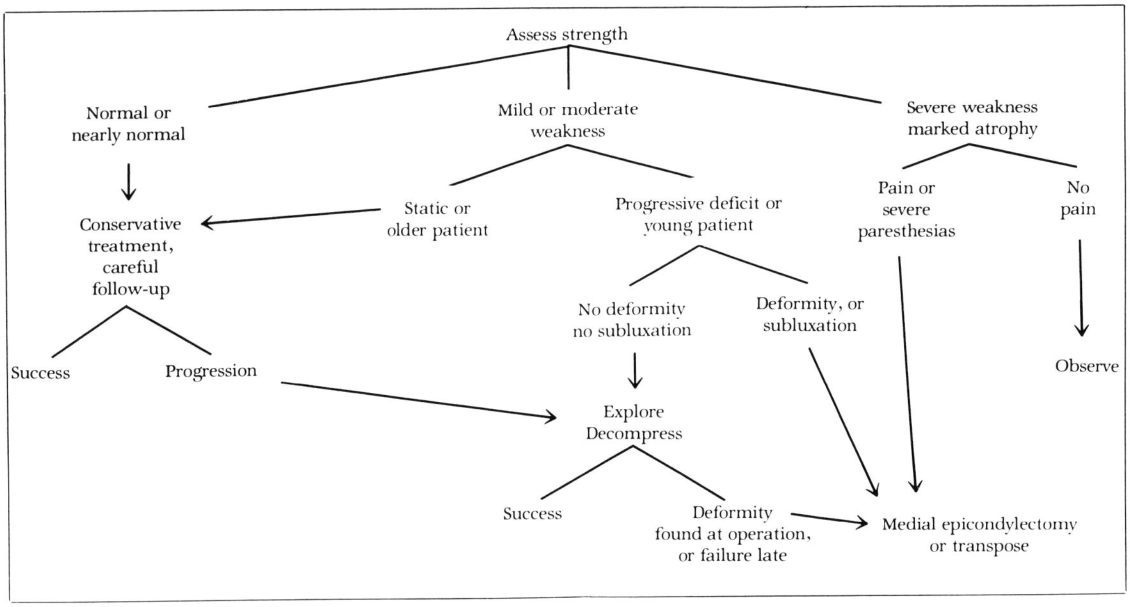

Figure 9-16 *(continued).*

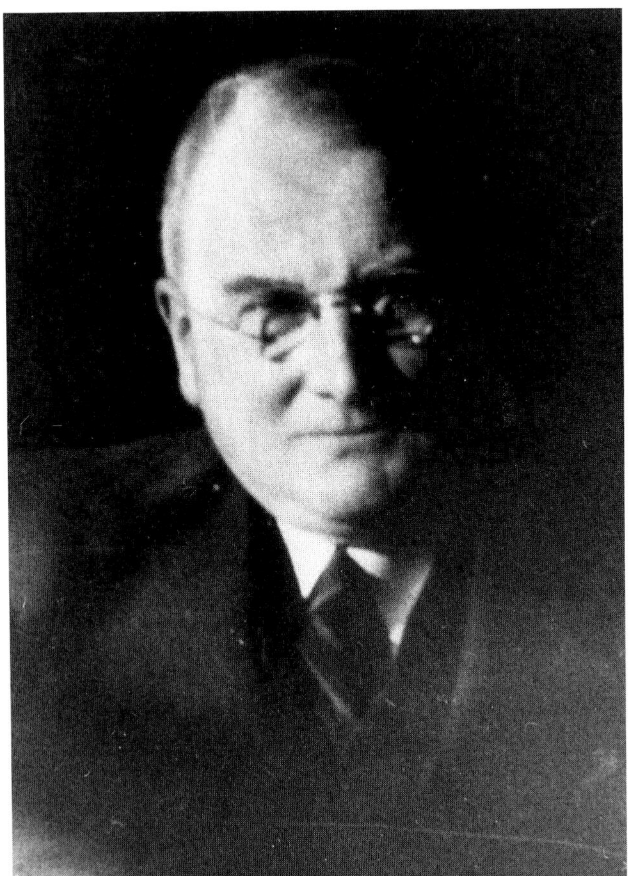

Figure 9-17. Sir James Learmonth, taken in 1949 when Learmonth was visiting professor at Queen's University, Kingston, Canada. (Photo courtesy of R. B. Lynn, M. D., cardiovascular surgeon. Photo by Knowles.)

this septum. As will be discussed in the "Results" section later, many of the reports with the use of submuscular placement still have a significant percentage of patients who do not achieve excellent results and who have persistent symptoms. The experience gained in carrying out the submuscular transposition has indicated that it must be done with meticulous detail so that there are no future proximal or distal sites of impingement as the nerve is moved into its new site. Simply decompressing the nerve is easily accomplished. Ensuring that the new location for the nerve will have no future sites for problems requires careful attention to surgical detail.

The modifications that have evolved in the use of this technique[83] include a step-cut lengthening of the flexor pronator muscle fascia, which lengthens this origin by approximately 1.5 cm, thereby ensuring that the new tunnel into which the ulnar nerve is placed, that is, the new attachment of the flexor pronator muscle mass, does not put presure against the underlying ulnar nerve. Additionally, it has been noted that the periosteal origin of the flexor carpi ulnaris head from the ulna, that is, distal to the medial humeral epicondyle, may serve as the same source for future entrapment, or failure, that the medial intermuscular septum serves proximal to the medial humeral epicondyle. Attention is therefore paid to protecting the ulnar nerve while placing tension on the flexor carpi ulnaris origin and dividing distally this periosteal origin. The common flexor origin is not only divided but also released distally, permitting the entire flexor-pronator muscle mass to slide distally, thus opening the space for the transposed ulnar nerve. Surgical technique is summarized in Figure 9-18 and is explained

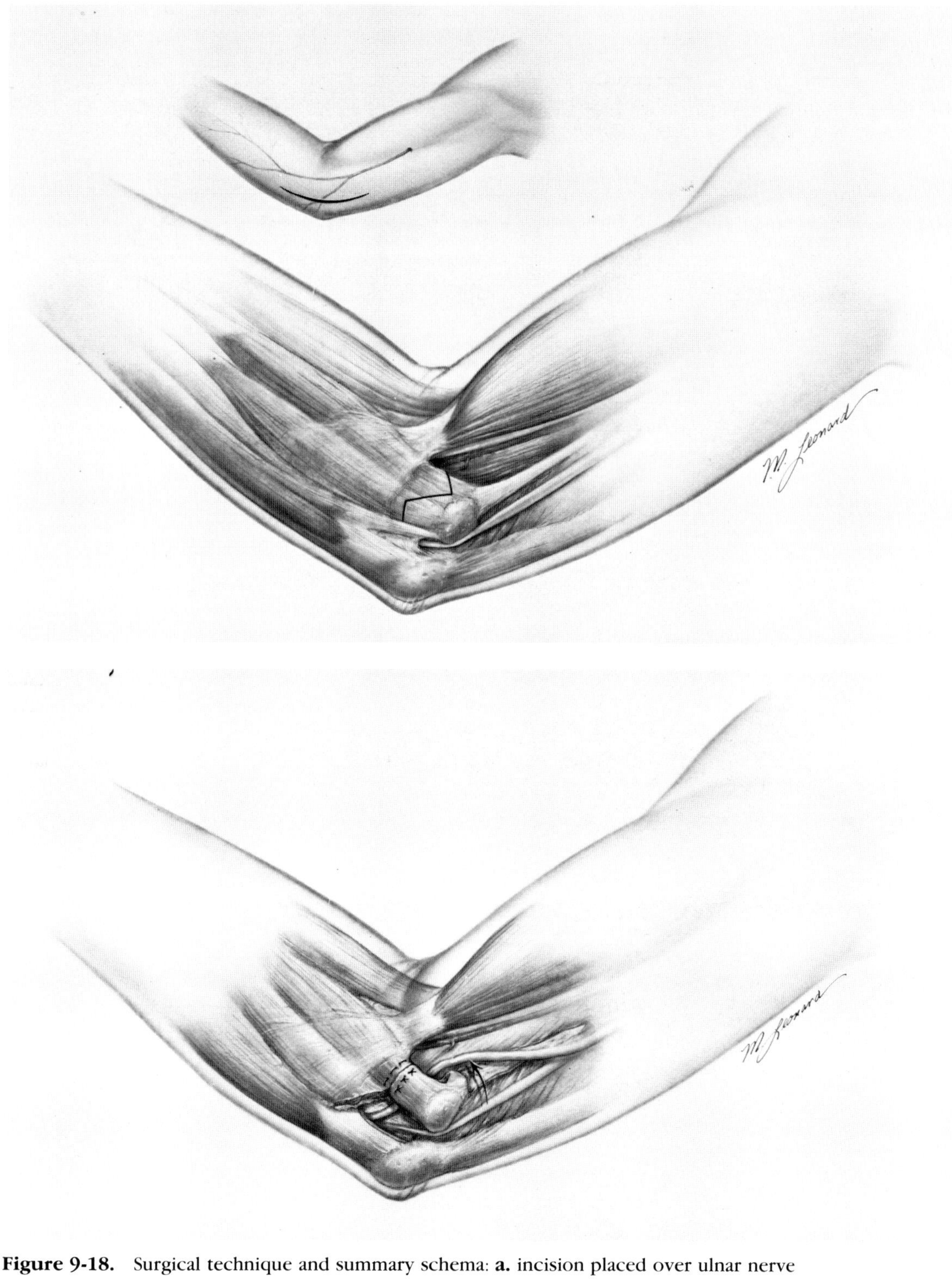

a

b

Figure 9-18. Surgical technique and summary schema: **a.** incision placed over ulnar nerve and medial antebrachial cutaneous nerve posterior branch (avoid injury to cutaneous nerve). Note proposed step-cut lengthening technique in flexor-pronator muscle fascia; **b.** ulnar transposed beneath lengthened muscle or fascia reconstruction, which avoids tightness in the new location. Note *excised* medial intermuscle septum and released periosteum of flexor carpi ulnaris head from ulnar. These two steps prevent proximal and distal kinking of transposed ulnar nerve.

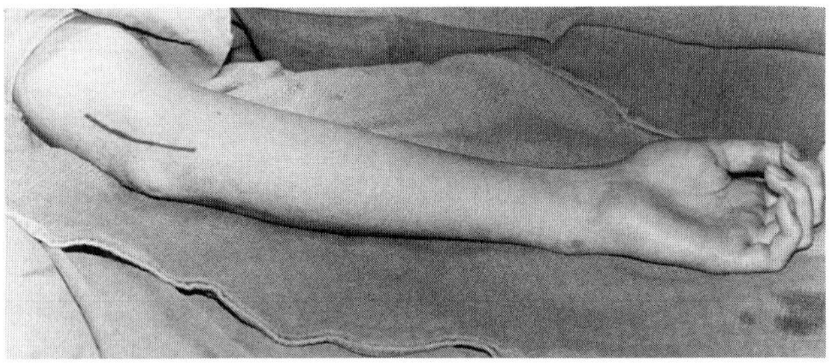
a

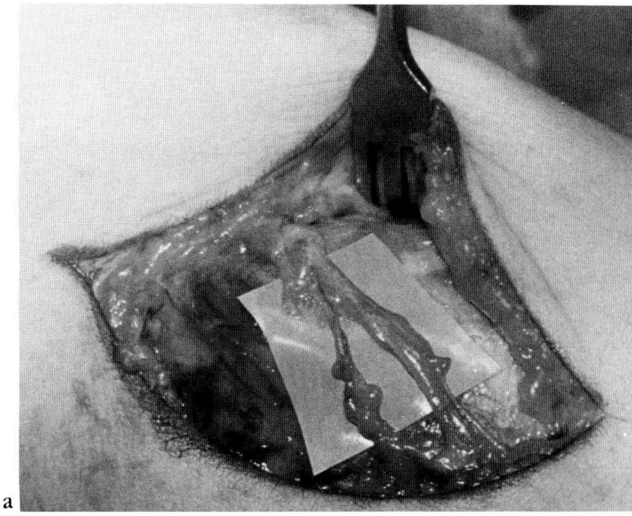
b

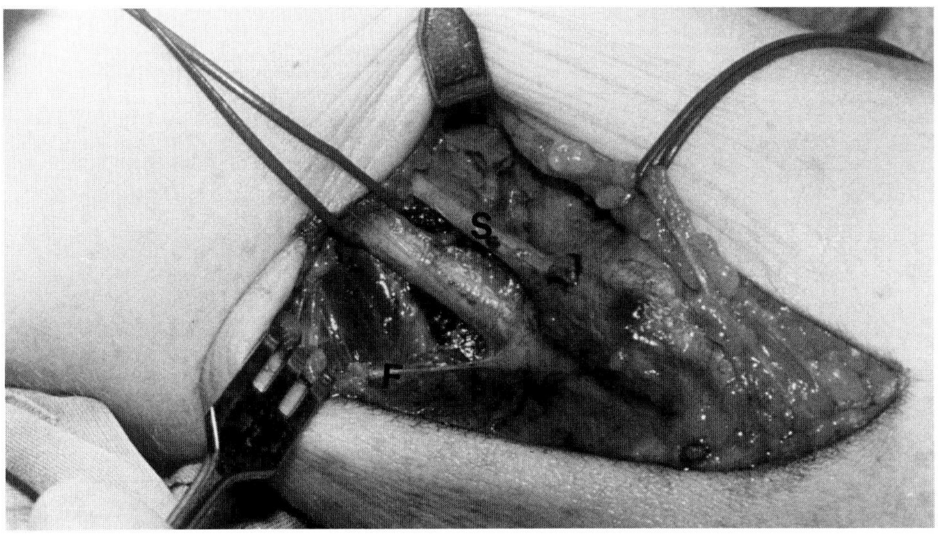

c

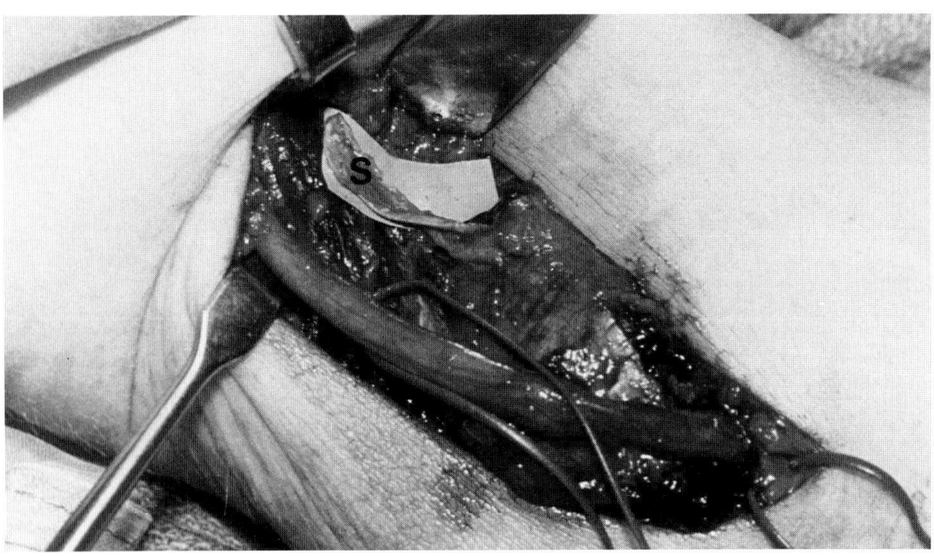

d

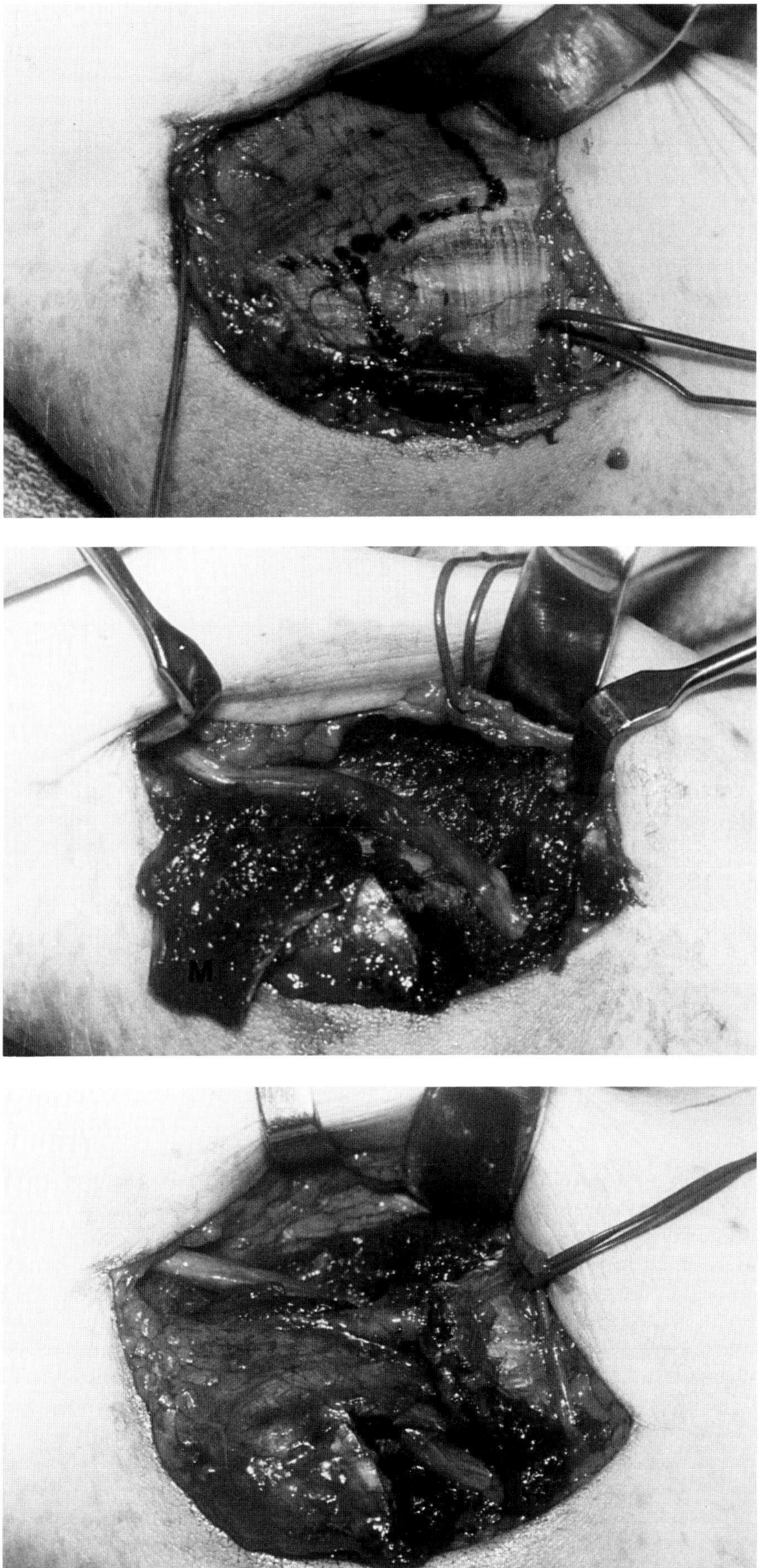

Figure 9-19. Surgical technique: intraoperative photograph sequence. **a.** Incision outlined; **b.** medial antebrachial cutaneous nerve identified and encircled with a vessel loop in **c**. In **c**, fascia from medial head of triceps (f) to medial intermuscular septum is incised, and the ulnar nerve encircled with a vessel loop. This fascia is released then for 8 cm proximally. **d.** The medial (s) intermuscular septum is excised; division of it is not sufficient. Then the roof of the cubital tunnel is split distally. The ulnar nerve may be lifted from the postcondylar groove and any proximal motor branches to the flexor carpi ulnaris are dissected distally and preserved to gain length for the transposition. An epineurectomy is done now and if necessary, an internal neurolysis also (see Figs 9-1, 9-4, 9-5). **e.** The step-cut to lengthen the flexor pronator muscle now is outlined and cut **(f)**. The common flexor tendon, which is the origin of the flexor digitorum sublimis muscle, must be completely divided deep and distal. The fascia is back-cut laterally and distally if needed. This distal piece will be sutured to the proximal, medial one left attached to the medial humeral epicondyle (m). The periosteal origin of the flexor carpi ulnaris from the ulnar is released distally while protecting the ulnar nerve. The ulnar nerve is transposed anteriorly to lie on the brachialis muscle **(g)**. The flexor pronator muscle fascia is reconstructed with three horizontal mattress sutures of 3-0 nonabsorbable braided suture. The new tunnel freely admits the surgeon's finger.

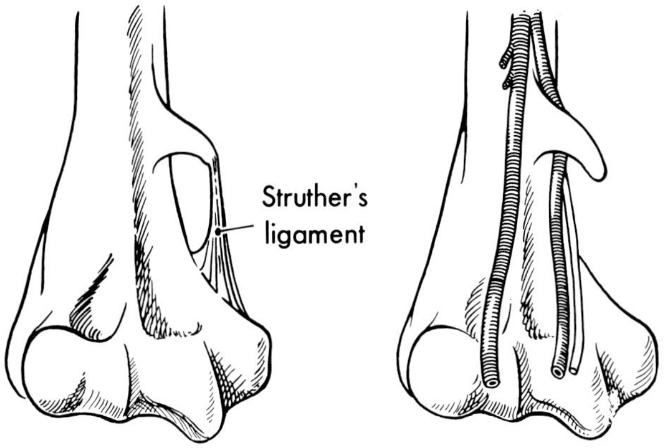

Figure 9-20. Struther's ligament occuring in less than 1% of people (left) may be associated with a medial course of the median nerve and brachial artery (right).

in detail in the photographic sequence in Figure 9-19.

With the patient in the supine position and under satisfactory anesthesia, administered either as a general anesthesia or usually a brachial block, the patient's arm is prepared and draped in an appropriate manner on an arm board. A pneumatic tourniquet has been placed before the preparations. (It is usually not always necessary to use a sterile tourniquet, depending on the build of the patient.) The tourniquet is placed as high toward the axilla as possible, leaving at least 16 cm above the medial humeral epicondyle for the postoperative dressing, which may be applied while the tourniquet is still inflated. The incision is outlined over the course of the ulnar nerve in the postcondylar groove and varies in length from 4 to 8 cm, depending on the bulk of the patient's arm. The incision is deepened through the subcutaneous tissue and then care is taken to identify branches of the medial antebrachial cutaneous nerve. There may be one to three separate branches, which arise from the posterior branch of the medial antebrachial cutaneous nerve and may cross anywhere from the proximal to the distal length of the incision. When these are identified, they are encircled with vessel loops to avoid their being injured, which may result in neuroma formation. Occasionally, a nerve in the very proximal aspect of the wound coming from more posteriorly will represent a branch of the medial brachial cutaneous nerve, and this should be protected also. Then the ulnar nerve is palpated in the postcondylar groove between the medial humeral epicondyle and the olecranon with the elbow in extension.

Observations are made now as to whether or not there are any congenital abnormalities, such as an epitrochleoanconeus muscle, or subluxation of the ulnar nerve as the elbow is flexed, whether there are inflammatory changes around the medial humeral epicondyle consistent with ulnar nerve subluxation, whether there has been excessive thickness and scarring of the subcutaneous tissue during the approach that would identify previous trauma, whether there is a palpable pseudoneuroma on the ulnar nerve or a ganglion, lipoma, or other mass in the cubital tunnel, and whether or not there is an Osborne's band present. Such observations will be recorded in the operative note.

A scissors is inserted into the fascia between the medial head of the triceps and the medial intermuscular septum. This fascia is slit proximally for 8 cm. A vessel loop is placed to encircle the ulnar nerve and its accompanying superior ulnar collateral vessels. The medial intermuscular septum is clearly separated from the ulnar nerve and the medial intermuscular septum is excised proximally. Next, the ulnar nerve is released from the cubital tunnel. The overlying roof of the cubital tunnel is identified, and, with the scissors, this is released distally until muscle between the two heads of the flexor carpi ulnaris is reached. In order for the transposition to be carried out, any proximal branches innervating the flexor carpi ulnaris must be dissected by intramuscular dissection distally. There will be small accompanying blood vessels that will require cauterization. The internal neurolysis may now be done if it is required (see next paragraph). The flexor pronator fascia now is outlined for the step-cut lengthening. This is a form of a Z-lengthening. Approximately 2 cm is left attached in length to the medial humeral epicondyle. The width of this first step is approximately 1.5 cm but may be larger in a larger person. From the tip of the step, the dissection is then made toward the proximal lateral aspect of the medial humeral epicondyle. Deep dissection is done here with scissors to avoid injury to an anomalous median nerve, that may be located quite medially if a Ligament of Struthers is present (Fig. 9-20). From here, the step goes directly across the flexor pronator fascia, where it joins the lacertus fibrosis. This incision may need to be curved distally and laterally to allow this tissue to be completely released and extend distally. This back-cut fascia is on the distal end of the flexor pronator muscle mass that will become sutured to the step of fascia and muscle that was left attached to the medial humeral epicondyle. The common flexor tendon, which is the thick fibrous tissue that runs from the medial humeral epicondyle into the flexor pronator muscle mass and which is primarily the origin of the flexor digitorum sublimis, must be divided down to the surface of the elbow joint and then cut at its junction with this, so it is completely released and allowed to move distally. If this is not done, there will remain fibrous strands that will lie beneath the transposed ulnar nerve. The ulnar nerve is gently reflected away from the wound distally, while the flexor carpi ulnaris is lifted outward and upward from the wound. This delineates the periosteal origin of the flexor carpi ulnaris head from the ulna. This periosteal band will present a site for future impingement of the ulnar nerve distally once it is transposed. This periosteal origin must be divided distally for 1.5 to 2 cm to allow the ulnar nerve to make a smooth transposition. Now the ulnar nerve is transposed to lie on top of the brachialis muscle. The elbow is flexed and extended and the examiner's finger explores proximally. There may be large veins that will serve as a proximal site of impingement now running from the deeper muscle layer into the subcutaneous flap. These veins must be cauterized and divided. Any proximal fibrous bands of the medial intermuscular septum not released before may now be identified and released. The distal transposition site is also explored and checked. Then the flexor pronator muscle mass is sutured in the advanced position with three horizontal mattress sutures of nonabsorbable suture material. After completion of the reconstruction of the flexor pronator muscle mass, the examiner's finger may be placed in the tunnel beneath the muscle and above the ulnar nerve. If there is concern the tourniquet may be deflated to ensure hemostasis. The skin is closed with interrupted 4-0 absorbable synthetic intradermal sutures and a similar suture for a subcuticular skin closure. The dressing is xeroform over the incision, two rolls of soft roll, with a posterior plaster splint holding the elbow in 90° of flexion, the forearm pronated, and the wrist in neutral position. This is held in place with kling, paper tape, stockinette, and a 4-inch wide tensor wrap. The tourniquet is then let down. Operative time averages 1 hour.

In all cases, the epineurium is opened and the fascicles are identified. An internal neurolysis may be added when the ulnar nerve is sufficiently exposed. The fascicles should be soft with good perineurial markings (bands of Fontana). If this is not the case, or if there are discrete areas of firmness palpated, an intraneural neurolysis, that is, an internal neurolysis, is carried out as described in Chapter 5. Examples may be seen in Figures 9-3, 9-10, 9-12, 9-14. Preoperative suspicion of the need for an internal neurolysis is the presence of severe degrees of nerve compression as manifested by persistent sensory change, atrophy, or abnormal two-point discrimination.

The operative technique just described can be modified to carry out synovectomies of the elbow joint, resection of hypertrophic osteoarthritic bone spurs that may cause pain in the elbow joint, excision of ganglion, division or excision of an epitrochleoanconeus muscle, and others. The median nerve at the antecubital crease and in the proximal forearm sometimes can be released through this incision, which may require extension of the incision (see Chapter 7).

Postoperative Care

The patient is seen 1 week after surgery and the dressing and sutures are removed. The patient is kept in a sling for 1 additional week. The wound is steristripped. The patient begins elbow flexion and carries out wrist and finger flexion. He may get the wound wet during this second week. During the first 2 weeks, the flexor pronator muscle mass is healing in its new lengthened position but movement is begun so that the ulnar nerve may slide through the operative field and not become scarred in this new location.[60] The patients are instructed to start gentle finger flexion exercises. During the third week, the patient is begun on heat to the incisional area, gentle massage, and gradual elbow extension, so that by the time the patient is seen in the office at 1 month after surgery, the elbow is expected to be completely extended. At this time, strengthening exercises are instituted. If the elbow has not become completely extended, the patient may be referred for physical therapy. At 6 to 12 weeks after surgery, if the scar becomes thickened or is painful, a steroid cream (betamethasone valerate) is massaged into the incision for 1 to 2 minutes, three to four times a day. A steroid impregnated tape may otherwise be used. (A more detailed description of postoperative care that is suitable to be given to the patient is presented in Appendix B)

After internal neurolysis, there is often a burning sensation along the ulnar aspect of the forearm, palm, and into the little finger. The patient is "reassured" by being told that this is the "pain of neural regeneration," it is a "good sign," and will lessen over the next 3 to 12 weeks. This "good pain", however, may require medication with either analgesics or atarax.

Postoperative Complications

The most common complication after ulnar nerve surgery at the elbow has been, in our experience, the various effects of injuring branches of the medial antebrachial cutaneous nerve's posterior branch[84] (Fig. 9-3). For example, in a series of 26 patients with recurrent ulnar nerve problems at the elbow requiring exploration, we found that 24 of these patients had injuries to this nerve. The posterior branch of the medial antebrachial cutaneous nerve (as described in "Surgical Anatomy") crosses the line of incision and may be injured. Types of injury range from complete transsection, in which case there is usually a painful scar with an anesthetic area distal to the scar, to an intact cutaneous nerve that has been simply entrapped in scar, in which case there may be paresthesias or dysesthesias distal to the scar and in the tender area within the scar. The diagnosis can be made by preoperative nerve blocks, which should eliminate the pain. The diagnosis also can be made by the fact that the pain in the scar when it is tapped does not radiate into the little and ring fingers but radiates into the posterior elbow region or the medial aspect of the forearm. The treatment is massage and topical cortisone cream, and ultimately reexploration with resection of the neuroma to a more proximal level may be required so that it lies in the subcutaneous tissue or implantation of the nerve into the triceps muscle (see Chapter 16). These postoperative complications are the most common we have observed in our series of patients undergoing anterior ulnar nerve transposition for the first time, as well as those in whom exploration is done for persistent or recurrent ulnar nerve compression problems. An injury to this nerve in one patient was reported by Richards in 1945.[85] MacNichol[71] noted numbness about the elbow in 50% of the patients postoperatively. Eaton et al[80] and Leffert[3] each has cautioned the surgeon to be aware of this nerve and to prevent its injury during their operative approach to the ulnar nerve. Otherwise, we have been unable to find reference to this nerve in the extensive literature of ulnar nerve surgery.

The next most common complication that we have encountered[22] in an extensive series of ulnar nerve transpositions relates to bleeding. Bruising is frequent and is generally minor in degree. It can be treated with topical heat applications and massage and generally has resolved by 2 weeks. Two patients from a series of more than 400 have had a hematoma drain spontaneously through the incision site during the second week. No patient has been reexplored for bleeding. One patient, in whom draining did not occur spontaneously, had the hematoma resolve slowly over a month, leaving significant fibrosis. This caused compression on the ulnar nerve and prevented complete recovery, requiring subsequent reexploration. There have been no cases of postoperative infection. In more than 500 cases of internal neurolysis of the ulnar nerve, there have been no cases of postoperative reflex sympathetic dystrophy. One patient who had made an excellent recovery after an internal neurolysis and an anterior submuscular transposition returned to work 6 months after surgery. While at work on the first day, he was required to carry out 2300 repetitive movements with the elbow as he transferred meat in a meat packing plant. That evening his arm and hand became swollen and he developed a sympathetic mediated pain syndrome (reflex sympathetic dystrophy) (see Chapter 16). He had partial response to stellate ganglion block and partial response to physiotherapy over the next 6 months. However, he lost all sensation in the little and ring fingers and had profound weakness. He was reexplored and an internal neurolysis carried out again. He has had only protective sensation return to his fingers and remains profoundly weak in pinch and grip strength. He has no intrinsic atrophy. He does manifest a curling of the little and ring fingers, which can be passively and actively extended, and this persists despite attempts at splinting. A similar finding of curling-in of the little and ring fingers was noted in a patient with a deep band compressing the underside of the ulnar nerve in the cubital tunnel (Fig. 9-12).

Perhaps in the truest sense, persistent or recurrent ulnar nerve symptomatology after ulnar nerve surgery should be considered a complication of the operation (Figs. 9-21 through 9-25). This is because these persistent or recurrent symptoms are usually found at reexploration to be due to some technical aspect of the initial procedure. The usual problems are persistence of the medial intermuscular septum, tethering of the ulnar nerve back into the postcondylar groove by branches of the flexor carpi ulnaris not dissected far enough distally, the distal periosteal origin of the flexor carpi ulnaris head from the distal ulna, a tight reconstruction of the flexor pronator muscle mass (the earliest,[9,82] as well as the most recent,[58,87] illustrations show this tight reconstruction), or tightness of the subcutaneous check-rein type ligaments that are reconstructed to hold the anterior subcutaneously transposed ulnar nerve in place. As indicated in the "Results" section, persistent or recurrent or worsening symptoms comprise at least one-quarter of most series and up to a third of other reported series of surgical results. As with most complications, these are best dealt with initially by prevention. The surgical technique described herein for anterior submuscular transposition, with meticulous attention to the new position of the ulnar nerve, is the most effective way of dealing with this complication. That is, "prevention is the best form of treatment."

Once the complication has been diagnosed as persistent or recurrent ulnar nerve compression at the elbow, and once at least 12 months has been allowed to elapse to ensure that the condition is not improving on its own, reexploration with internal neurolysis of the ulnar nerve and submuscular positioning is the treatment of choice (see "Results"). This course of treatment, however, is recommended with extreme caution in persons who are over the age of 60 years and especially in those who have had more than two previous ulnar nerve operations, because additional surgery of this type may cause irreversible ischemia with infarct of the ulnar nerve. We had this situation occur in two patients in this age group with multiple previous operations for the ulnar nerve, in whom we have carried out this operation with disastrous sequelae. A third patient identical to this has been reported to us. These patients lost complete ulnar nerve function and regained only some protective sensation and strength by 2 years after their repeat surgery. One of these patients now has persistent pain in the distribution of the ulnar nerve. These ischemic symptoms come from repeated surgery on an already injured nerve. In this regard, two articles have reported the use of silicone sheaths interposed between the compressed ulnar nerve and a scarred bed.[87,88] As is noted in Chapter 2, the nerve compression models require wrapping nerves with silicone. Silicone causes loss of vascular ingrowth to these nerves and may minimize the nerve's ability to gather any segmental supply from its new bed. Furthermore, the silicone may engender its own fibrous response about the nerve and over a period of time contribute to compression. As noted in "Results," with the techniques of silicone sheeting a significant percentage of patients do not improve and have persistent symptoms. Therefore the use of silicone should be contraindicated. Age, in and of itself, is not a contraindication to surgery in these patients, and successful internal neurolysis in the elderly has been reported.[81] We have patients in our series who are octogenarians who have done well after anterior submuscular transposition of the ulnar nerve with internal neurolysis.

Results

> Excellent clinical judgment requires optimal decision-making. Many of the decisions that physicians make in their practices involve little uncertainty and little risk: these routine choices need no special contemplation because they are "tried and true practices." But for each routine problem, there are several for which no easy solution is at hand; use an algorithm developed for such patients; use the problem-oriented approach to data gathering and hope that the solution to the problem will emerge; or ask for the help of one or more consultants. The frustrations encountered with all these approaches are familiar to all.[89]

It is clear that decision analysis for the patient with ulnar nerve compression at the elbow must be placed on a more scientific basis. To do this requires obtaining data that can be used to give information for each point in the decision-making process. Attempts to do this, taking either patient symptomatology (Fig. 9-16) or cause of compression (Fig. 9-16) have been elaborated.[51,90] This information has not been obtainable, however, from the vast array of data on ulnar nerve compression that has been reported. The reasons for this are that the surgical literature on the results of treatment of ulnar nerve compression at the elbow is generally comprised of reports by individual surgeons utilizing their favorite technique. The reports are generally characterized by groups of patients who have not been preoperatively staged as to the degree of compression and for whom postoperatively some criteria for success are enumerated. Only six reports have directly measured, or implied that they measured, two-point discrimination.[25,72,78,80,91,92] There has been a general absence of standardization for any reporting techniques. Only five reports have utilized statistical analysis to compare groups of patients operated on by different techniques.[70,71,73,79,93] The patients were rarely of comparable preoperative stage and never randomized into treatment groups. No reports have demonstrated a significant advantage of one technique over another.

It is not that there is a lack of information about ulnar nerve compression at the elbow. It is more a problem that the information that exists has not been obtained in a manner that is useful to solving the decisions we must make: How should the patient with ulnar nerve compression at the elbow be treated? To begin to solve this decision analysis problem, the following must be agreed on: How to make the diagnosis of ulnar nerve compression at the elbow? (this was described previously), How to stage patients so that patients with equal degrees of ulnar nerve compression at the elbow may be treated in a similar manner (a staging system was described earlier, see also Table 9-10). The results of the different methods of treatment must be analyzed and compared with some common basis or denominator (this will be done in the remainder of this section). These factors may then be utilized to arrive at a decision analysis based on the most currently available data analyzed in a scientific manner.

In an attempt to establish some order from this surgical literature, the classification given in Table 9-10 has been applied to the previously reported patient groups.[93] Where conflict might occur, the "benefit" was given to the original article's author in terms of having achieved better results. If the initial surgeon had called his patient's result "normal," this was considered as normal and was considered "excellent." A "good" result reported by an author, however, was not equated to "normal" or "excellent." "Improved," in general, was considered "good" because the authors generally contrasted this with patients who did not improve. Since virtually no authors established a category for persistent or recurrent ulnar nerve problems, the category of "not improved" was equated to this category. Those patients listed as "recurrent" were accepted as "recurrent." Recurrent cases were deleted from groups of patients and placed into a separate category. Weakness was not considered as equivalent to atrophy. The revised data from previous reports are presented in tabular form for each series with a separate table for nonoperative treatment (Table 9-12), simple decompression procedures (Table 9-13), medial epicondylectomy procedures (Table 9-14), anterior subcutaneous transposition (Table 9-15), anterior intramuscular transposition (Table 9-16), anterior submuscular transposition (Table 9-17), and a separate table for the treatment of recurrent ulnar nerve entrapment (Table 9-18). An additional table is presented in which a given author has attempted to compare the results of different operative techniques in his own series of patients (Table 9-19). The tables are then summarized (Table 9-20).

Table 9-12. Results of Nonoperative Treatment for Ulnar Nerve Compression at Elbow

Reference	No. Patients	Mean Follow-up (Mo)	Staging: Degree	Staging: No. Patients	Total Relief (%)	No Atrophy (%)	Normal Strength (%)	Normal 2PD (%)*	No Paresthesias (%)	Worse (%)	Recurrent (%)
Paine[79] 1970	7	18	Minimal		56	—	14	—	—	—	44
Payan[92] 1970	2	6	Moderate	1	0	—	—	—	—	0	0
			Severe	1	—	—	—	—	—	—	100
Eisen and Dannon[26] 1974	30	22	Minimal		90	—	—	—	—	—	10
Wadsworth[94] 1977	14	40	Minimal	4	25	—	—	—	—	—	75
			Moderate	8	—	—	—	—	—	—	87
			Severe	2	—	—	—	—	—	—	100
Lister 1985	76	9†	—								
Dellon[22] 1988	100	24	Minimal		50						50

*2PD: two-point discrimination.
†"86% improved."

Table 9-13. Results of Decompression Treatment for Ulnar Nerve Compression at Elbow

Reference	No. Patients	Mean Follow-up (mo)	Staging: Degree	Staging: No. Patients	Total Relief (%)	No Atrophy (%)	Normal Strength (%)	Normal 2PD (%)*	No Paresthesias (%)	Worse (%)	Recurrent (%)
Osborne[21] 1957	13	—	—								
Feindel and Stratford[20] 1958	3	13	Severe		100						
Osborne[65] 1966	100	12–60	Minimal/moderate		98						2
Vanderpool et al[31] 1968	38	2–84	Minimal/moderate	36	60						6
			Severe	2		50			100		50
Paine[79] 1970	20	18	Moderate/severe			21			31	8	15
Wilson and Krout[67] 1973	14	7	Minimal	3					33		
			Moderate	10			50		50		
			Severe	1		100			100		
Hagstrom[95] 1977	13	60	—						60		15
Fannin[96] 1978	27	6–72	Severe			8	30		30	0	50
MacNichol[71] 1979	63	51	Moderate		5					0	30
Clark[69] 1979	135	—	Minimal						100		
			Severe			0					
Foster and Edshage[70] 1981	29	50	Minimal	6	50						
			Moderate	18	33						12
			Severe	5	0						
Osborne[66] 1982	46	—	Minimal	9			100		100		
			Moderate	19			74		74		0
			Severe	18		5			39		16
Benit et al[88] 1987	70	13	—		3					7	27

*2PD: two-point discrimination

Table 9-14. Results of Medial Epicondylectomy Treatment for Ulnar Nerve Compression at Elbow

Reference	*No. Patients*	*Mean Follow-up (mo)*	*Staging: Degree*	*Staging: No. Patients*	*Total Relief (%)*	*No Atrophy (%)*	*Normal Strength (%)*	*Normal 2PD (%)**	*No Paresthesias (%)*	*Worse (%)*	*Recurrent (%)*
King and Morgan[104] 1950	16	—	—	—	0	0		0			
Gore and Larson[102] 1966	14	—	Minimal	2	100						
			Moderate	12	33		33				
Neblett and Ehni[101] 1970	14	4–108	Severe			79			93	0	7
Jones & Gaunt[84] 1979	22	6–17	Moderate/severe		0						35
Laha and Panchal[100] 1979	8	—	Minimal	3					100		
			Moderate	4			50		100		
			Severe	1		0			0		
Craven and Green[78] 1980	30	22	Minimal	6					100		
			Moderate/severe	24			55		75		
Froimson and Zahraw[103]	30	60	Minimal	12	100						
			Moderate	12			67		67		33
			Severe	6							100
Culver[81] 1987	26	46	Moderate		19						54

*2PD: two-point discrimination.

Table 9-15. Results of Anterior Subcutaneous Transposition Treatment for Ulnar Nerve Compression at Elbow

Reference	*No. Patients*	*Mean Follow-up (mo)*	*Staging: Degree*	*Staging: No. Patients*	*Total Relief (%)*	*No Atrophy (%)*	*Normal Strength (%)*	*Normal 2PD (%)**	*No Paresthesias (%)*	*Worse (%)*	*Recurrent (%)*
Curtis[13] 1898	1	—	—								
Sheldon[19] 1921	15	20	Severe		47	40			53		33
McGowan[25] 1950	46	12–24	Minimal	6	100						
		12–60	Moderate	27			41	74	45		11
		12–48	Severe	13	7		80				40
Paine[79] 1970	11	30	Moderate/severe		18				27	9	9
Payan[92] 1970	11	14	Moderate	8	0					25	37
			Severe	3		33		33		33	33
Harrison and Nurick[91] 1970	23	72	Moderate	2	100		100				
			Severe	21		5	15	10	45	5	40
Ho and Marmor[41] 1971	2	9	Moderate	1	100						
			Severe	1	100						
Levy and Apfelberg[105] 1972	2	5	Moderate	1	0				0		
			Severe	1	100	100					
Hagstrom[95] 1977	69	60	Minimal/moderate	40			31		31		13
			Severe	29		46	31	78	31	9	13
Lugnegard et al[72] 1977	25	19	Minimal	7	100						
			Severe	18	33	33		33			22
Laha and Panchal[100] 1979	42	—	Minimal	6					100		
			Moderate	30			73		80		27
			Severe	6		16			33	16	50
Eaton et al[80] 1980	16	18	Minimal/moderate	12	100						
			Severe	4			75	75			25
Foster and Edshage[70] 1981	19	50	Minimal	4	50						0
			Moderate	4	25						25
			Severe	11	27						10

*2PD: two-point discrimination.

Table 9-16. Results of Anterior Intramuscular Transposition Treatment for Ulnar Nerve Compression at Elbow

Reference	*No. Patients*	*Mean Follow-up (mo)*	*Staging*		*Total Relief (%)*	*No Atrophy (%)*	*Normal Strength (%)*	*Normal 2PD (%)**	*No Paresthesias (%)*	*Worse (%)*	*Recurrent (%)*
			Degree	*No. Patients*							
Adson[14] 1918	3	—	Severe	—	0						
Platt[9] 1928	>100	—	—	—		"Most gratifying"					
Davidson and Horowitz[10] 1935	—	—	—	—	47	40			53	33	
Gay and Love[106] 1947	76	—	Severe	—	7						70

*2PD: two-point discrimination.

Table 9-17. Results of Anterior Submuscular Transposition Treatment for Ulnar Nerve Compression at Elbow

Reference	*No. Patients*	*Mean Follow-up (mo)*	*Staging*		*Total Relief (%)*	*No Atrophy (%)*	*Normal Strength (%)*	*Normal 2PD (%)**	*No Paresthesias (%)*	*Worse (%)*	*Recurrent (%)*
			Degree	*No. Patients*							
Learmonth[82] 1942	0	—	—	—							
Richards[85] 1945	12	16	Moderate	2	100					0	
			Severe	10	20					30	
Sunderland[11] 1946	14	≥ n8	—	—	13				42	29	29
Seddon[2] 1972	"12"	—	Minimal	4	100						
			Moderate	4			50		75		
			Severe	4		"Some"			50		
Levy and Apfelberg[105] 1972	7	37	Moderate	5	80						20
			Severe	2	50	50					50
MacNichol[71] 1979	47	51	Moderate/severe		4					0	30
Leffert[3] 1982	24	23	Minimal	1	100						
			Moderate	20	60		85		75		
			Severe	3	67						33

*2PD: two-point discrimination.

Table 9-18. Results of Treatment for Recurrent Ulnar Nerve Compression at Elbow

Reference	*No. Patients*	*Mean Follow-up (mo)*	*Staging*		*Total Relief (%)*	*No Atrophy (%)*	*Normal Strength (%)*	*Normal 2PD (%)**	*No Paresthesias (%)*	*Worse (%)*	*Recurrent (%)*	*Comment†*
			Degree	*No. Patients*								
Gay and Love[106] 1947	1	—	Severe	—	100	—	—	—	—	—	—	SM + IN
McGowan[25] 1950	6	—	—	—	100	—	—	—	—	—	—	SM
Campbell et al[87] 1974	7	46	Severe		—	—	42	—	70	—	28	SM + IN
Lluch[109] 1975	1	—	Severe		100							SM + IN
Broudy et al[110] 1978	10	14	Moderate/severe				60		70			
Leffert[3] 1982	14	23	Moderate	8			63		63			SM + EN
			Severe	3		100	67		67			

*2PD: two-point discrimination.

†IN: internal neurolysis; SM: submuscular.

Table 9-19. Results of Studies Comparing Different Treatment Methods

Treatment 1 / Treatment 2	Nonoperative	Anterior Transposition* SQ	IM	SM
Nonoperative		Equal for minimal degree[21]		
Nonoperative		"Good" non: 50% SQ: 36% Not staged[92]		
Decompression		Equal 30% excellent Moderate[79]		Equal 5% excellent 30% recurrent Moderate-severe[71]
Decompression		Equal excellent Minimal: 50% Moderate: 30%[70]		
Medial Epicondylectomy		Equal 80% good Not staged[100]		
Anterior submuscular		Good SM: 86% SQ: 59% Not staged[108]		
Anterior submuscular		Excellent SM: 70% SQ: 100% Minimal moderate[105]		
Decompression		Excellent / persistent: / worse SM/IM 18 / 15 / 3 Decompression 30 / 15 / 3 Moderate-severe[73]		
Decompression	Equal 100% recurrence Moderate-severe[94]	Equal 100% recurrence Moderate-severe[94]		
Decompression		Excellent / Worse 14 / 42 23 / 18 Moderate-severe[127]		Excellent / Worse 14 / 42 25 / 37 Moderate-severe[127]

*SQ: subcutaneous; IM: intramuscular; SM: submuscular.

Nonoperative

The results of treating ulnar nerve compression at the elbow by nonoperative technique is outlined in Table 9-12 for six separate series that have addressed this problem[22,26,66,79,92,94] and these series are summarized in Table 9-20. The technique for nonoperative management as we practice it is given earlier. An example of a splint that might be used in this type of technique is demonstrated in Figure 9-16. The literature does not record even the suggestion that ulnar nerve compression at the elbow may be treated by nonoperative approach until 1970[79,92] because, as already discussed, before this the importance of trauma in the cause of ulnar nerve compression at the elbow, and therefore the degree of injury to the nerve, was such that spontaneous recovery was rarely noted. It may be concluded from this literature review (Table 9-20) that for preoperative staging of minimal degree of nerve compression, 50% of the patients may be anticipated to achieve excellent results, whereas 42% of the patients will not have improvement and will demonstrate persistence of their ulnar nerve compression problems requiring further treatment. There has been very little experience gained in applying this type of nonoperative management to those with either moderate or severe degree of nerve compression. The few reports that deal with this subject[92,94] have demonstrated that 77% of those with moderate and 100% of those with severe degree of nerve compression have had persistence of their problem requiring further treatment.

Decompression

The results of treating ulnar nerve compression at the elbow by a decompression technique are presented for

Table 9-20. Summary by Degree of Compression of Treatment for Ulnar Nerve Compression at the Elbow

				Percent Achieving				
Treatment	*Stage*	*Reference*	*No.*	*No Atrophy (%)*	*Normal Strength (%)*	*No Paresthesia (%)*	*Worse (%)*	*Recurrence (%)*
Nonoperative	Minimal	22,26,79,94	141			58		42
	Moderate	92,94	9		0			77
	Severe	92,94	3	0				100
			Total 153					
Decompression	Minimal	31,65–67,69,70	216			94		1
	Moderate	31,66,67,70,71,95	141		33	33		16
	Severe	20,31,66,67,69,70, 79,88,96,124,125,129	210	25		30	3	19
			Total 567					
Medial epicondylectomy	Minimal	78,100,102,103	35			100		
	Moderate	78,81,100,102,103	78		41	50		23
	Severe	84,100,101,103	43	25		30		35
			Total 156					
Anterior subcutaneous transposition	Minimal	25,70,72,80,100	35			94		0
	Moderate	25,41,70,91,92,95, 100,105	113		43	71	2	15
	Severe	19,25,41,70,72,79, 80,91,92,95,100,105	133	30		53	5	25
			Total 281					
Anterior intramuscular transposition	Severe	14,106	79		6	6	67	
Anterior submuscular transposition	Minimal	2,3	5			100		
	Moderate	2,3,85,86	31		81	77		3
	Severe	2,3,85,71,105	66	12		14		30
			Total 102					
Recurrent (anterior submuscular transposition)	Moderate	3	8		63	63		6
	Severe	3,25,87,106,109,110	31	15		52		
			Total 39					
Total patients reviewed			1377					

the series that have directly addressed this problem in Table 9-13.[20,21,31,66,67,70,71,79,88,95,96] This technique has been most commonly reported in the surgical literature and 567 cases reported in these series are summarized in Table 9-20. Osborne's[21] article in 1957 represented the first description of the concept that simply decompressing the ulnar nerve where it was trapped beneath the thickened distal end of the cubital tunnel might be enough surgery to treat this problem. His initial concept was simply splitting the roof of the cubital tunnel. He described this again in 1959.[97] He became sufficiently interested in the problem of nerve compression that with Weissl,[98] he developed a model to evaluate nerve compression in the rat. He banded the rat sciatic nerve with silicone bands. This was the forerunner of a technique we ultimately developed to evaluate nerve compression (see Chapter 2). Osborne, however, primarily created a model with significant compression by narrowing the nerves by 20 to 50%, thereby creating a situation of more acute degeneration than chronic compression. Nevertheless, this technique demonstrated that the more peripheral fascicles are more significantly affected than the more central fascicles; he demonstrated increased vascularity by microinjection techniques that suggested that inflammation played a role in chronic compression, and he confirmed the observations of others that myelin thinning was related to the pathophysiologic changes of nerve compression. Osborne had two recurrences in his early series that he believed were related to reattachment of the divided roof of the cubital tunnel. He therefore modified his technique[65] to include suturing the divided edges of the cubital tunnel posterior to the nerve in this postcondylar groove. He restated these observations in 1970.[99] Only his initial paper in 1957 and his book chapter in 1966 contained a mention of the number of patients. He described a classification for ulnar nerve compression preoperative staging in this book chapter[65] and subsequently modified this (Table 9-11). His classification included four separate categories. His type of classification, which included both sensory and motor changes, is the forerunner of the classification we have adopted. However, his stage III and stage IV both contained patients with muscle wasting and therefore conceptually are the same degree of compression in terms of pathophysiologic changes and treatment, as reflected in the staging system we utilize (Table 9-10). In response to a written request, Osborne wrote in March of 1982[66] and gave the postoperative results of 46 patients based on this preoperative staging system. These previously unpublished results are given in Table 9-13. By these results, Osborne was the first to take patients staged preoperatively and then grade each patient based on the amount of postoperative change achieved. Osborne's results[66] clearly show that the patients who benefit the most from the decompression technique are those with the minimal degree of nerve compression. Few, if any, excellent results are achieved once significant weakness or muscle atrophy has occurred. Three of the series of patients[88,95,96] added an external neurolysis to the simple decompression. It may be concluded from the summary Table 9-20 that 94% of patients with a minimal degree of nerve compression can achieve excellent relief of their sensory symptoms by a decompression technique. When the degree of compression has progressed to moderate, just 33% of the patients achieve normal strength and normal sensation, with 16% having persistence of their preoperative symptoms and physical findings. When the degree of compression has progressed to severe, just 25% of the patients achieve recovery of atrophied muscles, just 30% achieve excellent sensory recovery, 3% have their preoperative symptoms and signs worsen and 19% have their preoperative symptoms and signs persist (Fig. 9-21). The technique of simple decompression does not address any intrinsic pathologic conditions present within the nerve or the problem of the relationship of the nerve with its nerve bed. Therefore, as discussed in the final paragraph of this section, the technique cannot be recommended by us except for the most minimal degree of nerve compression where there is no associated direct trauma to the nerve or pathologic state in the postcondylar groove, and to be utilized only in patients who are willing to accept a second, more extensive procedure should the simple decompression technique not prove successful.

Medial Epicondylectomy

The results of the treatment for ulnar nerve compression at the elbow by medial epicondylectomy are presented for a series of articles that directly dealt with this problem in Table 9-14.[78,81,84,100–104] The results are summarized in Table 9-20. The technique of medial epicondylectomy was described by King and by Morgan, who were aware of each other's work and collaborated but who essentially wrote small separate papers adjoined to each other and published in 1950[104] and again in 1959.[104a] The technique was described primarily as an alternative to the more extensive and complicated anterior transposition procedures, many of which were not yielding excellent results for the patients so treated. A technique was developed so that the nerve, itself, would not be directly treated. Morgan cautioned: "The nerve should not be explored nor its branches handled." He described his technique as being "easier and quicker to perform, requiring less technical skill." King agreed, indicating that this was a "simple operation that appeared to avoid the dangers of a fibrociccatrical contracture which occurred when nerve is embedded in the flexor muscles." This concept was echoed by Neblett and Ehni,[101] who indicated that the "natural bed of the ulnar nerve should not be disturbed" and added that "a neurolysis will only result in unwanted ciccatrical change in the nerve." Craven and Green[78] indicate in their abstract that all their patients achieved relief. However, in the text, two patients, in fact, were noted to have no relief and their data have been altered by these two patients, as reflected in Table 9-14. King and Morgan reflected the thinking of their time that ulnar nerve compression was progressive and that if a patient did not improve but at least got no worse, he was considered as having had a successful operation. For example, they wrote, "Results were satisfactory: gross signs either improved or progressed no further." In addition to the medial epicondylectomy, Froimson and Zahraw[103] excised the medial intermuscular septum and carried out an external neurolysis of the ulnar nerve. Jones and Gaunt[84] also carried out an external neurolysis of the ulnar nerve but did not excise or incise the medial intermuscular septum. Many of the authors differ in the extent of bone resection carried out, with the most aggressive procedures including a portion of the humerus as it extends out to form the medial humeral epicondyle. The concept is to allow the nerve to come to lie in a position where it is not stretched around or over the medial humeral epicondyle. The drawback to the procedure is that it does not directly treat the pathologic state within the nerve, nor does it prevent kinking of the nerve on either the medial intermuscular septum or between the two heads of the flexor carpi ulnaris. When surgeons who have achieved the best results with this procedure, such as Craven and Green,[79] perform the procedure, they will do more than a simple medial epicondylectomy. They will treat the medial intermuscular septum proximally and neurolyze the nerve externally between the two heads of the flexor carpi ulnaris. The results achieved in the minimal degree of nerve compression are 100% relief of the patient's sensory symptoms. In those with a moderate degree of nerve compression, there is a 41% recovery of normal strength and 50% of the patients recover normal sen-

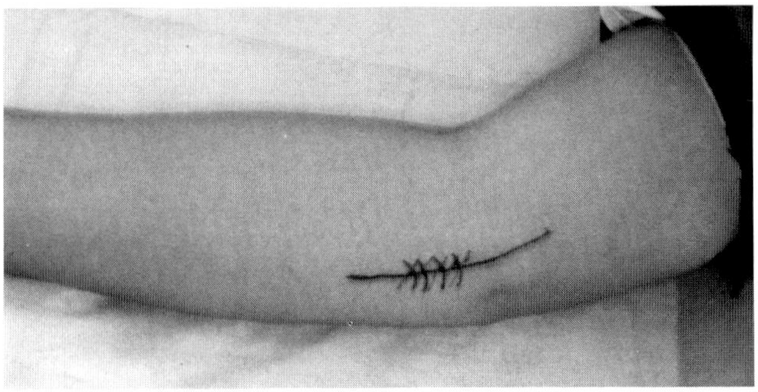

a

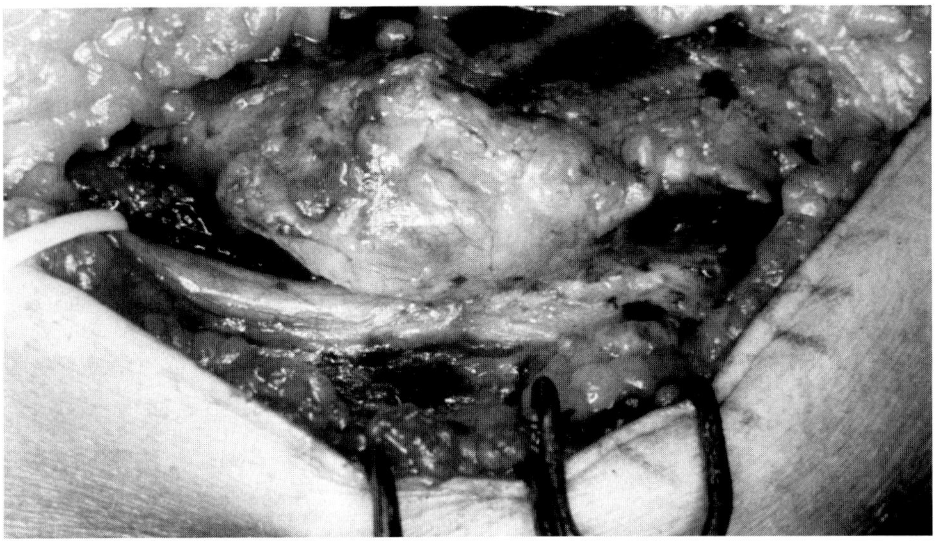

b

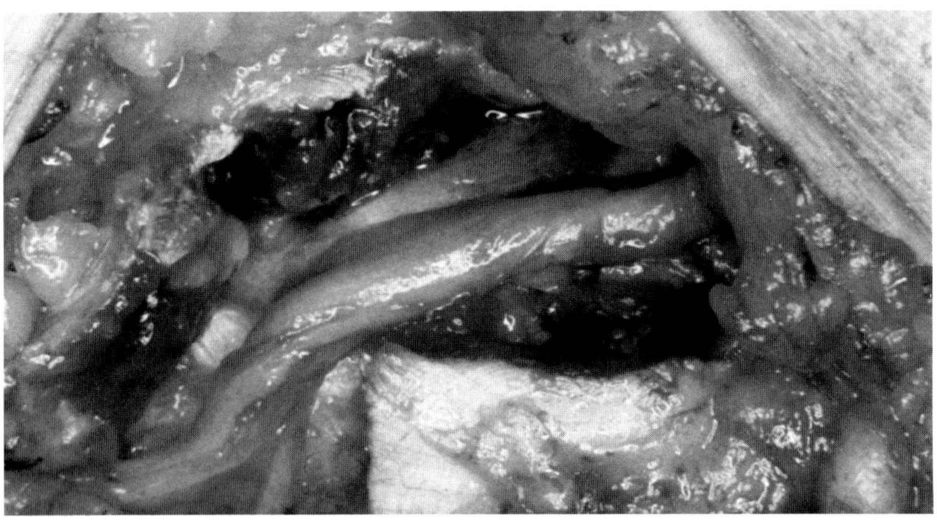

c

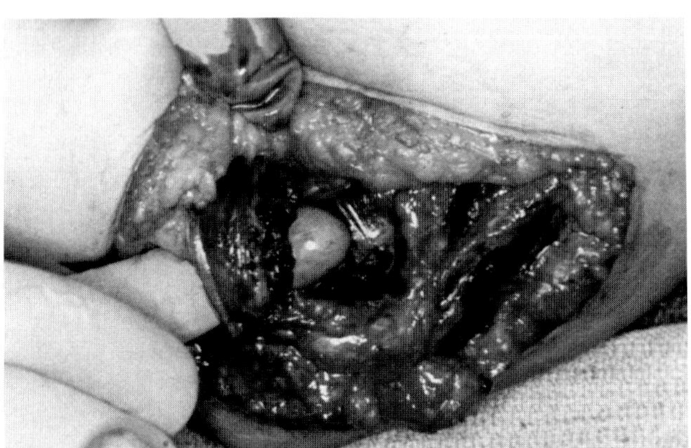

d

Figure 9-21. Recurrent ulnar nerve entrapment after decompression alone **(a)**. **b.** Note scarring of nerve into postcondylar groove. **c.** After neurolysis, ulnar nerve lies on brachialis muscle. **d.** Submuscular transposition completed, and new tunnel size is demonstrated.

sation. However, 23% of the patients have persistence or recurrence of their preoperative sensory and motor symptoms. When the degree of nerve compression is severe, 25% of the patients achieve recovery of muscle atrophy, 30% only recover normal sensation, and 35% of the patients have either persistence or recurrence of their preoperative sensory and motor function. Because of the long-term problems with persistence and recurrence of the preoperative symptoms and because in order to achieve even the results already stated, more than a simple epicondylectomy must be carried out, it is our preference to move the nerve into a submuscular position and directly treat the pathologic condition within the nerve by internal neurolysis when indicated.

Anterior Subcutaneous Transposition

The results of treatment of ulnar nerve compression at the elbow by an anterior subcutaneous transposition are given for the series of articles that directly report this technique in Table 9-15[13,19,25,41,70,72,79,80,91,92,95,100,105] and are summarized in Table 9-20. The first report of this technique by Curtis[13] in 1898 was of just one patient, and he indicated that the result were "surprisingly satisfactory." The technique was described for a larger series of patients by Sheldon in 1921,[19] who did not illustrate the technique, but whose patients were of a severe degree of nerve compression, and he included an "internal neurolysis" in the patients' treatment. The most commonly quoted series is that by McGowan in 1950.[25] The description of McGowan's operative technique indicates that the dissection was extremely extensive. The medial intermuscular septum was resected, as had been recommended by Learmonth.[82] McGowan cut a "little groove" in the flexor pronator muscle fascia but did not truly place the nerve intramuscularly because a subcutaneous tissue was fashioned to maintain the ulnar nerve in its transposed position rather than closing the flexor pronator muscle fascia over the nerve. The distal dissection was very extensive. McGowan was the first to report a preoperative staging system, which, however, ignored the role of sensory changes. Among subsequent authors writing about anterior subcutaneous transposition, the medial intermuscular septum was resected and an external neurolysis carried out by Hagstrom[95] and by Eaton et al.[80] An internal neurolysis was carried out, in addition to Sheldon as described previously by Ho and Marmor.[41] In order to keep the nerve in an anterior position, rather than falling back into the postcondylar groove, various types of slings were fashioned either from slips of fascia from the flexor pronator muscle mass or from surrounding subcutaneous tissues. These attempts to maintain their advanced position frequently, and especially when the more proximal sites of compression over the medial intermuscular septum are not dealt with, are the source of the nerves becoming compressed against the medial humeral epicondyle in its new transposed position, and this is the most common cause for this procedure's failures. From Table 9-20 it is clear that, with a minimal degree of nerve compression, 94% of the patients achieve excellent relief of their preoperative sensory symptoms. With a moderate degree of nerve compression, 43% of the patients achieve normal strength, 71% of the patients achieve normal sensation, 2% of the patients are made worse, and 15% of the patients have persistence or recurrence of their preoperative motor and sensory symptoms. With a severe degree of nerve compression, 30% of the patients achieve normal muscle function with reversal of their preoperative atrophy, 53% achieve normal sensory function, and 5% are made worse, with 25% of the patients having persistence or recurrence of their preoperative sensory and motor symptoms (Figs. 9-22, 9-23). Because of the problem with the sling that must be fashioned to maintain the nerve in this anterior subcutaneous position and because in order to achieve excellent results with this technique the medial intermuscular septum must be excised and extensive dissection carried out distally, the technique of submuscular transposition with internal neurolysis when indicated is preferred by us over this technique.

Anterior Intramuscular Transposition

The results of treating ulnar nerve compression at the elbow by an anterior intramuscular transposition are described in Table 9-16 for those series of patients directly reported to have been treated by this technique.[9,10,14,106] The results are summarized in Table 9-20. The initial description of this technique by Adson in 1918 is important for describing the presence of interstitial neuritis with definite thickening in the nerve as a result of its trauma. He described the development of "neuromas with intraneural fibrous tissue." His technique for maintaining the nerve in the anterior transposed position was to cut a groove into the muscle. He did not describe careful complete division of the common flexor tendon. He maintained the nerve in this position by taking a sheath of fascia lata, placing it about the nerve, suturing one end deep into the muscle and the other end more superficial but attempting not to constrict the ulnar nerve. He described his results as being "most gratifying," with no additional notations. When Platt described his technique in 1928, he described, "more than 100 patients" but did not stage the degree of severity nor quantitate the results except also by stating that his results were "most gratifying." His description of the technique, however, clearly de-

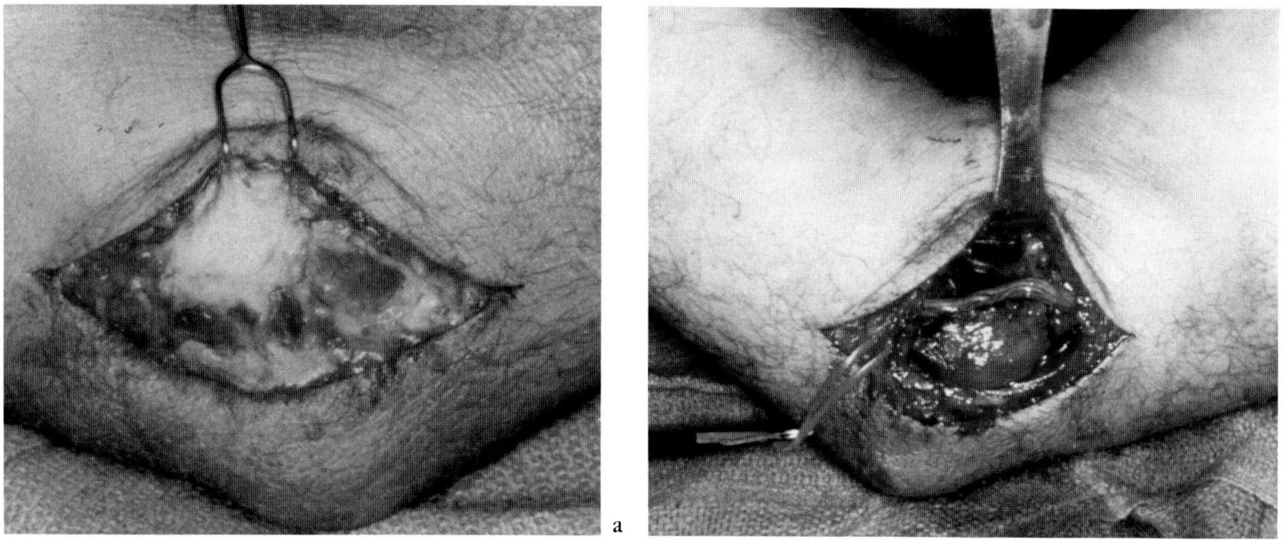

Figure 9-22. Recurrent ulnar nerve entrapment after subcutaneous transposition. **a.** Note scar binding nerve to medial humeral epicondyle; **b.** After neurolysis and before submuscular transposition.

scribed a deep intramuscular positioning with a complete division of the common flexor tendon noted in his drawings. He also excised the medial intermuscular septum. Thus, his dissection technique closely approximated that which would be described by Learmonth as a submuscular technique.[82] Gay and Love[106] indicated that they carried out an internal neurolysis on 54% of their patients with a severe degree of nerve compression. However, the internal neurolysis in the absence of appropriate releases of the nerve proximally, that is, at the medial intermuscular septum and directly in the muscle mass (over the common flexor tendon), will not permit the nerve to have sufficient excusion to prevent the internal neurolysis from scarring back down into this bed. A location of the nerve adjacent to cut muscle fibers, if the nerve is allowed to glide in the postoperative period, will not, in and of itself, cause severe scarring of the nerve.[52] Indeed, it is our belief that those investigators who have discussed good results from an intramuscular anterior transposition must carry out a sufficiently deep intermuscular transposition so that the common flexor tendon is completely released and carry out an extensive enough proximal and distal dissection so that, in essence, they have performed a submuscular rather than an intramuscular transposition. The results of this technique can only be judged in two series,[14,106] comprising just 79 patients who had a severe degree of nerve compression. Just 6% achieved normal motor and sensory function, with 67% of the patients having persistence or recurrence of their preoperative sensory and motor function (Figs. 9-24, 9-25). An intramuscular placement that does not release the common flexor tendon or extensively dissect the ulnar nerve distally and resect the medial intermuscular septum proximally is doomed to failure, as has already been described. This technique is generally not indicated for the treatment of ulnar nerve compression.

Anterior Submuscular Transposition

The results of the treatment of ulnar nerve compression at the elbow by an anterior submuscular transposition are listed in Table 9-17 for those series directly reporting this technique.[2,3,11,71,82,85,105] The results are summarized in Table 9-20. This is the technique that we prefer and was described extensively in the Surgical Technique section. Two reports of patients treated by this procedure are not included in Table 9-17 because insufficient information was available. The article by Hartel[107] indicates that 70% of the patients achieved excellent results. This translation ws obtained from Sunderland.[11] Gerl and Thorwith[108] were also quoted by Sunderland as having 86% excellent relief in 22 patients. The results of patients with anterior submuscular transposition and with a minimal degree of nerve compression have only been reported for five patients, in whom 100% excellent relief was obtained (Table 9-20). For patients with a moderate degree of nerve compression, 81% recovered normal strength and 77% recovered normal sensation with persistence of the sensory and motor symptoms occurring in just 3% of the patients. For patients with a severe degree of nerve compression, the available literature review indicates that just 12% recovered normal muscle when atrophy existed preoperatively and that just 14% achieved normal sensation, with 30% of the patients having persistence or

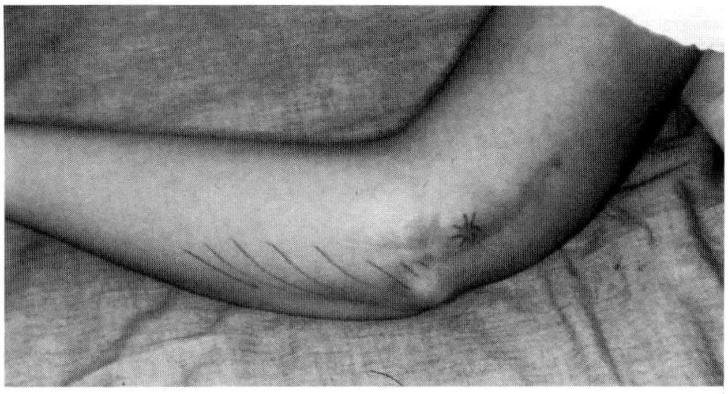

a

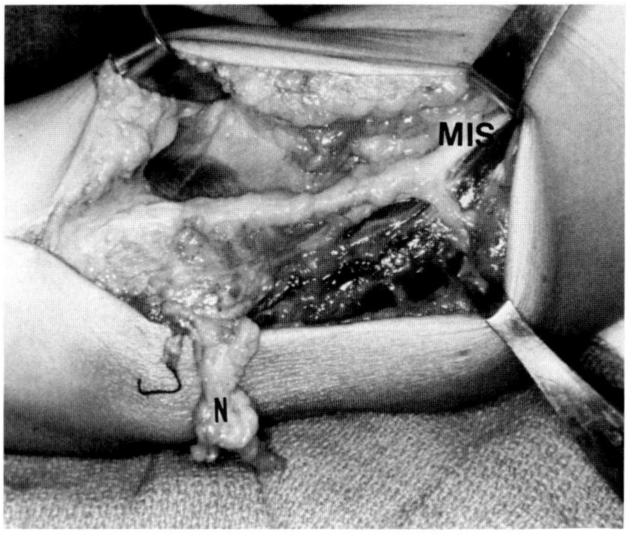

b

Figure 9-23a. Recurrent ulnar nerve entrapment after subcutaneous transposition with associated neuroma of medial antebrachial cutaneous nerve: Cross-hatched area of decreased sensation, Tinel's sign proximal to this. **b.** Ulnar nerve scarred into medial humeral epicondyle with neuroma still attached (N). **c.** After neurolysis and before transposition. Note excised medial intermuscular septum (MIS). **d.** Close-up of pseudoneuroma after neurolysis. Note plexus formation.

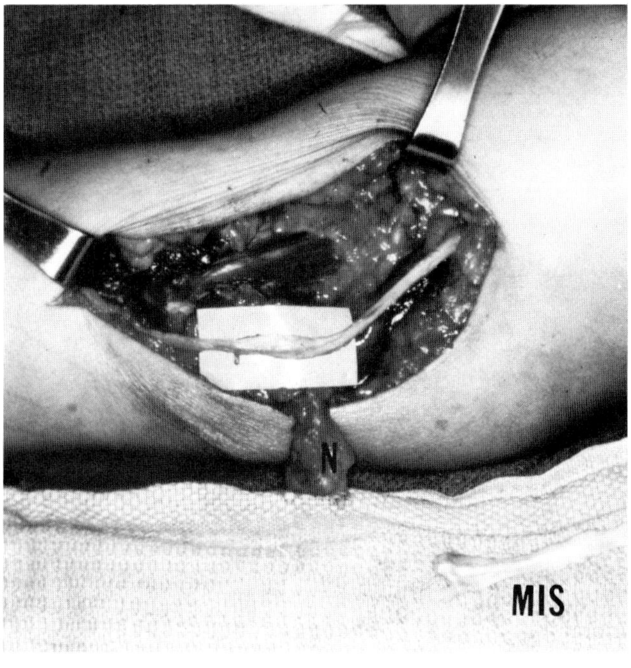

c

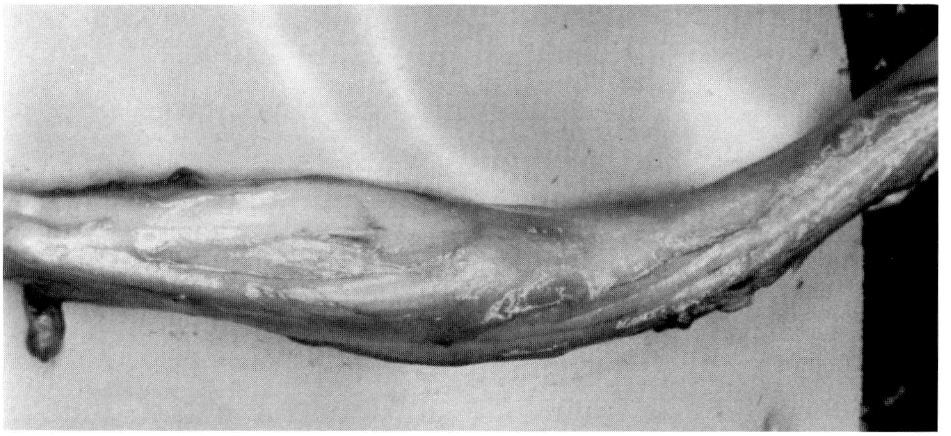

d

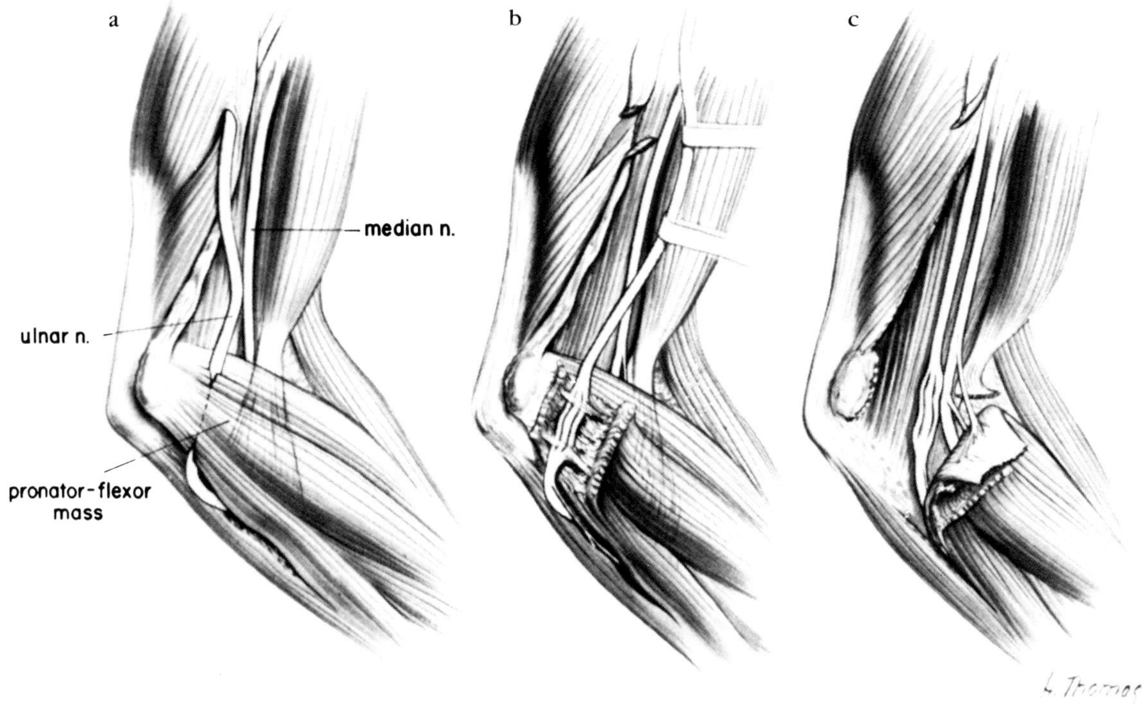

Figure 9-24. Recurrent ulnar nerve entrapment after intramuscular transposition. **a.** Note tight closure of fascia over transposed nerve; **b.** nerve compressed against common flexor tendon; **c.** deep, submuscular positioning. (Reproduced with permission from Spinner.[47])

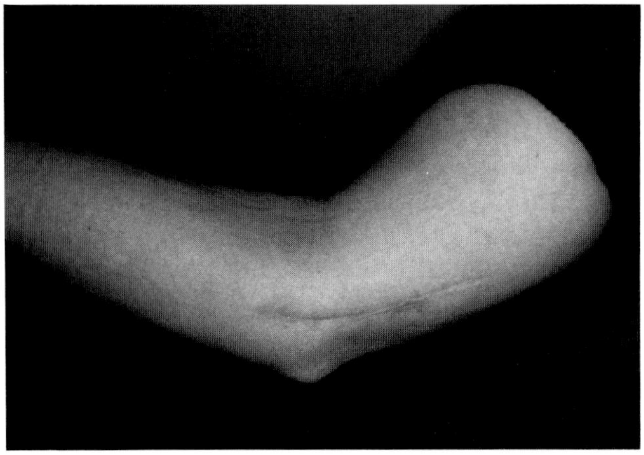
a

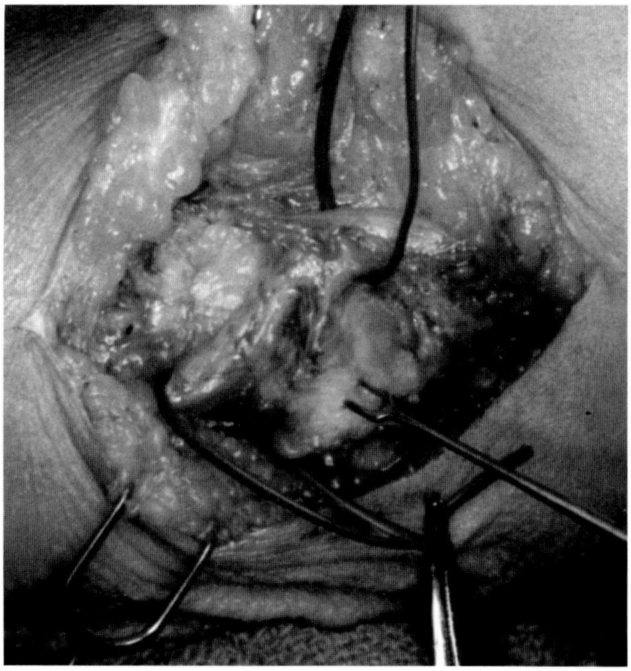
b

Figure 9-25. Recurrent ulnar nerve entrapment after intramuscular transposition. **a.** Note nerve forming two right angle turns as it enters and leaves flexor pronator muscle mass; **b.**

recurrence of their sensory and motor symptoms. It must be noted that the reported series of patients here treated by anterior submuscular transposition did not include an internal neurolysis in the patients with a severe degree of nerve compression. In Dellon's personal series when an internal neurolysis is added in the severe degree of nerve compression, approximately 80% of the patients achieved excellent recovery of motor function in terms of reversal of muscle wasting and achieved recovery of normal moving two-point discrimination. As already described, in this personal series there is a less than 2% recurrence rate as judged by reoperation in more than 400 patients. This is our preferred technique. In this technique, patients with minimal or moderate degree of nerve compression, in whom internal neurolysis is not carried out, 90 to 100% relief of sensory symptoms and 90% recovery of normal strength is anticipated.

Recurrent Ulnar Neuropathy

When recurrent ulnar nerve compression at the elbow is treated by surgery, the results for those series that have directly discussed this problem are listed in Table 9-18[3,25,87,106,109,110] and the results summarized in Table 9-20. The surgical technique used to treat the patients with recurrent ulnar nerve compression at the elbow, the majority of which have been treated previously either by simple decompression or by subcutaneous or intramuscular anterior transposition techniques, has been a submuscular transposition with either external neurolysis[3] or internal neurolysis.[87,106,109] In the eight patients who may have been judged to have a moderate degree of nerve compression at the time they were reoperated on, 63% achieved normal strength and 63% achieved normal sensation. In those with a severe degree of nerve compression at the time they were reoperated on, 15% achieved reversal of their muscle atrophy, 33% achieved normal strength, 52% achieved normal sensation, and 6% had persistence of their preoperative sensory and motor problems. Our personal approach to these patients is to carry out an anterior submuscular transposition and internal neurolysis of the ulnar nerve. As already described, it is cautioned that if a patient is being operated on for the second or third time and they are more than 60 years of age, the nerve may be sufficiently ischemic that further internal neurolysis may result in an infarction of the ulnar nerve and, accordingly, surgery in this group of patients must be undertaken with extreme caution and with appropriate preoperative advice to the patient. Indeed, an internal neurolysis in this select group of patients may be contraindicated.

There have been 11 studies reported[21,70,71,73,79,92–94,100,105,108] that have attempted to address the problem of which type of surgical technique is better than another for the treatment of ulnar nerve compression at the elbow. These are reviewed in Table 9-19. The problem with these studies has already been described. The studies' most common methodologic failure was not comparing groups that were of equivalent stages preoperatively and in not applying statistical analysis. Although there are exceptions to these methodologic flaws, the overall conclusion from Table 9-19 is that none of these articles has demonstrated clearly the superiority of one surgical technique over any other surgical technique. The basis for choosing the surgical technique at the present time therefore must be related to the pathophysiologic condition of the ulnar nerve compression, an understanding of the cause of the nerve compression in the patient's particular case, and the various methods and potential technical drawbacks of the various operative procedures that have been outlined. This choice is further described in the concluding paragraphs to follow.

Postoperative Electrodiagnostic Testing

A note of caution must be included about doing electrodiagnostic studies in the patient who has had anterior transposition of the ulnar nerve. This problem has been recently discussed.[111] The electrodiagnostic studies have been found to be altered in their results based on the elbow position.[112] When the ulnar nerve is in the pretransposition location, which is in the postcondylar groove, nerve conduction velocities are increased when the elbow is flexed. Thus, it becomes critical in determining the postoperative electrodiagnostic studies to place the elbow in a position that is appropriate. Once the nerve has been transposed to lie anteriorly, then the effect of elbow flexion on the ulnar nerve will be altered. Furthermore, if skin markings are measured posterior to the elbow, as is usually done in a preoperative situation, these distances are increased when the elbow is flexed and decreased when the elbow is extended. If an anterior skin marking position is to be used in the postoperative position because the ulnar nerve has been transposed anteriorly, then the reverse situation exists, that is, the distances are longer when the elbow is extended than when the elbow is flexed (Fig. 9-15). A series of patients was measured in the operating room before and after ulnar nerve transposition. The skin markings were made with the elbow flexed and extended. The distance of the ulnar nerve, itself, was directly measured in the pre- and post-transposition positions and the electrodiagnostic testing was done in the pre- and postoperative positions. The latency obtained across the elbow was related to the various skin markings and the different conduction velocities obtained are outlined in Table 9-21. This study demonstrates that,

Table 9-21. Variation in Conduction Velocity of the Ulnar Nerve Across the Elbow Due to Parameters of Elbow Flexion and Skin Marking, Intraoperative Conduction Velocities (m/sec)*

	Pretransposition		*Post-transposition*				
	1	*2*	*3*	*4*	*5*	*6*	*7*
Patient No.	*Skin, posterior,† elbow flexed*	*Nerve,† elbow flexed*	*Skin, posterior,† elbow flexed*	*Skin, posterior,† elbow extended*	*Skin, anterior,† elbow flexed*	*Skin, anterior,† elbow extended*	*Nerve,† elbow extended*
1	33	35	42	33	44	46	31
2	36	38	48	36	42	55	38
3	44	42	50	44	42	51	42
4	50	57	64	50	57	78	57
5	48	60	60	48	60	65	60
6	48	48	75	59	58	59	52
7	50	39	49	48	41	52	40
8	54	39	54	45	41	47	40

*Reprinted with permission from Dellon et al.[111]

†Distance measured.

depending on the skin marking chosen and the position of the elbow, the conduction velocity found in evaluating a patient after anterior transposition of the ulnar nerve may vary by as much as 10 m/s, thereby making the difference between determining whether the patient has been improved by surgery or has failed to improve by surgery. The recommendations of this study are that the patient be tested by the same person who did the preoperative study when possible. If possible, the skin marking distance that was used preoperatively should be used postoperatively, and the preoperative marking position should be defined in the reports, ideally with the elbow in the flexed position. Postoperatively, the elbow should be studied in the extended position using the skin marking that was utilized in the preoperative testing.

Conclusion

If surgery is elected as the method of treatment for ulnar nerve entrapment at the elbow, it must be realized that there is no prospective, randomized study of patients treated by different surgical techniques that gives guidance as to which surgical procedure provides the best results. Those surgeons listed in Table 9-19, that attempted to compare techniques even if methodologically without flaw, showed no significant difference in the techniques they compared. It may be concluded from a review of the literature that simple decompression techniques can give good to excellent results for patients whose etiology does not include trauma, tumor, or a repetitive work disorder, for patients with a minimal degree of nerve compression, and for whom the findings at surgery are the presence of an Osborne's band or a similar congenital anomaly, such as an epitrochleoanconeus muscle or snapping triceps tendon. For any other situation, the results with simple decompression have not been shown to be as successful as other reported techniques (see Table 9-20). Medial epicondylectomy is not considered as a surgical alternative by us because it does not treat the basic pathophysiologic condition, and long-term recurrence rate is high.[93] The more extensive techniques that may be joined to the medial epicondylectomy approach are those recommended by us, which are an anterior submuscular transposition with an internal neurolysis of the ulnar nerve when such is indicated. When these are done, as described above, the medial epicondyle need not be removed. The anterior *intra*muscular transposition yielded the fewest excellent results with the highest recurrence rate, and we therefore believe this is never the procedure of choice. Statistical analysis by chi-square of the data in Table 9-20 for moderate degree of compression demonstrated that the anterior submuscular transposition gave a significantly greater percentage of excellent results than all other surgical techniques.[93] For a severe degree of nerve compression, the best results were obtained when an internal neurolysis was added to a submuscular transposition in the treatment of the subgroup of recurrent ulnar nerve compression. It is this technique, anterior submuscular transposition with internal neurolysis, as described in this chapter, that we recommend for the treatment of the severe degree of ulnar nerve entrapment at the elbow.

References

1. Diamond ML, Lister GD: Cubital tunnel syndrome treated by long-arm splintage. (Abstr.) J Hand Surg [Am] 10:430, 1985.
2. Seddon H: Surgical Disorders of the Peripheral Nerves. Williams & Wilkins, Baltimore, 1972.
3. Leffert, RD: Anterior submuscular transposition of the ulnar nerves by the Learmonth technique. J Hand Surg 7:147–155, 1982.

4. Kline DG: Comments on "Neurolysis combined with the application of a Silastic envelope for ulnar nerve entrapment at the elbow." Neurosurgery 20:597–598, 1987.
5. Panas J: Sur une cause peu connue de paralysie du nerf cubital. Arch Gen Med 2:5–22, 1878.
6. Broca A, Mouchet A: Complications nervuses des fractures de l'extermite inferieure de l'humerus. Rev Chir (Paris) 19:701, 1899.
7. Mouchet A: Paralysies tardives du nerf cubital a la suite des fractures du condyle externe de l'humerus. J Chir (Paris) 12:437, 1914.
8. Platt H: The pathogenesis and treatment of traumatic neuritis of the ulnar nerve in the post-condylar groove. Br J Surg 13:409–431, 1926.
9. Platt H: On the peripheral nerve complications of certain fractures. Surg Gynecol Obstet 47:822–825, 1928.
10. Davidson AJ, Horowitz MT: Late or tardy ulnar paralysis. J Bone Joint Surg 17:844–856, 1935.
11. Sunderland S: Nerves and Nerve Injuries, 2nd ed. Churchill Livingstone, 1978, pp 780–795.
12. Mouchet A, Sille G: Paralysie tardive du nerf cubital et accident du travail. Presse Med 57:197, 1949.
13. Curtis BF: Traumatic ulnar neuritis—transplantation of the nerve. J Nerv Ment Dis 25:480–481, 1898.
14. Adson AL: The surgical treatment of progressive ulnar paralysis. Minn Med 1:455–460, 1918.
15. Earle H: Cases and observations illustrating the influence of the nervous system in regulating animal heat. Med Chir Trans 7:173–185, 1816.
16. Calder FWG: Effects of a division of the ulnar nerve. Lancet 1:489–490, 1833.
17. Sherren J: Remarks on chronic neuritis of the ulnar nerve due to deformity in the region of the elbow joint. Edinb Med J 23:500–509, 1908.
18. Andrae H: Uber traumatische Luxation des Nervus ulnaris am Ellenbogen. Inaugural dissertation: Greifswald, 1889.
19. Sheldon WD: Tardy palsy of the ulnar nerve. Med Clin North Am 5:499–509, 1921.
20. Feindel W, Stratford J: The role of the cubital tunnel in tardy ulnar palsy. Can J Surg 1:287–300, 1958.
21. Osborne GV: Surgical treatment of tardy ulnar neuritis. (Abstr.) J Bone Joint Surg 39B:782, 1957.
22. Dellon AL: Think nerve in upper extremity reconstruction. Clinics Plastic Surg 16:617-627, 1989.
23. Morrey BF, Askew LJ, An KN, Dobyns JH: Rupture of the distal tendon of the biceps brachii. J Bone Joint Surg 67A:418–421, 1985.
24. Brook DM: Editorial. J Bone Joint Surg 32B:291–292, 1950.
25. McGowan AJ: The results of transposition of the ulnar nerve for traumatic ulnar neuritis. J Bone Joint Surg 32B:293–301, 1950.
26. Eisen A, Dannen J: The mild cubital tunnel syndrome. Neurology (Minneap) 24:608–613, 1974.
27. Eisen A: Early diagnosis of ulnar nerve palsy: An electrophysiologic study. Neurology (Minneap) 24:256–262, 1974.
28. Dellon AL: Clinical use of vibratory stimuli to evaluate peripheral nerve injury and compression neuropathy. Plast Reconstr Surg 65:466–476, 1980.
29. Fine EJ, Wongjirad C: The ulnar flexion maneuver. (Abstr.) Muscle Nerve 8:612, 1985.
30. Dellon AL: Prospective study of the non-operative treatment of minimal degree of ulnar nerve compression at the elbow. J Hand Surg, 1990. Submitted.
31. Vanderpool DW, Chalmers J, Lamb DW, Whitstson TB: Peripheral compression lesions of the ulnar nerve. J Bone Joint Surg 50B:792–802, 1968.
32. Apfelberg DB, Larson SJ: Dynamic anatomy of the ulnar nerve at the elbow. Plast Reconstr Surg 51:76–81, 1973.
33. Dellon AL: Musculotendinous variations about the medial humeral epicondyle. J Hand Surg [Br] 11:175–181, 1986.
34. Pechan J, Julis I: The pressure measurement in the ulnar nerve: A contribution to the pathophysiology of the cubital tunnel syndrome. J Biomech 8:75–79, 1975.
35. Sunderland S: The intraneural topography of the radial, median and ulnar nerves. Brain 68:243–253, 1945.
36. Chang KSF, Low WD, Chan ST: Enlargement of the ulnar nerve behind the medial humeral epicondyle. Anat Rec 145:149–153, 1963.
37. Rolfsen L: Snapping triceps tendon with ulnar neuritis. Acta Orthop Scand 41:74–76, 1970.
38. Dreyfus D, Kessler J: Snapping elbow due to dislocation fo the medial head of the triceps. J Bone Joint Surg 60B:56–58, 1978.
39. Reis ND: Anomalous triceps tendon as the cause for snapping elbow in ulnar neuritis. J Hand Surg 5:361–362, 1980.
40. Hayashi Y, Kojima T, Kohno T: Case of cubital tunnel syndrome caused by the snapping of the medial head of the triceps brachii muscle. J Hand Surg [Am] 9:96–99, 1984.
41. Ho KC, Marmor L: Entrapment of the ulnar nerve at the elbow. Am J Surg 121:355–356, 1971.
42. Nicolle FV, Woolhouse FM: Nerve compression syndromes of the upper limb. J Trauma 5:313–315, 1965.
43. Hirasawa Y, Sawamura H, Sakakida K: Entrapment neuropathy due to bilateral epitrochleoanconeus muscles: A case report. J Hand Surg 4:181–184, 1979.
44. Kane E, Kaplan EB, Spinner M: Observations on the course of the ulnar nerve in the arm. Ann Chir 27:470–496, 1973.
45. Spinner M, Spencer PS: Nerve compression lesions of the upper extremity: A clinical and experimental review. Clin Orthop 104:46–68, 1974.
46. Spinner M, Kaplan EB: The relationship of the ulnar nerve to the medial intermuscular septum in the arm and its clinical significance. Hand 8:239–242, 1976.
47. Spinner M: Management of nerve compression lesions in the upper extremity. In Omer GE Jr, Spinner M, eds: Management of Peripheral Nerve Problems. WB Saunders Co, Philadelphia, 1980.
48. Struthers J: On a peculiarity of the humerus and humeral artery. Month J Med Sci 28:264–267, 1848.

49. Struthers J: On some points in the abnormal anatomy of the arm. Br For Med Chir Rev 14:170–179, 1854.
50. Dellon AL, Mackinnon SE: Injury to the medial antebrachial cutaneous nerve during cubital tunnel surgery. J Hand Surg [Br] 19:33–36, 1985.
51. Dawson DM, Hallet M, Millender LH: Entrapment Neuropathies. Little, Brown, Boston, 1983, p 109.
52. Dellon AL, Mackinnon SE, Hudson AR, Hunter DA: Effect of submuscular versus intramuscular placement of ulnar nerve: Experimental model in the primate. J Hand Surg [Br] 11:117–119, 1986.
53. Amadio PC, Beckenbaugh RD: Entrapment of the ulnar nerve by the deep flexor-pronator aponeurosis. J Hand Surg [Am] 11:83–87, 1986.
54. Inserra A, Spinner M: An anatomic factor significant in transposition of the ulnar nerve. J Hand Surg [Am] 11A:80–82, 1986.
55. Neary D, Eames RA: The pathology of ulnar nerve compression in man. Neuropathol Appl Neurobiol 1:69–88, 1975.
56. Neary D, Ochoa J, Gilliatt RW: Subclinical entrapment neuropathy in man. J Neurol Sci 24:283–298, 1975.
57. Mackinnon SE, Dellon AL, Hudson AR, Hunter DA: Chronic human nerve compression: A histologic assessment. Neuropathol Appl Neurobiol 12:547–565, 1986.
58. Dellon AL, Mackinnon SE: Human ulnar nerve compression: Clinical, Electrophysiological and morphometric assessment. J Reconstr Microsurg 4:179–187, 1988.
59. Dellon AL: Tinel or not Tinel? J Hand Surg [Br] 9:216, 1984.
60. Dellon AL: The vibrometer. Plast Reconstr Surg 71:427–431, 1983.
61. Checkles NS, Russakov AD, Pareo DL: Ulnar nerve conduction velocity: Effect of elbow position on the measurement. Arch Phys Med Rehabil 52:362–365, 1971.
62. Froment MJ: La paralysie de l'adductur du pouce et le signe de la prahnsion. Rev Neurol (Paris) 28:1236–1240, 1915.
63. Wartenberg R: A sign of ulnar palsy. JAMA 112:16–88, 1939.
64. Steadman's Medical Dictionary. 21st ed. Williams & Wilkins, Baltimore, 1966.
65. Osborne G: The elbow and forearm. In Rob C, Smith R, eds: Clinical Surgery. Butterworths, London, 1966, pp 417–454.
66. Osborne G: Personal communication, March, 1982.
67. Wilson DH, Kraut R: Surgery of ulnar neuropathy at the elbow in sixteen cases treated by decompression without transposition. J Neurosurg 38:780–785, 1973.
68. Gilliatt RW, Thomas PK: Changes in nerve conduction with ulnar lesions at the elbow. J Neurol Neurosurg Psychiatry 23:312—320, 1960.
69. Clark CB: Cubital tunnel syndrome. JAMA 241:801–802, 1979.
70. Foster RJ, Edshage S: Factors related to the outcome of surgically managed compressive ulnar neuropathy at the elbow level. J Hand Surg 6:181–192, 1981.
71. MacNichol MF: Results of operations for ulnar neuritis. J Bone Joint Surg 61B:159–164, 1979.
72. Lugnegard H, Waldheim G, Wenberg G: Operative treatment of ulnar nerve neuropathy in the elbow region. Acta Orthop Scand 48:168–176, 1977.
73. Chan RC, Paine KW, Varughese G: Ulnar nerve at the elbow: Comparison of subcutaneous decompression and anterior transposition. Neurosurgery 7:545–550, 1980.
74. Wright EA, McQuillen MP: Hypoexcitability of ulnar nerve in patients with normal motor and nerve conduction studies. Neurology (Minneap) 23:78–83, 1973.
75. De Jesus PV, Stiner JC: Spontaneous recovery of ulnar neuropathy at the elbow. Electromyogr Clin Neurophysiol 16:239–248, 1976.
76. Miller RG: Cubital tunnel syndrome: Diagnosis and precise localization. Ann Neurol 6:56–59, 1979.
77. Brown WF, Yates SK: Percutaneous localization of conduction abnormalities in human extremities. Can J Neurol Sci 9:391–400, 1982.
78. Craven RR, Green DP: Cubital tunnel syndrome: Treatment by medial epicondylectomy. J Bone Joint Surg 62A:986–990, 1980.
79. Paine EW: Tardy ulnar palsy. Can J Surg 13:255–261, 1970.
80. Eaton RG, Crowe JF, Parkes JC III: Anterior transposition of the ulnar nerve with a non-compressing fasciodermal sling. J Bone Joint Surg 62A:820–825, 1980.
81. Culver JE: Compression neuropathy at the elbow treated by medial humeral epicondylectomy. Long term follow-up. J Bone Joint Surg. 1988. In press.
82. Learmonth JR: Technique for transplantation of the ulnar nerve. Surg Gynecol Obstet 75:792–793, 1942.
83. Dellon AL: Operative technique for submuscular transposition of the ulnar nerve. Contemp Orthop, 16:17–24, 1988.
84. Jones RE, Gauntt C: Medial epicondylectomy for ulnar nerve compression syndrome at the elbow. Clin Orthop 139:174–178, 1979.
85. Richards RL: Traumatic ulnar neuritis: The results of anterior transposition of the ulnar nerve. Edinb Med J 52:14–21, 1945.
86. Spinner M: Injuries to the Major Branches of the Peripheral Nerves of the Forearm, 2nd ed. WB Saunders, Philadelphia, 1980, p 240.
87. Campbell JB, Post KD, Marantz RA: A technique for relief of motor and sensory deficits occurring after anterior ulnar transposition. J Neurosurg 40:405–409, 1974.
88. Benoit BG, Preston DN, Atack DM, Da Silva VF: Neurolysis combined with the application of a Silastic envelope for ulnar nerve entrapment at the elbow. Neurosurgery 20:594–598, 1987.
89. Pauker SG, Kassier JP: Decision analysis. N Engl J Med 316:250–258, 1987.
90. Stewart JD: Focal Peripheral Neuropathies. Elsevier, New York, 1987.
91. Harrison MJG, Nurick S: Results of anterior transposi-

tion of ulnar nerve for ulnar neuritis. Br Med J 1:27–29, 1970.

92. Payan J: Anterior transposition of the ulnar nerve: an electrophysiological study. J Neurol Neurosurg Psychiatry 33:157–165, 1970.
93. Dellon AL: Review of treatment results for ulnar nerve entrapment at the elbow. J Hand Surg 14A:688—700, 1989.
94. Wadsworth TG: The external compression syndrome of the ulnar nerve at the cubital tunnel. Clin Orthop 124:189–204, 1977.
95. Hagstrom P: Ulnar nerve compression at the elbow. Scand J Plast Reconstr Surg 11:59–62, 1977.
96. Fannin TF: Local decompression in the treatment of ulnar nerve entrapment at the elbow. J R Col Surg Edinb 23:362–366, 1978.
97. Osborne G: Ulnar neuritis. Postgrad Med J 35:392–396, 1959.
98. Weisl H, Osborne GV: The pathological changes in rat's nerves subject to moderate compression. J Bone Joint Surg 46B:297–305, 1964.
99. Osborne J: Compression neuritis of the ulnar nerve. Hand 2:10–14, 1970.
100. Laha RK, Panchal PD: Surgical treatment of ulnar neuropathy. Surg Neurol 11:393–398, 1979.
101. Neblett C, Ehni G: Medial epicondylectomy for ulnar palsy. J Neurosurg 32:55–62, 1970.
102. Gore D, Larson S: Medial epicondylectomy for subluxing ulnar nerve. Am J Surg 111:851–853, 1966.
103. Froimson AI, Zahraw IF: Treatment of compression neuropathy of the ulnar nerve at the elbow by epicondylectomy and neurolysis. J Hand Surg 5:391–395, 1980.
104. King T, Morgan FP: Treatment of traumatic ulnar neuritis. Aust NZ J Surg 20:33–42, 1950.
104a. King T, Morgan FP: Later results of removing the medial humeral epicondyle for traumatic ulnar neuritis. J Bone Joint Surg 41B:51–55, 1959.
105. Levy DM, Apfelberg DB: Results of anterior transposition for ulnar neuropathy at the elbow. Am J Surg 123:304–308, 1972.
106. Gay J, Love J: Diagnosis and treatment of tardy paralysis of the ulnar nerve. J Bone Joint Surg 29B:1087–1097, 1947.
107. Hartel R: Munch Med Wochenschr 113:1580–1582, 1971.
108. Gerl A, Thorwith V: Ergebnisse der Ulnarisver Lagering. Acta Neurochir (Wien) 30:227–246, 1974.
109. Luch AL: Ulnar nerve entrapment after anterior transposition at the elbow. NY State J Med 75:75, 1975.
110. Broudy AS, Leffert RD, Smith RJ: Technical problems with ulnar nerve transposition at the elbow: findings and results of reoperation. J Hand Surg 3:85–89, 1978.
111. Dellon AL, Schlegel RW, Mackinnon SE: Validity of nerve conduction velocity studies following anterior transposition of the ulnar nerve. J Hand Surg 12A:700–703, 1987.
112. Nelson MR: Effects of elbow position on motor conduction velocity of the ulnear nerve. Phys Ther 60:780–783, 1980.
113. Pulkki T, Vainio K: Compression of the ulnar nerve due to rheumatoid arthritis at the elbow. Ann Chir Gynecol Fenn 51:327–330, 1962.
114. DeAndrade JR, Casagrende PA: Ulnar nerve entrapment in rheumatoid arthritis. Arthritis Rheuma 8:294–301, 1965.
115. Moore JR, Weiland AJ: Bilateral attritional rupture of the ulnar nerve at the elbow. J Hand Surg 5:358–360, 1980.
116. Ash EN, Hurst EM: Anatomical factors in etiology of ulnar neuropathy. Can Med Assoc J 87:159–163, 1962.
117. Childress HM: Recurrent ulnar nerve dislocation at the elbow. J Bone Joint Surg 38A:978–984, 1956.
118. Wadsworth TG, Williams RM: Cubital tunnel external compression syndrome. Nurs Times 73:1357–1359, 1977.
119. Ekerot L: Post-anesthetic ulnar neuropathy at the elbow. Scand J Plast Reconstr Surg 11:225–229, 1977.
120. Alvine FG, Schurrer ME: Postoperative ulnar nerve palsy. J Bone Joint Surg 69A:255–259, 1987.
121. Woltman HW: Pressure as a factor in the development of neuritis of the ulnar and common peroneal nerves in bedridden patients. Am J Med Sci 179:528–532, 1930.
122. Gilliatt RW, Wilson RG: Peripheral nerve conduction in diabetic neuropathy. J Neurol Neurosurg Psychiatry 25:11–16, 1962.
123. Frazier DM, Campbell IW, Ewing DJ, Clark BF: Mononeuropathy in diabetes mellitus. Diabetes 28:96–101, 1979.
124. Dyck PJ, Thomas PK, Asbury AK, Winegrad AI, Porte D Jr: Diabetic Neuropathy. WB Saudners, Philadelphia, 1987, p 171.
125. Weingarden SI, Weingarden HP: Spasmodic torticollis as a cause of ulnar nerve entrapment. Neurosurgery 14:332–334, 1984.
126. Carayon A: Investigations on physiopathology of the nerve in leprosy. Int J Leprosy 81:278–294, 1971.
127. Adelaar RS, Foster WC, McDowell C: The treatment of cubital tunnel syndrome. J Hand Surg [Am] 9:90–95, 1984.

10

Radial Sensory Nerve Entrapment in the Forearm

Historical Review

Entrapment of the radial sensory nerve in the forearm was first described in 1932 by Robert Wartenberg.[1] Wartenberg was a neurologist at the University of Freiberg in Germany. He was a keen clinical observer who relied primarily on the physical examination to arrive at his diagnosis. He reported a series of five patients who had complaints of areas of pain or numbness over the dorso-radial aspect of the hand. Each of these patients had a tender area to palpation over the course of the superficial sensory branch of the radial nerve. These patients had functional impairment in their hand, particularly with pinch or grip movements, although no muscle weakness could be detected on their physical examination. With forceful ulnar deviation of the wrist, a shooting pain was produced, radiating into the dorso-radial aspect of the hand. The patients' symptoms were worsened with pronation of the forearm. Although Wartenberg, in fact, went on to describe in each of these patients some type of predisposing factor to entrapment of the radial sensory nerve in the forearm, he, nevertheless, believed he was describing a mononeuritis or an inflammatory disorder of this peripheral nerve. Subsequent descriptions of this clinical problem have been referred to in the neurologic literature as "Wartenberg's disease".[2,3] Perhaps it is because Wartenberg's original description was in German that the subsequent neurologic, neurosurgical, orthopedic, and hand surgery literature has been essentially devoid of careful descriptions or further investigations of this peripheral nerve entrapment syndrome. Recently, a translation of Wartenberg's article has appeared.[4] From this translation, it is clear that one of Wartenberg's patients had sustained an injury to one of the peripheral branches of the radial sensory nerve, another patient was a diabetic, another appeared to have had, in fact, multiple peripheral nerve entrapments, one patient had a tight wristwatch band as the initiating problem, and another patient had a work-related problem with the hand. Wartenberg carefully reviewed the previous literature with respect to other causes of mononeuritis. A previous description of radial sensory nerve entrapment due to a watchband compression has been recorded by Matzdorf.[5] There have been seven other cases of radial sensory nerve entrapment due to wristwatch bands.[2,3,5–7] The reference, often misquoted, is that of Stopford,[8] which was not to a radial sensory but a dorsal cutaneous branch of the ulnar nerve, which was compressed at the wrist by a watchband. The most recent descriptions of radial sensory nerve entrapment have been case reports related to "handcuff neuropathy."[9–11] The vast majority of these localized nerve entrapments from band appliances about the wrist have responded to removing the offending band. None of Wartenberg's patients were operated on and none of his patients recovered. The majority of the individual case reports just referred to were of shorter duration than Wartenberg's patients, and most lacked a Tinel's sign over the radial sensory nerve. These earlier reports did not record whether or not patients had persistent sensory discomfort in the area or had abnormal two-point discrimination over the dorsoradial aspect of their hand.

Surgical Anatomy

The radial sensory nerve lies beneath the brachioradialis muscle in the forearm and is superficial to the radial artery. The nerve transits from below fascia to the subcutaneous plane by emerging between the tendons of the extensor carpi radialis longus and the brachioradialis tendon at about the juncture of the distal third and the middle third of the forearm. The fascia at this point of transition bridges the tendon and musculotendinous juncture of the brachioradialis muscle joining this tendon to the tendon of the extensor carpi radialis longus. The nerve may make its exit point anywhere from as far distally as a few centimeters proximal to the radial styloid to approximately the mid-portion of the forearm. In those persons in whom the nerve emerges more distally, the nerve lies in close proximity to the radial styloid, which may make it more likely to receive compressive forces from external bands, such as wristwatches and handcuffs.

In the most proximal regions of the forearm, the nerve lies in a location in which it is in jeopardy of being impinged on by metallic pins from external fixation devices. It is in the juncture between the distal third and middle third, however, that the nerve is most commonly found to exit, where it has a natural predisposition to entrapment from certain anatomically related situations. When the forearm is supinated, the location of the radial wrist extensor is such that it becomes separated from the brachioradialis tendon. During pronation of the wrist, the axis of the wrist extensor shifts to become more closely related to the brachioradialis tendon, thereby causing a natural pinching or compression of the radial sensory nerve as it exits between these two tendons. The radial sensory nerve lies along the dorsoradial border of the wrist. In this location, when the wrist is radially deviated and hyperextended, the nerve is relaxed, but when the wrist is flexed and ulnar deviated, as it is with most types of hammering movements of the wrist, then the radial sensory nerve is stretched. Thus, any action that causes either repeated supination and pronation or radial extension and ulnar deviation, or in the most provocative position, that of hyperpronation of the forearm and ulnar deviation of the wrist, the radial nerve becomes compressed and stretched. There are thus compressive forces against the nerve in its normal anatomic location and shearing forces. These combine to give repetitive, multiple trauma to the nerve in this location sufficient to cause the syndrome[12] (Fig. 10-1).

The radial sensory nerve begins to branch only after it has become subcutaneous in its location. Its distal branches most commonly go to the dorso-radial aspect of the thumb to the level of the interphalangeal joint, to the web space between the thumb and index finger, to the proximal interphalangeal level of the dorsal aspect of the index and middle fingers and portions of the ring finger. It has been repeatedly observed in patients who have even high division of the radial sensory nerve that sensibility over the dorso-radial aspect of the hand may remain completely intact and that there appears in many persons to be only a small, if any, so-called autonomous zone for this nerve. If there is, it lies over the dorsoradial aspect of the thumb and index finger.

There appears to be extensive overlap from dorsal cutaneous branches of the ulnar nerve and most significantly by branches of the lateral antebrachial cutaneous nerve.[13] The lateral antebrachial cutaneous nerve has been found in a dissection of 94 hands to have in one-third of these a high split, so that at the level at which the radial sensory nerve begins to exit, there is an overlap with the lateral antebrachial cutaneous nerve. Between overlap patterns of this nerve proximal and distal with the radial sensory nerve, altogether 75% of hands have either a partial or complete overlap of these two nerves over the dorsoradial aspect of the hand (Fig. 10-2; see also Chapter 17). This anatomic arrangement, in particular, makes electrodiagnostic studies of the radial sensory nerve in the forearm difficult because a normal, noncompressed nerve, the lateral antebrachial, may overlay the compressed radial sensory nerve.[15]

The existence of nerve compression in the location described for radial sensory nerve has been documented by histologic examination of this nerve. The radial sensory nerve contained pathologic changes ranging from epineurial thickening, both extra- and intrafascicular, to perineurial thickening and loss or thinning of myelin, Wallerian degeneration, and neural regener-

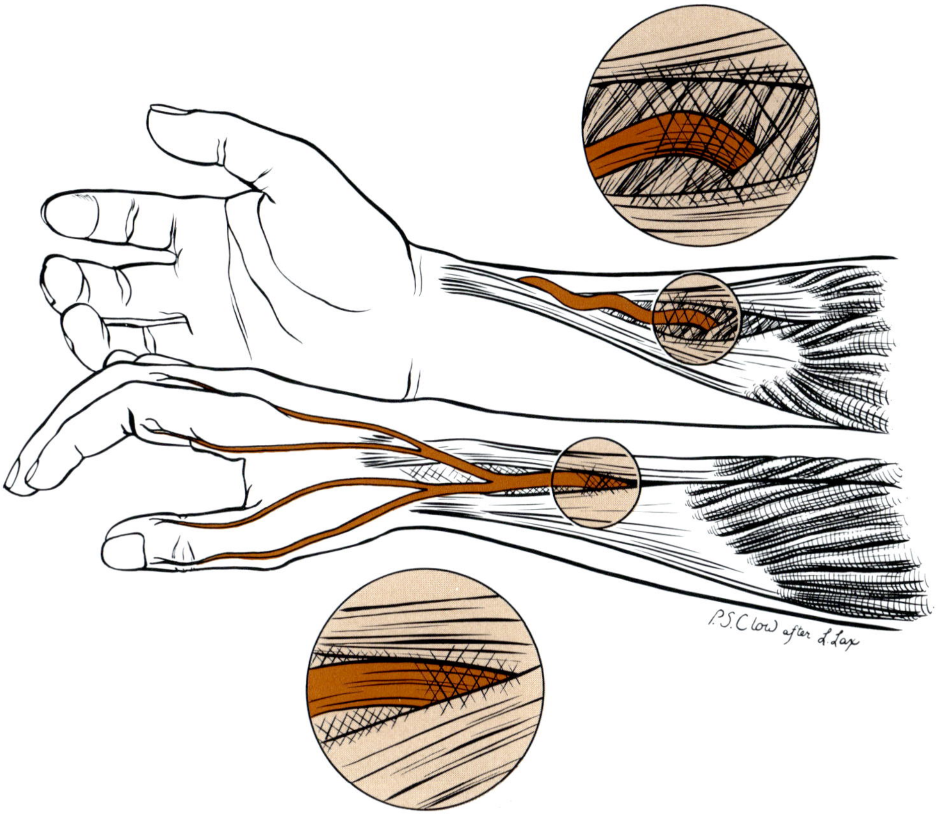

a

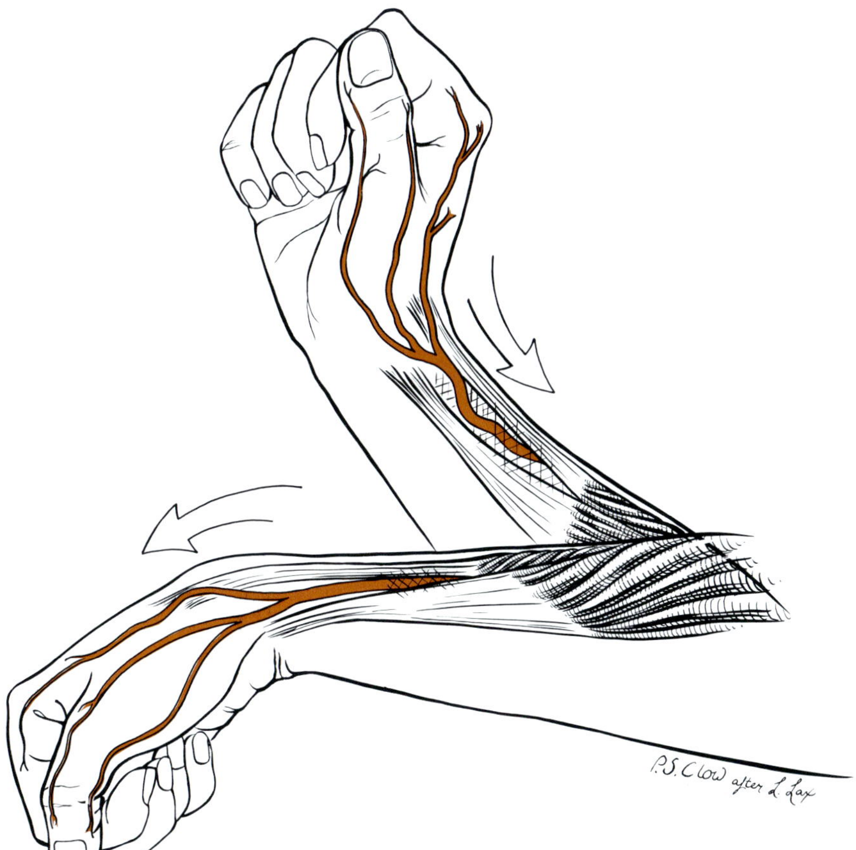

b

Figure 10-1a. Diagrammatic illustration of mechanism of radial sensory nerve entrapment. With the forearm supinated, the superficial branch of the radial nerve lies beneath the fascia but without compression between the tendons of the brachioradialis and the extensor carpi radialis longus. When the forearm pronates, the extensor carpi radialis longus tendon pulls proximally, crossing beneath the brachioradialis tendon, creating a scissoring or pinching of the superficial branch of the radial nerve. **b.** In the arc of motion from dorsal extension to ulnar flexion, the radial nerve is placed on stretch, with tension causing shearing forces at this same locus. (Reproduced with permission from Dellon et al.[12])

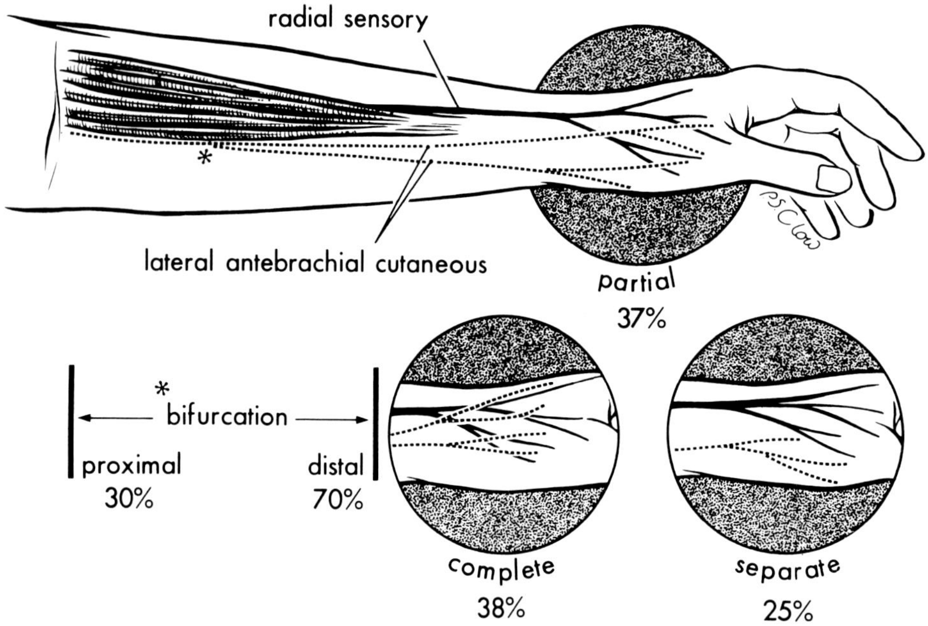

Figure 10-2. Schematic diagram of overlap pattern of superficial sensory radial nerve and lateral antebrachial cutaneous nerve. (Reproduced with permission from Mackinnon et al.[13])

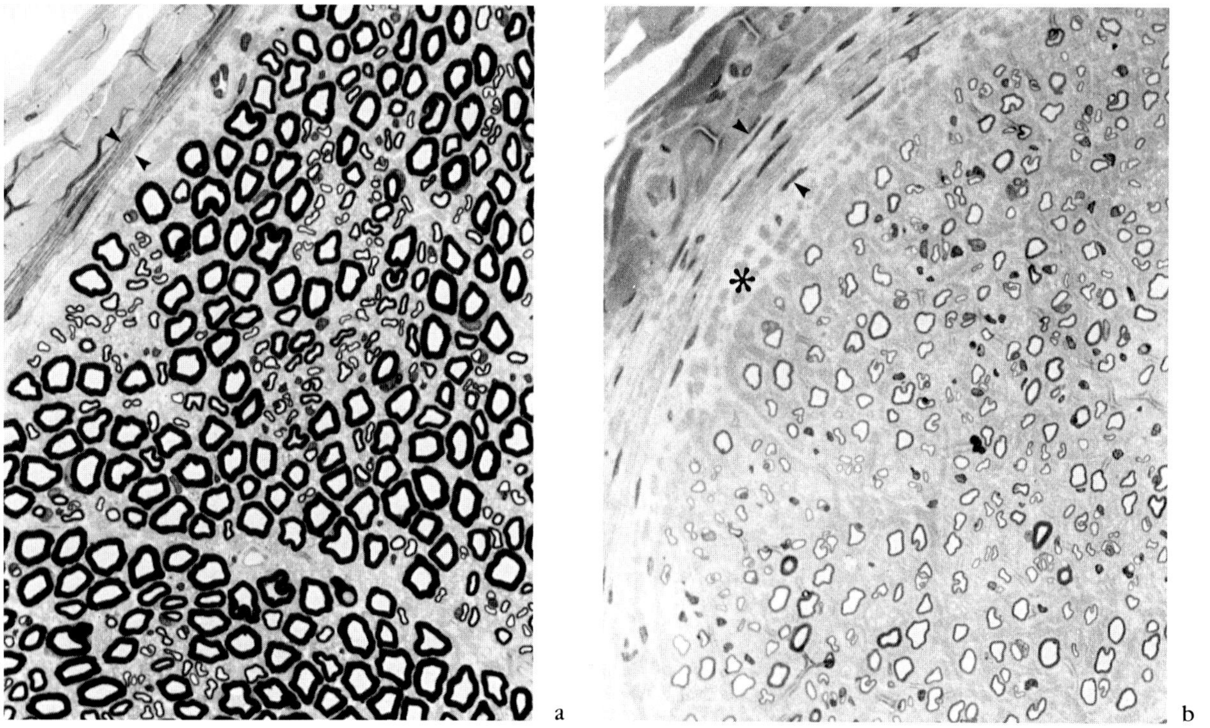

Figure 10-3a. A normal myelinated fiber population, as well as perineurium (arrow), are shown **b.** In the region of maximum compression, marked thickening is seen of the perineurium (arrow). Some subperineurial edema is also seen (*). Most of the large myelinated fibers demonstrate profound thinning of the myelin. (Toluidine blue stain, ×512.) (Reproduced with permission from Mackinnon et al.[14])

ation. Severity of pathologic alterations was related to the degree of clinical symptoms.[14,16] (Fig. 10-3; see also Chapter 2).

Diagnosis

The diagnosis of radial sensory nerve entrapment is made by combining the history with the physical examination. The history characteristically begins with complaints of pain over the dorsoradial aspect of the hand. Less commonly, the patient will complain of numbness or tingling or burning over the dorsoradial aspect of the hand. Another group of patients will not complain of sensory changes over the back of the hand initially but will indicate that their hand hurts when writing or pinching or gripping. There is often a history of trauma, such as a fall on the arm, a twisting motion of the forearm, or something else striking the dorsoradial aspect of the forearm. The work-related conditions that bring on this clinical entrapment may be sought in the history-taking. Assembly line work or using pneumatic tools or carpentry work where repetitive supination and pronation movements, especially with the wrist held in an ulnar flexed position or going from radial extension to ulnar flexion, predispose to this. This seems to occur also in chefs, bookkeepers, and dishwashers.

Associated diseases that are related to the occurrence of this nerve entrapment are diabetes and rheumatoid arthritis.

Physical examination generally reveals a Tinel's sign along the course of the radial sensory nerve. When the thumb is grasped between the fingers and the wrist moved into an ulnar flexed position, pain is elicited along the course of the radial sensory nerve. This physical finding was described by Finkelstein[17] as being indicative of first dorsal extensor tenosynovitis. However, Finkelstein's sign is also positive for radial sensory nerve entrapment, and this finding was clearly described by Wartenberg.[1] Wartenberg described pronation of the arm as inducing or aggravating these symptoms. More recently, a provocative test designed to bring out this compression has been described.[18] This position requires the patient to place his arm in front of him, hyperpronating the forearm with the wrist in ulnar flexion (Fig. 10-4). This provocative test within 1 minute generally brings on numbness and tingling over the dorsoradial aspect of the hand. This is interpreted as a positive finding. Ulnar wrist flexion simultaneous with forearm hyperpronation puts increased tension on the radial sensory nerve, but in patients who have an associated carpal tunnel, this position will, of course, put pressure on the median nerve in the wrist also, and symptoms of numbness and tingling will also occur over the volar aspect of the fingers. This should be sought by questioning the patient to distinguish the origin of the symptoms with this provocative test. The dorsoradial aspect of the hand subjected to careful moving touch testing will demonstrate a difference between the two hands. Moving two-point discrimination will become abnormal in the more advanced cases. In particular, the first dorsal extensor compartment over the radial styloid should not be tender, extension of the thumb should not produce tenderness, and resisted thumb extension should not produce pain, which would occur if there were tenosynovitis in the first dorsal extensor compartment.

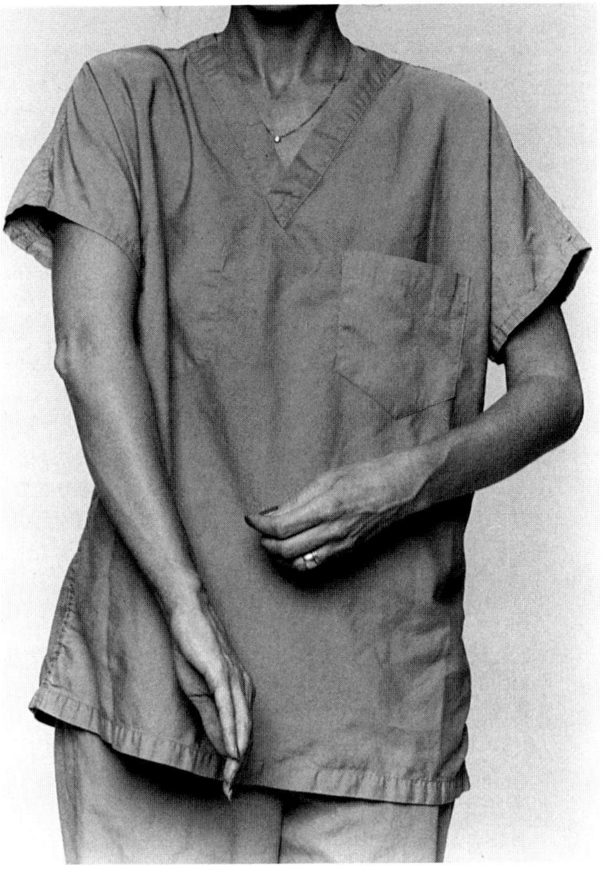

Figure 10-4. Provocative test for radial sensory nerve entrapment. The forearm is placed in hyperpronation with the wrist held in neutral. Within 1 minute, symptoms of dorsoradial burning, paresthesias, or tightness demonstrate a positive test for this nerve entrapment. Pressure over the intersection zone of the two tendons (brachioradialis, extensor carpi radialis longus) will augment symptoms as will wrist ulnar flexion.

Electrodiagnosis

With the extensive overlap of the lateral antebrachial cutaneous nerve, special electrodiagnostic studies are helpful in establishing the diagnosis of radial sensory nerve entrapment. The most commonly used methods have employed recording of the sensory nerve action potential from the web space between the thumb and index finger or from the thumb. Stimulation of the superficial branch of the radial nerve has been done in the distal forearm. While these techniques have proven very useful, they do not examine radial nerve function in the proximal forearm. To determine normal function, superficial radial sensory nerve conduction studies were performed bilaterally in 30 subjects with no evidence of neurologic disease.[15] Conduction was also examined in the lateral antebrachial cutaneous nerve in each arm (Table 10-1). Subjects ranged in age from 20 to 74, with a mean age of 39. Skin temperature at the wrist was maintained greater than 31°C in all patients. Radial sensory nerve action potentials were recorded from the web space between the thumb and index finger. The proximal recording disc electrode was placed over a palpable branch of the radial sensory nerve where it crosses the extensor pollicis longus tendon. The distal recording electrode was placed 4 cm distally over the thumb. Distal stimulation was performed supramaximally over the radius at a point ten cm proximal to the proximal recording electrode. The radial nerve was also stimulated in the antecubital fossa along the medial border of the brachioradialis. Surface stimulation of the nerve at this point was adequate in all control subjects. However, in very obese or heavily muscled patients, needle stimulation at the elbow may be necessary. All latencies were measured from the onset of the stimulus to the onset of the negative phase of the action potential. Conduction velocity in the distal segment was determined by dividing the ten cm distance by the distal latency. Forearm conduction was determined by dividing the distance between the two stimulus sites by the difference between the proximal and distal latencies. Peak-to-peak sensory nerve active potential amplitudes were measured. Sensory conduction in the lateral antebrachial cutaneous nerve was performed by stimulating the nerve at the biceps tendon at the elbow with recording of the sensory nerve action potential twelve cm distally. Since the radial sensory and lateral antebrachial cutaneous nerves are rather closely spaced at the elbow, following stimulation of either nerve at the elbow, recording was made from both these nerves distally to look for overlap patterns or spread of the stimulus to the adjacent nerve.

Diagnosis of radial sensory nerve entrapment in the presence of an overlapping normal lateral antebrachial cutaneous nerve is then possible by comparison of the values obtained for each of these nerves with each other and with the normative data in Table 10-1.

Table 10-1. Normal Radial and Lateral Antebrachial Cutaneous Sensory Conduction Velocities[15]

Nerve	*Segment*	*Mean Velocity ± SD (m/sec)*	*Range*
Radial	Wrist–1st web space	56.4 ± 4.0	48–67
Radial	Elbow–wrist	61.4 ± 3.1	54–70
Radial	Right–left difference	1.8 ± 1.6	0–7.0
LACN	Elbow–wrist	61.7 ± 2.9	56–70
LACN–Radial	Difference–same side	1.9 ± 1.6	0–7.0
Nerve	*Segment*	*Mean Amplitude ± SD (uv)*	*Range*
Radial	Wrist–1st Web Space	30.5 ± 5.9	20–50
Radial	Elbow–1st Web Space	19.2 ± 6.4	10–30

Surgical Technique

The operation can be done under regional anesthesia. The patient's position is supine. An upper arm penumatic tourniquet is placed. The hand is prepared with povidone-iodine and draped in the appropriate manner. A 3 to 4 cm incision is made over the volar radial aspect of the forearm and centered on the point of the patient's positive Tinel sign, which should approximate the point at which the radial sensory nerve transits from deep to superficial. The incision is carried down through the subcutaneous tissue to the level of the antebrachial fascia. This approach goes between the two branches of the lateral antebrachial cutaneous nerve if the nerve has the proximal split variation or adjacent to it if the nerve has not split proximally. Therefore care must be taken to avoid injury to this nerve by gentle retraction. At the level of the fascia, the dissection continues dorsally. Hemostasis is obtained throughout with the bipolar coagulator. The tendon of the brachioradialis will be identified at this point, with the muscle belly being more proximal. The fascia attaching the brachioradialis tendon to the extensor carpi radialis longus tendon is usually somewhat edematous, with the nerve bulging in this area (Fig. 10-5).

It will be of interest to the surgeon before incising the deep fascia to observe the relationships, previously described, as the two tendons change position when the forearm moves from supination to pronation and then to watch the tension on the radial sensory nerve after

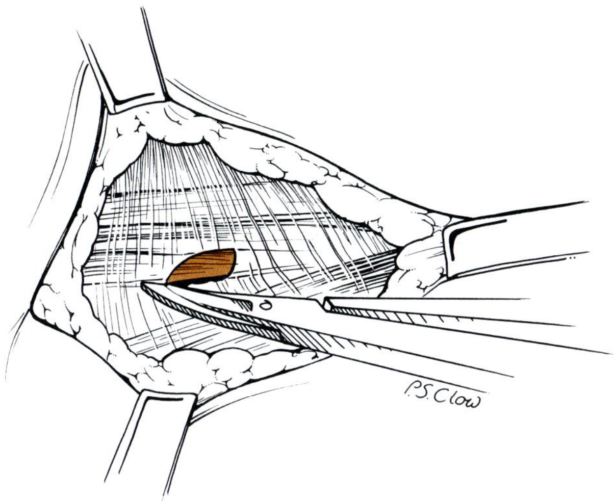

a

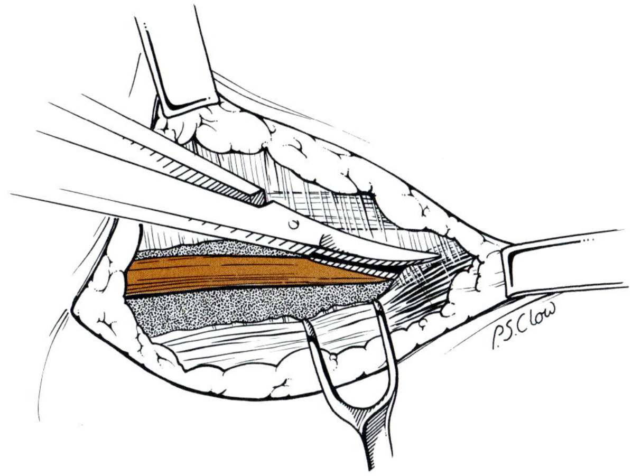

b

Figure 10-5. Operative technique. Note the proposed line of incision on the volar radial aspect of the forearm at a point paralleling the positive Tinel's sign at which the radial sensory nerve makes its transit from deep to superficial (Fig. 10-1A). **a.** The fascia between the brachioradialis tendon and the extensor carpi radialis longus is slit and the brachioradialis tendon is reflected. **b.** This fascia is released distally to the insertion of the brachioradialis tendon and proximally, completely separating the fascial attachments of these two tendons. **c.** The radial sensory nerve is separated from the underlying scarring in its bed and an internal neurolysis carried out if required. (Hand is toward left.) (Reproduced with permission from Dellon et al.[18])

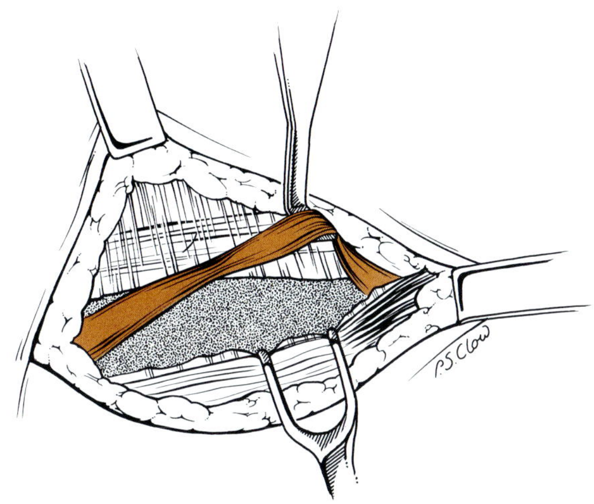

c

the fascia is incised as the wrist goes from radial extension to ulnar deviation and flexion (Fig. 10-6).

The tight fascia is carefully lifted and incised. A double hook is placed beneath the tendon of the brachioradialis and the tendon is pulled in a volar direction. This relieves pressure on the nerve, which lies beneath it (Fig. 10-5). The tips of a scissors are now used to incise the fascia proximally between the two tendons, going approximately 6 to 8 cm proximal to the proximal extent of the incision. The fascia of the brachioradialis tendon is then incised distally down to the level of the tendon's insertion into bone. Now the tendon can be pulled completely away from the radial sensory nerve. The radial sensory nerve is gently separated from the underlying tissues. The pathologic features at this time generally show a narrowing of the nerve at the point of transition, with the nerve being more swollen proximally. A subtle finding is that the vessels on the surface of the nerve may have become obliterated at this point of transition (Fig. 10-7). The nerve, itself, has a grayer, more edematous appearance in this region than it does proximally or distally. In severe cases, the nerve may be grossly narrowed.[16] The nerve is elevated from its bed gently and maintained in this position with a right-angle retractor. Now the nerve is separated proximally from all surrounding subcutaneous tissue. Its branches are dissected distally until they lie completely loose in the subcutaneous tissue. This completes the decompression portion of the radial nerve.

Now microsurgical instruments and technique are used. The epineurium of the nerve is opened very gently and any intraneural fibrosis is treated with a gentle, yet meticulous, intraneural neurolysis. Generally, between five and eight small fascicles may be seen. The dissection is carried out until there is a good fascicular pattern and perineurial markings. Usually no plexus formation is noted (Fig. 10-7). The nerve is returned to its bed. The wound is irrigated with sterile saline. Interrupted intradermal absorbable sutures are placed and then a continuous intradermal or skin suture is placed. The inci-

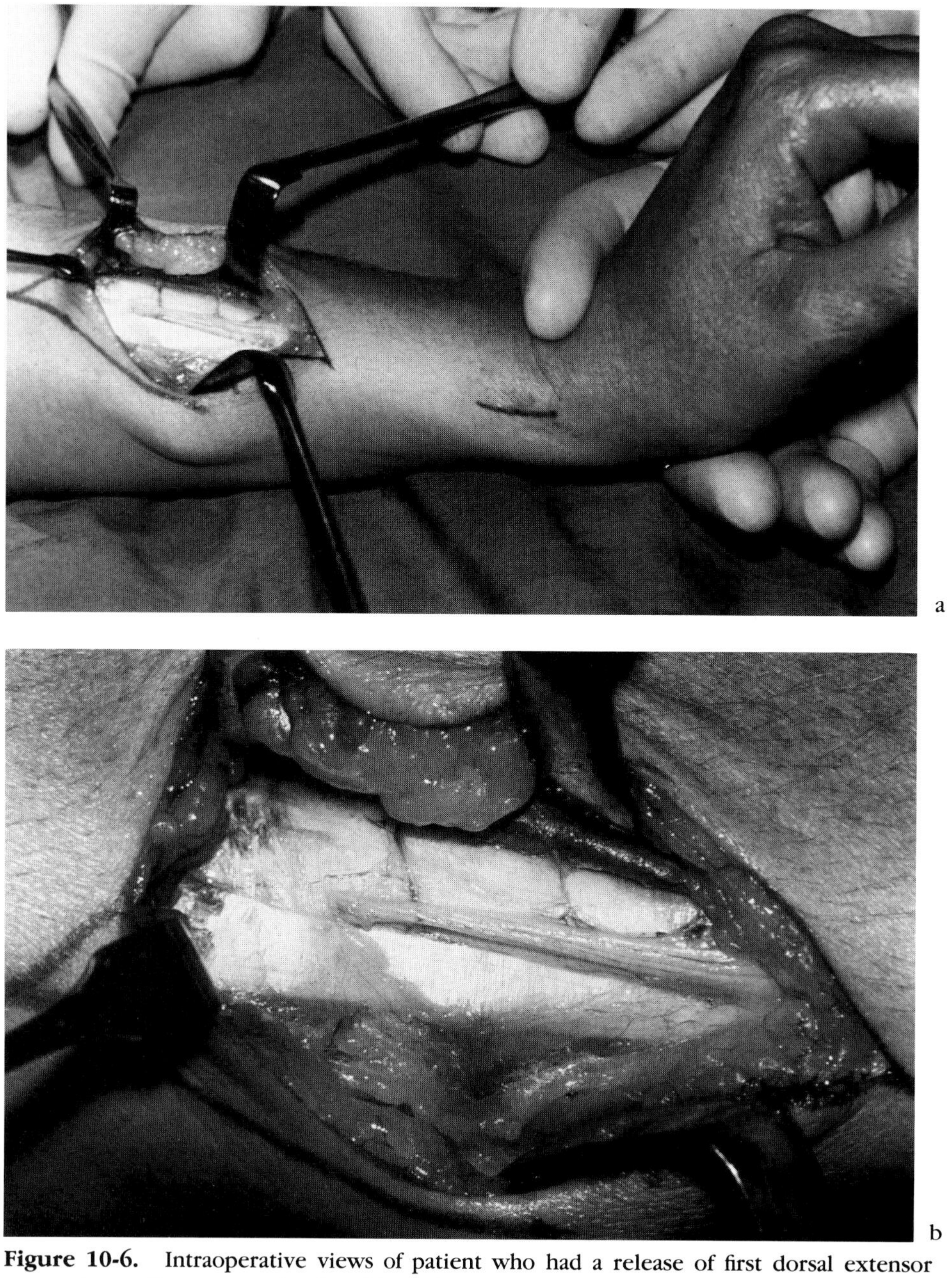

Figure 10-6. Intraoperative views of patient who had a release of first dorsal extensor compartment 2 years previously without improvement in symptoms. At surgery, with the forearm pronated (**a**), note radial sensory nerve compressed between the brachioradialis and the extensor carpi radialis longus as the nerve transits from deep to superficial through the fascia. With forearm supinated (**c**), the tendons move apart and the radial sensory nerve is less compressed. Photographs **b** and **d** are close-ups of **a** and **c**. Note **d** is immediately after release of fascia.

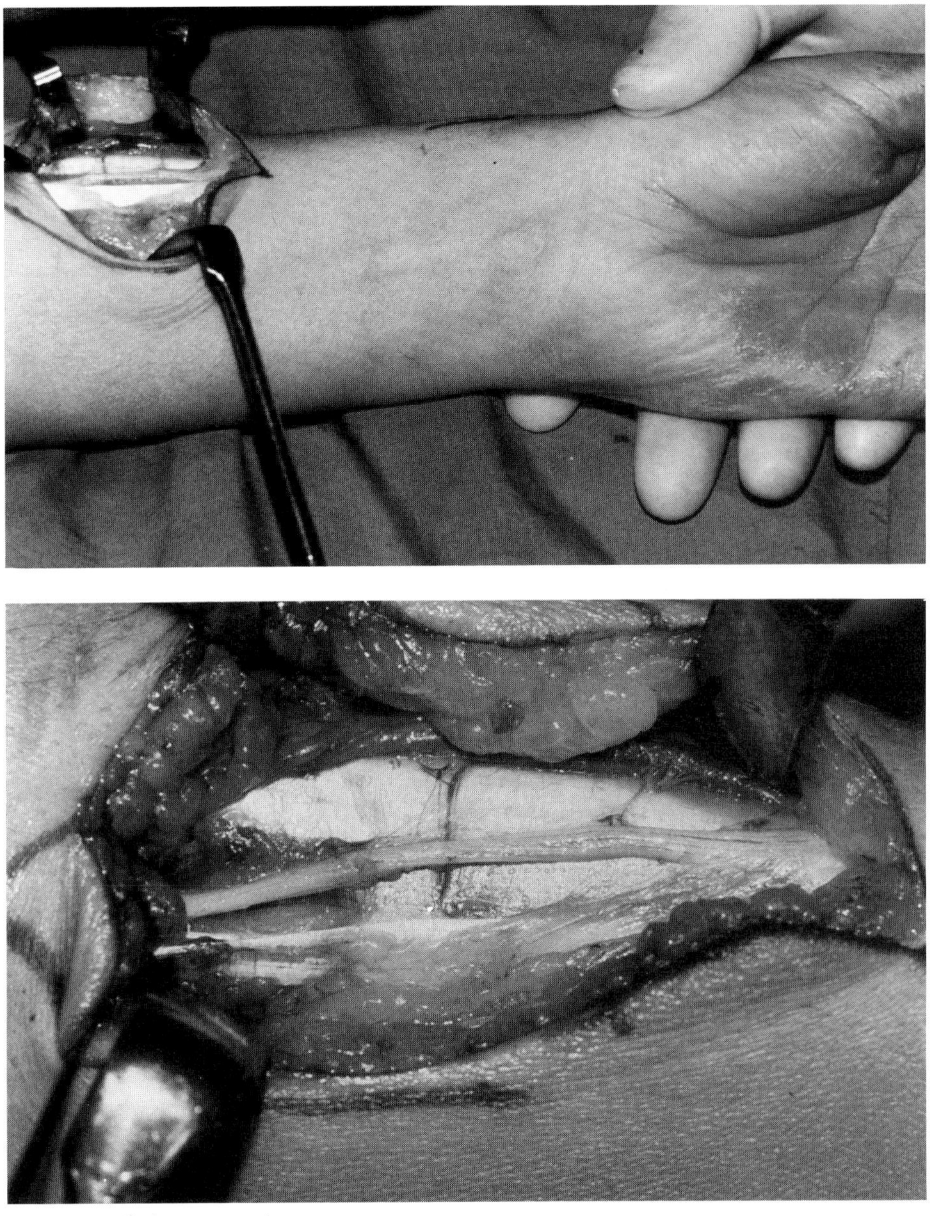

c

d

Figure 10.6. (*continued*).

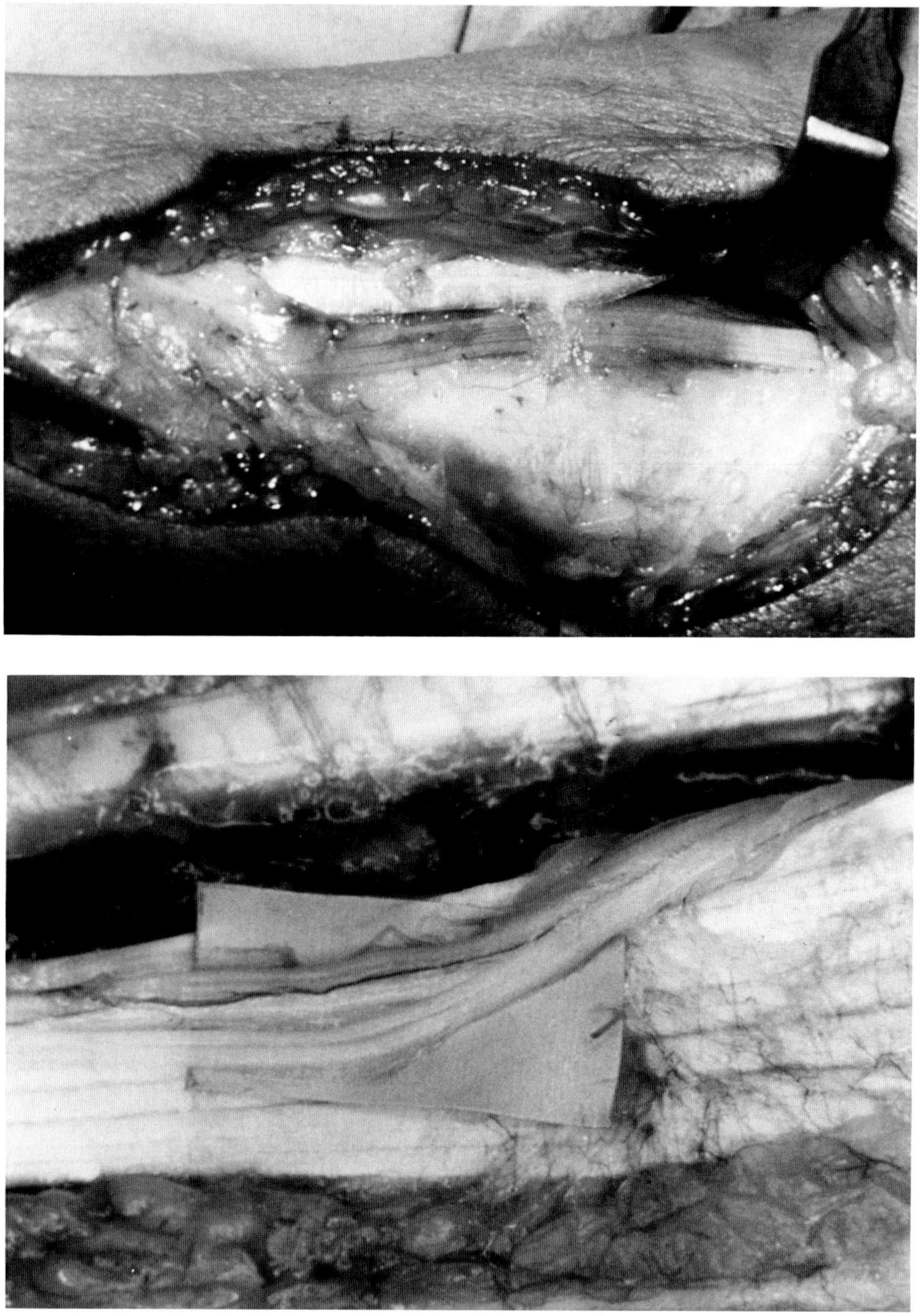

a

b

Figure 10-7. Intraoperative view of radial sensory nerve entrapment. Fingers are to the left. **a.** Note change in vascular pattern and color of nerve and color along the surface of the nerve. **b.** After decompression and after microsurgical internal neurolysis. Note good fascicular pattern and preservation of longitudinal intrinsic blood supply to the nerve.

sion lies on an area more volar than the location of the radial sensory nerve.

The dressing is nonadherent gauze, fluffs, soft roll, and a volar plaster splint, holding the wrist in neutral position. This is held in place with kling, paper tape, stockinette, and an elastic wrap. The tourniquet is then let down. The operative time is generally 1 hour.[18]

Postoperative Care

The dressing is removed on the eighth postoperative day. Any sutures are removed. The wound is steri-stripped for an additional 7 days if the forearm is not hair-bearing. Beginning with the second postoperative week, the patient begins gentle wrist ulnar flexion, clenching and unclenching the fingers, to encourage gliding of the nerve through the operated tissues. At the third week, the patient begins twice daily scar massage with a moisturizing cream. If at the follow-up visits the scar begins to hypertrophy, steroid cream is prescribed for the twice daily massage. The goal of the massage is to loosen the skin from the underlying nerve.

Complications

The most common complication in our experience has been scar hypertrophy due to the relative tightness of the skin in this region and the underlying muscle belly volume changes during hand activity. There were no postoperative complications related to the internal neurolysis. In particular, there were no postoperative causalgias. There was often a period postoperatively, lasting up to 6 weeks, in which hypersensitivity occurred. There were no complications directly related to the operative procedure, itself.

Results

The first surgical report related to radial sensory nerve entrapment in the forearm was a single case by Linscheid[7] in 1965 in which he reported a "neurolysis" of the radial sensory nerve. Braidwood,[19] in 1975, described nine patients who fit the clinical description by Wartenberg. Four of these patients recovered without treatment, and two recovered after a "steroid injection" that was placed where the nerves felt "thickened" about the region of the radial styloid. Three patients were operated on, and they had an excision of the radial sensory nerve, with the level of the resection being beneath the brachioradialis tendon.

One additional series of patients was reported by Rask[20] in 1978. Rask reported on three patients whose symptoms would have conformed to those described by Wartenberg. These symptoms were in association with a de Quervain's stenosing tenosynovitis. Rask indicated that he believed there were postinflammatory or secondary changes about the radial sensory nerve overlying the first dorsal extensor compartment and that, with relief of the tenosynovitis, there occurred a resolution of the neuritis.

The only mention in a surgical text is the chapter by Eversmann[21] in Green's text. In this chapter, the entrapment of the radial sensory nerve is listed and a technique for decompression of the nerve is described that includes an excision of a portion of the brachioradialis tendon. A specific number of treated patients or results are not described.[21]

A review therefore of the world literature through 1985 contains just 28 previously reported cases of radial sensory nerve entrapment. Twenty-four of these were managed by nonsurgical means. Of these 24 patients, seven did not and 17 did improve. Of the 17 who were improved, 12 did so spontaneously. Three improved after release of the first dorsal extensor compartment. Two improved after steroid injection in the region of the radial styloid. All four patients managed surgically, one by neurolysis and three by resection of the radial sensory nerve, improved.

The operative technique described in this chapter has been reported in 32 patients with 35 involved hands.[18] At the time of that report, these patients ranged in follow-up from 3 to 26 months postoperatively, with a mean of 7 months. Relief of pain, as judged by the patient and surgeon, was excellent in 37% of these patients, good in 49%, and fair in 6%. Only 8% had no improvement after the operation. Forty-three percent of this group of patients returned to their regular job and another 20% were either in vocational rehabilitation or working at a different job. The remaining 35% were grouped either as not working or remaining disabled due to associated injuries. This improved hand function was further documented by improvement in pinch and grip strength and improved range of motion at the wrist.

Among the group of 28 patients, 20 hands were severe enough to require an internal neurolysis. This group of patients was distinguished by having either persistent sensory discomfort or an abnormal moving two-point discrimination in the first dorsal web space. Moving two-point discrimination has a wide range in this region, 6 to 15 mm. Abnormal moving two-point discrimination was taken as being either greater than 15 mm or more than 5 mm greater than the measurement in the contralateral hand.

Comment

Entrapment of the radial sensory nerve is surely more common than the few previous reports in the world literature would lead one to suspect. The clinical entity of radial sensory nerve entrapment is most commonly misdiagnosed, we believe, as de Quervain's extensor tenosynovitis (Fig. 10-6) (see further discussion at the end of this chapter). It may be possible, as described by Rask,[20] that the two may be associated because inflammation about the extensor tenosynovium may induce inflammatory symptomatic change in the radial sensory nerve. Nevertheless, perhaps many cases of remaining pain after release of the first dorsal extensor compartment are due to undiagnosed entrapment of the radial sensory nerve. Most likely, many cases of radial sensory nerve entrapment are believed to be related to "sprains" of the wrist after falls. Indeed, many patients with these complaints may be labeled, as Wartenberg described in 1932, as having a "work neurosis," which may occur in Workmen's Compensation situations where physical findings may be totally inappropriate for the extent of the physical complaints, making the patients appear to be malingerers. As awareness of this clinical entity spreads, we believe that many patients on reexamination will prove to have this entrapment syndrome.

Diagnostic nerve blocks are extremely helpful in proving the existence of this problem. First preinjection pinch and grip strength measurements and range of wrist motion measurements are obtained. Then the radial sensory nerve may be blocked in the region of the positive Tinel's sign. Within a few minutes, there should be an improvement in pinch and grip strength and range of motion, as well as relief of the patient's symptoms. The Finkelstein's sign becomes negative.

We have observed three cases in which the volar pad of the thumb is innervated totally by the radial sensory nerve (Fig. 10-8). These patients have presented as unusual variants of carpal tunnel syndrome, with persistent sensory change over the thumb pulp and normal electrodiagnostic findings for the median nerve at the wrist. One patient already was noted as a "failed carpal tunnel release." Diagnostic nerve block of the radial sensory nerve in the contralateral forearm resulted in loss of sensation in that hand's thumb pulp, confirming the anomalous radial sensory innervation of thumb pulp. Neurolysis of the radial sensory nerve in the forearm resulted in sensory recovery in the thumb pulp of all three of these patients. Similarly, we have two patients in whom pain in the thumb along the radial or ulnar mid-lateral border after laceration was related to injury of both the thumb volar digital nerve and a branch of the radial sensory nerve. In these cases of anomalous

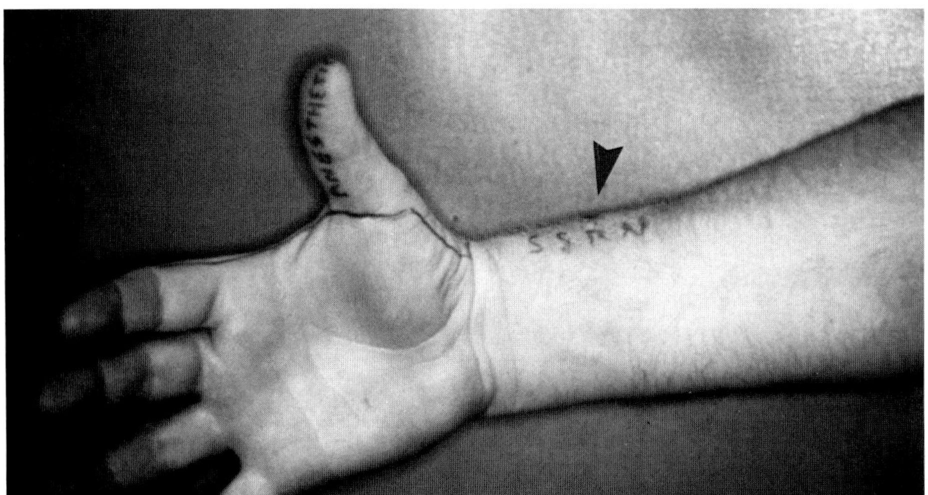

Figure 10-8. Clinical views of hand and forearm of man who had a crush injury to this area and subsequently was operated on for carpal tunnel syndrome, which presented as abnormal sensation in the thumb, with loss of two-point discrimination in the thumb pulp, but normal median nerve electrodiagnostic studies. Diagnostic nerve block demonstrated that his radial sensory nerve innervated his entire thumb pulp. The arrow indicates site of nerve block. The area of anesthesia after the nerve block is shown.

thumb pulp innervation by the radial sensory nerve, diagnostic nerve blocks are critical to making the correct diagnosis.

Radial sensory nerve entrapment can exist in the presence of and be associated with a neuroma of the radial sensory nerve distally. It is possible that the same injury that caused the direct damage to the radial sensory nerve branch was responsible for swelling or traction to produce the site of entrapment. Another common mechanism is the misdiagnosis of radial sensory nerve entrapment, release of a nonexisting first dorsal extensor tenosynovitis, and injury during this surgical procedure of branches of the radial sensory nerve. In these situations, the diagnostic nerve block is critical. If pain remains distally after the nerve block, then evaluation of the lateral antebrachial cutaneous nerve must also be undertaken with an additional nerve block. In these situations, the patient should be brought back a second time and the order of the nerve blocks reversed, blocking the lateral antebrachial cutaneous nerve first and carrying out this block at a much more proximal level, in the region of the antecubital fossa to be sure that the lateral antebrachial is blocked without blocking an adjacent radial sensory nerve.[13,22] (See Chapter 17.)

Among the alternatives for surgical treatment, we have found that there is often sufficient scarring within and about the radial sensory nerve to require both an internal and an external neurolysis of the nerve. Although the nerve still exits from beneath the brachioradialis tendon, the separation of the linkage between the brachioradialis tendon and the extensor carpi radialis tendon permits the nerve now to find a new resting position between these tendons for any given position of pronation and supination of the forearm. Thus, it was not found necessary in this series of 28 surgical patients[18] to excise any portion of the brachioradialis tendon. Should, however, the operative technique described fail, then it may be that division of the brachioradialis tendon would be helpful in eliminating a compressive course over the radial sensory nerve. For failure of the technique described, resection of the radial sensory nerve would represent a final alternative with implantation of the nerve proximally into the brachioradialis muscle.[22–24] In cases in which there is coexistence of a peripheral neuroma and proximal entrapment of the radial sensory nerve, resection of the radial sensory nerve and muscle implantation would be the treatment of choice.

In order to explore further the inter-relationship of nerve entrapment, neuroma formation, and extensor tenosynovitis, we did a retrospective review of our own patients.[25] Between 1982 and 1986, 71 patients were treated for radial sensory nerve entrapment and 82 patients were treated for neuromas of the sensory branches of the dorsoradial nerves at the wrist (radial sensory and lateral antebrachial cutaneous nerves). In the group of patients with radial sensory nerve entrapment, 17 patients had previously been diagnosed as having de Quervain's disease. Five of these 17 patients had developed neuromas of the dorsoradial sensory nerves following release of the first extensor compartment (Table 10-2). In the second group of patients with dorsoradial wrist neuromas, 24 patients had previously been diagnosed as having de Quervain's disease. None of these patients had improved following surgical release of the first extensor compartment, and all of them had developed neuromas of the dorsoradial wrist nerves. Diagnosis of radial sensory nerve entrapment as de Quervain's disease will lead to predictable failure after surgical release of the first dorsal compartment. This surgery may well be complicated by an injury to the dorsoradial wrist nerves (radial sensory and/or lateral antebrachial cutaneous nerves).

Table 10-2. Clinical Data[25]

	Radial Sensory Nerve Entrapment	*Dorsoradial Wrist Neuromas*
Patients (No.)	71	82
Male/female	33/38	40/42
WCB	37	60
Previous trauma	59	55
Diabetes	9	2
Previous diagnosis: de Quervain's disease	17	24
Previous surgery: de Quervain's disease	5	24

References

1. Wartenberg R: Cheiralgia Paresthetica (Isolierte Neuritis des Ramus Superficialis nerve radialis). Z Ges Neurol Psychiatr 141:145–155, 1932.
2. Sprofkin BF: Cheiralgia paresthetica—Wartenberg's disease. Neurology (Minneap) 4:857–862, 1954.
3. Sprofkin BF, Isom JB: Sensory mononeuropathy. Am Pract Digest Treat 11:745–759, 1960.
4. Ehrlich W, Dellon AL, Mackinnon SE: Cheiralgia paresthetica (entrapment of the radial sensory nerve). J Hand Surg [Am] 11:196–198, 1986.
5. Matzdorf P: Zivei seltene Falle von Peripherer Sensibler Lahmung. Klin Wochenschr 5:1187, 1926.
6. Bierman HR: Nerve compression due to a tight watch band. N Engl J Med 261:237–238, 1959.
7. Linscheid RL: Injuries to radial nerve at the wrist. Arch Surg 91:942–946, 1965.
8. Stopford JSB: Neuritis produced by a wristlet watch. Lancet 1:993–994, 1922.
9. Dorfman LJ, Jayram AR: Handcuff neuropathy. JAMA 239:957, 1978.

10. Massey EW, Pleet AB: Handcuffs and cheiralgia paresthetica. Neurology (NY) 28:1312–1313, 1978.
11. Smith MS: Handcuff neuropathy. Ann Emerg Med 10:668, 1981.
12. Dellon AL, Mackinnon SE: Susceptibility of the superficial sensory branch of the radial nerve to form painful neuromas. J Hand Surg [Br] 9:42–45, 1984.
13. Mackinnon SE, Dellon AL: The overlap pattern of the lateral antebrachial cutaneous nerve and the superficial branch of the radial nerve. J Hand Surg [Am] 10:522–526, 1985.
14. Mackinnon SE, Dellon AL, Hunter DA: Histopathology of compression of the superficial radial nerve in the forearm. J Hand Surg [Am] 11:206–209, 1986.
15. Spindler HA, Dellon AL: Nerve conduction studies in the superficial radial nerve entrapment syndrome. Muscle and Nerve 13:1—5, 1990.
16. Mackinnon SE, Dellon AL, Hudson AR, Hunter DA: Histopathology of chronic human nerve compression. Neuropath Appl Neurobiol 12:547–565, 1986.
17. Finkelstein H: Stenosing tendovaginitis at the radial styloid process. J Bone Joint Surg 12A:509–539, 1930.
18. Dellon AL, Mackinnon SE: Radial sensory nerve entrapment in the forearm. J Hand Surg [Am] 11:199–205, 1986.
19. Braidwood AS: Superficial radial neuropathy. J Bone Joint Surg 57B:380–383, 1975.
20. Rask MR: Superficial radial neuritis and de Quervain's disease: Report of three cases. Clin Orthop 131:176–178, 1978.
21. Eversmann WH Jr: Entrapment and compression neuropathies. In Green DP, ed: Operative Hand Surgery. New York, Churchill Livingstone, 1982, pp 990–992.
22. Mackinnon SE, Dellon AL: Results of treatment of recurrent dorsal-radial wrist neuromas. J Ann Plast Surg, 19:54–61, 1987.
23. Mackinnon SE, Dellon AL, Hudson AR, Hunter DA: Alteration of neuroma formation by manipulation of neural environment. Plast Reconstr Surg 76:345, 1985.
24. Dellon AL, Mackinnon SE: Treatment of the painful neuroma by neuroma resection and muscle implantation. Plast Reconstr Surg 77:427–436, 1986.
25. Saplys R, Mackinnon SE, Dellon AL: The relationship between nerve entrapment versus neuroma. Complications and the misdiagnosis of de Quervain's Disease. Contemp Ortho 15:51–57, 1987.

11

Radial Nerve Entrapment in the Proximal Forearm and Brachium

Radial nerve injuries may be subdivided into those due to direct trauma and those due to compression. Seddon[1] has reviewed the largest series of traumatic injuries to the proximal radial nerve (Table 11-1) (Monteggia fracture).[2] Injury due to associated fractures of the humerus is the most common cause (Fig. 11-1). It has been generally agreed that in the closed fracture it is appropriate to wait 3 months with a transverse or spiral fracture of the humerus before surgical exploration. Repeat clinical and electrodiagnostic testing will determine whether radial nerve function has occurred. This will be determined by recovery of function into the brachioradialis muscle,[1] an advancing Tinel's sign, or electrodiagnostic findings of reinnervation. If it is a compound fracture or the wound requires exploration for open reduction of the fracture, then the radial nerve certainly should be explored. Classically, the radial nerve may be either entrapped in the fracture site in the spiral groove of the humerus or divided by the fracture, itself, in this region. Seddon provides one of the earliest descriptions of treatment of this injury by direct repair of the radial nerve[3] (Figs. 11-2, 11-3). A similar time frame has been noted by Omer,[3] who found recovery in isolated nerve lesions above the elbow in 11 fracture and stretch injuries to occur by 2 to 4 months after the fracture. In terms of incidence, it should be noted that Barton[4] found 16% of the fractures of the shaft of the humerus to be complicated by immediate radial nerve palsy.[5] In a series of 23 radial nerve palsies in which immediate exploration was carried out, Garcia and Maeck[6] found just one case of radial nerve division.

Table 11-1. Causes of Radial Nerve Injuries (Noncompressive)*

Lacerations	13
Missile wounds	68
Iatrogenic	16
Associated with skeletal injury	74
Traction injury	2
Other (ischemia, tumor, injection)	37
Total	210

*Reprinted with permission from Seddon.[1]

The second most common cause for radial nerve injury after those associated with fractures of the humerus is due to gunshot wounds (Table 11-1). The mechanism of injury involved disruption in nerve function over a length that is related to the velocity of the

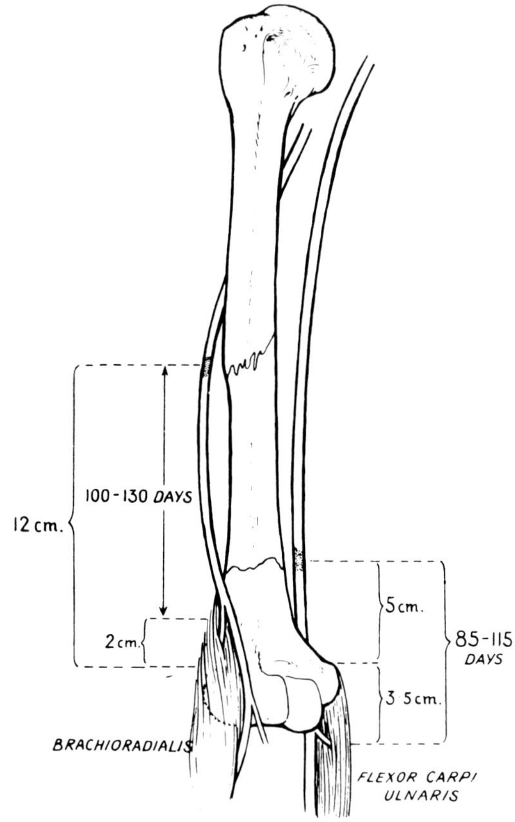

Figure 11-1. Most common cause of radial nerve injury is a humerus fracture. The first muscle to be reinnervated after a high radial nerve palsy is the brachioradialis, which receives its innervation 2 cm proximal to the lateral humeral epicondyle. By calculating the length from the area in which the radial nerve may be injured by either a transverse humerus fracture (left) or an oblique fracture (right) to the brachioradialis muscle, estimated time for radial nerve recovery can be derived. (Reproduced with permission from Seddon.[1])

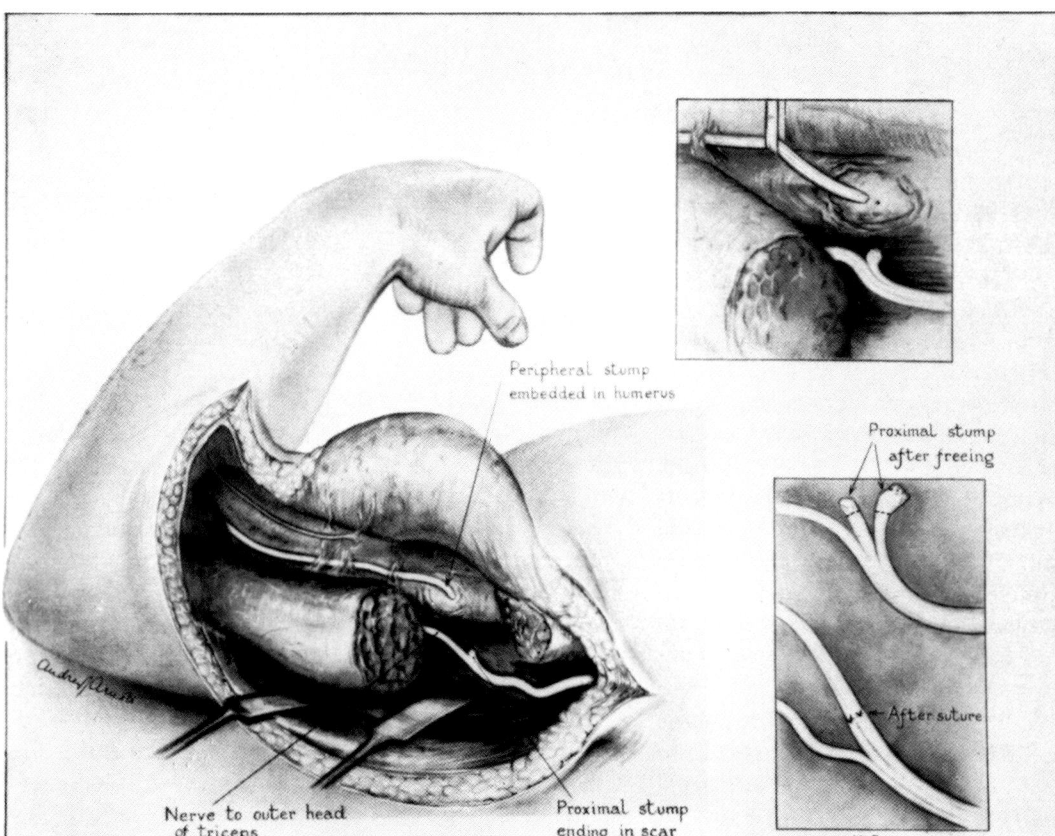

Figure 11-2. Historical illustration of site of radial nerve injury with humeral fracture, and treatment by nerve suture. (Reproduced with permission from Seddon.[2])

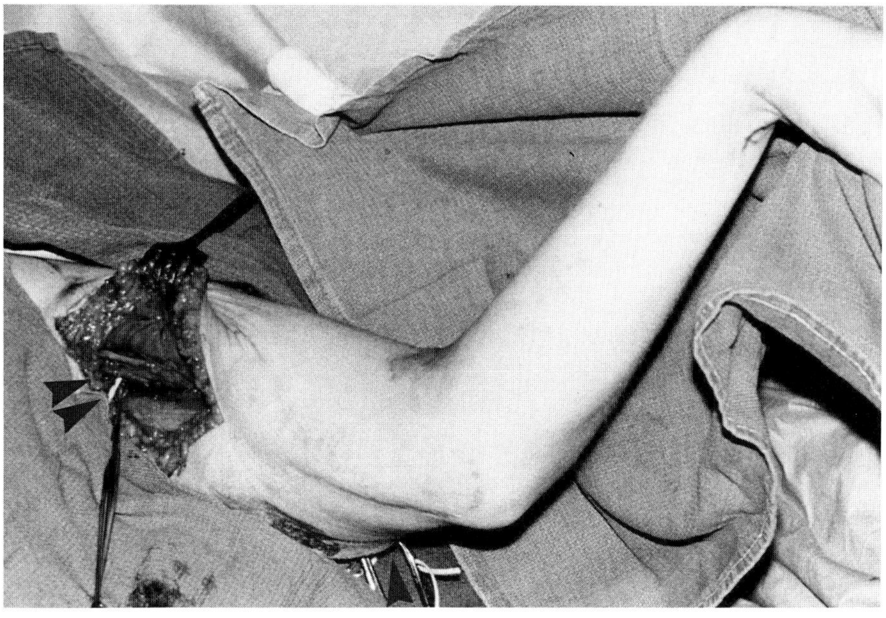

Figure 11-3. Clinical example of radial nerve injury (nerve in vessel loop) associated with humerus fracture. Note wrist drop. Nerve is explored distally at elbow (arrow) and proximally at axilla (double arrow).

missile, but, in general, nerve paralysis after gunshot wounds has a favorable prognosis. The most thorough study of this is the one reported in 1974 by Omer.[3] Sixty-nine percent of 331 patients with low velocity gunshot wounds and 69% of 264 patients with high velocity gunshot wounds recovered good clinical function spontaneously. The time frame for this recovery was longer, however, than for the fractures, 4 to 7 months being necessary in low velocity and 3 to 6 months being necessary in high velocity gunshot wounds in isolated nerves located above the elbow. Thus, with radial nerve injuries due to fracture or gunshot wounds, surgical exploration to evaluate the nerves is indicated if more than 3 months has elapsed after the former and more than 5 months has elapsed after the latter mechanism of the injury.

Injury to the radial nerve can be caused not only by direct injection-type injuries, but also from scar tissue secondary to the drug, itself.[7–9] The causes of compression neuropathy of the radial nerve in the brachium are numerous, and crush, pressure against the humerus, compression of the nerve against the bone by the edge of a chair or table or the edge of an operating room table, stretcher, or traction device, and compression of the radial nerve beneath the pneumatic tourniquet utilized during an operative procedure have all been described in detail.[10–17] Discrete anatomic structures that may cause compression of the radial nerve have been described in three patients after physical activity that caused traction on the upper arm where the radial nerve crosses the lateral intermuscular septum,[18] and, additionally, compression of the radial nerve within the triceps muscle, itself, has been described.[19] In general, the compression palsies of the radial nerve due to these high sites of compression in the brachium resolve spontaneously and do not require surgical intervention. When the nerve has been directly damaged by the substance injected in an injection injury, no recovery may occur even with surgical exploration. The patient reported by Manske[19] and surgically explored failed to recover.

Radial nerve injury in the region of the elbow and proximal forearm is most commonly due to nerve compression. Although lacerations in this region can certainly cause direct injury to the nerve and dislocation or fracture of the radial head can damage the overlying posterior interosseous nerve, the vast majority of clinical problems related to radial nerve injury in this area are due to compression of the nerve at several distinct anatomic sites. Traditionally, these sites have included "pure motor paralysis" due to the "posterior interosseous nerve syndrome." The associated sensory complaints are primarily those of pain in this region without distal sensory loss. More recently, this entity has been described and termed the "radial tunnel syndrome." The description of these syndromes will be given more fully under "Diagnosis," with particular reference to distinguishing them from tennis elbow. The concept, as described in Chapter 14, of the multiple crush syndrome with multiple anatomic sites within a single anatomic region applies to the radial nerve in the proximal forearm and elbow region. As will be noted later, the same surgical approach to releasing all compressive sites will be recommended regardless of the clinical presentation. The presentation will be determined by the site most intimately related to the site of most compression. Radial sensory nerve compression that results in purely sensory symptoms and changes is

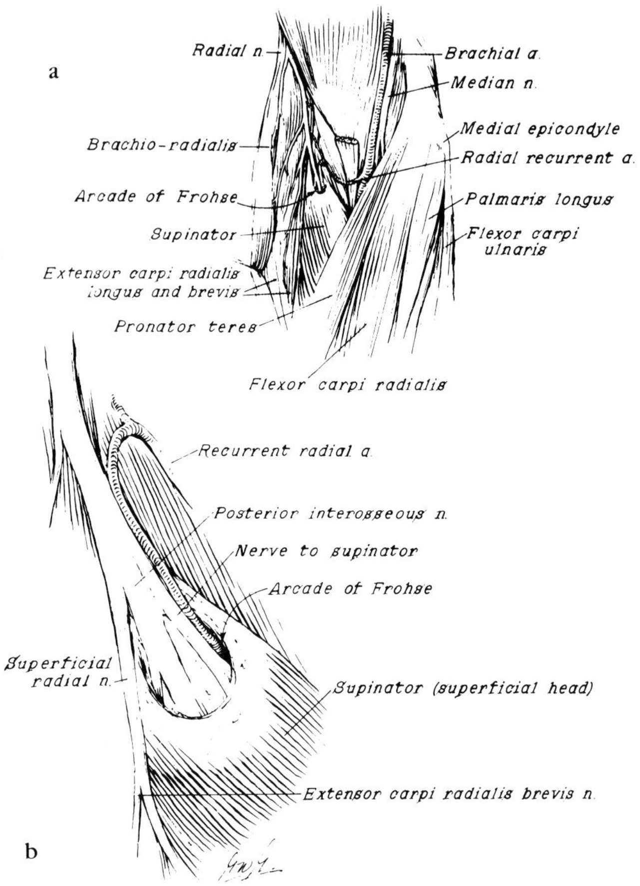

Figure 11-4. Illustration of the radial nerve dividing into its superficial and deep components at the level of the elbow, the region of the radial tunnel **(a)**, and the site of the deep branch entrapment beneath the arcade of Froshe, which produces the posterior interosseous nerve syndrome **(b)**. (Reproduced with permission from Spinner.[25])

most likely due to entrapment in the distal third of the forearm (Fig. 11-4) (see Chapter 10).

Surgical Anatomy

The radial nerve is the largest terminal branch of the posterior cord of the brachial plexus. Variations in this termination have been reported in approximately 20% of cadaver dissections by Kerr in 1918,[20] the variation being the absence of the posterior cord with a common radial-axillary nerve being formed by the union of the posterior divisions of the upper and middle trunks. At a more distal level, the radial nerve received the posterior division contributions from the lower trunk. More rarely, the axillary nerve was formed completely from divisions of the upper and middle trunks, with the posterior division of the lower trunk forming the radial nerve, receiving a more distal communication of the axillary nerve. The nerve may penetrate an anomalous muscle in the posterior wall of the axilla, the so-called accessory scapularis-teres-latissimus muscle.[21] Traditionally, the most common anatomy has the radial nerve containing cervical root contributions from C5, C6, C7, and C8. The formation of the radial nerve goes from posterior to the axillary artery behind or posterior to the humerus, through the muscle bellies of the triceps muscle, and, at this location, gives off the posterior cutaneous nerve of the arm and the posterior cutaneous nerve of the forearm, which become subcutaneous at this point. The radial nerve continues deep, crossing the musculospiral groove, and then enters the anterior portion of the arm by piercing the lateral intermuscular septum at a site that is usually 10 cm proximal to the lateral humeral epicondyle. Approximately 2 to 3 cm proximal to the lateral humeral epicondyle, the nerve lies lateral to the brachialis muscle and the biceps tendon and medial to the origin of the brachioradialis muscle. This anatomic relationship is useful in identifying the nerve at surgery. At this level, the radial nerve gives off the lower branches to innervate the brachioradialis and the extensor carpi radialis longus. Then, at a site that may vary over the next 5 cm, the radial nerve bifurcates into the sensory or superficial radial nerve and the motor, or deep radial nerve components. This deep motor branch is termed the "posterior interosseous nerve."[22] The nerve to the extensor carpi radialis brevis is a distinctly separate nerve originating from a more proximal portion of the radial nerve in the region of the sensory and motor bifurcation. It can, thus, occasionally appear to divide from the sensory nerve. The nerve to the extensor carpi radialis brevis always appears to lie superficial to the posterior interosseous nerve proximal to the entrance of the posterior interosseous nerve into the supinator muscle. The region of the supinator muscle is of particular anatomic interest. The German anatomist Fröhse with Frankel described in 1908 an arch where the two heads of the supinator muscle arose from the lateral and medial edges of the lateral humeral epicondyle.[23] Entrapment of the posterior interosseous nerve in this region had been noted, prompting Spinner[24] to carry out anatomic investigations of this region in 50 adult cadavers. He found that 30% of the adult specimens contained a fibrous arch in this region, which he termed the arcade of Fröhse. The thickness of this fibrous arch varied (Fig. 11-4). Spinner[24] has noted that, once the posterior interosseous nerve enters the supinator beneath the arcade of Fröhse, it divides into multiple branches that resemble the cauda equina, with the main pattern consisting of two major components, one supplies the more superficial layer of muscles (the extensor digitorum communis, extensor digiti quinti, and the extensor carpi ulnaris) and the second goes to the deeper of the muscles (the abductor pollicis longus, the extensor pollicis longus and brevis, and extensor indicis propius). Branches occur after the posterior interosseous nerve has passed through the length of the supinator muscle. Proximal to these divisions, the radial nerve may pass in 25% of the patients across a so-called bare area[26] of the radius. In this area, which lies posterior to the bicipital tuberosity, the nerve is likely to be injured either directly in fractures or by placement of plates to correct fractures. Examples of such injuries to the posterior interosseus nerve have been nicely documented photographically by Spinner.[25]

The extensor carpi radialis brevis muscle frequently has a fibrous edge that may compress the posterior interosseus nerve just at the region of its entrance beneath the arcade of Fröhse.

After innervating the last of the extensor muscles, the posterior interosseous nerve continues to provide innervation to the dorsal wrist capsule and intercarpal ligaments. Its course proceeds along the interosseus membrane and then along the most radial side of the fourth extensor compartment adjacent to Lister's tubercle. It lies adjacent to the terminal branches of the anterior interosseous artery. In this location, it may be covered by a fascial sheath and therefore not be apparent when the fourth extensor compartment is inspected in a cursory fashion.[27] The posterior interosseous nerve's terminal branch may be blocked for diagnostic purposes in terms of wrist pain and may be resected in the treatment of dorsal wrist pain, carrying out a partial dorsal wrist denervation procedure.[28] When the accessory muscle to the fingers, the extensor brevis manus, exists, it is innervated by a branch from this terminal portion of the posterior interosseous nerve.[29] The muscle mass may simulate a symptomatic ganglion.

There may be variations in the muscles in the elbow and proximal forearm region. One variation described is a solitary muscular head arising from the medial portion of the lateral humeral epicondyle. In this instance, the posterior interosseous nerve lies on top of the supinator muscle instead of passing between it. Fusions of the brachioradialis and brachialis muscles have been noted. These may, in fact, be failures of segmentation of this muscle group. When this occurs, it may form part of the compressive forces over the radial nerve at the proximal aspect of what has been called the radial tunnel syndrome.[25]

Diagnosis

The diagnosis of injury to the radial nerve occurring in the proximal forearm, elbow region, and brachium relies on distinguishing sensory loss in the distribution of the radial sensory nerve, partial or complete paralysis of the muscles innervated by the posterior interosseous nerve, and partial or complete paralysis in the brachioradialis muscle, and partial or complete paralysis of the most proximally located group, the triceps muscle. Loss of sensation in the posterior aspect of the forearm and the posterolateral surface of the brachium would suggest injuries to the posterior cutaneous nerve of the forearm and posterior cutaneous nerve of the brachium, suggesting injuries to the radial nerve at a level at the exit of this nerve from the axilla and at its takeoff from the posterior cord of the brachial plexus. Caution must be maintained in the sensory evaluation in that complete lesions of the radial nerve still may have a very small, if not absent, autonomous area of innervation. The most reliable area would be over the dorsal radial aspect of the second metacarpal or the dorsal ulnar aspect of the first metacarpal. In contrast, an extended distribution has been described by Learmonth[30] in which the radial sensory nerve innervates the dorsal ulnar aspect of the hand, as well as the dorsal radial aspect. Another variation in the radial nerve that may cause confusion in the differential diagnosis is the so-called Froment-Ruber nerve. Spinner[25] has the best historical review of this anomaly and notes that Bichat was the first to actually note this connection in 1802 between the terminal branch of the posterior interosseous nerve and the deep branch of the ulnar nerve. This anomaly causes the radial nerve to innervate the first dorsal interosseous muscle. Froment described this in 1846 and it was further described and clearly depicted in 1865 by Ruber. In the differentiation of the sensory loss over the back of the hand from a C7 radiculopathy, consider that in the radiculopathy generally the palmar aspect of the middle finger is involved, as well as the dorsal aspect. A C7 root lesion causes weakness primarily in the triceps and the wrist and finger extensors but will also cause weakness in some of the median innervated muscles, such as the pronator teres and the flexor carpi radialis, the flexor digitorum superficialis, and the flexor pollicis longus. Lesions in the brachial plexus posterior cord would have an accompanying partial to complete radial nerve paralysis, weakness in the axillary nerve innervated muscles, such as the deltoid, and in those innervated by the thoracodorsal nerves, such as the latissimus muscle. The posterior interosseous nerve, with loss of extension of the fingers, may be confused with tendon ruptures to the fingers and to the thumb, as commonly seen in rheumatoid arthritis.[31] In this instance, when tendons have ruptured, there is a loss of the tenodesis effect, so that when the wrist is flexed, normally the fingers become extended, and when the wrist is extended, the fingers become flexed. The tenodesis effect is still present in the posterior interosseous nerve lesion. Electromyography is, of course, helpful in differentiating the location of these lesions.

The diagnosis of a complete posterior interosseous nerve lesion, regardless of cause, should be clear. The description has become classic due to the multiple reports of this problem.[24,32–46] The patient's hand is held with the fingers flexed at the metacarpophalangeal joints without ability to extend the metacarpophalangeal joints of any finger, yet with the ability preserved to extend the interphalangeal joints due to the intrinsic muscles. In the same fashion, the thumb lies volar to the plane of the second through fifth metacarpals due to lack of ability to extend the first metacarpal from paralysis of the abductor pollicis longus and the extensor pollicis brevis. The extensor pollicis longus tendon, although paralyzed, still does not prevent the interphalangeal joint of the thumb from being extended to at least a neutral position by the median and ulnar innervated thumb intrinsics. However, the thumb cannot be hyperextended at the interphalangeal joint. The wrist can be extended but only to the radial side due to remaining innervation of the extensor carpi radialis longus, since its intervention comes proximal to the arcade of Fröhse, whereas the extensor carpi ulnaris is innervated distal to the arcade. The extensor carpi radialis brevis is innervated just in the region of the arcade, and thus it may or may not be innervated, depending on the nature of the pathologic alterations.

With partial paralysis of the posterior interosseous nerve, there may be inability to extend the little and ring fingers. This gives the situation that has been described as the "pseudoclaw hand."[47,48] Careful evaluation, however, will reveal clinically that there is no hyperextension at the metacarpophalangeal joints of the little and ring fingers, which would be present with the ulnar claw hand. Depending on the location of the compression of the posterior interosseous nerve, other muscles may be partially paralyzed or not paralyzed at all. In these circumstances, electromyography is helpful. In a rare case in which the radial wrist extensors are innervated by the posterior interosseous nerve and thereby paralyzed, posterior interosseous nerve paralysis has been reported.[37] In all cases of pure posterior interosseous nerve compression, sensation is maintained in the radial nerve distribution. A systemic toxic neuropathy occurs with lead poisoning, which classically has been described to involve the entire radial nerve but preserve radial sensory function.[49] The diagnosis of posterior interosseous nerve problems when associated with trauma that has occurred directly to this region should not present a problem in the differential diagnosis.[22,50–54] The cause of posterior interosseous nerve compression can, of course, be due to other than traumatic problems and to anatomic structures compressing the nerve. For example, this palsy has been reported to be due to a ganglion,[55] to rheumatoid arthritis with synovitis coming from the surrounding joints,[56–59] and from lipomas.[60–62]

In order to evaluate and diagnose radial nerve injuries appropriately, we must be able to determine whether a nerve is regenerating appropriately. With radial nerve injuries, the sequence in which recovery should occur is: brachioradialis muscle, then the extensor carpi radialis longus, then the extensor carpi radialis brevis. This is the sequence in which these muscles are innervated proximal to the elbow. Once the posterior interosseous nerve has separated from the radial nerve, the average distance the nerve must travel before it innervates the remaining muscles has been recorded by Packer et al.[5] These distances are listed in Table 11-2. Continuing the sequence of reinnervation, the muscles to be reinnervated are: the extensor carpi ulnaris, then the extensor digitorum communis, and then the extensor digiti quinti. The nerve then must travel proximally 4 cm more before innervating the so-called outcropping muscles. The first to be reinnervated is the abductor pollicis longus, then the extensor pollicis brevis, and the extensor indices proprious. The last to be reinnervated is the extensor pollicis longus (Fig. 11-5). Lister has illustrated the clinical evaluation of these muscles.[63]

The radial tunnel syndrome was described in 1972 by Roles and Maudsley from England.[64] The stimulus to their description of this nerve compression syndrome was the inability to relieve discomfort in patients with lateral humeral epicondylitis (tennis elbow). They reasoned that entrapment of the radial nerve in this region might give rise to symptoms similar to those caused by tennis elbow. They described what, in fact, is not really a tunnel but a region through which the radial nerve passes (Fig. 11-6). The distinction between the anatomy that gives rise to the radial tunnel syndrome and that which gives rise to the posterior interosseous nerve syndrome overlaps in the region of the arcade of Fröhse. The radial tunnel region begins just after the takeoff of the motor branches to the brachioradialis, extensor carpi radialis longus and brevis, so that at the entrance

Table 11-2. Distances from Posterior Interosseous Nerve Division to Muscle Innervation: A Guide to Order of Recovery of Function*

Extensor carpi ulnaris	1.25 cm
Extensor digitorum communis	1.5 cm
Extensor digiti quinti	1.8 cm
Abductor pollicis longus	5.6 cm
Extensor pollicis brevis	6.8 cm
Extensor indicis proprious	6.8 cm
Extensor pollicis longus	7.5 cm

*Reprinted with permission from Packer et al.[5]

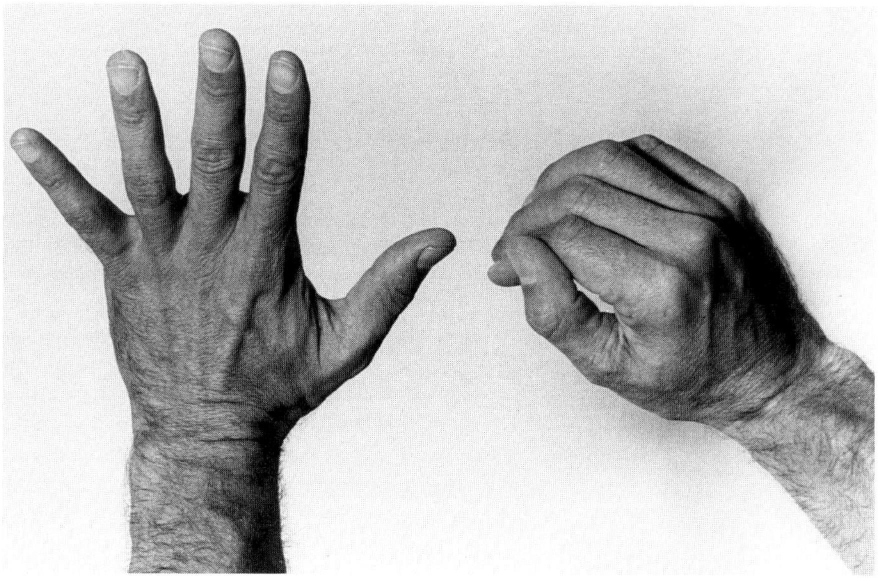

Figure 11-5. Diagnosis of posterior interosseous nerve syndrome. With wrist extension, the affected side (right) deviates radially. Extensor carpi radialis longus is innervated normally and inserts on the radial side of the wrist (second metacarpal). Also, all fingers remained flexed at metacarpophalangeal joints, but the normal hand (left) can actively extend.

to this region, the radial nerve is bordered medially by the brachialis muscle and the biceps tendon, laterally by the origin of the brachioradialis muscle and posteriorly by the lateral humeral epicondyle. As the radial nerve progresses distally, it becomes crossed by the extensor carpi radialis brevis, whose muscle belly may be large enough to compress the nerve against the underlying capitellum. The extensor carpi radialis longus originates from inferior or posterior to the nerve and does not contribute in compression. In some cases, the extensor carpi radialis brevis has a fibrous arch that, as the radial nerve divides into the posterior interosseous nerve, may compress the radial nerve against the arcade of Fröhse in this more distal portion of the radial tunnel region. The radial nerve may pass through a region of fibrous adhesions, possibly induced by the inflammatory process from the lateral humeral epicondylitis as it crosses over the radial head.

Roles and Maudsley[64] thought that the recurrent radial artery and vein contributed to compression in the distal area just as the posterior interosseous nerve entered into the arcade of Fröhse, and they also found in their cases that the arcade of Fröhse was compressing the radial nerve. However, their patients did not have motor paralysis. Therefore, although there is an anatomic overlap between the structures that can compress the radial nerve in the radial tunnel syndrome and the posterior interosseous nerve syndrome, there is no motor paralysis in the radial tunnel syndrome. This syndrome is characterized by aching pain in the proximal portion of the forearm. Pain may be worsened with use of the arm. There are no sensory changes distally in the distribution of the radial sensory nerve. Roles and Maudsley described the provocative test that duplicates the patient's syndrome when the examiner resists the patient's attempt to extend his middle finger (Fig.

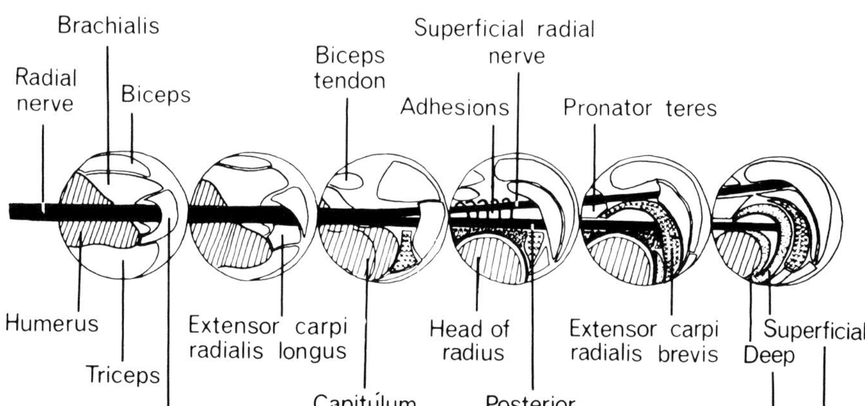

Figure 11-6. Schematic representation of the "radial tunnel," along the course of which the radial nerve may become compressed to give rise to the radial tunnel syndrome. (Reproduced with permission from Roles and Maudsley.[64])

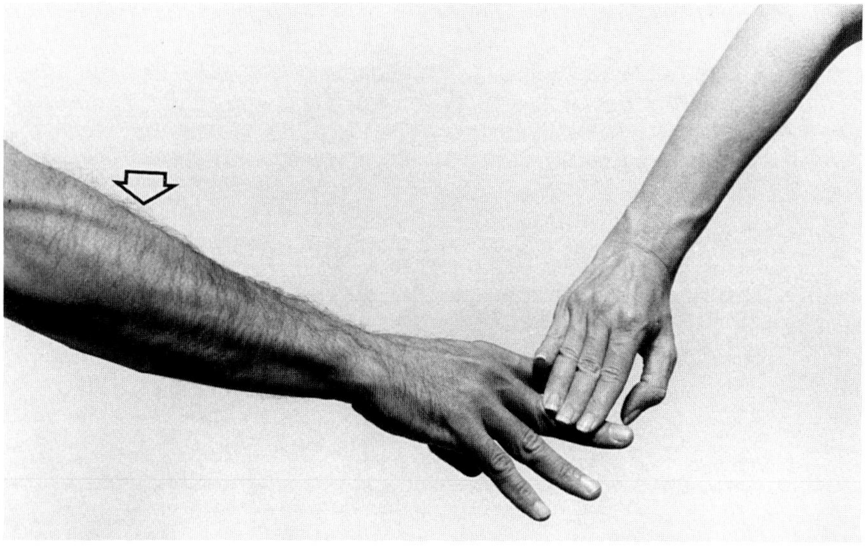

Figure 11-7. Diagnosis of radial tunnel syndrome. Resisted middle finger extension causes more pain to be referred to an area beneath the mobile muscle wad (arrow) than does resisted extension of the little or ring finger. Mechanism of symptom induction is compression of the nerve by extensor carpi radialis brevis origin. The extensor carpi radialis brevis inserts at the base of the third ("middle") metacarpal.

11-7). Lister[63] has noted that the middle finger extension when resisted creates more pain than does resistance to the index, ring, or little finger, which in tennis elbow may cause pain referred to this general area also. One important distinguishing feature as described by Lister is that the referral of pain is not to the lateral humeral epicondyle, but rather to an area beneath the mobile muscle wad over the radial head. Resisted forearm supination causes pain to be referred beneath the mobile muscle wad. With lateral humeral epicondylitis, resisted finger extension or wrist extension causes pain to be produced at the lateral humeral epicondyle rather than beneath this mobile muscle wad. The radial nerve is tender to palpation in the region of this muscle mass (Figs. 11-7, 11-8).

After initial descriptions, subsequent articles have reported other similar cases of radial tunnel syndrome. In addition to the 36 cases reported initially,[64] Lister et al[65] in 1979 reported 20 cases, Sponseller and Engber[66] in 1983 reported two cases. Moss and Switzer[67] also in 1983 reported 15 cases. These 73 cases in total created a uniform series of symptoms that can be distinguished on clinical examination from tennis elbow. Two of the structures that may compress the radial nerve in this vicinity that have been referred to by Sponseller and Engber[66] have added a distal site within the supinator muscle.

We would take exception, however, to Sponseller and Engber's use of the term "double entrapment radial tunnel syndrome." They attempted to say that the cases they were describing were examples of the double crush syndrome.[68] However, as discussed in Chapter 14,

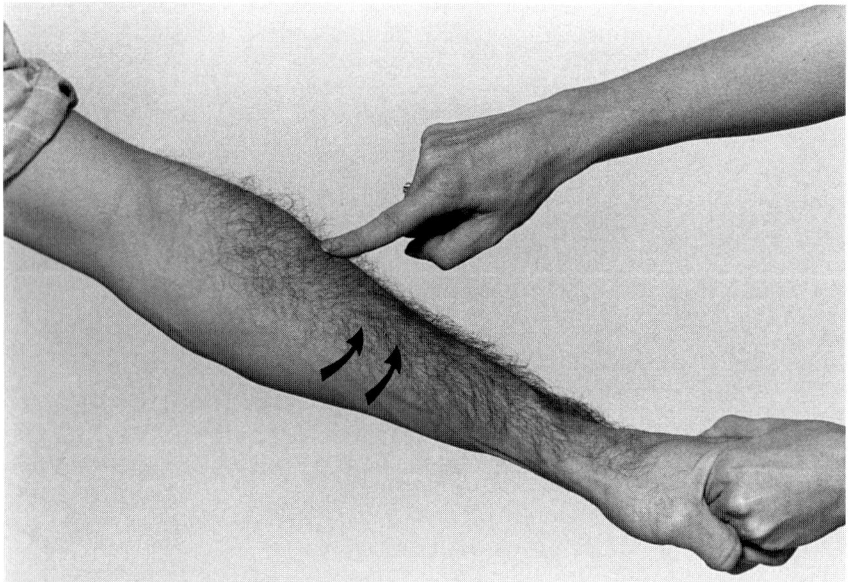

Figure 11-8. Diagnosis of the radial tunnel syndrome. Resisted supination creates pain referred to the mobile muscle wad (indicated). Palpation of radial nerve in this region causes pain. (The lateral humeral epicondyle, which is tender with tennis elbow, is where resisted wrist and finger extension produce pain with lateral humeral epicondylitis, tennis elbow.)

what they really have been demonstrating is that the radial nerve in this anatomic region can be crossed by many anatomic sites, each of which may, in and of itself, be insufficient to create the symptoms. Since it is not clear which of these sites may be the more offending, it is essential to release every potential site of entrapment in this entire anatomic region. Thus, we term this syndrome the "multiple crush syndrome" (see Chapter 14).

This anatomic region is notable in that again it represents an example in which vessels in close proximity to a nerve may contribute to the nerve entrapment. We have discussed this in relationship with vessels along the course of the median nerve in the proximal forearm, and it has been well-described in relationship to intracranial compression of cranial nerves V and VII in production of trigeminal neuralgia (tic douloureux) and hemifacial spasm, respectively (see Chapter 14). Along with the concept of needing to require every potential site of compression to be released when doing a nerve decompression, Sponseller and Engber noted that of the four patients in Roles' series and the one in Lister's series who did not obtain good relief from their operations, some may have had this more distal fibrous band that was not released.

Problems that can affect the lateral humeral epicondyle and give pain in this region, which may be confused with radial nerve entrapment, include those related to what has been traditionally termed "tennis elbow." A recent review of the history of this problem notes the addition of the term "tennis elbow" to the many other athletic problems, such as jogger's toe, cyclist palsy (see Chapter 7), football ankle, jumper's knee, billiard player's finger, bowler's thumb, racquet player's pisiform, musher's knee, and hooker's elbow.[69] These descriptive terms generally do not reflect the anatomic site of the problem. It is therefore of interest that the first article reporting tennis elbow, in 1882, referred to it as "lawn tennis arm".[70] The writer described the problem during the backhand of tennis due to rapid pronation and referred to medial humeral epicondylitis. It was not until the game became played much more extensively that problems referrable to the lateral humeral epicondyle were described. By the early 1900s, classic descriptions were recorded.[71,72] The cause of lateral humeral epicondylitis continues to be debated, but the prevailing theory was put forward by Goldie[73] with continued confirmation by Nirschel and Pettrone[74] as an inflammation at the origin of the extensor radialis brevis and also of the communis from the lateral humeral epicondyle, resulting in granulation tissue forming about the base of these tendons. Thus, the physical diagnosis shows pain over the lateral humeral epicondyle and pain referred there with resisted wrist extension and finger extension. The treatment is nonoperative and is successful in more than 70% of the cases and requires topical cold or heat applications, oral anti-inflammatory medication, and cortisone injection. Only after failure of conservative therapy is a surgical approach taken. There are a variety of surgical techniques, all of which seem equally successful. In common, they have the concept of releasing or lengthening these extensor tendons, either at their origin or further down in the forearm with subsequent later muscle strengthening. It is clear that the attention directed toward this region may result in additional fibrous tissue or scarring around the radial nerve as it passes through this area. Thus, cases of so-called resistive tennis elbow may, in fact, have been cases of tennis elbow that responded but in the process of treatment have subsequently produced radial nerve entrapment. Thus, the physical examination as described in the paragraph above and in Figures 11-6, 11-7, and 11-8, and the possible dual existence of the problems, must be taken into account in the examination of the patient.

Surgical Technique

The operation is begun by first marking the site for the incision for an approach to the posterior interosseous nerve. The patient's forearm is resisted as the patient

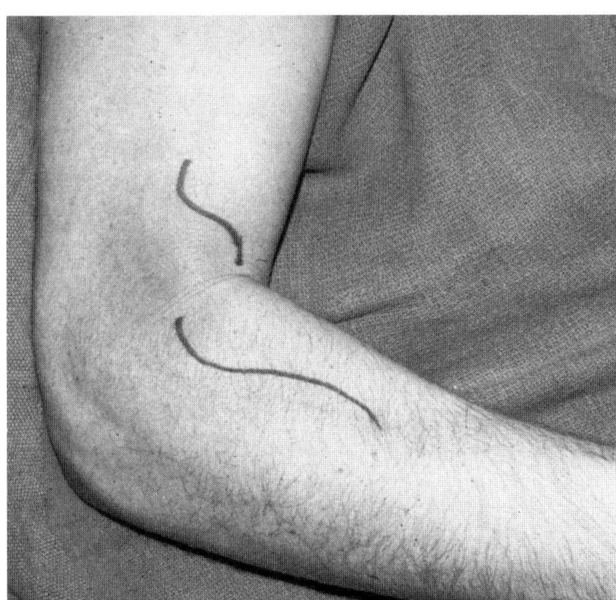

Figure 11-9. Operative approach to the posterior interosseous nerve. The incision is outlined as a lazy S in the interval between the brachioradialis and extensor carpi radialis longus. This interval is identified easily when the elbow is flexed against resistance, with the forearm in the neutral position.

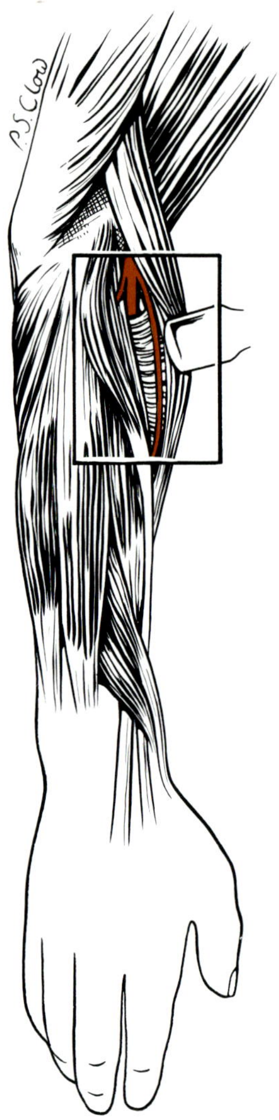

a

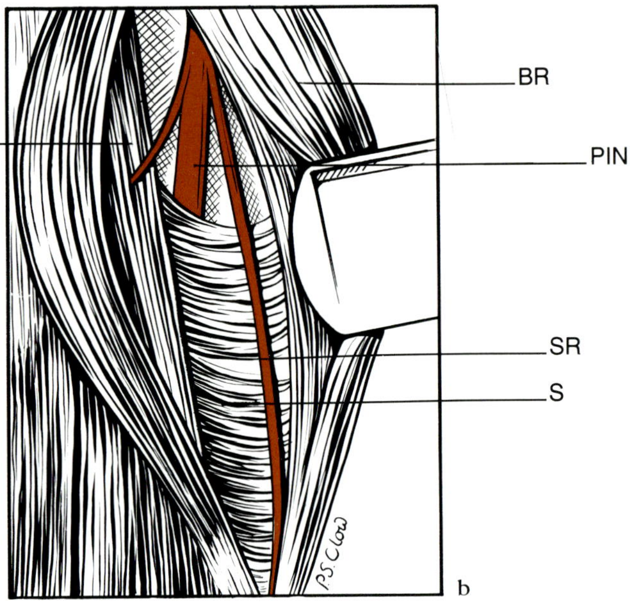

b

Figure 11-10a. Operative approach to the posterior interosseous nerve. Surgical anatomy demonstrated in full arm view. **b.** In close-up view, the brachioradialis (BR) is retracted away from the extensor carpi radialis longus. This reveals the extensor carpi radial brevis (ECRB) crossing the supinator (S). Here each of these muscles is shown without a fibrous edge, and the ECRB is shown being innervated from a branch of the posterior interosseous nerve (PIN), in contrast to Figure 11-4, which shows this branch coming off the superficial sensory radial nerve (SR). (Reproduced with permission from Hall et al.[75])

attempts to flex it. The forearm is kept in a neutral position. This reveals the interval between the brachioradialis muscle and the extensor carpi radialis longus. A lazy "S" incision is made over this area (Fig. 11-9). A second separate lazy "S" incision is made over the internal between the brachioradialis and the biceps tendon. The patient is placed under satisfactory regional or general anesthesia with a pneumatic tourniquet placed over the upper arm, which is protected by soft roll. The hand is prepared and draped in the appropriate manner. The tourniquet is inflated to 100 mm above systolic pressure and the lower incision is opened. This brings the surgeon down upon the region of the posterior cutaneous nerve of the forearm, which usually overlays the interval between the brachioradialis muscle and the extensor carpi radialis longus. The fascia is released and the extensor carpi radialis longus is reflected laterally and by blunt dissection the interval between this muscle and the brachioradialis is dissected (Figs 11-10, 11-11). The surgeon will next note the vessels of the recurrent radial artery and its accompanying veins. Ligature ties or small hemoclips are necessary to divide these vessels. The surgeon will now identify the extensor carpi radialis brevis. In those patients in whom the brevis has a fibrous edge or the extensor carpi radialis brevis is exceedingly bulky, the fibrous edge will need to be completely divided and the muscle bulk partly divided to release the underlying posterior interosseous nerve appropriately. When the extensor carpi radialis brevis muscle is either divided, as just described, or reflected further laterally, the radial nerve will be identified at the proximal aspect of the wound giving off the superficial sensory branch of the radial nerve. Radial sensory nerve will continue beneath the belly of the brachioradialis muscle. The posterior interosseous nerve will continue beneath the proximal edge of the superficial head of the supinator. The separate smaller nerve to the extensor carpi radialis brevis will be just superficial to the pos-

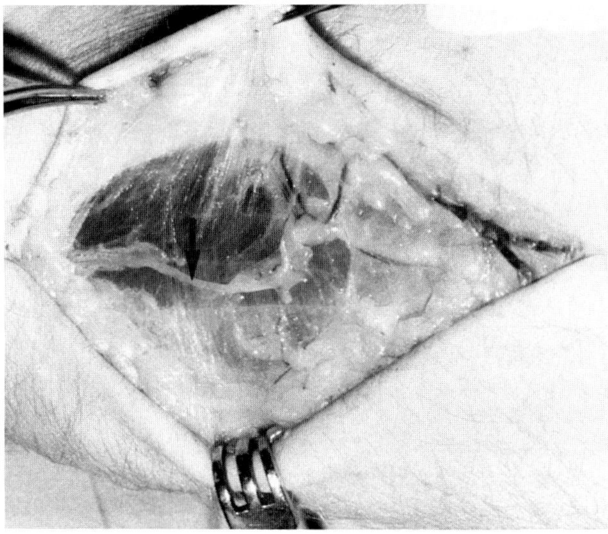

a

Figure 11-11a. Intraoperative view of posterior interosseous nerve decompression; hand toward right elbow toward left the posterior cutaneous nerve (arrow) is identified and protected. **b.** Dissection carried out bluntly between the brachioradialis (BR) and extensor carpi radialis longus (ECRL) reveals (**c**) the extensor carpi radialis brevis muscle (here without a fibrous edge) overlying the posterior interosseous nerve (PIN). Radial collateral vessels (1) must be resected because they compress the nerve and partially divided if necessary (preserving its innervation (2) to reveal the (**d**) supinator (SUP) muscle with the fibrous proximal edge (arcade of Frohse). After division of this arcade (**e**), the PIN is shown released. An internal neurolysis may now be added if necessary. Note the superficial radial branch (S) beneath the BR. (Reproduced with permission from Hall et al.[75]) (*Figure continues.*)

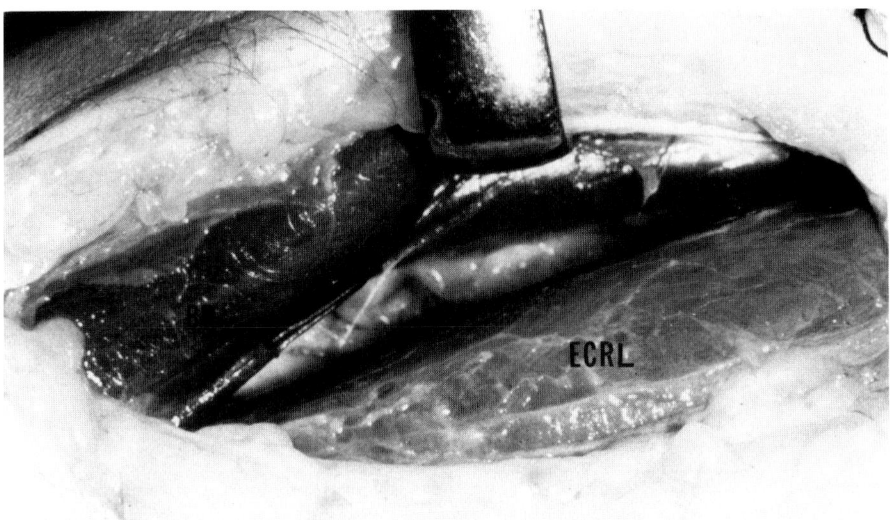

b

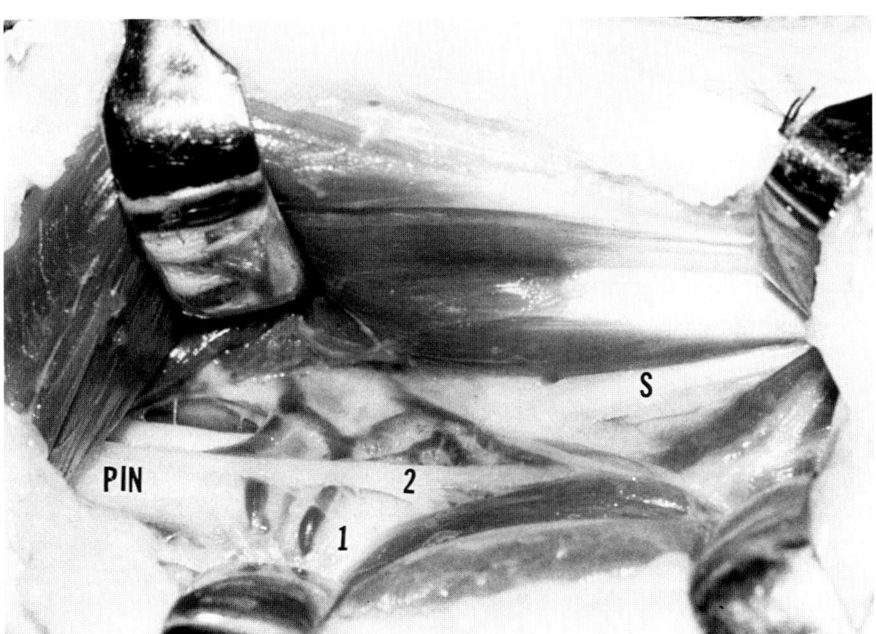

c

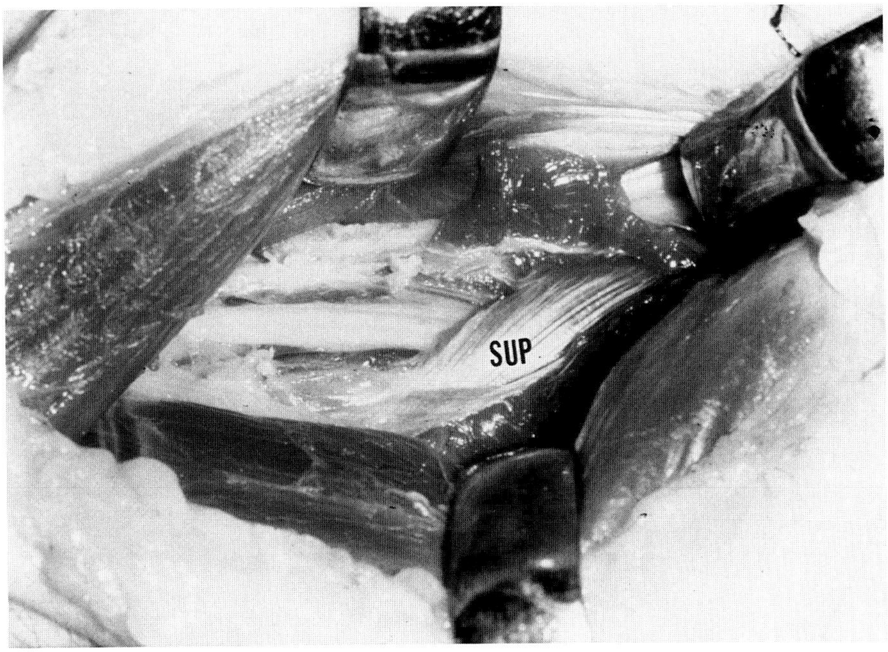

d

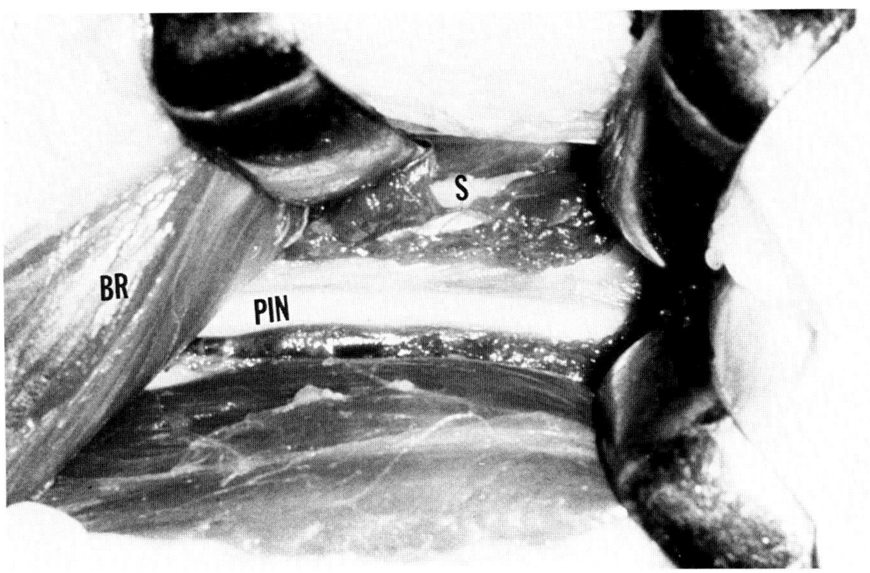

e **Figure 11-11** (*continued*) **d, e.**

terior interosseous nerve. In those cases in which this is fibrous in origin (the arcade of Fröhse), the fibrous arcade will need to be completely divided. The supinator muscle frequently has a striped appearance because of the alternation of the fibrous bands and the muscle, itself. The operative approach is continued in our practice by placing a finger along the course of the posterior interosseous nerve and following it completely through the supinator muscle until it exits from the distal portion. Additional fibrous bands may be present in the body of the supinator or its distal edge that may require resection. The entire superficial head of the supinator will usually require division. The operative approach is continued and the supinator sufficiently divided or retracted until the multiple divisions of the posterior interosseous nerve into the small branches that will innervate the extensor carpi ulnaris, the extensor digitorum communis and the extensor digiti quinti, are identified. The long terminal branch, which will supply the outcropping muscles and the wrist joint, are identified.

If the clinical presentation is anything other than a completely pure posterior interosseous nerve palsy, then the second more proximal incision is opened, that is, if there is significant pain in the proximal forearm or weakness of the brachioradialis or extensor carpi radialis longus or sensory abnormalities on the dorsum of the hand, or if pressure over this proximal site induces symptoms.

When the preoperative physical examination and history are compatible with radial nerve compression in the radial tunnel, that is, when paralysis of the muscles innervated by the posterior interosseous nerve are not part of the preoperative picture, then the incision is made more proximally, and although still a lazy S, it extends more over the muscle mass of the brachioradialis muscle coming proximally toward the lateral humeral epicondyle. Here, the incision is carried down to the brachioradialis muscle and the muscle mass, itself, is bluntly dissected with the examiner's finger probing to find the radial head. The radial head is identified after the brachioradialis muscle fibers are dissected and at this point the radial nerve is revealed before it divides into the sensory and deep motor portions. Here the surgeon can directly release fibrous adhesions that bind the radial nerve to the radial head, release under direct vision any fibrous bands or excessive muscle bulk of the brachioradialis muscle, the extensor carpi radialis longus, or the extensor carpi radialis brevis, which may be compressing the radial nerve against the distal portion of the humerus. From this approach, the examiner can guide his finger proximally along the course of the radial nerve about the humerus. In this most proximal region of the so-called radial tunnel, there may be cojoined fibers of the brachioradialis and the brachialis muscle that need to be released. After this, proximal release is carried out and the sensory portion is clearly identified to run easily beneath the brachioradialis muscle. The radial collateral artery and vein crossing the posterior interosseous nerve are divided and then the fibrous edge of the supinator, if present, is divided. Through the distal portion of the incision, entrance may be gained farther distally along the course of the posterior interosseous nerve, and the distal portion of the supinator muscle, if necessary by muscle retraction on the supinator or complete division of the superficial head of the supinator, the terminal portions of the posterior interosseous nerve where it divides into its multiple fine branches, may be observed directly.

An internal neurolysis is indicated when complete paralysis occurs for any of the muscles innervated by the posterior interosseous nerve or when extreme weakness is present, since it may be difficult preoperatively to detect wasting in these muscles. It is also indicated if the electromyogram has demonstrated denervation of potentials in these muscles. During the internal neurolysis, the branch to the extensor carpi radialis brevis can be identified and separated from the main posterior interosseous nerve, and the main division of the posterior interosseous nerve into those fascicles that will go to the more proximally innervated muscles from those that will go to the more distally innervated muscles can be completed. With the radial tunnel syndrome, a neurolysis may be required in the radial nerve overlying the radial head, and in both syndromes it may be required beneath the radial collateral vessels. The neurolysis is continued until there is a good fascicular pattern with good perineurial markings.

Postoperative Care

The patient is placed into a dressing made of well-padded dressings, fluff, soft roll, and a posterior plaster splint holding the elbow in 60 to 90° flexion with the forearm in a neutral position. This is placed and then covered with elastic wrap and the tourniquet is deflated.

The patient wears this dressing for 7 to 10 days, after which the dressing is removed and any sutures are removed. Even with the dressing in place, the patient is encouraged to move the wrist, fingers, and elbow within the limitation of the dressings. The patient is begun on wrist movement, elbow flexion and extension in the second week postoperatively to allow the nerve to glide through the operative plane. This is critical in preventing adhesions from forming between the nerve and the tissues that have been extensively released.

In the third postoperative week, the patient is encouraged to use gentle massage to the operative area and is begun on gentle resisted exercises of the thumb, fingers, wrist, and forearm.

In the sixth week, a cortisone cream is given to the patient to apply to the wound if scar hypertrophy has begun.

In those patients who have paralysis of the muscles innervated by the posterior interosseous nerve, a dynamic splint has been prepared preoperatively and the patient is placed in this after removal of the cast, in which case the cast has been prepared to place the wrist for a radial nerve palsy with the wrist being extended and the fingers being extended at the metacarpophalangeal joints. This dynamic splint is worn throughout the day and replaced by a static radial nerve palsy splint at night. The patients with radial tunnel syndrome have no need of this splinting.

Complications

The complications of this operation are scarring of the forearm, the potential for bleeding, infection in the postoperative period, and direct injury to the innervation of the extensor carpi radialis brevis, the superficial radial nerve, and the posterior interosseous nerve. If an internal neurolysis is done during the operative procedure, there may be a period of increased sensitivity, either to hot or cold or normal touch stimuli in the postoperative period. In the reported cases of the posterior interosseous nerve syndrome and the radial tunnel syndrome, few complications have been described.

Results

A review of the overall resuls of all the articles describing the posterior interosseous nerve syndrome has not been done. Of the 73 cases reported with the radial tunnel syndrome,[64,67] all but six patients achieved excellent results after the decompression of the nerve. There was 92% good to excellent results.

Results of radial nerve repair in the brachium are generally discussed as being good, because it is a short distance to reinnervate the wrist extensors. Little reported information, however, is actually available. Sunderland[76] lists three cases of repair to the radial nerve, two after laceration and one after a gunshot wound; one with a level of injury 12.5 cm above the lateral humeral epicondyle and the other two with levels of repair at 4 to 5 cm proximally. All three recovered function in the extensor pollicis longus tendon by 40 to 45 weeks after the repair, but the strength of the muscle recovery and whether sensation recurred were not noted.

References

1. Seddon H: Surgical Disorders of the Peripheral Nerve. Williams & Wilkins, Baltimore, 1972.
2. Seddon H: Nerve lesions complicating certain closed bone injuries. JAMA 135:691–694, 1947.
3. Omer GE Jr: Injuries to the nerves of the upper extremities. J Bone Joint Surg 56A:1615–1624, 1974.
4. Barton NJ: Radial nerve lesions. Hand 5:200–208, 1973.
5. Packer JW, Foster RR, Garcia A, Grantham BA: The humeral fracture with radial nerve palsy: Is exploration warranted? Clin Orthop 88:34–38, 1972.
6. Garcia A Jr, Maeck BH: Radial nerve injuries and fractures of the shaft of the humerus. Am J Surg 99:625–627, 1960.
7. Kim LYS: Compression neuropathy of the radial nerve due to pentazocine-induced fibrous myopathy. Arch Phys Med Rehabil 68:49–50, 1987.
8. Broadbent TR, Odom GL, Woodhall B: Peripheral nerve injuries in the administration of penicillin. Report of four clinical cases. JAMA 140:1008–1010, 1949.
9. Ling CM, Loong SC: Injection injury of the radial nerve. Injury 8:60–62, 1976.
10. Sunderland S: Traumatic injuries of peripheral nerves: Simple compression injuries of the radial nerve. Brain 68:56–72, 1945.
11. Dhuner KG: Nerve injuries following operations: A survey of cases occurring during a six-year period. Anesthesiology 11:289–293, 1950.
12. Weston B: Prevention of upper limb nerve injuries in Trendelenburg position. Acta Chir Scand 108:61–68, 1954.
13. Parks BJ: Postoperative peripheral neuropathies. Surgery, 74:348–357, 1973.
14. Eckhoff NL: Tourniquet paralysis: A plea for the extended use of the pneumatic tourniquet. Lancet 2:343–345, 1931.
15. Moldauver J: Tourniquet paralysis syndrome. Arch Surg 68:136–144, 1954.
16. Rudge PE: Tourniquet paralysis with prolonged conduction block: Electrophysiological study. J Bone Joint Surg 56B:716–720, 1974.
17. Bolton CF, MacFarland RM: Human pneumatic tourniquet paralysis. Neurology (NY) 28:787–793, 1978.
18. Lotem M, Fried A, Levy M, Solzi P, Najensoss T, Nathan H: Radial palsy following muscular effort: A nerve compression syndrome possibly related to a fibrous arch of the lateral head of the triceps. J Bone Joint Surg 53B: 500–506, 1971.
19. Manske PR: Compression of the radial nerve by the triceps muscle. A case report. J Bone Joint Surg 59A:835–836, 1977.
20. Kerr AT: The brachial plexus nerves in man, the variations in its formation and branches. Am J Anat 23:285–395, 1918.
21. Kameda Y: An anomalous muscle (accessory scapularis-tres-latissimus muscle) in the axilla penetrating the brachial plexus in man. Acta Anat 96:513–533, 1976.
22. Spinner M, Freundlich BD, Ticher J: Posterior interosseous nerve palsy as a complication of Monteggia fracture in children. Clin Orthop 58:141–145, 1968.
23. Fröhse F, Frankel M: Die Muskeln des Menschlichen Armes. Bardeleben's Hendbuch der Anatomie des Menschlichen. Fisher, Jena 1908.
24. Spinner M: The arcade of Fröhse and its relationship to posterior interosseous nerve paralysis. J Bone Joint Surg 50B:809–812, 1968.
25. Spinner M: Injuries to the Major Branches of Peripheral Nerves of the Forearm, 2nd ed. WB Saunders, Philadelphia, 1978.
26. Davies F, Laird M: The supinator muscle in the deep radial (posterior interosseous) nerve. Anat Rec 101:243–250, 1948.
27. Dellon AL, Seiff SS: Neuroma of the posterior interosseous nerve simulating a recurrent ganglion: A case report and anatomical dissections relating the posterior interosseous nerve to the carpus. Etiology of dorsal ganglion pain. J Hand Surg 3:326–332, 1978.
28. Dellon AL: Partial dorsal wrist denervation: Resection of distal posterior interosseous nerve. J Hand Surg [Am] 10:527–533, 1985.
29. Kaplan EB: Functional and Surgical Anatomy of the Hand, 2nd ed, JB Lippincott, Philadelphia, 1965.
30. Learmonth JR: Variation of the radial branch of the musculospiral nerve. J Anat 53:371–372, 1919.
31. Vaughan-Jackson OJ: Rupture of the extensor tendons by

attrition at the inferior radioulnar joint. J Bone Joint Surg 30B:528–530, 1948.
32. Gullain G, Courtellemont R: L'action du muscle court supinator dans la paralysie du nerf radial. Presse Med 13:50–52, 1905.
33. Woltman HW, Learmonth JR: Progressive paralysis of the nervous interosseous dorsalis. Brain 57:25–31, 1934.
34. Hobhouse N, Heald CB: A case of posterior interosseous paralysis. Br Med J 1:841, 1936.
35. Grigoresco D, Iordanesco G: Une cas rare de paralysie partielle du nerf radial. Rev Neurol (Paris) 32:102–104, 1937.
36. Silverstein A: Progressive paralysis of the dorsal interosseous nerve. Report of a case. Arch Neurol Psychiatry 38:885–886, 1937.
37. Otenasek FJ: Progressive paralysis of the nervus dorsalis: Pathological findings in one case. Bull Johns Hopkins Hosp 81:163–167, 1947.
38. Kruse F, Jr: Paralysis of the dorsal interosseous nerve not due to direct trauma. A case showing spontaneous recovery. Neurology (Minneap) 8:307–308, 1958.
39. Whitely WH, Alpers BJ: Posterior interosseous palsy with spontaneous neuroma formation. Arch Neurol I:226–229, 1959.
40. Capener N: Posterior interosseous nerve lesions. Proceedings of the Second Hand Club. J Bone Joint Surg 46B: 361, 1964.
41. Capener N: The vulnerability of the posterior interosseous nerve of the forearm. J Bone Joint Surg 48B:770–773, 1966.
42. Goldman S, Honet JC, Sobel R, Goldstein AS: Posterior interosseous-nerve palsy in the absence of trauma. Arch Neurol 21:435–441, 1969.
43. Mulholland RC: Non-traumatic progressive paralysis of the posterior interosseous nerve. J Bone Joint Surg 48B: 781–785, 1966.
44. Sharrard WJW: Posterior interosseous neuritis. J Bone Joint Surg 48B:777–780, 1966.
45. Bryan FS, Miller LS, Panijaganond P: Spontaneous paralysis of the posterior interosseous nerve. A case report and review of the literature. Clin Orthop 80:9–12, 1971.
46. Nielson HO: Posterior interosseous nerve paralysis caused by fibrous band compression at the supinator muscle. A report of four cases. Acta Orthop Scand 47:304–307, 1976.
47. Marie P, Meige H, Patrikios R: Paralysie radiale dissociee simulant une griffe cubitale. Rev Neurol (Paris) 24:123–124, 1917.
48. Roussy G, Branche J: Deux cas de paralysies dissociees de la branche posterieure du radial a type de pseudo-griffe cubitale. Rev Neurol (Paris) 24:312–314, 1917.
49. Woltman HW, Kernohan JW: Disease of peripheral nerves. In Baker AB (ed): Clinical Neurology. Hoeber-Harper, New York, 1955, p 1629.
50. Dharapak C, Minberg GA: Posterior interosseous nerve compression. Report of a case caused by traumatic aneurysm. Clin Orthop 101:225–228, 1974.
51. Lichter R, Jacobsen T: Tardy palsy of the posterior interosseous nerve with Monteggia fracture. J Bone Joint Surg 57A:124–125, 1975.
52. Morris AH: Irreducible Monteggia lesion with radial-nerve entrapment. J Bone Joint Surg 56A:1744–1746, 1974.
53. Stein F, Grabias SL, Deffer PA: Nerve injuries complicating Monteggia lesions. J Bone Joint Surg 53A:1432–1436, 1971.
54. Strachan JCH, Ellis BW: Vulnerability of the posterior interosseous nerve during radial head resection. J Bone Joint Surg 53B:320–323, 1971.
55. Bowen TL, Stone KH: Posterior interosseous nerve paralysis caused by a ganglion at the elbow. J Bone Joint Surg 48B:774–776, 1966.
56. Marshall SC, Murray WR: Deep radial nerve palsy associated with rheumatoid arthritis. Clin Orthop 103:157–162, 1974.
57. Marmor L, Lawrence JF, Dubois E: Posterior interosseous nerve paralysis due to rheumatoid arthritis. J Bone Joint Surg 49A:381–383, 1967.
58. Millender LH, Nalebuff EA, Holdsworth DE: Posterior interosseous nerve syndrome secondary to rheumatoid synovitis. J Bone Joint Surg 55A:753–757, 1973.
59. Popelka S, Vainio D: Entrapment of the posterior interosseous branch of the radial nerve in rheumatoid arthritis. Acta Orthop Scand 45:370–372, 1974.
60. Moon N, Marmor L: Parosteal lipoma of the proximal part of the radius. J Bone Joint Surg 46A:608–614, 1964.
61. Richmond DA: Lipoma causing a posterior interosseous nerve lesion. J Bone Joint Surg 35B:83, 1953.
62. Phalen GS, Kendrick JI, Rodriguez JM: Lipomas of the upper extremity. Am J Surg 121:298–306, 1971.
63. Lister G: The Hand: Diagnosis and Indications. Churchill Livingstone, Edinburgh, 1977.
64. Roles NC, Maudsley RH: Radial tunnel syndrome: Resistant tennis elbow as a nerve entrapment. J Bone Joint Surg 54B:499–508, 1972.
65. Lister GD, Belsole RB, Kleinert HE: The radial tunnel syndrome. J Hand Surg 4:52–59, 1979.
66. Sponseller PD, Engber WD: Double-entrapment of radial tunnel syndrome. J Hand Surg 8:420–423, 1983.
67. Moss SH, Switzer HE: Radial tunnel syndrome: A spectrum of clinical presentations. J Hand Surg 8:414–419, 1983.
68. Upton ARM, McComas AJ: The double crush in nerve entrapment syndromes. Lancet 2:259–362, 1973.
69. Emery SE, Gifford JF: One hundred years of tennis elbow. Contemp Orthop 12:53–58, 1986.
70. Morris H: The rider's sprain. Lancet 2:133, 1982.
71. Marshall CF: Tennis elbow. Br Med J 1:559, 1907.
72. Couse WP: Epicondylitis (Franke) or tennis elbow. Boston Med Surg J 170:461, 1914.
73. Goldie I: Epicondylitis lateralis humeri. Acta Chir Scand [Suppl] 339:7, 1964.
74. Nirschel RP, Pettrone FA: Tennis elbow and the surgical treatment of lateral epicondylitis. J Bone Joint Surg 61A: 832–839, 1979.
75. Hall HH, Mackinnon SE, Gilbert RW: An approach to the posterior interosseous nerve. Plast Reconstr Surg 74:435–437, 1984.
76. Sunderland S: Nerves and Nerve Injuries, 2nd ed. Churchill Livingston, Edinburgh, 1978, p 837.

Tarsal Tunnel Syndrome

12

Historical Review

The term "tarsal tunnel syndrome" was introduced by Keck in 1962.[1] Although the prevalence of tarsal tunnel syndrome must be much greater, there have been 315 cases reported through 1984.[1–25] The majority of these articles represent individual case reports. The reports in general seem to be in agreement that the tarsal tunnel syndrome is the result of compression of the posterior tibial nerve in its course through the tarsal tunnel. The tarsal tunnel in these articles is generally described as a tunnel having as its roof the flexor retinaculum (previously called the lancinate ligament) bridging the space between the calcaneus and the medial malleolus. The floor of the tunnel contains the fibro-osseous coverings of the tendons of the posterior tibialis, the flexor hallucis, and the flexor digitorum longus. The contents of the tarsal tunnel, beside the posterior tibial nerve and its branches, are the posterior tibial artery and its accompanying veins. Articles written by the electrodiagnosticians have been concerned with standardizing recording techniques for the medial and lateral plantar nerves and the posterior tibial nerve in this region.[7,17–19,22] The published surgical reports describe treatment as being successful in approximately 90% of the cases, with this treatment consisting of division of the flexor retinaculum.[1–6,8–10,12,13] There are occasional references extending to the release more distally over the course of the medial and lateral plantar nerves, but this particular suggestion is neither documented nor areas of constriction in these distal regions described. There is general agreement that the area of symptoms includes the plantar aspect of the foot, and there is variable incorporation of the heel into the symptom complex. There appears to be a consensus that the most common cause of tarsal tunnel syndrome is injury to the ankle region with disruption of ligaments, swelling, and subsequent fibrosis. The occurrence of tarsal tunnel syndrome in patients with arthritis has been documented.[11,21] In one study of 40 patients with rheumatoid arthritis, 15% were found to have peripheral neuropathy as determined by delayed nerve conduction velocity in the posterior tibial nerve. In addition to these patients, an additional 5% were found to have increased latencies in the medial or lateral plantar nerves.[21] As with the carpal tunnel syndrome, with increased awareness of this problem, more and more related causes will be reported. For example, recently tarsal tunnel syndrome has been reported with regional migratory osteoporosis[20] and with hyperlipidemia.[24] Tarsal tunnel syndrome being due to the presence of a ganglion in the tarsal tunnel has been reported.[15] Varicosities of the veins accompanying the posterior tibial artery have also been previously cited as a cause of tarsal tunnel syndrome.[1,2,12]

Our experience with the tarsal tunnel syndrome, however, has raised several areas of controversy and areas requiring further study. These concern the anatomic branch patterns in the posterior tibial nerve, the potential sites for chronic compression, including tunnels for the medial and lateral plantar nerves, the relationship of the tunnels in the foot and ankle to those of the hand, and the technique for surgical release.

Surgical Anatomy

The only anatomic study of which we are aware that directly deals with variations in the posterior tibial nerve is that by Horwitz in 1938.[26] Horwitz observed the following:

> The terminal plantar nerves are formed 1½ inch (1.3 cms.) above and behind the tip of the internal malleolus. The smaller posterior division immediately gives off the medial calcaneal branch or branches. In four cases, this branch arose from the posterior tibial nerve directly and in three coming off one inch (2.5 cms.) and in the fourth, 3 inches (7.5 cms.) above the site of terminal division. In four instances, the posterior tibial nerve was split for a distance of 2 inches (5 cms.), three to four inches above the internal malleolus by a small twig off the posterior tibial artery.

In order to define these relationships better, anatomic dissections were carried out in 31 feet in 20 cadavers.[27] The bifurcation into medial and lateral plantar nerves occurred within 1 cm of the malleolar-calcaneal axis in 90% of the feet. Seven of 11 bilateral specimens were bilaterally symmetrical in the bifurcation location: three varied within 1 cm between sides, and in the fourth cadaver, one side bifurcated at 3 cm and the other at 5 cm proximal to the axis (Fig. 12-1). The calcaneal nerve showed great variability; in seven cadavers it arose within, in eight cadavers, proximal to, and in five cadavers there were multiple branches arising both proximal to and within the tarsal tunnel (Fig. 12-2). Recently we have observed a calcaneal branch to arise from the medial plantar nerve within the tarsal tunnel. This branch crosses superficial to the lateral plantar nerve to enter the heel and is very easily injured during release of the flexor retinaculum, resulting in postoperative "heel pain."[35]

With respect to the tarsal tunnel, the roof is formed by a thickening in the deep lower leg fascia. This thickens to become the flexor retinaculum going between the medial malleolus and the calcaneus. Distal to this thickening is an area of subcutaneous tissue. The posterior tibial nerve enters the tarsal tunnel between the overlying flexor retinaculum and the underlying tendon sheaths of the posterior tibialis, the flexor hallucis, and the flexor digitorum longus. The posterior tibial nerve then bifurcates into the medial and lateral plantar nerves. In just one of 20 normal adults, the nerve will bifurcate proximal to the flexor retinaculum; a greater incidence of high split of the posterior tibial nerve may be present in patients with the tarsal tunnel syndrome. If this anomaly predisposes to nerve compression once the nerve has split into the medial and lateral plantar nerves, these nerves then each enter separate anatomic tunnels.[28] The roof for both of these tunnels is formed by fibrous origins that will become the plantar aponeurosis, for the roof of the lateral plantar nerve, and the origin of the abductor hallucis brevis muscle for the medial plantar nerve. The fibrous origins of this common roof are from the calcaneus. Superficial or more plantar to this band is the abductor hallucis brevis muscle. The division between the medial and lateral plantar tunnels is a fibrous septum that originates from the fibro-osseous canal of the flexor hallucis longus tendon or directly from the calcaneus. The entire tarsal tunnel, therefore, may be viewed as a cone, whose narrow inlet begins on the medial aspect of the lower leg proximal to the malleolus and extends distally in a

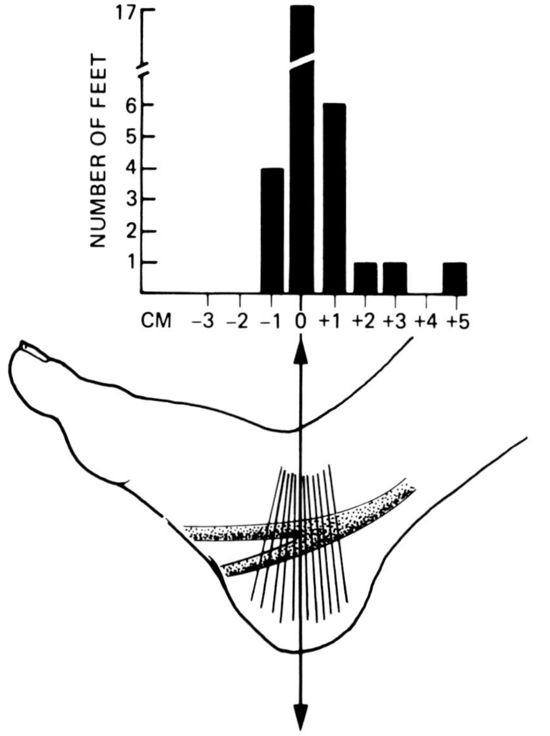

Figure 12-1. Distribution of location of bifurcation of posterior tibial nerve with respect to the malleolar-calcaneal axis. (Reproduced with permission form Dellon and Mackinnon.[27])

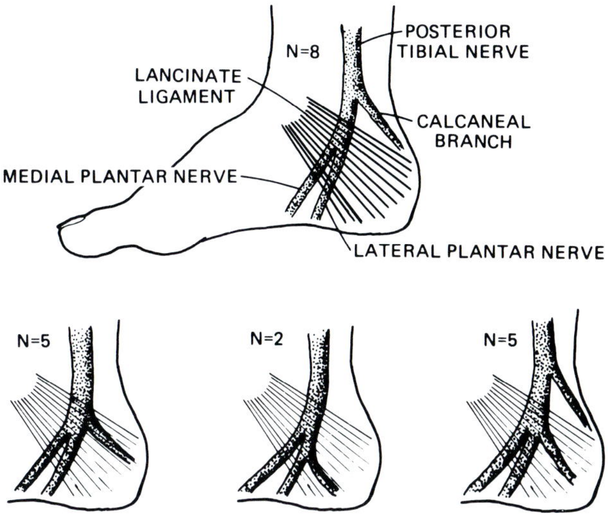

Figure 12-2. Patterns of origin of medial calcaneal nerve from tibial nerve in 20 patients. (Reproduced with permission from Dellon and Mackinnon.[27])

widening fashion, entering the plantar aspect of the foot (Figs. 12-3, 12-4).

In an article in 1960 on peripheral entrapment neuropathies and neuropathies of the lower extremity, Kopell and Thompson[29] described the possibility of entrapment of the posterior tibial nerve in the region of the ankle and the foot. Although they did not specifically describe the tarsal tunnel syndrome, their Figure 5 demonstrates the medial and lateral plantar nerve entering into separate fibrous tunnels beneath the abductor hallucis muscle. This is the closest representation of these two separate tunnels of which we are aware in the literature.[29] Spalteholz'[30] *Atlas,* from 1906, contains one plate that illustrates the existence of these two tunnels.

The appropriate analogies between the tarsal tunnel and the carpal tunnel are as follows:[28] the carpal tunnel is analogous to the tunnel in which just the medial plantar nerve lies. The hamate dividing the carpal tunnel from Guyon's canal is analogous to the septum arising from the calcaneus adjacent to the fibro-osseous canal of the flexor hallucis tendon. The roof of Guyon's canal is analogous to the roof over the lateral plantar

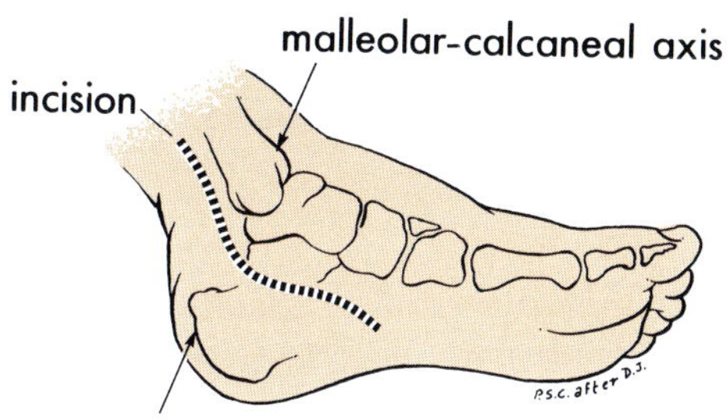

a

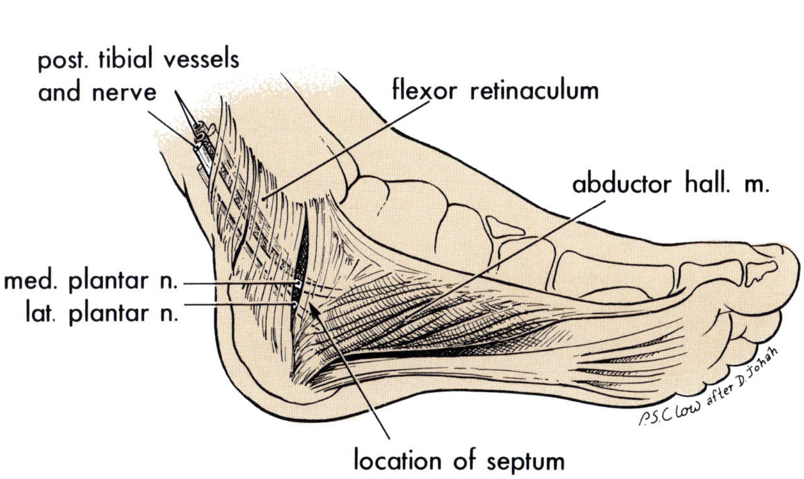

b

Figure 12-3. Sites of posterior tibial nerve compression extending from proximal to the medial malleolus onto the plantar aspect of the foot. Note posterior tibial nerve entering the tarsal tunnel at its narrow proximal end, splitting into the medial and plantar nerves, which then go through two separate tunnels. (Reproduced with permission from Mackinnon and Dellon.[28]) (*Figure continues.*)

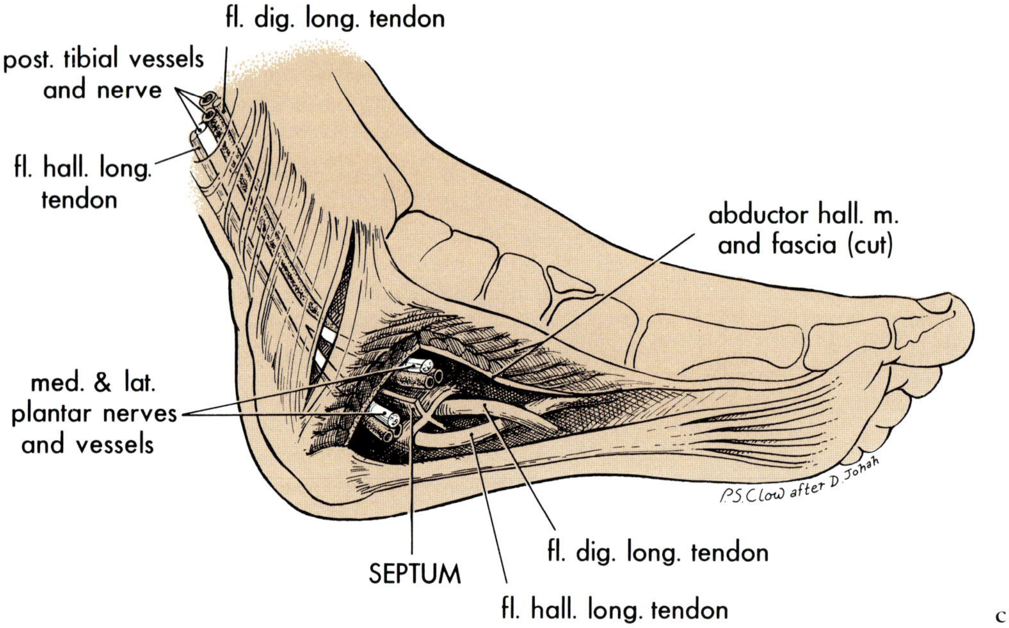

Figure 12-3 (*continued*).

nerve. The roof of the medial plantar tunnel and the origin of the abductor hallucis from this roof is analogous to the transverse carpal ligament and the origin of the thenar muscles from the transverse carpal ligament. The posterior tibial nerve beneath the flexor retinaculum is most analogous to the wrist region proximal to the carpal tunnel and to Guyon's canal, where the antebrachial fascia thickens and begins to blend into the transverse carpal ligament. It follows that just as a release of the forearm fascia is not sufficient to release the medial nerve from beneath the transverse carpal ligament, so then would a release of just the flexor retinaculum over the posterior tibial nerve not be sufficient to release the medial or lateral plantar nerves from compression in their respective tunnels (Table 12-1).

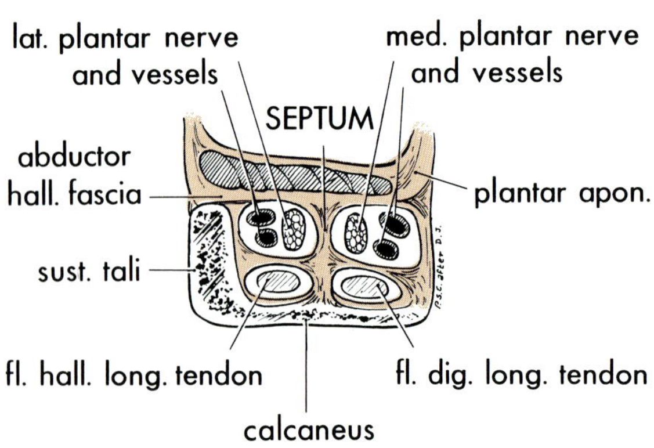

Figure 12-4. Cross-section through distal portion of the tarsal tunnel demonstrating the separate tunnel for the medial plantar and lateral plantar nerves. Note roof of tunnel comprised of ligamentous origin from the calcaneus of the fascia giving rise to the abductor hallucis and that over the lateral plantar nerve continuing distally as the plantar aponeurosis. (Reproduced with permission from Mackinnon and Dellon.[28])

Histopathology of Tarsal Tunnel Syndrome

There is only one report of an examination of a human posterior tibial nerve from a patient with a tarsal tunnel syndrome.[25] In that excised posterior tibial nerve, the anatomic variation of the calcaneal branch was such that it came off proximal to the tarsal tunnel and therefore lay at the periphery of the multiple fascicles that were compressed. Histologic examination of the excised nerve demonstrated that the axons within the calcaneal branch were the best preserved of all the fascicles. This provides an explanation of why some patients may have preservation or relative sparing of the sensation in the heel when the rest of the foot is severely affected by the tarsal tunnel syndrome.

The experimental model for peripheral neuropathy that bears directly on the tarsal tunnel syndrome is that of the hind foot of the caged guinea pig. Gilliott and Fullerton's model[31] is "developmental" in that as the caged guinea pig matures and accrues increasing "mileage" in its cage, the posterior tibial nerve exposed to a varying amount of repetitive trauma over time develops chronic nerve compression. In individual guinea pigs with advanced compression, significant electrodiagnostic and morphometric changes occur related to myelin, axon, and supporting connective tissues. However, the model is unpredictable in producing a defined degree of histopathologic or electrophysiologic change in a given percentage of animals in the aged guinea pig population.

Diagnosis

The patient with a tarsal tunnel syndrome usually presents with complaints of burning, tingling, numbness, or pain in the plantar aspect of the foot, usually in the toes or beneath the metatarsal heads. Symptoms can extend to the heel. Rarely, complaints related to the heel will be the presenting signs. When they are, they suggest compression of a calcaneal branch and may mimic complaints from a calcaneal bone spur. These spurs may exist coincidentally in the population over age 50 years (Fig. 12-5). The aching discomfort from the tarsal tunnel syndrome can shoot up into the calf region. The symptoms do not extend to the dorsal aspect of the foot, although an isolated report of this has been presented.[32] Tarsal tunnel symptoms are worsened by walking, standing, and may be worse at night. The symptoms are relieved by rest and elevation. Associated medical illnesses are chronic lower leg edema due to venous stasis or renal or cardiovascular problems, lower leg trauma, hypothyroidism, diabetes, and alcoholism (Fig. 12-5). There are rarely complaints related to weakness in the foot, although patients may complain of cramping in their feet, or of their toes "curling."

The physical examination demonstrates frequently a swelling posterior to the medial malleolus, a positive Tinel's sign along the course of the posterior tibial nerve as it enters beneath the flexor retinaculum, a separate Tinel's sign over the medial and over the lateral plantar nerves as they enter their separate distal tunnels. The Tinel's sign over the medial plantar nerve is referred to the big toe. That over the lateral plantar nerve is referred to the little toe. There will be diminished vibratory perception in the toes compared with the opposite foot. There may be abnormal two-point discrimination present in the toes. This is difficult to test in the little toe. In the big toe, it is easier to test; for the moving two-point discrimination test, the test

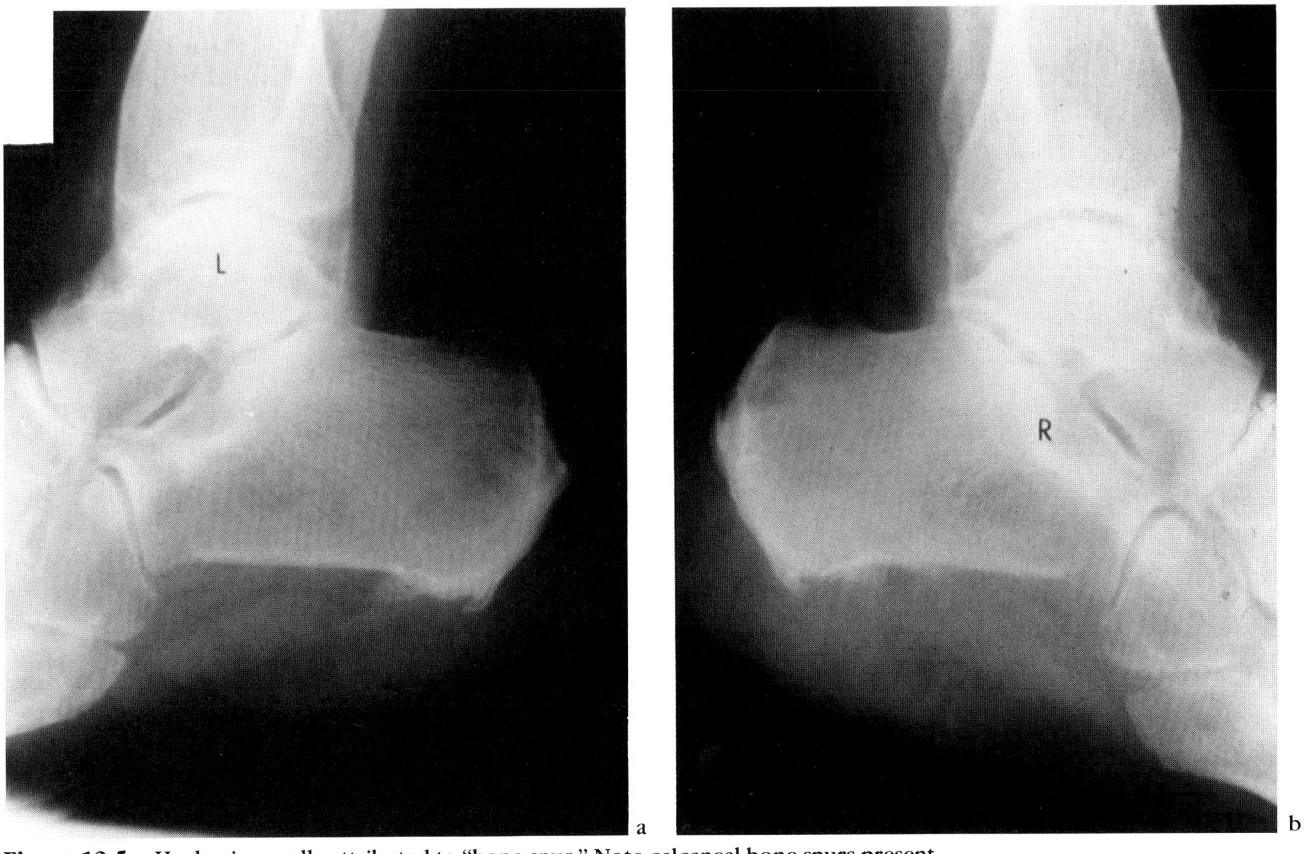

a b

Figure 12-5. Heel pain usually attributed to "bone spur." Note calcaneal bone spurs present bilaterally in 68-year-old diabetic woman. Only left foot (a) was symptomatic. There was an entrapped calcaneal nerve. Cortisone injection about the calcaneal nerve relieved the pain, permitting her to dance the anniversary waltz at her 50th anniversary.

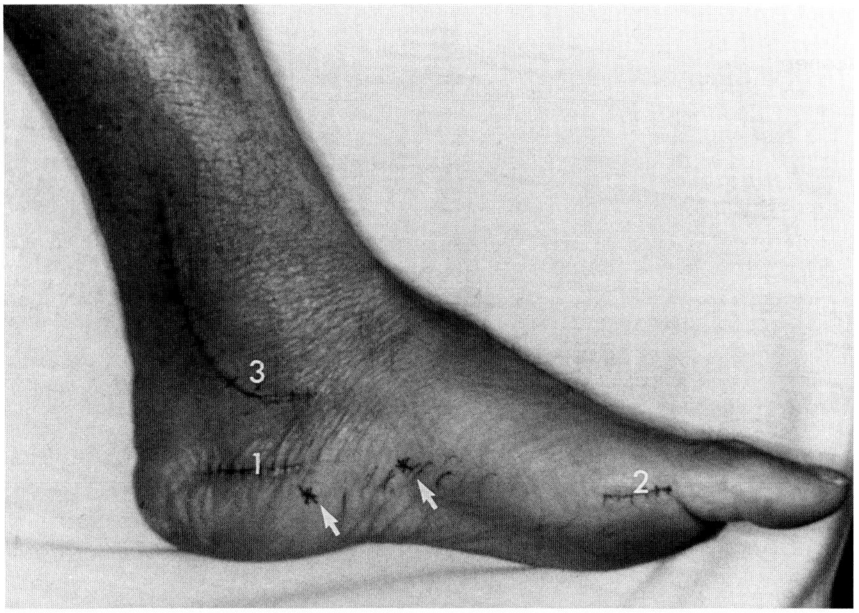

Figure 12-6. Misdiagnosis or inadequate treatment in patients with tarsal tunnel syndrome: plantar fascitis (1), Morton's neuroma (2), and inadequate previous tarsal tunnel release (3). Arrows indicate sites of remaining entrapment of medial and lateral plantar nerves.

instrument is moved from proximal to distal. Normal moving two-point discrimination in the big toe is 5 to 7 mm. Normal static two-point discrimination in the big toe has been reported to vary from 5 to 8 mm.[33] There may be weakness of the abductor hallucis. Frequently, there is wasting of the abductor hallucis and this can be directly determined by palpation of the thickness of the muscle bulk (Fig. 12-5). Due to intrinsic muscle weakness from the lateral plantar nerve compression, there may be clawing of the toes. This is frequently mistaken for hammer toes (Fig. 12-5). There will often be an associated pes planus. It is common to see patients with tarsal tunnel syndrome who previously were misdiagnosed as plantar fasciitis, dorsal sensory neuromas, Morton's neuroma, or failure of previous tarsal tunnel release that was inadequate (Fig. 12-6).

There are usually good posterior tibial and dorsalis pedis pulses present, unless there is an associated vascular problem. This should be documented because often the patient's initial complaint is one of "circulation problems" in the foot.

Surgical Technique

With the patient in the supine position and under either general or spinal anesthesia, the leg and foot is prepared with povidone-iodine. A pneumatic leg tourniquet is placed proximal to the knee over padding. The leg is elevated and exsanguinated with an elastic bandage and the tourniquet inflated to 300 mmHg pressure. The incision begins 3 cm proximal to a line drawn from the medial malleolus to the calcaneus and directly over the course of the posterior tibial nerve (Figs. 12-7 to 12-12). It extends distally between the medial malleolus and the calcaneus and then curves gently to approach the plantar aspect of the foot, terminating just before the plantar aspect of the foot. The incision is well posterior to the malleolus to avoid injury to terminal branches of the saphenous nerve. The incision is deepened into the subcutaneous tissue. Hemostasis is obtained throughout with the bipolar coagulator. The posterior tibial nerve is identified proximal to the tarsal tunnel. Vessel loops are placed about the posterior tibial artery and accompanying veins. The nerve is dissected distally until the flexor retinaculum is reached. The flexor retinaculum is divided under direct vision and completely until the fat distal to it is reached. The origin of the calcaneal nerve is noted, and the calcaneal nerve is dissected toward the heel, releasing any sites of compression in the plantar fascia. Releasing the flexor retinaculum from proximal to distal aids in identifying the not infrequent accessory calcaneal branch, which we have identified arising from the medial plantar nerve (Figs. 12-8, 12-10) and crossing superficial to the lateral plantar nerve to enter the heel. Injury to this nerve will result in a painful scar with radiation to the heel.[35] Any pathologic condition within the proximal region of the tarsal tunnel is noted. Ganglion or varicosities (Fig. 12-8), if present, are removed. Synovitis from the joint about the ankle is removed. Any scarring about the nerve grossly from previous trauma is removed. Surrounding veins and the medial and lateral plantar arteries are protected throughout this portion of the procedure. If large tortuous veins are considered contributory to the compression, they are excised (Figs. 12-6, 12-8, 12-9). Then the abductor hallucis

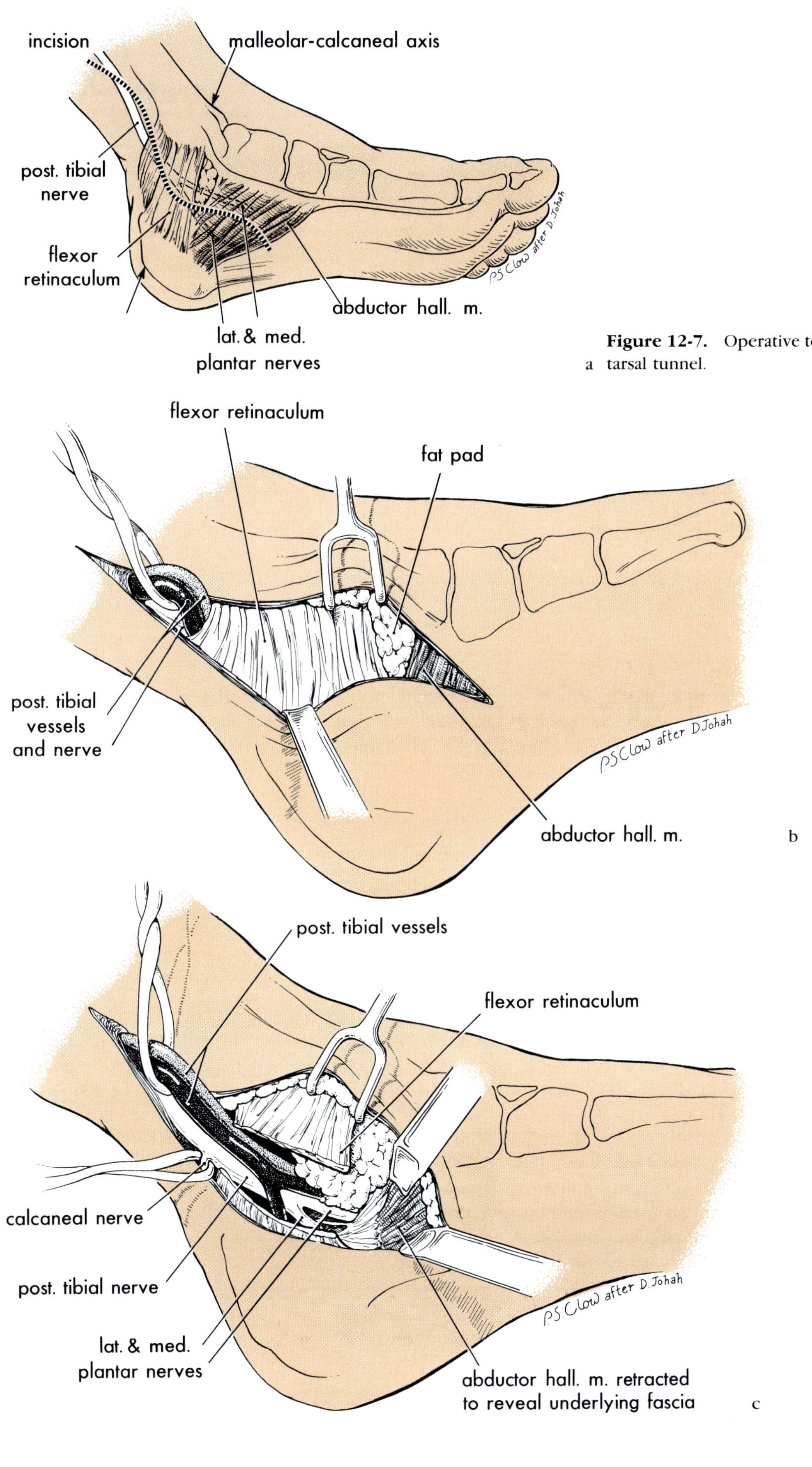

Figure 12-7. Operative technique for release of tarsal tunnel.

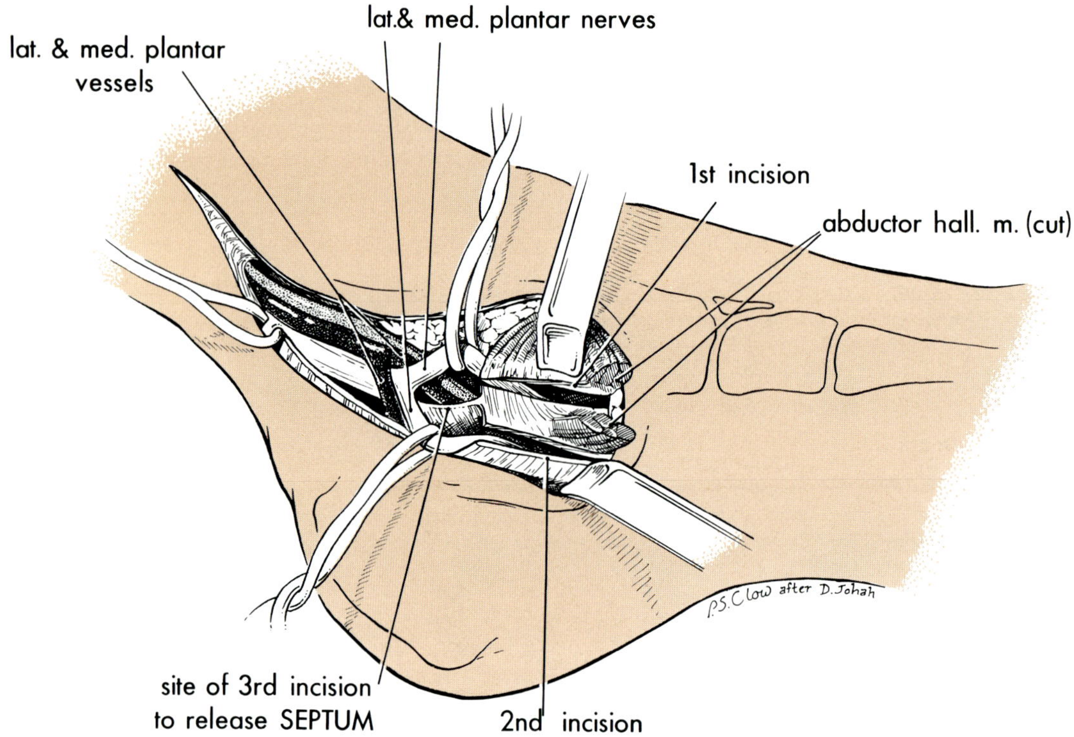

Figure 12-8. Operative technique for release of tunnels of the medial plantar and lateral plantar nerves.

muscle is retracted and the underlying fascial origin of the muscle that forms the roof of the medial plantar tunnel is identified. A clamp is placed alongside the course of the medial plantar nerve going into the medial plantar tunnel to confirm for the surgeon the confines of this tunnel. Then a scissors is placed superficial to the nerve and directly across the fascial roof and the tunnel opened by dividing this fascia, is continued distally until the distal edge of the band is reached. The examiner's finger is now admitted onto the plantar aspect of the foot. A similar maneuver is then carried out for the lateral plantar nerve. The fascial origin here from the calcaneus is divided and the division is carried distally until the examiner's finger can be inserted along the course of the lateral plantar nerve onto the plantar aspect of the foot. Now the septum between the medial and lateral plantar tunnels remains. This is divided at its origin, creating a common large tunnel for the medial and lateral plantar nerves, giving total release of these two nerves (Figs. 12-7 to 12-11). Now the epineurium of the posterior tibial and medial and lateral plantar nerves is opened and, if required, an intraneural neurolysis (Figs. 12-8B, 12-10C) is carried out as described in Chapter 5. The wound is irrigated with sterile saline and the skin is closed with several interrupted 4-0 intradermal sutures and continuous 5-0 nylon suture. The foot is dressed with nonadherent gauze fluff, soft roll, and then a "Robert Jones" cotton splint is applied, held in place with kling, and finally an elastic wrap. The tourniquet is then let down.

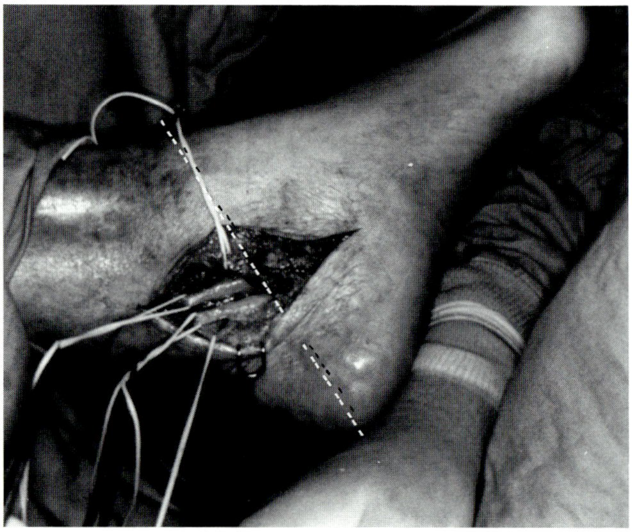

Figure 12-9. Intraoperative view, tarsal tunnel syndrome. Note high division of posterior tibial nerve into medial and lateral plantar nerve, here 3 cm proximal to the malleolar-calcaneal axis (dotted lines).

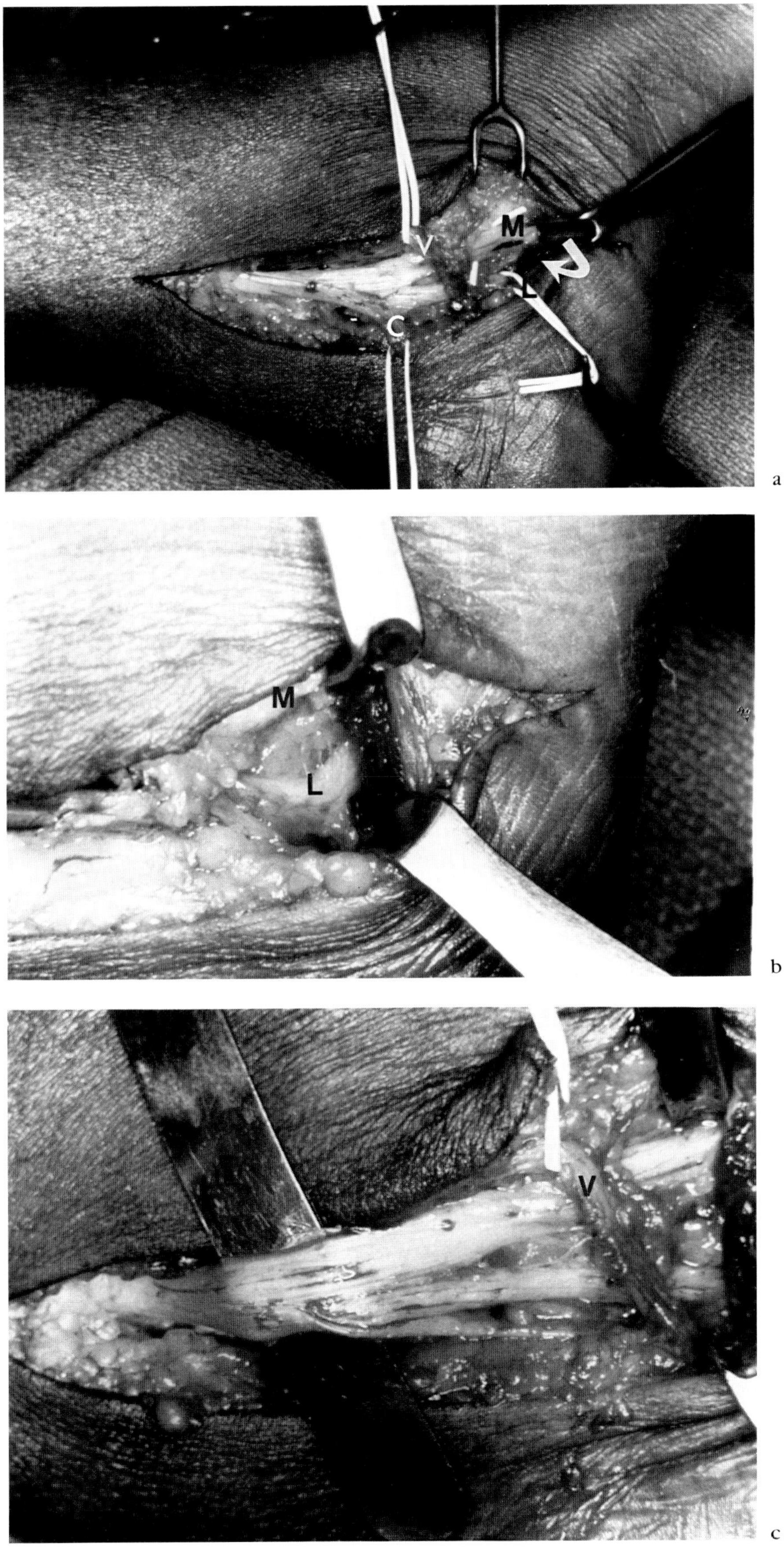

Figure 12-10. Intraoperative view of tarsal tunnel syndrome. **a.** Rubber loops isolate calcaneal branch (c), vessels (v) within tarsal tunnel, and medial (m) and lateral (l) plantar nerves as they enter distal tunnels. Note the abductor hallucis at the distal tunnel (arrow). **b.** The abductor hallucis is retracted to reveal the medial (M) and lateral (L) plantar tunnels. **c.** After internal neurolysis of all entrapped nerves. (V): vessels.

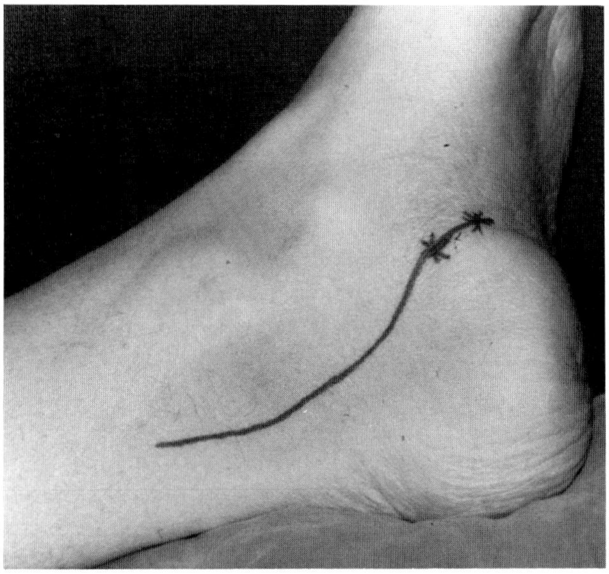

a

Figure 12-11. Intraoperative view, tarsal tunnel syndrome, emphasizing preoperative localization of Tinel sign (*) over medial and lateral plantar tunnels (**a**). Note incision is well posterior to malleolus; closer incisions are often painful due to saphenous nerve injury. Intraoperative view of nerves (**b**) entering medial (M) and lateral (L) plantar tunnels and the interfascicular septum (S).

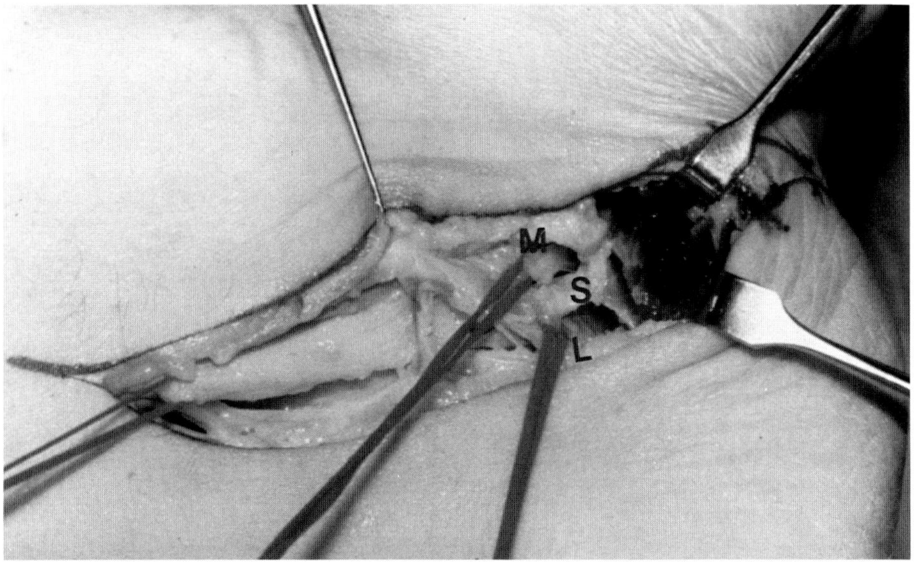

b

Postoperative Care

The patient is kept at bedrest 3 to 4 days and then allowed crutch or cane walking with minimal weight-bearing on the foot. For diabetics, the entire postoperative recovery is lengthened to 3 weeks, with their being asked to remain largely at bedrest for 2 weeks after surgery and the sutures being left for 3 weeks. Beginning at the second postoperative week, the incision is massaged for 5 minutes twice a day and ankle movement regained.

Complications

The most common complication of the operation in our hands, in our first 50 tarsal tunnel surgeries,[35] has been failure of the wounds to heal. The patients with this problem have largely been diabetic, with one patient requiring a skin graft to achieve wound closure after failure to get healing after 3 months of outpatient management. One patient had a soft tissue loss over the Achilles' tendon and the posterior aspect of the heel due to tightness of a posterior plaster splint. This wound subsequently required skin grafting, and since then a "Robert Jones" cotton wrap immobilization of the ankle instead of plaster is used for the dressing. No patient

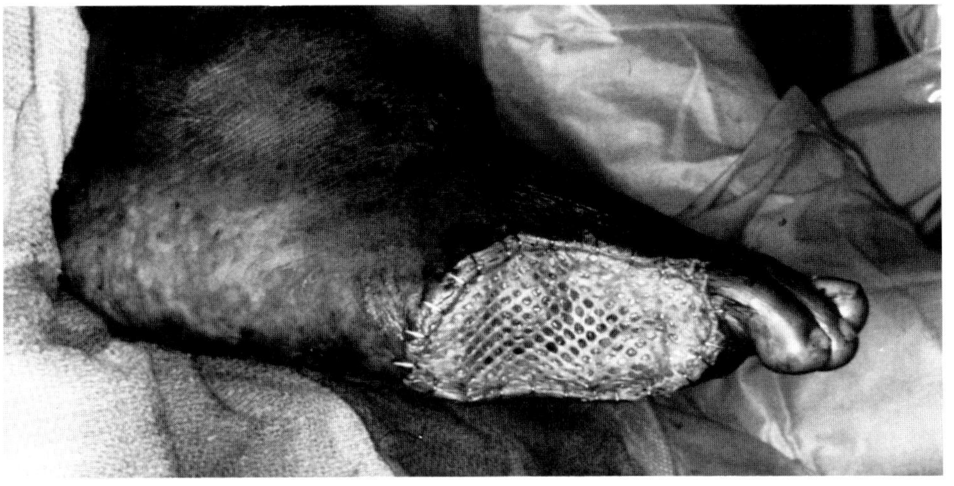

a

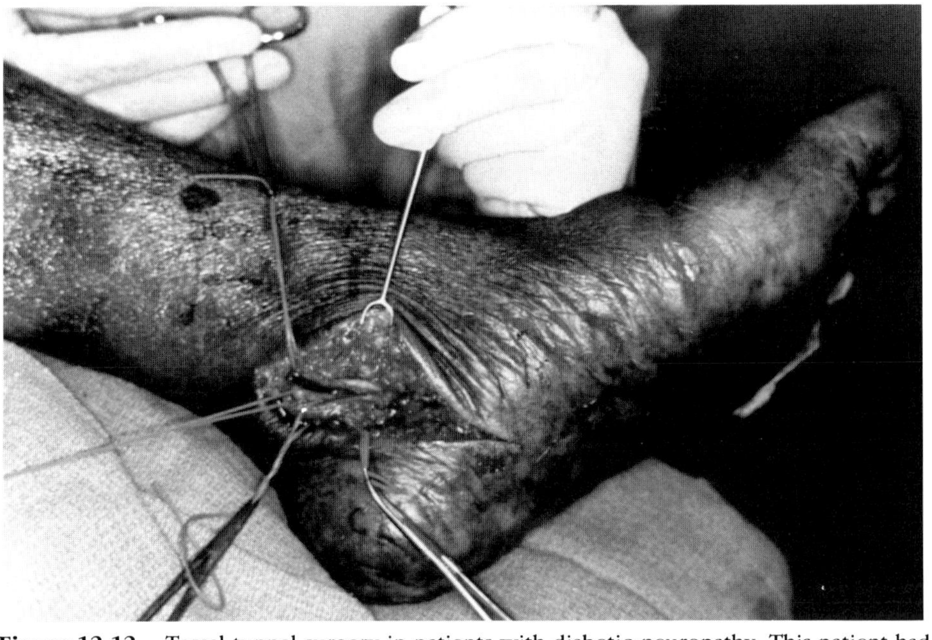

b

Figure 12-12. Tarsal tunnel surgery in patients with diabetic neuropathy. This patient had vascular supply reestablished by popliteal endarterectomy, then was referred for soft tissue coverage of his anesthestic foot. Simultaneously with the skin grafting procedure (**a**), the tarsal tunnel was decompressed to restore sensation to his remaining three toes **b**. At 1 year after neurolysis, two-point discrimination having been recovered in his big toe.

has developed causalgia. Patients who have had symptoms for more than a year before surgery have had prolonged time for recovery of sensibility and several have had dysesthesia postoperatively. The dysesthesia is characterized by increasing symptoms of heat or burning sensations in the plantar aspect of the foot. These are attributed to reinnervation of the foot and the problem responds to increased analgesics, massage of the scar, desensitization of the foot, and emotional support and encouragement of the patient during the months for which this problem may last. One patient has an area of decreased sensation to the medial aspect of the heel due to injury to a calcaneal branch. Two of the diabetic patients have postoperative weakness of ankle inversion, which may be due to associated worsening of a diabetic amyopathy.

Results

A recent report of tarsal tunnel release in 51 feet of 34 patients found excellent results in 26%; good results in

Table 12-1. Homologies Between Carpal and Tarsal Tunnels

Carpal Tunnel	*Tarsal Tunnel*
Antebrachial fascia	Flexor retinaculum (lacinate ligament)
Carpal tunnel	"Tunnel" for medial plantar nerve
Transverse carpal ligament	Fascial origin of abductor hallucis muscle
Guyon's canal	"Canal" for lateral plantar nerve

53%; fair results in 12%; and no improvement in 8%. Excellent results are defined as "complete relief (but) with symptoms returning after strenuous activity"; and good defined as "marked improvement with some symptoms returning with moderate activity." A microsurgical internal neurolysis was not done in these patients.[34]

Although most case reports and the few small series in the literature suggest that the vast majority of patients recover after tarsal tunnel syndrome, none of these investigators has staged the patient preoperatively in terms of presence or absence of abnormal two-point discrimination or muscle wasting. In general, the symptoms of the patient have been relieved. Muscle wasting has rarely been improved. None of the previous surgical reports has utilized internal neurolysis in the posterior tibial nerve.

Our series of patients comprised 50 feet with tarsal tunnel syndrome.[35] In this series of patients, there have been three who have failed to recover. Two were among the first few patients operated on and each had had symptoms for more than 10 years. They had no two-point discrimination present. They had muscle wasting and the nerves were markedly compressed at the time of surgery. One diabetic, who had been using insulin for 41 years, failed to improve. With the exception of these three patients, all patients, including those with diabetes, have improved after the extensive surgical procedure previously described, including internal neurolysis for those patients with abnormal two-point discrimination, persistent sensory discomfort in the feet, or muscle wasting. These patients have recovered two-point discrimination to normal values, the intrinsic muscle wasting has reversed. The length of time for this to occur has varied from 6 months to 2 years, with those patients being past 50 years of age, those with symptoms present for more than a year, and those with diabetes taking longer to recover.

It is especially noteworthy that those patients with even type I diabetes whose numbness in the feet was attributed to diabetic neuropathy alone and for whom no treatment was thought possible by their other physicians did respond with excellent recovery to the surgical procedure. Those juvenile diabetics whose symptoms had been present for less than 2 years responded within a few weeks. One patient with symptoms present for 40 years responded, although much more slowly. It is possible that there exists a cause for optimism for the symptoms of diabetic neuropathy[36] in that perhaps a significant portion of the symptomatology may be due to peripheral nerve compression (Figs. 12-12, 12-13).

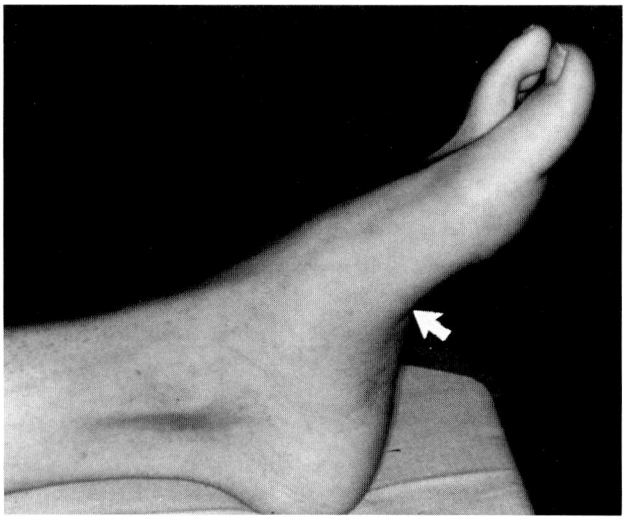

Figure 12-13. Physical findings in patient with advanced tarsal tunnel syndrome related to juvenile diabetes. Atrophy of abductor hallucis brevis muscle (arrow) and clawing of toes often mistaken for "hammer toes." Patients may describe "higher" instep with development of abductor atrophy.

References

1. Keck C: The tarsal-tunnel syndrome. J Bone Joint Surg 44A:180–182, 1962.
2. Lam SJS: A tarsal-tunnel syndrome. Lancet 2:1354–1355, 1962.
3. Moloney S: Tarsal tunnel syndrome pain abated by operation to relieve pressure. Calif Med 101:378–379, 1964.
4. Muenthaler V. Probst C, Muenthaler A, Weber EG, Schnyder J: Das tarsal tunnel Syndrome. Schweiz Med Wochenschr 94:373–382, 1964.
5. Goodgold J, Koeppel HP, Sprelholz NI: The tarsal tunnel syndrome: Objective diagnostic criteria. N Engl J Med 173:742–745, 1965.
6. Barba GE: Burning foot syndrome: Bilateral occurrence with radical cure. Med J Aust 1:764–765, 1965.
7. Johnson EW, Ortez PR: Electrodiagnosis of tarsal tunnel syndrome. Arch Phys Med Rehabil 47:776–780, 1966.
8. Lam SJS: Tarsal-tunnel syndrome. J Bone Joint Surg 49B: 878–892, 1967.
9. Ijkelenstam PA: Compression of the posterior tibial nerve (the tarsal tunnel syndrome). Arch Chir Neeland 20:1–6, 1968.

10. Edwards WG, Lincoln R, Bassett FH, Goldner JL: Tarsal tunnel syndrome. JAMA 207:716–720, 1969.
11. Lloyd K, Agarwal A: Tarsel tunnel syndrome, a presenting feature of rheumatic arthritis. Br Med J 3:32, 1970.
12. Linsheid RL, Burton RC, Fredericks EJ: Tarsal tunnel syndrome. South Med J 63:313–316, 1970.
13. Mann RA: Tarsal tunnel syndrome. Orthop Clin North Am 5:109–115, 1971.
14. Guiloff RJ, Sagratt RM: Sensory conduction in medial plantar nerve. J Neurol Neurosurg Psychiatry 40:1168–1181, 1977.
15. Phor WH, Raszid D: A ganglion causing tarsal tunnel syndrome: Report of a case. Aust NZ J Surg 48:96–97, 1978.
16. Wilemon WK: Tarsal tunnel syndrome: A fifty year survey of world literature and report of two new cases. Orthop Rev 8:111–117, 1979.
17. Oh SJ, Sarala PK, Kuba T, Elmore RS: Tarsal tunnel syndrome: Electrophysiological study. Ann Neurol 5:327–30, 1979.
18. Fu R, DeLiso JA, Kraft GH: Motor nerve latencies through the tarsal tunnel in normal adult subjects. Arch Phys Med Rehabil 61:243–248, 1980.
19. Kaplan PE, Kernahan WT: Tarsal tunnel syndrome: An electrodiagnostic and surgical correlation. J Bone Joint Surg 63A:96–99, 1981.
20. Byrd JW, Ricciardi JM, Jun BI: Regional migratory osteoporosis in tarsal tunnel syndrome. Clin Orthop 157:164–169, 1981.
21. Grablis M, Puentes J, Lidski M: Tarsal tunnel syndrome in rheumatoid arthritis. Arch Phys Med Rehabil 62:401–403, 1981.
22. Saeed MA, Gatens PF: Compound nerve action potential of medial and lateral plantar nerves through the tarsal tunnel. Arch Phys Med Rehabil 63:304–307, 1982.
23. Radinel EL: Tarsal tunnel syndrome. Clin Orthop 181:167–170, 1983.
24. Ruderman MI, Palmer RH, Olarte MR, et al: Tarsal tunnel syndrome caused by hyperlipidemia: Reversal after plasmaphoresis. Arch Neurol 40:124–125, 1983.
25. Mackinnon SE, Dellon AL, Daneshvar A: Tarsal tunnel syndrome: Histopathological examination of a human posterior tibial nerve. Contemp Orthop 9:43–47, 1984.
26. Horwitz MT: Normal anatomy and variations of the peripheral nerve of the leg and foot. Arch Surg 36:626–636, 1938.
27. Dellon AL, Mackinnon SE: Tibial nerve branching in the tarsal tunnel. Arch Neurol 41:645–646, 1984.
28. Mackinnon SE, Dellon AL: Homologies between the tarsal and carpal tunnels: Implications for surgical treatment in the tarsal tunnel syndrome. Contemp Orthop 14:75–78, 1987.
29. Kopell HP, Thompson WAL: Peripheral entrapment neuropathy of the lower extremity. N Engl J Med 262:56–60, 1960.
30. Spalteholtz W: Hand Atlas of Human Anatomy. Barker LF, Translator of Fourth German edition. JB Lippincott, Philadelphia, 1906, pp 360, 361, 757.
31. Fullerton PM, Gilliatt RW: Pressure neuropathy in the hind foot of the guinea pig. J Neurol Neurosurg Psychiatry 30:18–25, 1967.
32. Walpin LA: Anomalous tibial nerve innervation of the dorsum of the foot: A factor complicating the diagnosis of tarsal tunnel syndrome. (Abstr.) American Congress of Rehabilitation Medicine, 1984, p 230.
33. Dellon AL: Sensory recovery in replanted digits and transplanted toes. J Reconstr Microsurg 2:123–129, 1986.
34. Sydney SV, Byank RP: Tarsal tunnel syndrome. Presented at Foot and Ankle Society Meeting, February 1988, Atlanta, Georgia.
35. Dellon AL: Tarsal tunnel syndrome: Results of surgical treatment including internal neurolysis. J Bone Joint Surg, submitted, 1988.
36. Dellon AL. A cause for optimism in diabetic neuropathy: Ann Plastic Surg 20:103–105, 1988.

13

Other Lower Extremity Nerve Entrapments

Nerve entrapments in the lower extremity are not rare. They are being recognized with increasing frequency. In our overall series of operative nerve decompressions in the past 10 years, lower extremity entrapment neuropathies represent 10% of our patients. As confidence in examining the nerves in the lower extremity increases, and as the surgeon's experience for peripheral nerve surgery grows, there will be increasing opportunity for evaluation of lower extremity problems. We are finding now an increasing percentage of our practice being devoted to treatment of nerve injuries in the lower extremity. As this occurs, we recall Joplin's opening remarks from his presidential address in 1971 to the First Annual Meeting of the American Orthopedic Foot Society:[1]

> A rare opportunity awaits the young surgeon who is interested in foot problems, because in this special field which remains almost unexplored, he has a choice to exert his ingenuity, as in no other branch of surgery that I know of today. There are patients everywhere waiting to be treated ... and twice as many feet as there are people.

The most common lower entrapment neuropathy is that of the posterior tibial and medial and lateral plantar nerves in the tarsal tunnel, as described in Chapter 12. The next most common entrapments with which we have dealt are those of the peroneal nerves. The description of these syndromes, the anatomic relationships of the nerves, and the surgical technique will be described for both common peroneal nerve entrapment at the knee and deep peroneal nerve entrapment over the dorsal aspect of the foot and ankle. Less common entrapment neuropathies of the lower extremity also will be described briefly in this chapter. The techniques for examining any peripheral nerve, as described in Chapter 3, and the techniques for internal neurolysis of peripheral nerves, as described in Chapter 5, are equally applicable to lower extremity nerves.

Perhaps the most common cause of not diagnosing lower extremity entrapment neuropathies is the lack of familiarity of most physicians with the nerves in the lower extremity. Perhaps, the second most common reason is that many of the patients' complaints related to lower extremity nerve entrapments appear to have a vascular cause, leading to referrals to vascular surgeons or to home remedies or medication to improve circulation in the feet. The literature on lower extremity nerve entrapments is commensurate with the general lack of familiarity of most physicians with these problems. Although an extensive literature exists on the nerves and nerve entrapments in the upper extremities, only recently has a textbook appeared devoted to the anatomy of the foot and ankle, containing extensive descriptions of the nerves from the mid calf down.[2] The lower extremity nerve injuries, as distinct from nerve compressions, have been described well in general works on nerve injuries[3–5] and a small portion of these works is allocated to lower extremity entrapment neuropathies. The most recent book related to entrapment neuropathies contains a better description of the clinical features of the lower extremity nerve compression sites but deals superficially with the anatomy and makes no reference to techniques for surgical decompression.[6] Much of the writing on lower extremity nerve injuries[3–5] is, in fact, not related to nerve compression but describes sharp injuries to nerves and the results of nerve repair in the lower extremities. (Our experience with nerve repair and grafting in the lower extremity is described in Chapter 4.) The subject of Morton's neuroma, which has its cause in nerve compression rather than the result of end-bulb neuroma formation after nerve transection, will be discussed in this chapter.

Common Peroneal Nerve Entrapment

Historical Review

The common peroneal nerve is particularly prone to injury by virtue of the combination of its superficial location and its peculiar anatomic tethering. Lying in a subcutaneous location over the fibular head, it is easy to palpate and therefore equally susceptible to compression by various forces, from complications of surgery, such as adhesive strapping,[7] to pressure with the stirrups during obstetric and gynecologic procedures,[8] to more mundane problems, such as sitting with the legs crossed or in various occupations where the knees may be acutely flexed and the buttocks rested on the heels.[9,10] The critical motor function carried through the deep branch of the common peroneal nerve is readily noted by the patient in terms of his foot dragging or inability to extend the toes, since these bring the problem with this nerve to his attention dramatically. Less commonly does the patient become aware of unusual sensations over the side of his calf and the top of his leg or muscle problems referable to isolate superficial peroneal motor palsy (loss of foot eversion). For example, common peroneal palsy has been described as a sudden painless foot drop in strawberry pickers who must squat while working,[11] and it has been described in persons after yoga.[12] Relationship of the common peroneal nerve to the tibiofibular joint has led to early awareness of injury to this nerve not only with fractures of the neck of the fibula,[13] but also with dislocations of this joint.[14] Indeed, a complete division of the common peroneal nerve has been recorded with medial dislocations of the knee.[15] Due to the tethering of the common peroneal nerve beneath the peroneus longus muscle over the fibular neck, forceful ankle inversion causes a sudden stretch with traction injury to the common peroneal nerve.[16] An extensive literature has been published concerning ganglion arising from the tibiofibular joint as a source of compression of the common peroneal nerve.[17] These may appear to be intramuscular or intraneural and may require intraneural dissection if they have been present for a significant amount of time and have forced a separation of the common peroneal into its multiple fascicles. As new operations are developed in the lower extremity, such as total knee arthroplasty, so too will new complications of these procedures occur. Rose et al[18] have reported an incidence of 0.88% for peroneal palsy after total knee arthroplasty (23 cases in 2626 operations between 1974 and 1980). The largest group of patients with common peroneal nerve palsy whom we are seeing today for treatment, however, are those in whom compression is due to anatomic structures about the fibular head. Compression by the tendon of the biceps femoris, at the hip, has been described.[19] The most common anatomic area of compression, suggested by Kopell and Thompson[20] on anatomic grounds in 1963 and confirmed with electrodiagnostic techniques more recently,[21] is the area that has been termed the fibular tunnel.

Surgical Anatomy

The common peroneal nerve departs from the sciatic nerve in the popliteal fossa to cross the lateral head of the gastrocnemius and soleus muscles at the fibular head. From here, the common peroneal nerve crosses the fibular neck to enter a tunnel that is formed by the two heads of the peroneus longus muscle. The superficial head of the peroneus muscle arises from the tibial plateau and as it crosses the fibular head has a fibrous border beneath which the common peroneal nerve passes. This narrow region, which has at its deep surface the fibular neck and the fibrous origin of the deep head of the peroneus longus, represents an area where the nerve must pass before entering the lower leg. The anatomic and physiologic studies of Sunderland and Bradley[22,23] are pertinent with regard to the predisposition of the common peroneal nerve to injury in this region. In ten cadavers, the number of fascicles at various levels along the common peroneal were counted and compared with those in the posterior tibial nerve. Similar assessment was done at the region of the fibular neck. The mean number of fascicles in the popliteal region for the common peroneal nerve was 7.8, whereas at the fibular neck this mean number of fascicles increased to 16.1. Thus, at least a twofold increase in the number of fascicles on the average occurs as the common peroneal nerve goes through an area of narrowing. The posterior tibial nerve in contrast has a mean number of 27.9 fascicles in the popliteal fossa and at the level of the fibular neck has a mean of 26.8, essentially undergoing no increase in number of fascicles across the same anatomic region. Analysis of the cross-sectional area of these nerves demonstrates that the peroneal nerve has 51% connective tissue in the popliteal fossa. This increases to 68% in the region of the neck of the fibula. There is no change in this percentage (65%) in the posterior tibial nerve in these two different regions. These observations have been confirmed by Shizhen et al[24] in independent investigations done in China. Thus, the common peroneal nerve as it enters an area of anatomic narrowing or entrapment not only on an average doubles its number of fascicles, but increases its percentage of connective tissue. The maximum load that the common peroneal nerve may sustain before reaching its elastic limit and rupturing is less than that of the tibial nerve in this same region. This finding again suggests that the common peroneal nerve subjected to the same force is more susceptible to injury than the posterior tibial in the same location.[22,23]

The common peroneal nerve divides underneath the peroneus longus and its fibers then are at risk for compression beneath another fibrous arch, the origin of the extensor digitorum longus. In this short interval of 1 cm, the deep peroneal nerve and its branches become separated from the superficial peroneal nerve and its branches. The superficial peroneal nerve under cover of the peroneus longus innervates this muscle and continues descending distally to innervate the peroneus brevis, becoming superficial in the distal third of the lower leg. The deep peroneal nerve immediately after passing beneath the fibrous lateral edge of the peroneus longus gives off geniculate branches and branches to the tibialis anterior, which act to tether the deep peroneal branch more so than the superficial peroneal nerve in this same region. The deep peroneal nerve then continues innervating the extensor hallucis longus and then, through a separate long branch, the extensor digitorum longus, and then continuing distally, innervates the peroneus tertius muscle. The peroneus tertius muscle represents, in essence, a distal portion or head of the extensor digitorum longus. The deep peroneal nerve then enters a more superficial region over the dorsal portion of the ankle. Further descriptions of the superficial peroneal and the deep peroneal nerves will continue in subsequent sections.

The clinical importance of an understanding of the functional topography is no longer debated in upper extremity peripheral nerve surgery. Of equal importance to the surgeon during the common peroneal decompression is a knowledge of the internal topography of the nerve in this region. Two extensive works are

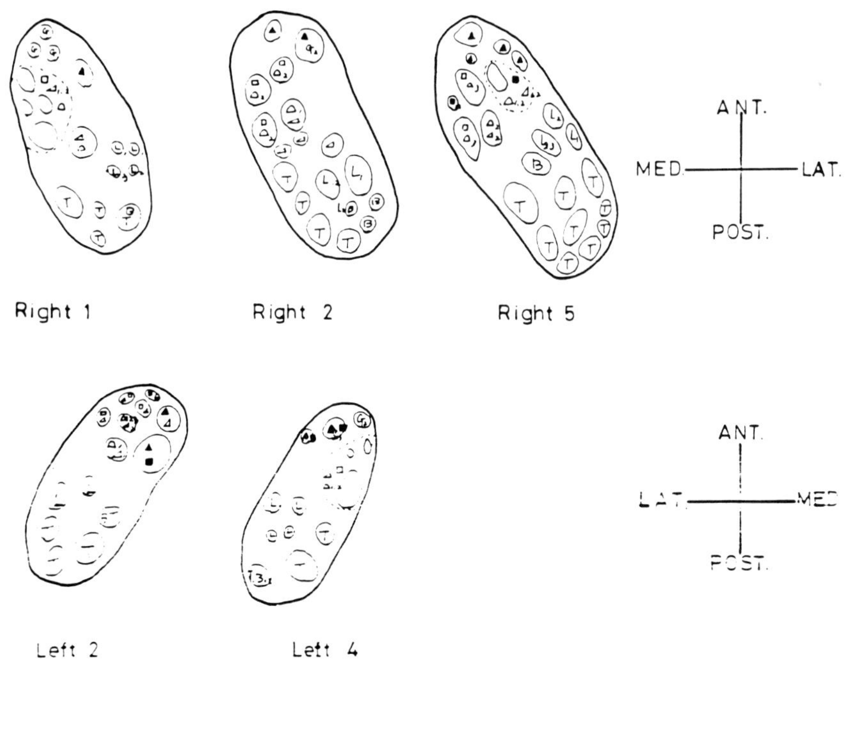

Figure 13-1. Intraneural topography of the common peroneal nerve at the fibula neck in five specimens. Note that in each case the deep peroneal division is anterior (open and filled figures) whereas the superficial division is posterior (letters). In the anterior group of fascicles (deep peroneal nerve), the most anterior fascicles go to the knee joint (G: geniculate), and the anterior tibialis (▲). It was difficult at this level to distinguish the purely sensory (■) terminal branches of the deep peroneal from those innervating the toe extensors (△, □). In the posterior group of fascicles (superficial peroneal nerve), the most posterior fascicles were the terminal (T) sensory branches, and the motor branches to the peroneus longus (L) were the more anterior of this grouping, and those to the peroneus brevis (B) were intermediate in location. (Reproduction with permission from Urushidani.[26])

available.[25,26] Unfortunately, these references are in disagreement precisely in the region of the neck of the fibula. The description by Urushidani[26] closely resembles our surgical experience and is depicted in Figure 13-1. The symbols in Figure 13-1, which Urushidani uses, are identical to those used by Sunderland and Ray in the earlier study in 1948. Review of Sunderland and Ray's drawing suggests the discrepancy between these investigators is in two factors: The diagram for posterior, anterior, lateral, and medial is 90° out of phase with the drawing in Sunderland and Ray's text, and the fascicles that go to the terminal sensory portions of the superficial peroneal nerve are represented in a more superficial or more anterior location with respect to the deep peroneal nerve than they are in the drawings of the Japanese adults. Both studies, as well as the longitudinal dissections reported in Chinese adults,[24] agree that, several centimeters proximal to the fibular neck, the common peroneal nerve may be dissected to demonstrate the group of fascicles that are most anterior and that will become the deep peroneal nerve and a group of fascicles that is most posterior that will become the superficial peroneal nerve and that, as these fascicles approach the peroneus longus, *the most superficial group of fascicles will remain anterior and have immediate recurrent branches divide to innervate the joints and the anterior tibialis muscle.* The larger of the fascicles in this anterior group continues to become the terminal sensory branches of the deep peroneal nerve with the next most immediate group of small fascicles innervating the extensor hallucis longus. The next fascicle to come from this most anterior group will innervate the extensor digitorum longus, and the adjacent large fascicle will continue more distally as the terminal sensory fibers. In the more posterior group of fascicles, those destined to become the superficial peroneal nerve, the largest group of fascicles, which appears to be the most posterior in the group, will continue as the terminal sensory fibers. The multiple smaller fascicles which are more anterior or superficial in this group, will innervate the overlying peroneus longus and then the peroneus brevis muscles (Figs. 13-1, 13-3, and 13-4). Importantly, it is the superior fascicles that recur immediately around the fibular head that innervate the anterior tibialis muscle.

Diagnosis

The diagnosis of common peroneal palsy centers on a knowledge of the sensory and motor functions of this nerve and differentiating entrapment of the nerve at the knee level from problems more proximal or distal that may present in a similar manner. Berry and Richardson[10] give a good review of the clinical and electrodiagnostic testing techniques and review 75 cases of common peroneal palsy. The deep peroneal nerve function is tested by manually assessing anterior tibialis function by resisted ankle dorsiflexion. Long toe extension is easily tested. It is helpful to compare the strength of these muscles with those of the opposite leg, because frequently the patient presents with weakness, not complete palsy. The toe extensors to the second, third, fourth, and fifth toes may also be reliably tested. The extensor digitorum brevis palpable over the lateral aspect of the foot is not a reliable muscle to test in diagnosing common peroneal palsy, because weakness of this muscle may be caused by a more distal site of entrapment, as will be discussed later. If the extensor digitorum brevis is weak or wasted, in addition to the muscles mentioned, the common peroneal nerve as the entrapment site may be considered. There will be loss of sensation in the area over the entire aspect of the dorsum of the foot, with the possible exception of the fifth toe, which can be innervated through the sural nerve. There will be weakness of the ankle everters from involvement of the superficial peroneal nerve at the fibular neck. There will be loss of sensation over the lateral aspect of the calf if the lateral cutaneous nerve of the calf or the communicating branch of the sural nerve is entrapped in an area close to the common peroneal nerve, as will be discussed in the section "Operative Technique." After blunt trauma to the knee, if common peroneal function has not returned, surgical exploration is indicated.[10] The patient may be tested by measuring two-point discrimination in the first web space between the first and second toes dorsally. Electrodiagnostic studies are important to rule out problems at the L4 or L5 root level, or to rule out a generalized neuropathy or motor neuron disease, or to follow patients after blunt trauma. With lesions at the spinal level from a herniated lumbar disc or spinal stenosis, there are frequently complaints of back pain and pain radiating down the whole of the leg. With diffuse neuropathy and motor neuron disease, the patient will commonly have bilateral symptoms. If the sciatic nerve is involved, there will additionally be problems in the posterior tibial nerve distribution. If any uncertainty exists as to whether the symptoms are due to a localized problem at the fibular neck versus more proximal lesions, additional neurologic consultation is encouraged.

Surgical Technique

The operation is done under general or spinal anesthesia with the patient in a supine position and with a pneumatic tourniquet over the thigh with appropriate padding. The foot is prepared, elevated, and exsanguinated with an elastic bandage and with the foot on the table so the knee is flexed and elevated off the table. This position is maintained either by an assistant holding the foot on the table and the knee in an appropriate position or with the additional help of a sterile sandbag placed at the foot to brace it in this position. An S-shaped incision is made beginning distally and longitudinal along the fibular neck with the S-shaped portion coming posteriorly and then curving proximally over the biceps tendon insertion, so that the transverse limb lies at the distal popliteal fossa crease. The incision is deepened into the subcutaneous tissue. The leg may be flexed and extended as needed. The fascial expansion from the biceps tendon and the iliotibial tract into the deep fascia of the calf is incised and a search is made for branches of the lateral cutaneous nerve of the calf or the sural communicating branch from the common peroneal nerve (Fig. 13-2). These are frequently encountered but coming at right angles or obliquely through the fascia in areas where they, too, may be entrapped with leg movements and tightening of the fascial bands. This can be demonstrated by extending the knee. Nerves found in this area are released by dividing these fascial sites of potential entrapment. The common peroneal nerve is identified in the popliteal fossa and encircled with a vessel loop. It is then dissected distally to encounter a thick fascial covering that is contiguous with the fibrous lateral edge of the peroneus longus. This fibrous edge is incised for 1 cm, revealing the fleshy muscle of the peroneus longus. A right angle retractor is placed here and the peroneus longus muscle elevated. Immediately, a fibrous edge to the flexor digitorum longus is seen and this also is divided (Figs. 13-3, 13-4). The examiner's finger can be placed along the course of the common peroneal nerve, having divided into the superficial peroneal and deep peroneal branches, so that the examiner's finger can pass beneath the peroneus longus and down into the proximal third of the calf. Then microsurgical instruments and technique are used, fat is removed, and the fascicles gently spread until the division into the deep peroneal and superficial peroneal nerve

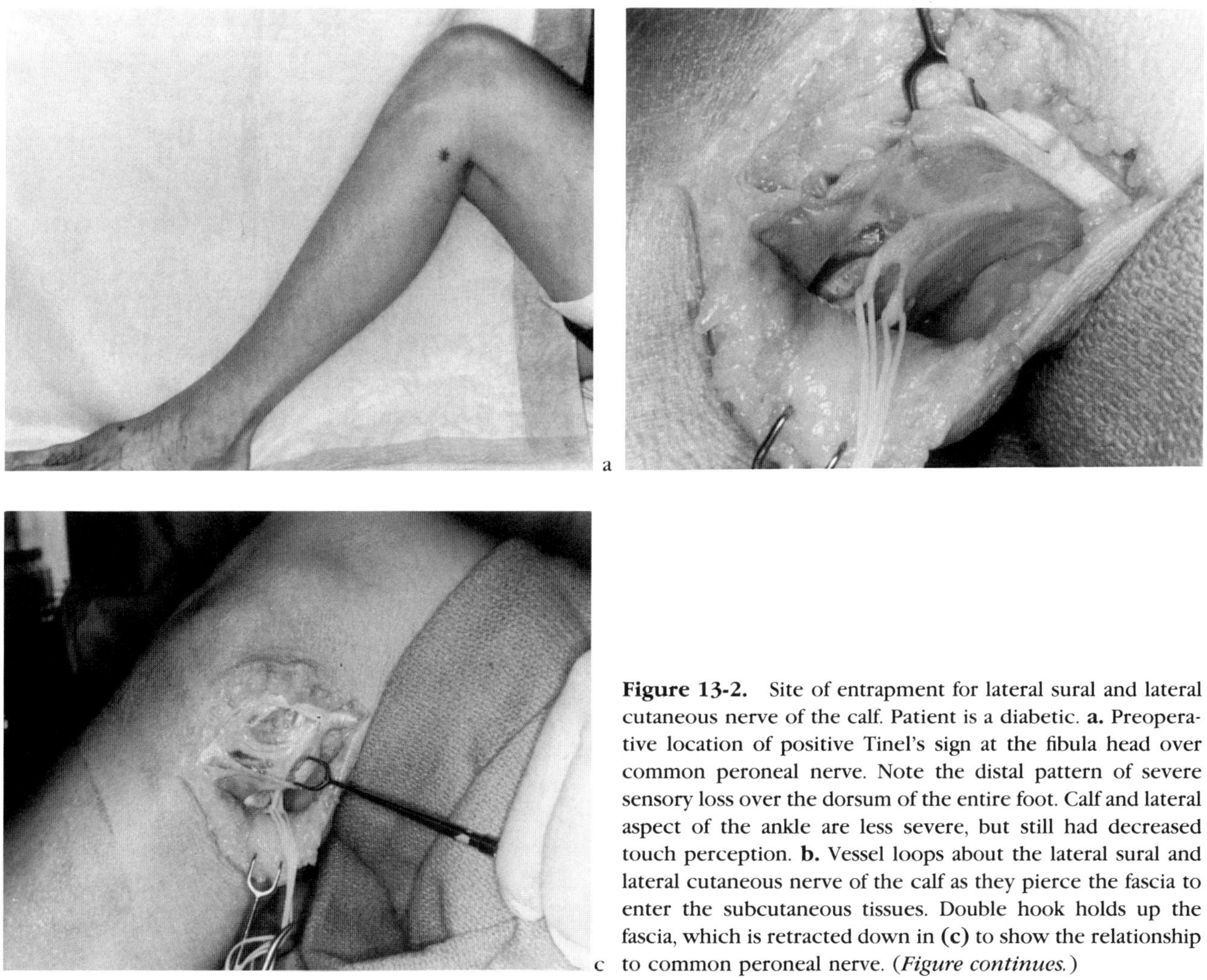

a b c

Figure 13-2. Site of entrapment for lateral sural and lateral cutaneous nerve of the calf. Patient is a diabetic. **a.** Preoperative location of positive Tinel's sign at the fibula head over common peroneal nerve. Note the distal pattern of severe sensory loss over the dorsum of the entire foot. Calf and lateral aspect of the ankle are less severe, but still had decreased touch perception. **b.** Vessel loops about the lateral sural and lateral cutaneous nerve of the calf as they pierce the fascia to enter the subcutaneous tissues. Double hook holds up the fascia, which is retracted down in **(c)** to show the relationship to common peroneal nerve. (*Figure continues.*)

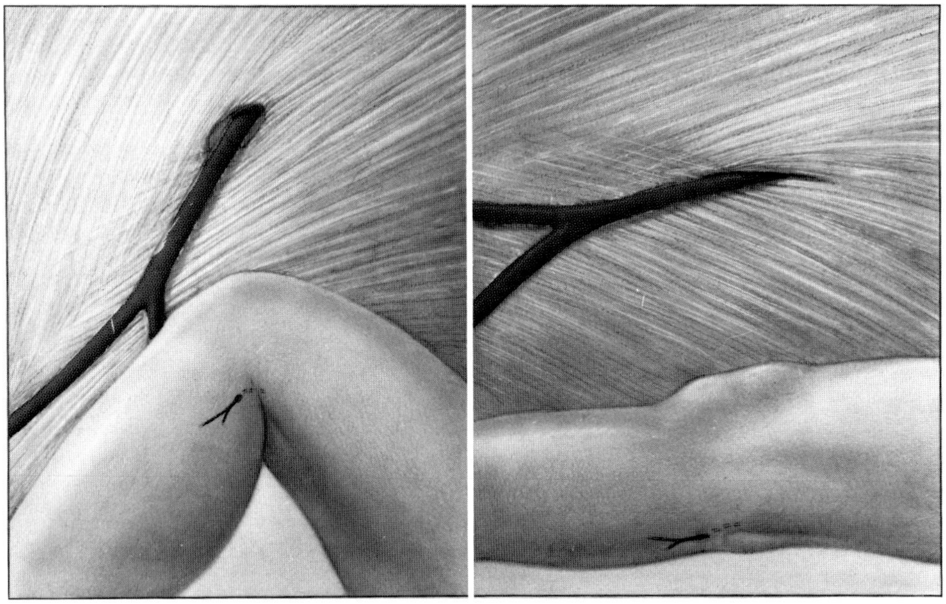

d

Figure 13-2. (*continued*) **d.** Artist's illustration of fascia tightening about these branches, which innervate the lateral side of the lower leg and ankle, demonstating the round opening with knee flexed constricting these nerves with leg extension as the fascia tightens into oval slits.

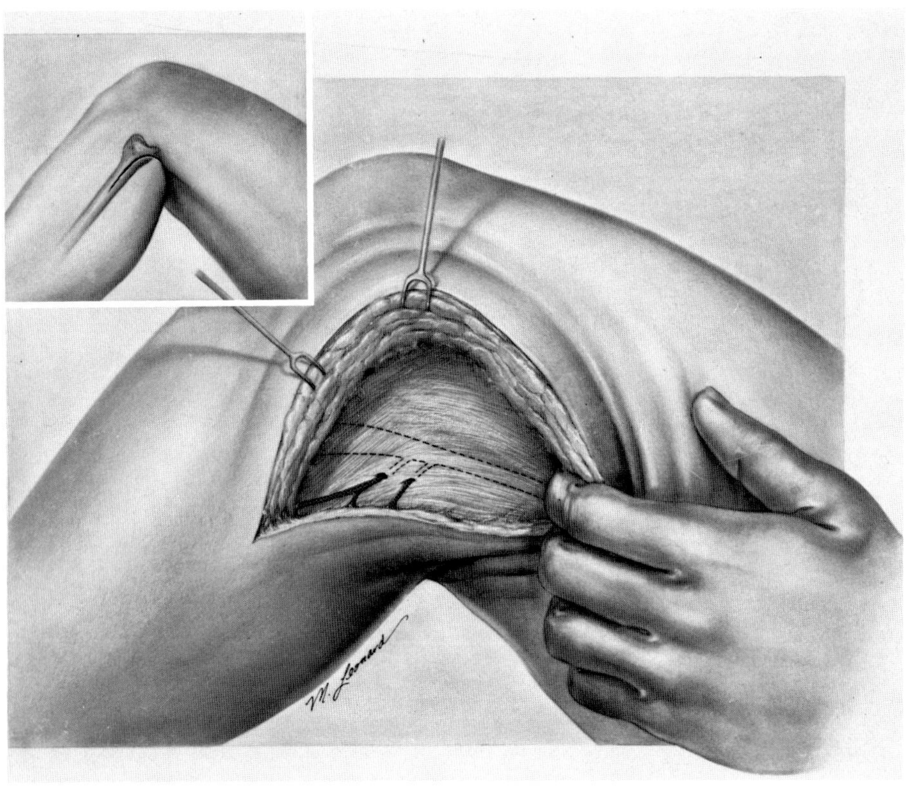

a

Figure 13-3a. (*Figure continues.*)

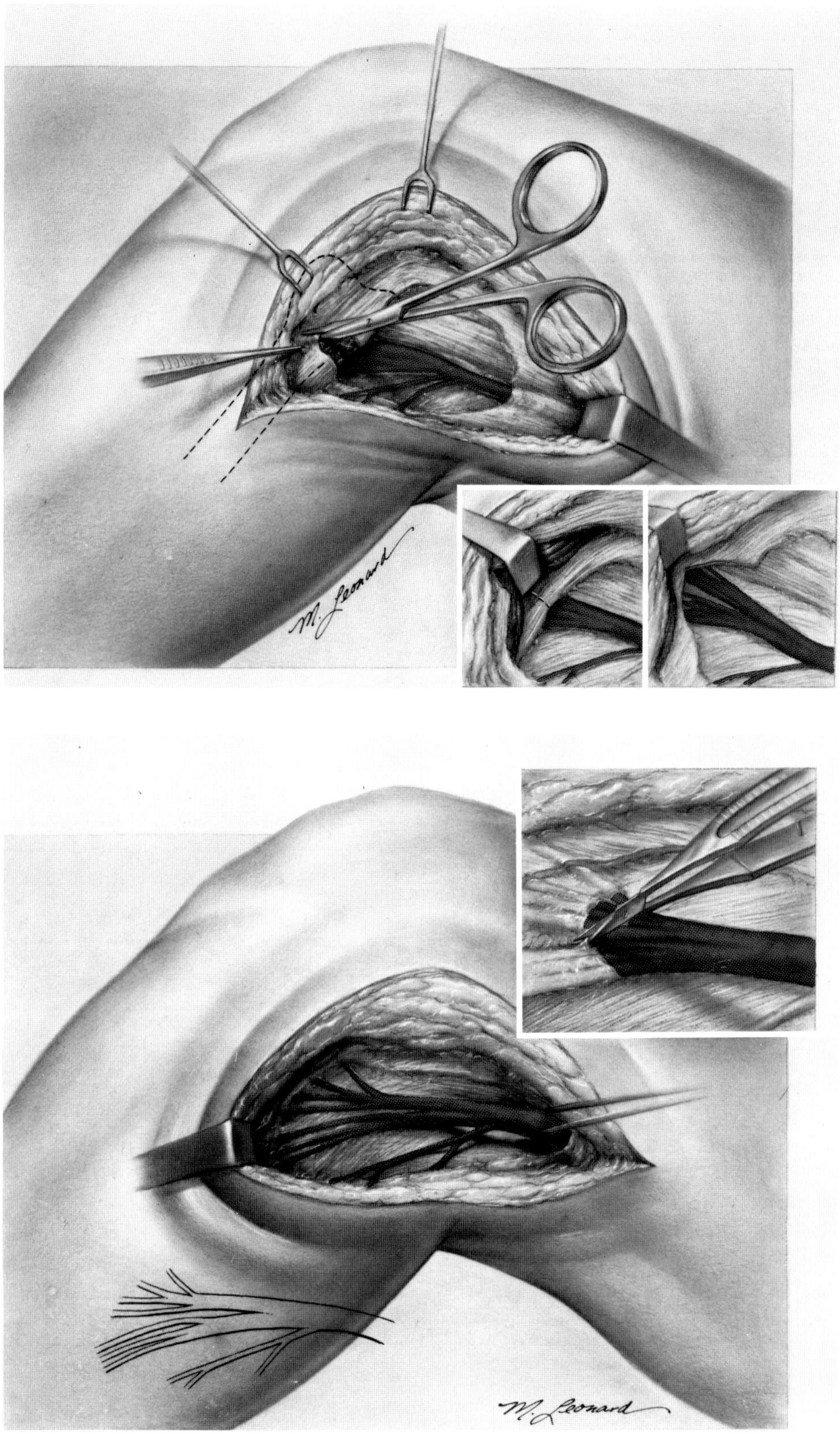

b

c

Figure 13-3. Operative technique for common peroneal nerve. An S-shaped incision is made centered over the fibular neck. The fascial extension from the iliotibial tract and biceps femoris to the deep fascia of the calf is incised and sensory branches to the lateral leg (lateral sural, lateral cutaneous nerve of the calf) are identified and released from this fascia. **a.** The fibrous edge of the peroneus longus is divided, its muscle retracted. The fibrous edge of the extensor digitorum longus of the extensor digitorum longus is divided to release the common peroneal and its superficial and deep divisions (**b**). An internal neurolysis is done (**c**).

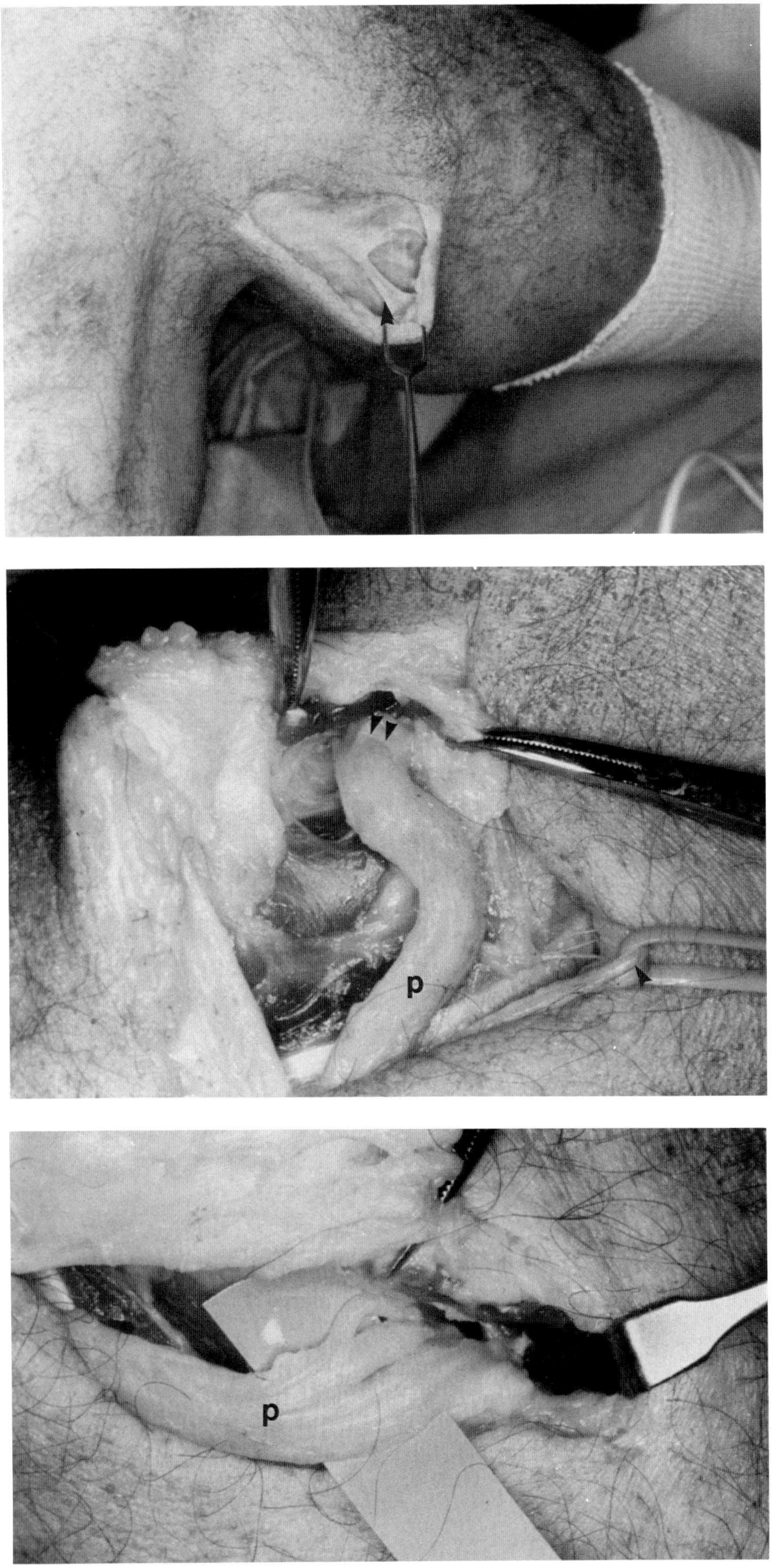

a

b

c

Figure 13-4. Intraoperative view of release of common peroneal nerve in a right leg (right views). The lateral sural and lateral cutaneous nerves of the calf are encircled by a vessel loop in (a) and (b) (arrow). Note entrapment site for these branches in **a** as they pierce the deep fascia. The fascia of the peroneus longus and extensor digitorum longus is released at clamps (double arrow). Then an intraneural dissection of common peroneal (p) into deep and superficial peroneal nerves, and of each of their component fascicles, is done (**c**). (See also Fig. 5-7c.)

is observed clearly. Each of these nerves is then dissected distally until its branching pattern becomes clear and it is obvious that no additional fibrous bands are pressing on these fibers. If good perineurial markings are not easily seen or if the multiple fascicles are adherent to each other with intraneural fibrosis, an internal neurolysis is done as described in Chapter 5. A disposable nerve stimulator may be utilized to demonstrate motor from sensory fascicles. The epineurium is submitted for pathologic examination and additional sources of compression, such as ganglion and tumor, are searched for. In the absence of such additional pathologic conditions, the wound is closed with 4-0 intradermal absorbable sutures and the skin closed with continuous absorbable sutures. The dressing is soft roll, gauze, kling, and a elastic wrap is applied. The tourniquet is deflated. The elastic bandage is removed 1 hour after the procedure. The patient is allowed ambulation as soon as he is comfortable.

Results

The results of common peroneal nerve release are difficult to find in the literature. The textbooks that describe common peroneal paralysis indicate that if the nerve is released before muscle wasting, a generally good result can be expected. In their seven reported cases of work-related, repetitive trauma-induced peroneal palsy, Sandhu and Sandberg[11] released the fibrous peroneus longus arch and noted six of the seven recovered excellent function. Just one of seven, or 14%, had a poor result. Berry and Richardson[10] reported a series of 15 patients explored surgically for common peroneal palsy. Two of the 15 were found to have nerve divisions. Of the 13 patients with the nerve in-continuity, a neurolysis of the common peroneal nerve was done: One (8%) had an excellent result, six (46%) had good results, five (38%) had poor results (no improvement), and one (8%) was lost to follow-up.[9] These results did not correlate with the patient's preoperative electrodiagnostic and electromyographic staging. The largest reported surgical series consists of 32 operative procedures in patients with leprosy.[27] In these patients, an external neurolysis was done from the sciatic nerve down into the anterolateral component of the leg. When intraneural microabscesses were suspected, multiple epineurotomies were done. An internal neurolysis was not done due to concern over blood supply. Contraindication to surgery was painless, longstanding paralysis, usually found in tuberculoid leprosy, in which the intraneural scarring, or necrosis, was severe. Pain was the main indication for surgery. Overall, 100% received significant pain relief, and 38% had improved motor function.

We have had experience in common peroneal nerve release, primarily in patients with underlying neuropathy, such as diabetes. This should be among the worst categories, because the surgical procedure cannot be anticipated to correct the neuropathy, itself. The assumption is that the neuropathy acts to diminish nerve function and particularly axoplasmic flow in some degree but may not be sufficient at the time of the surgical procedure to be giving the patient all their symptoms. The ischemia due to the superimposed nerve compression is the cause of the symptoms. The neuropathy predisposes the nerve to additional compression, which occurs in natural areas of narrowing. This represents a manifestation of the double crush hypothesis (described in Chapter 14) and the surgery relieves the mechanical component of the double crush. In patients who have this type of situation, entrapment of the common peroneal nerve at the knee, especially if there is a significant contribution of the lateral sural or sural communicating branch from the common peroneal, which is also entrapped, combined with entrapment of the posterior tibial nerve at the ankle, can result in circumferential sensory changes consistent with the so-called stocking distribution (Fig. 13-5).

Our experience in diabetics with ten common peroneal nerve releases had been excellent in nine and a failure in one. The one failure was a patient who had insulin-requiring diabetes for 41 years. In this patient, although sensation improved in the distribution of the common peroneal nerve, there was minimal improvement in strength of ankle dorsiflexion and great toe extension. In the remaining nine patients, five had severe weakness in the extensor hallucis longus and the tibialis anterior, and they recovered to near normal strength with return of sensation to the dorsum of the foot and the lateral side of the foot and calf area. Seven of the nine had improvement in two-point discrimination in the web space between the first and second toes.[28] (See Diabetic neuropathy, Chapter 14.)

The other large group of patients we have treated have had a peroneal nerve palsy develop after soft tissue and bony trauma to the lower extremity. The mechanism of injury in these patients is the same as that which occurs in patients who develop carpal tunnel syndrome after major forearm injury. Unfortunately, the same surgeon who recognizes nerve entrapment in the upper extremity fails to recognize the same condition in the lower extremity. Thus, patients are often referred late and with very severe nerve entrapment.

Complications

We have had one complication related to the series of common peroneal nerve releases, weakness in ankle eversion in a diabetic with a 41 year history, described above.

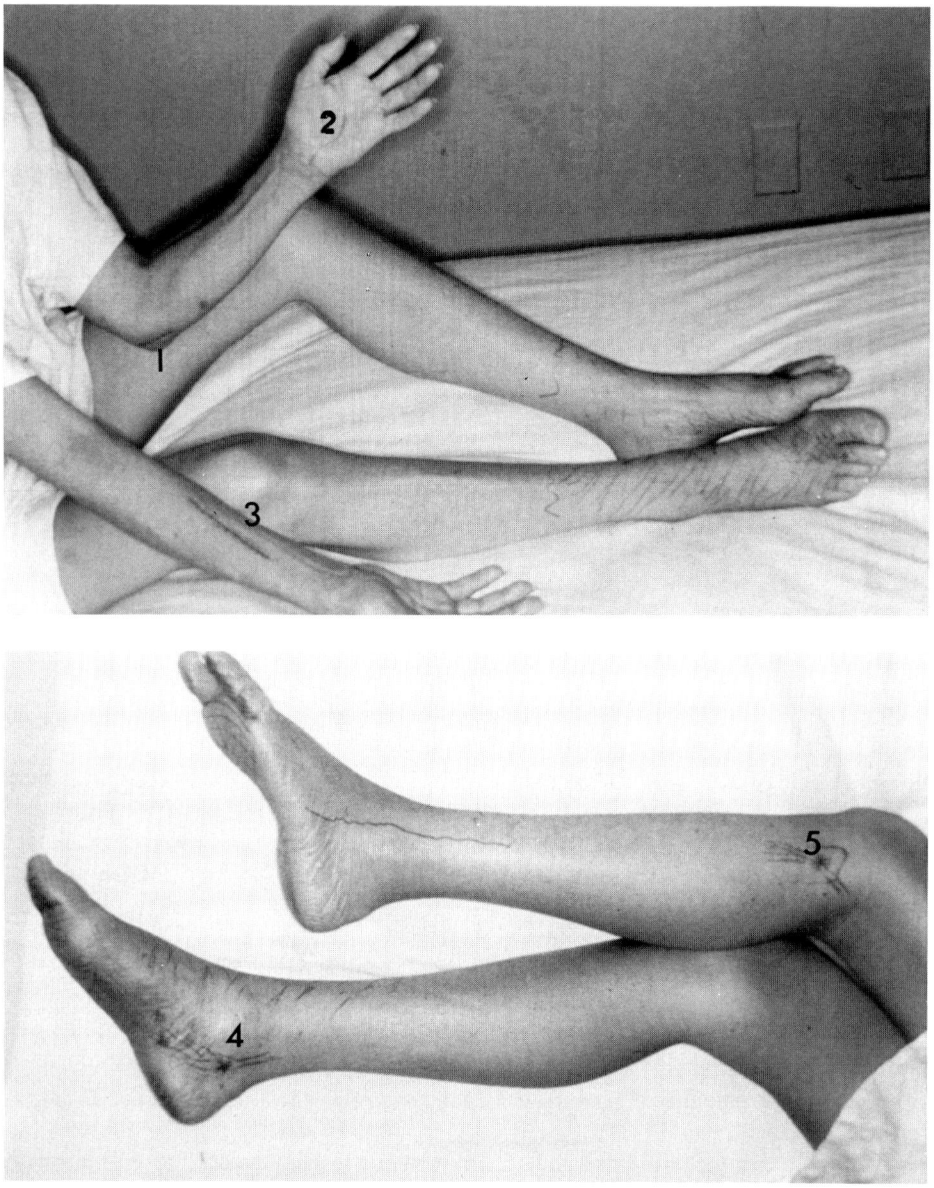

a

b

Figure 13-5. Multiple peripheral nerve entrapments present as stocking and glove distribution. **a.** This patient with a 41 year history of insulin-requiring diabetes first had release of cubital (1) and carpal (2) tunnels and radial sensory (3) nerve entrapment syndromes in each upper extremity with successful recovery of sensation and strength in hands. **b.** This approach was then attempted in her lower extremities. The posterior tibial nerves (4) and common peroneal nerves (5) were released.

Deep Peroneal Nerve Entrapment

Historical Review

Entrapment of the deep peroneal nerve in the region of the ankle is an entrapment neuropathy only recently described and, as such, remains poorly recognized among clinical problems. Remembering that the tarsal tunnel syndrome, entrapment of the posterior tibial nerve beneath the flexor retinaculum over the medial aspect of the ankle, was described only as recently as 1962 (see Chapter 12), it was not until 1968 that Marinacci[29] described an entrapment beneath the extensor retinaculum over the anterior aspect of the ankle with entrapment of the deep peroneal nerve. He termed this the "anterior tarsal tunnel syndrome."[29] Although Kopell and Thompson[20] recognized the possibility of entrapment of this nerve in this location in 1963, the syndrome was not clearly differentiated until the reports by Marinacci, which also included the electrodiagnostic approach for this entrapment.[30] Review of the literature through 1984 includes less than a dozen reported cases of the anterior tarsal tunnel syndrome.[31–34] Our experience personally has included 20 cases and has suggested an additional site of entrapment of the deep peroneal nerve's medial (sensory) branch at a site more distal than that already described. This site is over the junction of the first and second cuneiform bones with the metatarsal bones, where the nerve is bound down by the deep fascia and crossed by the extensor hallucis brevis tendon.[35] It is anticipated that with greater awareness of this problem, an increasing number of patients with compression of the deep peroneal nerve in the ankle and dorsum of the foot will be identified in the future.

Surgical Anatomy

There have been several anatomic studies related to the superficial and deep peroneal nerves. Two hundred and twenty-nine cadavers were dissected by a combined committee from Great Britain and Ireland and the observations reported in 1892,[36] particularly with respect to the patterns of innervation in the dorsum of the foot. A similar study was reported by Kosinski in 1926 of 118 feet.[37] A study of 100 legs was done by Horowitz and reported in 1938.[38] Recently, Kenzora[39] has studied sensory loss after lidocaine block of the deep peroneal nerve at the ankle in 24 patients (Fig. 13-6).

The deep peroneal nerve exits from beneath the extensor hallucis longus muscle belly in a location averaging 2.5 cm above the ankle, at which point it lies lateral to the tendon of the extensor hallucis longus and medial to the tendon of the extensor digitorum longus and, in approximately 98% of the cases, lateral to the

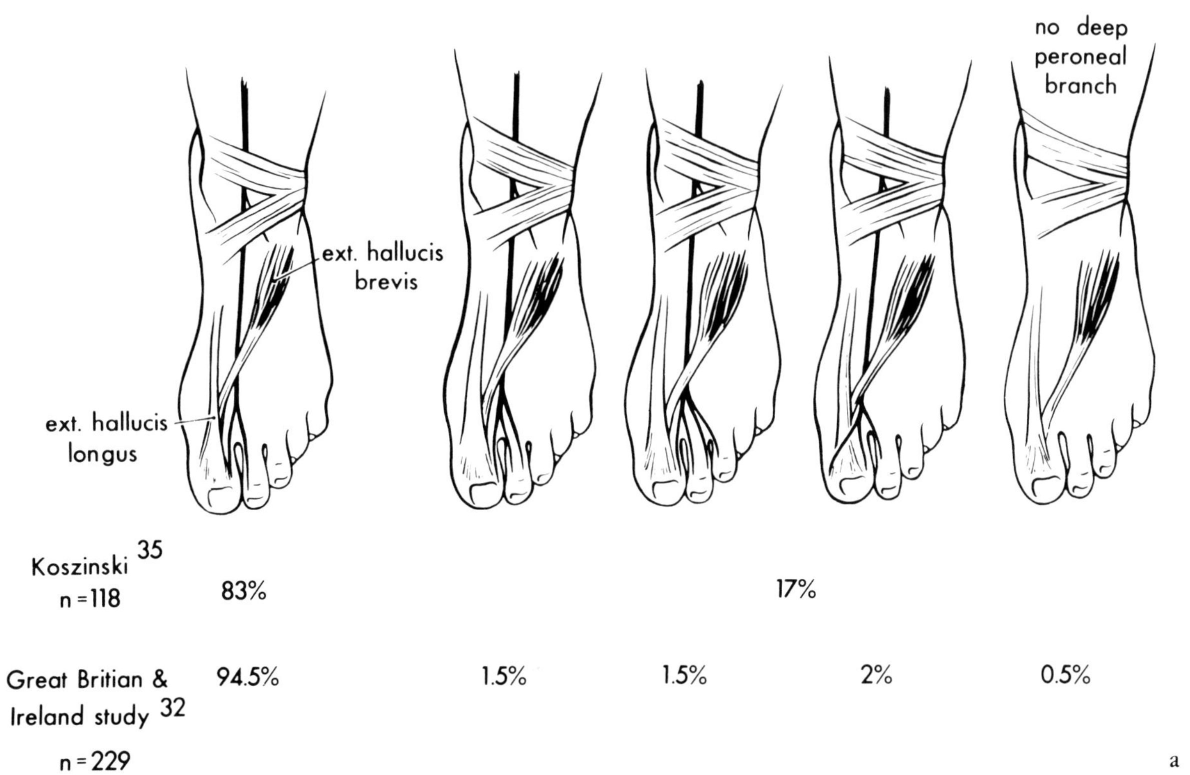

Figure 13-6. Composite illustration of variations found in cadaver dissections of sensory branches of deep peroneal nerve (**a**) and superficial peroneal nerve (**b**). (*Figure continues.*)

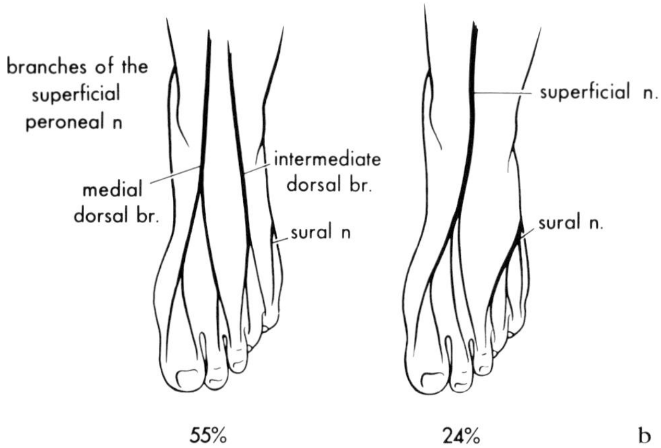

Figure 13-6. *(continued)*

anterior tibial artery. The nerve then passes beneath the superior and then the inferior limb of the extensor retinaculum. During this transition over the dorsum of the foot, the deep peroneal nerve divides into a medial and a lateral branch. The medial branch continues as a sensory branch lying adjacent to the dorsalis pedis artery and accompanies this artery distally. The lateral branch crosses beneath the inferior limb of the extensor retinaculum to innervate the extensor digitorum brevis muscle. It enters this muscle on its deep surface.

In reviewing anatomy texts, the extensor hallucis brevis is always depicted as a separate muscle, yet there is no description of the nerve that innervates the extensor hallucis brevis muscle. It is clear on careful review of the anatomic drawings that the extensor hallucis brevis represents one slip of the extensor digitorum brevis muscle. Thus, the lateral branch of the deep peroneal nerve as it crosses to enter the extensor digitorum brevis innervates the extensor hallucis brevis muscle. The extensor digitorum brevis sends tendinous slips to the big toe and the second, third, and fourth toes. It does not send a slip to the fifth toe. Of interest is the anomalous nerve innervation of the extensor digitorum brevis, which, when present, is associated with a tendinous slip from the peroneus tertius muscle that inserts as an additional extensor tendon to the fifth toe. The peroneus tertius muscle effectively is an extensor of the fifth toe at the base of the fifth metatarsal. The peroneus tertius as described in the section on the common peroneal nerve represents an accessory head of the extensor digitorum longus and is the most distal muscle to be innervated by the superficial peroneal nerve, except when the anomaly of the accessory deep peroneal nerve exists.

An accessory deep peroneal nerve was described by Bryce in 1901.[40] It has been described further by Winkler[41] in 1934 in seven patients, investigated by electrodiagnostic testing by Lambert[42] in 1969 in 50 patients, and also has been described more recently.[43] The accessory deep peroneal nerve was found by Lambert to occur in 22% of the 50 cases he studied by electrodiagnostic testing. Thus, this nerve represents a significant variation. When it exists, it represents a remaining motor branch from the superficial peroneal nerve that pierces the peroneus tertius muscle and extends laterally across the ankle to innervate the extensor digitorum brevis. Its significance clinically is that an entrapment of the deep peroneal nerve at the level of the ankle may exist without electromyographic studies demonstrating denervation potentials in the extensor digitorum brevis muscle or, as in the case reported by Gutmann,[43] there may be wasting of the extensor digitorum brevis muscle without compression of the deep peroneal nerve.

The sensation over the dorsum of the foot that is supplied by the deep peroneal nerve has been evaluated by the diagnostic nerve blocks done proximal to the ankle by Kenzora.[39] He found that in all 24 patients, there was loss of sensation from the junction of the first and second metatarsals distally to include the adjacent areas of the first and second toes. In some cases this area extended medially to the entire dorsum of the big toe and laterally to the entire dorsum of the second toe, but that in no patients did the third toe lose sensation.[39] The cadaver studies that are illustrated in Fig. 13-6 show that the vast majority of patients, approximately 90%, had the deep peroneal nerve emerge in the web space between the first and second toes and sent a single branch to the adjacent surfaces of the big toe and the second toe. Although Kosinski found that 14% of the patients had a branch of the deep peroneal nerve going to the web space between the second and third toes, this was found in only 3 of the 229 cases dissected during the combined British and Irish investigations. That combined study found one specimen with no deep peroneal nerve.

The extensor retinaculum beneath which the deep peroneal nerve passes is best described as a Y-shaped structure beginning on the lateral malleolus and has its stem extending onto the dorsum of the foot where it splits into a superior and inferior segment. These are appropriately called the superomedial and the inferomedial limbs of this extensor retinaculum. The entire retinaculum with this "Y" shape has been classically termed the inferior extensor retinaculum. The superior retinaculum, however, rather than being a separate retinacular structure, represents a thickening in the distal end of the deep fascia of the lower leg and is accordingly therefore not described here as a separate retinacular system. Beneath the inferomedial limb of this inferior retinaculum is the talonavicular joint where the deep peroneal nerve may become compressed most significantly when the foot is plantar flexed in women wearing high-heeled shoes. Our observation has also been that shoes with straps that cross the dorsum of the foot more distally cross at the juncture of the first and second metatarsal bones with the first and second cuneiform bones. It is in this location where an additional more distal site of entrapment for the purely sensory fibers of the deep peroneal nerve can occur (Fig. 13-7).[35]

Diagnosis

Diagnosis of entrapment of the deep peroneal nerve depends on identifying sensory and motor changes consistent with the problem with this nerve and without additional sensory or motor loss in distribution of other nerves. Patients' main complaints are those of aching and discomfort in the dorsal aspect of the foot, and there may be actual complaints of pain. These are usually worse with walking and the symptoms are relieved with rest. The moving touch sensation is diminished in the distribution of the deep peroneal nerve with more normal sensation being preserved on the medial and lateral aspects of the foot and dorsum away from the first and second web spaces. Moving and static two-point discrimination will be different in more advanced cases in the affected foot than in the contralateral foot. There will always be tenderness to pressure over the deep peroneal nerve either beneath the inferior extensor retinaculum and against the underlying talonavicular joint or distally at the apex of the first and second web spaces where the first and second metatarsals join the first and second cuneiform bones. A positive Tinel's sign may be elicited at the distal site. The extensor digitorum brevis muscle may be weak or diminished in bulk or obviously atrophied when toe extension is resisted during manual muscle testing. This is done by having the patient extend the toes and this toe extension is resisted by the examiner. The muscle belly is easily palpated over the lateral aspect of the foot. Its bulk and location may be compared with the opposite foot. Confirmatory electrodiagnostic testing is recommended with the appropriate

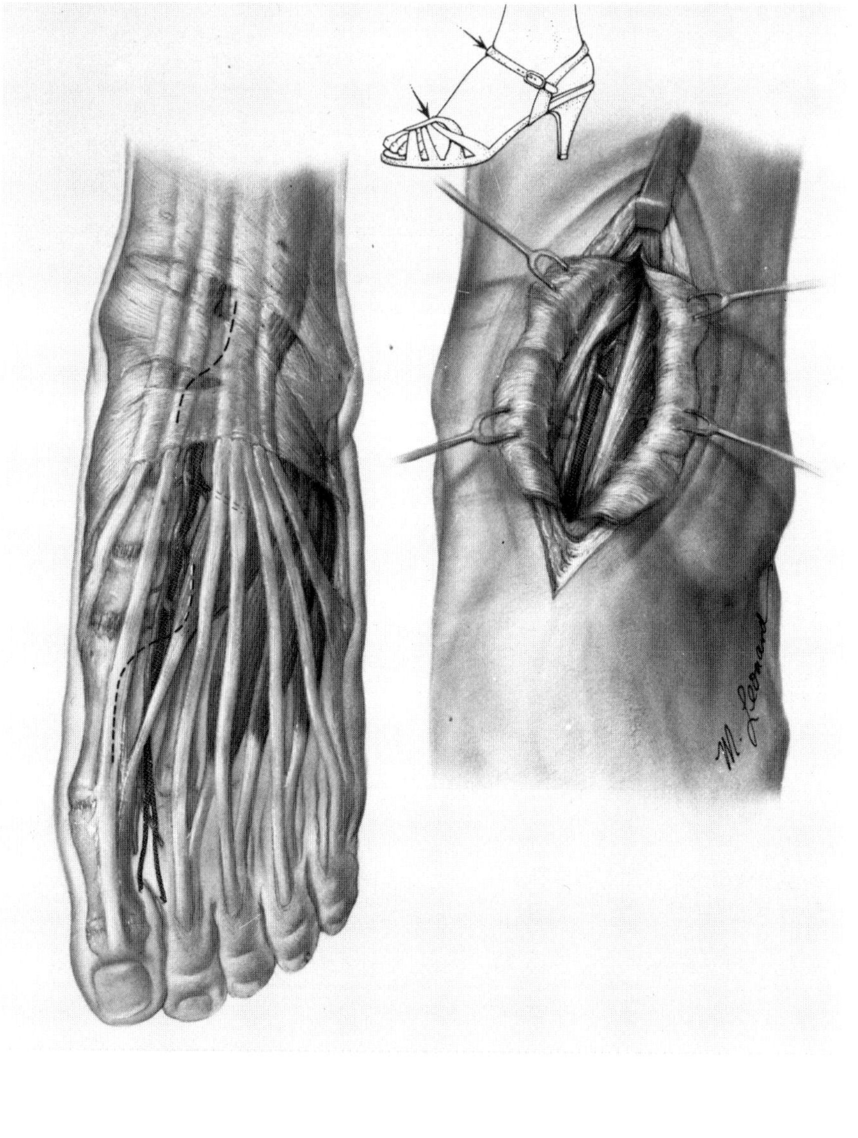

a

Figure 13-7. Operative technique for the deep peroneal nerve. **a.** The incisions for the release over the dorsal ankle and mid dorsum of the foot are outlined. **a.** The distal lower leg fascia (superior extensor retinaculum) is released, as are the two limbs (superomedial and inferomedial) of the inferior extensor retinaculum to revel the deep peroneal nerve. (*Figure continues.*)

caution that the examiner is aware of the possibility of an accessory deep peroneal nerve being present in approximately one-fifth of the patients tested. The examination must eliminate a more proximal source of entrapment in the common peroneal nerve with only a partial lesion being manifest. In these cases, which are rare, additional sensory change over the rest of the dorsum of the foot is evident and there is weakness in the long toe extensor, foot dorsiflexion, and foot eversion.

Most helpful is a diagnostic nerve block.[35] In patients in whom the Tinel is directly over the first and second metatarsal and first and second cuneiform regions, we have carried out a block with 3 ml of 1% lidocaine without epinephrine instilled just proximal to this area. After 15 minutes, the patient should be able to walk and stand on his toes without pain. This suggests that the site of entrapment is primarily here. If this treatment is ineffective in completely relieving the pain, a more proximal block can be carried out, coming 2 cm proximal to the ankle and injecting between the tendons of the extensor hallucis longus and the extensor digitorum longus. When there is obvious physical evidence of the extensor digitorum brevis being involved or electromyographic signs of denervation in this muscle, then the site of entrapment must be considered to be at the ankle level rather than on the mid dorsum of the foot, or both.

Surgical Technique

The operation is carried out with the patient in the supine position under general or spinal anesthesia and a pneumatic tourniquet is placed over the thigh. The foot is prepared with antiseptic solution, elevated, and exsanguinated with an elastic bandage and tourniquet

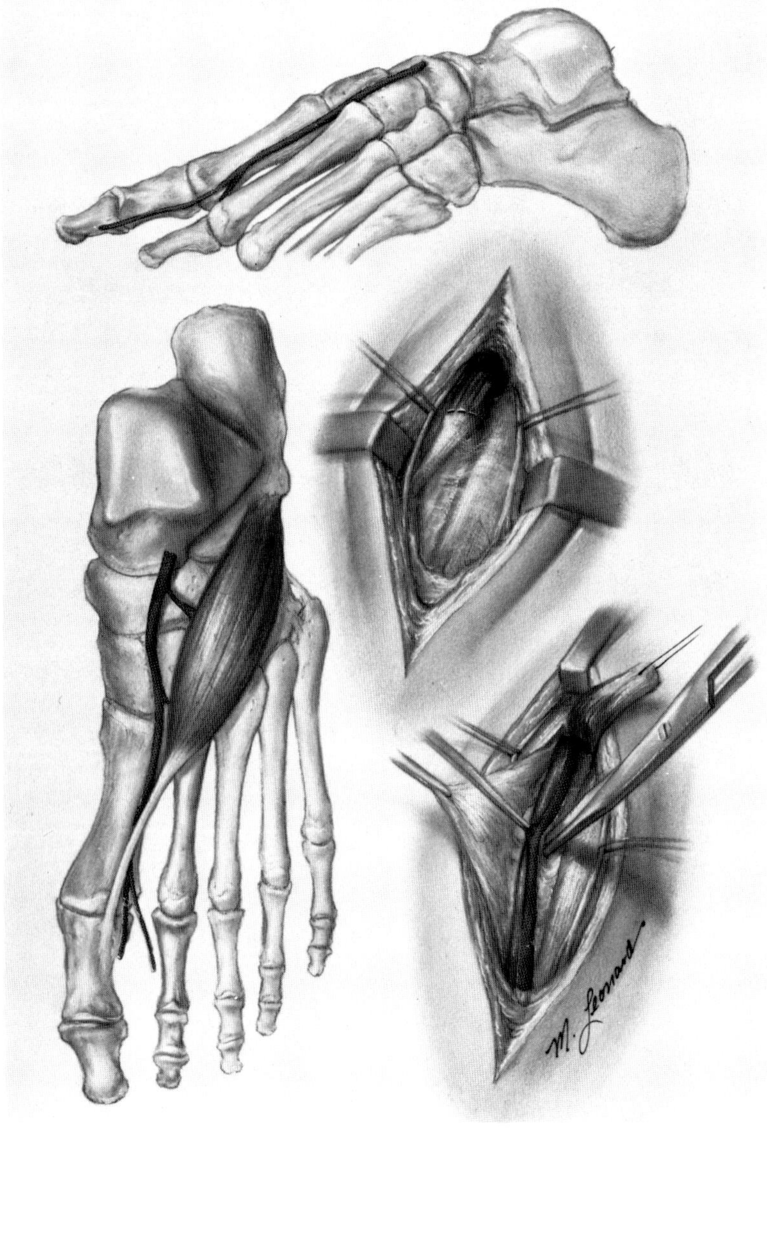

b **Figure 13-7** (*continued*) **b.** Over the juncture of the first and second metatarsals with the first and second cuneiform bones, the deep fascia is released, crossing branches of the superficial peroneal nerve are preserved. The extensor hallucis brevis tendon is excised. The fascia binding the sensory branch of the deep peroneal nerve to the bone is released and neurolysis completed.

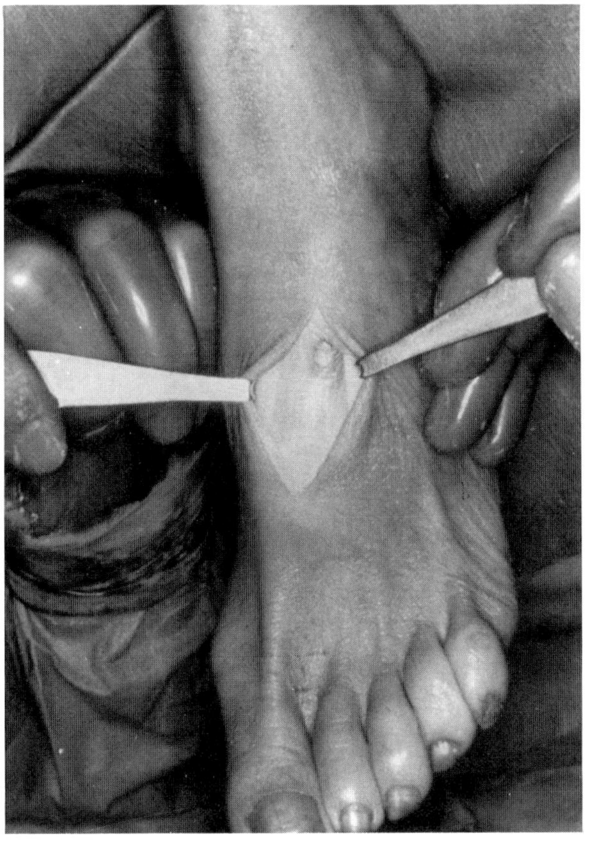

a

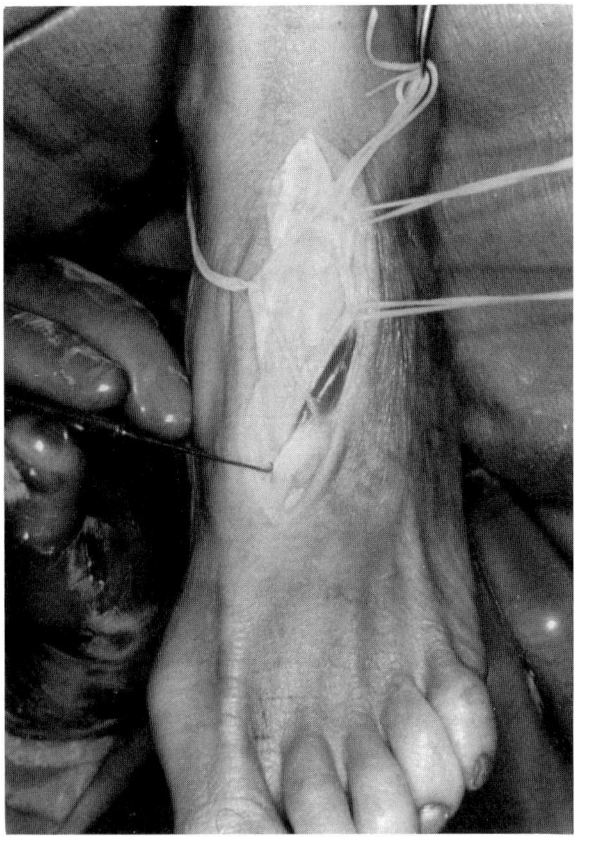

b

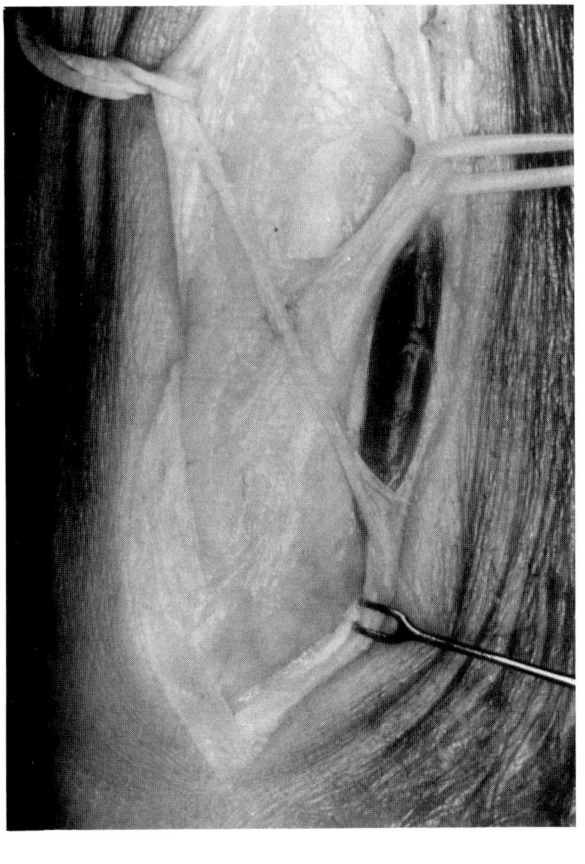

c

Figure 13-8. **a**. Intraoperative views of deep peroneal nerve release over the foot. **b**. The muscle belly of the extensor hallucis brevis is seen, its tendon with a single hook, noting site where it entraps the deep peroneal nerve, and retraced off the nerve with double hook (**c**) before excising the tendon. In (**c**) the vessel loop protects superficial peroneal nerve branches, and the thickened scar about the deep peroneal nerve is demonstrated by other vessel loop.

inflated to 300 to 400 mmHg pressure. An incision is made approximately 4 cm in length over the mid dorsum of the foot centered between the extensor hallucis longus and the extensor digitorum longus tendons. The incision is deepened into the subcutaneous tissue. Care is taken in case an anomalous course of the superficial peroneal nerve is encountered or of its medial branch. The distal lower leg fascia is incised. The superomedial and inferomedial limbs of the inferior extensor retinaculum are divided. The deep peroneal nerve and anterior tibial artery are identified. A search is carried out for structures arising from the joint, such as ganglia or bone spurs or adhesions between the nerve and adjacent tendons. Whatever structures might be compressing the nerve are excised or removed. Utilizing microsurgical instruments and technique, the epineurium is opened. If there is intraneural fibrosis present, an internal neurolysis is carried out. The incision is closed with interrupted intradermal absorbable sutures and the skin with continuous nonabsorbable sutures (Figs. 13-7, 13-8).

In patients with evidence of more distal entrapment, combined with the more proximal site or with just distal entrapment alone, an S-shaped incision is made beginning medially over the first metatarsal and crossing over the area between the first and second metatarsal bones and the first and second cuneiforms and coming proximally. This incision is deepened into the subcutaneous tissue and adjacent branches of the superficial peroneal nerve are identified and their integrity preserved. The fascia is opened and the extensor hallucis brevis tendon is found crossing the nerve at this juncture. The tendon is divided distally and then excised. A deep fascial covering will now be found compressing the deep peroneal nerve and dorsalis pedis artery to the underlying bony structures. This fascia is opened, the artery identified, and a separate branch of the nerve may be found on both the medial and lateral sides of the artery, depending on the anatomic variations in the deep peroneal nerve that are present. A release of this deep fascia proximally is carried out for an additional 1 to 2 cm and an internal neurolysis of the one or more branches of the deep peroneal nerve carried out as indicated. The closure is made with absorbable sutures in the deep dermis and continuous sutures in the skin. The dressing is nonadherent gauze and soft roll and then a large cotton bulky dressing is wrapped about the foot. This is held in place with kling and an elastic bandage, after which the tourniquet is deflated (Figs. 13-7, 13-8, 13-9).

Postoperatively, the patient is allowed ambulation with a cane or a crutch but, in general, for 2 weeks is urged to remain off the foot as much as possible. Any sutures are removed 2 weeks after surgery.

Results

Of the cases in the literature of deep peroneal nerve entrapment at the ankle, only the one reported by Borges et al[33] was treated surgically and that patient improved. Four patients treated by Gessini et al[34] and one patient treated by Borges et al[33] improved after cortisone injection. Other patients reported improvement after altering the shoes they were wearing. All previous investigators suggest that with the failure of conservative therapy, surgery is indicated.

In the 20 patients operated on for deep peroneal nerve entrapment more distally, only one did not improve after surgical release over the dorsum of the foot.[35] That patient had electromyographic evidence of denervation in the extensor brevis muscle and the entrapment should have been released more proximally also. The remaining 19 patients, released at the junction of the first and second metatarsals with the first and second cuneiforms have had good to excellent relief of pain and recovery of two-point discrimination. Of interest is that two of these patients had preexisting fractures of the second metatarsal, after which the pain began. One patient had had a crush-avulsion injury to the foot resulting in loss of the distal phalanges of the first and second toes. Four patients had a crush injury to the entire foot. In one patient, the symptoms were related to a peripheral neuropathy in a setting of collagen vascular disease,[35] and in 4 patients in association with diabetic neuropathy (see Chapter 14). In these 5 patients with an associated neuropathy, the deep peroneal nerve was released in conjunction with releases to the posterior tibial and medial and lateral plantar and the common peroneal nerves.[35]

Complications

We have had no complications after surgery for nerve entrapment at this site.

Superficial Peroneal Entrapment

Historical Review

Entrapment of the superficial peroneal nerve is usually not considered in the discussion of lower extremity entrapments.[2,3,5] Superficial peroneal entrapment is mentioned in a cursory fashion by Kopell,[44] who suggests that "the superficial peroneal pierces the deep fascia in the distal portion of the leg. The opening (in the fascia) may provide the opportunity for a muscle hernia. The symptomatology attributed to the hernia may be the result of nerve compression rather than muscle compression." Kopell makes a point that symptoms of

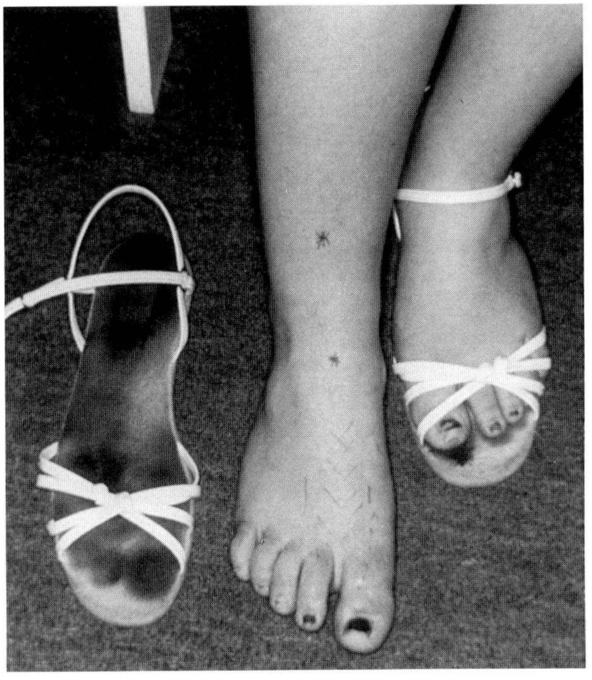

Figure 13-9. Relationship of woman's shoe strappings to deep peroneal nerve entrapment. The pattern of sensory loss if noted, as well as sites of positive Tinel's sign. The electromyogram demonstrated denervation of the extensor digitorum brevis muscle.

aching in the lower leg were thought to be due to muscle herniation, and the treatment by closing the fascia over the palpable muscle bulge would worsen the symptoms, which, in fact, were due to nerve compression, not due to the constricted muscle in the hernia. It has become clear that increased pressure in the anterolateral compartment of the leg can cause compression of the superficial peroneal nerve by the muscles bulging at sites where the superficial peroneal nerve exits from the fascia. This can present not only in acute compartment syndromes with fibula fractures or bleeding in the compartment, but has now been reported to occur in athletes. This type of exertional compartment syndrome has been well-documented.[45] The general subject area of compartment syndromes recently have been reviewed extensively.[46] As awareness of the potential for entrapment of the superficial peroneal nerve increases, it may be anticipated that additional cases will be reported, not only in those with exertional causes but other cases in which symptoms may now be recognized as being related to the superficial peroneal nerve and the diagnosis confirmed with electrodiagnostic studies.[47]

Surgical Anatomy

The superficial peroneal nerve leaves the cover of the peroneus brevis muscle and pierces the deep fascia of the lower leg where it divides into a medial and intermediate dorsal cutaneous nerve that will extend onto the dorsum of the foot. In studying 100 legs, Horowitz[38] found that in 90% the fascia was pierced 12.5 cm proximal to the lateral malleolus. In 1%, it arose more proximal than this, and in 2% it arose 10 cm proximal from the lateral malleolus, in 5%, 7.5 cm proximal to the lateral malleolus, and in the remaining, it arose even more proximally. Kosinski[37] noted in 118 legs that the superficial peroneal nerve pierced the deep fascia 10 cm above the lateral malleolus in 75% of the specimens, and in the remaining it pierced it at a higher level. Accordingly, it is clear that the site of exit of the superficial peroneal nerve is variable, with the majority of cases arising approximately 10 to 12 cm proximal to the lateral malleolus.

The distribution of the superficial peroneal nerve is the dorsum of the foot, with the exception of that area supplied by the deep peroneal nerve. The exact distribution of the superficial peroneal nerve is in some direct relationship to that area covered by the sural nerve. In Kosinski's[37] series, 17% of the dissections had the sural nerve contributing to sensation over the fifth, fourth, and part of the third toes. In the study of 229 cadavers by the Anatomic Society of Great Britain and Ireland, 26% of the specimens contained sural nerve contributing branches to the fifth, fourth, and portion of the third toes. In one of the specimens from this latter series, the saphenous nerve contributed significantly to sensation over the dorsal aspect of the big toe. In consideration of the sural nerve's contribution to the dorsal aspect of the foot, the older nomenclature called the sural nerve the lateral dorsal cutaneous nerve in the foot, whereas the superficial peroneal contributed, by its two main terminal divisions, the medial and the intermediate dorsal cutaneous nerves of the foot. Present nomenclature considers the superficial peroneal nerve to have a medial and intermediate branch. In the dissections by the Anatomic Society of Great Britain,[36] 4% of the specimens, in fact, did not have this branching at the level of the dorsal aspect of the foot. There was a single branch of the superficial peroneal that did not begin its branching until dorsally over the foot. The branching of the superficial peroneal into its medial and intermediate divisions generally occurs just after it pierces the superficial fascia, and thus it exists as two separate branches in 76% of the specimens at the level of the inferior retinacular ligaments.

Diagnosis

The diagnosis of superficial peroneal nerve entrapment rests on identifying the source of the patient's discomfort as being due to involvement of the sensory innervation of the superficial peroneal nerve. The sources of entrapment that might affect the peroneus brevis and longus would occur high enough that the site of compression would probably be at the level of the common peroneal nerve. Accordingly, the only abnormality identifiable on physical examination is decreased sensation in the distribution of the superficial peroneal nerve, mainly the dorsal aspect of the foot, with the exception of the web space between the first and second toes and with the exception of the dorsal aspect of the fifth toe. Recently, we have noticed that forceful inversion of the foot will cause the patient pain, similar to the positive Finkelstein test in radial sensory nerve entrapment (see Wartenberg's traction neuritis in Chapter 10) as the branches of the superficial peroneal nerve are stretched in the maneuver against the restraint of the proximal fascial opening. The patient's complaints do not begin until he is carrying out some type of strenuous or repetitive activity. The physical examination may show no sensory abnormalities at the time of the examination. In patients whose sensory changes are persistent in nature or the problem is long-standing, there may be sensory changes demonstrable between one side of the foot and the other side and, between one leg and the other leg. Sensory testing may also be done with a tuning fork. Vibratory testing with tuning forks is effective in the upper extremity for diagnosis of peripheral nerve entrapment,[48] and we have found it to be effective in evaluation of nerve entrapments in the lower extremity also (Chapter 3).

Recently, an evaluation of compartment pressures in the lower extremity in volunteers demonstrated that at the time the pressure in the compartment was approximately 30 mmHg less than diastolic, at which time the patients began to experience discomfort and complain of sensory changes in their toes, the first sign that could be demonstrated on physical examination was abnormal perception of the 256 cps vibratory stimulus.[49] Thus, for chronic and acute entrapment of the nerve, vibratory testing is recommended as an adjunct to the clinical evaluation.

The physical examination may also demonstrate a bulge of muscle, either the extensor digitorum longus or the peroneus tertius in the distal third of the anterolateral compartment of the leg at the fascial site or where the superficial peroneal nerve transits from deep to superficial. This bulge becomes more prominent with resisted ankle eversion and toe extension. Numbness and tingling may be described or pain frequently radiates up the lateral aspect of the leg, where proximal evaluation over the fibular head does not demonstrate a positive Tinel's sign. There may be a positive Tinel's sign or pain directly over the site where the superficial peroneal nerve is compressed beneath its fascial ring. Electrodiagnostic studies are useful in demonstrating a change in the sensory latency of the superficial peroneal nerve and failing to demonstrate local conduction defect over the common peroneal nerve at the fibular head. There should be normal function in the extensor digitorum brevis and preserved sensation in the web space between the first and second toes.

Nerve blocks are also valuable in the diagnosis of this nerve entrapment as a source of pain. Lidocaine can be infiltrated approximately 10 to 12 cm proximal to the lateral malleolus or at the point of muscle herniation or at the point of positive Tinel's sign, and the patient may carry out some exertional activity to see if some of the pain is blocked. Use of this technique has been reported in cases in which it has been difficult to ascertain whether a sural nerve or peroneal nerve has been involved in a patient with an unusual case of causalgia.[50] The placement of the wick catheter to measure directly compartmental pressures, as described by Garfin et al,[45] is also recommended in cases in which the diagnosis is difficult to obtain by other techniques.

Surgical Technique

The same general operative approach is used as described for the common peroneal and deep peroneal nerve explorations. An S-shaped incision is made, centered over the muscle bulge or fascial defect. If no muscle bulge is noted, it is centered over a site approximately 10 cm proximal to the lateral malleolus, since this is the most common site for the superficial peroneal nerve to exit. Subcutaneous tissue is entered and the branches of the superficial peroneal nerve identified. The fascia is released 2 cm distal and 2 cm proximal, making a wide generous opening for the superficial peroneal nerve. In cases in which there is aching throughout the entire anterolateral compartment with exertional activities and, especially if symptoms during exertional activities extend to involve weakness in muscles innervated by the superficial peroneal nerve and deep peroneal nerve, suggesting that they are also being entrapped, the recommended treatment is to release the fascia over the entire anterolateral compartment. If there is intraneural fibrosis present, an internal neurolysis is carried out (as described in Chapter 5). The incision is closed with interrupted absorbable intradermal sutures and the skin with continuous absorbable suture. A bulky dressing is applied and an elastic bandage. The tourniquet is deflated and the elastic bandage is removed 1 hour later. The patient is started on early ambulation.

Results

We have been able to find only six reported cases of surgically treated superficial peroneal nerve entrapment. One case was reported by Garfin et al,[45] four cases were reported by Mackey et al,[51] and one case was reported by Sridhara and Izzod.[47] All of these cases made a complete recovery after surgical release of the entrapped superficial peroneal nerves and no complications have been reported.

Sural Nerve Entrapment

Historical Review

An anatomic site of entrapment of the sural nerve has not been described previously. An isolated report of four patients with entrapment of the terminal branch of the sural nerve at the ankle secondary to an injury and scarring has been recorded.[52] Indeed, the sural nerve is routinely biopsied for diagnostic purposes in cases of unusual neuropathies. The assumption here is that the sural nerve reflects what is going on in the peripheral nervous system and that any pathologic condition found is not related to a more proximal site of nerve compression. The sural nerve, as will be described in the section to follow, has two potential sites of nerve entrapment where it passes through fascial windows. Entrapment of the sural nerve may therefore contribute to patients' symptoms and may cause some ambiguity in the interpretation of sural nerve biopsies. This subject has been reviewed recently with respect to the situation in diabetic neuropathy.[53] The human material on which the histopathologic study of diabetic neuropathy was described originally was from sural and radial sensory nerve biopsies. Those biopsies demonstrate histopathologic states that are consistent with peripheral nerve compression, as well as the basic diabetic axonopathy. The changes in the sural nerve consistent with chronic compression are those which have been demonstrated in the experimental models for experimental peripheral nerve compression (see Chapter 3) and in human radial sensory nerve compression from which specimens have now been evaluated (see Chapter 10).[53,54] It is therefore possible that compression of the sural nerve, superimposed on diabetic neuropathy, may have been in part responsible for the histopathologic condition observed in the specimens of nerve obtained from patients with diabetes and previously attributed to diabetes alone. An awareness of the potential sites for sural nerve entrapment may lead to a greater awareness in identification of this problem in patients with the appropriate symptoms.

Surgical Anatomy

The sural nerve, as it is usually called, is, in fact, the common sural nerve. The medial sural nerve, coming from the posterior tibial nerve in the popliteal fossa and extending between the two heads of the gastrocnemius, enters the distal leg approximately 16 cm proximal to the lateral malleolus. This nerve is joined in 75% of patients[55] by a lateral sural nerve. This nerve may join it just after the contribution from the posterior tibial nerve has exited from the deep fascia or may join it deep to the fascia. The lateral sural contribution can be equal to or larger in size than the contribution from the posterior tibial nerve. This study was done in 30 fresh cadavers and highlighted a problem with nomenclature.

The common peroneal nerve, several centimeters proximal to the fibular neck, gives off either one or two branches that will ultimately supply sensation to the lateral aspect of the calf from the fibular head down to the side of the fifth toe. The branches may not join with the sural nerve at all and these branches are appropriately termed the lateral cutaneous nerve of the calf.[55] The branch that joins the medial sural nerve is clearly appropriately named the lateral sural nerve. In cases in which there is not a lateral sural nerve, which may also be called the sural communicating nerve, the posterior tibial nerve is the only supplier to the final sural nerve and therefore to the region about the lateral portion of the ankle, the lateral portion of the heel, and the fifth toe. A variable contribution to this area extending this far distally may come from the lateral cutaneous nerve of the calf. In a patient in whom it is critical to learn the distribution, a block may be carried out approximately 16 cm proximal to the malleolus or the common peroneal nerve or a block may be placed in the popliteal fossa just proximal and posterior to the fibular head in an attempt to elucidate the different territories.

Our explorations of the common peroneal nerve have identified sites where the lateral cutaneous nerve of the calf and the lateral sural or communicating sural nerve may be entrapped as they go from the popliteal fossa through the thick fascial sheath that joins the iliotibial tract to the deep fascia of the leg (Figs. 13-2, 13-4, 13-5). This site of entrapment may combine with pressure in the distal calf and potentially summate to give sufficient pressure to cause symptoms in the sural nerve distribution, especially in the patient who may have a predisposition to compression neuropathies, like the diabetic.

Results

There is no published study by which the results of sural nerve compression alone can be evaluated. Our experience has been sural nerve in conjunction with other peripheral nerve releases. In this section we would like to draw an analogy between peripheral nerve entrapments and the clinical appearance of stocking and glove sensory loss. Particularly in peripheral neuropathies, such as diabetes, the appearance of the patient is with sensory changes that may be mapped out to give entire

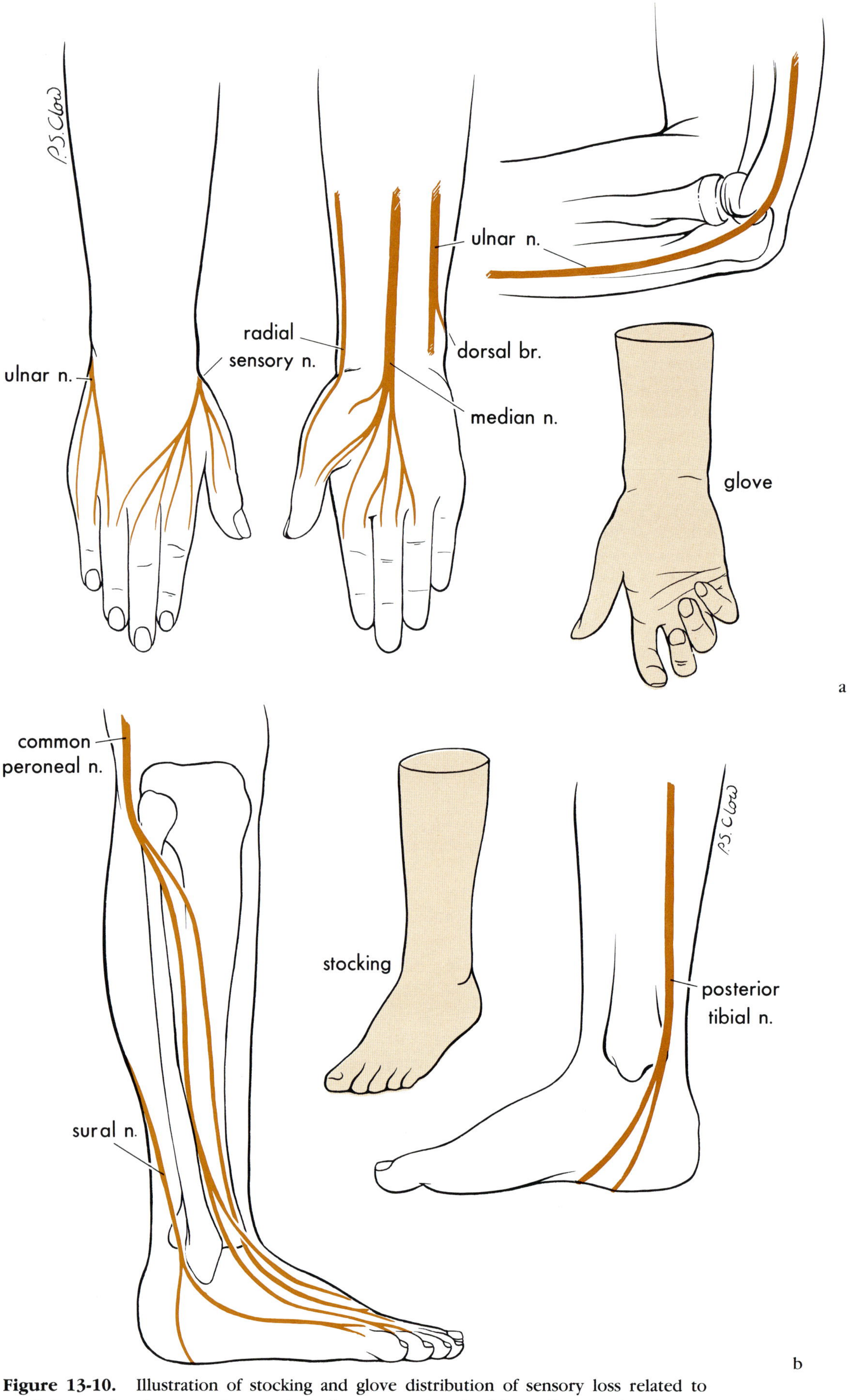

Figure 13-10. Illustration of stocking and glove distribution of sensory loss related to multiple peripheral nerve entrapments. In the upper extremity (a), median at wrist, ulnar at elbow, and radial sensory in forearm combine to give a glove pattern. In the lower extremity (**b**), common peroneal, lateral sural, and lateral cutaneous nerves of calf, posterior tibial, and deep peroneal contribute to the stocking pattern.

limb sensory losses. In the leg, in patients with diabetic neuropathy, we have released posterior tibial and included its medial and lateral plantar branches, the common peroneal nerve and therefore its terminal superficial and deep peroneal branches. When the common peroneal nerve gives off a lateral sural communicating branch or a lateral cutaneous nerve to the calf, these branches have also been decompressed in and about the region of the knee. We have not made separate fascial incisions in the calf, but more distal releases of these nerves. In these patients, sensation has been improved not only over the dorsal and plantar aspects of the foot, but also over the lateral aspect in areas innervated by the sural nerve, confirming the hypothesis that this nerve is involved in the double crush concept, multiple crush syndromes, (see Chapter 14) and contributes to the stocking appearance of the sensory loss in patients with multiply entrapped peripheral nerves superimposed on the underlying neuropathy. The same situation exists in the arm where entrapment of the radial sensory nerve in the forearm, median and ulnar nerves at the wrist, and the ulnar nerve at the elbow contribute to a glove-type distribution (Fig. 13-10) (see Diabetic neuropathy, Chapter 14).

Plantar Nerve Compression (Morton's Neuroma)

Historical Review

Compression of a common plantar digital nerve was among the earliest of chronic compression neuropathies to be described. It was described in 1876[56] and its original description has been confirmed frequently in clinical experience. The problem is more common in women than in men and is more common in adults than in adolescents. Generally, there is a pain that occurs with walking that is between the third and fourth toes, with the fourth toe being the more painful. Taking off shoes and elevating the foot and massaging the base of the foot is frequently helpful. Wearing high-heeled shoes or shoes that compress the metatarsal bones together will compress the nerve and aggravate the problem. Increased physical activity aggravates the problem. The pain is often lightening-like and may shoot into the toes, causing the patient to cease activity. Commonly, the feet have no physical problems that can be detected, although the examiner can frequently provoke the pain by holding the foot and compressing the first and fifth metatarsals together.

Of historical interest is Morton's[56] actual description of the problem and his treatment. Morton describes in detail the history of 11 patients with this problem. Their worst symptoms involved the fourth and fifth toes and thus, unlike current experience that implicates the common plantar digital nerve to the third and fourth web spaces, Morton believed that the fourth and fifth web space nerve was the most frequently involved. Morton also is quoted uniformly as treating his patients by resection of the fourth metatarsal head. Careful reading of Morton's own reported operative procedures, however, reveals that "in the surrounding soft parts (of the fourth metatarsal head), the nerves distributed about the joint were also necessarily excised." For example, in another description, Morton notes that beside the fourth metatarsal head, "the base of the first phalanx was also removed.... The adjacent soft parts were dissected away to insure the excision of all surrounding nerve branches." Thus, Morton did neurectomies of the plantar digital nerves.

The problem of Morton's neuroma that is interesting in terms of neuropathologic studies and surgical treatment is that no other human nerve compression is treated by excision of the nerve. The current operative technique for Morton's "neuroma" as most commonly practiced is to resect the involved nerve. Clearly, after resection of a nerve, a neuroma will form. The paradox is that Morton's neuroma, which is not a neuroma, is treated as if it were a neuroma, with the consequence that a neuroma, in fact, forms. Yet this treatment is generally successful in relief of the pain. Also of interest is why this particular affliction occurs between the third and fourth toes so much more commonly than between other toes. This answer may be related to the surgical anatomy.

Surgical Anatomy

The common plantar digital nerve to the web space between the third and fourth toes may be formed entirely from a branch from the lateral plantar nerve, which goes about the lateral aspect of the flexor digitorum brevis slip to the fifth toe. However, most commonly, just proximal to the space between the second and third metatarsals, this main contributory branch from the lateral plantar nerve to the common plantar digital nerve to the third and fourth web spaces is joined by a communicating branch from the medial plantar nerve, which also crosses the flexor digitorum brevis, but from its medial aspect. With toe flexion, these contributory branches to the common plantar digital nerves to the third and fourth web spaces are pulled proximally or tethered against a distal pulling force. The common plantar digital nerve crosses plantar or superficial to the intermetatarsal ligament between the third and fourth metatarsal heads and then divides into its terminal branches to the adjacent surfaces of the third and fourth toes. With foot plantar flexion and weight being borne on the metatarsal heads, which dorsiflexes the toes, the common plantar digital nerve is pulled distally by the

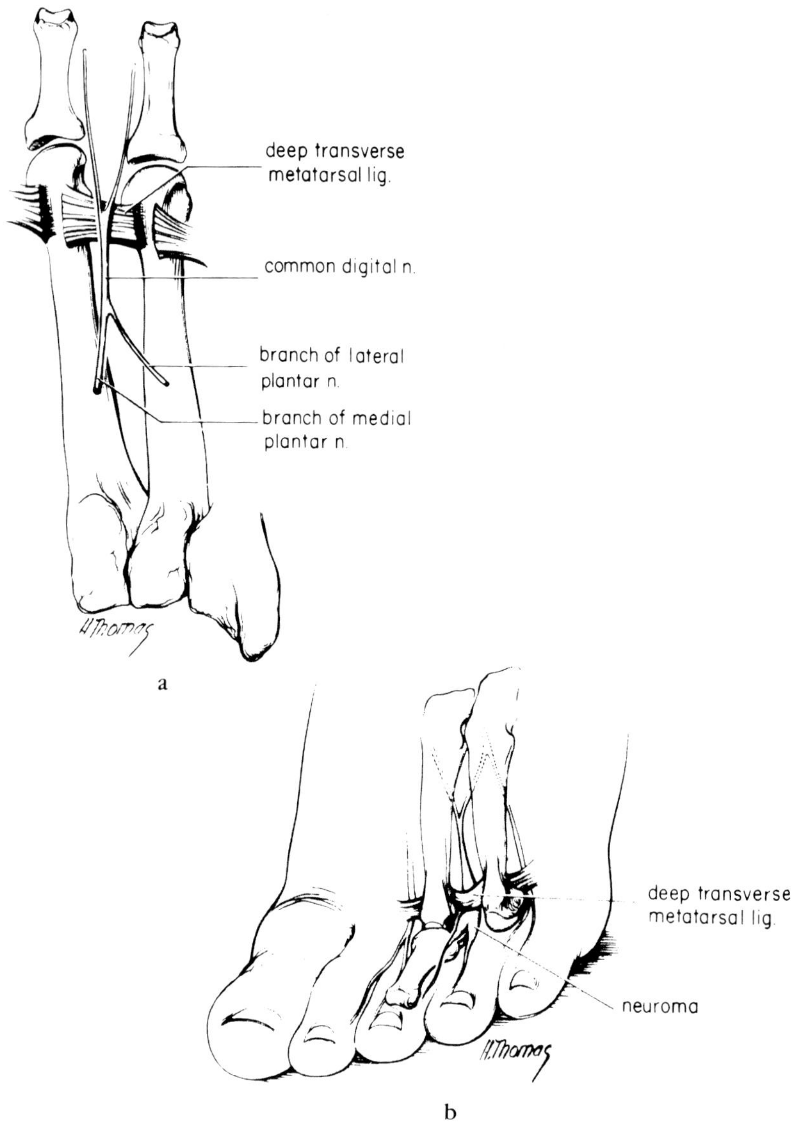

Figure 13-11. Illustration of pathomechanics of chronic nerve compression of the common plantar nerve to the third and fourth web spaces that results in Morton's metatarsalgia. Note a proximal tethering of the nerve by its contributing branches (from the medial and lateral plantar nerves) as they pass around the flexor digitorum brevis, which pulls upon them during toe flexion. Note that with foot plantar flexion and weight bearing on the metatarsal heads, the common plantar digital nerve is stretched distally by the toes, while being compressed by the overlying intermetatarsal ligament, which is the site of the repetitive trauma to the nerve, as it is also intermittently compressed on each side by the metatarsal heads. (Reproduced with permission from Kopell.[44])

toes' extension while being tethered proximally about the flexor digitorum brevis. This mechanism for the pathomechanics of the cause of Morton's neuroma was put forward by Betts in 1940[57] and is illustrated in Figure 13-11. Accompanying the common plantar digital nerve in this location is the common plantar digital artery, thickening and occlusion of which was noted by Nissen in 1948,[58] who proposed that ischemia to the nerve was responsible for the symptoms. The location of the common plantar digital nerve just inferior to but between the metatarsal heads of the third and fourth metatarsals places the nerve in position to be compressed by these bones if the foot is squeezed during walking. Thus, tight shoes would keep the first and fifth metatarsals restrained from lateral movement while pressure on the foot would allow descent of the remaining metatarsals into the space between the first and fifth metatarsals, resulting in inward movement of the third and fourth metatarsal heads. It is this mechanism that was believed to be the source of the nerve problem by Morton[56] and continued to be believed as the source of the problem by researchers much more recently, such as Mulder in 1951,[59] who also believed that a metatarsal bursa in this location may play a role in the mechanism of injury.

The mechanism proposed by Betts,[57] with proximal tethering and distal stretching of the nerve during certain foot actions, is similar to that we have proposed for the susceptibility of the radial sensory nerve to injury and peripheral nerve entrapment (as described in Chapter 11). The radial sensory nerve exits from deep to superficial through the fascia along the side of the brachioradialis tendon. It is proximally tethered it at this location, and it becomes subject to stretch and shearing forces with ulnar flexion of the wrist and gripping and pinching movements of the fingers because the nerve is required to carry out a significant excursion during these motions. Additionally, the radial sensory nerve can be compressed between the two tendons, the brachioradialis and extensor carpi radialis longus, during supination and pronation, just as the common plantar digital nerve may be compressed between the two metatarsal heads. Thus, shearing and stretching forces, as well as intermittent direct compression, can contribute to a repetitive trauma disorder of a peripheral nerve resulting in significant symptoms and histopathologic changes.

The intraoperative findings are suggestive of an in-continuity neuroma (Figs 13-10 to 13-12). In reality, however, the pathologic findings as described by King in 1946,[60] and more recently by Lassman et al in 1976,[61] demonstrate that a classic neuroma is not present (Fig. 13-12b). Instead, the individual fascicles within the common plantar nerve are surrounded by markedly thickened perineurium and interfascicular epineurium. There is Wallerian degeneration and loss of the large myelinated fibers in varying degrees, depending on the degree of the compression. There is not a disorganized mass of randomly oriented regenerating neural units, as would be seen in a classic neuroma (see Chapter 17). Lassman et al constructed nerve fiber histograms on the excised "neuromas" and found by morphometric analysis that the specimens more resembled the reported cases of chronic human nerve compression.[61]

Diagnosis

The diagnosis of a Morton's neuroma is based on a history compatible with pain with walking, centered about the metatarsal heads and most commonly between the third and fourth metatarsal heads, which shoots into the toes, most commonly the third or fourth toe, with relief when the foot is rested or elevated. There is usually no worsening of pain during the night. There is, on physical examination, pain elicited by pressure in the web space between the metatarsal heads with the pain most commonly directed toward the fourth, but also toward the third, toe. Mulder[59] has described a physical finding in which compression on the medial and lateral aspects of the foot can produce a clicking sound with a palpable bulge in the web space between the third and fourth toes on its plantar aspect as the neuroma is forced plantarward by the metatarsal heads coming together, with reproduction of the patient's symptoms. Gauthier[62] has noted pain with forced extension of either the metatarsal or interphalangeal joint, and relief with joint flexion. There may be a detectable sensory change in the web space between the third and fourth toes in comparison with the opposite foot. A diagnostic nerve block with lidocaine in the web space should remove the patient's symptoms and permit the patient to walk without the occurrence of pain. Electrodiagnostic studies may be useful in ruling out more proximal sites of compression, such as the medial and lateral plantar nerves in the tarsal tunnel.

Surgical Technique

There appears to be today a general consensus that the appropriate treatment for Morton's neuroma is excision of the involved nerve. Historically, however, this has certainly not been the case nor is this treatment in conformity with our general approach to the problem of nerve compressions elsewhere in the body. Morton[56] believed that the problem was initiated by pressure from the metatarsal head against the common plantar nerve, and therefore he recommended resection of the fourth metatarsal head. This was his treatment of choice and was the treatment practiced for almost a half century. When his original writing is carefully read for each case report, it is clear, however, that in addition to resecting the metatarsal head, he also resected the common plantar nerve and the accompanying compressed "soft parts" adjacent to the bone. With the description by King[60] of pathologic changes in the common plantar nerve that resembled grossly a neuroma, attention was directed to the nerve, itself, and resection of the common plantar nerve to a level proximal to the intermetatarsal ligament was recommended. Betts[57] in 1940 may have been the first to recommend this treatment. Nissen[58] recommended a plantar approach for the neurectomy, but at the present time, despite the more difficult exposure, a dorsal approach seems to be the one most commonly in use. The digital nerve should be divided proximal to the intermetatarsal ligament and is usually resected at the point where the swelling is observed in the nerve. An approach that is more consistent with the mechanism of the nerve compression is described by Gauthier,[62] in 1979, and in his experience with more than 200 patients, demonstrates that division of the intermetatarsal ligament alone may be successful in relief of the pain from Morton's neuroma.

Our approach to Morton's metatarsalgia is based upon that outlined for any compressed peripheral nerve. A period of nonoperative management, attempting to alter the patient's activities, orthotics, or appropriate change in footwear and general patient awareness of the problem. After 3 months of this to improve the patient's symptoms, cortisone injection between the metatarsal heads would appear warranted. Failing this, in a patient whose symptoms have not been of an extremely long duration and who is not totally incapacitated by pain, would appear to be a surgical approach through a dorsal incision with simple division of the intermetatarsal ligament. At that time, an intraneural

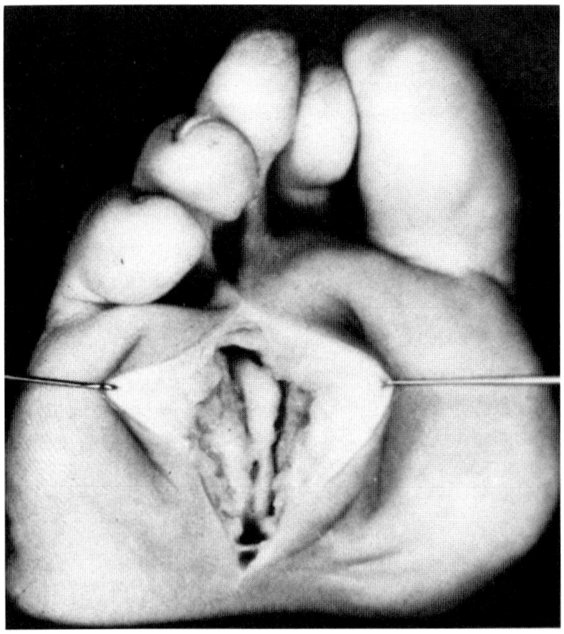

a

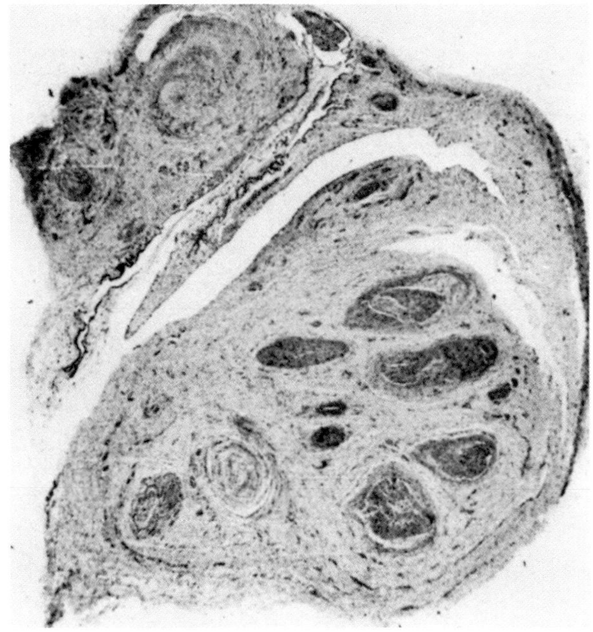

b

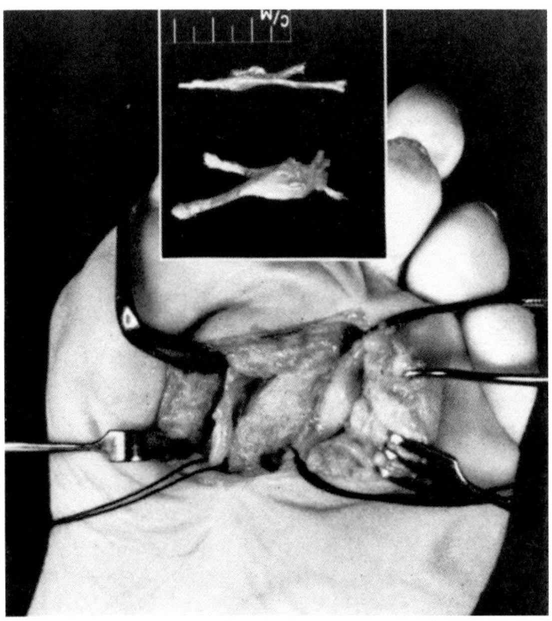

c

Figure 13-12. Intraoperative view of Morton's neuroma on common plantar digital nerve to the third and fourth web spaces, viewed through a plantar approach. **a.** Most common finding, a fusiform swelling on the nerve. **b.** Histopathologic study of excised neuroma shows not a neuroma but multiple small fascicles each surrounded by dense intraneural fibrosis. Within the fascicles there is Wallerian degeneration and loss of nerve fibers, rather than a degeneration and loss of nerve fibers, rather than a disorganized mass of randomly regenerating neural units as seen in classic neuromas. **c.** Example of multiple plantar nerve involvement with excised "neuromas" shown in inset. Note upper one has two nerves (from right) contributing to the common plantar (medial and lateral plantar), whereas the specimen from the second and third web spaces (below) has just one contributing. Toward the left in each specimen are the two branches to the adjacent sides of toes in the web space. (Reproduced with permission from Seddon.[2])

neurolysis should be carried out of the plantar digital nerve. If radiographically there are signs of bone problems with the metatarsal head or if other orthopedic reasons seem appropriate, a metatarsal head resection might be done. This approach attempts to relieve the compressive and shear forces that are operative in this distal region of direct compression. No surgical approach is taken to relieve the proximal tethering of the plantar nerves about the flexor digitorum brevis. If the intraneural dissection suggested severe damage to the fascicles, so that there were no perineurial markings and so that the nerve was translucent, suggestive of severe Wallerian degeneration, and if the surgical exposure was such that a good proximal level of resection could be obtained, then a primary resection of this severely damaged nerve might be warranted at this time. Resection of the involved plantar digital nerve, however, might be more appropriately reserved for patients in whom relief of the compressive forces and neurolysis has failed. Resection of a proximal neuroma, as described in the preceding paragraph, would be recommended as the treatment of choice for a "recurrent" metatarsalgia in which

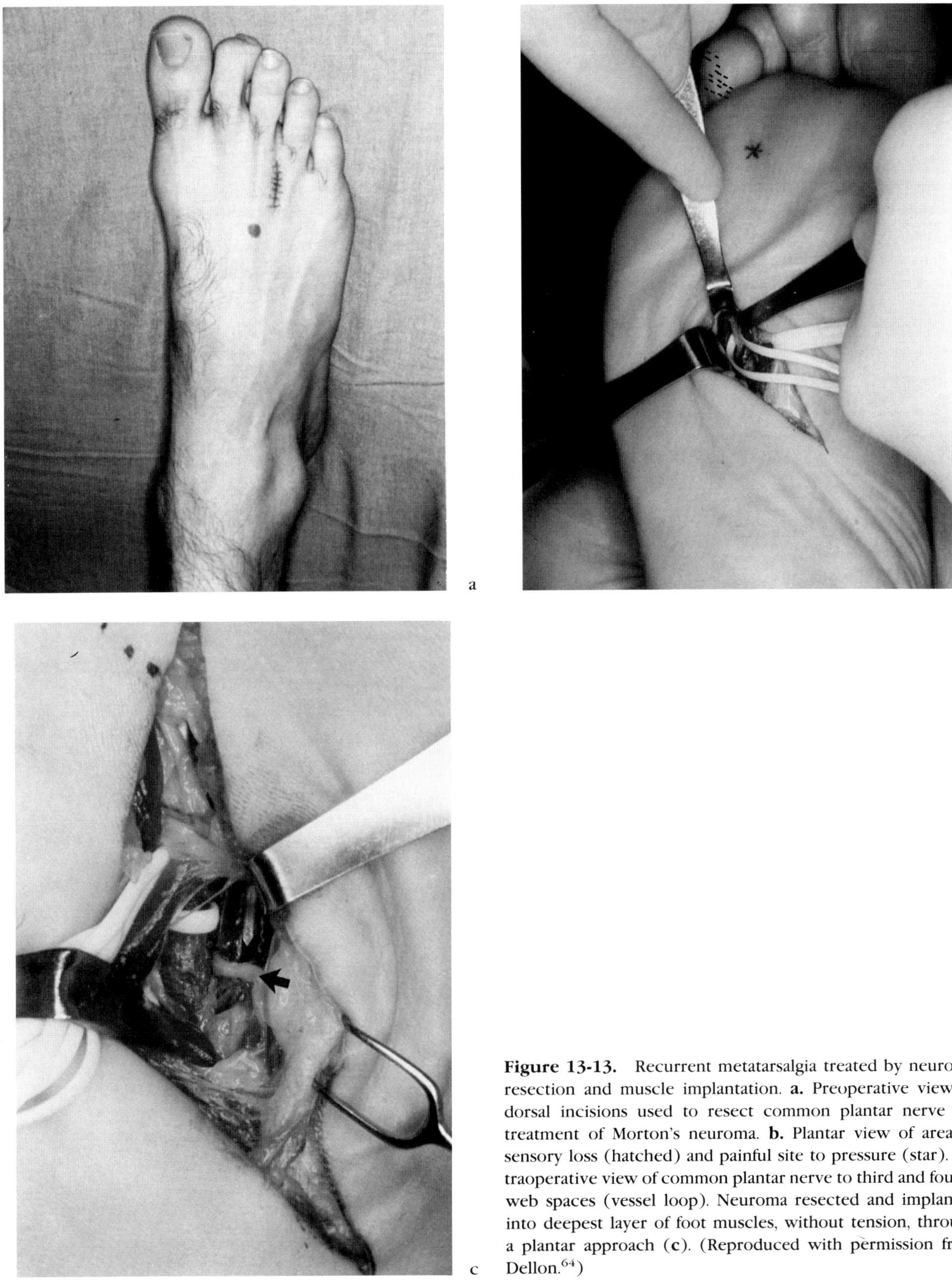

a

b

c

Figure 13-13. Recurrent metatarsalgia treated by neuroma resection and muscle implantation. **a.** Preoperative view of dorsal incisions used to resect common plantar nerve for treatment of Morton's neuroma. **b.** Plantar view of area of sensory loss (hatched) and painful site to pressure (star). Intraoperative view of common plantar nerve to third and fourth web spaces (vessel loop). Neuroma resected and implanted into deepest layer of foot muscles, without tension, through a plantar approach (**c**). (Reproduced with permission from Dellon.[64])

the initial operation was resection and the subsequent recurrence of pain was due to a true neuroma at the proximal site where the nerve had regenerated distally.

Results

There are few studies on the long-term results of treatment of Morton's neuroma despite the fact that the problem is so common and has been recognized for so long. Betts,[57] in 1940, operated on 19 patients with 100% excellent results. Nissen,[58] in 1948, subdivided his patients into those with a "recent" or "early" presentation versus those who presented "late" for treatment. Ten of 11 in his "early" group and 15 of 16 in his "late" group had excellent results with no pain. In contrast to these results with neuroma resection stands Gauthier's[62] report in 1979 of 304 neuromas in 204 patients treated by release of the intermetatarsal ligament. Although there was no neuroma resection, he did do an epineurectomy. His results were 83% excellent, 14% improved, 3% no change with a mean follow-up of 21 months. His results were determined by a second, independent observer.[62]

The great surprise is that so many persons have been helped by a treatment that resects the chronically compressed nerve, leaving its proximal end to form, in the natural course of nerve healing, a neuroma. If the proximal extent of resection is not sufficiently proximal, then the neuroma will grow and in its attempt to reinnervate its distal denervated plantar skin, will regenerate distally, causing branches to become again in contact with compressive and stretching forces. Thus, it would seem that a likely result after resection of a common plantar digital nerve would be some remaining pain in a significant portion of persons and significant pain in a smaller portion of persons from the subsequent neuroma formation. In the most recent extensive report given at the February 1988 meeting of the Foot and Ankle Society, excellent results were reported following "neuroma" resection, thus supporting the position that neural regeneration with recurrent symptoms must occur more commonly than previously described.[63]

Complications

We have encountered two patients with recurrent pain after Morton's neuroma resection. The first was in a teenage male runner, who had been approached through a dorsal incision and then reapproached through the dorsal incision and then finally had to give up running. Based on the experience with treatment of upper extremity neuromas by muscle implantation, this young runner was approached through a plantar incision. A muscle of minimal excursion and stretch was sought and the neuroma identified and resected (this treatment is outlined in Chapter 17 for the upper extremity neuromas). The proximal portion of the nerve was then implanted into the deepest layer of the foot muscles, the adductor hallucis. The result obtained was such that the patient has been able to resume competitive running (Fig. 13-13).[64] A similar successful outcome was obtained with another patient who was sufficiently crippled by her recurrent metatarsalgia pain that she required a wheelchair because she could not ambulate. After the neuroma resection and implantation into the adductor hallucis, she is able to walk without a crutch.

References

1. Joplin RJ: The proper digital nerve, vitallium stem arthroplasty and some thoughts about foot surgery in general. Clin Orthop 76:199–212, 1971.
2. Sarrafian SK: Anatomy of the Foot and Ankle. JB Lippincott, Philadelphia, 1983.
3. Seddon H: Surgical Disorders; of the Peripheral Nerves. Williams & Wilkins, Baltimore, 1972.
4. Sunderland S: Nerves and Nerve Injuries. Churchill Livingston, Edinburgh, 1978.
5. Omer GE Jr, Spinner M: Management of Peripheral Nerve Problems. WB Saunders, Philadelphia, 1980.
6. Dawson DM, Hallet M, Millendes LH: Entrapment Neuropathies. Little, Brown, Boston, 1983.
7. Selig S: Peroneal paralysis due to compression by adhesive plaster. J Bone Joint Surg 20:222–223, 1938.
8. Burkhardt FL, Daly JW: Sciatic and peroneal nerve injury: A complication of vaginal operations. Obstet Gynecol 28: 99–101, 1966.
9. Woltman HW: Crossing the legs as a factor in the production of peroneal palsy. JAMA 93:670–672, 1929.
10. Berry H, Richardson PM: Common peroneal nerve palsy: A clinical and electrophysiological review. J Neurol Neurosurg Psychiatry 39:1162–1171, 1962.
11. Sandhu HS, Sandberg BS: Occupational compression of the common peroneal nerve at the neck of the fibula. Aust NZ Surg 46:160–163, 1976.
12. Chusid JG: Yoga foot drop. JAMA 217:827–828, 1971.
13. Perrin E, Labry R: La fracture de l'asophyse, styloide, du Peronee. Rev Orthop 13:325–331, 1926.
14. Lyle HHM: Traumatic luxation of the head of the fibula. Ann Surg 82:635–639, 1925.
15. Ferguson JA, Allen L: Complete medial dislocation of the knee joint with division of the common peroneal nerve. J Bone Joint Surg 21:1012–1014, 1939.
16. Meals RA: Peroneal nerve palsy complicating ankle sprain. J Bone Joint Surg 59A:966–968, 1977.
17. Muckart RD: Compression of the common peroneal nerve by intramuscular ganglion from the superior tibiofibular joint. J Bone Joint Surg 58B:241–244, 1976.
18. Rose HA, Hood RW, Otis JC, Ranawat CS, Insall JN: Peroneal nerve palsy following total knee arthroplasty. J Bone Joint Surg 64A:347–351, 1982.
19. Aasar YH: A peculiar relation of the femoral head of the bicep femoris to the common peroneal nerve. J Anat 72:305, 1938.

20. Kopell HP, Thompson WAL: Peripheral Entrapment Neuropathies. Williams & Wilkins, Baltimore, 1963.
21. Brown WF, Ferguson GG, Jones MW, Yates SK: The location of conduction abnormalities on human entrapment neuropathies. J Can Sci Neurol 3:111–114, 1976.
22. Sunderland S, Bradley KC: The cross-sectional area of peripheral nerve trunks devoted to nerve fibres. Brain 72: 428–449, 1949.
23. Sunderland S, Bradley KC: Stress-strain phenomena in human peripheral nerve trunks. Brain 84:102–119, 1961.
24. Shizhen A, Xiangluo T, Muzhi L: The microanatomy of peripheral nerves. In Shizhen Z, Yongjain H, Wenchum Y, eds: Microsurgical Anatomy. MTP Press, Lancaster, 1985, pp 299–350.
25. Sunderland S, Ray LJ: The intraneural topography of the sciatic nerve and its popliteal divisions in man. Brain 71: 242–273, 1948.
26. Urushidani H: The funicular pattern of the sciatic nerve in Japanese adults. Arch Jpn Chir 43:254–275, 1974.
27. Chaise F, Roger B: Neurolysis of the common peroneal nerve in leprosy. J Bone Joint Surg 67B:426–429, 1985.
28. Dellon AL: A cause for optimism in diabetic neuropathy. Ann Plast In Surg 20:103–105, 1988.
29. Marinacci AA: Neurological syndromes of the tarsal tunnels. Bull Los Angeles Neurol Soc 33:90–100, 1968.
30. Marinacci AA: Applied Electromyography. Lea & Febiger, Philadelphia, 1968.
31. Krause KH, Witt T, Ross A: The anterior tarsal tunnel syndrome. J Neurol 217:67–74, 1977.
32. Rash MR: Entrapment of the anterior tibial nerve: Report of a case treated surgically. J Neurol Orthop Surg 1:153, 1980.
33. Borges LF, Hallett M, Selkoe DJ, Welch K: The anterior tarsal tunnel syndrome. J Neurosurg 54:89–92, 1981.
34. Gessini L, Jandols B, Pietrangeli A: The anterior tarsal tunnel syndrome. J Bone Joint Surg 66A:786–787, 1984.
35. Dellon AL: Entrapment of the deep peroneal nerve over the dorsum of the foot. Foot Ankle, Oct., 1990.
36. Anatomical Society of Great Britain and Ireland: Report of Committee of Collective Investigation on the Distribution of Cutaneous Nerves on the Dorsum of the Foot. J Anat Physiol 26:89–90, 1892.
37. Kosinski C: The course, mutual relations and distribution of the cutaneous nerves of the metagional region of the leg and foot. J Anat 60:274–297, 1926.
38. Horowitz MT: Normal anatomy and variations with the peripheral nerves of the leg and foot. Arch Surg 36:626–636, 1938.
39. Kenzora JE: Symptomatic incisional neuromas on the dorsum of the foot. Foot Ankle 5:2–15, 1984.
40. Bryce TH: The long muscular branch of the musculo cutaneous nerve of the leg. J Anat 31:5–12, 1896.
41. Winckler G: Le nerf peronies accessorie profound: Etude d'anatomie comparee. Arch Anat (Strasbourg) 18:181, 1934.
42. Lambert EH: The accessory deep peroneal nerve: A common variation in innervation of the extensor digitorum brevis. Neurology (Minneap) 19:1169–1176, 1969.
43. Gutmann L: Atypical deep peroneal neuropathy in the presence of accessory deep peroneal nerve. J Neurol Neurosurg Psychiatry 33:453–456, 1970.
44. Kopell HP: Lower extremity lesions, In Omer GE Jr, Spinner M: Management of Peripheral Nerve Problems. WB Saunders, Philadelphia, 1980.
45. Garfin S, Mubarak SJ, Owen CA: Excertional anterolateral compartment syndrome. Case report with a fascial defect, muscle herniation and superficial peroneal nerve entrapment. J Bone Joint Surg 59A:404–405, 1977.
46. Matsen FA III: Compartmental Syndromes. Grune & Stratton, New York, 1980.
47. Sridhara CR, Izzo KL: Terminal sensory branches of the superficial peroneal nerve: An entrapment syndrome. Arch Phys Med Rehabil 66:789–792, 1985.
48. Dellon AL: Clinical use of vibratory stimuli to evaluate peripheral nerve injury and compression neuropathy. Plast Reconstr Surg 65:466–476, 1980.
49. Beatty SE, Phillips JE, Mackinnon SE, Dellon AL, O'Brien J: Vibratory sensory testing in acute compartment syndrome: A clinical and experimental study. Plast Reconstr Surg 79:796–801, 1987.
50. Hoffert MJ, Greenberg RP, Walshee PJ, Gracely RH, Werdzeh PR, Vinayakom K, Dubner R: Abnormal collateral innervations of sympathetic and peripheral sensory fields associated with causalgia. Pain 20:1–12, 1984.
51. Mackey D, Colbert DS, Chater EH: Musculocutaneous nerve entrapment. Ir J Med Sci 146:100–102, 1977.
52. Pringle RM, Protheroe K, Mukherjee SK: Entrapment neuropathy of sural nerve. J Bone Joint Surg 56B:465–468, 1974.
53. Mackinnon SE, Dellon AL, Hudson AR, Hunter DA: Histopathology of compression of the superficial radial nerve in the forearm. J Hand Surg [Am] 11:206–209, 1986.
54. Mackinnon SE, Dellon AL, Hudson AR, Hunter DA: Chronic human nerve compression: A histologic assessment. Neuropathol Appl Neurobiol 12:547–565, 1986.
55. deMaura W, Gilliert A: Surgical anatomy of the sural nerve. J Reconstr Microsurg 1:31–39, 1984.
56. Morton TG: A peculiar and painful affection of the fourth metatarsophalangeal articulation. Am J Med Sci 71:37–45, 1876.
57. Betts LO: Morton's metatarsalgia: Neuritis of the fourth digital nerve. Med J Aust 1:514–515, 1940.
58. Nissen KI: Plantar digital neuritis: Morton's metatarsalgia. J Bone Joint Surg 30B:84–94, 1948.
59. Mulder JD: The causative mechanism in Morton's metatarsalgia. J Bone Joint Surg 33B:94–95, 1951.
60. King LSL: Note on the pathology of Morton's metatarsalgia. Am J Clin Pathol 16:124–128, 1946.
61. Lassman G, Lassman H, Stockinger L: Morton's metatarsalgia: Light and electron microscopic observations and their relation to entrapment neuropathies. Virchow's Arch [A] 370:307–321, 1976.
62. Gauthier G: Thomas Morton's disease: A nerve entrapment syndrome. Clin Orthop 142:90–92, 1979.
63. Parr J, Johnson K: Interdigital neuroma treated by neuroma resection. Presented at the Foot and Ankle Society meeting, February 1988, Atlanta, Georgia.
64. Dellon AL: Treatment of recurrent metatarsalgia by neuroma resection and muscle implantation. Microsurg 10:256–259, 1989.

Multiple Crush Syndrome

14

Historical Review

Multiple crush syndrome is a symptom complex due to compression of a peripheral nerve at more than one site of entrapment. In its simplest form, this syndrome was described on a purely theoretical basis by Upton and McComas in 1973.[1] They had made the clinical observation that 70% of their patients had either carpal tunnel syndrome or ulnar neuropathy associated with evidence of cervicothoracic root lesions. Additionally, they had observed that there appeared to be an increased association between patients with metabolic neuropathy, such as diabetes, and carpal tunnel syndrome. They hypothesized that serial constraints on axoplasmic flow, each insufficient by itself to cause a symptomatic nerve compression syndrome, could summate to cause symptomatic neural dysfunction (Fig. 14-1). Thus, in cervical arthritis, the neural foramin would serve as one site of nerve entrapment, and this proximal site would cause the more distal portion of the peripheral nerve, contributed to by this cervical root, to be more susceptible to nerve compression. This susceptibility would be based on the decreased axoplasmic flow induced by the proximal site of compression, creating a situation, for example, in which carpal tunnel syndrome would occur at the site where the median nerve is compressed by the transverse carpal ligament at the wrist. An area of compression across the brachial plexus, such as at the thoracic outlet, would create a decrease in axoplasmic flow that would make the more peripheral portions of the nerve susceptible to a more distal nerve compression, such as the ulnar nerve in the cubital tunnel. Subsequent to this first report by Upton and McComas, which was published in the "Hypothesis Section" of *The Lancet,* other researchers began to publish series of patients confirming the frequent association of a proximal and a distal nerve compression syndrome. The term coined by Upton and McComas, "the double crush syndrome," thereby entered our medical terminology.[2,3]

Massey et al,[2] in 1981, reported on 19 patients who had a coexisting carpal tunnel syndrome and cervical radiculopathy, most commonly at C6 or C7. They also reported on four patients with brachial plexus compression and coexisting carpal tunnel syndrome. Their patients had radiographic and electrodiagnostic studies confirming the cervical radiculopathy and cervical arthritis and clinical and electrodiagnostic studies confirming the plexopathy and the carpal tunnel syndrome. In their discussion of the double crush syndrome, they attempted a theoretical explanation: (1) Underlying susceptibility of the peripheral nerves in some persons to pressure; (2) a proximal axon lesion rendering the distal nerve more vulnerable to pressure by impairing distal energy metabolism;[4] (3) proximal interruption of lymphatic or venous drainage, rendering the distal nerves more vulnerable to entrapment; (4) endoneurial edema at either the proximal or distal site,

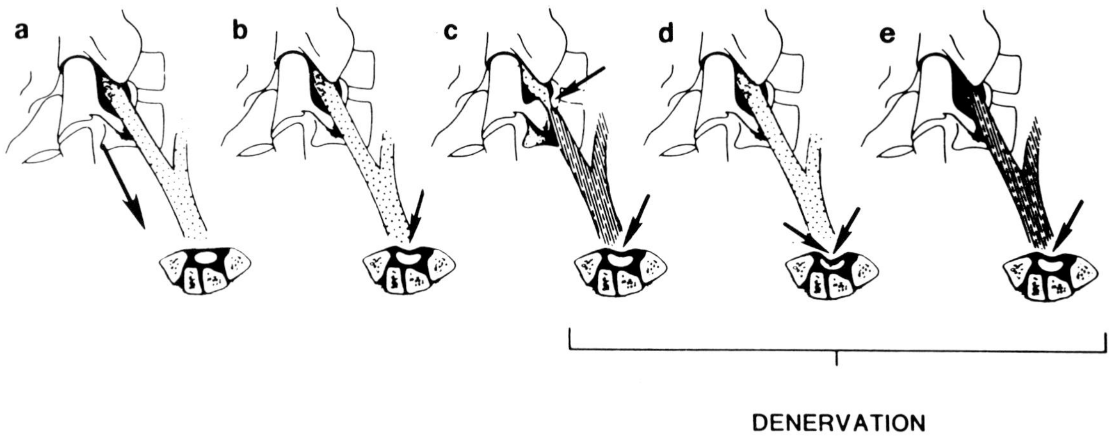

Figure 14-1. Diagrammatic representation of the double crush syndrome. The normal spine, median nerve, and carpal tunnel. The large black arrow represents the antegrade axoplasmic flow. **a.** Note the normal appearance of the exit of the root from the cervical spine and the normal configuration of the transverse carpal ligament and median nerve. **b.** The symptomatic threshold, that is, denervation, has not been reached, despite the fact that there is mild median nerve compression at the level of the carpal tunnel (small black arrow). **c.** There is impingement of the cervical root (upper black arrow) with abnormal axoplasmic flow as exemplified by the parallel lines in the nerve with distal mild carpal tunnel syndrome noted at the lower black arrow. A combination of the proximal and distal impingements with the associated impairment of axoplasmic flow by the proximal lesion results in denervation and symptoms because the symptomatic threshold has been surpassed. **d.** Cervical roots are normal, axoplasmic flow is normal, but there is a severe distal carpal tunnel syndrome (at the double black arrow) and the result is symptomatic carpal tunnel syndrome secondary to denervation. **e.** Abnormal axoplasmic flow is diagrammatically represented by the parallel lines in the nerve. This, combined with mild carpal tunnel impingement at the black arrow, results in denervation, and once again symptoms, because the safety margin has been surpassed by the combination of the peripheral neuropathy, such as diabetes, plus the mild carpal tunnel syndrome. (Reproduced with permission from Hurst et al.[3])

rendering axons or sheath at the other site more vulnerable to negligible trauma;[5] or (5) connective tissue abnormality to both conditions.[6] The most careful clinical study attempting to determine whether there was a statistically significant increased relationship of a proximal and distal nerve entrapment syndrome is the study by Hurst et al.[3] Published in 1985, this study reviewed a previously reported series of patients by Carroll and Hurst,[7] to compare the occurrence of bilateral carpal tunnel syndrome (1000 cases in 888 patients) with the occurrence of bilateral carpal tunnel syndrome in those patients in the series with diabetes mellitus and those with cervical arthritis. Eleven percent of the 888 patients in their series had cervical arthritis and in this subgroup, 41% had bilateral carpal tunnel syndrome; a correlation of bilateral carpal tunnel syndrome with cervical arthritis is significant at the $p < .005$ level. The diabetic patients in that series represented 7% of the 888 patients (compared with an incidence of diabetes in the general population of 1.7%[8]), and of this population with diabetes in the Hurst et al series,[3] 34% had bilateral carpal tunnel syndrome. In contrast, the next largest subgroup in their series, those patients with previous distal radius fracture (9% of their 888 patients), only four (5%) had bilateral carpal tunnel syndrome. Hurst et al conceptualized diagramatically the serial constraints that result when a proximal site of entrapment, or a metabolic neuropathy, results in decreased axoplasmic flow, thereby predisposing the nerve to symptomatic dysfunction (which they termed "denervation") (Fig. 14-1). They postulated a "safety margin" existing to "denervation," which when surpassed leads to these clinical symptoms. In their discussion, Hurst et al[3] suggest that the bilateral incidence of carpal tunnel syndrome noted with cervical arthritis would have a basis in the almost universal incidence of bilateral cervical arthritis noted in persons above the age of 50 years.[9,10] They also suggested that this proximal site of compression may be one of the explanations for the failure of some patients to respond to the usually effective surgical decompression of the carpal tunnel, and used the double crush syndrome as an explanation for other workers' early observation that there is frequently electrodiagnostic evidence of neural dysfunction proximal to the site of a distal nerve entrapment.[11]

The first experimental study to test the double crush hypothesis was reported in 1983.[12] In that study, the rat sciatic nerve model for chronic nerve compression[13,14] was extended to a series of two bands, one placed proximal to the sciatic nerve trifurcation and one placed about the posterior tibial nerve just distal to the trifurcation. The proximal band was placed bilaterally in these rats (Fig. 14-2). Four months later, the second, distal, band was placed. Four months after placement of the second band, electrodiagnostic studies were carried out directly from the nerves, stimulating proximal to the first band and recording bilaterally from both sciatic nerves at the same site distal to the second nerve entrapment location on the posterior tibial nerve. The results demonstrated a significant prolongation of motor latency between the double crush side and its contralateral, nonbanded, control side (1.85 versus 1.28 msec, $p < 0.001$) and between the now 8 months, single-banded, sciatic nerve (1.85 versus 1.54 msec, $p < 0.05$). There was no significant difference between the latency of the 8 months', single-banded and its control, contralateral, nonbanded sciatic nerve. There was a significant decrease in amplitude between the 4 months' double-crush and its control, nonbanded, contralateral sciatic nerve (6.7 versus 13.5 mv, $p < 0.025$) and the 8 months' single-banded sciatic nerve (6.7 versus 9.6 mv, $p < 0.05$). These results suggested that the presence of a proximal area of nerve compression in a rat, insufficient to produce changes in electrical activity of the sciatic nerve by itself, rendered the nerve more likely to develop significant electrical changes when a second band was placed distally than if the single band were left in place twice as long (Fig. 14-2).

Further basic biologic explanations for the double crush syndrome and the so-called reverse double crush syndrome were given by Lundborg.[15] Writing in a correspondence newsletter to the members of The Amer-

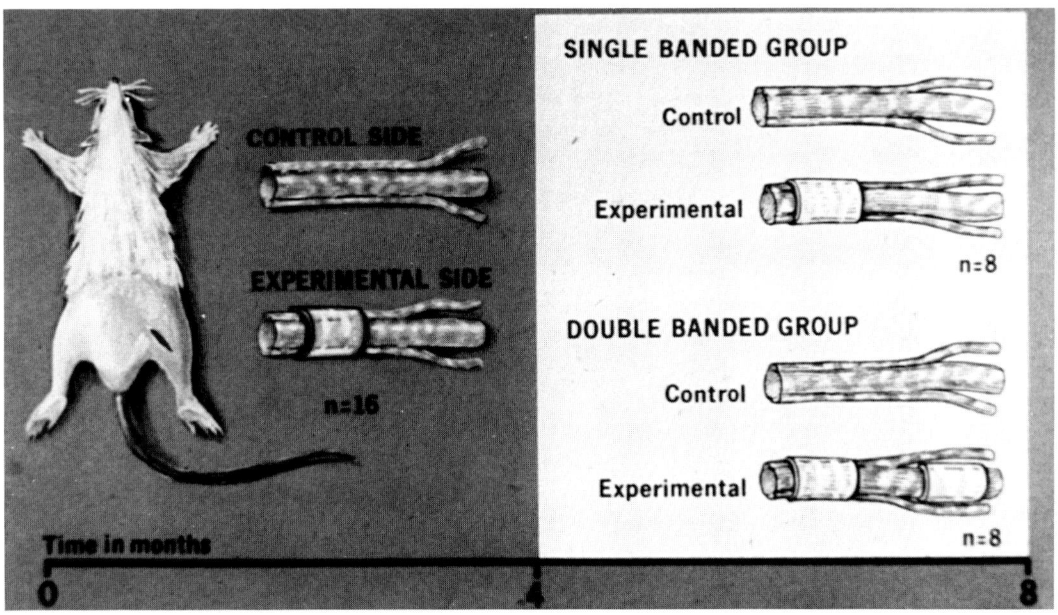

Figure 14-2. Diagrammatic representation of protocol for the first experimental study providing evidence for existence of the double crush syndrome. On each animal, the left side served as a nonbanded control, although the sciatic nerve on the right side of the rat was singly banded in all animals at the start of the procedure. After 4 months, by which time no electrical changes had occurred (a proximal single crush had been created that caused impairment of axoplasmic flow but had not created symptoms), a second band was placed distal to the sciatic nerve trifurcation in half of the animals. After another 4 months, the electrodiagnostic studies were carried out (see text for results). (Reproduced with permission from Seiler et al. [12])

ican Society for Surgery of the Hand in October, 1985, Lundborg confirmed that clinically he had noticed not only cases in which proximal nerve compressions were followed by distal nerve compressions, as Upton and McComas had hypothesized, but that there were cases in which a distal nerve entrapment preceded the subsequent development of a proximal nerve entrapment. "A typical example is a patient subjected to wrist trauma resulting in signs and symptoms indicating an ulnar nerve compression lesion in Guyon's canal. After some time, the same patient starts complaining of medial elbow pain, and that clinical examination shows weakness of the profundus muscle to the little finger, numbness of the dorsal ulnar aspect of the hand, signs typical for ulnar nerve compression at the elbow level." Lundborg's explanation for the original double crush syndrome is similar to that of Upton and McComas in that a very limited compression of a nerve may partially block axonal transport and jeopardize the necessary supply of materials to the distal parts of the axon. The result is obvious: "Alterations in structure and function of distal axonal portions make this part of the nerve less resistant to trauma and a limited local increase in tissue pressure might result in a (distal) entrapment syndrome at this level. This may serve as a good explanation of why cervical root problems can predispose for development of carpal tunnel syndrome." Lundborg gives a hypothetical explanation for the reverse double crush syndrome: "The interaction between the cell body and its target organ, the constant balance interaction between center and periphery. The cell body is under a constant trophic influence from its innervation territory. These trophic factors are transported retrogradely in the axon to the cell body. With a distal compression of the nerve, this retrograde axonal transport might be compromised and the metabolic machinery of the nerve's cell body may be jeopardized. A sick nerve cell body cannot manage the antegrade axonal transport and for this reason also the proximal portion of the axons will suffer from lack of material required to keep the axonal membrane in proper function. For these reasons, these axons may become less resistant to compression, and the distal entrapment has thereby predisposed to a more proximal compression lesion."

An experimental model that tested both the proximal effect on subsequent distal susceptibility to entrapment and of initial distal entrapment on the subsequent proximal susceptibility to further entrapment and compared single entrapment to simultaneous double entrapment has been completed (Fig. 14-3).[16] In this study, the model for banding of rat sciatic nerve[13,14] was utilized. At the initial time period, one group of rats had a single band placed proximally, another group of rats had a single band placed distally to the sciatic nerve

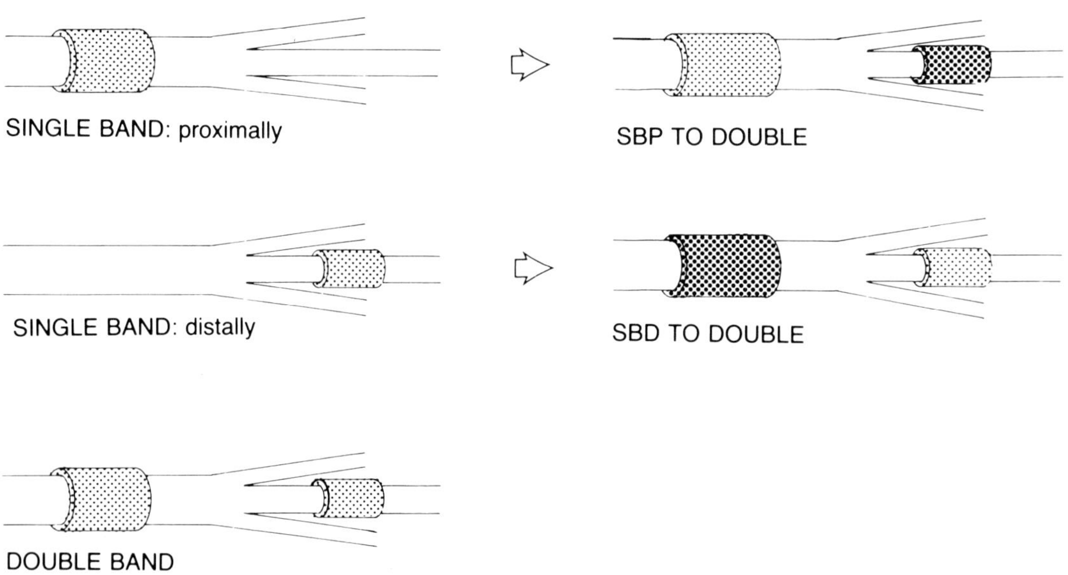

Figure 14-3. Schematic diagram protocol for a double crush syndrome experiment evaluating both proximal and distal initial sites of compression. In the left, three separate groups of rats were banded, with the single banding being either proximal (SBP), or distal (SBD), and in another group of animals, two bands were placed simultaneously. At a later time (see Fig. 14-4), a second band was placed distal to the sciatic trifurcation or proximal to the sciatic trifurcation to complete the double banding in the first two groups of rats. (Reproduced with permission from Dellon and Mackinnon.[16])

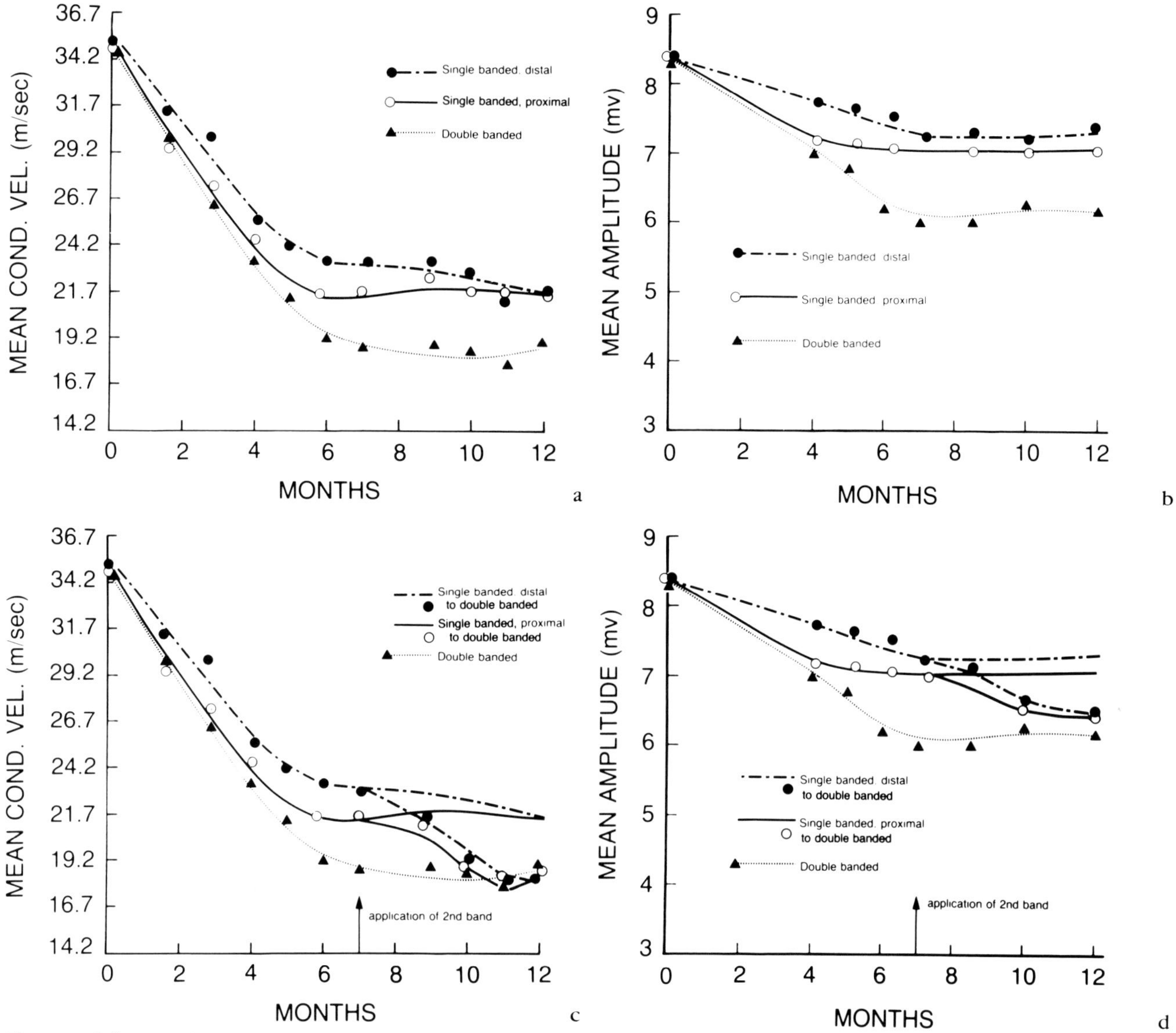

Figure 14-4. Results of double crush experiment with results expressed in terms of conduction velocity (a, c) and amplitude of the compound action potential (b, d). **a, b.** Demonstration of electrical changes for the three groups that were banded either singly, proximally, or distally, or doubly banded simultaneously from the start of the experiment. The changes plateaued by 6 months. **c, d.** At 7 months, a second band was added to complete the proximal or distal banding. Note that within 2 to 3 months of banding there were further changes in conduction velocity (c) and amplitude (d), demonstrating that the single banding, either proximal or distal, creates a situation in which the nerve is susceptible to a second site of compression, quickly causing significant changes in the nerve. The top figures also demonstrate that two bands placed simultaneously create a more significant degree of electrical changes than a single band. Thus, this study confirms the double crush hypothesis. (Reproduced with permission from Dellon and Mackinnon.[16])

trifurcation, and the third group of rats had both areas banded simultaneously. These animals were followed on a monthly basis with electrodiagnostic studies recording the conduction velocity and the amplitude of the compound action potential. After 6 months of banding, the degree of neural dysfunction had plateaued and the simultaneously double-banded group had a significantly greater reduction in the conduction velocity and in the amplitude of the compound action potential than did either of the singly banded groups (Fig. 14-4). The group that had the single proximal band placed had a more rapid onset of electrical dysfunction and to a more significant degree than did the group with the single band placed distally, but by 6 months, this difference was no longer significant. At 7 months into the study, a second band was placed in the previously single-banded groups to convert them into a double-banded situation. Within 2 to 3 months, each of these single-banded groups rapidly achieved the level of dysfunction of the simultaneously double-banded group, confirming that the existence of either a proximal or a distal single area of nerve entrapment predisposed the peripheral nerve to a second site of entrapment (Fig. 14-4). There is now good clinical, as well as experimental, evidence to support Upton and McComas' original double crush hypothesis.

Our own clinical observations necessitate that the double crush hypothesis or syndrome be enlarged. For example, patients have been referred with the diagnosis of "triple crush" or "quadruple crush." The patients have situations such as brachial plexopathy and carpal and cubital tunnel syndromes. Utilizing Upton and McComas' classification, these patients perhaps should be called "multiple double crush syndrome." For the patient who has compression at the cervical root level, the thoracic outlet level, and either the carpal or cubital tunnel level, the appropriate extension of Upton and McComas' concept might best be the "triple crush syndrome." If the problem were cervical, thoracic outlet, cubital tunnel, and entrapment in Guyon's canal, then perhaps a "quadruple crush" might be most appropriate. Clearly the future will be increasingly cumbersome with this terminology. Furthermore, the patient with a metabolic neuropathy may have entrapment at multiple anatomic sites. Additionally, as will be described later, in a given anatomic area, such as the antecubital area, a single nerve, or what is commonly considered a single site of nerve entrapment, may, in fact, be due to multiple discrete areas of entrapment, each of which the surgeon must addrress in the operating room; for example, the lacertus fibrosis, the crossing vascular structures, the fibrous arches at the pronator teres, and the flexor sublimis for median nerve compression. In this case, we have multiple areas of anatomic compression in the same region. Therefore we suggest the term, "multiple crush syndrome." The multiple crush syndrome would include two or more areas of axoplasmic flow decrease, but one of these may be a systemic metabolic neuropathy. The multiple crush syndrome would include widely disparate or separated areas, such as the cervical spine and the thoracic outlet and the elbow region and the wrist region, as well as it would include multiple closely connected anatomic areas of entrapment, such as those just described in the antecubital region for the median nerve (Table 14-1). Multiple crush syndrome must be distinguished from multiple separate nerve entrapments.

Table 14-1. Multiple Crush Syndromes

A. Multiple anatomic regions along a peripheral nerve
B. Multiple anatomic structures across a peripheral nerve within an anatomic region
C. Superimposed on a neuropathy
D. Combinations of the above

The patient who has a carpal tunnel syndrome coexisting with a cubital tunnel syndrome does not have a multiple crush syndrome. This patient has multiple peripheral nerve entrapments. If the patient has a carpal tunnel syndrome, a cubital tunnel syndrome, and cervical radiculopathy, he would have multiple nerves entrapped at multiple anatomic regions along each of these nerves and would have a multiple crush syndrome and multiple nerve entrapments.

The multiple crush syndrome is a spectrum of clinical symptoms due to more than one site of nerve compression. (For a layperson explanation and example of this problem, see the Appendix C.) Each of these sites of peripheral nerve compression is sufficient to produce a decrease in axoplasmic flow but may be insufficient in and of itself to create clinical symptoms. The sequential effect of multiple constraints on axoplasmic flow summates to create an overall axonal dysfunction capable of giving clinical symptoms. If the time course of this serial constraint on axoplasmic flow is sufficiently long, any one of the sites, but most probably the more distal of the sites, will have sufficiently severe pathophysiologic and irreversible changes. Structural changes within the peripheral nerve and with its individual nerve fibers may occur, so that relief of symptoms is only possible through a surgical release of the site of nerve compression. This multiple crush hypothesis implies that a time exists, before the occurrence of these irreversible changes, in which release of just one of the multiple sites of compression may be sufficient to relieve the entire clinical symptoms. The multiple crush hypothesis implies that there will be a point in time when irreversible changes occur at more than one of the sites, so that the relief of pressure at only one of the sites will be insufficient to relieve the clinical symptoms. A clinical example of this sequence of events would be the patient with a carpal tunnel syndrome, whose symptom complex includes aching or pain that goes up the arm into the shoulder and neck area. Although radiographically there may be cervical arthritis, there is no radiculopathy demonstrated by electrodiagnostic studies, and movements of the patient's head and neck do not reproduce the pain, so that clinically the diagnosis only includes carpal tunnel syndrome. In fact, the neck and shoulder symptoms may represent compression at the neural foramen proximally due to the more severe and long-standing distal carpal tunnel syndrome. When the carpal tunnel is released, the neck and shoulder symptoms improve because the proximal dysfunction had not been present sufficiently long to cause irreversible changes at that area. A similar sequence is seen in the patient 1 or 2 years after a rear-end automobile accident, in whom diffuse aching in the neck and shoulder region is clinically believed to be related to brachial plexus compression. There is, as well, a carpal tunnel or cubital tunnel syndrome. Because the physical examination suggests that either the cubital tunnel or carpal tunnel syndrome is more severe, this distal peripheral nerve compression is surgically treated. Shortly thereafter, symptoms in the upper arm and shoulder and neck region are gone. Although such a sequence has been interpreted[7] to suggest that there never was a more proximal site of compression and, in fact, that the thoracic outlet syndrome as a diagnosis is "elusive at best," the multiple crush hypothesis offers the alternative explanation that brachial plexus compression beneath either the anterior scalene or between the clavicle and the first rib existed as a proximal site of compression but had as yet not reached the irreversible stage pathophysiologically. Thus, symptoms from this proximal site were relieved by treatment of the more distal, more severe site of compression.

The multiple crush hypothesis lends itself to additional experimental investigation. The model already described[16] could be utilized to investigate therapeutic possibilities. For example, once the second band has been placed either proximally or distally, and after a sufficient period of time has elapsed, just one of the two bands could be removed to determine the effect on the electrical dysfunction, that is, would removing one site of compression permit improvement in nerve function despite the remaining presence of the second band. The relevant time course for the therapeutic possibilities could also be investigated: after what period of time would removal of this second banded site not permit improvement in the electrical parameters studied? The multiple crush syndrome provides the explanation for the need in patients to carry out more proximal nerve releases, such as the thoracic outlet when proximal symptoms remain after distal nerve release, that is, irreversible changes have already occurred at the proximal nerve entrapment site.

The multiple crush syndrome provides the theoretical framework for understanding complex anatomic sites of nerve compression, such as the so-called thoracic outlet syndrome. This syndrome, the diagnosis of which continues to be doubted by some,[7] is difficult to establish, even by those who do believe in its existence.[17] This thoracic outlet syndrome has no general agreement for method of treatment, with first rib resection being recommended by many but the individual approach varies (transaxillary, posterior thoracotomy, or supraclavicular). Indeed, some have questioned whether first rib removal is necessary, some carry out an anterior scalenectomy in addition to a first rib resection, and some now recommend a neurolysis of the plexus, itself (see the following section). The multiple crush hypothesis provides the framework for understanding this by suggesting that the entire clinical spectrum associated with what has previously been called the thoracic outlet syndrome may be contributed to by individual anatomic structures along the course of the brachial plexus, including the anatomic abnormalities of the scalene muscles, cervical rib, congenital bands, scarring in the brachial plexus itself, the omohyoid muscle, and the actual thoracic outlet between the first rib and the clavicle. Thus, patients who have had a transaxillary first rib resection but who have persistent neck and shoulder symptoms and who have been referred to in the past as an upper thoracic outlet syndrome, may find relief by having, in addition to the previously removed first rib, a resection of the anterior scalene.[18] Patients who still have persistent symptoms after first rib removal and scalenectomy may have this on the basis of persistent scarring within the brachial plexus. The multiple crush syndrome further provides the framework for understanding patients with clinical symptoms with an underlying metabolic neuropathy. This will be discussed later in the sections on diabetic neuropathy.

The multiple crush syndrome may serve as a new testing point to evaluate theoretical constructs, such as the original double crush hypothesis did in 1973. One area for investigation is the problem of superimposed nerve compression on an underlying neuropathy. Frequently, the electrodiagnostic findings in a patient with a metabolic neuropathy are diffuse involvement of motor and sensory nerves without identifying an area of discrete pressure. The clinical results of nerve decompression in these situations, even without electrodiagnostic evidence of localized compression (as will be discussed in the section on metabolic neuropathy), have shown that many patients improve when the peripheral nerve is decompressed. Is it possible that neural function may be so compromised by a metabolic neuropathy that our electrodiagnostic techniques are not capable of discerning an area of superimposed compression? This could be evaluated by combining the model for peripheral nerve compression with models of metabolic or toxic axonopathies. Another question is whether enough serial sites of compression could occur that these multiple sequential areas could summate to give, when electrical testing is done over the most distal segment, findings in the most distal segment that are consistent with a distal axonopathy, when, in fact, what has occurred are serial chronic nerve compressions? This could be directly tested by placing serial bands along a peripheral nerve and following electrically what occurs. This would be analogous to findings that have been reported in which multiple areas of compression were placed along peripheral nerves in a diabetic primate[19] (see section on metabolic neuropathy).

Multiple Anatomic Regions Along a Peripheral Nerve

Of the possible situations in which a multiple crush syndrome can occur, the easiest to describe, and the ones within most people's experience, are the syndromes related to multiple anatomic regions of compression along a given peripheral nerve (Table 14-1). The most common series of anatomic regions for compression are: (1) Cervical neural foramina for C5-C6-C7, the brachial plexus upper trunk, the median nerve in the forearm, the median nerve in the carpal tunnel; (2) cervical neural foramina for C8-T1, the lower trunk of the brachial plexus, the ulnar nerve in the cubital tunnel, the ulnar nerve in Guyon's canal; and (3) neural foramina for L5-S1, the sciatic nerve beneath the pyriformis muscle and at the sciatic notch, the common peroneal nerve at the fibular head, and the posterior tibial nerve and its medial and lateral plantar branches at the series of tunnels at the medial side of the ankle and beneath the abductor hallucis brevis muscle. With so many persons being subjected to trauma in our high-speed society, the physician managing post-traumatic pain syndromes will see an increase in patients with diffuse upper extremity or lower extremity and neck or back, shoulder, and head concurrent complaints; symptoms that have occurred after the accident and seem not to be relieved during the first 6 to 12 months of conservative management.[17] These are examples of the multiple crush syndrome in which multiple anatomic regions are involved along the course of one or more peripheral nerves.

The diagnosis of a multiple crush syndrome due to multiple anatomic regions along the peripheral nerve will require a careful and detailed physical examination, as described in Chapter 3. Inherent in the multiple crush syndrome is the concept that the individual anatomic regions may have a nerve compression that, in and of itself, may be insufficient to cause the patient clinical symptoms. The examiner must use provocative tests, must apply pressure to the site of nerve entrapment, and must record threshold changes (vibratory testing) and muscle strength (weakness). These entrapments may not, in and of themselves, cause sufficient compression to create Wallerian degeneration and therefore muscle wasting and abnormal two-point discrimination may not be present. The examiner must have confidence in his examination techniques. As discussed in the preceding chapters for the individual nerves, nerve compression may be staged. Frequently in the multiple crush syndrome with multiple anatomic regions along a peripheral nerve, the degree of compression is not severe at any one site. Because of the summating nature of the serial constraints on axoplasmic flow, the more distal anatomic regions of compression may manifest more severe symptoms and physical findings than the more proximal sites. This has implications in determining treatment. As discussed in theoretical comments in the introductory section to this chapter, it may be possible that by relieving the most severely compressed of the anatomic regions symptoms induced at the more proximal anatomic regions of compression will also be alleviated. Accordingly, the treatment site is therefore selected based first on the examiner attempting to determine which site is the more severely compressed, and then considering which surgery has the least complications and greatest chance for success in the individual patient. It follows from this discussion that electrodiagnostic testing may not demonstrate abnormalities at any of the anatomic regions of compression along the peripheral nerve; that the more distal regions of compression along the peripheral nerve may show electrodiagnostic changes, whereas the more proximal area does not; that electrodiagnostic testing, such as the F wave, which is dependent on distal stimulation and distal recording with the electrical impulse traveling up the arm and then back down along the arm, may be prolonged; and that, although this delay is frequently taken to mean there is a problem at the brachial plexus, any of the multiple sites, or more than one of the multiple sites, may contribute to delay in this F wave.

Multiple crush syndrome after trauma, especially work-related or litigation-associated motor vehicle trauma, is difficult to manage. Frequently, these patients have lived with discomfort, uncertainty, and disability, becoming chronic pain patients and frequently carrying the reputation of "malingerers." Further complicating the situation is the fact that the patient may have had one or more operative procedures that have not been successful. It may help to manage this group of patients with a team.[17] The team should include consultation by a psychiatrist interested in chronic pain as well as a rheumatologic consultation. Expertise from orthopedic surgery, neurosurgery and hand surgery is useful. Frequently, additional diagnostic help from a neurologist is necessary. A physiatrist is a valuable member in terms of preoperative management of the patient and design of the overall therapy program for muscle strengthening. Under their care, or else at the direct order of the surgeon involved, occupational and physical therapy may be required. Expertise in electrodiagnostic testing is critical. A member skilled at management of the "myofascial syndrome" and giving trigger point injections is helpful.[20]

Because these patients commonly carry with them a diagnosis of "reflex sympathetic dystrophy" or various other unusual pain conditions it may be useful to do additional diagnostic testing, such as thermography,[21] which by demonstrating areas of coolness may show increased sympathetic tone or by demonstrating areas of heat may indicate an underlying inflammatory process. More recently, three-phase radionuclide bone scanning has been demonstrated to be both specific and sensitive in the diagnosis of reflex sympathetic dystrophy.[22] In patients who do have a sympathetic dystrophy, the third phase demonstrates diffuse increased uptake of technetium-99 material.

Many patients with multiple crush syndromes have been living with chronic pain and have developed secondary mechanisms that make their care and pain assessment difficult. Because it is difficult for the surgeon to sort out patients with preinjury psychiatric problems, who may have difficulty coping with their surgical therapy, it becomes meaningful to have a preoperative screening test to suggest which patients are having an appropriate response to their pain and identify those patients with a significant functional overlay. Toward this end, the Hendler Chronic Back Pain Questionnaire[23] has been modified for use with upper extremity pain patients.[24] This enables the surgeon to identify patients preoperatively who will benefit from psychiatric counseling in their postoperative period. (See Appendix C, and Chapter 17.)

A frequent clinical presentation in patients with multiple crush syndrome is the patient who has had the more obvious or most common nerve entrapment site already released and still has persistent symptoms. Such a patient is illustrated in Figure 14-5. This patient had a carpal tunnel syndrome treated twice but still had significant symptoms in the hand. The physical examination with attention to more proximal potential sites of nerve compression, demonstrated that with resisted middle finger sublimis function, an aching pain occurred in the forearm. With pressure over the median nerve in the proximal portion of the forearm, the patient's symptoms of numbness in the median nerve distribution and deep aching in the forearm were reproduced. On resisted forearm pronation, there was aching in the forearm. Individual manual muscle testing suggested weakness of the flexor pollicis longus and flexor digitorum profundus to the index finger. Electrodiagnostic testing, however, did not reveal a proximal site of median nerve compression. Forearm exploration was carried out and it was found that the median nerve, as well as its anterior interosseus nerve, was compressed beneath two separate fibrous arches, one from the superficial and deep head of the pronator teres, and a second more distal beneath the flexor digitorum sublimis. Release of these fibrous arches and neurolysis of the median nerve resulted in complete relief of the patient's symptoms.

The results of a cadaver study have demonstrated that the median nerve can be compressed along multiple sites in the forearm (see Chapter 7, as well as the section to follow). In essence, this study demonstrated that a series of fibrous arches can occur in this anatomic region proximal to the anatomic region at the wrist and therefore can serve as a separate anatomic site along the same peripheral nerve.[25] As increasing awareness of these multiple crush syndromes at multiple anatomic sites along peripheral nerves occur, additional investigators also are identifying these patients. For example, at The American Society for Surgery of the Hand meeting in 1985, Breidenbach et al,[26] from the hand surgery group in Louisville, Kentucky, identified 21 patients in a 2-year period who had both carpal tunnel syndrome and proximal median nerve compression in the forearm. Fourteen of these 21 had confirmatory electrodiagnostic studies at both levels.[26]

Multiple Anatomic Structures Across a Peripheral Nerve Within an Anatomic Region

Multiple crush syndrome as a concept can be applied to a given anatomic region where it is possible that multiple sites within the region can cause compression of the nerve. This is extremely significant for the median nerve in the forearm, the brachial plexus, and the radial nerve in the forearm. Although the median nerve in the forearm is discussed extensively in Chapter 7 and the radial nerve in the mid forearm and proximal forearm is discussed in Chapters 10 and 11, it is worthwhile, in order to demonstrate the concept of the multiple crush syndrome, to discuss briefly the median nerve in the forearm and then discuss extensively how the multiple crush syndrome allows an enlightened approach to the treatment of brachial plexus compressions.

One of the main sources of failure of peripheral nerve decompression surgery is the fact that the surgeon is guided by the name of the syndrome he is supposedly decompressing in the search for a particular site for nerve compression in the anatomic region. Thus, when approaching the median nerve in the forearm, the surgeon may look specifically for a problem in the pronator teres muscle, since he believes he is treating the

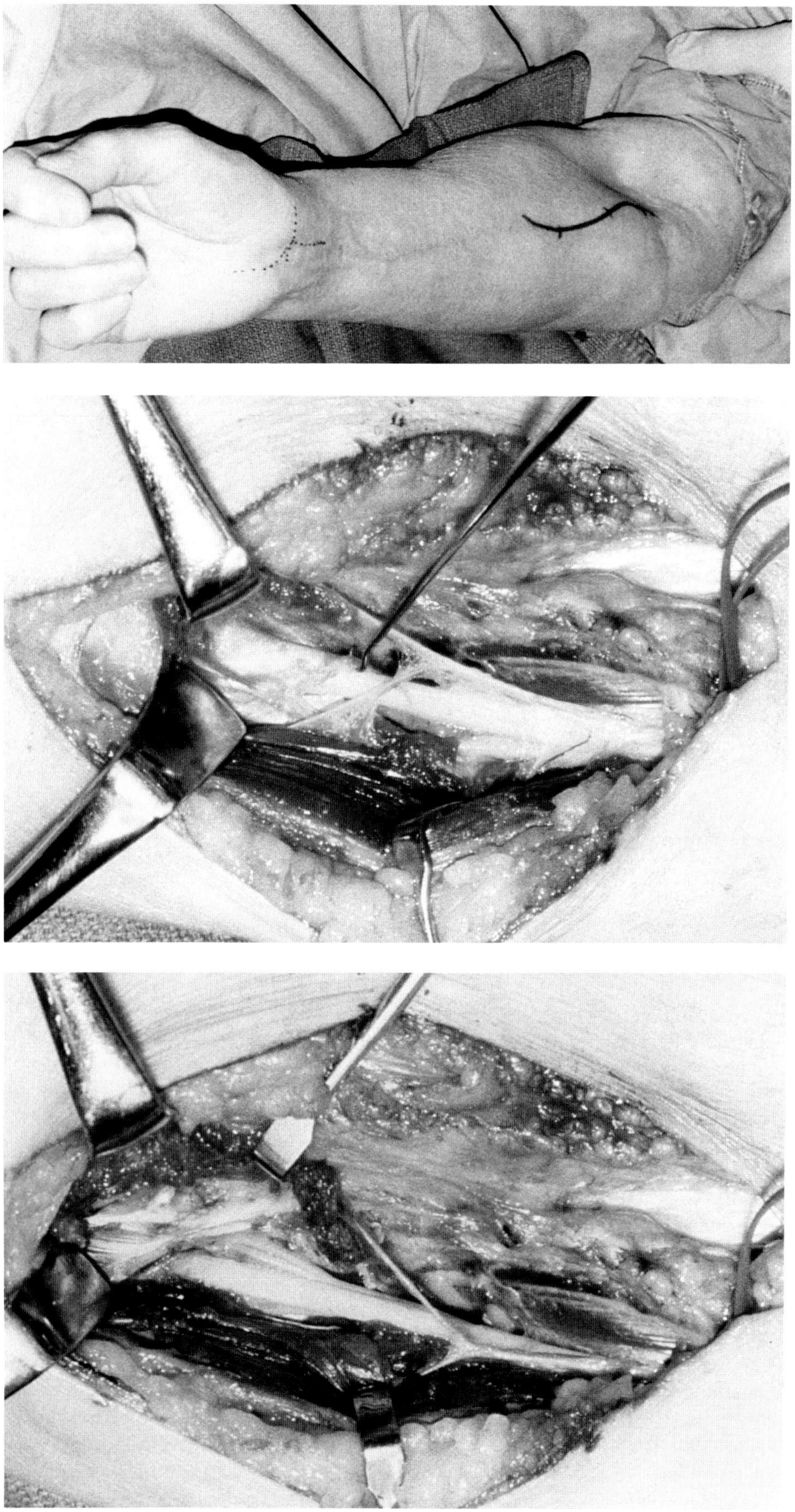

a

b

c

Figure 14-5a, b, c. (*Figure continues.*)

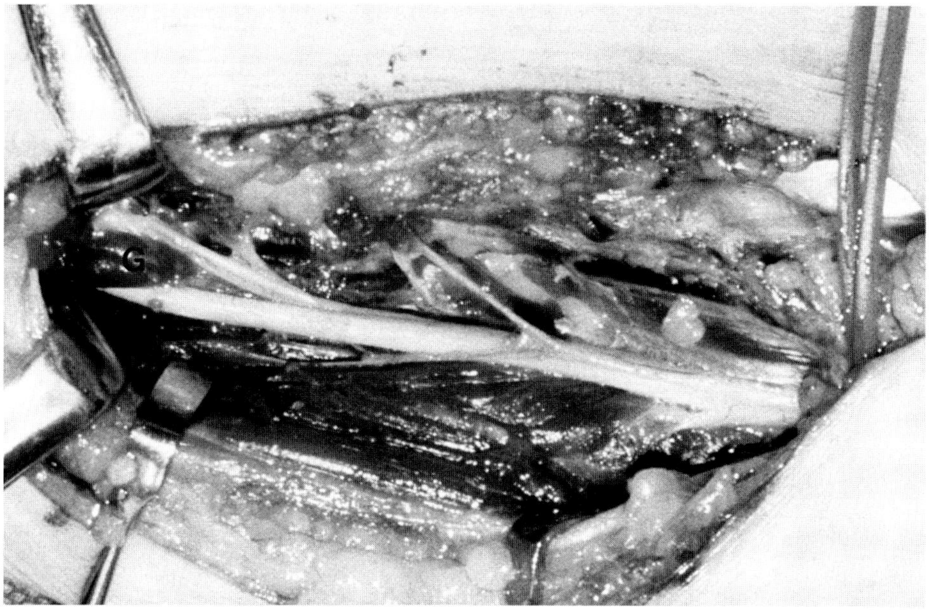

d

Figure 14-5. Clinical example of a patient with multiple crush syndrome due to multiple anatomic regions of compression along a peripheral nerve. **a.** The dotted lines indicate incision where two previous carpal tunnel releases had failed to relieve all of the patient's symptoms in this upper extremity. Careful physical examination suggested additional site of compression in the forearm. Note the "prominence" of the pronator teres muscle. Intraoperative sequence demonstrating (**b**), with the distal portion of the median nerve toward the left and the radial or lateral surface of the arm toward the top, that the superficial head of the pronator teres has been reflected down and the deep head of the pronator teres partially released in its muscular portion to leave the deep fibrous arch between the deep and superficial heads crossing the median nerve and lifted by the skin hook. **c.** The fibrous arch from the pronator group has been released and a second distal fibrous arch crosses the median nerve from the humeral head of the flexor digitorum superficialis to the superficialis head arising from the interosseous membrane. This crosses both the median nerve and the anterior interosseous nerve arising on the radial aspect of the median nerve. **d.** All structures crossing the median nerve in this anatomic region have been released and a neurolysis of the median nerve carried out. Note Gantzer's muscle (G) (The arrangement of arches in b and c may be appreciated with reference to Figure 14-6 a, and Gantzer's muscle with reference to Figure 14-6 b.)

pronator syndrome, and, in a similar fashion, the surgeon seems only to question which approach he should use to remove the first rib when he is treating a brachial plexus compression because he is directed toward the thoracic outlet.

Median Nerve Compression in the Forearm

For the median nerve in the forearm, the surgeon's approach should be one of attempting to release every possible anatomic site within this region where the median nerve can be compressed. Unfortunately, the surgeon usually does not approach the problem with this in mind. Since the description of median nerve entrapment by the pronator teres was described as the pronator syndrome by Seyffarth[27] in 1951, the surgeon treating the pronator syndrome often stops at median nerve release just in this one location. For example, in the most recent clinical series of nine patients with a pronator syndrome treated by Werner et al[28] in 1985, excellent results were obtained in only five of the nine patients. Good results were obtained in three and no improvement was found in one patient. These surgeons "followed the median nerve through the pronator teres muscle. Observations of the local anatomy were noted. The median nerve was dissected free to the sublimis arcade but the arcade was not divided."[28] As described

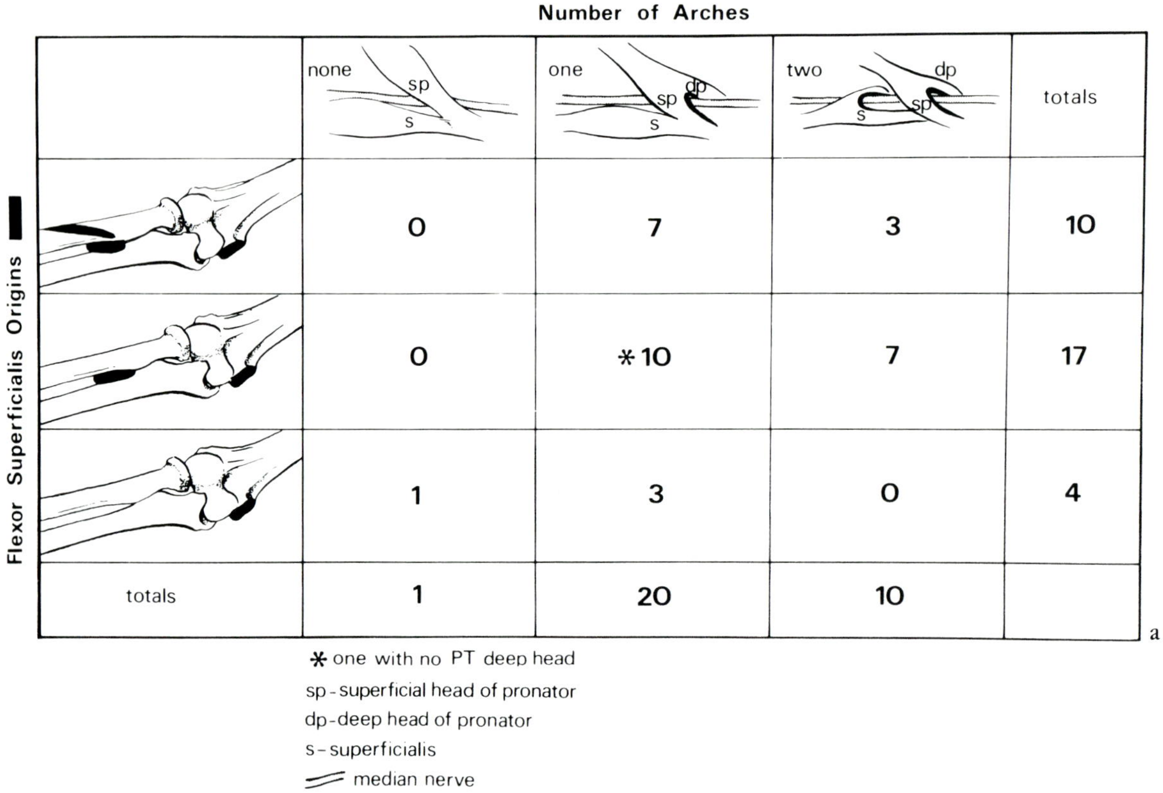

Flexor Superficialis Origins	none	one	two	totals
	0	7	3	10
	0	*10	7	17
	1	3	0	4
totals	1	20	10	

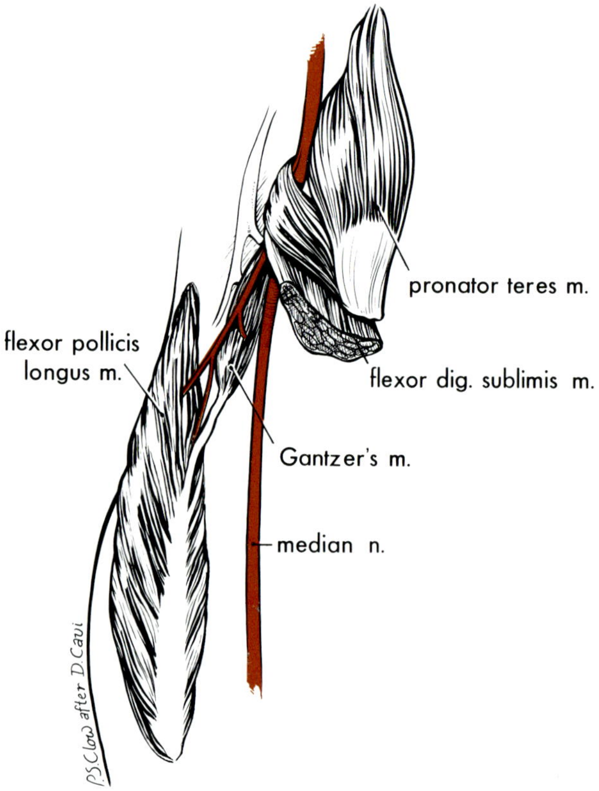

Figure 14-6. Multiple crush syndrome due to multiple anatomic structures across a peripheral nerve within an anatomic region is illustrated for the median nerve in the forearm. Above **a** is a chart from the anatomic dissections that demonstrated that across the median nerve in the forearm there may be either no arches, one arch, or two arches related to whether the pronator teres and the flexor superficialis have a deep head arising from the interosseous membrane and whether these deep heads cojoin with the superficial heads to form a single arch or whether they are separate in space, forming two distinct arches (see Fig. 15-5 for example of double arch across the median nerve. **b.** Gantzer's muscle represents an accessory head of the flexor pollicis longus. This muscle arises from the flexor pronator muscle mass from the medial humeral epicondyle and therefore is in a relationship to the median nerve and the anterior interosseous nerve such that it may contribute to compression of these nerves in this anatomic region (further description of Gantzer's muscle is given in Chapter 7). (Reproduced with permission from Dellon and Mackinnon.[25])

in the previous section and as noted in Figures 14-5 and 14-6, the deep head of the flexor sublimis arising from the interosseous membrane can form a separate independent fibrous arch over the median nerve and this can be a site of nerve entrapment.[25] Perhaps the failure to achieve excellent results in the remaining four patients in Werner et al's series was due to the fact that they did not release the sublimis arcade. The clinical diagnosis of multiple crush syndrome, as discussed in the preceding paragraph, implies that each individual anatomic site in the region may be insufficient in and of itself to cause clinical dysfunction and therefore insufficient to cause physical findings or electrodiagnostic findings to pinpoint the discrete anatomic site. Thus, in Werner et al's series, although the patients showed a positive response to resisted forearm pronation and had tenderness over the median nerve distal to the elbow, they had normal two-point discrimination, only slightly weakened grip, and normal electrodiagnostic studies. Since provocative tests can stress the nerve and create temporary ischemia, and therefore symptoms, so too may provocative tests be combined with electrodiagnostic testing. In Werner et al's report, an electrodiagnostic test done with the elbow at 30° flexion and isometric forearm pronation gave a positive test in four of their patients, implicating the pronator muscle. If, in addition, resisted sublimis muscle function had been added to their provocative testing, further delays in the motor conduction latency might have been demonstrated. Utilization of the pressure provocative test (direct pressure over the median nerve in the proximal forearm for 1 to 2 minutes) would also improve the "pickup" on electrodiagnostic testing. Although these provocative procedures have not been reported in the electrodiagnostic literature, we have found them useful in identifying the underlying entrapment at the second arch.

The anterior interosseus nerve theoretically can be compressed just distal to the site of the median nerve compression by the pronator teres muscle and thereby give symptoms purely of anterior interosseous nerve compression. Certainly, as described in 1952 by Kiloh and Nevin,[29] this can occur with a classic pattern of muscle weakness or palsy. However, with the concept of multiple crush syndrome due to multiple sites within the anatomic region, it is clear that varying degrees of compression at different sites along this small area of the median nerve can give relatively different presentations of these syndromes. Indeed, various forms of "incomplete anterior interosseous nerve palsies" have been described.[30] Recently, electrodiagnostic studies have attempted to distinguish between the pronator tunnel syndrome and the anterior interosseous nerve syndrome.[31] In 188 normal patients, there was a latency difference of 0.7 ms between the motor conduction of the median nerve across the elbow. In ten patients with the pronator tunnel syndrome, this motor latency was between 0.8 and 2.4 ms longer than in the opposite extremity and in six patients with the anterior interosseous nerve syndrome, direct stimulation of the flexor pollicis longus produced interphalangeal joint flexion but alternating current did not. The concept of the multiple crush syndrome implies that it is not necessary to attempt finer and finer electrodiagnostic differentiation in this anatomic region.

The multiple crush syndrome implies simply that the surgeon must release every potential site of median nerve compression from just proximal to the elbow to just distal to the flexor digitorum sublimis arch. Spinner[31] has clearly listed this series of structures (Table 14-2)[32] and to his list may be added a high origin of the superficial head of the pronator teres from the humerus.[33] This condition, present in 20% of normal persons can cause compression of the median nerve against the trochlear process of the humerus (see Chapter 7 for further description). Thus, the multiple crush syndrome as applied to multiple anatomic sites across a given anatomic region, as just exemplified, suggests that when the physical examination and the electrodiagnostic testing, even if incomplete and inconclusive, are suggestive that the median nerve is entrapped in the proximal forearm, the surgical approach must begin by releasing the lacertus fibrosis, releasing any fibrous arch related to the pronator or superficialis muscles that cross the median nerve, looking for any crossing arteries or veins or other anatomic variant structures that may compress the nerve in this area, and recognizing that the relationship of the anterior interosseous nerve to the median nerve and to the fibrous arches may predispose it to additional compression.[25] Clinical cases of incomplete recovery or failure to recover after lesser procedures suggests that reexploration be carried out with this extensive series of releases.

Table 14-2. Multiple Crush Syndrome due to Multiple Anatomic Structures Across the Median Nerve in the Proximal Forearm*

1. A tendinous origin of the deep head of the pronator teres
2. A tendinous origin of the flexor superficialis
3. Thrombosis of crossing ulnar collateral vessels
4. An accessory muscle and tendon from the flexor superficialis to the flexor pollicis longus
5. An accessory head of the flexor pollicis longus (Gantzer's muscle)
6. An aberrant radial artery
7. A tendinous origin of variant muscles, such as palmaris profundus or flexor carpi radialis brevis
8. An enlarged bicipital bursa encroaching on median nerve near region of the origin of the anterior interosseous nerve
9. A high origin of the pronator teres superficial head from the humerus[32]

*Modified from Spinner.[31]

Brachial Plexus Compression (Thoracic Outlet Syndrome)

The multiple crush syndrome, when applied to multiple sites of compression in the anatomic region between the neck and the clavicle, helps structure our understanding of this controversial region. As already discussed several times, multiple crush syndrome suggests that there may be individual sites within a given anatomic region, each of which may be insufficient in and of itself to cause symptoms, but which may summate to give overall symptomatic dysfunction. As discussed, the fact that a particular syndrome has an anatomic name attached to it seems to direct surgeons to carry out a very specific operative procedure to relieve this syndrome. If, in fact, the patient is not improved after this discrete surgical procedure, and this is frequently the case in procedures carried out in the anatomic region to be described here, the entire original diagnosis may come into question. In this anatomic region, the physical examination and electrodiagnostic techniques available frequently do not give "hard data" to demonstrate a nerve compression as, for example, they do for median nerve compression at the wrist. Given the fact that many patients with problems in this anatomic region may have vague symptoms, diffuse symptoms, or may have a history of work-related repetitive trauma disorder or some other accident involved in a litigation process, the issue is further complicated and confused.

We have chosen to call this condition brachial plexus compression, because this describes an anatomic region rather than a specific site. The term "brachial plexus compression" will indicate to the surgeon, within the context of the multiple crush syndrome, that every structure crossing the brachial plexus that may possibly be implicated in compression should be released, beginning at the neural foramen and going distally to the clavicle. This syndrome further implies that not all such structures need be released. It may be possible that sufficient relief of compression of the brachial plexus can be achieved by decompressing multiple anatomic sites, so that a remaining anatomic site, for example, the first rib, may not need to be resected.

How different, then, is the approach suggested by the multiple crush syndrome than that which has developed historically? The first description of symptoms related to a supernumerary cervical rib was given by Wilshire in 1860[33] and the first rib resection carried out by Coote in 1861.[34] Murphy,[35] in 1906, suggested the anterior scalene muscle could produce symptoms of upper extremity discomfort, and Adson and Coffey,[36] in 1927, in a article entitled, "Cervical Rib," suggested, in fact, that the anterior scalene muscle could be sectioned instead of removing the first rib in order to relieve symptoms. Subsequent publications of Ochsner et al[37] and by Naffziger and Grant[38] enshrined the "scalenus anticus" syndrome as another example of a diagnosis in which the surgeon is anatomically goal-directed. To these two anatomic sites of compression across the brachial plexus, that is, cervical rib and scalenus anticus muscle, were added by Adson[39] the possibility of an adjunctive cervicothoracic sympathectomy and the necessity to remove an anomalous formation of a first rib. For these observations, he built on the earlier observations by Jaboulay,[40] who first performed a periarterial sympathectomy in this region in 1861. Bramwell[41] observed in 1903 that a normal first rib might contribute to problems in this area and the first rib was removed through a supraclavicular approach for the first time in 1910 in Australia.[42] Attention was further directed to compression, primarily of the vascular as well as the nerve structures between the first rib and the clavicle, by Lewis and Pickering in 1934[43] and by Eden in 1939.[44] Their suggestion of compression at this site was ultimately termed the "costoclavicular syndrome" in 1943 by Falconer and Weddell.[45]

An additional site for compression near this anatomic region was described by Wright[46] in 1945 by his use of the term "hyperabduction syndrome," in which he believed that the pectoralis minor muscle compressed the brachial plexus just before it inserted on the coracoid process. A surgical approach suggested for the costoclavicular syndrome, as might be expected, had at least one advocate for resection of the clavicle, described by Lord in 1953.[47] The "thoracic outlet syndrome" as a term was described by Peet et al in 1956,[48] and they made a major contribution in describing a nonoperative approach to managing this group of patients. In 1962, giving the Presidential Address at The American Association of Thoracic Surgeons, Clagett[49] lent support to the concept of first rib resection. He also suggested the posterior approach for this purpose. The subsequent increased performance of anterior scalenotomies and scalenectomies, with or without a cervical rib resection when one was present, led to a significant number of patients who were not improved. This name switch to "thoracic outlet syndrome" took such hold on surgical thought, primarily due to the writings of Roos and Owens[50] and Urschel and Razzuk,[51] that the problem resolved itself not into what operative procedure should be done to decompress the entrapped nerves in this area, but which approach should be taken to remove the first rib, that is, transaxillary,[50,51] posteriorly through a parascapular approach for the thoracotomy,[49,52] or the more recently described approach through the supraclavicular region.[53–55] As Adson, on seeing the subclavian artery so severely compressed and indeed thrombosed by the anterior scalene, questioned whether the cervical rib, which was not in direct conjunction with the compressed subclavian artery in that particular patient, required cervical rib resection, so, too, have more recent observers of this complex problem questioned the need to resect the first rib for relief of the thoracic outlet syndrome.[56,57]

Among the other observations that suggested that not every structure that might compress the brachial plexus needs to be removed is the type of observation made by Halsted in 1916[58] in which a series of 716 patients with cervical ribs (Fig. 14-14A) were examined and just 35% found to have vascular symptoms. In a similar fashion, Hemple et al,[53] who performed pectoralis minor tendinotomies, stopped doing this after their first 19 patients as they began to appreciate that removal of other anatomic sites of compression along the brachial plexus would suffice to relieve their patients' symptoms. Additional anatomic factors that can be removed as they cross the brachial plexus are the omohyoid muscle, which Adson described as "taut" in his patients,[39] and at least seven varieties of congenital bands or anomalies associated with cervical and first rib and the scalene muscles as described by Roos.[59] One additional muscular structure that has been described is the scalenus minimus (muscle of Albinus), which may go from the transverse process of C7 compressing the lower trunk where the C8-T1 roots meet, as the muscle inserts on the inner half of the first rib[60] (Fig. 14-7).

Telford and Mottershead[60] also depicted variations in insertion of the scalenus anticus where a widened lateral fibrous insertion narrows or overlaps with the scalenus medius, narrowing the area of exit of the brachial plexus and subclavian artery between the scalenus anticus, scalenus medius and the curvature of the first rib (Figs 14-7, 14-14B). These investigators additionally describe a fibrous undersurface to the subclavius muscle that can compress the brachial plexus and vascular structures against the first rib rather than this compression being done by the clavicle, itself, which in this location has its convexity turned outward.

In summary, it is clear that the neurovascular structures crossing this anatomic region can have a multitude of anatomic structures crossing them, each or a combination of which, but not necessarily all, may be responsible for the clinical symptoms (Figs. 14-17, 14-8).

There remains an additional anatomic site within this region in which compression can occur with respect to the brachial plexus. That area is within the brachial plexus itself. This realization has come from our clinical experience with approximately 50 patients over the last 4 years.[75] These patients were referred for evaluation of thoracic outlet syndrome. All patients had a history of trauma. When the writings of thoracic outlet syndrome are reviewed historically, one is impressed by the fact that trauma contributed little to the number of cases reported earlier. For example, Telford and Mottershead[60] reported their experience with 122 cases

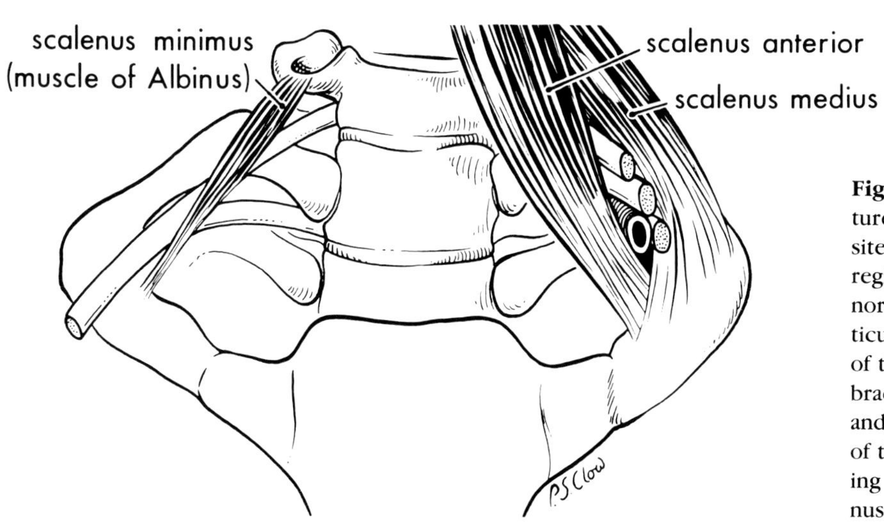

Figure 14-7. Examples of anatomic structures that may contribute to the multiple sites of compression in a given anatomic region in the multiple crush syndrome. Abnormalities in insertions of the scalenus anticus and scalenus medius create narrowing of the triangular region through which the brachial plexus traverses across the first rib and beneath the clavicle (right). Example of the scalenus minimus muscle compressing the first thoracic root (muscle of Albinus) (left).

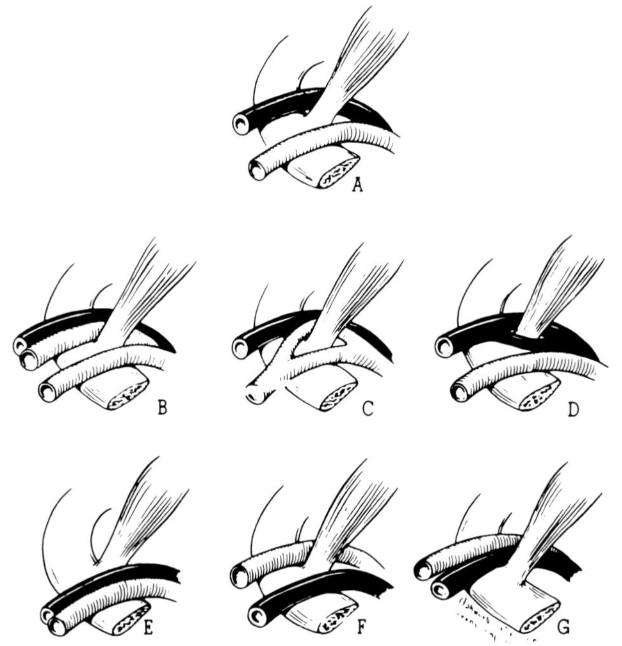

Figure 14-8. When the exposure is carried down to the level of the anterior scalene, the various relationships of the brachial artery (black) and subclavian vein (white) must be taken into account during the resection of scalene muscle. (Reproduced with permission from Nichols.[74])

operated on between 1908 and 1948. Of their 105 cases in which they classified the findings at operation, 70 had a cervical rib, 12 had a fibrous band, 8 had an abnormal disposition of the scalene muscles, 2 had a cancellous osteoma, 8 had a deformed thoracic outlet with pressure of the clavicle on the first rib, and 5 had no obvious causes found. These investigators from the Department of Surgery and the Department of Anatomy at the University of Manchester in England, and especially working with a group of patients with no history of trauma, had little basis for exploration within the plexus, itself. Yet, from the variety of their caseload and their intraoperative findings, they wrote, "It is clear from this analysis that the causes of pressure on the neurovascular bundle are many and varied. No one explanation, such as costoclavicular pressure, can account for all cases."[60] In an age when there was significantly less trauma than we have today, Adson[39] postulated that among the causative factors responsible for the symptoms in his patients was the "anatomic structure of the neck is different from that of normal persons. The cervical portion of the spinal column is longer and this same congenital defect accounts for the high lying second division of the subclavian artery at the base of the posterior cervical triangle which runs parallel with the superior border of the clavicle which shortened the width of the base and the distance between the posterior surfaces of the scalenus anticus, the scalenus medicus and the scalenus posticus muscles likewise are generally shorter or perhaps it should be called lowers, the space through which the artery and the cords of the brachial plexus must pass is decreased." Adson continues, "The second factor, which is concerned more with the onset of symptoms, probably is associated with the descent of the shoulder girdle. This process begins in early adult life. The descent or sagging of the shoulders possibly could add sufficient traction on the brachial cords to precipitate symptoms when the congenital abnormality of the lower part of the neck had already reduced the normal freedom of movement."[39] With trauma playing an increasing role in the mechanisms of injury, the percentage of patients presenting with vascular symptoms decreased from the high of 20 to 30% in some early series to that of just 3% arterial and 4% venous symptoms among the 433 operations in 358 patients between 1964 and 1975.[53]

The concept of the multiple crush syndrome due to multiple anatomic sites of compression in a given anatomic region, as described here for the brachial plexus, was anticipated by Telford and Mottershead,[60] who concluded their classic analysis by stating:

> Having decided on clinical grounds, radiographic evidence and the failure of conservative treatment that operation is indicated in the frankly *exploratory* approach through an adequate incision. To operate with no more purpose than to carry out a preconceived plan, such as anterior scalenotomy, is to invite failure.

Shortly thereafter, Raft[61] published his results in which fewer than 50% of patients had good results after having a scalenotomy or scalenectomy plus cervical rib resection. Although Roos and Owens[50] and Urschel and Razzuk[51] reported transaxillary first rib resection results with a 90% success rate, these patients included a small percentage of those with trauma and a high percentage of those with congenital anomalies. These investigators have discussed the failure of the transaxillary first rib resection to improve outcome in their patients.[18,52] A typical report by Hemple et al[53] in which the lessons of the past have been incorporated into an approach still report only 58% excellent results in a series of patients in whom the anterior scalenectomy and a supraclavicular approach for first rib resection were used. They had an additional 27% of their patients achieve good results for an overall 84% satisfactory results in a series of 366 patients. Other series of first rib resections through transaxillary approach has yielded, in general, a 20% failure rate.[62,63] Another series[64] reported a 27% failure rate when first rib resection was carried out, but their rate of failure varied, depending on the particular approach used. Thus, when a posterior "thoracoplasty" was done, they had 5 of 11 failures. When a supraclavicular approach was done, they had 9 of 18 failures. When a transaxillary approach was done, they had no failures.

The one area that was ignored by all of these approaches directed at first rib resection is potential scarring within the brachial plexus itself. Scarring within the brachial plexus is approachable through the technique of neurolysis (see Chapter 5). Two major studies, a decade apart,[65,66] have reported the operative experience with traumatic lesions of the brachial plexus. Both of these studies include a significant number of severe trauma cases, so that many of the patients had complete disruption of the brachial plexus, a degree of trauma several orders of magnitude different from those normally referred for diagnostic workup of the thoracic outlet syndrome. These two studies observed a significant amount of scarring within the brachial plexus where the plexus remained in-continuity. Lusskin et al[65] commented, "The use of an electrical nerve stimulator is of value during the dissection. Once neurolysis is completed, stimulation may elicit a satisfactory muscle contraction not previously present, thereby demonstrating that encumbrance of the brachial plexus by cicatrix can create a reversible conduction block." They noted that "neurolysis was followed by significant improvement in thirteen of seventeen patients." Kline and Judice[66] found, for example, that among brachial plexus injuries caused by gunshot wounds, after intraneural dissection of the plexus, 57 of 63 nerves that were spared because intraoperative nerve action potentials were demonstrated were found to have recovered function after treatment by neurolysis alone.

It has been our personal theoretical construct that if the journey for the brachial plexus exploration is considered as a tunnel, then the treatments at the level of the anterior scalene would be at the entrance of the tunnel and those directed at the first rib removal, regardless of approach, would be directed at the end of the tunnel. According to this construct, failures or recurrences, in particular in those cases in which the cause has not been due to congenital anomalies but due to trauma, are due to scarring within the brachial plexus itself, that is, within the tunnel. This represents an untreated problem. If this were to be true, then the appropriate approach, we reasoned, would be to carry out a supraclavicular approach for the brachial plexus exploration. The transaxillary approach allows removal of the first rib and treatment of congenital bands but does not allow an approach to the plexus neurolysis. In a similar fashion, the posterior approach allows cervical and first rib resection during approaches for patients with recurrent symptoms believed to be due to a remaining posterior segment of the first rib, but this posterior approach does not allow neurolysis of the plexus. In contrast, a supraclavicular approach allows a neurolysis of the plexus from the cervical roots to the area beneath the clavicle, rendering perhaps only first rib resection to be somewhat more difficult in this approach.[75]

Complications after supraclavicular first rib resection have been reported in 37 of 145 operations[54] (pleura opened, 24, temporary numbness and weakness in hand, 4, temporary phrenic nerve palsy, 4, thoracic duct leak, 1, long thoracic nerve injury, 2, and postoperative bleeding requiring reoperation, 2). Yet, as already described, first rib resection has been reported to have been done successfully through the supraclavicular approach (Fig. 14-9).[53–55] Should difficulty arise in removing the first rib by the supraclavicular approach, then combining a transaxillary or infraclavicular approach with the supraclavicular approach, as has been described for vascular reconstruction,[67] can be used as a general approach to this problem (Fig. 14-11).[63,67] The most recent literature also seems to support these constructs and conclusions.[68]

Our current personal approach to patients' symptoms and diagnosis of the multiple crush syndrome in the brachial plexus region must now be reviewed. The patient's symptoms most commonly include aching pain, discomfort, or heaviness in the neck and shoulder and upper arm region, followed next by discomfort or numbness and tingling down the inner aspect of the arm to the little and ring fingers, followed by abnormal sensory perceptions in the anterior chest and axillary region, all of which are accompanied by a feeling of tightness in the neck, and posterior cervical and occipital headaches. There may be nighttime awakening and this may, on questioning, be related to the patient sleeping in the prone position with the arms outstretched about a pillow, rather than the type of nocturnal paresthesias related to carpal tunnel syndrome. The symptom complex is usually brought on quickly with any attempt to work with the arm elevated at the level of the shoulder, such as when a woman attempts to hang clothes, wash or set the hair, put dishes on a shelf, or with persons working with their arms outstretched, such as painters, plasters, assembly line workers. When the symptoms have come on at a relatively early age and are not associated with direct trauma, congenital anomalies should be highly considered. When the patient has a history of trauma, either by repetitive work disorder or through a direct crushing accident to the neck or chest area, or, most commonly, a history of a modified stretch injury, such as occurs in motor vehicle accidents that are not as severe as the motorcycle injuries, then the post-traumatic situation discussed with scarring within and about the brachial plexus must be considered. The diagnostic workup must rule out associated causes for similar symptoms, primarily cervical disk disease.

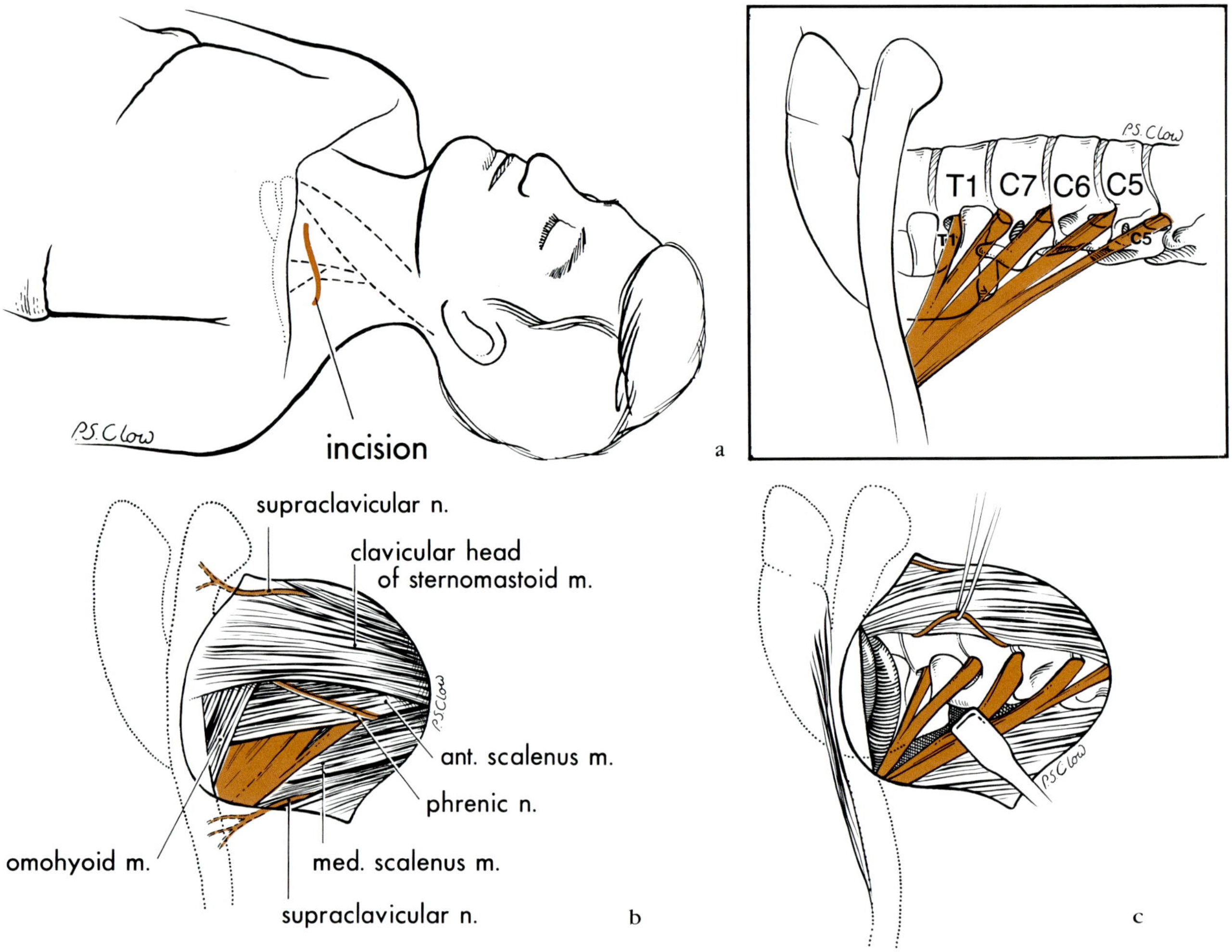

Figure 14-9. Illustration of the initial steps in the supraclavicular approach to brachial plexus decompression in the multiple crush syndrome. The operative incision is marked. The bone and nerve relationships are noted (**a**, a insert). The supraclavicular approach requires division of the cleido head of the sternocleidomastoid muscle. Resection of the omohyoid muscle, as well as complete release of the cervical fascia (shaded black area) beneath the scalene fat pad. The scalene fat pad is reflected posteriorly. Then the anterior scalene muscle is resected, identifying and preserving the phrenic nerve. **b.** The muscle may be divided by cautery with appropriate protection for the subclavian artery. If required, the first rib can be removed by division at its central portion and then continued removal posteriorly and anteriorly (**c**). Note that the anterior portion of the first plays little, if any, role in compression of the plexus against the clavicle.

A protocol with which we are currently working[69] includes cervical radiographs and a computer tomography (CT) scan with contrast media. CT scans (from C4 to the second rib at 0.05 cm cuts) without contrast will help define a prolonged transverse process of C7, cervical ribs, and tendinous bands within the scalene muscles. For those patients with significant pain that may be radicular or from direct nerve injury, diagnostic nerve blocks are carried out, usually by an anesthesiologist. The shoulder is extensively evaluated by a separate member of the team, usually an orthopedic surgeon, and may require in addition to radiographs, arthroscopy, steroid injection into the subacromial bursa, steroid treatment of any associated bicipital tendinitis, in order to evaluate pain originating from the shoulder region. The workup for specific peripheral nerve entrapments, such as the ulnar nerve at the cubital tunnel and the median nerve at the wrist, are carried out (see Chapters 3, 6, 7, and 9).

Electrodiagnostic testing for brachial plexus compression generally has had a lack of success. Diagnostic studies traditionally done, including conduction times measured from Erb's point, ulnar nerve conduction across the brachial plexus, F wave testing, may reveal a difference between the affected side and the other side but may not be helpful in bilateral problems. Newer approaches, including somatosensory evoked responses, offer some increased measure of diagnostic aid. For example, a recent study has found 9 of 13 patients with abnormal somatosensory evoked potentials in the affected side versus the nonaffected side.[70] This subject has been recently reviewed.[71] In essence, we obtain these electrodiagnostic studies. If they are within normal limits, given the concept of the multiple crush syndrome, a normal study does not serve as a contraindication to exploration if the symptom complex is appropriate, if the other diagnostic possibilities have been eliminated, and if the appropriate physical examination findings are present.

The most significant findings on physical examination, if brachial plexus compression is present, are: (1) a positive Tinel's sign or tenderness of the brachial plexus beneath the scalene muscles; a finding first described by Ochsner et al;[37] (2) a positive hyperabduction test, in which the forearm and arm are held at a 90° angle to the body and in less than a minute the patient's symptom complex is reproduced; first described by Roos and Owens[50] and termed a "positive Roos' sign" by us; (3) positive pressure provocative test in which direct pressure over the brachial plexus just posterior to the anterior scalene muscle for 10 to 60 seconds will reproduce the patient's symptoms and usually produce numbness in the hand; (4) elevation-induced stress test in which holding the arms directly above the head produces profound fatigue and discomfort in the affected upper extremity; and (5) vibratory threshold measurements in which quantitative measurement of vibration thresholds with a vibrometer (constant frequency, variable amplitude) allows measurement of baseline vibratory thresholds. After provocation with maneuvers 2, 3, and 4, these thresholds are significantly increased, that is, a greater threshold of vibration stimulation is required before the patient perceives a vibratory stimulus than was required before provocation.[72]

Once the diagnosis has been established, the patient must have had at least 6 months, and in all of our cases has had more than a year, of nonoperative management. Such a program, as initially described by Peet[48] and as carefully outlined by Jaeger et al,[73] is essential, since the vast majority of patients with this symptom complex may find improvement by the appropriate physical therapeutic modalities, trigger point injections, strengthening shoulder girdle muscles, resting the involved structures, among others. In the absence of the patient specifically complaining of vascular symptoms, such as extreme coldness in the hand or physical findings of swelling of the hand, bluish discoloration, or vascular insufficiency at the tips of the fingers with an absent radial pulse, little diagnostic weight is given to any of the classic signs for changes in the pulse with respirations or with movements of the head, neck or of the arm. The major series in which these vascular signs have been reviewed and compared with nonsymptomatic populations has demonstrated anywhere from a 30 to 50% false-positive findings in the normal population for the so-called Adson and Allen maneuvers.[69,53,60]

The surgical approach we favor[69] for the brachial plexus decompression is carried out with the patient under general anesthesia with the entire arm prepared free for movement within the operative field, the head turned to the opposite side, and utilizing general endotracheal anesthesia. A 6 to 8 cm incision is made 2 cm proximal to the clavicle beginning over the cleido head of the sternocleidomastoid muscle. The incision is deepened into the subcutaneous tissue and hemostasis obtained throughout with the bipolar coagulator. The platysma muscle is divided. Crossing branches of the supraclavicular nerves are identified and their integrity preserved. The cleido head of the sternocleidomastoid muscle is completely divided. This gives access to the medial area where the dissection of the cervical fascia is begun. The cervical fascia essentially is divided anteriorly and the scalene fat pad reflected posteriorly and left attached. During this dissection, crossing branches of the suprascapular or transverse cervical artery or vein, which may be enormous at times, must be doubly tied and divided. The omohyoid muscle is excised in the portion that crosses the wound. Then the anterior scalene muscle is identified and the phrenic nerve is identified and encircled with a vessel loop. The scalene muscle is divided approximately 2 cm before it inserts into the first rib and the division is carried as far medially until the muscle is completely divided (Fig. 14-9). The lateral and posterior surface of the anterior scalene muscle may be quite fibrotic and this is noted. The fascia overlying the anterior scalene, the cervical fascia of the scalene fat pad and its attachments to the clavicle and the underlying brachial plexus form one continuous layer. After trauma this thin layer becomes scar that, in the resting state, may not cause compression but in the mechanics of moving the arm, this fascial sheath may be found to become tight and compress the underlying brachial plexus (Fig. 14-10). A complete anterior scalenectomy is carried out resections to the transverse processes of C5 and C6. During this maneuver, the upper trunk and its contributing C5 and C6 roots are identified in the area where there was compression beneath the anterior scalene muscle. With microsurgical instruments and technique, utilizing in many instances, a DeBakey forceps and a Jamison scissors, the epineurium is resected from the upper trunk and the C5 and C6 roots. Going distally, the suprascapular nerve is identified and the anterior and posterior divisions of the upper trunk are identified going to the level of the clavicle. The epineurium is resected and submitted for pathologic examination. The contribution of C5 to the phrenic nerve can be observed. Any vascular problem between the subclavian artery or vein and the anterior scalene muscle will have been identified at this point. A cervical rib, if present, can be excised (Fig. 14-11). The C7 root and medial trunk of the plexus now may be found either scarred to the C6 root and the upper trunk or separated beneath an interposed anomalous muscle located from the anterior to the medial scalene muscles (Fig. 14-10). The C7 root and its middle trunk are then neurolysed, the same as for the upper trunk from the transverse process of the spine to the clavicle. Then the lower trunk of the plexus is identified. There is frequently dense scar tissue or anomalous muscle or fibrous band interposed between the middle and lower trunk of the plexus. Care must be taken to keep the subclavian artery from injury and in the dissection to avoid injuring the pleura. The first rib can be palpated in its posterior segment as a guide and generally the beginning portion of the lower trunk is adherent by scar tissue or muscle bands to the first rib at this location. This is where C8 from above and T1 from below cross the posterior portion of the first rib to form the lower trunk. The T1 root can be compressed here by the scalenus minimus. When the neurolysis is completed in this area and then carried gently distally, it will be found, after a resection of the epineurium, that the entire brachial plexus, including its five roots and three trunks, lays loosely within the wound. Clearly, these structures have been decompressed. The neurolysis has demonstrated fascicles with good fascicular formation and good perineurial markings. The examiner's finger now goes along the brachial plexus and beneath the clavicle. Generally, there is a great deal of room beneath this concave portion of the clavicle, so that the examiner's finger runs into the subclavius muscle. Once dissection of the fibrous undersurface of the

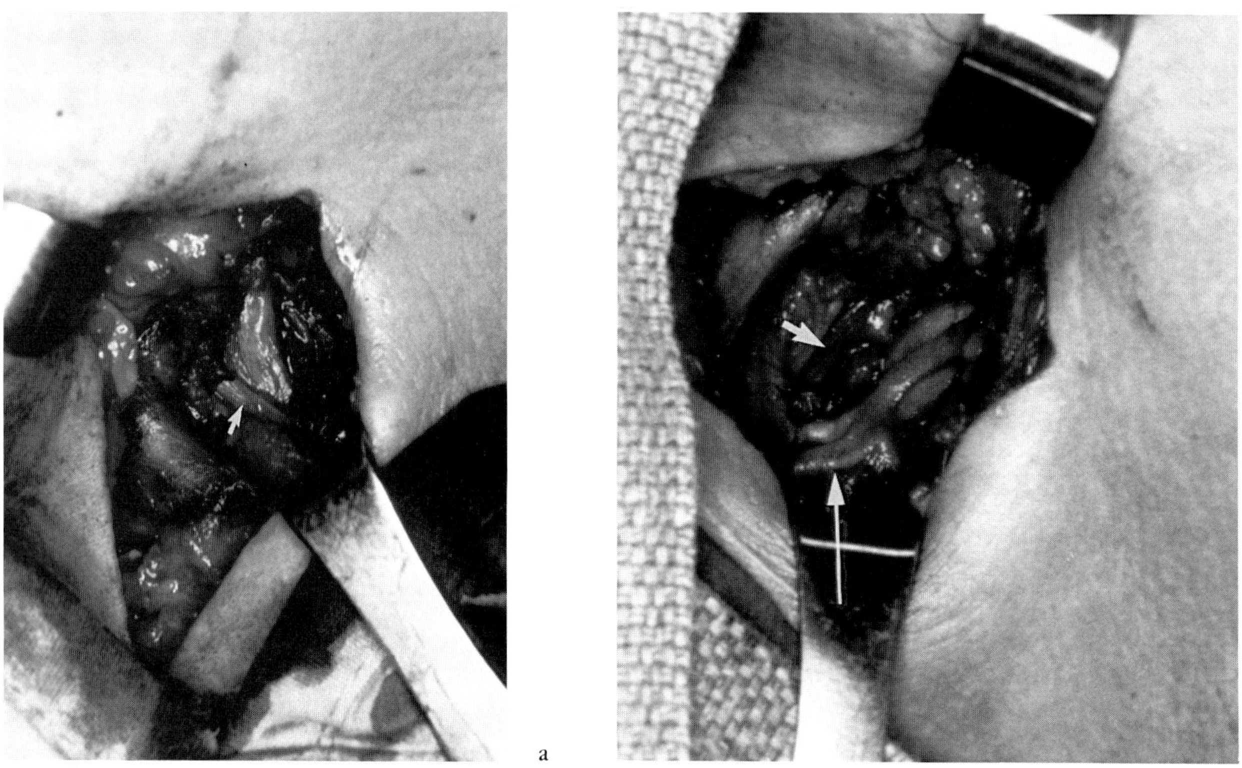

a b

Figure 14-10. Intraoperative views of patient with this supraclavicular approach. **a.** Note anterior scalene muscle (white arrow) and scar compressing upper trunk of plexus. **b.** After anterior scalenectomy and neurolysis of upper trunk, note indentation in upper trunk (long white arrow), and anomalous scalene muscle slip compressing middle trunk of plexus (short white arrow).

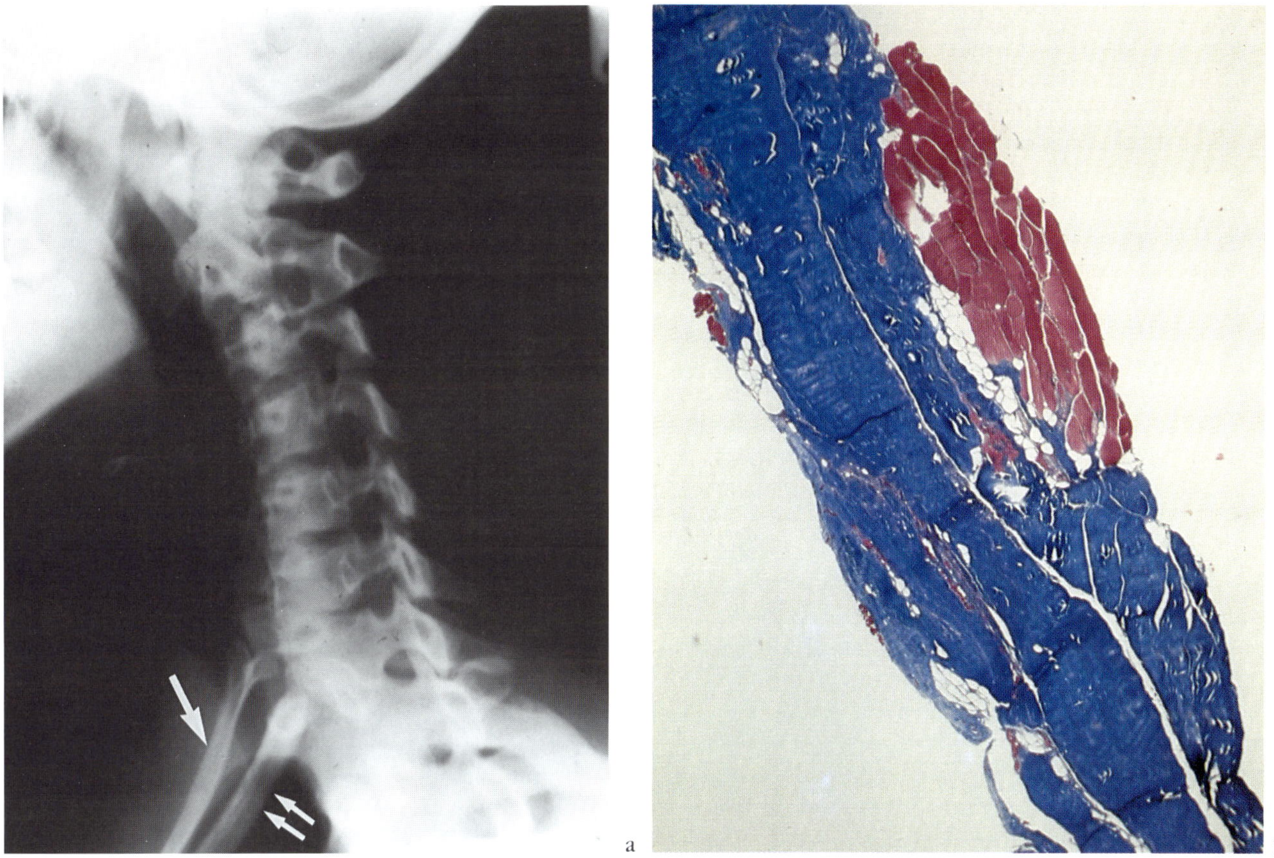

Figure 14-11. Brachial plexus compression can be due to a cervical rib (arrow), noted in this oblique view of cervical spine and by compression of the plexus against the first rib (double arrow). The plexus will pass between these two bony structures (**a**) by fibrous bands within the anterior scalene muscle (**b**). Note with Mallory stain the muscle is red, and the fibrous band's collagen is blue. (Photomicrograph courtesy of Doctor William Nelems, University of British Columbia, Vancouver.).

subclavius muscle and its muscle fibers are separated from the plexus, the plexus will be found not to be compressed between the anterior portion of the first rib and the clavicle. After this dissection, the examiner's finger is put between the plexus and the clavicle, while the arm is taken through a range of motion. If, in fact, the plexus is found to be compressed between some anomalous formation of the first rib or wider more lateral extent of the first rib and the clavicle, then a first rib resection may be done through the supraclavicular approach (Fig. 14-9). To do this, the subclavian artery is encircled with a vessel loop and maneuvered medial or lateral as necessary. A subperiosteal resection is carried out. A side-biting rongeur can divide the first rib at its wide portion in its central aspect and then a rongeur is used to go posteriorly to the facet with the transverse process and anteriorly to the sternum. Posteriorly, the roots from C8 and T1 must be carefully maneuvered so that their injury is avoided. In general, it will be found that in the vast majority of cases, the removal of the overlying compressive structures allows the plexus to come up off the first rib and the removal of scar tissue allows the trunks of the plexus to slide sufficiently when the arm is abducted at the shoulder. The plexus is not compressed beneath the first rib and the clavicle. Thus, in general, the first rib should not have to be removed in the cases of post-traumatic brachial plexus compression. Just one of our first 25 cases of supraclavicular neurolysis as described above, for brachial plexus compression, has required a secondary operation for first rib resection.

At the completion of the procedure, the wound is

filled with saline and the lungs hyperinflated to look for air leaks. A drain is placed in the wound. The scalene fat pad is sutured anteriorly to the stump of the clavicular head of the sternocleidomastoid muscle to interpose fat between plexus and the overlying skin. The platysma and dermis are closed and the skin is closed. A dry sterile dressing is applied.

The patient in the postoperative period is instructed to turn the head hourly to the opposite side from surgery, shrug the shoulders to attempt gentle movement of the shoulder and the neck so that the plexus glides through the operative field, preventing it from adhering to any of the dissected structures. The patient is instructed to anticipate swelling in the cervical region and some bruising. There may be some numbness in the distribution of the supraclavicular nerves. There may be occasional numbness in the fingers after the neurolysis procedure. In general, by the first postoperative visit on the seventh or eighth day, the patient may hold the arm abducted at the side without the same degree of symptoms being induced. Over the next 2 to 3 weeks, as the swelling in the neck subsides, aided by application of warm showers or local heat and as the gentle range of motion is continued, there is symptomatic improvement (Fig. 14-10).[75]

With this approach in 15 patients over 3 years, the following was found. The supraclavicular approach to the brachial plexus permits the surgeon to explore this multiple crush syndrome with multiple areas of potential anatomic compression in a single anatomic region. This approach may permit preservation of the first rib in the majority of patients.The approach requires physical examination and diagnostic techniques appropriate for multiple crush syndrome, understanding that each site may contribute to the overall dysfunction. The supraclavicular approach eliminates the complications of the transaxillary approach, which include irritation or frank neuromas of the intercoastal brachial nerves, and corrects the main limitation of the transaxillary approach, namely, that a neurolysis cannot be carried out. The supraclavicular approach leaves a more acceptable scar than the long posterior approach and additionally gives the potential for access to each of the structures that may be a cause for independent compression in the anatomic region.[75] The only disadvantage of the supraclavicular approach is that it may be more difficult to remove the first rib, in which case, if a rib removal is considered necessary, the transaxillary approach can be done either at the same time or later should symptoms still persist. In some very difficult patients (Workmen's Compensation, litigation, tertiary referral with several previous unsuccessful operative attempts), it has been found appropriate to decompress the brachial plexus and remove the first rib at the same operation. The reason is that the clinical situation is such that the patient deserves one surgical procedure and later operations for persistent symptoms in these patients would be inappropriate.[69]

Multiple Crush Syndrome Superimposed on a Neuropathy

The primary distinction in this section from the multiple crush syndromes discussed in the previous sections is that a metabolic neuropathy will act as an underlying "crush." In these instances, the diseased peripheral nerve has a susceptibility to compression imposed on it by the neuropathy. Although the surgeon cannot change this basic neuropathy, he can relieve any superimposed compression effects. At any area of normal anatomic narrowing, this peripheral nerve will be receiving pressure. Since the nerve is susceptible to pressure, each of these anatomic sites will serve as a potential new site for a superimposed compression on the underlying neuropathy. In the simplest situation, for example, a person with diabetes who has an associated carpal tunnel syndrome has this type of multiple crush syndrome, that is, a basic neuropathy with a superimposed nerve compression. This becomes a multiple crush syndrome because the entire length of the peripheral nerve, from the neural foramen and at every additional anatomic site, is receiving some small additional site of compression. Whichever anatomic site imposes the most significant compression becomes the most symptomatic, for which the patient generally seeks treatment. Distinguishing between symptoms due to the neuropathy and symptoms due to a superimposed nerve compression may be difficult, if not impossible. The usual situation is that electrodiagnostic testing in the clinical situation is interpreted as showing a diffuse symmetrical peripheral neuropathy. The person doing the study may not find evidence of a superimposed nerve compression, in which case the study is frequently reported as, "No evidence of radiculopathy or nerve compression is noted." According to the concepts of the multiple crush syndrome outlined previously, and those to be developed further later, it will be clear that such an electrodiagnostic study does not rule out the presence of superimposed nerve compression. Indeed, a surgical decompression of the nerve with subsequent clinical follow-up may be the only way in which truly to determine whether the patient's symptoms were due to the superimposed nerve compression or what part, for example, that remains after surgery was due or contributed by the underlying neuropathy. (The entire subject of peripheral neuropathy has been covered in an encyclopedic fashion by Dyck et al.[76])

The essential difference between the entrapment

neuropathies (compression neuropathies) and the toxic and metabolic neuropathies is that in an entrapment neuropathy, a normal nerve fiber is subjected to mechanical compression that induces changes first in the connective tissue wrappings of that nerve, such as the epineurium and perineurium, and secondarily in the myelin portion of the peripheral nerve. Finally, with more severe degrees of compression, actual axonal degeneration can occur (see Chapter 3). In contrast, the metabolic neuropathies begin with an abnormal axon and subsequent to this axonopathy changes may occur in the myelin, but changes that are different from the segmental demyelination associated with nerve entrapment. In the metabolic neuropathies, the epineurial and perineurial thickening noted in entrapment neuropathies are lacking.

In 1964, Cavanagh[77] introduced the concept of the "dying-back" process and continued to describe this.[78] The concept of the dying-back process as originally conceived was that the cell body, the perikaryon, in, for example, the dorsal spinal ganglion for the sensory nerve, would be affected by the disease. Since this nucleus generates the metabolites and structural proteins that are carried by axoplasmic flow to the distal segments of the nerve, those nerves that were largest in diameter and longest would have a clear deficiency of critical functioning proteins or trophic substances that would be felt most severely at the distal segment. Therefore the axon would undergo distal segment dysfunction. This would result in changes that were worse distally and not so severe proximally. This theory helped explain many clinical situations, as well as the pathologic and electrophysiologic findings. The pathogenesis of this was elucidated by Spencer and Schaumberg[79] in work published in 1976, in which they began the use of the term "central-peripheral distal axonopathy." On further consideration, it became clear that many of the toxic neuropathies had the toxin circulating in the blood and therefore available to affect the axon along its entire length. Furthermore, it became clear that at certain sites, for example, the nodes of Ranvier or at the terminal sensory receptors, the axon was particularly vulnerable to neurotoxic agents and not just at its nucleus. Lowndes and Baker[80] have clearly described the potential sites for various toxins, such as isoniozid and organophosphates. These concepts were formalized into a classification by Spencer and Schaumberg[81] and include the types of nerve fiber de-

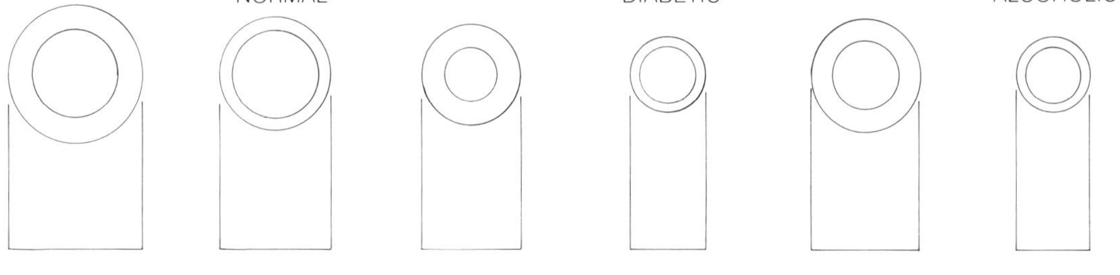

	NORMAL	COMPRESSED NORMAL	DIABETIC	COMPRESSED DIABETIC	ALCOHOLIC	COMPRESSED ALCOHOLIC
Axon/Myelin Ratio	.6	1.7	.6	1	.6	.9
Fiber Diameter (μ)	6.7	4	7.2	4.7	7.2	4.2
Wallerian Degeneration		±		+		+ +

Figure 14-12. Schema of morphometric changes in myelin due to chronic compression and axonopathy due to diabetes and alcoholism. Chronic compression results in segmental demyelination with calculated increase in axon-myelin ratio. Axonopathy is manifested by axonal dwindling, with secondary myelin shrinkage or knuckling and calculated decrease in axon-myelin ratio. Axonopathy with superimposed compression will have, theoretically, a decrease in myelin and axoplasm and the ratio may be unchanged, but the nerve fiber diameter will decrease. Endoneurial edema will decrease the nerve fiber density. In advanced disease, Wallerian degeneration occurs, but these cells are traditionally not included in measurement of fiber density. Degenerating myelin forms due to Wallerian degeneration can be expressed with respect to the fiber density.

generation encountered in laboratory models. The scheme was based on the study of pathologic changes after toxic insult with descriptors of the primary categories: neuronopathy, myelinopathy, axonopathy. A common situation was the central-peripheral distal axonopathy type, which forms the basis of the large majority of the clinically noted symmetrical peripheral neuropathies. Asbury and Brown[82] have given a clear description of the histopathologic changes that demonstrate in the axonopathy that there is axonal "dwindling" with preservation of the myelin, subsequent myelin adjustments to this narrowing of the axoplasm, subsequent either degeneration or regeneration with remyelination (Fig. 14-12).

Why should an axonopathy predispose to nerve compression? With an entrapment neuropathy or a chronic nerve compression, it has been demonstrated (as discussed in Chapter 3) that the earliest changes are altered permeability of the perineurial and endoneurial microvessels with subsequent subperineurial edema, and endoneurial edema (edema between the nerve fibers within the fascicles).[13,14] The increase in edema gives rise to increased endoneurial fluid pressure.[83] This pathophysiologic sequence, edema leading to increased endoneurial fluid pressure, is the same noted in the axonopathies, and perhaps the best study experimentally has been the axonopathy associated with diabetes. In a series of experiments extending over a decade, Jakobsen[84,85] demonstrated that giving a rat streptozocin, which damages the beta islet cells in the pancreas and induces an insulin-requiring type I diabetes, results in a typical distal axonopathy. This axonopathy is characterized by early permeability changes[86] leading to endoneurial edema (Fig. 14-13).[87] The increase in endoneurial fluid pressure results in alterations in axoplasmic flow.[88,89] As it became clear that the earlier hypotheses regarding the pathogenesis of diabetic neuropathy, such as vascular causes, would not be tenable,[90] the observation of increased water content of the peripheral nerves was viewed with new interest. The glucose enters into the nerve directly, since there is no blood–nerve barrier to glucose. The glucose is metabolized into polyols. These are hydrophilic and help to pull water into the endoneurial space. This concept has been reformulated with newer biophysical structural concepts recently to give additional support to the mechanisms of the pathogenesis of diabetes neuropathy.[91]

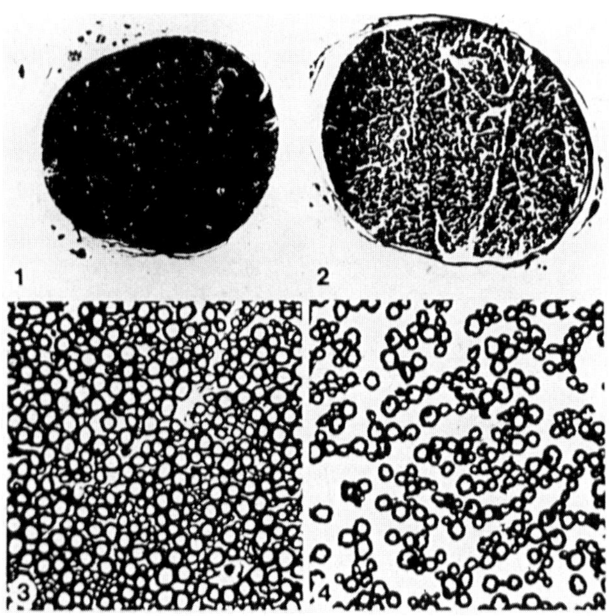

Figure 14-13. Endoneurial and subperineurial edema in streptozocin-induced diabetes mellitus in the rat sciatic nerve. 1, normal; 2, diabetic; 3 and 4 are the corresponding higher magnification reviews of 1 and 2, respectively. (Reproduced with permission from Jakobsen et al.[86])

Galactosemia is a disease similar to diabetes in that there is a high serum sugar content. There is also no blood–nerve barrier to galactose. These observations led to the study of an experimental model for galactosemia with the identification of nerve conduction defects,[92] structural changes in the peripheral nerves,[93,94] and ultimately the identification of endoneurial edema and increased endoneurial fluid pressure. In lead neuropathy, animals are given a diet containing 4% lead carbonate. After a period of time, the nerves can be evaluated. In addition to the abnormal nerve conductions that may be obtained and alterations in axoplasmic flow, there is a striking finding of endoneurial edema[95] (Fig. 14-14). With increasing edema comes increased endoneurial fluid pressure, and this is associated with myelin changes in this model also. Lead intoxication, however, has been frequently described as a model of primary segmental demyelination.[96] The mechanism appears to be first alterations in the blood–nerve barrier induced directly by the lead, leading to the endoneurial edema. Other research has demonstrated that meylin changes can occur secondary to an underlying axonopathy.[97,98] The particular mechanism for demyelination in lead intoxication has been demonstrated to be that once the blood–nerve barrier alters, lead directly enters into the endoneurial space and has a direct toxic effect on Schwann's cells, with subsequent alterations in myelin.[99,100] Thus, it has been demonstrated in the few good experimental models of neuropathy that the events leading to the axonopathy begin with endoneurial edema and increased endoneurial fluid pressure. Since these are the same events that initiate the process in entrapment neuropathies, it appears clear that a common mechanism exists in each of these two conditions and therefore the preexistence of endoneurial edema and increased endoneurial fluid pressure in a metabolic neuropathy should predispose the nerve to chronic nerve compression.

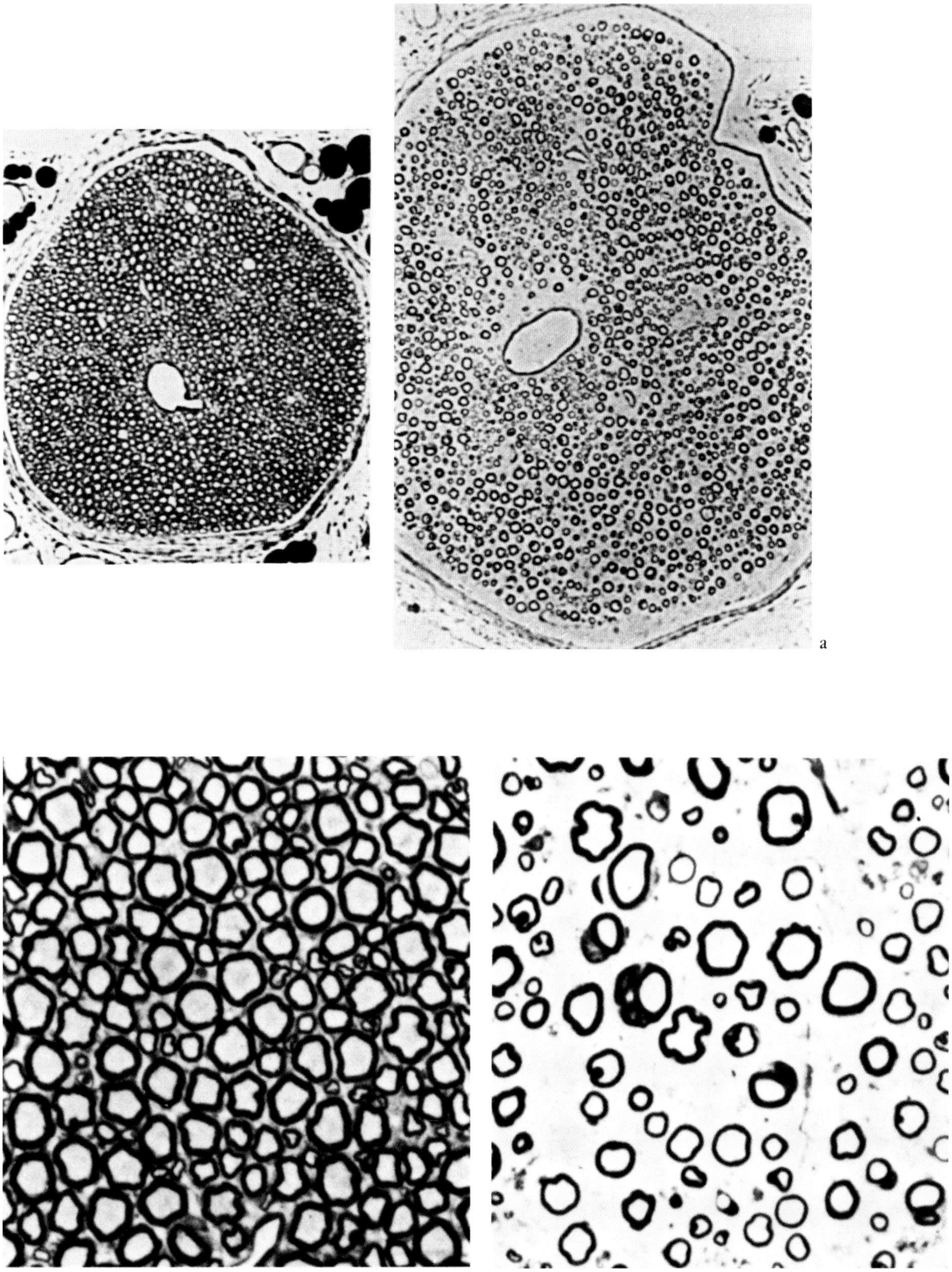

a

b

Figure 14-14. Histopathologic features of lead-induced neuropathy. The earliest change is subperineurial and endoneurial edema induced by direct toxic effect of lead on the vascular permeability of vessels in the perineurium and endoneurium. Normal rat views (left) and lead neuropathy (right) are same magnification in low power (**a**) and high power views (**b**). (Reproduced with permission from Ohniski et al. [96])

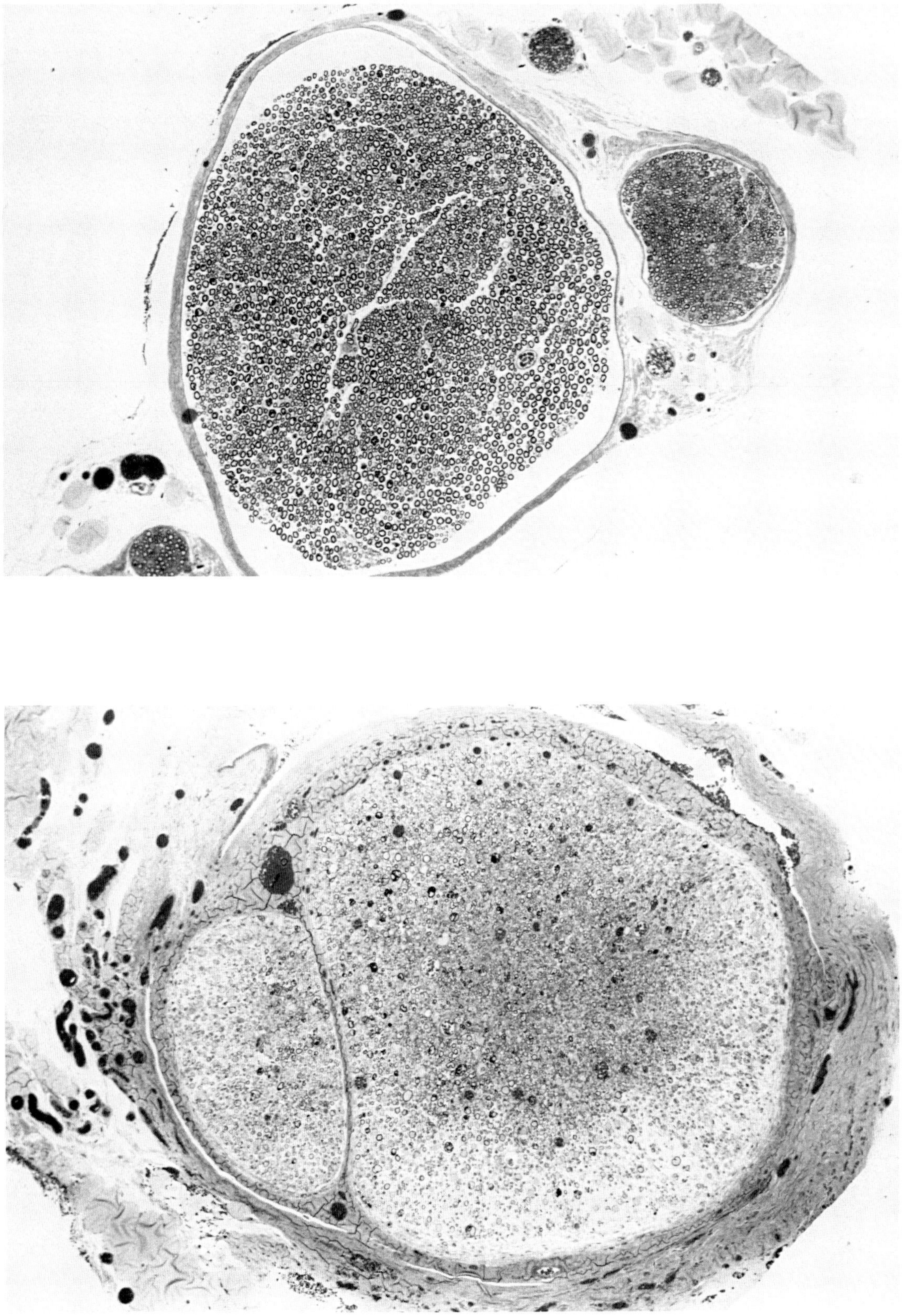

a

b

Figure 14-15a, b. (*Figure continues.*)

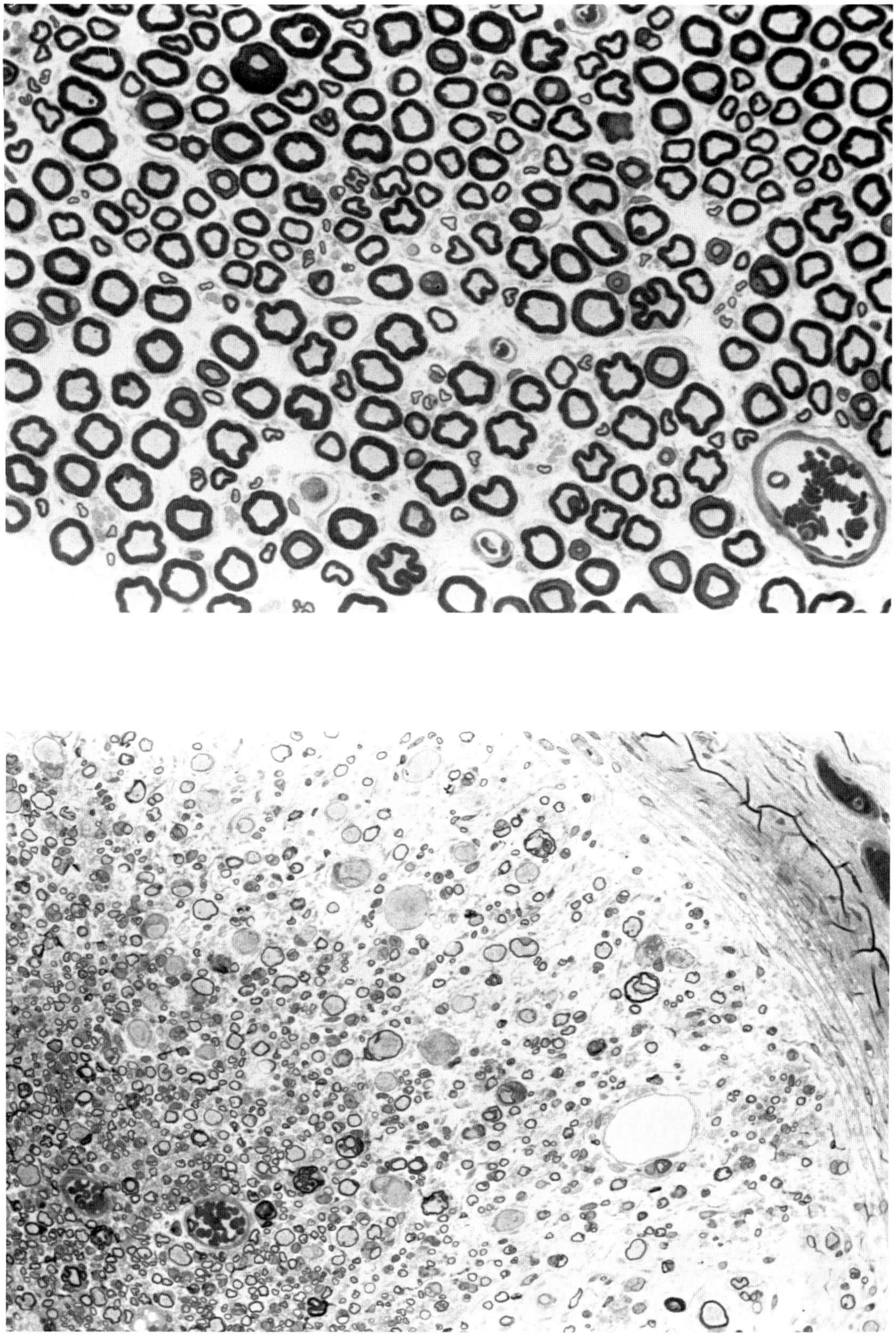

c

d

Figure 14-15. Histopathologic features of diabetic rat sciatic nerve (**a, c**) with superimposed nerve compression for 6 months (**b, d**). In the diabetic nerve note the subperineurial edema (**a**), the axonopathy is manifested by axonal dwindling myelin and knuckling (**c**). The superimposed compression has induced perineurial thickening (**b**) and myelin thinning and Wallerian degeneration (**d**). (Reproduced with permission from Mackinnon and Dellon.[105])

Table 14-3. Susceptibility of Diabetic Rat Sciatic Nerve to Chronic Compression*

Groups	*No. Sciatic Nerves*	*Conduction Velocity (m/sec)*	*Amplitude (mv)*
Nondiabetic, nonbanded	17	35.0 ± 1.8	8.5 ± 0.6
Nondiabetic, 6-month banded	17	22.3 ± 1.4	7.4 ± 0.4
Diabetic, nonbanded	11	25.7 ± 1.2	8.1 ± 0.4
Diabetic, 6-month banded	11	18.3 ± 1.4†	6.2 ± 0.3

*Reprinted with permission from Dellon et al.[104]

†$p < 0.001$ (for nondiabetic banded versus diabetic banded).

A body of literature is building that demonstrates that the peripheral nerve in the presence of a neuropathy is susceptible to chronic nerve compression. For example, the classic study of streptozocin-induced diabetes that purports to demonstrate structural changes in the peripheral nerve due to experimental diabetes, in fact may be interpreted as demonstrating increased susceptibility of the diabetic nerve to chronic compression. In that study, Brown et al[101] evaluated the plantar digital nerves in their diabetic animals. Subsequently, Sharma et al[102] studied the same nerves in the same animal model. The changes they found were demyelination in addition to the subperineurial edema and axonopathy. It is well-known, however, that the plantar nerves must pass through the tarsal tunnel, a well-documented site of chronic nerve entrapment (see Chapter 12). Thus, the changes these researchers found demonstrated that the nerve in a diabetic animal could undergo changes that have been described with chronic nerve entrapment[13,14] superimposed on the underlying neuropathy. Recently, in a model of acute nerve compression, the streptozocin-induced diabetic rat had a 30 mmHg force applied for 3 hours to the sciatic nerve and the fast component of axoplasmic transport was measured.[103] Accumulation of axonally transported proteins was significantly higher in the acutely compressed diabetic nerve than in the nondiabetic nerve. We have demonstrated, also in the streptozocin-induced diabetic rat, that in chronic nerve compression, utilizing the model previously described,[13,14] the diabetic nerve is more susceptible to compression.[104] In this study, nondiabetic rats had one sciatic nerve banded and one sciatic nerve in the diabetic rat, induced by streptozocin, was also banded. Six months after banding, at which time only minimal changes occur in the nondiabetic rat (Table 14-3), significant changes had occurred in the diabetic rat, related to the diabetes alone (the nonbanded sciatic nerve in the diabetic rat), whereas the most significant changes in conduction velocity and amplitude had occurred in the banded nerve in the diabetic rat ($p < 0.001$) (Fig. 14-15). These results suggest that in the presence of hyperglycemia, the peripheral nerve is more susceptible to chronic compression. The histopathologic findings from this study clearly demonstrate that the axonopathy results only in subperineurial and endoneurial edema, with axonal dwindling and myelin knuckling, whereas compression induces demyelination, connective tissue changes and Wallerian degeneration (Fig. 14-15)[105] (Table 14-4).

Table 14-4. Morphometric Assessment of Rat Sciatic Nerve in Diabetes*

	Normal	*Diabetic Noncompressed*	*Diabetic Compressed*
Axon/myelin ratio	0.6	0.6	1.0
Nerve fiber diameter (μ)	6.7	7.2	4.7
Wallerian degeneration	none	none	some

*From Mackinnon and Dellon.[105]

Alcoholic Neuropathy

The clinical approach to the treatment of persons with symptomatic neuropathy increasingly will become based on the observations outlined. For the most common cause of peripheral neuropathy, diabetic neuropathy, the situation will be described extensively in the next section. Another common cause of peripheral neuropathy is alcoholic polyneuropathy. There still exists considerable debate as to whether the neuropathy is related to a toxic effect of the alcohol itself or to nutritional factors.[106] Shields[107] has noted that the "institution of a nutritionally balanced diet constitutes the principal therapy for alcoholic neuropathy, however significant improvement following such therapy is not frequently seen." In contrast, Hillbom and Wennberg[108] have noted a more favorable prognosis. Interestingly, their work seems to favor a toxic effect of the alcohol in that "three patients who continued drinking in our series were given adequate vitamin therapy but despite this their signs and symptoms were not markedly improved. On the other hand, four of the eight patients who managed to abstain (from alcohol) and who did not receive vitamins at all, nevertheless recovered."

Nerve entrapment that can occur clinically in patients with alcoholic neuropathy has been noted by many but, in particular, one study[109] compared the results of the treatment of ulnar nerve compression at the

Table 14-5. Results of Ulnar Nerve Transposition Related to Alcohol Abuse*

Symptoms or Signs	*No.*	*Motor Function Improved*	*Improved Sensibility*
Alcohol abuse	6	1/4 (25%)	1/5 (20%)
No alcohol abuse	19	5/8 (63%)	10/13 (77%)

*Reprinted with permission from Lugnegar et al.[109]

elbow in alcoholics and nonalcoholics (Table 14-5). These researchers showed that among 25 patients, those with alcohol abuse had improvement in only 25% in terms of motor function and 20% in terms of sensibility recovery versus 63 and 73% for the group that did not abuse alcohol. The problem with this study's conclusion, which would be that alcoholics do not do well after clinical nerve decompression, is that the technique used for transposition was not a submuscular transposition and, in addition, their patients did not have an internal neurolysis (see next section for current treatment of diabetic neuropathy with superimposed nerve compression). Furthermore, the investigators did not state whether the patients had refrained from alcohol abuse in the postoperative period.

The existence of a diet described by Lieber et al[110,111] permits the induction of alcoholism with a nutritionally balanced diet by feeding the animals a certain percentage of their calories as alcohol. We have utilized this diet to create alcoholic rats and then after 5 months, when liver biopsies have demonstrated fatty infiltration, the rats had their sciatic nerves banded.[13,14] After 6 months of banding and electrophysiologic recordings, it was demonstrated that, as described for the diabetic rat,[112] the alcoholic rat's sciatic nerve had increased susceptibility to chronic nerve compression (Fig. 14-16; Table 14-6).

In alcoholism, the histopathologic examination demonstrated some subperineurial edema and little else. However, the banded alcoholic sciatic nerve showed marked myelin thinning and perineurial and epineurial thickening. The toxic effect of the alcohol, predisposing the nerve to compression, is most evident by the large number of fibers with Wallerian degeneration (Table 14-6; Fig. 14-15).

Table 14-6. Morphometric Assessment of Rat Sciatic Nerve in Alcoholism

	Normal	*Alcoholic Noncompressed*	*Alcoholic Compressed*
Axon/myelin ratio	0.6	0.6	0.9
Nerve fiber diameter (μ)	6.7	7.2	4.2
Wallerian degeneration	none	none	moderate

*From Dellon and Mackinnon.[112]

It may be inferred, then, that the symptoms of alcoholic neuropathy may be related to chronic nerve compression and perhaps a more aggressive approach to attempting nerve decompression in these patients, as outlined for diabetics, would be worthwhile.

Uremic Neuropathy

As continuing experimental models are developed, this same approach may be related to patients with symptoms of uremic neuropathy. Although a model for uremic neuropathy was not available in the past,[77] a model has recently been developed.[113,114] The morphometric studies indicating the susceptibility of uremic nerves to compression have yet to be carried out; however, the approach to the treatment of symptoms in these patients by nerve decompression has been reported.[115] All 20 of the cases reported in this series had successful release, and intraoperatively the median nerve was markedly narrowed beneath the transverse carpal ligament, was adherent to the transverse carpal ligament, and had proximal pseudoneuroma formation. In these patients, the roof of Guyon's canal (see Chapter 8) also was opened and the ulnar nerve appeared "compressed and constricted by the thickened ligament."

Further complicating the etiology in the uremic patients may be the coexistence of amyloid. Amyloid was present in the median nerve epineurium in 19 of the 20 hands operated on (11 patients). This study contains a good description of the problems in attempting to diagnose a superimposed nerve entrapment on an underlying neuropathy by electrodiagnostic criteria alone. Some help may be available in this dilemma by utilization of the new technique comparing the F wave.[116] In this study, which evaluated 30 normal, 30 diabetic, and 30 uremic patients, the conduction in the proximal and distal median and ulnar nerve segments were evaluated. Further refinements and modifications continue to be reported to aid in diagnosis of these entrapments.[117]

Other Nondiabetic Neuropathies

Another clinical area of importance concerns patients with vasculitis. Patients commonly encountered are those with rheumatoid arthritis, scleroderma, polyarteritis, or other forms of vasculitis. These patients have diffuse neuropathies that are frequently symptomatic. A model has been described of inducing a chronic inflammatory polyneuropathy.[118] In that study, patients had a plasmapheresis done and had symptomatic improvement during this treatment. The plasma was passively transferred to monkeys who subsequently developed an inflammatory polyneuropathy. The mechanism of the neuropathy as documented electrophysiologically was not determined. The controversy of the role of ischemia in neuropathy, as initially reported by Eames and Lang,[119] has been recently discussed.[120] The current concept is that in a vasculitic neuropathy, with a predisposition for distal symptoms, the basis for the symptoms is ischemia with nerve infarct, as had been described in the diabetic with oculomotor problems[121] and ischemic mononeuropathy.[122]

Parry[120] has made the point that in "rheumatoid arthritis and systemic lupus erythematosis, there is a propensity for individual nerve deficits to be quite insignificant and that the neuropathy comes to light only when these deficits become confluent, by which time the multifocal nature of the disorder becomes apparent." This comment by Parry reflects the concept of this chapter, of the multiple crush syndromes in which the underlying neuropathy predisposes to multiple sites of anatomic compression. There has been a recent report of carpal tunnel release in patients with diffuse peripheral neuropathy.[123] Of the 44 patients, 14 had diabetes, two had rheumatoid arthritis, two had hypothyroidism, one had hyperthyroidism and the cause of the generalized peripheral neuropathy was not determined in 22. Symptomatic improvement was obtained in 92% of the patients and complete relief in 72%.[123]

There is not supposed to be a neuropathy associated with hyperuricemia. Four patients with gout have been operated on by us for peripheral nerve compression. The compression was not found to be due to pressure from tophi. It seemed to us that an alternative might be a neuropathy secondary to the patient's medical treatment for gout, that is, colchicine or allopurinol. Since colchicine is a classic toxin, used to arrest cell division in metaphase and to injure neural microtubules in experimental models, this seemed likely. No known mechanism for allopurinol in neural toxicity has been described, but perhaps it has not been tested directly. This could be done by placing animals on a diet containing allopurinol and adding a sciatic nerve compression, in a manner analogous to that described for diabetes[104] and alcoholism.[112] Recently, in fact, clinical examples of colchicine neuropathy have been described.[124] These patients have an associated weakness due to direct toxic effect of the colchicine on muscle. This would be critical to ascertain (by elevated serum creatinine kinase levels) for evaluating recovery of strength, for example, after ulnar nerve decompression at the elbow.

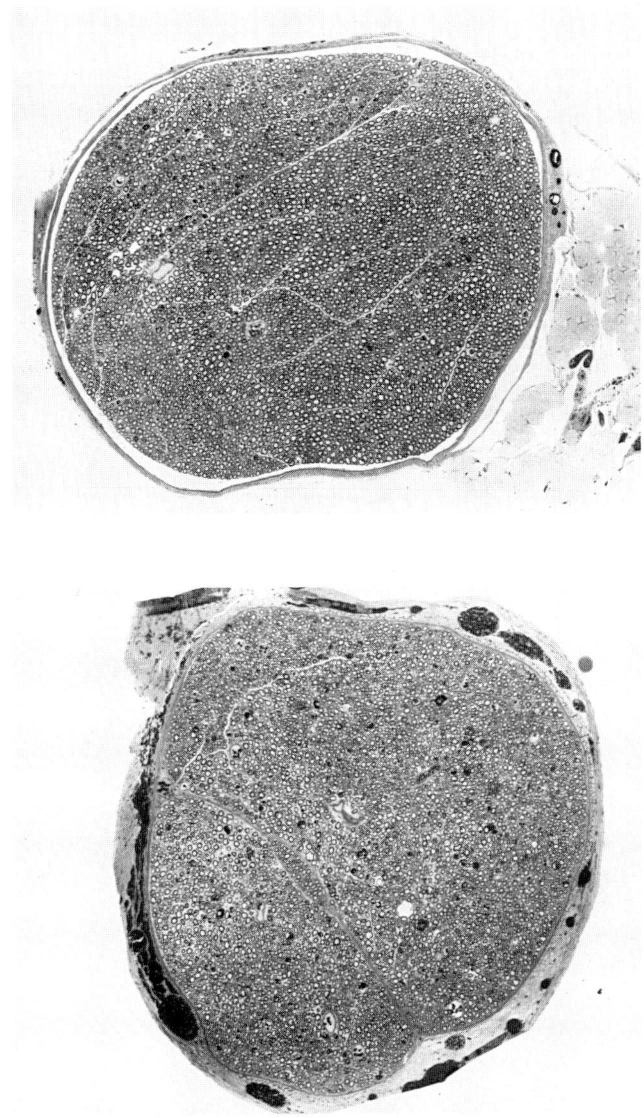

a

b

Figure 14-16. Histopathologic features of alcoholic rat sciatic nerve (a, c) with superimposed nerve compression for 6 months (b, d). In alcoholic neuropathy in this model, there is subperineurial edema (a), with preservation of the myelin and little axonopathy measurable. (*Figure continues.*)

Diabetic Neuropathy

In diabetes, there has long been disagreement and controversy over the definition of terms and diagnostic criteria, as well as over the safety and efficacy of recommended therapeutic modalities ... the most genuine controveries result from inadequate knowledge. The field of diabetes mellitus is awash with controversies that need to be resolved by carefully designed and executed epidemiologic, clinical and basic research. After

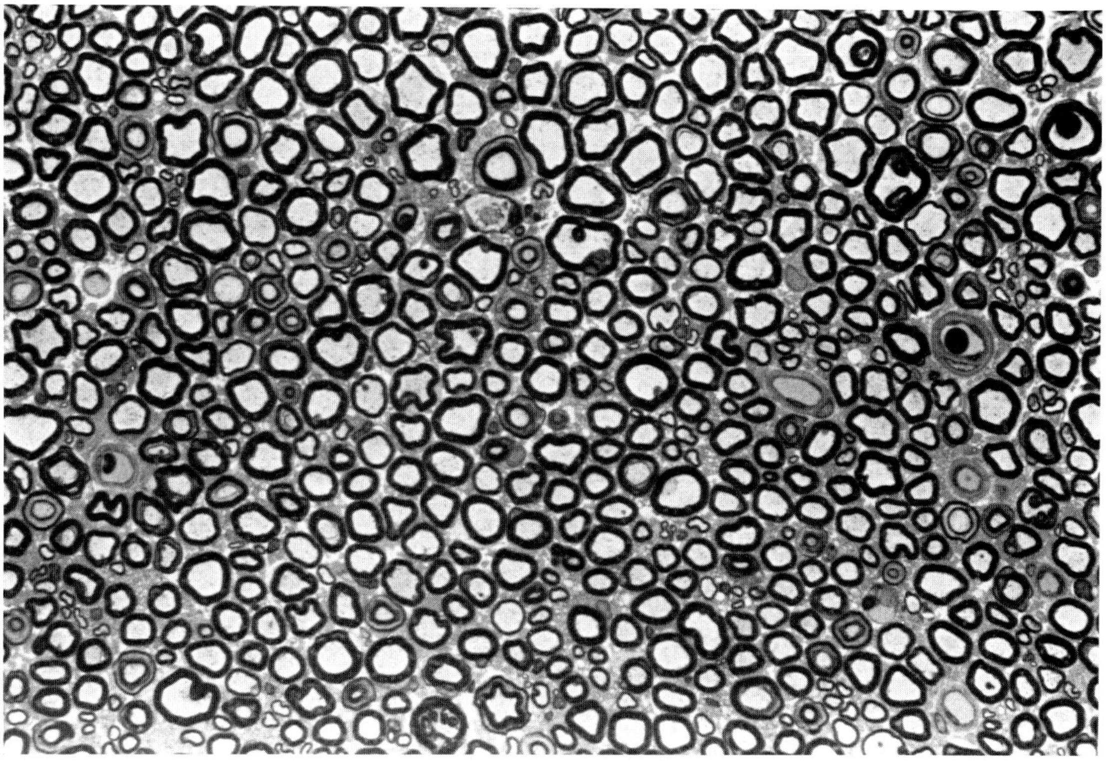

c

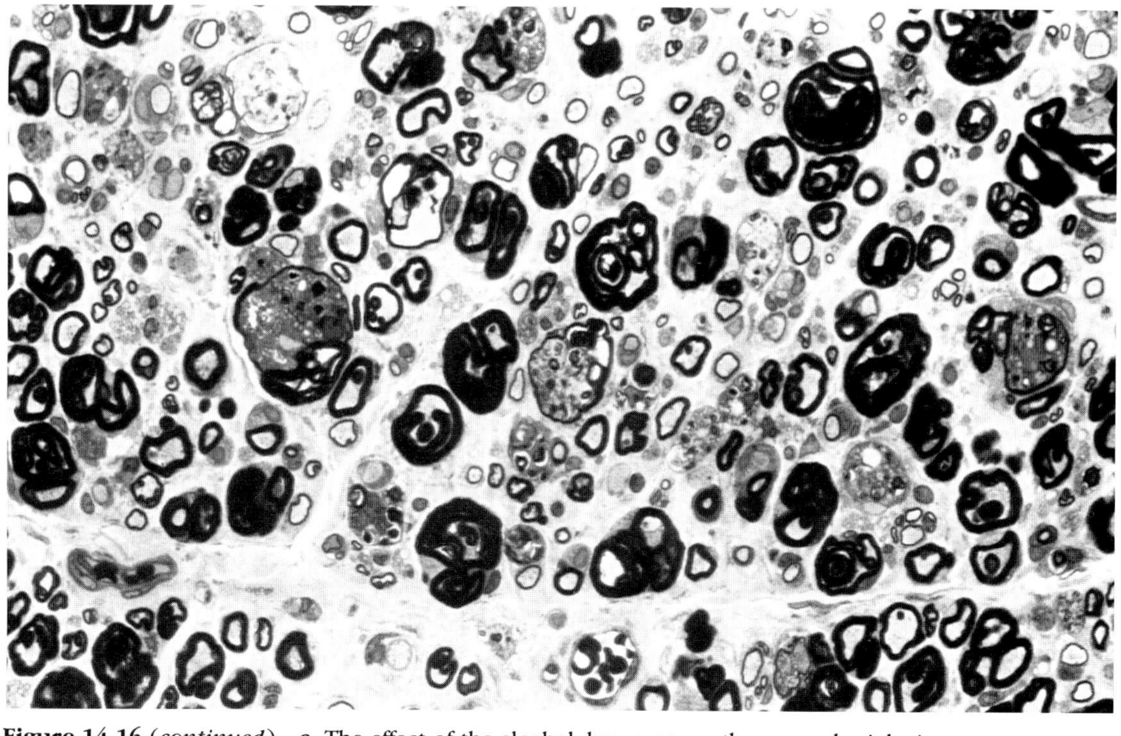

d

Figure 14-16 (*continued*) **c.** The effect of the alcohol, however, on the neurophysiologic state, despite this lack of structural change, is clear when mild compression is placed about the nerve. There is epineurial and perineurial thickening (**b**), as well as myelin thinning and Wallerian degeneration (**d**). The alcoholic nerve is extremely susceptible to nerve compression. Compare "alcoholic" nerve (**c**) to compressed alcoholic nerve (**d**). (Reproduced with permission from Dellon and Mackinnon.[112])

> the needed research is completed, most of the controversies almost certainly will recede into the fog of history.[125]
>
> As is often the case in medicine, physicians are called upon to make decisions that are based on fragmentary and inconclusive evidence, and that may have a profound influence on patients ... as heretical as it may sound, my feeling is that much of the information in textbooks and review articles on diabetes mellitus is not pertinent to these kinds of clinical decisions.[126]

The cost to our society from diabetic neuropathies is enormous. For example, there are 11 million diabetics now, with the prevalence increasing at 6% per year, to an estimated 20 million by the year 2000. The incidence of diabetes neuropathy is approximately 10% at onset of diabetes, increasing to 90% by 25 years' duration of diabetes, and the diabetic population is increasing in age. Half are over the age of 50 years. Amputations are performed on more than 35,000 diabetics per year. Twenty percent of diabetics enter hospitals because of foot problems, whose basis is usually neuropathy.[127]

In a recent treatise on the treatment of peripheral neuropathies, Hallet et al[128] reviewed 336 articles. They indicate no role for surgical decompression in the treatment of peripheral neuropathy. This is not surprising, since the classic teaching has been that diabetic neuropathy is an irreversible, progressive disease.[77,126,129] However, based on the multiple crush syndrome concepts outlined in the preceding sections and the basic science studies just outlined, it became clear that cause for optimism in diabetic neuropathy might exist.[130] We proceeded with clinical work; the hypothesis being that symptoms of diabetic neuropathy may be due to multiple peripheral nerve entrapments. This concept was elucidated as segments of related book chapters.[131–133] In 1988, this cause for optimism appeared as an editorial,[134] accompanying our basic research article on the increased susceptibility of the diabetic nerve to compression.[135]

During this time, the opportunity developed to evaluate a case of insulin-requiring diabetes that developed spontaneously in an aged cynomolgus monkey.[19,134] Electrophysiologic studies in this animal demonstrated findings consistent with classic diabetic neuropathy.[136] Following these baseline studies, one upper extremity was subjected to a series of Silastic bands, utilizing the technique previously described in our model for chronic nerve compression in the primate.[137] After just 4 months of banding, there was significant deterioration in the electrophysiologic findings. In the model for chronic compression in the primate, this degree of electrical change was not present until the nerves had been banded for 1 year, thus confirming the susceptibility of this primate diabetic nerve to compression. The histopathologic findings (Fig. 14-17) demonstrated that in the nonbanded side where the nerve was not subjected to normal anatomic narrowing in its compression, the nerve had subperineurial edema and axonopathy. As this nerve crossed a normal set of anatomic narrowings, such as the elbow with Osborne's band, it underwent significant thinning of the myelin with findings of epineurial and perineurial thickening, such as was found in the model for chronic nerve compression. In a more distal site of anatomic narrowing, such as the carpal tunnel, the morphometric findings were more severe. On the side with the banding, there were sequential worsenings of all morphometric measurements as multiple sites of anatomic compression were summated (Table 14-7).[19]

These observations in the diabetic primate confirmed the observations of the diabetic rat nerve susceptibility to compression and suggested that published earlier reports of "pure" human diabetic neuropathy[138] (Fig. 14-18) were, in fact, examples of the histopathologic evidence of diabetic neuropathy with superimposed chronic nerve compression. The biopsies of human nerves came from radial sensory and sural nerves,[138] sites that we know can have compression (Chapters 10 and 13). Furthermore, the published biopsies (Fig. 14-17) resembled our experimental compression models (Figs. 14-14, 14-17) and human nerve compression,[139,140] than they do experimental diabetes (Figs 14-13, 14-17). Thus, the stage was set for clinical investigation.

The results of the treatment of 84 entrapped peripheral nerves in 33 patients with symptomatic dia-

Table 14-7. Morphometric Assessment of Diabetic Primate Radial Nerve with Multiple Crush Syndrome*

Radial Nerve	*Mean Fiber Diameter (μ)*	*Percent Neural Tissue (%)*	*Axon to Myelin Ratio*
Nonbanded side			
Proximal to elbow	6.6	34	0.36
Banded side			
Proximal to elbow (no band)	6.7	41	0.34
2 cm distal to elbow (band)	5.4	32	0.33
Mid forearm (band)	5.2	25	0.43
At distal forearm fascial transit site	4.2	21	0.38
At radial styloid	3.8	20	0.63

*From Mackinnon and Dellon[19]

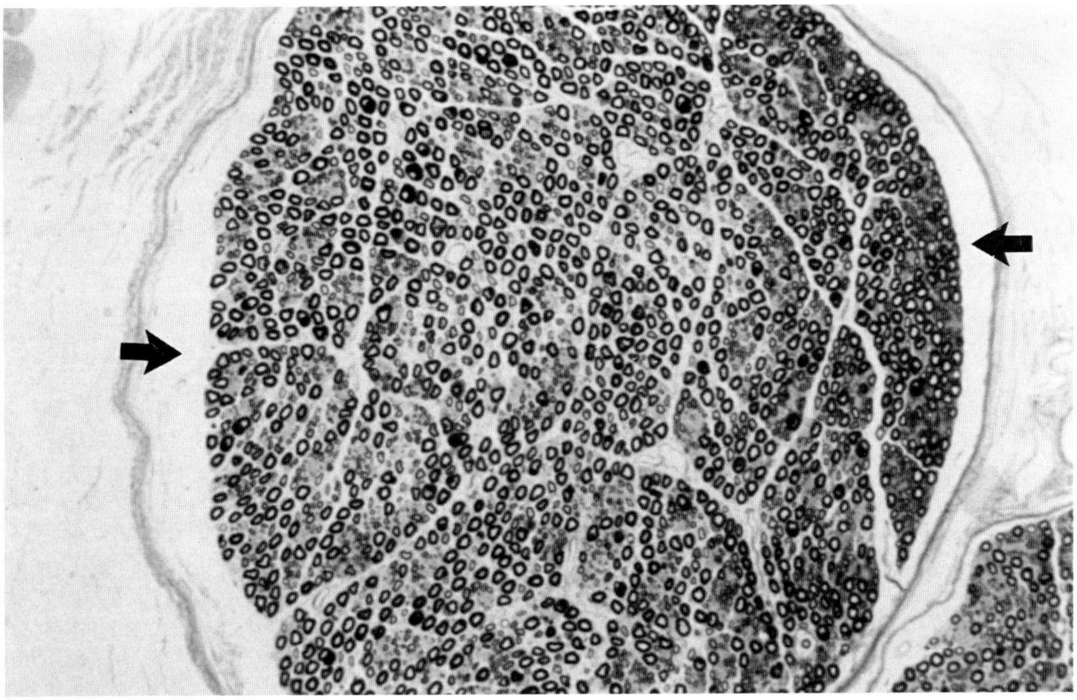

a

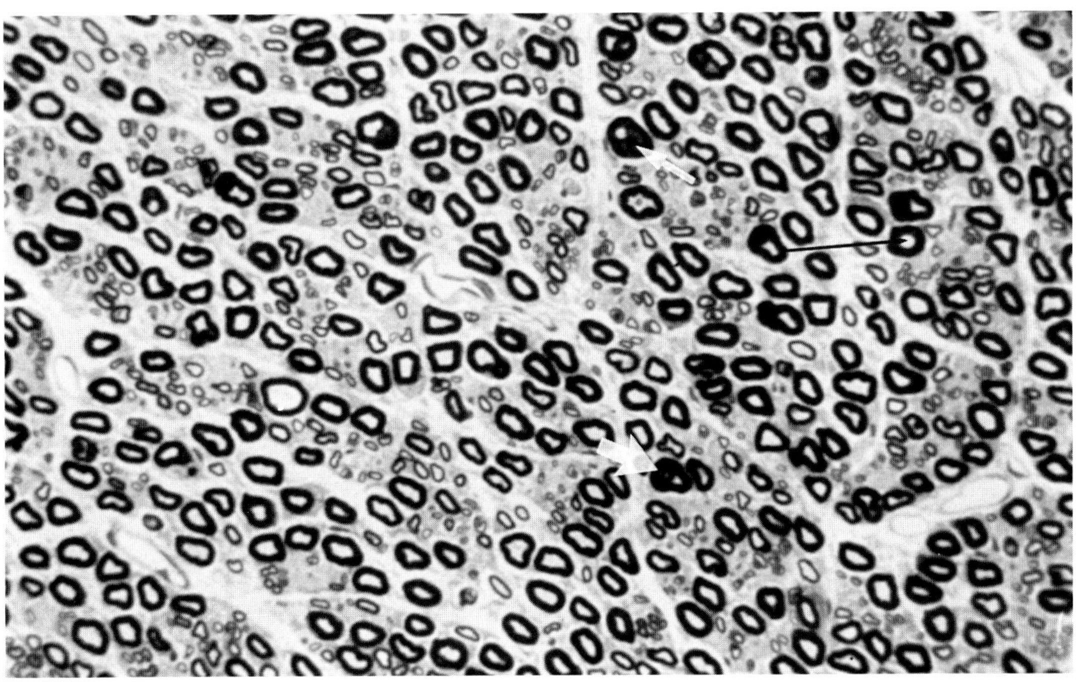

b

Figure 14-17. Histopathologic features of diabetic primate, spontaneously type I. Low power (**a, c, e**) and higher power (**b, d, f**) views of ulnar nerve in upper arm (**a, b**), ulnar nerve in cubital tunnel beneath Osborne's band (**c, d**), and median nerve in carpal tunnel (**e, f**). Without compression, the primate peripheral nerve in type I diabetes shows subperineurial edema (**a**) (arrows), endoneurial edema, axonopathy (note axonal dwindling [thin black arrow] and myelin knuckling [thick white arrow]), (**b**) without connective tissue change or myelin thinning. As compression is added to the diabetic neuropathy by normal anatomic structures, such as Osborne's band (**c, d**) and the transverse carpal ligament (**e, f**), there is increased epineurial thickening (**c**) (thick white arrows), both extra- and intrafascicular, increased perineurial thickening, and thinning of the myelin (**d**) (thin arrows), progressing to Renaut (r) bodies (**e**) and Wallerian degeneration (**f**) (open arrow). (Reproduced with permission from Mackinnon and Dellon.[19]) *(Figure continues)*

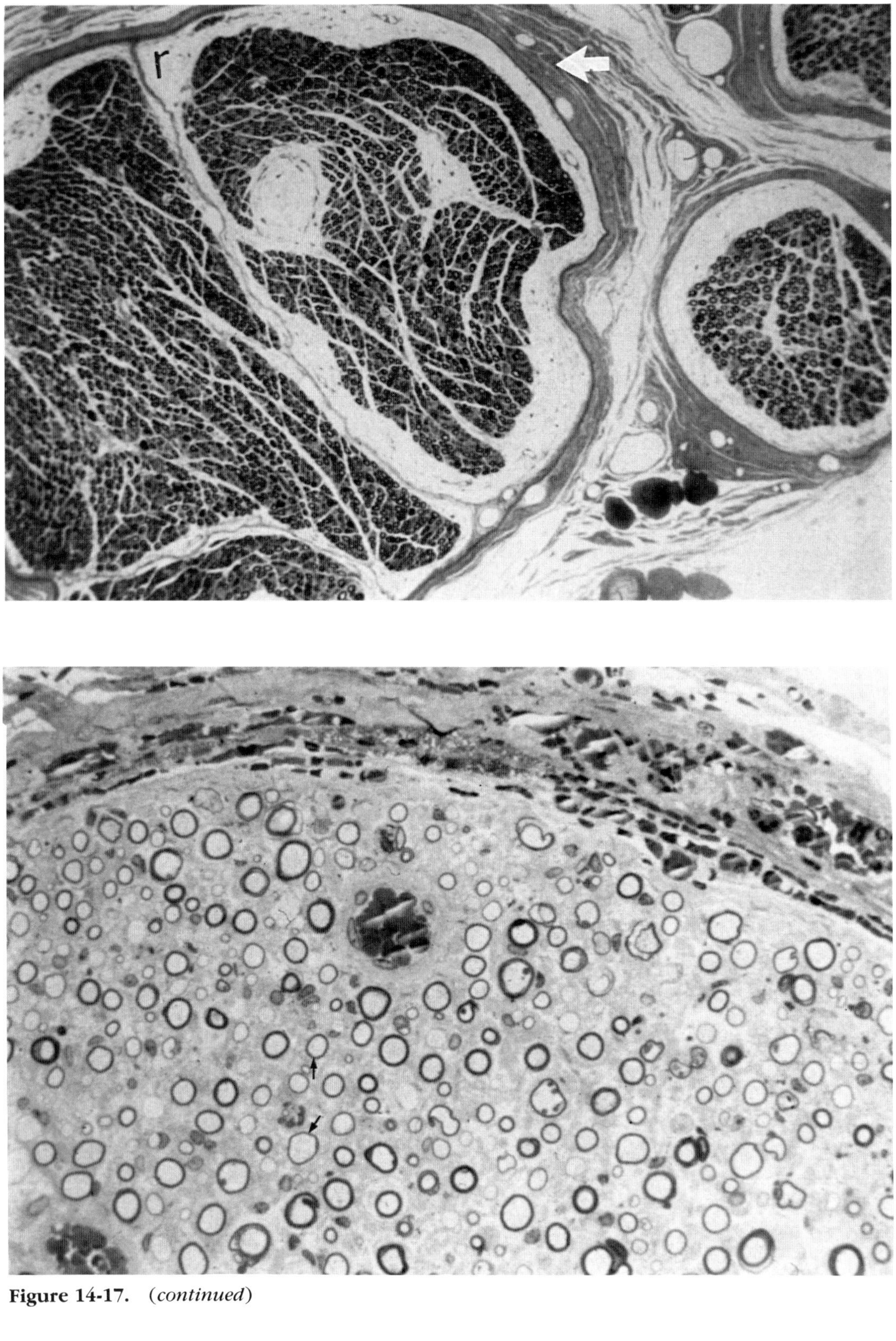

c

d

Figure 14-17. (*continued*)

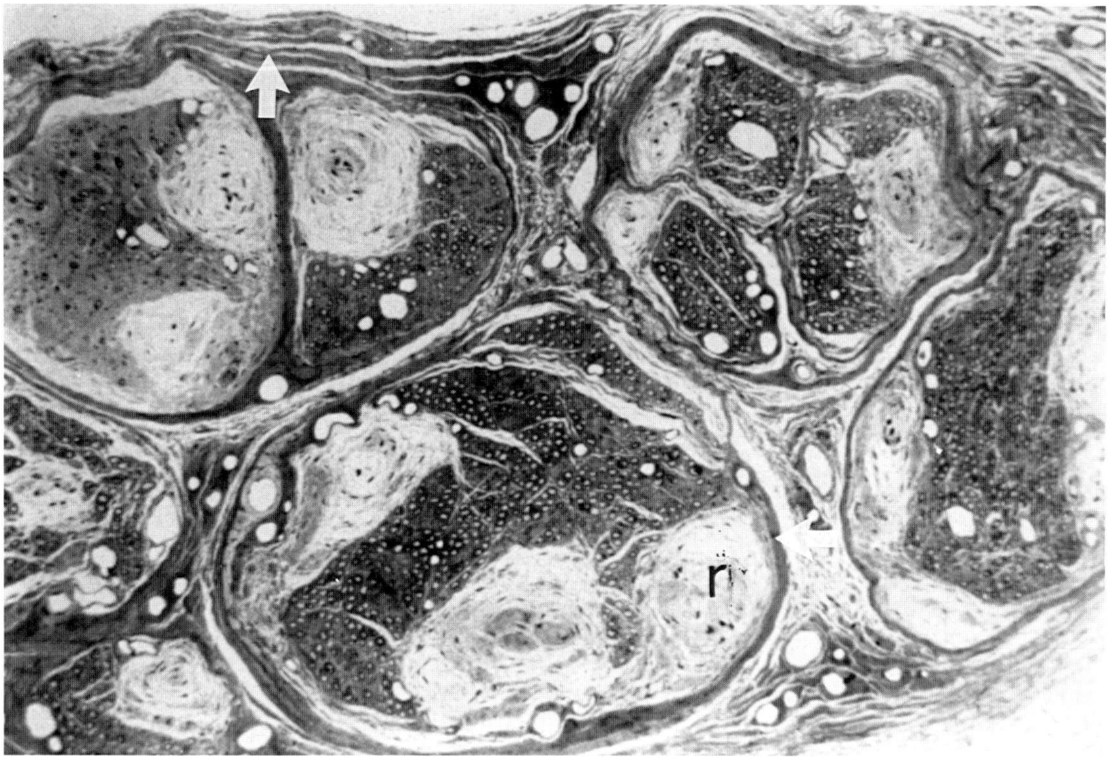

e

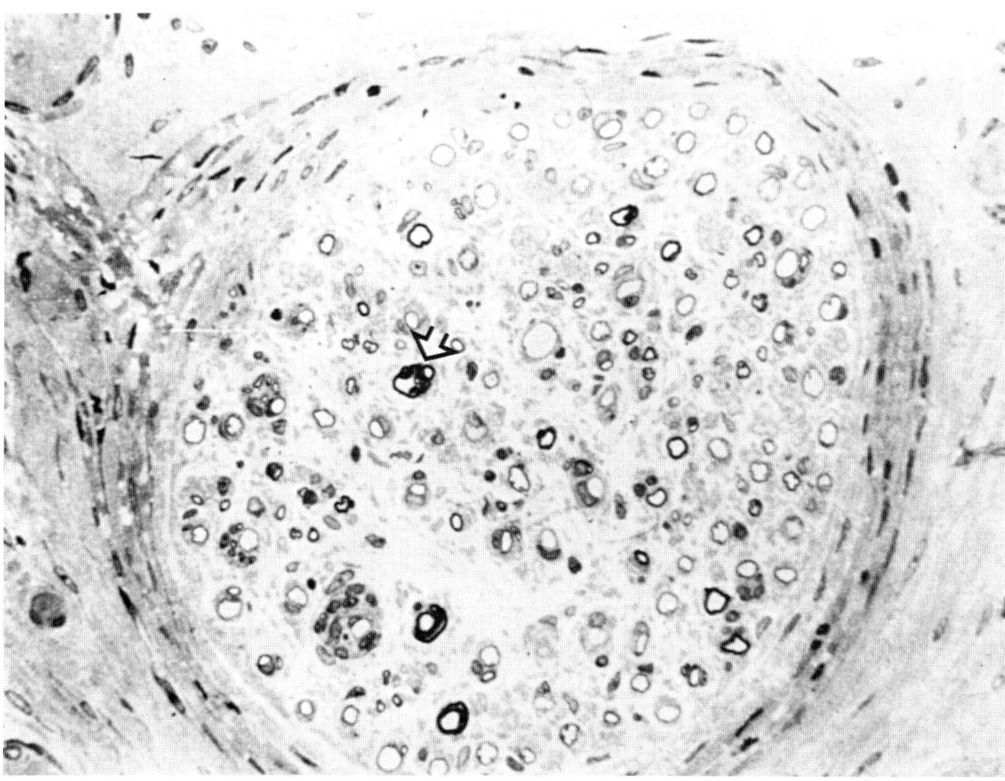

f

Figure 14-17. (*continued*)

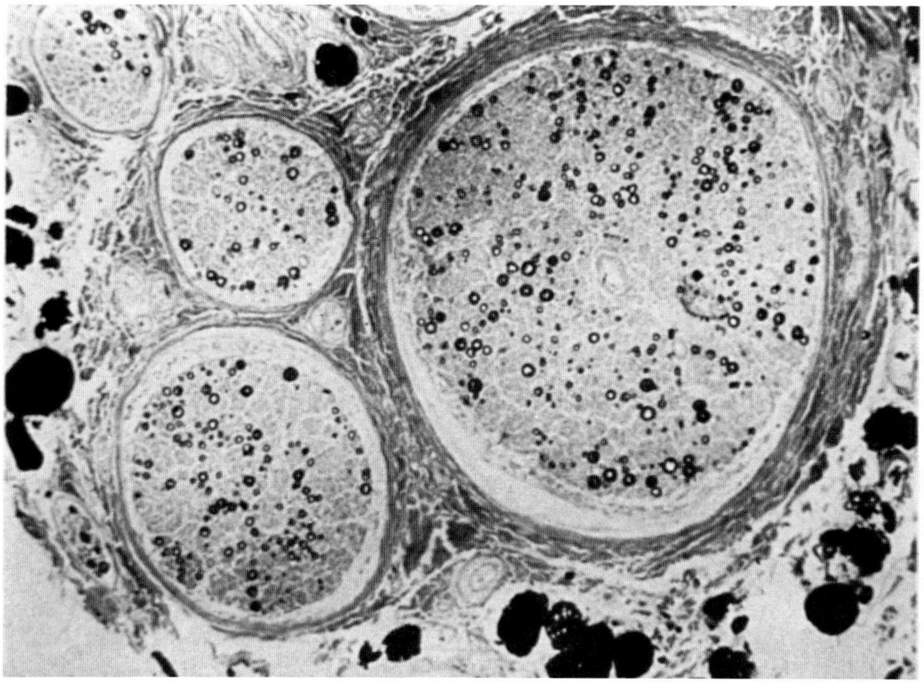

Figure 14-18. Reported changes in human diabetic neuropathy. This biopsy of a human radial nerve from a diabetic shows the subperineurial edema characteristic of diabetes, and some axonopathy, but the predominant pattern is thickening of epineurium and perineurium, marked thinning and loss of myelin, changes most consistent with superimposed nerve compression (see text for further comparison with experimental and human nerve compression). (Reproduced with permission from Thomas and Lascelles et al. [138])

betic neuropathy were reported before The American Association of Plastic Surgery in 1987.[141,142] The mean follow-up was 17.2 months. Operative sites were median nerves at the wrist (Chapter 6), ulnar nerves at the elbow (Chapter 9), radial sensory nerves in the forearm (Chapter 10), posterior tibial, medial, and lateral plantar nerves in the tarsal tunnel (Chapter 12, and Figs. 12-12, 12-13), common peroneal nerve at the knee (Chapter 13), and deep peroneal nerve over the dorsum of the foot (Chapter 13). The operation was a release of external compressive structures, such as Osborne's band and the flexor retinaculum, remembering that multiple peripheral nerve entrapments in a single extremity can give a clinical picture resembling a "stocking" or "glove" sensory loss (Figs. 13-2, 13-5, 13-10). For each severely compressed nerve, a microsurgical internal neurolysis was included (Chapter 5). A microsurgical internal neurolysis can be done without creating additional scarring[143] and yields better results than simple decompression alone in a model of severe chronic nerve compression[144] (Table 14-8). The results were evaluated by the surgeon's subjective analysis, by detailed sensory and motor final evaluations (Tables 14-9, 14-10), by comparisons of the preoperative versus the postoperative sensory and motor changes (Table 14-11), and by preoperative and postoperative electrodiagnostic studies (Table 14-12). Results of this study

Table 14-8. Surgical Treatment of Symptomatic Diabetic Neuropathy: Nerve Distribution*

Nerve Distribution	*Type I Diabetes*	*Type II Diabetes*	*Total*
Upper extremity			
Median at the wrist	14	14	28
Ulnar at the elbow	8	12	20
Radial sensory, forearm	5	1	6
Subtotal	27	27	54
Lower extremity			
Posterior tibial, ankle	13	7	20
Common peroneal, knee	6	2	8
Deep peroneal, foot	1	1	2
Subtotal	20	10	30
Total	47	37	84

*Reprinted with permission from Dellon.[141]

Table 14-9. Surgical Treatment of Symptomatic Diabetic Neuropathy: Upper Extremity Preoperative and Postoperative "Final" Grading Scales*

Sensory†					*Motor*		
Vibratory	*m2PD (mm)*	*s2PD (mm)*			*Pinch (lb)*	*Grip (lb)*	*Wasting (%)*
Normal	≤3	≤6	Excellent	Female	≥15	≥40	1+
				Male	≥20	≥60	
↑ or ↓	4–5	7–14	Good	Female	10–14	26–39	2+
				Male	13–19	31–59	
↓	6–8	15–29	Fair	Female	6–9	15–25	3+
				Male	6–12	15–30	
↓ ↓	≥9	≥30	Poor		≤5	≤15	4+

*Reprinted with permission from Dellon.[141]

†m2PD: moving two-point discrimination; s2PD: static two-point discrimination; ↑: increased; ↓: decreased.

Table 14-10. Surgical Treatment of Symptomatic Diabetic Neuropathy of Other Areas: Sensory Grading Scales*

	Moving Two-Point Discrimination (mm)		
Grade	*Big Toe*	*Dorsal Foot Web*	*Dorsal Radial Hand*
Excellent	≤6	≤6	≤6
Good	7–9	7–12	7–9
Fair	10–13	13–19	10–15
Poor	≥14	≥20	≥15

*Reprinted with permission from Dellon.[141]

Table 14-11. Surgical Treatment of Symptomatic Diabetic Neuropathy: Preoperative to Postoperative "Change" Grading Scales*

Degree of Change	*Grade*
No change from preoperative status	No change
Any down-grading from before surgery	Worse
Upgrading of one degree	Good
Upgrading of two degrees	Excellent

*Reprinted with permission from Dellon.[141]

demonstrated that 80% of the patients received good to excellent results regardless of which evaluation technique was utilized (Figure 14-19; Tables 14-13, 14-14). In particular, 76% of the patients with postoperative

Table 14-13. Surgical Treatment of Symptomatic Diabetic Neuropathy: Results by Clinical Assesment*

	Criteria (%)				
		Sensory		*Motor*	
Results	*Subjective*	*Final*	*Change*	*Final*	*Change*
Excellent	64	62	39	46	32
Good	30	21	54	38	50
Fair or no change	6	17	7	12	16
Poor or worse	0	0	0	4	2

*Reprinted with permission from Dellon.[141]

Table 14-14. Surgical Treatment of Symptomatic Diabetic Neuropathy: Results by Electrodiagnostic Criteria*

	Number of Patients with Preoperative Diagnosis			
	Neuropathy Only	*Neuropathy and Superimposed*	*Nerve Compression Only*	*Total*
	No. of Patients			
Improved	7	8	5	20
No change	6	1	0	7
Worse	3	0	0	3
Total	16	9	5	30

*Reprinted with permission from Dellon.[141]

Table 14-12. Surgical Treatment of Symptomatic Diabetic Neuropathy: Preoperative Electrodiagnostic Studies*

		Preoperative Diagnosis						
Normal		*Neuropathy*		*Nerve Compression*		*Nerve Compression Superimposed on Neuropathy*		
No.	*%*	*No.*	*%*	*No.*	*%*	*No.*	*%*	*Total*
11	14	36	46	17	22	14	18	78

*Reprinted with permission from Dellon.[141]

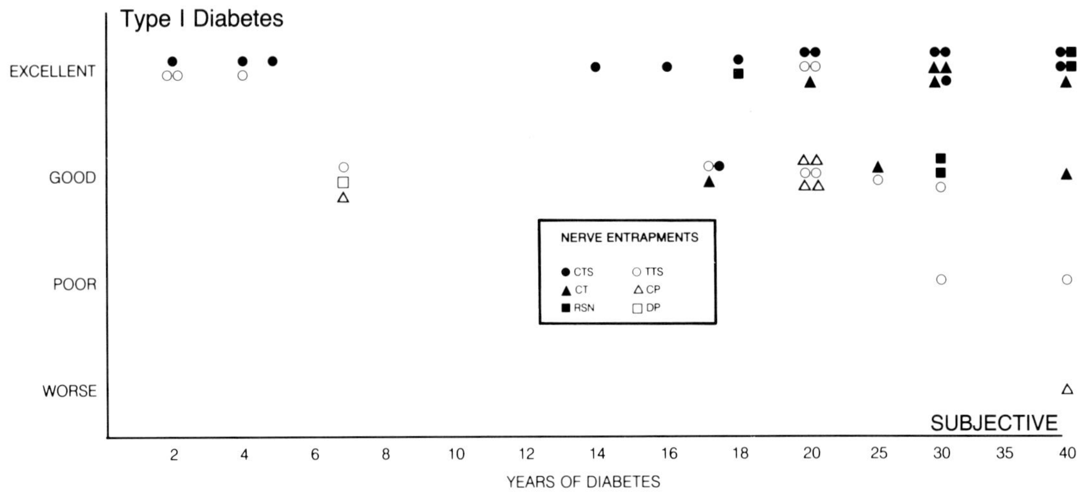

a

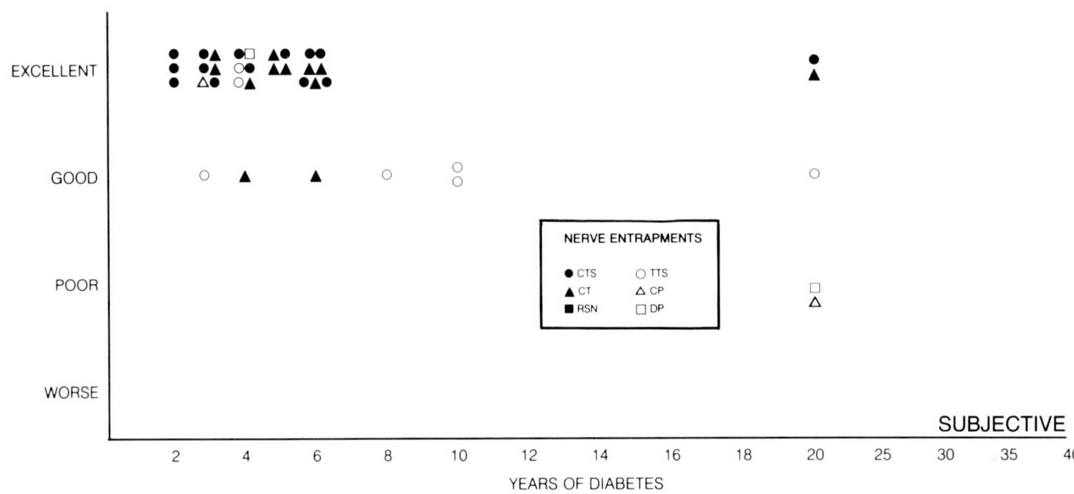

b

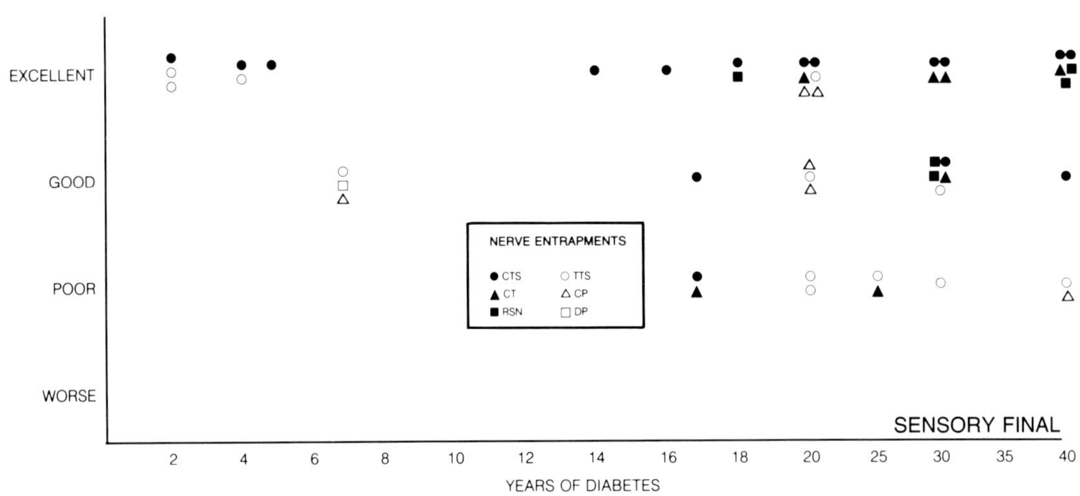

c

Figure 14-19. Results of surgical treatment of symptomatic diabetic neuropathy depicted by a scattergram for each of the five different evaluation schemes: subjective (**a, b**), sensory final (**c, d**), sensory change (**e, f**), motor final (**g, h**), motor change (**i, j**) for both type I (a, c, e, g, i) and type II (b, d, f, h, j) diabetics. The degree of success of the operation is plotted against the duration of each patient's diabetes, so each dot represents one patient. *(Figure continues.)*

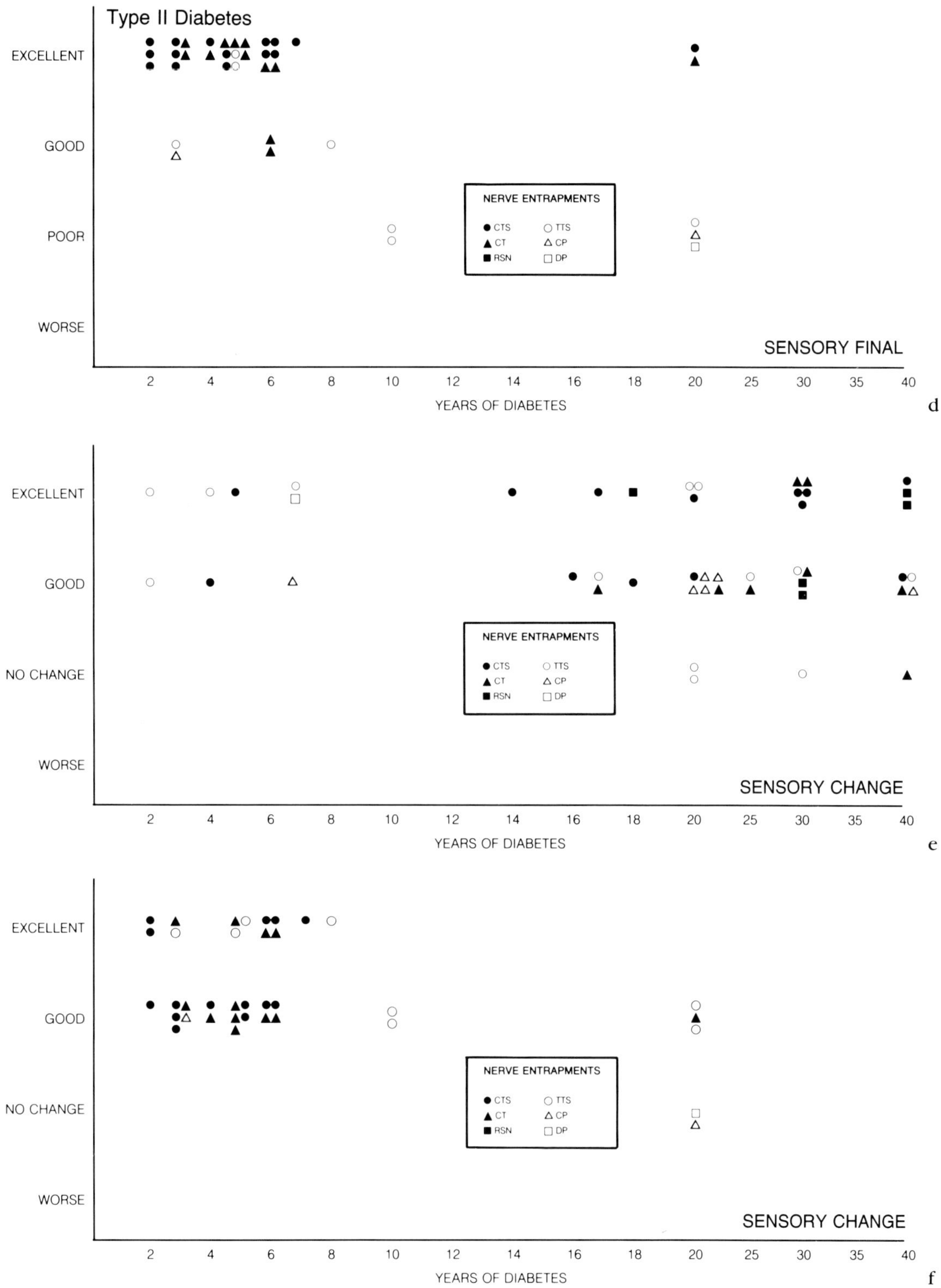

Figure 14-19 (*continued*). The shape of the patient representation (circle, square, etc.) indicates which nerve was treated, with upper extremity nerves being represented by open and lower extremity by filled-in characters. By any evaluation criteria, greater than 80% of the patients achieved good to excellent results from the surgery (see also Table 14-13). (Reproduced with permission from Dellon.[141]) *(Figure continues)*

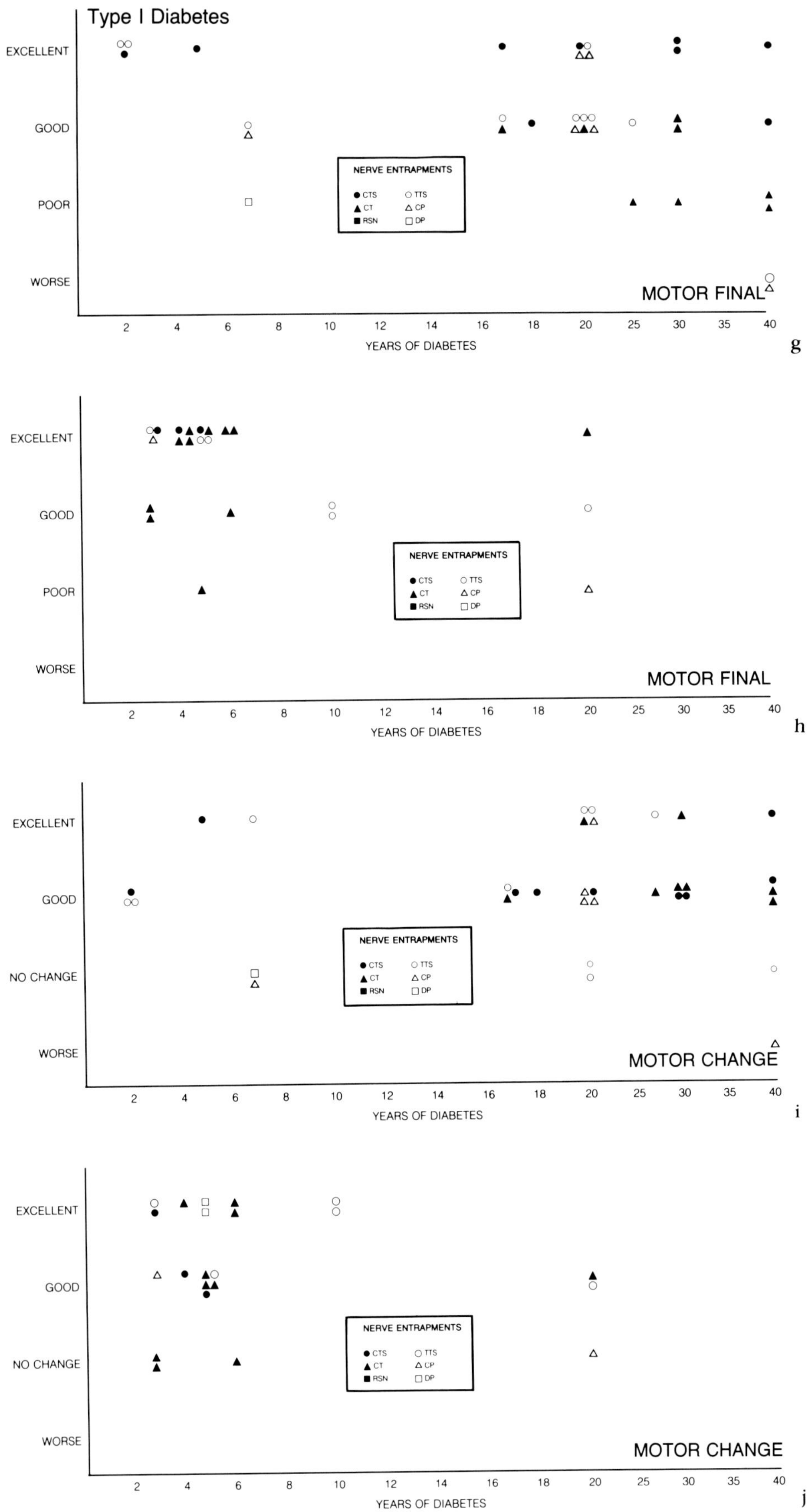

Figure 14-19. *(continued)*

P.G. 27 Y.O. FEMALE TYPE I DIABETES, 4 years

Carpal tunnel syndrome	m2PD (mm)	grading systems: clinical		grading systems: electrical	latency (msec)
1/84	4	Good	↓ Good	↓ Excellent	5.1
4/86	2	Excellent			4.4
Tarsal tunnel syndrome					
1/84	11	Fair	↓ Excellent	↓ None	none
4/86	5	Excellent			none

Figure 14-20. Case study. Surgical treatment of symptomatic diabetic neuropathy from median nerve compression at wrist and posterior tibial nerve compression at ankle in a 27-year-old with type I diabetes of 4 years' duration. At follow-up 27 months after surgery, two-point discrimination had improved in the hand and foot. The final sensory and sensory change gradings are noted. The electrical studies showed improvement in distal sensory latency to the index fingers, but for the big toe, where preoperatively there was no obtainable sensory response to stimulation, there was no postoperative improvement. This case highlights the different reportable results possible for the same operation, same patient, depending on the grading system utilized. (Reproduced with permission from Dellon.[141])

D.E. 55 year old Type II Diabetic of 4 years

R carpal tunnel syndrome	Clinical: Sensory			Motor pinch	Motor grip			Electrical: latency motor	latency sens.	C.V.	amplitude	
9/85	persist	G	↓ G					4.6	5.2		3000	1
3/86	normal	E						3.0	3.6		6000	7
R cubital tunnel syndrome												
9/85	persist	G	↓ G	15	20	F	↓ E	9.1		52	5000	
3/86	normal	E		20	60	E		8.0		69	6000	

Figure 14-21. Case study. Surgical treatment of symptomatic diabetic neuropathy from median nerve compression at the wrist and ulnar nerve compression at the elbow in a 55-year-old with type II diabetes of 4 years' duration. In contrast to the case in Figure 14-20, this patient's analysis included motor function because the ulnar nerve was involved at the elbow level. Note that at follow-up at 6 months after surgery, pinch strength increased from 15 to 20 pounds and grip strength from 20 to 80 kg, an excellent result by both motor final and motor change assessment techniques. Note, too, that electrically there is not only improved sensory latencies for the median nerve at the wrist, but also improved sensory amplitude. Motor evaluation by nerve conduction improved from 52 to 69 m/s after surgery, and the motor latency improved, too (9.1 to 8.0 ms.). (Reproduced with permission from Dellon.[141])

SURGERY

L.M. 59 TYPE I DIABETES, 2 years

Carpal tunnel syndrome	m2PD	symptoms	grading clinical		electrical
2/84	3	persistent	Good	Good	4.9 msec
4/86	3	gone	Excellent		4.5
Tarsal tunnel syndrome					
5/84	10	persistent	Fair	Excellent	5.2 msec
4/86	5	gone	Excellent		3.9

a

NO SURGERY

L.M. 59 TYPE I DIABETES, 2 years

Carpal tunnel syndrome	symptoms	electrical
R sural		3.6 mse
11/81	persistent	no response
8/85	persistent	
R peroneal		
11/81	persistent	4.7 msec
8/85	persistent	no response

b

Figure 14-22. Case study. Surgical treatment of symptomatic diabetic neuropathies from tarsal and carpal tunnel syndrome in a type I diabetic, whose diabetes onset was 2 years previously. In addition to the sensory final and change grading systems discussed in Figure 14-24 and the text, note that there was improved electrical functioning in each treated nerve by 26 months postoperatively. **a.** In this same patient, two other nerves were not treated surgically, the sural and the peroneal. Please note that postoperatively the electrical response of these two, nonoperated nerves worsened, whereas the same test in the treated nerves improved during this same time period (**b**). (Reproduced with permission from Dellon.[141])

electrodiagnostic studies showed improvement, and greater than 80% of patients achieved good to excellent results by any other criteria used. The lower extremities, as well as the upper extremities, achieved these results, but it took longer to achieve this level in the lower extremities. Type I diabetics did as well as type II diabetics. Results were achieved even in patients requiring insulin for as long as 30 years. Just one patient was made worse by the operative procedure, a patient requiring insulin for 41 years, who had loss of the foot everters after common peroneal release. Individual case studies are instructive (Figs. 14-20 to 14-22). The overall conclusion is that *there is an optimism for the treatment of the symptoms of diabetic neuropathy* by the surgeon carrying out a decompression and internal neurolysis of multiple entrapped nerves in each extremity. It should be clear that the surgeon, while not being able to treat the underlying neuropathy, can decompress the nerve at points of entrapment.

References

1. Upton ARM, McComas AJ: The double crush in nerve entrapment syndromes. Lancet 2:359–362, 1973.
2. Massey EW, Riley TL, Pleet AB: Co-existent carpal tunnel syndrome and cervical radiculopathy (double crush syndrome). South Med J 74:957–959, 1981.
3. Hurst LC, Weissberg D, Carroll RE: The relationship of the double crush to carpal tunnel syndrome (an analysis of 1,000 cases of carpal tunnel syndrome). J Hand Surg [Br] 10:202–204, 1985.
4. Spencer PS, Sabri MI, Schaumburg HH, et al: Does a defect of energy metabolism in the nerve fiber underlie axonal degeneration in polyneuropathies? Ann Neurol 5:501–507, 1979.
5. Powell HC, Myers RR, Costello ML, et al: Endoneurial

fluid pressure in Wallerian degeneration. Ann Neurol 5:550–557, 1979.
6. Liveson JA, Spielholz NI: Peripheral Neurology. FA Davis, Philadelphia, 1979, p 20.
7. Carroll RE, Hurst LC: The relationship of thoracic outlet syndrome and carpal tunnel syndrome. Clin Orthop 164: 149–153, 1982.
8. Traisman HS, Newcomb AL: Management of Juvenile Diabetes. CV Mosby, St Louis, 1965, pp 1–25.
9. Bland JH, Nakano KK: Neck pain. In Edgar S, Kelly WN, Harris ED, Ruddy S, Sledge CCB, eds: Textbook of Rheumatology. WB Saunders, Philadelphia, 1981, pp 411–446.
10. Rothman HR, Simeone FE: The Spine. WB Saunders, Philadelphia, 1975, pp 387–433.
11. Cseuze KA, Thomas JE, Lambert EH, Love JG, Lipscomb PR: Long-term Results of operation for carpal tunnel syndrome. Mayo Clin Proc 41:232–241, 1966.
12. Seiler WA, Schlegel R, Mackinnon SE, Dellon AL: The double crush syndrome: Experimental model in the rat. Surg Forum 34:596–598, 1983.
13. Mackinnon SE, Dellon AL, Hudson AR, Hunter D: Chronic nerve compression—an experimental model in the rat. Ann Plast Surg 13:112–120, 1984.
14. O'Brien JP, Mackinnon SE, MacLean AR, Dellon AL, Hudson AR, Hunter DA: A model of chronic nerve compression in the rat. Ann Plast Surg 19:430–435, 1987.
15. Lundborg G: The theory of the double crush syndrome. Correspondence Newsletter #9, American Society of Surgery of the Hand, Oct 24, 1985.
16. Dellon AL, Mackinnon SE: Verification of the double crush hypothesis. Ann Plast Surg 1990. In press.
17. Dellon AL, Hendler N, Hopkins JET, Karas AC, Campbell JN: Team management of patients with diffuse upper extremity complaints. Md Med J 35:849–852, 1986.
18. Roos DB: The place for scalenectomy and first rib resection in thoracic outlet syndrome. Surgery 92:1077–1085, 1982.
19. Mackinnon SE, Dellon AL: Morphometric assessment of banded and non-banded nerves in Type I diabetic primate. In preparation. 1990.
20. Hendler N, Fink H, Long D: Myofascial syndrome: Response to trigger point injections. J Acad Psychosom Med 24:990–999, 1983.
21. Hendler N, Uematesu S, Long D: Thermographic validation of physical complaints in psychogenic "pain" patients. J Acad Psychosom Med 23:4–9, 1982.
22. Mackinnon SE, Holder LE: Use of three-phase radionuclide bone scanning in the diagnosis of reflex sympathetic dystrophy. J Hand Surg [Am] 9:556–563, 1984.
23. Hendler N, Biernstein M, Gucer RP, Long D: A preoperative screening test for chronic back pain patients. J Acad Psychosom Med 20:801–808, 1979.
24. Mackinnon SE, Dellon AL, Hendler N: Modification of a screening test for chronic back pain for application in upper extremity pain patients. In preparation.
25. Dellon AL, Mackinnon SE: Musculoaponeurotic variations along the course of the median nerve in the proximal forearm. J Hand Surg [Br] 12:359–363, 1987.
26. Breidenbach W, Tsai T, Manstein C: Ipsilateral pronator teres and carpal tunnel compression of the median nerve. (Abstr.) J Hand Surg [Am] 10:432, 1985.
27. Seyffarth H: Primary myoses in the M. pronator terres as causive lesion of the M. medianus (the pronator syndrome). Acta Psychiatr Neurol [Suppl] 74:1, 1951.
28. Werner CO, Rosen I, Thorngren KG: Clinical and neurophysiologic characteristics of the pronator syndrome. Clin Orthop 197:231–236, 1985.
29. Kiloh LG, Nevin S: Isolated neuritis of the anterior interosseus nerve. Br Med J 1:850–851, 1952.
30. Hill NA, Howard FM, Huffer BR: The incomplete anterior interosseous nerve syndrome. J Hand Surg [Am] 10A:4–16, 1985.
31. Spinner M: Injuries to the Major Branches of the Peripheral Nerves of the Forearm, 2nd ed. WB Saunders, Philadelphia, 1978, p 162.
32. Dellon AL: Musculotendinous variations about the elbow. J Hand Surg [Br] 11:175–181, 1986.
33. Willshire WH: Supernumerary first rib: Clinical records. Lancet 2:633, 1860.
34. Coote H: Pressure on the axillary vessels and nerve by an exostosis from a cervical rib: Interference with the circulation of the arm. Removal of rib and exostosis: Recovery. Med Times Gaz 2:108, 1861.
35. Murphy JB: The clinical significance of cervical ribs. Surg Gynecol Obstet 3:515–520, 1906.
36. Adson AW, Coffey JR: Cervical rib: A method of anterior approach for relief of symptoms by division of the scalenus anticus. Ann Surg 85:839–857, 1927.
37. Ochsner S, Gage M, DeBakey M: Scalenus anticus (Naffziger's syndrome). Am J Surg 28:669–695, 1935.
38. Naffziger HC, Grant WT: Neuritis of the brachial plexus. Mechanical in origin: The scalenus anticus syndrome. Surg Gynecol Obstet 67:722–730, 1938.
39. Adson AW: Surgical treatment for symptoms produced by cervical ribs; in the scalene anticus muscle. Surg Gynecol Obstet 85:687–696, 1947.
40. Jaboulay, 1899. Cited by Kirtley JA, Riddell DH, Stoney WS, Wright JK: Cervicothoracic sympathectomy in neurovascular abnormalities of the upper extremities: Experience in 76 patients with 104 sympathectomies. Ann Surg 165:869–879, 1967.
41. Bramwell E: Lesion of the first dorsal nerve root. Rev Neurol Psychiatr 1:299, 1903.
42. Murphy T: Brachial neuritis caused by pressure of the first rib. Aust Med J 15:582, 1910.
43. Lewis T, Pickering G: Observations upon maladies in which the blood supply to the digits ceases intermittently or permanently. Clin Sci 1:327–366, 1934.
44. Eden KC: The vascular complications of cervical ribs in first thoracic rib abnormalities. Br J Surg 27:111–139, 1939–40.
45. Falconer MA, Weddell G: Costoclavicular compression of the subclavian artery and vein in relations to the scalenus anticus syndrome. Lancet 2:539–544, 1943.
46. Wright IS: Neurovascular syndrome produced by hyperabduction of the arm. Original communication. Heart J 29:1–19, 1945.
47. Lord JW Jr: Surgical management of shoulder girdle syndromes. Arch Surg 66:69–83, 1953.

48. Peet RM, Hendrickson JD, Anderson TP, Martin GM: Thoracic outlet syndrome: Evaluation of a therapeutic exercise program. Staff Meet Mayo Clinic 31:281–287, 1956.
49. Clagett OT: Presidential Address: Research and prosearch. J Thorac Cardiovasc Surg 44:153–166, 1962.
50. Roos DB, Owens JC: Thoracic outlet syndrome. Arch Surg 93:71–74, 1966.
51. Urshel HC, Razzuk MA: Management of the thoracic outlet syndrome. N Engl J Med 286:1140–1143, 1972.
52. Urshel HC, Razzuk MA, Albers JE, et al: Reoperation for recurrent thoracic outlet syndrome. Ann Thorac Surg 21:1–9, 1976.
53. Hempel GK, Rusher AH Jr, Wheeler CG, Hunt DG, Bukhari HI: Supraclavicular resecton of the first rib for thoracic outlet syndrome. Am J Surg 141:213–215, 1981.
54. Sanders RJ, Raymer S: The supraclavicular approach to scalenectomy and first rib resection: Description of technique. J Vasc Surg 2:751–756, 1985.
55. Swinson WM, Vigesaa RE, Hieb RE, James EC: Thoracic outlet syndrome: The supraclavicular approach to first rib resection. Surg Rounds, 73–78, Sept 1986.
56. Stalworth JM, Quinn GJ, Aiken AF: Is first rib resection necessary for relief of thoracic outlet syndrome: Ann Surg 185:581–589, 1979.
57. Stalworth JM, Horn JB: Diagnosis and management of thoracic outlet syndrome. Arch Surg 119:1149–1151, 1984.
58. Halsted WS: An experimental study of circumscribed dilation of an artery immediately distal to a partially occluding band, and its bearing on dilation of the subclavian artery observed in certain cases of cervical rib. J Exp Med 24:271–290, 1916.
59. Roos DB: Congenital anomalies associated with thoracic outlet syndrome. Am J Surg 132:771–778, 1976.
60. Telford ED, Mottershead S: Pressure at the cervicobrachial junction: An operative and anatomic study. J Bone Joint Surg 30B:249–263, 1948.
61. Raff J: Surgery for cervical rib and scalenus anticus syndrome. JAMA 157:219–223, 1955.
62. Batt M, Griffet JE, Scotti LE, Bas P: Thoracic outlet syndrome: Report of 112 cases toward a more defined tactical approach [translation from French]. J Chir (Paris) 120:687–691, 1983.
63. Qvarfordt PG, Ehrenfeld WK, Stoney RJ: Supraclavicular radical scalenectomy and transaxillary first rib resection for the thoracic outlet syndrome. A combined approach. Am J Surg 148:111–116, 1984.
64. Martens V, Bugden C: Thoracic outlet syndrome: A review of 67 cases. Can J Surg 23:357–358, 1980.
65. Lusskin R, Campbell JB, Thompson WAL: Post-traumatic lesions of the brachial plexus: Treatment by transclavicular exploration and neurolysis or autograft reconstruction. J Bone Joint Surg 55A:1159–1176, 1973.
66. Kline DG, Judice DJ: Operative management of selected brachial plexus lesions. J Neurosurg 58:631–649, 1983.
67. Martin J, Gaspar DJ, Johnston PW, Kohl RD, Jr, Dietrick W: Vascular manifestations of the thoracic outlet syndrome and surgical urgency. Arch Surg 111:779–782, 1976.
68. Pang D, Wessel B: Thoracic outlet syndrome: Review article. Neurosurg 22:105–121, 1988.
69. Dellon AL, Mackinnon SE, Campbell J, Patterson GA: Throacic outlet diagnostic protocol, prospective study. In preparation. 1990.
70. Siivoli J, Sulg I, Pokela R: Somatosensory evoked responses as a diagnostic aid in thoracic outlet syndrome. A preoperative study. Acta Chir Scand 148:647–652, 1982.
71. Huffman JD: Electrodiagnostic techniques for and conservative treatment of thoracic outlet syndrome. Clin Orthop 207:21–23, 1986.
72. Mackinnon SE, Nelems W: The use of the vibratory stress test in the diagnosis of thoracic outlet syndrome. In preparation. 1990.
73. Jaeger SH, Read R, Smullens SN, Breme P: Thoracic outlet syndrome: Diagnosis and treatment. In Hunter JM, Schneider LH, Macken EJ, Callahan AD, eds: Rehabilitation of the Hand, 2nd ed. CV Mosby, St Louis, 1984, pp 378–389.
74. Nichols HM: Anatomic structures of the thoracic outlet. Clin Orthop 207:13–20, 1986.
75. Dellon AL: Brachial plexus compression versus thoracic outlet syndrome: An example of the multiple crush syndrome. In preparation. 1990.
76. Dyck PJ, Thomas PK, Lambert EH, Bunge R: Peripheral Neuropathy, vol. 1 & 2; 2nd ed. WB Saunders, Philadelphia, 1984.
77. Cavanagh JB: The significance of the "dying back" process in experimental and human neurologic disease. Int Rev Exp Pathol 3:219–267, 1964.
78. Cavanagh JB: The dying back process. A common denominator in many naturally occurring and toxic neuropathies. Arch Pathol Lab Med 103:659–664, 1979.
79. Spencer PS, Schaumberg HH: Central-peripheral distal axonopathy: The pathogenesis of dying back polyneuropathies. In Zimmerman H, ed: Progress in Neuropathy, vol 3. Grune & Stratton, New York, 1976, p 253.
80. Lowndes HE, Baker T: Toxic site of action in distal axonopathies. In Spencer PH, Schaumberg HH, eds: Experimental and Clinical Neurotoxicology. Williams & Wilkins, Baltimore, 1980, pp 193–205.
81. Spencer PS, Schaumberg HH: Classification of neurotoxic disease. In Spencer PS, Schaumberg HH eds. Experimental and Clinical Neurotoxicology. Williams & Wilkins, Baltimore, 1980, p 92.
82. Asbury AK, Brown MJ: The evolution of structural changes in distal axonopathies. In Spencer PS, Schaumberg HH eds. Experimental and Clinical Neurotoxicology. Williams & Wilkins, Baltimore, 1980, p 179.
83. Lundborg G: Structure and function of the intraneural microvessels as related to trauma, edema formation and nerve function. J Bone Joint Surg 57A:938–948, 1975.
84. Jakobsen J: Axonal dwindling in early experimental diabetes. I. A study of cross-section nerves. Diabetologia 12:539–546, 1976.
85. Jakobsen J: Axonal dwindling in early experimental diabetes. II. A study of isolated nerve fibers. Diabetologia 12:547–553, 1976.
86. Jakobsen J, Malgrin L, Olsson Y: Permeability of blood-

nerve barrier in the streptozotocin diabetic rat. Exp Neurol 60:277–285, 1978.

87. Jakobsen J: Peripheral nerves in early experimental diabetes. Expansion of the endoneurial space as a cause of increased water content. Diabetologia 14:113–119, 1978.
88. Jakobsen J, Sidenius P: Decreased axonal flux of retrogradally transported glycoproteins in early experimental diabetes. J Neurochem 33:1055–1060, 1979.
89. Jakobsen J, Sidenius P: Decreased axonal transport of structural proteins in streptozotocin diabetic rats. J Clin Invest 66:292–296, 1980.
90. Powell HC: Pathology of diabetic neuropathy: New observations and new hypotheses. Lab Invest 49:515–518, 1983.
91. Eaton RP: The collagen hydration hypothesis: A new paradym for the secondary complications of diabetes mellitus. J Chron Dis 39:763–766, 1986.
92. Gabbay KH, Snider JJ: Nerve conduction defect in galactose-fed rats. Diabetes 21:295–300, 1972.
93. Sharma AK, Thomas PK, Baker RW: Peripheral nerve abnormalities related to galactose administration in rats. J Neurol Neurosurg Psychiatry 39:794–802, 1976.
94. Powell HC, Meyers RR: Schwann cell changes and demyelination in chronic galactose neuropathy. Muscle Nerve 6:217–218, 1983.
95. Meyers RR, Powell HC: Galactose neuropathy: Impact of chronic endoneurial edema on nerve-blood flow. Ann Neurol 16:587–594, 1984.
96. Ohnishi A, Schilling K, Brimijoin WS, Lambert EH, Fairbanks VF, Dyck PJ: Lead neuropathy. I. Morphometry, nerve conduction and cholinacetyle transferase transport: New finding of endoneurial edema associated with segmental demyelination. J Neuropathol Exp Neurol 36: 499–518, 1977.
97. Clark AW, Griffin JW, Price DL: The axonal pathology in chronic IDPN intoxification. J Neuropathol Exp Neurol 39:42–55, 1980.
98. Dyck PJ, Lais AC, Karnes JL, Sparks MS, Hunder H, Low PA, Windbank AG: Permanent axotomy, a model of axonal atrophy in secondary segmental dymyelination and remyelination. Ann Neurol 9:575–583, 1981.
99. Windbank AJ, McCall JT, Hunder HG, Dyck PJ: The endoneurial content of lead related to the onset and severity of segemental demyelination. J Neuropathol Exp Neurol 39:692–699, 1980.
100. Windbank AJ, Dyck PJ: Kinetics of 210 Pb and entry into the endoneurium. Brain Res 225:67–73, 1981.
101. Brown MJ, Somner AJ, Greene DA, Diamond SM, Asbury AK: Distal neuropathy in experimental diabetes mellitus. Ann Neurol 8:168–178, 1980.
102. Sharma AK, Bajada S, Thomas PK: Influence of streptozotocin-induced diabetes in myelinated nerve fiber maturation and body growth in the rat. Acta Neuropathol (Berl) 53:257–261, 1981.
103. Dahlin LB, Meiri KF, McEan WG, Rydevik B, Sjostind J: Effects of nerve compression on fast axonal transport and streptozotocin-induced diabetes mellitus. Diabetologia 29:181–185, 1986.
104. Dellon AL, Mackinnon SE, Seiler WA IV: Susceptibility of diabetic nerve to chronic compression. Ann Plast Surg 20:117–119, 1988.
105. Mackinnon SE, Dellon AL: Morphometric assessment of the diabetic rat sciatic nerve with and without superimposed peripheral nerve compression. In preparation. 1990.
106. Victor M: Polyneuropathy due to nutritional deficiency and alcoholism. In Dyck PJ, Thomas PK, Lambert EH, Bunge R, eds: Peripheral Neuropathy, vol 1 & 2; 2nd ed. WB Saunders Co., Philadelphia, 1984, p 1899–1940.
107. Shields RW Jr: Alcoholic polyneuropathy. Muscle Nerve 8:183–187, 1985.
108. Hillbom M, Wennberg A: Prognosis of alcoholic peripheral neuropathy. J Neurol Neurosurg Psychiatry 47:699–703, 1984.
109. Lugnegar DH, Walhein G, Wennberg A: Operative treatment of ulnar nerve neuropathy in the elbow region. A clinical and electrophysiologic study. Acta Orthop Scand 48:168–176, 1977.
110. Lieber CS, Jones DP, Mendlison J, DeCarli LM: Fatty liver, hyperlipemia and hyperuricemia produced by prolonged alcohol consumption despite adequate dietary intake. Trans Assn Am Physic 76:289–300, 1963.
111. Lieber CS, DeCarli LM: Feeding of alcohol and liquid diets: Two decades of applications. A 1982 update. Alcoholism (NY) 6:523–531, 1982.
112. Dellon AL, Mackinnon SE: Susceptibility of the nerve in chronic alcoholism to chronic compression. Ann Plast Surg. In press. 1990
113. Tegner R, Brismar T: Experimental uremic neuropathy. Part I (Decreased nerve conduction velocity in rats). J Neurol Sci 65:29–36, 1984.
114. Brismar T, Tegner R: Experimental uremic neuropathy. Part II (Sodium permeability decrease and inactivation in potential clamped nerve fibers). J Neurol Sci 65:37–45, 1984.
115. Minami A, Ogino T: Carpal tunnel syndrome in patients undergoing chemodialysis. J Hand Surg [Am] 12:93–97, 1987.
116. Fierro B, Modica A, D'Arpa A, Santangelo R, Raimondo D: Analysis of F wave in metabolic neuropathies: A comparison study in uremic and diabetic patients. Acta Neurol Scand 75:179–185, 1987.
117. Katims JJ, Naviasky EH, Rendell MS, Ng LKY, Bleeker ML: Constant current sine wave transcutaneous nerve stimulation for the evaluation of peripheral neuropathy. Arch Phys Med Rehabil 68:210–213, 1987.
118. Heininger K, Liebert UG, Toyka KV, Hanivoll FT, et al: Chronic inflammatory polyneuropathy: Reduction of nerve conduction velocities in monkeys by systemic passive transfer of immunogobulin G. J Neurol Sci 66:1–14, 1984.
119. Eames RA, Lange LS: Clinical and pathological study of ischemic neuropathy. J Neurol Neurosurg Psychiatry 30:215–226, 1967.
120. Parry GJG: Mononeuropathy multiplex. Muscle Nerve 8:493–498, 1985.
121. Asbury AK, Aldredge H, Hirshberg R, Fisher CM: Oculomotor palsy in diabetes mellitus: A clinicopathological study. Brain 93:555–560, 1970.

122. Raff M, Asbury AK; Ischemic mononeuropathy and mononeuropathy multiplex in diabetes mellitus. N Engl J Med 279:17–22, 1968.
123. Clayburgh RH, Beckenbaugh RD, Dobyns JH: Carpal tunnel release in patients with diffuse peripheral neuropathy. J Hand Surg [Am] 12A:380–383, 1987.
124. Kuncl RW, Duncan G, Watson D, Alderson K, Rogawaski MK, Peper M: Colchicine myopathy and neuropathy. N Engl J Med 316:1562–1568, 1987.
125. Davidson JK, ed: Clinical Diabetes Mellitus. Thieme, New York, 1986, p xvii.
126. Davidson MB: Diabetes Mellitus: Diagnosis and Treatment, 2nd ed. John Wiley & Sons, New York, 1986, p x.
127. Levin ME: Pathophysiology of diabetic foot lesions. In Davidson JK, ed: Clinical Diabetes Mellitus. Thieme, New York, 1986, pp 381–396.
128. Hallett J, Tandon D, Berardelli A: Treatment of peripheral neuropathies. J Neurol Neurosurg Psychiatry 48: 1193–1207, 1985.
129. Walker HK: Peripheral neuropathy. In Davidson JK, ed: Clinical Diabetes Mellitus. Thieme, New York, 1986, pp 416–425.
130. Dellon AL: Unpublished letters.
131. Morain WD, Dellon AL, Mackinnon SE, Colen LB: Reconstructive surgery in the diabetic extremity. Adv Plast Surg 4:1–36, 1987.
132. Dellon AL, Mackinnon SE: Basic scientific and clinical applications of peripheral nerve regeneration. In Nyhus LM, ed: Surg Annual. Appleton, Lange, Norwalk, CT, 1987, pp 59–100.
133. Dellon AL: Interruption of nerve function. In Marsh J, ed: Current Therapy in Plastic and Reconstructive Surgery. BC Becker, Inc., Toronto, 1988.
134. Dellon AL: A cause for optimism in diabetic neuropathy. Ann Plast Surg 20:103–105, 1988.
135. Dellon AL, Mackinnon SE, Seiler WA IV: Susceptibility of the diabetic nerve to chronic compression. Ann Plast Surg 20:117–119, 1988.
136. Cornblath DR, Dellon AL, Mackinnon SE: Electrodiagnostic evaluation of peripheral nerves in Type I diabetic primate. Muscle Nerve, 12:233—235, 1989.
137. Mackinnon SE, Dellon AL, Hudson AR, Hunter DA: Primate model for chronic nerve compression. J Reconstr Microsurg 1:185–196, 1985.
138. Thomas PK, Lascelles RG: Pathology of diabetic neuropathy. Q J Med 35:449–456, 1966.
139. Mackinnon SE, Dellon AL, Hudson AR, Hunter DA: Histopathology of compression of the superficial radial nerve in the forearm. J Hand Surg [Am] 11:199–205, 1986.
140. Mackinnon SE, Dellon AL, Hudson AR, Hunter DA: Chronic human nerve compression: A histologic assessment. Neuropathol Appl Neurobiol 12:547–565, 1986.
141. Dellon AL: Optimism in diabetic neuropathy. Diabetes 37:139A Suppl. (abstr #550), 1988.
142. Dellon AL: Results of the treatment of symptomatic diabetic neuropathy by internal neurolysis of the upper and lower extremity. Presented at American Association of Plastic Surgeons meeting, Nashville, Tennessee, May 1987. In preparation. 1988.
143. Mackinnon SE, Dellon AL: Evaluation of microsurgical internal neurolysis in a primate median nerve model of chronic nerve compression. J Hand Surg. In press. 1990.
144. Mackinnon SE, O'Brien JP, Dellon AL, MacLean AR, Hudson AR, Hunter DA: An assessment of the effects of internal neurolysis, on a chronically compressed rat sciatic nerve. Plast Reconstr Surg 81:251–256, 1988.

Facial Nerve Injury

15

The muscles of the cheek (affected) side are wasted and there appears to remain nothing but the thin integument, which hangs upon the side of the face as if dead without having any action in them or wrinkles, as in the (opposite) cheek; and when he speaks this (paralyzed) cheek is alternately puffed out and then collapsed, the air first distending it as if it were a bag and then escaping at the angles of the mouth. His whole mouth is drawn to the (non-paralyzed) side, thus producing the most remarkable distortion of the face. Whatever action there is in the mouth is altogether owing to the contraction of the muscles on the non-paralyzed side; the paralyzed angle of the mouth hangs loose and it is quite passive; and the saliva is allowed to flow constantly out of the lower lip on this side.

Charles Bell, 1821[2]
London

The eye cannot close and constantly weeps. The mouth dribbles, the speech is interfered with and mastication impaired. The delicate shades of continence are lost. Joy, happiness, sorrow, shock, surprise, all the emotions have for their common expression the same blank stare.

Sterling Bunnell, 1927[3]
San Francisco

In the management of facial palsy, the struggle to re-establish mimetic integrity and natural emotional expression will go on for some time. A perfect rehabilitation will probably never be attainable, but in almost all cases, some degree of improvement is a justifiable hope.

John Conley, 1984
New York

Judged in relation to organic life, paralysis of the seventh cranial nerve is a minor accident. It is, however, an affliction which is difficult to endure, fixing half the face in total, limp inertia, and rendering any attempt at normal expression both grotesque and ridiculous.

Michael Portmann, 1984[11]
Bordeaux

Facial palsy is a truly devastating problem that knows no social or economic boundaries. People interact with fear that the condition is contagious; the simple amenities of handshaking and cheek kissing become embarrassing situations. The patient shuns reflective surfaces, public dining and conversing with strangers. In the marketplace, they may be viewed as handicapped; employers and co-workers may be concerned about their mental ability, wrongfully equating intelligence with facial dysfunction. The inability to show facial expression will cause even the strongest self-esteem to wither. Compassion for those afflicted with facial palsy can only emanate from a true sense of personal vulnerability, an understanding that "this can happen to me."

Annette Rubin, 1986
Long Island

Historical Review

Restoration of function to the face after facial nerve injury has as its ideal goal the restoration of normal facial nerve function. This ideal goal has been pursued for more than a century and a half and yet to be achieved. The facial nerve has a multitude of functions. It carries not only motor fibers to the muscles of facial expression, but also the parasympathetic efferent fibers and the afferent taste fibers, as well as motor fibers to accessory auditory and masticatory muscles (Table 15-1; Figs. 15-1, 15-2[1]). The concept of attempting to restore facial nerve function probably began shortly after Sir Charles Bell first demonstrated, in 1821, the loss of facial expression that occurred with transsection of the seventh cranial nerve.[2] Of historic interest is the first attempt to suture the facial nerve within the temporal bone by Sterling Bunnell in 1927,[3] whose experience in repairing "over 100 small nerves in the hand" by that time enabled him to try this repair, and report

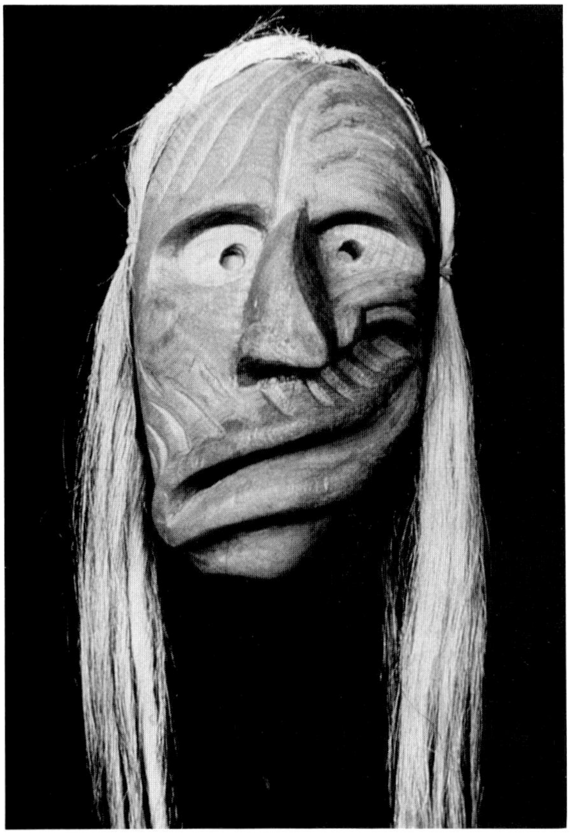

Figure 15-1. "Broken Nose," a Canadian (Ojibway) Indian mask that demonstrates all the classic deformities associated with facial palsy. Note loss of forehead wrinkling, the deviation of the nose and mouth to the nonparalyzed side, sagging of the paralyzed side with loss of nasolabial crease, and the rounder right eye suggesting lagophthalmos.

Table 15-1. Facial Nerve Functions

- I. Motor
  - A. Accessory auditory
    (via nerve to stapedius muscle; loss causes hypercussis)
  - B. Accessory masticatory
    (via branches to posterior belly of digastric and to stylohyoid muscle; loss is not noticeable)
  - C. Facial expression
    1. Frontalis
    2. Ear group
    3. Orbicularis occuli
    4. Zygomaticus group
    5. Nasal group
    6. Cheek group
    7. Orbicularis oris
    8. Lower lip depressor group
    9. Platysma
- II. Secretory
  (via efferents from superior salivatory nucleus)
  - A. Lacrimal gland
  - B. Parotid gland
  - C. Submandibular-sublingual glands
- III. Afferent from taste fibers
  - A. Anterior two-thirds of tongue (via chordotympany and lingual nerve)
  - B. (?)Face ("motor afferents" from muscles of facial expression)

excellent results 17 months later. Unfortunately, such "excellent" results are often not obtained. Frequently, attention to the nerve injury, with repair or grafting, will fail to restore facial nerve function. The goal for the reconstructive surgeon is to reestablish the function of the muscles of facial expression. Evidence of the growing interest in facial nerve problems is the increasing publication of monographs on the facial nerve and its surgery;[4–7] almost 200 pages of text devoted to facial paralysis in our classic plastic surgery texts;[8,9] the appearance of a monograph on reanimation of the paralyzed face;[10] and the Triennial Meeting of the International Symposium on the Facial Nerve published as its Proceedings.[11]

This vast accumulated experience has demonstrated the limits of direct or indirect nerve repair techniques and that the goal of the reconstructive surgeon may be more narrowly defined toward restoration of facial expression. Regardless of the anatomic level of the nerve injury (in its intracranial portion, its intratemporal bone portion, or its extracranial portion), at-

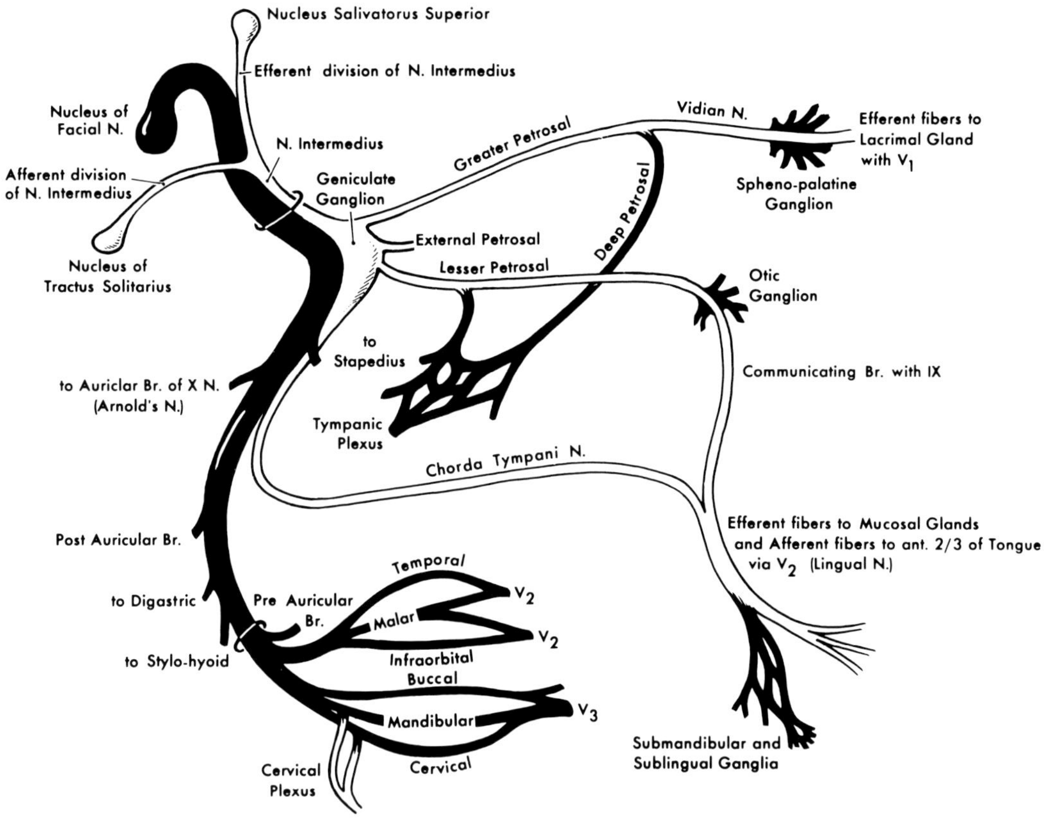

Figure 15-2. Communications of facial nerve with cranial nerves V (trigeminal and divisions of V_1, V_2, V_3), IX (glossopharyngeal), and X (vagus) and with cervical plexus (greater auricular and transverse cervical branches). (Modified with permission from Gray's *Anatomy*.[1])

tempts to rehabilitate the face after facial nerve injury have been directed at three major areas: restoration of protective function to the eyelids to prevent corneal exposure; reconstruction of oral continence to the lower lip; and, most importantly, restoration of smile function. Traditionally, operative procedures involving the muscles of facial expression have been thought of as attempts to restore balance to the face when the facial muscles are either active or at rest (Fig. 15-3). The concept of restoring balance to the face incorporates procedures that work not only on the paralyzed side, but also to relax the overactivity of the nonparalyzed side.

In this chapter, we will not attempt to describe all operative procedures that try to restore balance to the face, since these have been well-described and depicted in the past,[8–10] nor will we attempt to delineate the physical examination and electrodiagnostic studies of the facial nerve or possible causes of facial nerve palsy, since these, too, have been well-described.[5–7,9] Rather, this chapter will attempt to outline our current approach to reanimation of the face based on the use of

Table 15-2. Surgical Approaches to Rehabilitation After Facial Nerve Injury

- **I. Nonmicrosurgical approaches**
  - A. Static procedures
    1. Fascial slings to eyelids, mouth
    2. Metal springs and weights to eyelids
    3. Cosmetic procedures (such as rhytidectomy, creation of nasolabial folds, browlifts, Z-plasty to lip)
  - B. Dynamic Transfers
    Muscle
      a. Temporalis
      b. Masseter
  - C. Muscle plication for partial paralysis[12]
  - D. Contralateral procedures
    1. Myotomy
    2. Selective denervation
- **II. Microsurgical approaches**
  - A. Nerve transfers
    1. Voluntary control (nonfacial nerve input)
      a. Hypoglossal nerve to facial
      b. Trigeminal nerve to facial
    2. Involuntary (spontaneous emotional) control (facial nerve input); cross-facial nerve grafts
  - B. Muscle transfers
    1. Grafts, e.g., extensor digitorum brevis
    2. Free microvascular muscle transfers
  - C. Combination of A-2 followed by B-2
  - D. Combination of A-1 followed by A-2 (the "babysitting" procedure)

the newer microsurgical procedures, enhancing the effects of the microsurgical procedures by the more traditional techniques as needed (Table 15-2). This chapter will also review the results that can be expected from the classic approaches to facial nerve repair and grafting and the decompression procedure being utilized to treat hemifacial spasm.

Anatomic Basis for Surgical Strategies

A normal facial expression requires a conscious or unconscious thought to initiate the impulse through the normal intact nerve that will produce contraction in a normal muscle. For the remainder of this chapter, it is assumed that the facial nerve paralysis is not due to a central inability to initiate the neural impulse that generates activity from the motor nucleus. The surgeon must assess the status of the facial nerve injury and muscle injury. Rarely is the cause of facial palsy one in which only muscle is missing. Congenital absence of a particular group of facial muscles might rarely occur; a tumor might require ablation of a particular group of facial muscles; direct severe facial trauma, as seen in motor vehicle accidents or gunshot wounds to the face, will present a need to replace muscle, as well as restore nerve function. Fortunately, the problem facing the reconstructive surgeon is often one in which muscles are present. The surgeon must decide if these muscles have sufficient remaining activity to permit them to be reinnervated, or whether these muscles must be replaced. The nucleus to the individual muscle cells remains alive. The facial muscle following loss of facial nerve input undergoes, in time, atrophy of the muscle fibers themselves and fibrosis of the supporting connective tissue, so that generally by 1 year after denervation, these muscles cannot be reinnervated. For practical purposes, a muscle that has been denervated for more than $1\frac{1}{2}$ years will not likely be successfully functionally reinnervated. In this instance, it will be necessary to replace muscle in the overall reconstructive strategy.

The placement of small slips of muscle, as muscle

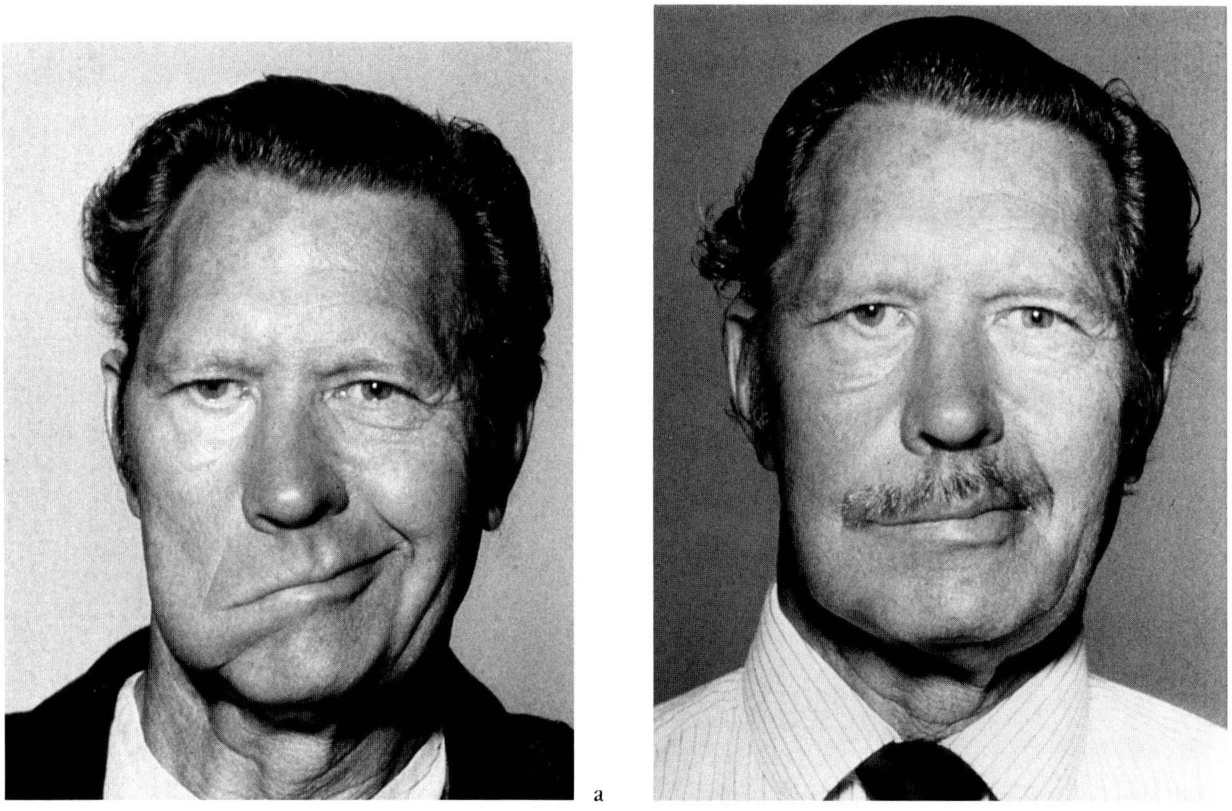

a b

Figure 15-3. Example of tensor fascia lata used as a static sling. **a.** Preoperative view of patient with right-sided facial paralysis. **b.** Postoperative view 1 year later. Note improved appearance of face at rest due to raising of right oral commissure. **c.** Harvested tensor fascia lata from donor site and on cheek (**d**) before insetting. (*Figure continues.*)

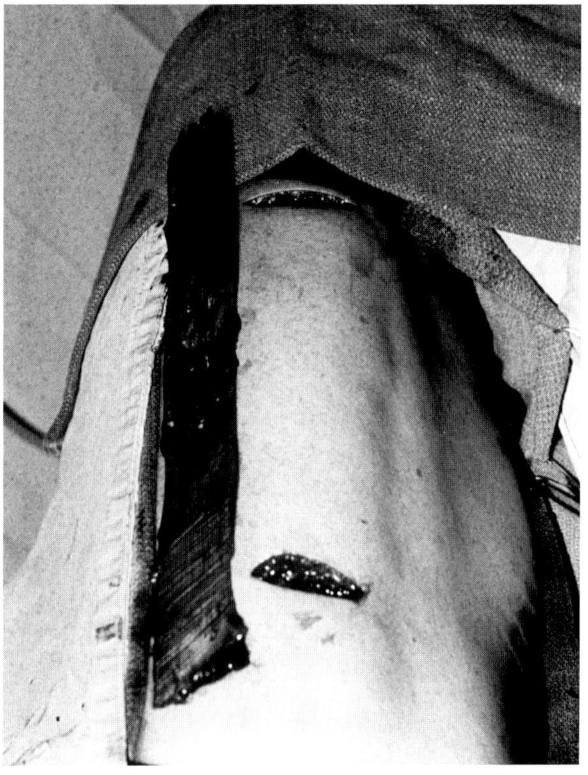

c

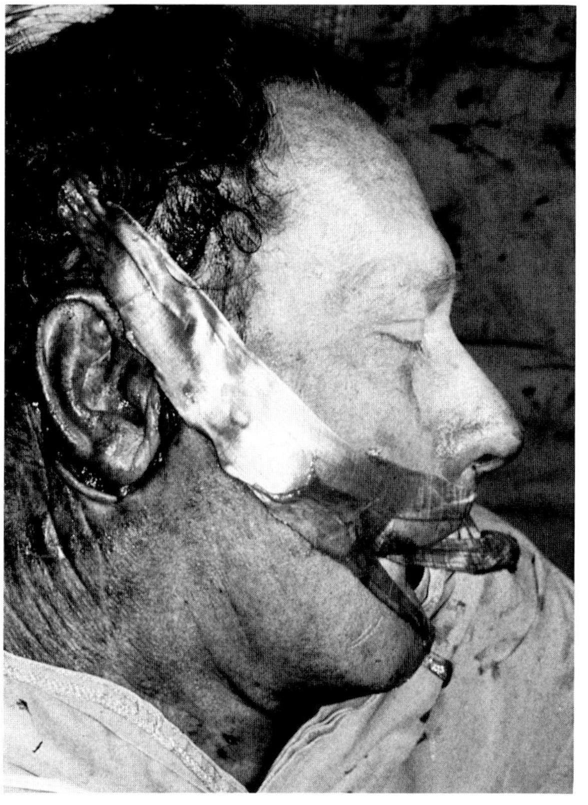

d

Figure 15-3 (*continued*).

grafts, into the face in the positions desired for restoration of facial function has been described.[13] Although it has been demonstrated that pieces of muscle can be implanted into the face and survive, the function that occurs from these muscles relies on random revascularization from the grafting bed, possible reinnervation from underlying other cranial nerves, such as the trigeminal nerve, motor portions of which might extend through temporalis or masseter muscles, the result in general being less than satisfactory for a reliable standard approach. Provision of a larger muscle mass was made possible by the description of the microsurgical transfer with vascular anastomosis of muscles by Tamai et al in 1970.[14] It thus became technically feasible to resupply the face with a muscle, in any given location, to restore whatever given facial function might be desired. Tamai's group demonstrated that a nerve repair could be added to the microvascular repair in this free muscle transfer so that muscle function could be reestabished, and in 1976, Harii et al[15] described the first transfer of the gracilis muscle to the face with microneurovascular anastomoses to restore a particular facial function, raising the oral commissure for a smile. Subsequent experimental work has suggested the parameters for the harvesting and insetting of these muscles to achieve the appropriate length-tension relationships in the transfer.[16,17]

If a patient is referred for reconstruction of facial palsy between 6 and 9 months after the loss of facial nerve function, it may be possible to provide reinnervation of the facial muscle before it undergoes irreversible changes. Attempts to substitute another cranial nerve, such as the hypoglossal, to replace facial nerve function have been extensively described.[18] In general, these procedures can restore tone to the muscle and prevent atrophy of the muscle by providing appropriate neurotrophic impulses. This approach, however, never results in natural spontaneous and involuntary (emotional) expression. The patient must learn altered techniques to mimic facial expression, for example, moving the tongue forward or to the side to achieve a smile. With mastication, undesirable facial expressions occur. In a similar manner, when the 11th cranial nerve is used as a transfer, a spinofacial transfer, the patient must learn to shrug his shoulder or turn his head in order to achieve voluntarily a smile or eye closure. With physical activity, undesirable facial expressions occur when the head is turned or the shoulder elevated.[3]

Ideally and theoretically, the best results should occur if the function of the ipsilateral facial nerve can be restored. *Primary* repair of "clean" lacerations of the ipsilateral facial nerve will often yield an excellent result, as will repair of a branch of the facial nerve distal to the stylomastoid foramen. A branch, such as the buc-

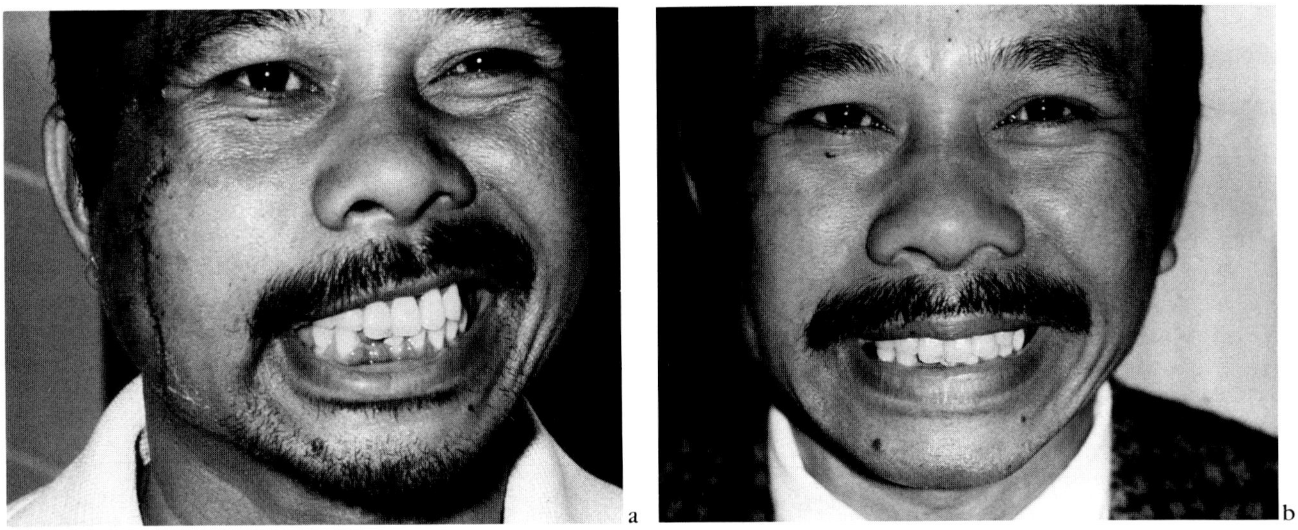

a b

Figure 15-4a. Primary repair of a peripheral branch of facial nerve (buccal) can restore good to excellent function by 1 year (**b**). (Photograph courtesy of Joesph S. Gruss, M. D., Toronto.)

cal branch or the zygomatic temporal branch, already has fibers that are clearly committed to a specific muscle group and repair of this nerve can restore good function in that facial group (Fig. 15-4). It is well-known that with facial nerve transsections more peripheral or more distal to the line drawn from the corner of the eye to the corner of the lip, to a line drawn from the zygomatic arch to the angle of the mandible, oftentimes recovery occurs without repair. An example of an extratemporal (peripheral) facial graft is given in Figure 15-5. Results of repairs and grafting to the facial nerve all along its course have been detailed and reviewed.[19,20] When a *delayed* repair or a nerve graft of the facial nerve is carried out, more proximally, topographic fascicular arrangement and vascular markings are no longer available as a reliable guide for the appropriate alignment of the nerve repair. Although function of facial muscles and facial muscle "tone" will be achieved after such ipsilateral nerve repair and nerve grafting procedures, the results, in general, are not satisfactory. The primary reason for unsatisfactory results is uncontrolled mass movements of various facial muscles, synkinesis or dyskinesis. Thus, with voluntary or involuntary facial expression attempts, the actual movements that occur are bizarre and distracting. The basis for this failure is not due to inability of nerves to regenerate long distances or of nerve grafting to succeed. It is rather a failure of a definite spatial orientation of the facial nerve from its intracranial position through its temporal bone passage, out to the individual peripheral nerve branches. An extremely large body of basic work has been devoted to attempting to identify the spatial orientation of these facial nerve fascicles.[21–29] The conclusion from this basic work, despite many conflicting results, and the conclusion from clinical observations of nerve repair work based supposedly on the spatial orientation of the facial nerve, is that there is *no* reliable fascicular orientation along the course of the facial nerve even as far distal as the stylomastoid foramen. Even relatively distal peripheral branches will occasionally carry "mixed" motor function, as demonstrated by direct electrical stimulation.[32]

Thus, while surgery on the ipsilateral facial nerve will reliably allow reinnervation of the facial muscles, because a precise spatial orientation of the facial nerve does not exist (Fig. 15-6), this reinnervation pattern will usually be characterized by dyskinesis. When attempting to restore innervation to facial musculature that is not characterized by this dyskinetic response, consideration must be given to cross-facial nerve grafting techniques (Fig. 15-6a) as the procedures of choice (Fig. 15-6b). This will be true whether that musculature be recently denervated and still *in situ* or new muscle brought in by microvascular transfer.

Many procedures have been recommended for the management of facial palsy. The surgeon will first consider whether it is possible to salvage the denervated facial musculature. If it is possible to reinnervate these muscles, they will obviously produce the best result as long as the nervous control is appropriate. The more distal the nerve repair or graft, the more likely will it be to produce a good result. When the graft is very proximal, dyskinesis or mass movement is likely. Certainly, if a neurotization procedure is required (such as

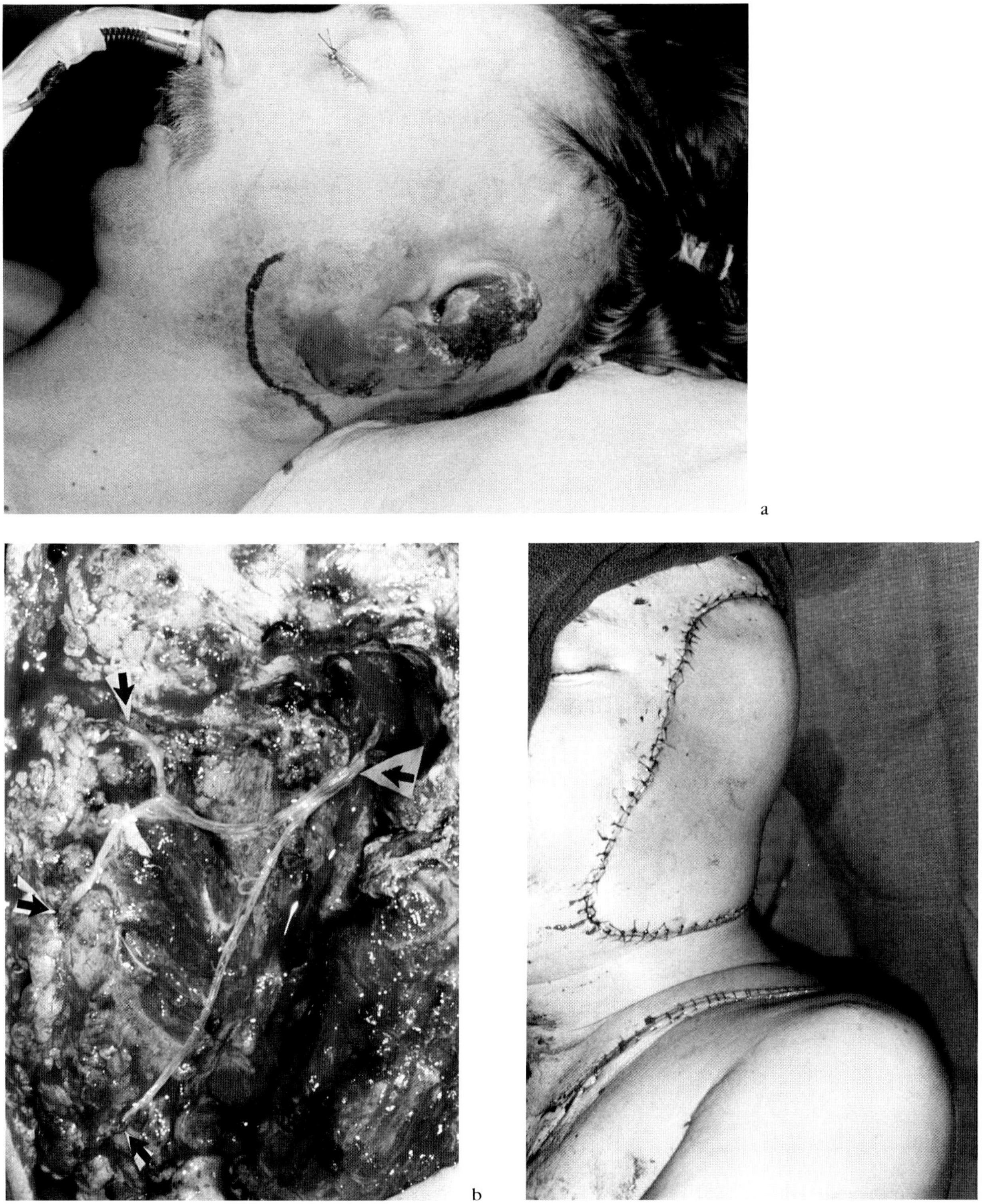

a b c

Figure 15-5. Facial nerve graft in extratemporal facial nerve for hemangioma. **a.** After tumor resection, long sural nerve grafts were used to reconstruct the facial nerve. **b.** The grafts are noted (arrows). **c.** Latissimus dorsi myocutaneous flap coverage. (*Figure continues.*)

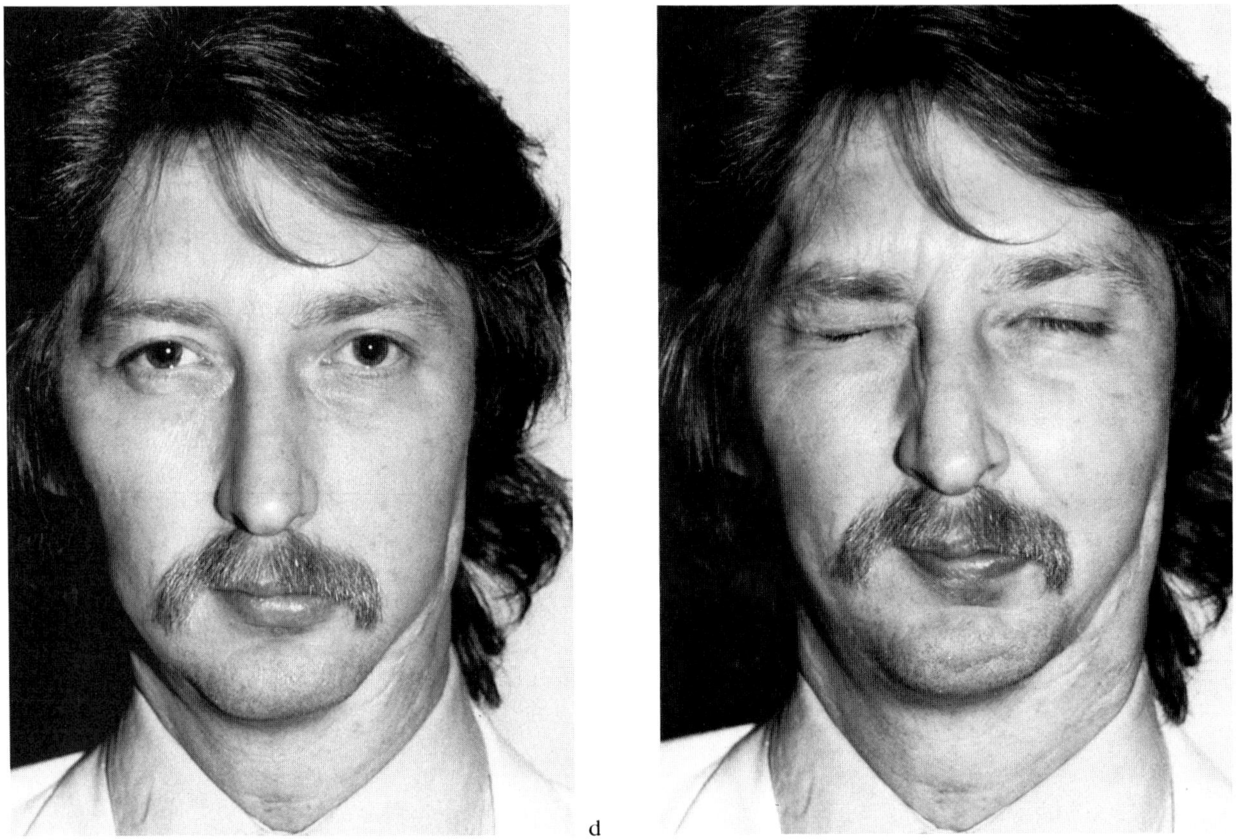

d e

Figure 15-5 (*continued*). **d.** Two years' postoperatively there is excellent symmetry at rest, and good facial muscle recovery (**e**), although dyskinesis and mass movement were noted.

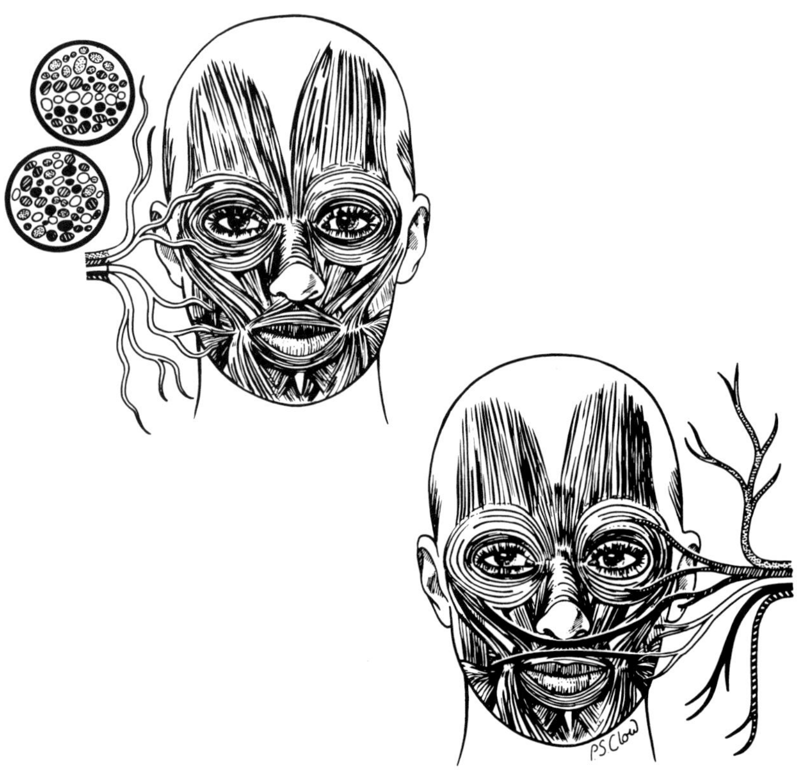

a

Figure 15-6a. Schemata of the desired spatial orientation of the facial nerve, which would permit ipsilateral nerve reconstruction techniques is seen in the top circle. Unfortunately, the internal topography of the proximal stump of the facial nerve presents a mixed motor pattern, so that when this portion of the nerve is used to motor the transferred muscle, a dyskinetic mass movement will result (above). Cross-facial nerve grafts from the peripheral portion of the contralateral facial nerve (below) will allow the muscle transfer to be innervated with axons that serve the same motor function rather than a mixed motor function (circles represent schematic internal topography from proximal facial nerve as the reconstructive surgeon "wishes" it were arranged (top circle) and as it actually is arranged (bottom circle). (*Figure continues.*)

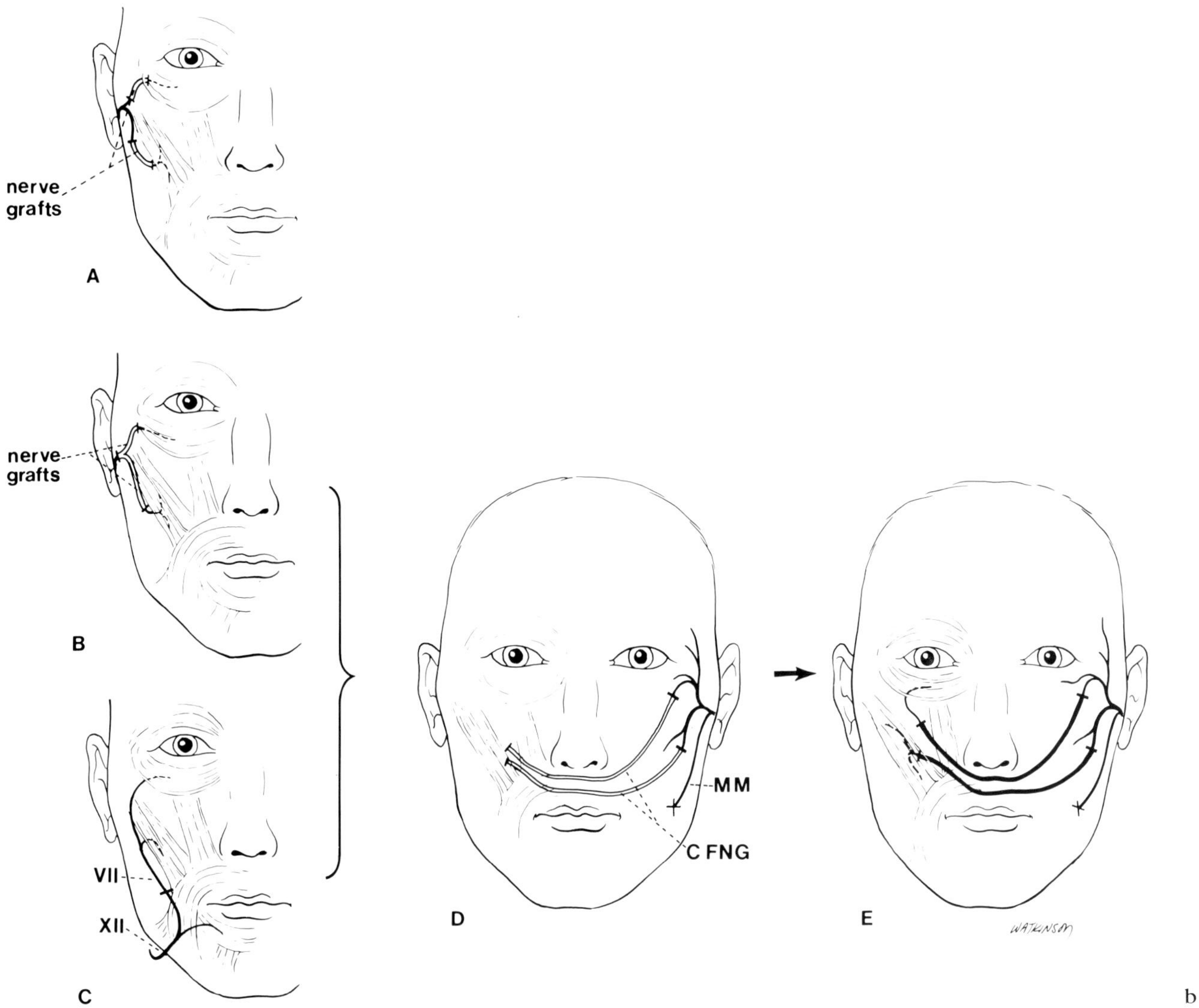

Figure 15-6 (*continued*). **b.** In (A) nerve grafts from distal branches of the seventh nerve should give a satisfactory result. Both procedures (B) and (C) may be the definitive operation or may just serve to "babysit" the facial muscles on a temporary basis until a cross-facial nerve graft can bring more appropriate and specific motor fibers from the peripheral branches of the contralateral facial nerve (D). After the nerves have traversed the graft, the "babysitting" procedures (B,C) are taken down and the distal portion of the cross-facial nerve graft is transferred to the distal branches of the ipsilateral facial nerve (E). CFNG: cross-facial nerve graft; MM: mandibular marginal (note this nerve has been ablated to improve symmetry of the lower face).

Table 15-3. Surgical Algorithm for the Management of Facial Palsy

Facial muscles →	Salvageable →	Neurotize* ⟹	CFNG† ⟹	TRANSFER CFNG to distal ipsilateral VII ⟹	ANCILLARY COSMETIC PROCEDURES§
		Neurotize* →		→	ANCILLARY COSMETIC PROCEDURES§
Facial muscles →	Nonsalvageable ⟹	CFNG ⟹	FREE MUSCLE ⟹	⟹	ANCILLARY COSMETIC PROCEDURES§
	Nonsalvageable →	Sling‡ →		→	ANCILLARY COSMETIC PROCEDURES§

*Partial XII, proximal ipsilateral VII.

†CFNG: cross facial nerve graft.

‡Dynamic or static.

§Such as face or brow lift.

⟹: Course chosen for the younger or highly motivated patient.

XII to VII), then, although motor return will occur, the movement will be controlled by the tongue, not facial movements. In these latter two situations, consideration will be given to using either of these two procedures simply to "babysit" the facial muscles providing trophic support of the facial muscles without "appropriate" control. Cross-facial nerve grafts will bring the "appropriate" motor function from the normal side of the face. Once these fibers have traversed the grafts, the original nerve repairs are taken down and the distal end of the sural nerve grafts are repaired to the distal facial nerve branches on the previously palsied side (Table 15-3).

Cross-facial nerve grafts were described by Anderl[30] in 1973 and modifications of these are now extensively utilized. The technique as originally described involved exposure of the branches of the buccal plexus in the area of the nasolabial crease. These distal nerve branches were used as the donor nerves. In general, these provided an insufficient neural input. The current approaches involve grafting from larger, more proximal branches of the facial nerve. This requires a thorough knowledge of the anatomy of the branches of the facial nerve; these have been well-described in anatomic dissections (Fig. 15-7).[31] These classic anatomic studies, as well as recent studies in the subhuman primate,[32] demonstrate that there are usually overlapping peripheral branches of the facial nerve to any given group of facial muscles. Thus, by electrical stimulation of carefully dissected facial nerve peripheral branches, choices can be made of which fascicles may be sacrificed to provide functionally defined neural input to the cross-facial nerve graft that will ultimately provide motor control for a desired facial expression. The sural nerve is used as the donor nerve for the nerve graft. This approach permits the central initiation of a particular facial expression, such as a smile, to be carried through the intratemporal facial nerve, along the contralateral peripheral nerve branch, and across the cross-facial nerve graft to the muscle on the paralyzed side. This approach avoids synkinesis and dyskinesis and, most importantly, facilitates spontaneous involuntary movement.

When the reconstructive surgeon is faced with the loss of both muscle and neural input on the injured side, then the approach must combine the cross-facial nerve graft technique with a microsurgical transfer of a muscle. The gracilis was the muscle first chosen by Harii et al.[15] This muscle has been extensively used and its technique reported by Manktelow, Zuker, and McKee.[33] Other muscle donor sites have been utilized and described: the latissimus dorsi,[34,35] the extensor digitorum brevis,[36] the pectoralis major,[37] the pectoralis minor,[38,39] and the serratus anterior.[40] Although many dif-

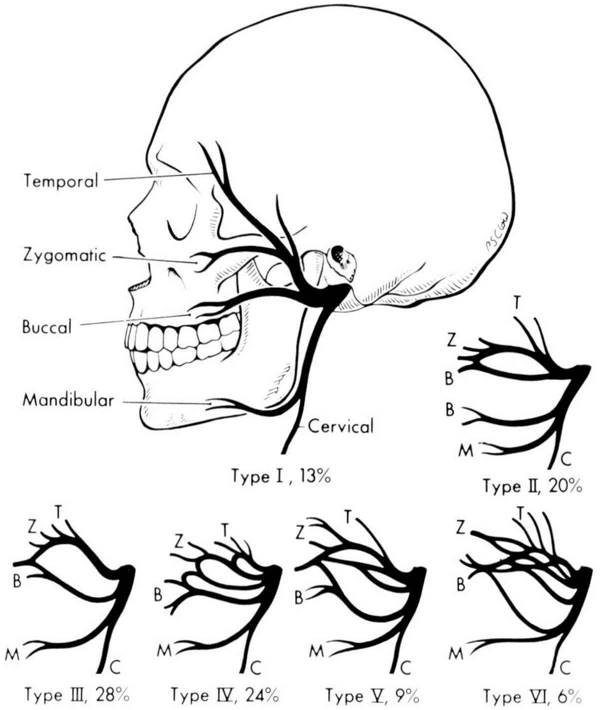

Figure 15-7. Patterns of the facial nerve's peripheral branching. (Modified with permission from Davis et al.[31])

ferent muscles have been chosen, there are drawbacks to many of these, such as difficult technical dissections, small vascular pedicles, or excessive bulk in the donor muscle.

Other factors may prove important in selecting the donor muscle for free muscle transfer, such as the predominance of slow versus fast twitch muscle fiber type. It has been determined that some muscles are primarily antigravity or support muscles, containing primarily slow twitch, or type II, muscle fibers like the soleus. In contrast, the gastrocnemius is a predominately fast twitch, type I, muscle. Although we are not aware of anyone reporting the fiber typing of facial muscles, it is of interest to speculate that they may be half and half, since an antigravity function with tone maintenance is required all the time in the face, but rapid movements are also required throughout eating, talking, and emotional expression. The muscles used for transfer also have not been typed yet. Of significance is that the type I muscle can hypertrophy greatly with exercise, whereas type II muscles do not. Such knowledge might make a difference in determining how much muscle bulk to transfer. This is an area for future study.

Clearly, each of the muscles previously transferred has replaced only one of the expressions of the facial muscles. The ideal muscle transfer would provide multiple muscle functions with a single vascular repair. Toward this concept, Manktelow and Zuker[41] have suggested muscle transplantation determined by fascicular territory. This approach allows electrical stimulation of the nerve to the gracilis muscle. Separate stimulation of the individual fascicles allows definition of separate muscle territories. An application of this approach is possible with the latissimus dorsi muscle. The anatomic basis for splitting the latissimus muscle into two separate large muscles has been reported.[42,43] Further anatomic dissections have demonstrated that the thoracodorsal nerve can be divided into several separate fascicles, each innervating well-defined segments of the latissimus dorsi muscle. This approach has allowed the transfer of multiply innervated muscle segments on a single vascular pedicle for reanimation of the face (Fig. 15-8).[44] This approach has allowed provision of muscle with a long vascular pedicle, a dissection technique that is readily mastered, and the ability theoretically to re-

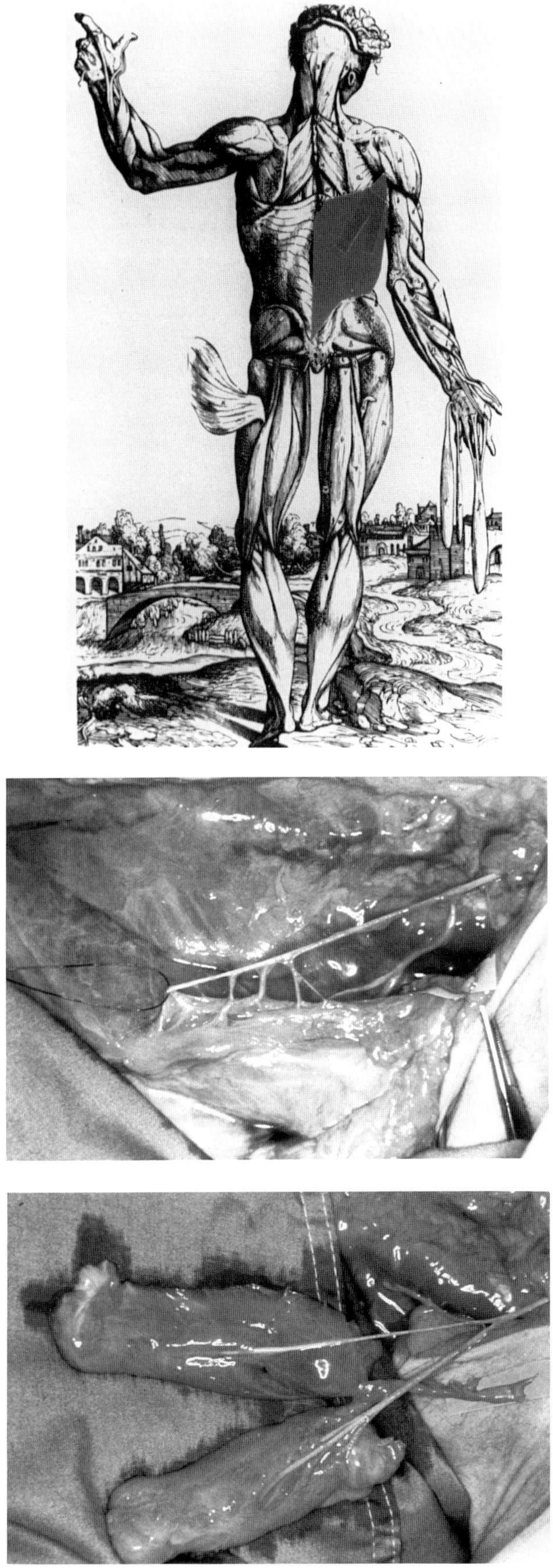
a
b
c

Figure 15-8. The latissimus muscle as the choice to replace facial muscles. Small segments can be designed from within this large muscle (**a**) so that separate branches of the thoracodorsal nerve innervate each segment (**b**). The resulting dissection yields multiple independently innervated muscle segments supplied by the single thoracodorsal arteriovenous pedicle (**c**). (Reproduced with permission from Dellon and Mackinnon.[44])

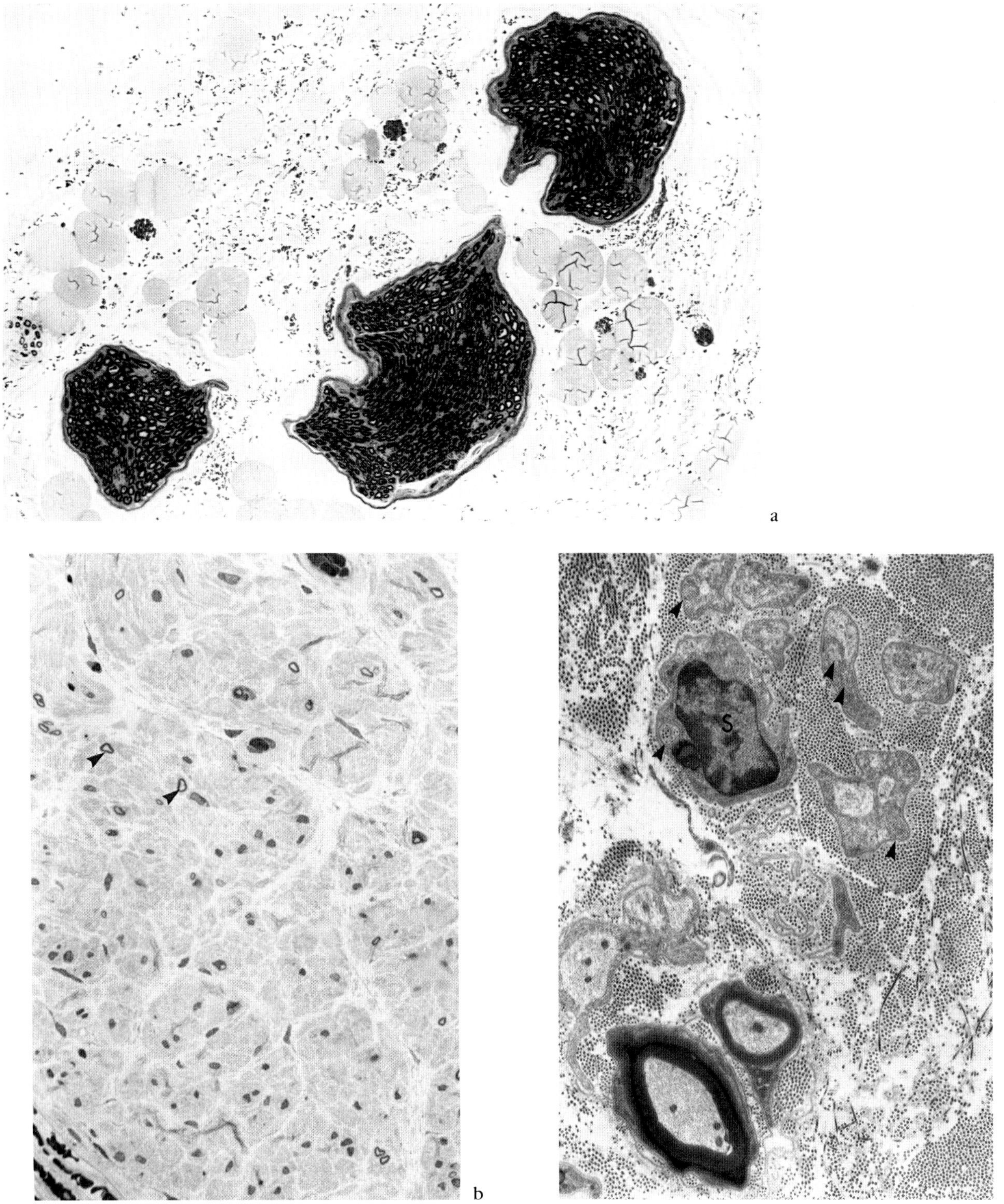

Figure 15-9. Transverse sections of (**a**) thoracodorsal nerve, which normally innervates the latissimus muscle and (**b**) of the sural nerve cross-facial graft 1 year after regeneration has occurred. Note the few myelinated axons (arrows) in the graft. (Toluidine blue staining; ×150 **b** and ×60 **a**). Electron microscopic section (**c**) of this cross-facial graft demonstrate two myelinated fibers and a population of unmyelinated fibers (arrow). Schwann cell nucleus is also shown (s). (Uranyl acetate; ×9, 200). Despite the few myelinated fibers present at the end of the graft, when the microneurovascular transfer was completed, the muscle developed excellent function (see Fig. 15-15). (Reproduced with permission from Dellon and Mackinnon.[44])

construct more than one paralyzed facial muscle group. It is this approach that will be described and illustrated in detail in the sections to follow.

A further anatomic consideration is the relationship between a muscle's ability to contract and the degree of contracture required to achieve a smile. The gracilis muscle has been demonstrated to have sufficient contractile power to permit finger flexion when transferred into the hand. The normal profundus muscle has a 7 cm requirement to permit full extension and full gripping of the finger.[33] Recently, Pately and Chaban, working with Manktelow, noted from cine studies of normal men and women that the average excursion of the oral commissure in smiling is 1.4 cm in a vector toward tragus (41° above the horizontal).[45] Is it possible that a muscle that normally carries out a long excursion may not be capable of a short excursion, or would the resting length at which it is inset need to be adjusted to some degree? This is another area for future study. An example of latissimus muscle 5 cm excursion in a segment dissected for transfer to the face is noted in Figure 15-15.

The relationship between the number of axons reinnervating the free muscle transfer from the cross-facial nerve graft and the final degree of muscle function remains to be determined. In Figure 15-9, note how the number of axons in the sural nerve cross-facial graft (center) is so much less than the number in the nerve that normally innervates the muscle (top); yet in the clinical case from which these specimens were taken, the muscle developed good bulk and function (2 cm excursion). Similar "paradoxically" good function from a reduced number of axons in facial reanimation has been noted also by Terzis.[46] Based on measured nerve fiber to muscle fiber ratios, she has found facial muscles to have a higher ratio (1 : 8) than other muscles (1 : 50), giving better control over the facial musculature normally. She has suggested therefore that better facial reanimation may occur if the cross-facial nerve graft were used to reinnervate innervated contralateral, such as frontalis or ipsilateral (digastric) anterior belly muscles, which could be transferred to provide ipsilateral eyelid and lower lip function, respectively.[46]

Diagnosis and Informed Consent: Preoperative Consultations

The surgical reconstruction of the patient with a facial palsy must take psychologic and emotional factors into consideration. The patient with a facial nerve palsy must cope with not only the physical disabilities but, very importantly, the emotional and psychologic components of this palsy. Unlike the withered hand or crippled foot, it cannot be hidden in a pocket or shoe. It is constantly on display. Each glimpse of their own image in a glass or mirror is a fleeting reminder of their disability. Each family photograph provides a permanent documentation of either their bizarre asymmetrical smiling image or, more commonly, a symmetrically but expressionless facies. At this "extreme" of the "cosmetic surgery" continuum, more than in many other types of surgery, informed consent is imperative for both the patient and the surgeon. Toward this goal, in this section the wording and phrasing are written largely for the patient in "layman's" terms.

During the preoperative consultation with the patient, a mirror should be present and the patient's face examined with him in the mirror. The stigmata of the completely paralyzed hemiface due to unilateral facial paralysis is striking. It is, however, important to address the patient's own main concerns. The patient must realize that his face will never have normal balance or symmetry. He must also be prepared for two or three operative procedures to achieve optimum results (Table 15-4). The first procedure involves exploration of the normal facial nerve combined with the cross-facial nerve graft. This operative procedure will take some of the strong contractions of the nonparalyzed side away, thereby weakening and beginning to help with facial symmetry. It is stressed to the patient that the overall imbalance in the face is due not only to the weakness on the paralyzed side, but the severe overcontraction that is usually present on the normal side. Deviation of the midline facial structures to the normal side is brought to the patient's attention to emphasize this point. The patient is told that in the initial postoperative period after the cross-facial nerve graft, there may be significant facial weakness on the normal side that may take several months to recover. Some weakness on the normal, nonparalyzed side, especially around the eye, may take 3 or 4 months to return to normal.

Table 15-4. Stages of Surgical Reconstruction for Rehabilitation of Patient with Facial Nerve Injury

When facial muscles cannot be reinnervated	
Stage I:	Exploration of normal facial nerve with cross-facial nerve graft
Stage II:	Free microneurovascular muscle transfer
Stage III:	"Touch-up" operation or operations to improve balance and symmetry of face
When facial muscles can be reinnervated	
Stage I:	Nerve tranfer to "babysit" facial muscles and cross-facial nerve graft
Stage II:	Transfer of cross-facial nerve graft to ipsilateral distal facial nerve branches
Stage III:	"Touch-up" operation or operations to improve balance and symmetry of face

During the initial consultation, it is critical to evaluate the dynamics of the patient's smile. The three common smile patterns are discussed with the patient. One shows the upper teeth with the pull primarily being lateral due to the zygomatic muscle group. This is present in approximately 65% of the population. Another smile has additionally a strong pull directly upward from the levator labii superioris. This often shows the canine teeth and is present in approximately one-third of the population. The remaining group has significant contribution to their smile from the depressor group of lower lip muscles and therefore show the lower teeth in their smile. The patient is made aware that when the muscle is placed at the second stage, the correct pull, either directly laterally or including insertions into the levator labii superioris area, will be chosen.[47] Most importantly, if their smile on the non-paralyzed side includes the depressor muscles, the patient must be made aware that during the first stage of their operative procedure, in order to further balance the smile, they may require partial or complete denervation or myotomies of the depressor anguli group of muscles. The bilateral preauricular and submental facial scars, the midline philtral incision, and the scar on the leg from the sural nerve donor site are explained to the patient. The risk of possible nerve donor site pain proximally where the sural nerve will form a neuroma and permanent numbness on the lateral aspect of the foot are explained to the patient. Preoperative videotaping of the patient's face provides not only a permanent record, but allows the surgeon to study in detail the dynamics of the patient's facial movements. The patient should be told at the initial consultation that the goals to be achieved in the first two stages of the procedure are provision of smiling, provision of protection to the cornea by attempting to provide some return of function to the lower lid, and a partial relaxation of the overcontraction on the contralateral side of the face. After the first stage, a period of approximately 9 months to 1 year will ensue, during which time the nerve will be regenerating across the face along the sural nerve graft. The significance of a progressive Tinel's sign in monitoring nerve regeneration along the graft is explained to the patient.

The second stage of the operation, which will be performed approximately 1 year after the first stage, will require donor site scars, usually in the axilla and side of the chest that is opposite the paralyzed side, since this permits the functioning of two teams during the microvascular transfer of the latissimus muscle. The well-muscled patient should be aware that it will alter his appearance from the back where the latissimus bulge may be significantly diminished. The nerve remaining, innervating the more posterior or lateral component of the latissimus, is saved and some function of this muscle is preserved. There is usually no noticeable functional loss from using this muscle.[48] The patient is told that the second stage of the operative procedure may last an average of 8 hours (compared with 3 to 4 hours for the cross-facial nerve graft) and require blood transfusions and several days postoperatively in the hospital. They will have a drain at the muscle donor site and at the facial area. Patients need to be aware that the success rate of microvascular transfers is approximately 90%. If postoperative monitoring of muscle viability is to be used, this is discussed with the patient. The patient should be told that, a portion of muscle may be left exposed without the wound being closed in order to determine its viability, or a small piece of skin graft may be placed over the muscle to attempt to monitor visually the muscle, since temperature monitoring and oxygen monitoring transcutaneously are currently not universally available for monitoring buried free-muscle transfers. They should be aware that techniques are now available that may require placement of electrical monitoring equipment within the muscle, such as described by Fasching and VanBeek,[49] or the placement of thermocouples about the anastomotic vessels as described by May et al,[50] and that these may require a brief second operative procedure to remove this hardware used to monitor the muscles. The patient is told that the initial postoperative period is devoted to helping the muscle learn to live in the new location and is accompanied by significant swelling of the face related to the surgery to implant the muscle. Over a 3-month period, the swelling decreases and some of the bulk of the muscle reduces due to lack of innervation of the muscle. The cross-facial nerve graft has been sutured to the thoracodorsal nerve that innervates the muscle and during this 3-month period will be regenerating into the muscle. The patient is told to expect small contractions in the muscle between 3 and 6 months after the second stage of the operation. These little twitches within the cheek may be perceived several months before actual elevation of the paralyzed side of the face. In particular, the bulk of muscle placed in the lower eyelid may cause partial occlusion of the eye for a short period of time. He should be aware that the normal eye musculature is circular, functioning like a diaphragm and a camera lens to cause eyelid closure and that, in fact, most of the muscle's function in the lower lid is not active contraction as much as a support for the lower lid. Placement of muscle in both the upper and lower eyelids to mimic normal sphinteric function has proved to be inappropriate. This muscle placement has resulted in such strong contraction as to prevent opening of the eyelids and thus necessitated removal or division of the "upper lid" muscle. It is stressed to the patient that only lower lid elevation and support, and possibly some movement during facial expression, are anticipated by the muscle implanted into the lower lid. As an incision is necessary in the medial canthal region to insert this muscle, the patient should be made aware of the need for a scar in that area. The patient should be advised that some surgeons preplace fascial slings about the mouth because they feel this facilitates insertion of the free muscle. In the approach described here, this is not done. A postoperative complication noted by other workers in the field has been wrinkling of the skin, either from fascia left attached to the muscle that becomes adherent to the implanted muscle or from the previously placed fascia from the temporalis to the orbicularis, or from previous sling placements. Thus, this approach is not utilized by us. Nevertheless, the patient should be appraised that some adherence of the dermis to the underlying muscle may cause wrinkling along the course of the implant in areas other than where it is most desired, such as in the attempt to recreate the nasolabial crease. If this wrinkling occurs, it can be loosened at the third stage of the operative procedure.

The third stage of the operative procedure is devoted to final balancing and adjustments and may include several small operations to establish symmetry if the patient's desire for continued adjustments is present.[51] The patient should be assured that the surgeon is willing to continue to work on him until the most that can be achieved has been achieved. Typically, the patient should be appraised that the muscle implanted will continue to improve in strength for 24 to 36 months and that the third stage will not occur until the muscle strength has plateaued. At that time, if the muscle implanted remains too bulky, it may be reduced. In this regard, technically, it should be noted that while most surgeons do the nerve and vessel surgery in a location that is superficial to the muscle, the approach described here will place these repairs and anastomoses deep to the muscle so that subsequent debulking may be done without fear of disrupting the nerve repair or the vessel anastomoses. At the third stage, the work on the depressor muscles on the normal side can be carried out, a further accentuation of a nasolabial crease can be made by the usual techniques of excision of an ellipse in a desired location with suturing to create a scar and the appearance of a nasolabial crease. If the nose still remains deviated to the nonparalyzed side, weakening of the levator labii superioris alaeque nasi can be carried out. If the eyebrow on the paralyzed side is drooping, an ellipse of skin can be taken from above the eyebrow to create a mini-lift in this area. In the older group of patients, an actual facelift on the nonparalyzed side may be helpful in adjusting balance.

The patient should be aware that during a third stage adjunctive procedure, attempting to convert a "good" result into an "excellent" result, complications can occur, in fact, converting the "good" to a "poor"

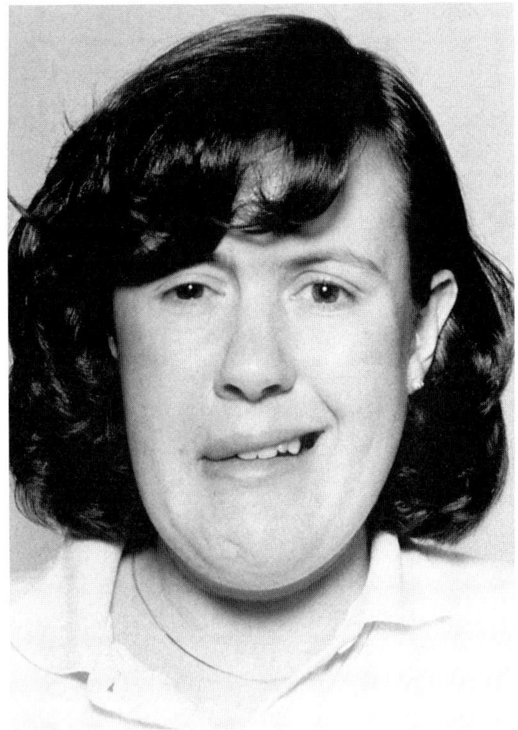

a

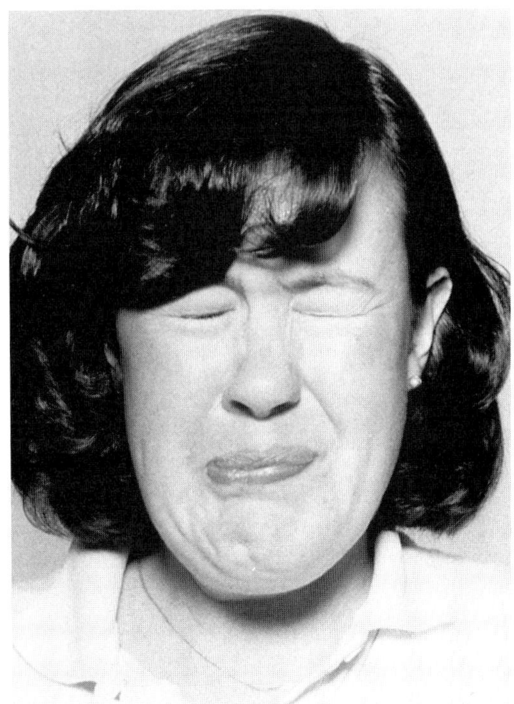

b

Figure 15-10. Example of the proximal 7th cranial nerve used to provide physiologic input to a denervated muscle. **a.** Smile **b.** Eyelid closure. When the patient closes her eyes there is an increased movement of the lower face because of inappropriate motor reinnervation. The proximal 7th has reinnervated the muscle to give good tone but not good control of the function. A cross facial nerve graft from the normal side will be done to improve motor control.

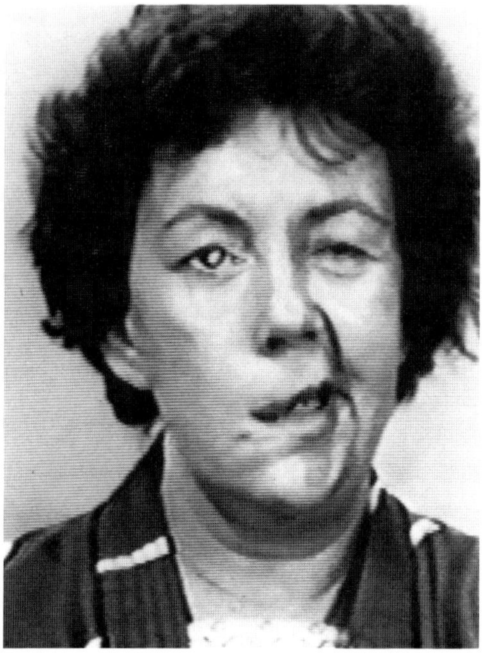
a

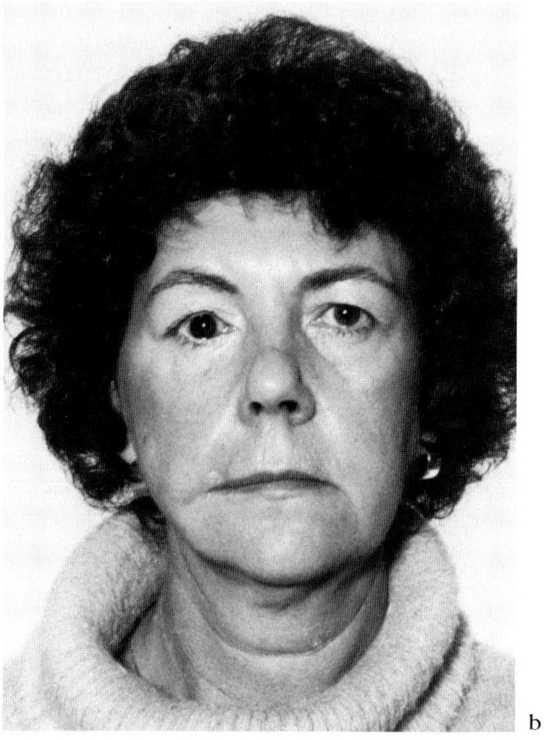
b

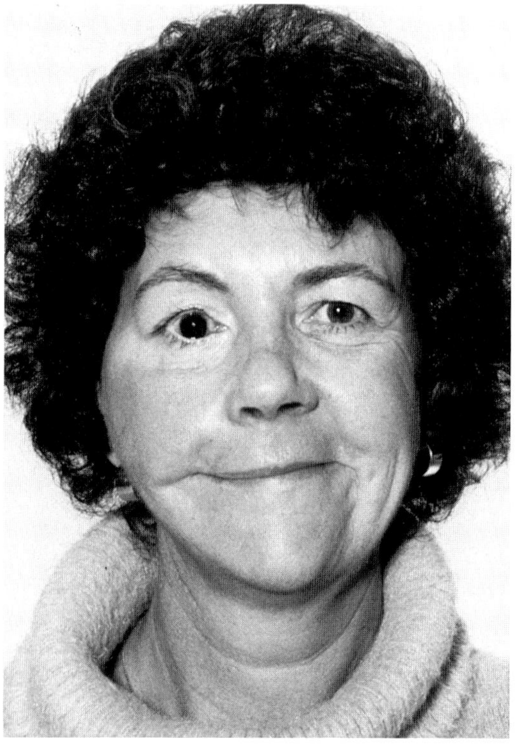
c

Figure 15-11. Before (**a**) and 2 years after (**b, c**) cross-facial nerve grafting and free-muscle transfer. At rest (**b**) and smiling (**c**). The opacified cornea is covered with a colored contact lens in the postoperative photographs. (Reproduced with permission from Mackinnon and Dellon.[74])

result. In two patients, we have injured the cross-facial nerve graft during such an adjunctive procedure. In one case, the nerve injury was noted at its occurrence and the nerve repaired. In the second, the injury was not recognized until the postoperative period when the transferred muscle no longer functioned. Three months postoperatively, with negative electromyographic results, the patient was reexplored, the injury found in the contralateral preauricular area of an adjunctive facelift procedure, and a partial 12th cranial to distal cross-facial nerve graft done to "babysit" the transferred muscle and regain tone (Fig. 15-10).

At some point in the patient's consultations and operative procedures, it may be valuable to enlist the aid of an ophthalmologist. Frequently, the patient will have an associated problem with the eye, such as corneal scarring or opacification. A corneal transplant if vision has been lost or a colored contact lens to remove the distracting appearance of the white cornea may be considered (Fig. 15-11). Patients with an esotropia or exotropia may be benefited by ocular muscle surgery. There may also be an associated dry eye syndrome due to loss of lacrimal gland function. An appropriate ophthalmologic consultation in terms of corneal protection, eye drop lubrication, among others, may prove valuable.

Operative Technique

Stage I: Cross-Facial Nerve Graft

With the endotracheal tube to the side of the paralyzed face, the surgical team will have complete access to both sides of the face. The head should be free to be turned to both the left and right. One leg is chosen for the sural nerve donor site and is prepared and draped to a level at the mid thigh. A tourniquet is optional. One surgical team may proceed with harvesting the sural nerve while another team begins with the facial nerve dissection. One or two cross-facial nerve grafts will be required, depending on the reconstructive goals. One graft may be needed to carry a defined function for eyelid and another a defined function for the smile. A 15 to 18 cm length of graft is appropriate for each of these two cross-facial nerve grafts and therefore the total length of the sural nerve that is required for harvesting will be 30 to 36 cm. Our preferred technique is to use a single longitudinal incision up the back of the leg in order not to damage any of the sural nerve branches, for with this technique the entire anatomy of the nerve is visualized. Occasionally, after preoperative discussion with the patient, an incision posterior to the lateral malleolus and multiple small transverse incisions are used. Even in this latter situation, we are prepared to make a longer incision in the region approximately 16 cm proximal to the malleolus where there is frequently (in three-fourths of the population) a major contribution from the lateral sural nerve to the main sural nerve.[52] If this is a significant branch, then it also must be dissected to the popliteal fossa, taking it from its origin from the common peroneal nerve. The sural nerve donor site is closed with interrupted 4/0 absorbable sutures placed in the dermis, a subcuticular absorbable suture and Steri-strips. The leg is wrapped with a tensor bandage. The sural nerve graft should be tagged with a suture at its proximal end. When the nerve graft is positioned, it will be reversed at the time of its insertion so that no regenerating axons will be lost through small branches. The nerve graft is placed in a separate colored towel or pan so that it is not lost or misplaced during the operative procedure.

The team working in the facial area outlines the proposed incision in the preauricular crease, curving posterior to the auricle and then extending downward below the angle of the mandible. This area is deliberately not infiltrated with an anesthetic solution because this infiltration may cause a conduction block of the facial nerve and thereby make the mapping of the facial nerve and, indeed, its localization difficult with the nerve stimulator. We will choose infiltration with epinephrine alone to minimize bleeding. Similarly, neuromuscular blocking anesthetic agents are not used. The skin flap is elevated in the subcutaneous plane. The facial nerve may be approached proximally at the main trunk of the facial nerve, as with a parotid dissection. It has been suggested that the facial nerve may be visualized during operative dissections by placement of a blue dye in the plane beneath the parotid gland.[53] Our preferred technique is to localize more peripheral branches of the facial nerve. Generally, we begin in the pretemporal region looking for branches of the zygomatic and temporal portion of the facial nerve. These will be visualized as small (less than 1 mm) white structures. Loupe magnification (3.5 power) and a disposable nerve stimulator will be required. The nerve stimulator will be used often in the initial dissections. When one of the small branches is found, the dissection is then carried proximally toward the facial nerve trunk. The search for peripheral branches of the facial nerve should be continued until one branch is found that will remain to cause elevation of the corner of the mouth on the nonparalyzed side. There usually remains one and more often two other branches that overlap and cause some elevation of the corner of the mouth and, more importantly, of the upper lip and corner of the nose. Since these are branches that usually are causing disfigurement and the facial imbalance, these are the ones most important to take as the donor nerves to attempt to motor the paralyzed corner of the mouth. Care should be taken not to include a branch here that causes lower lid movement. There is frequently one branch from the buccal branch that will cause both upper lip and lower eyelid movement. Most probably, unless this is a small branch, it should be included with the graft to the lip. Generally, only two branches can be found that cause lower eyelid contraction. There is usually one prominent branch that goes to upper and lower eyelids. This branch should be saved and branches that only go to the lower lid taken for the graft across to the opposite

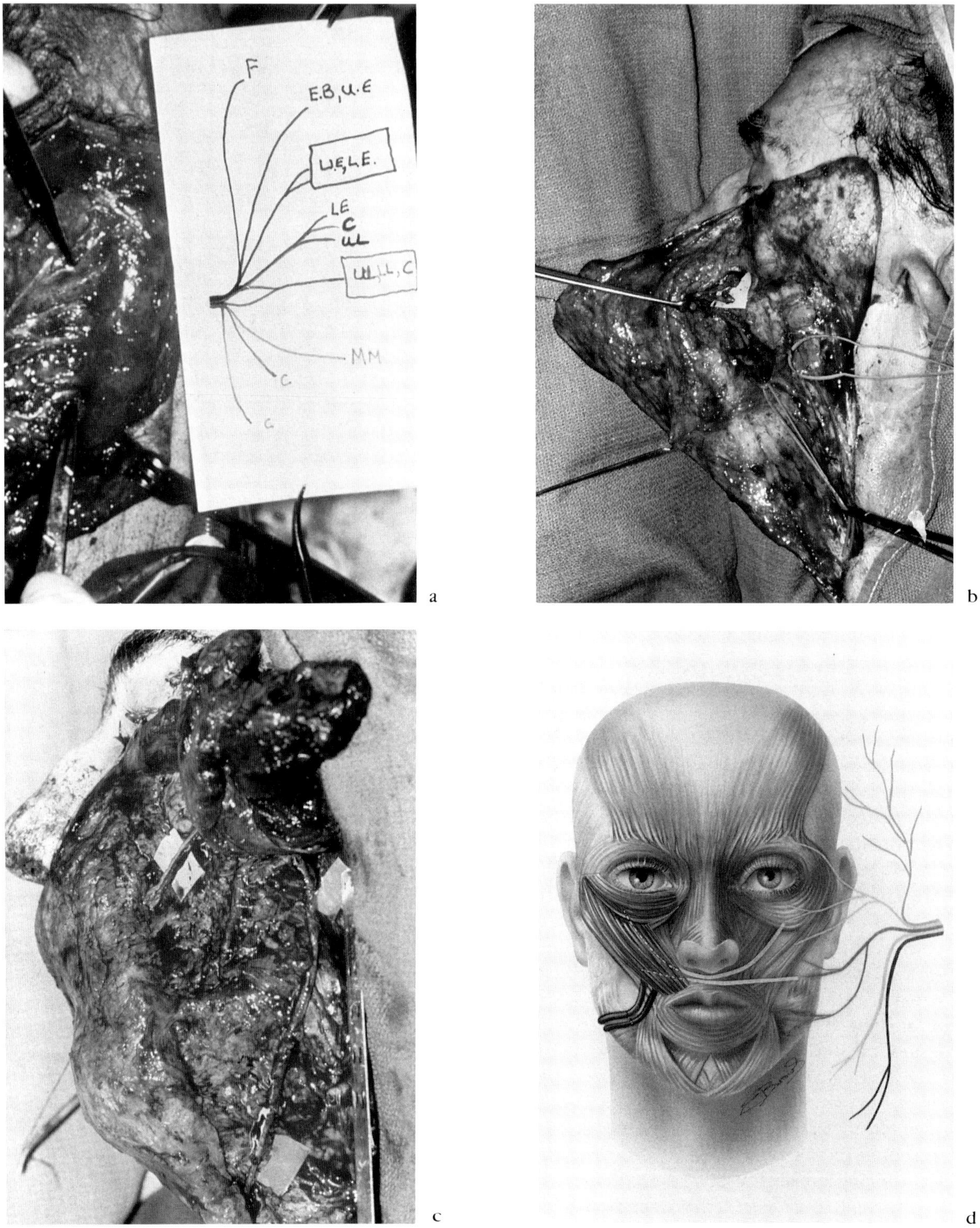

Figure 15-12a. At Stage I, the normal facial nerve is mapped with electrical stimulation to identify donor branches for eyelid (UE,LE) and smile function (UL,LL,C). F: frontalis; EB,UE: eyebrow and upper eyelid; UELE: upper eyelid and lower eyelid; UL,LL,C: upper lip and lower lip and commissure; MM: mandibular marginal and (**c**) cervical. **b.** Stage II, cross-facial nerve graft distal end is identified on visibility background. The vessel loops identify recipient artery and vein for muscle transfer. **c.** The muscle is reflected superiorly and nerve repairs and vessel anastomoses are done on the deep surface of the muscle, so that if muscle debulking is needed in stage III, it can be done safely without risk of nerve or vessel injury. **d.** A schema of hookups at end of stage II.

side of the face for innervation of the muscle slip to the paralyzed lower lid. The donor branches are dissected as proximally as possible to get the largest diameter of nerve (Fig. 15-12a). At this time we recommend ablation of the mandibular marginal branch of the facial nerve and/or the cervical branch if these nerves produce significant depression of the lower lip on the nonparalyzed side. Neurectomy at this stage is simple, safe, and will produce immediate improvement in lower facial symmetry. A tunnel is then made across the upper lip. Frequently, a small incision must be made in the location of the future nasolabial crease on the paralyzed side to facilitate passage of the graft to the paralyzed side of the face. A Penrose drain or Silastic Foley catheter is utilized to facilitate the passage of the nerve graft. The nerve grafts are placed in this tube and then the tube in pulled through the tunnel rather than pulling the nerve graft through the tunnel. This ensures a gentle passage of the nerve graft.[54] It is recommended that the sural nerve fascicle that will ultimately carry facial signals to the eye be tagged with a separate type of suture than the fascicle that will be used to motor the mouth. When these are located during the second stage, confusion may occur. The mnemonic that we utilize is to always place a w*i*re around the distal end of the fascicle to the *eye* (the *i* in wire sounding similar to the word *eye*).

The distal ends of the nerve graft on the paralyzed side of the face have traditionally been left to lie in the subcutaneous tissue. In order to investigate the potential neurotrophic effects on nerve regeneration from the distal nerve repair, a study has been carried out in primates[55] that has demonstrated that a greater number of nerve fibers will travel through a cross-facial nerve graft that is placed in-continuity with the terminal portions of the paralyzed facial nerve than will travel through a cross-facial nerve graft that is left to lie in the subcutaneous tissue (Fig. 15-13). Furthermore, the fibers that do regenerate that have been under the neurotropic influence have a larger diameter and a greater thickness of myelin than those left to lie simply in the subcutaneous tissue (Table 15-5). Accordingly, it is recommended that consideration be given to completing the distal neurorrhaphy between the nerve graft and the facial nerve on the paralyzed side of the face. A similar preauricular incision on the paralyzed side of the face facilitates this dissection. In terms of technically doing the nerve repair between the sural nerve and the donor nerve fascicles, it is frequently noted that there is significant size discrepancy that makes matching, and therefore suturing, of the sural nerve fascicles to the facial nerve fascicles quite difficult. This is especially true of the match between the nerve graft and the fascicles mediating eye function. A technique that can be

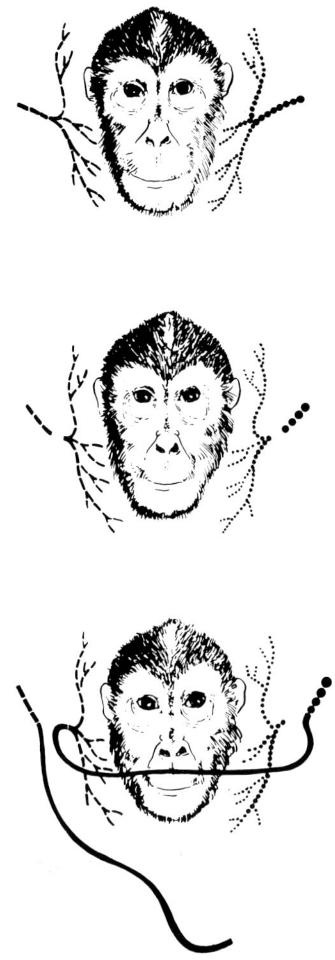

Figure 15-13. Experimental model to determine whether provision of an appropriate target end-organ (facial muscle) or subcutaneous tissue would result in better regeneration across a cross-facial nerve graft in the monkey (top). Schema showing one facial nerve prolonged via a sural nerve graft into the contralateral distal facial nerve and facial muscles, and the other facial nerve is prolonged via a sural nerve graft into the subcutaneous tissue of the neck and chest region. (Reproduced with permission from Mackinnon and Dellon.[55])

Table 15-5. Morphometric Assessment of Experimental Facial Nerve Graft*

Experimental Group (End-Organ Connection)	*Mean Fiber Diameter (μm ± SE)*	*Neural Tissue*
Present	3.1 ± 0.55	15.5%
Absent	2.3 ± 0.27†	10.6%‡

*Reprinted with permission from Dellon and Mackinnon.[51]

†$p < 0.02$.

‡$p < 0.001$.

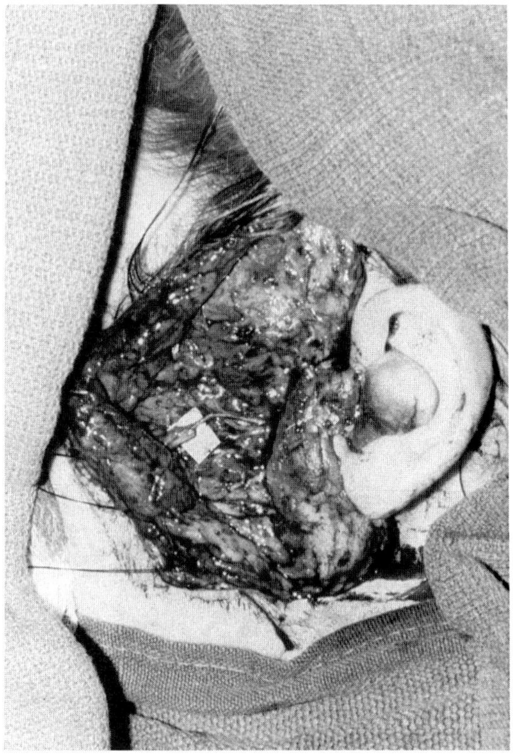

a

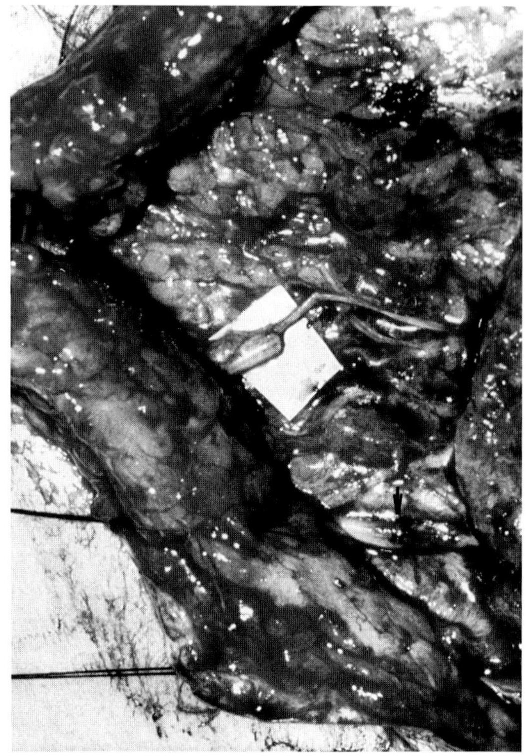

b

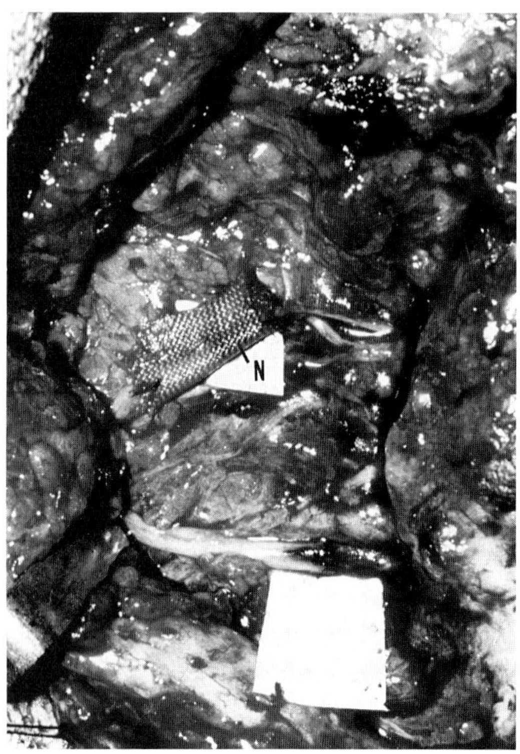

c

Figure 15-14. Intraoperative facial nerve dissection and cross-facial nerve grafting. **a.** At the time of the cross-facial nerve graft procedure, the normal facial nerve is isolated through a preauricular incision and branches that produce isolated eye and mouth contracture are identified. The sural nerve grafts are in position for the cross-facial transfer of these functions. **b.** At a closer view, it is apparent that although the "match" between the sural nerve graft and the large branch of the facial nerve to the commissure muscle is good (arrow), the "match" between the cross-facial sural graft and the branch carrying the eyelid function is poor (background). **c.** A "cone"-shaped Dexon mesh nerve conduit, (Davis and Geck) facilitates matching of this size discrepancy.

utilized to overcome this is to use a Dexon mesh sheet rolled into the shape of a cone and then heat-sealed (see Chapter 20).[56] The small facial nerve donor fascicles are placed into the small end of the cone and the sural nerve into the larger end of the cone, thereby facilitating this size matching (Fig. 15-14). The wounds are closed and Penrose drains are placed in the postauricular region. The patient is positioned in bed with the head elevated. The sutures are removed on the fifth postoperative day. Pre- and postoperative antibiotic coverage is the surgeon's choice. The patient is allowed ambulation. Elastic stockings during the postoperative period to minimize edema in the operated leg are recommended. The patient is seen in intervals postoperatively, and tapping along the cross-facial nerve grafts is carried out. A Tinel's sign will be elicited by which it may be determined that the nerve is regenerating across the face. It has become our practice to wait 3 months past the time at which the Tinel's sign is regenerated across to the opposite cheek before doing the second stage of the operative procedure.

Stage II: Free Muscle Transfer

The second stage is carried out with preparation of the anterior and posterior chest and arm on the side opposite to the side of the facial paralysis. The patient is positioned on his back with the arm abducted and a sandbag placed under his back. The thoracodorsal neurovascular pedicle can be easily identified and a muscle flap elevated in this position. The patient does not need to be positioned on his side. This supine position will facilitate a two-team operative approach. One team begins to identify the cross-facial nerve grafts on the paralyzed side of the face; the other team begins to harvest the donor muscle. In the face, the previous incision is opened and the dissection carried out peripherally, identifying the cross-facial nerve grafts. The facial artery and vein are dissected as the recipient artery and vein for the microvascular anastomosis. The superficial temporal artery and vein may be dissected as alternative vessels. In one patient with significant trauma and multiple previous surgeries, no recipient veins were identified in the entire side of the neck and an external jugular vein from the opposite side of the neck was required as a recipient vein. This required an interposition vein graft.

The latissimus muscle is harvested through a long incision beginning in the axilla and continuing along the mid axillary line. The latissimus muscle's free anterior edge is identified. With blunt dissection, the muscle is separated easily from the rib cage. Continuing this dissection in a superior direction will facilitate identification of the neurovascular bundle. Very careful identification must be made of what would appear to be the branch from the long thoracic artery to the thoracodorsal artery. There is normally a communication here. However, there is the occasional anatomic variation in which the thoracodorsal artery is closely applied to the serratus anterior muscles and then crosses to the latissimus muscle. In this instance, what may have appeared to be the communicating branches is, in fact, the main vascular supply to the latissimus muscle. Thus, before dividing this so-called serratus anterior communicating branch, the thoracodorsal artery must be dissected into the axilla to the axillary artery.

The thoracodorsal nerve is identified in the axilla and dissected distally. Two large branches can be identified. The posterior or medial nerve is frequently preserved. This will supply the corresponding posterior portion of the latissimus dorsi. The branch to the anterior or vertical portion is dissected into the muscle for a considerable way until it begins to divide into two or three separate branches. These, then, are stimulated with the nerve stimulator. Utilizing a marking pen, longitudinal sections of muscle are outlined in this lateral portion of the latissimus dorsi muscle that corresponds to areas that respond to electrical stimulation of the specific separate nerve branches. Depending on how many muscle branches are required, and the size match to the sural nerve grafts, portions or all of the posterior or medial aspect of the muscle may also be utilized. The required number of separate muscle slips of the desired width and length are dissected on a common vascular pedicle. Usually, two separate muscles are required (eye and mouth function). Silk sutures are placed at 2-cm intervals along the length of the muscle strip to identify the normal resting length of the latissimus dorsi muscle (Fig. 15-15). Having completed this dissection, and with the facial recipient vessels identified, the latissimus muscle segments are transsected distally and brought superiorly with the dissections so that the muscle slips are taken on a single artery and vein. The thoracodorsal nerve to the anterior or vertical segment being divided proximally, frequently leaving intact the branch to the posterior or medial segment of the muscle. The geometry is carefully determined before excision of the muscle flap, so that there is sufficient length of nerve and vascular pedicle to carry the nerve repairs superiorly toward the eye and inferiorly toward the corner of the mouth, with the neurovascular island positioned on the deep side of the transfer so that later adjustments in muscle bulk can be made without regard to denervating or devascularizing the muscle. The length of muscle to be cut is taken as the longest length being from the zygomatic arch to the nasolabial fold.

When two independent muscles are required for reanimation of the eye and mouth, we have found a reliable, satisfactory pattern to be one that uses the anterior section of the muscle for the reconstruction of the mouth and smile function and the posterior muscle territory for the muscle flap for eye closure. This will mean a 360° rotation of the muscle from its *in situ* position in the chest to the new position in the face. In the in situ position in the chest, the neurovascular structures are on the anterior surface of the muscle. In its new position in the face, these structures are placed "face down." This will facilitate debulking of the muscle as required without any injury to the neurovascular structures. The most proximal portion of the muscle or that located toward the axilla will be located in the

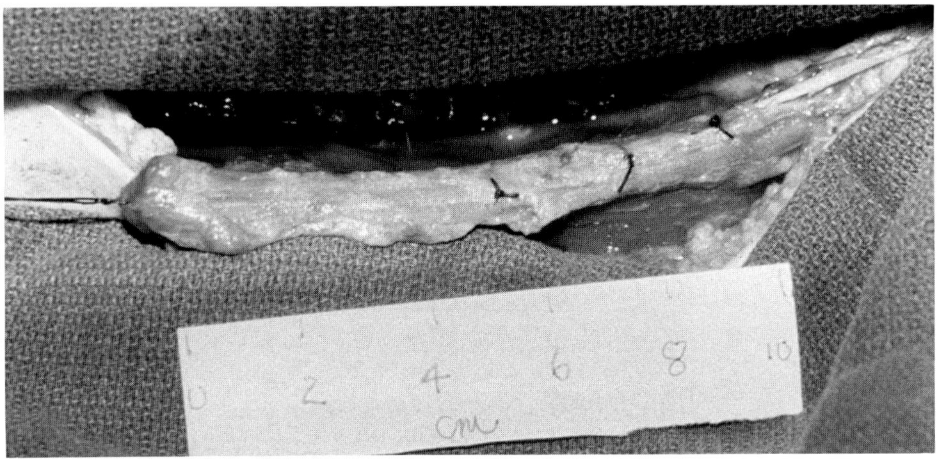

a

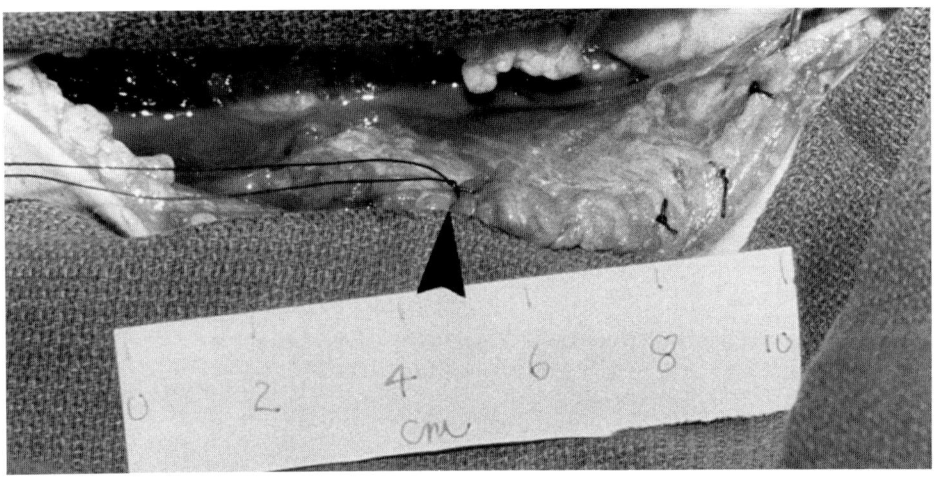

b

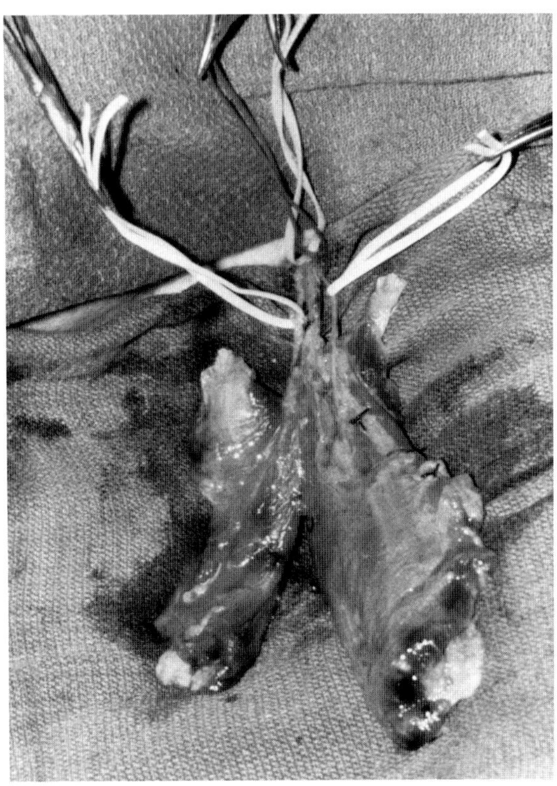

c

Figure 15-15. The latissimus dorsi muscle intraoperative dissection demonstrating marking of resting length (**a**) and degree of muscle contraction with electrical stimulation, note the nerve stimulator upper right **b.** A muscle transfer of independently innervated segments of muscle on a single vascular pedicle is then dissected (**c**).

region of the zygoma. The more distal portion of the muscle toward the free border of the latissimus will be placed in the region of the medial canthus and the nasolabial fold (Figs 15-16, 15-17).

As the two independent muscle paddles are dissected, any distal branches of the thoracodorsal nerves that are not maintained in the muscle territories will be dissected distally and then transposed proximally into the muscle in order to neurotize the muscle so that no motor fibers will be lost. Small muscle territories are fashioned so that the length of the muscle flaps in the resting position will be equal to that necessary to reconstruct the facial muscles from the zygoma to the nasolabial fold for the mouth and from the lateral to medial canthus for the eye. The muscle flaps can then be transferred to the face using the usual microvascular techniques. The insertion of the two muscle flaps is secured before the neurovascular repair and anastomosis. Sutures are made directly from the muscle into the undersurface of the dermis. The medial aspect of the muscle flap is sutured into the dermis to define a new nasolabial crease without the need for excising skin and dermis and creating a scar in this region. A 4-0 nonabsorbable braided suture material is used. The same suture material is used to suture the proximal end of the muscle to the fascia overlying the zygomatic arch and lateral aspect of the inferior orbital rim. The muscle is inset so that the distance between the silk sutures is the same as it was when the latissimus muscle was in situ. The bulk of muscle is twice the thickness of the normal facial musculature, thus allowing for some decreasing bulk in the postoperative period. There will generally be tightness in the attempt to close the skin over this muscle. The skin is closed therefore in the cervical region, but in the preauricular region a skin graft is used if needed. This skin graft will be taken from the side of the donor latissimus muscle site. This graft can be excised in the third stage of the procedure. A Penrose drain, rather than a suction catheter, is placed in the cervical portion of the incision.

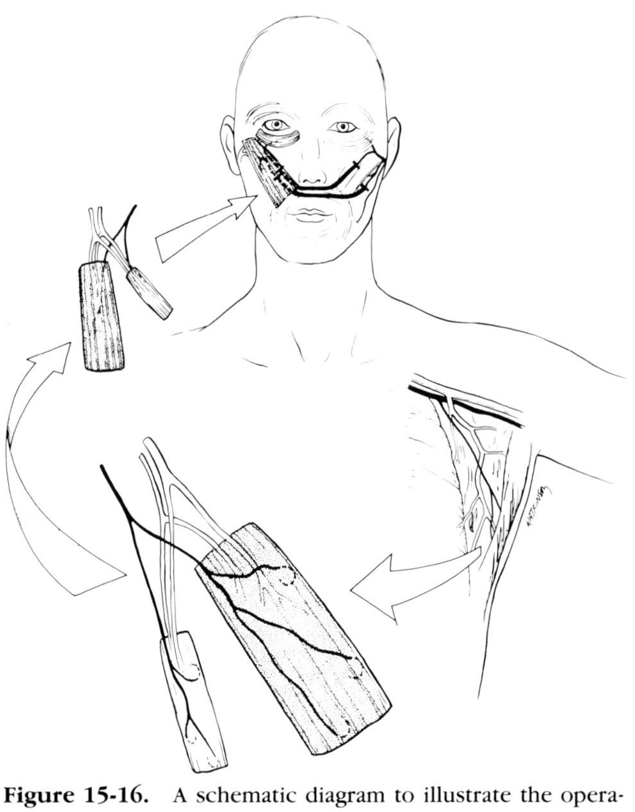

Figure 15-16. A schematic diagram to illustrate the operative technique of the free muscle transfer and the geometric planning of the two muscle flaps. (Reproduced with permission from Mackinnon and Dellon.[74])

In order to position the muscle slip for lower eyelid function, the flap is dissected from the lateral skin incision in the preauricular region dissecting in the plane between the lower eyelid skin and lower eyelid atrophied muscle. A separate incision is made in the medial canthal region and a small slip of the muscle is secured with figure-of-eight 4-0 nonabsorbable braided sutures to the medial canthal ligament. The muscle bulk here is carefully trimmed so that the eye does not appear closed during this stage of the operative procedure, knowing that swelling postoperatively may well cause closure of the eye. Postoperatively, the patient is positioned with the head slightly elevated with no dressings on the face. Significant facial swelling for several weeks is expected. The patient is monitored at intervals with the awareness that facial nerve function will not begin to be noticeable on physical examination until at least 4 to 6 months in the postoperative period. Observation of this early muscle contraction is facilitated by having the patient lie supine, eliminating the effect of gravity. Without the force of gravity for the muscle to overcome, the patient attempts various facial activities and the examiner's hand placed lightly on the cheek can perceive small contractions within the muscle. The patient is placed on biofeedback postoperatively, which can be done usually by the patient himself in front of a mirror, carefully monitoring his facial expressions, touching various aspects of his face and working on attempting to get the type of facial movements he desires. Muscle stimulators and transcutaneous muscle stimulation by electrical means in the postoperative period is used, using a low-frequency faradic stimulator (Eutrophic, Biomeds Corporation, Toronto, Ontario, Canada). This is commenced about 1 month postoperatively.

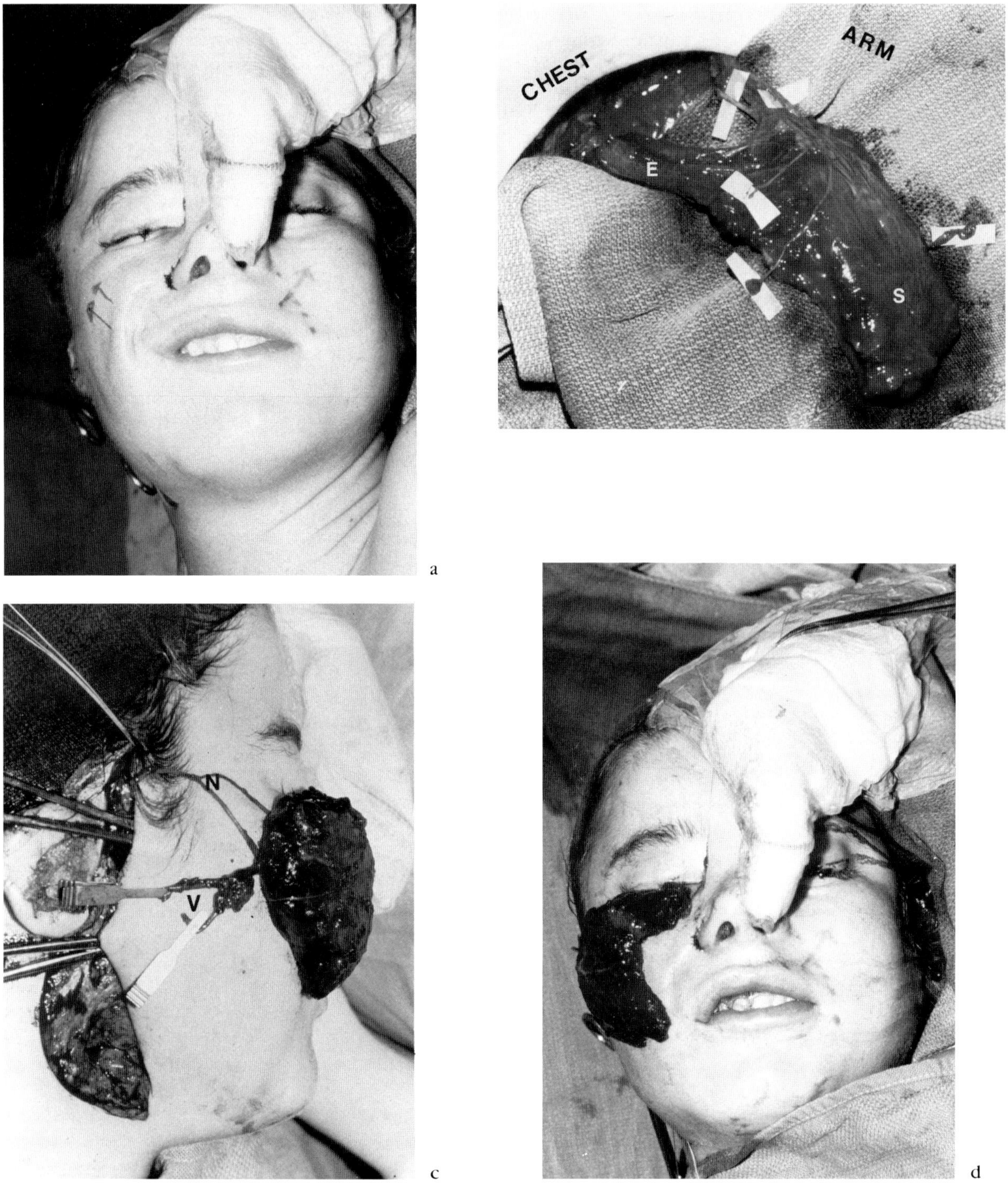

Figure 15-17a. Stage II, free muscle transfer. The dermal sutures in the nasolabial fold have been preplaced. Note the positioning of the nasotracheal tube. **b.** In the left axilla, the two independent muscle flaps (E for eye, S for smile) have been identified using electrical stimulation. Arm, top of photo, chest wall to the left. **c.** The two muscle flaps are positioned on face. V: vessels; N: thoracodorsal nerves. **d.** The two muscle flaps are seen placed on the face. (Reproduced with permission from Mackinnon and Dellon.[74])

Stage III: Ancillary "Touch-Up" Balancing Procedures

The third stage of the operative procedure is carried out at approximately 1½ to 2½ years after the second stage. The third stage does not imply a single operative procedure. A number of additional procedures may prove beneficial to improve facial asymmetry.[51] These, as already described, include tightening or debulking the transferred muscle, adjustments to the contralateral facial muscles either by myotomy or partial denervation, adjustments to the paralyzed eye in terms of contact lens utilization or extraocular muscle plication, additional cosmetic procedures, such as browlift on the paralyzed side with or without associated rhytidectomy on both sides. These techniques are all well-described in other publications. Any ancillary procedures that are in the region of the cross-facial nerve graft must be carried out with extreme care because damage to the nerve graft can occur.

The results achieved after the microneurovascular muscle transfer are enhanced by biofeedback reeducation techniques. We believe these results are superior to those obtained by the more traditional temporalis and masseter muscle transfers.[57] These can be done either by the patient, alone, manually, in front of a mirror, or assisted by a therapist with sophisticated electronic hardware.[58]

Results

In order to standardize reporting of the results not only of facial reconstruction by the reanimation schemes described, but also after facial nerve surgery, it is essential to have agreement on what constitutes degrees of facial nerve function. Toward this end, a committee met at the Fifth International Symposium on the Facial Nerve held in Bordeaux, France, in September, 1984. M. Portmann from France was the Chairman, with other members being U. Fisch of Switzerland, J. W. House of the United States, E. Stennert of Germany, and N. Yanagiharo of Japan. The conclusions of the committee,[59] the proposed rating system, are given in detail in Table 15-6. This system, modified from that described initially by House,[60] adds percentage of function to a rating scale determined by gross categories of facial function that independent observers can rate with good interobserver agreement.

Hemifacial spasm has been traditionally treated by destructive procedures to branches of the facial nerve. In this approach, used when medical treatment to control the unwanted facial movements, or hyperkinesia, has failed, branches of the extracranial facial nerve were cut or excised. This subject has been reviewed thoroughly,[61] and photographically documented long-term results of 80% good to excellent success in movement control can be obtained, but at the loss of facial nerve function. In 1966, Janetta[62] initiated a surgical treatment for hemifacial spasm based on the theory that vascular compression of the facial nerve at its intracranial root entry zone caused the irritation leading to the pathophysiologic state of facial nerve dysfunction. The early reports documented the gross findings of one or more variations of either the vertebral artery, the posterior or anterior inferior cerebellar artery compressing the seventh cranial nerve, as well as ultrastructural findings.[62–64] Janetta's[65] results of 229 intracranial decompressions at which Teflon felt strips were used to lift the vessels off the seventh nerve have been reported, along with diagrams of the operative technique and the abnormal anatomy. He reports 88% of patients with no spasm after the first operation, and an additional 5% of patients relieved after a second operation. An additional 5% had partial relief. Janetta's proposed mechanism for the spasm is that vascular compression leads to demyelination of the nerve fibers that permits ectopic impulse generation from one axon to an adjacent axon, without transmission across a synapse. This ephaptic conduction he demonstrated to exist by electrophysiologically recording the blink reflex before and after decompression intracranially. He demonstrated that such ephaptic transmission could be abolished in 73%, and made unidirectional in another 17% of patients.[66] These findings are probably universal, in the sense that any nerve can become compressed by an overlying vascular structure.

Table 15-6. Facial Nerve Grading Scale

Grade I: Normal (100%)
Normal facial function in all areas
Grade II: Mild dysfunction (99% to 75%)
Slight weakness noticeable only on close inspection. At rest: normal symmetry and tone. Motion: some to normal movement of forehead. Eye closure normal with minimal and maximal effort. Secondary defects: very slight synkinesis may be observed on close inspection. No contracture or hemifacial spasm
Grade III and IV: Moderate dysfunction (75% to 50%)
Obvious weakness or disfiguring asymmetry. Rest: normal symmetry and tone. Motion: no movement of forehead; inability to close eye completely with maximal effort; asymmetrical movement of corners of mouth with maximal effort. Patients with synkinesis, mass action, or hemifacial spasm severe enough to interfere with function are grade IV regardless of degree of motor activity
Grade V: Severe dysfunction (25% to 0%)
Only barely perceptible motion. At rest: possible asymmetry with droop of corner of mouth and decreased or absent nasal labial fold. Motion: no movement of forehead; incomplete closure of eye and only slight movement of lid with maximal effort; slight movement of corner of mouth. Synkinesis, contracture, and hemifacial spasm usually absent
Grade VI: Total paralysis (0%)
Loss of tone; asymmetry; no motion; no synkinesis, contracture, or hemifacial spasm

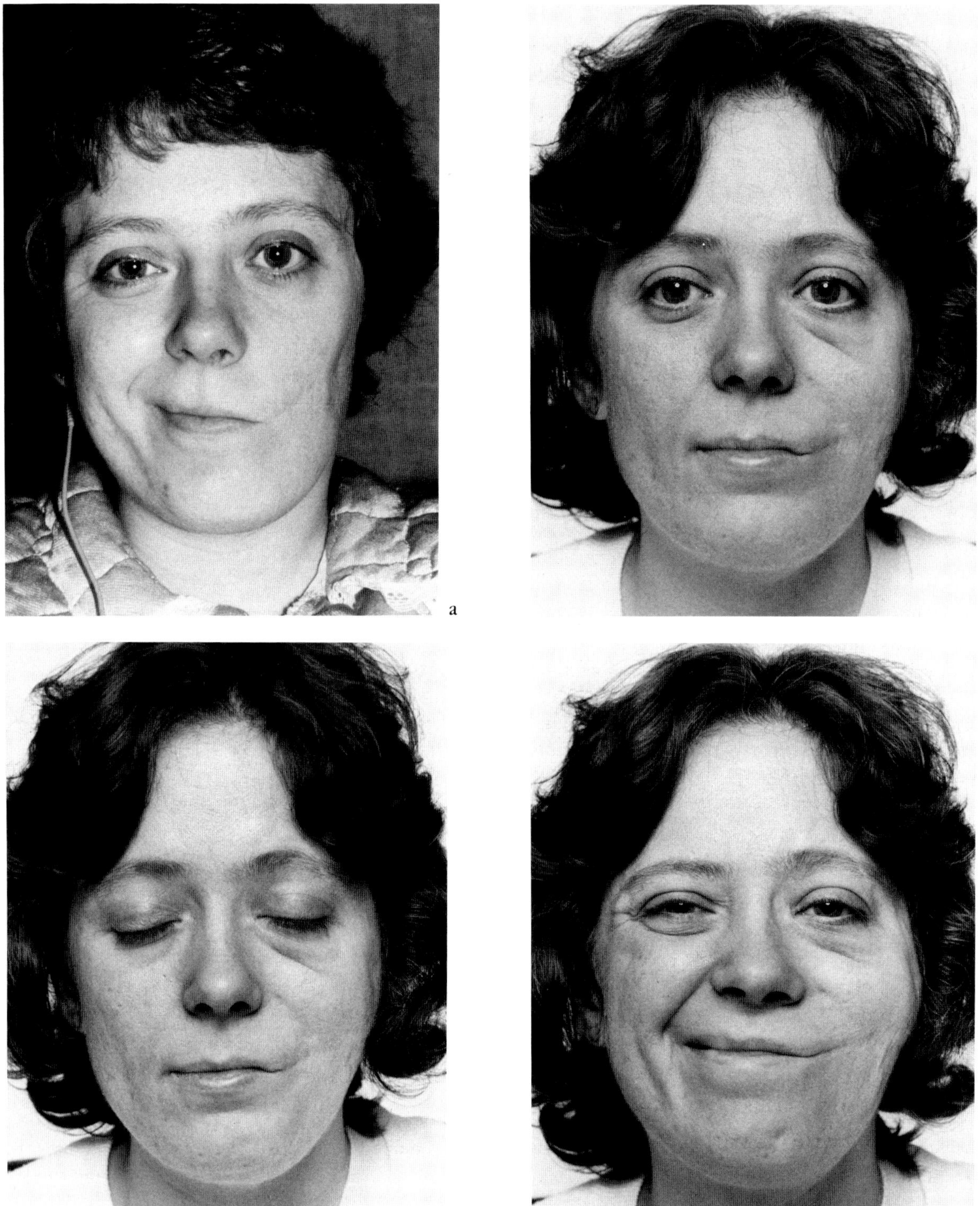

a b c d

Figure 15-18. Independent smile and eyelid closure obtained by a multiple innervation, multiple segment configured latissimus muscle transfer. At stage I, separate cross-facial nerve grafts were dedicated to eyelid closure and smile function. At stage II, independent muscle slips of the latissimus transferred on a single artery and vein were connected by separate branches of the thoracodorsal nerve to the appropriate cross-facial nerve grafts. Above, 9 months after stage II, there is independent function of these muscles. **a.** Preoperative with patient smiling. Note how left corner of mouth is drooping, and nostril and eyelid assymetry. Postoperative: **b.** Symmetry at rest. **c.** Closing eyes. **d.** Smiling. (Reproduced with permission from Mackinnon and Dellon.[74])

We note this in the forearm (Chapters 7 and 11), and Janetta has documented it for another cranial nerve, the trigeminal,[67–69] in the cause of facial pain, tic douloureux.

Continued study of the results of facial nerve injury and repair confirm the observations on peripheral nerve injury and repair discussed in detail in Chapters 2 and 4. For example, electron microscopic evaluation of 25 normal and 17 paralytic human facial muscle specimens has been reported.[70] Of interest was the observation that the spectrum of ultrastructural changes showed no dependence on the length of the denervation period, with the time periods studied being 1 month to 36 years postdenervation. An unusual variety of inclusion bodies was also noted. With regard to facial nerve repair and grafting, Miehlke[71] has reported his results and reviewed the literature through 1973, and Janeka and Conley[72] have updated this through 1987. The collective experience shows optimism with 80% good to excellent results when these nerve reconstructions are done in the peripheral branches of the seventh nerve.

Utilizing a surgical algorithm[73] for the management of facial palsy (Table 15-3), we anticipate improved results and continuing refinement of the surgical techniques described in this chapter.[74] The management of the patient with facial palsy is currently in a stage of rapid evolution. Utilization of the techniques described in this chapter can result in significant improvement in facial symmetry and even independent, spontaneous, and voluntary control of facial animation (Fig. 15-18).

References

1. Gray's Anatomy, 15th British ed. Bounty Books, New York, 401, 1977, p 743.
2. Bell C: On the nerves, giving an account of some experiments on their structure and functions, which leads to a new arrangement of the system. Trans R Soc Lond 3:398, 1821.
3. Bunnell S: Suture of the facial nerve within the temporal bone with a report of the first successful case. Surg Gynecol Obstet 45:7–12, 1927.
4. Miehlke A: Surgery of the Facial Nerve. WB Saunders, Philadelphia, 1973.
5. Diamond C: Facial nerve. Hofstra University Press, New York, 1979.
6. Green MD, House WF: Disorders of the Facial Nerve; Anatomy, Diagnosis and Management. Raven Press, New York, 1980.
7. May M: The Facial Nerve. Thieme, New York, 1986.
8. Converse JM: In Kazanjian VH and Converse JM, eds: Surgical Treatment of Facial Injuries, 3rd ed, Williams & Wilkins, Baltimore, 1974, pp 1235–1288.
9. Freeman BS: Facial Palsy. In Converse JM, ed: Reconstructive Plastic Surgery, 2nd ed. WB Saunders, Philadelphia, 1977, pp 1774–1868.
10. Rubin LR: Reanimation of the Paralyzed Face. CV Mosby, St. Louis, 1977.
11. Portmann M, ed: Facial Nerve, Proceedings of the Fifth International Symposium. Masson Publishing USA, New York, 1985.
12. Rubin LR, Lee GW, Simpson RL: Reanimations of the longstanding partial facial paralysis. Plast Reconstr Surg 77: 41–49, 1986.
13. Thompson N: Autogenous muscle grafts in the reconstruction of the paralyzed face. In Converse JM, ed: Reconstructive Plastic Surgery, 2nd ed. WB Saunders, Philadelphia, 1977, pp 1841–1848.
14. Tamai S, Komatsu S, Sakamoto H, et al: Free muscle transplants in dogs with microsurgical neurovascular anastomoses. Plast Reconstr Surg 46:219–225, 1970.
15. Harii K, Ohmori K, Toru S: Free gracilis muscle transplantation with microneurovascular anastomoses for treatment of facial paralysis. Plast Reconstr Surg 57:133–143, 1976.
16. Terzis JK, Sweet RC, Dykes RW, Williams HB: Recovery of function in free muscle transplants using microneurovascular anastomoses. J Hand Surg 3:37–59, 1978.
17. Frey M, Gruber H, Havel M, Sterner E, Freilinger G: Experimental free-muscle transplantation with microneurovascular anastomoses. Plast Reconstr Surg 71:689, 1983.
18. Baker DC, Conley J: Facial nerve grafting: A thirty year retrospective review. Clin Plast Surg 6:343–360, 1979.
19. Meissl G, Millesi H: Nerve suture and grafting to restore extratemporal facial nerve. Clin Plast Surg 6:335–342, 1979.
20. Samii M: Facial nerve grafting in acoustic neuroma. Clin Plast Surg 11:221–225, 1984.
21. Sunderland S, Cossar DF: The structure of the facial nerve. Anat Rec 116:147, 1953.
22. Miehlke A: Normal and anomalous anatomy of the facial nerve. Trans Am Acad Ophthalmol Otolaryngol 68:1030, 1964.
23. Harris WD: Topography of the facial nerve. Arch Otolaryngol 88:264–267, 1968.
24. White A, Verma PL: Spatial arrangement of facial nerve fibers. J Laryngol Otol 87:957–963, 1973.
25. May M: Anatomy of the facial nerve (spatial orientation of fibers in the temporal bone). Laryngoscope 83:1311, 1973.
26. Sade J: Facial nerve reconstruction and its prognosis. Ann Otol Rhinol Laryngol 84:695–698, 1975.
27. Crumley R: Spatial anatomy of facial nerve fibers—a preliminary report. Laryngoscope 90:274–280, 1980.
28. Kempe LF: Topical organization of the distal portion of the facial nerve. J Neurosurg 52:671–673, 1980.
29. Thomander L, Aldskogius H, Grant G: Motor fiber organization in the intratemporal portion of the cat and rat facial nerves studied with horseradish peroxidase technique. Acta Universitatis Upsaliensis. Abstr of Upsala Dissert Fac Med, #404 iii:1, 1981.
30. Anderl H: Reconstruction of the face through cross-face nerve transplantation in facial paralysis. In Converse JM: Reconstructive Plastic Surgery, WB Saunders, Philadelphia, 1977, pp 1848–1864.

31. Davis RA, Anson BJ, Puddinger JM, Kurth RE: Surgical anatomy of the facial nerve and parotid gland based upon study of 350 cervical facial halves. Surg Gynecol Obstet 102:385–412, 1956.
32. Seiler WA, Dellon AL, Mackinnon SE: Correlation of facial muscle anatomy and motor function in Maccaca fascicularis. Peripheral Nerve Repair Regeneration 1:41–48, 1986.
33. Manktelow RT, Zuker RM, McKee NH: Functioning free muscle transplantation. J Hand Surg 9A:32–39, 1984.
34. Ferreira MC, Marchese AT, Spinno Y: Injectos transfacia les des nervios en al tratamiento de la paralysis facial observaciones iniciales. Chir Plast Ibero Lat Am 3:301, 1977.
35. O'Brien B, Franklin JD, Morrison WA: Cross-facial nerve grafts and microneurovascular free muscle transfer for long-established facial palsy. Br J Plast Surg 33:202–215, 1980.
36. Mayou BJ, Watson JS, Harrison DH, Wynn-Parry CB: Free microvascular and microneural transfer of the extensor digitorum brevis muscle for the treatment of unilateral facial palsy. Br J Plast Surg 34:362–367, 1981.
37. Manktelow RF, McKee NH, Veltese T: Anatomical study of pectoralis major muscle as related to functioning free muscle transplantation. Plast Reconstr Surg 65:610–615, 1980.
38. Terzis JK, Manktelow RT: Pectoralis minor: A new concept in facial reanimation. Plast Surg Forum 5, 1982.
39. Harrison DH: The pectoralis minor vascularized muscle graft for the treatment of unilateral facial palsy. Plast Reconstr Surg 75:206–213, 1985.
40. Buncke HJ, Albert BS, Gordon L, et al: Free serratus anterior muscle transplantation for unilateral facial nerve paralysis. Paper presented at the American Association of Plastic Surgery, Annual Meeting, May, 1984.
41. Manktelow RT, Zuker RM: Muscle transplantation by fascicular territory. Plast Reconstr Surg 73:751–755, 1984.
42. Bartlett SP, May JW Jr, Yaremchuk MJ: The latissimus dorsi muscle: A free cadaver study of the primary neurovascular pedicle. Plast Reconstr Surg 67:631–636, 1981.
43. Tobin GR, Schusterman M, Peterson GH, et al: The intramuscular neurovascular anatomy of the latissimus dorsi muscle. The basis for splitting the flap. Plast Reconstr Surg 67:637–641, 1981.
44. Dellon AL, Mackinnon SE: Segmentally innervated latissimus dorsi muscle: Microsurgical transfer for facial reanimation. J Reconstr Microsurg 2:7–12, 1985.
45. Pately JL, Manktelow RT, Chaban R: The anatomy of the normal smile. Presented at the American Association of Plastic Surgeons meeting, Nashville, Tennessee, May, 1987.
46. Terzis J: Experience in restoring symmetrical expression. Presented at the American Association of Plastic Surgeons Meeting, Nashville, Tennessee, May, 1987.
47. Rubin LR: The anatomy of a smile—its importance in facial paralysis. Plast Reconstr Surg 53:384–387, 1974.
48. Laitung JKG, Peck F: Shoulder function following the loss of the latissimus dorsi muscle. Br J Plast Surg 38:375–379, 1985.
49. Fasching MC, VanBeek AL: Monitoring muscle viability using M Waves. Plast Reconstr Surg 75:217–272, 1985.
50. May JW, Lukash FN, Galico GG, Sterrat CR: Removable thermocouple probe microvascular patency monitor: An experimental and clinical study. Plast Reconstr Surg 72: 366, 1983.
51. Dellon AL, Mackinnon SE: Adjunctive procedures to facilitate facial symmetry after cross-facial nerve grafting and microneurovascular muscle transfer for facial paralysis. In preparation.
52. deMauro W, Gilbert A: Surgical anatomy of the sural nerve. J Reconstr Microsurg 1:31–40, 1984.
53. Kurihara K, Cohen M, Schultz RC: Nerve staining with leucomethylene blue: An experimental study. Plast Reconstr Surg 73:960–964, 1984.
54. Dellon AL, Mackinnon SE: Gentle passage of nerve grafts. J Hand Surg 8:108–109, 1983.
55. Mackinnon SE, Dellon AL: A histologic assessment of the effects of the distal nerve in determining regeneration across a nerve gap. Microsurgery 9:46–51, 1988.
56. Mackinnon SE, Dellon AL: An alternative to the management of the short nerve gap. Plast Reconstr Surg, November, 1988.
57. May M: Muscle transposition for facial reanimation. Arch Otol 110:184–189, 1984.
58. Brown DM, Nahai F, Wolf S, Basmajian JV: Electromyographic biofeedback in the re-education of facial palsy. Am J Phys Med 57:183–190, 1978.
59. Portmann M: Conclusions (of the Fifth International Symposium on the Facial Nerve regarding A Facial Nerve Grading System). In Portmann M, ed: Facial Nerve. Masson Publishing USA, New York. 1985, pp 43–44.
60. House JW: Facial nerve grading system. Laryngology 93: 1056–1069, 1983.
61. Fisch U: Extracranial surgery for facial hyperkinesis. In May M ed: The Facial Nerve. Thieme, New York, 1986, pp 509–523.
62. Janetta PJ: Microsurgical exploration and decompression of the facial nerve in hemifacial spasm. Curr Top Surg Res, 2:217–220, 1970.
63. Ruby JR, Janetta PJ: Hemifacial spasm. Ultrastructural changes in the facial nerve induced by vascular compression. Surg Neurol 4:369–370, 1975.
64. Janetta PJ, Abbosy M, Maroon JC, et al: Etiology and definitive microsurgical treatment of hemifacial spasm. Operative technique and results in 47 patients. J Neurosurg 47:321–328, 1977.
65. Janetta PJ: Microvascular decompression for hemifacial spasm. In May M, ed: The Facial Nerve. Thieme, New York, 1986, pp 499–508.
66. Nelsen VK, Janetta PJ: Pathophysiology of hemifacial spasm: III: Effects of facial nerve decompression Neurology (Cleve) 34:891–897, 1984.
67. Janetta PJ: Arterial compression of the trigeminal nerve and the pons in patients with trigeminal neuralgia. J Neurosurg 26:159–162, 1967.
68. Janetta PJ: Microsurgical approach to the trigeminal nerve for tic douloureux. Prog Neurol Surg 7:180–200, 1976.
69. Janetta PJ: Neurovascular compression in cranial nerve and systemic disease. Ann Surg 192:518–525, 1980.
70. Bardosi A, Goebel HH, Stennert E: The ultrastructure of normal and denervated human facial muscle. Plast Re-

cosntr Surg 79:171–176, 1987.
71. Miehlke A: The results of surgery of the facial nerve. In Miehlke A, ed: Surgery of the Facial Nerve. Urban & Schwarzenberg, Munich, 1973, pp 225–235.
72. Janeka IV, Conley J: Primary neoplasms of the facial nerve. Plast Reconstr Surg 79:177–185, 1987.
73. Mackinnon SE, Dellon AL: A Surgical algorithm for the management of facial palsy. Microsurgery 9:30–35, 1988.
74. Mackinnon SE, Dellon AL: Technical considerations of the latissimus dorsi muscle flap: a segmentally innervated muscle transfer for facial reanimation. Microsurg 9:36—45, 1988.

Brachial Plexus Injuries

16

The appropriate management of even a simple laceration to a single peripheral nerve presents a challenge to the reconstuctive surgeon. The management of a closed injury is equally demanding. It is not surprising, then, that the majority of surgeons perceive brachial plexus injury as a problem so formidable that they avoid becoming involved in its treatment. In these instances, it is not a single nerve that is involved, but a number of roots, trunks, cords, and divisions that are related in a complicated anatomic fashion. Within these multiple nerves, various nerve injury patterns usually occur, not at a discrete location, but along the longitudinal axis of the nerves for varying distances. To compound the problem, the injuries occur at such a proximal level that the regeneration distances challenge the time limits of the motor response (muscle end-organ) for reinnervation. Finally, the extensive nature of the injury is such that the patient's donor sites for nerve graft material are often exhausted, as is the surgeon's operative stamina for long microneurosurgical operations. By nature of the injury, the time between the initial traumatic event and the completion of all potential reconstructive procedures, including nerve grafts, muscle flaps, tendon transfers, and bony work, is often several years. This long-term commitment to the patient is demanding, especially in view of the fact that complete rehabilitation and recovery is usually impossible.

Of all peripheral nerve problems, brachial plexus injuries present some of the most interesting. It is the treatment of these devastating problems in a patient population of young persons who are just beginning their most productive years that provides the peripheral nerve surgeon with the continuous impetus for improvement of diagnostic, operative, and rehabilitative techniques. The room for improvement in functional results is so great that the management of these problems remains a therapeutic challenge.

This chapter will review and highlight the critical aspects of brachial plexus injuries, emphasizing the management of traumatic traction injuries. Recommended to the reader are the excellent review text of brachial plexus injuries by Leffert[1] and the multi-authored work edited by Terzis[2] of the microsurgical reconstruction of brachial plexus injuries. These recent texts present different but complementary approaches to the management of the patient with brachial plexus surgery. Both texts provide well over 200 pages each of important information for surgeons interested in this problem.

Historical Review

The relationship between brachial plexus injury and traumatic birth deliveries has been documented, with the first notation in 1768 by Smellie[3] who described a case of bilateral brachial plexus palsy after a difficult delivery. The classic upper plexus palsy described in 1872 by Duchenne[4] (and in adults by Erb[5] in 1874) is well recognized, as is the less common lower plexus palsy that Klumpke described in 1885.[6] In 1827, Flaubert[7] described a traction injury to the plexus after the closed reduction of a dislocated shoulder.

The earliest reports of the surgical management of brachial plexus injuries appeared around the turn of the 20th century. Thoburn[8] in 1903 described a surgical repair of an injury to the brachial plexus. Kennedy[9] in 1903 described a surgical repair of the brachial plexus for birth palsies and in the same year Harris and Low[10] described a neurotization procedure for reconstruction of patients with Erb's palsy. In 1913, Tuttle[11] described similar procedures in adults. In the early 1900s, Taylor presented a series of articles on the surgical results of plexus surgery.[12–15] Comparing 70 operative cases to 130 control nonoperative cases, he reported 1% spontaneous recovery in the nonoperative group and "marked improvement" in the operative group.[15] Similarly, Davis et al[16] reviewed the surgical treatment of brachial plexus injuries and suggested that significant functional improvement could be expected after surgery.

This initial enthusiasm for brachial plexus surgery in the early part of the century was followed by a pessimistic outlook as several reports documented poor results with brachial plexus surgery.[17–19] Even in 1963, Seddon[20] condemned brachial plexus surgery except for injury to the upper trunk.

Renewed enthusiasm for operative management of these injuries awaited the introduction of microneurosurgical technique and nerve grafting. Millesi[21,22] pioneered the use of nerve grafts to manage these injuries. With these improved techniques has come improved results. Kline and Nulsen,[23] Hudson and Tamner,[24] Narakas,[25–28] Gilbert and Tassin,[29] Brunelli,[30] Merle and Deburge,[31] Alnot et al,[32] Allieu,[33] Samii and Kahl,[34] Leffert,[1] Terzis et al,[35] and Kotani et al[36] have all made important contributions toward the operative management of plexus injuries.

Surgical Anatomy

The surgical anatomy of the brachial plexus has been well described[1] (Fig. 16-1). The fifth to eighth cervical and first thoracic nerve roots are the constant contributors to the brachial plexus. A "prefixed" plexus implies a significant contribution from the fourth cervical root with little if any contribution from T1. A postfixed plexus implies contribution from the second thoracic root with a small contribution from C5. The roots lie between the anterior and middle scalene muscles. Since there is not an eighth cervical vertebra, C5, C6, and C7 roots exit above their numbered cervical vertebra and C8 and T1 roots exit below the 7th cervical and first thoracic vertebra, respectively. This has significance in brachial plexus chronic compression (see Chapter 14) in that the first rib's posterior portion lies between the C8 and T1 root juncture, at which point they form the lower trunk of the plexus. The upper trunk is formed by the fifth and sixth cervical roots, the middle trunk is a continuation of the seventh cervical root. The eighth cervical and first thoracic root combine to form the lower trunk. The trunks lie in the lower part of the posterior cervical triangle.

The three trunks divide into anterior and posterior divisions at the level of the clavicle. The three posterior divisions unite to form the posterior cord (C5, C6, C7, C8, T1). The anterior divisions of the upper and middle trunks form the lateral cord, (C5, C6, C7). The anterior division of the lower trunk continues as the medial cord (C8, T1). The three cords are named to correspond to their position with respect to the axillary artery and are located just below the pectoralis minor muscle.

Most of the branches of the brachial plexus originate from the cords. The cords are distal to the clavicle and these branches may be termed "the infraclavicular plexus." Some supraclavicular branches will arise from the roots or trunks. Branches from the cords will not necessarily contain innervation from all roots that make up that cord (for example, the posterior cord, [C5, C6, C7, C8, T1] gives the subscapular branch [C5, C6]).

The medial cord continues as the ulnar nerve after giving a terminal branch to the medial head of the median nerve. The medial cord contributes the innervation of the intrinsic muscles supplied by the median nerve. The lateral cord continues as the musculocutaneous (C5, C6, C7) nerve after giving a terminal branch to the lateral head of the median nerve. Thus, the lateral cord contributes the innervation of the sensory component of median nerve. The posterior cord continues as the radial nerve after giving a terminal branch, the axillary nerve (C5, C6). The axillary nerve travels through the quadrangular space with the circumflex humeral (axillary) vessels. As the nerve courses posteriorly through this space, it will be subject to a secondary traction injury superimposed on the original brachial plexus stretch injury. The boundaries of the space are the teres minor and major muscles above and below and the surgical neck of the humerus laterally and the long head of triceps medially. This anatomical arrangement renders the axillary nerve susceptible to greater nerve injury with stretch brachial plexus injuries, and an isolated entrapment can occur here, the quadrangular space syndrome.

Of the three branches from the nerve roots, two of these are clinically important. The long thoracic

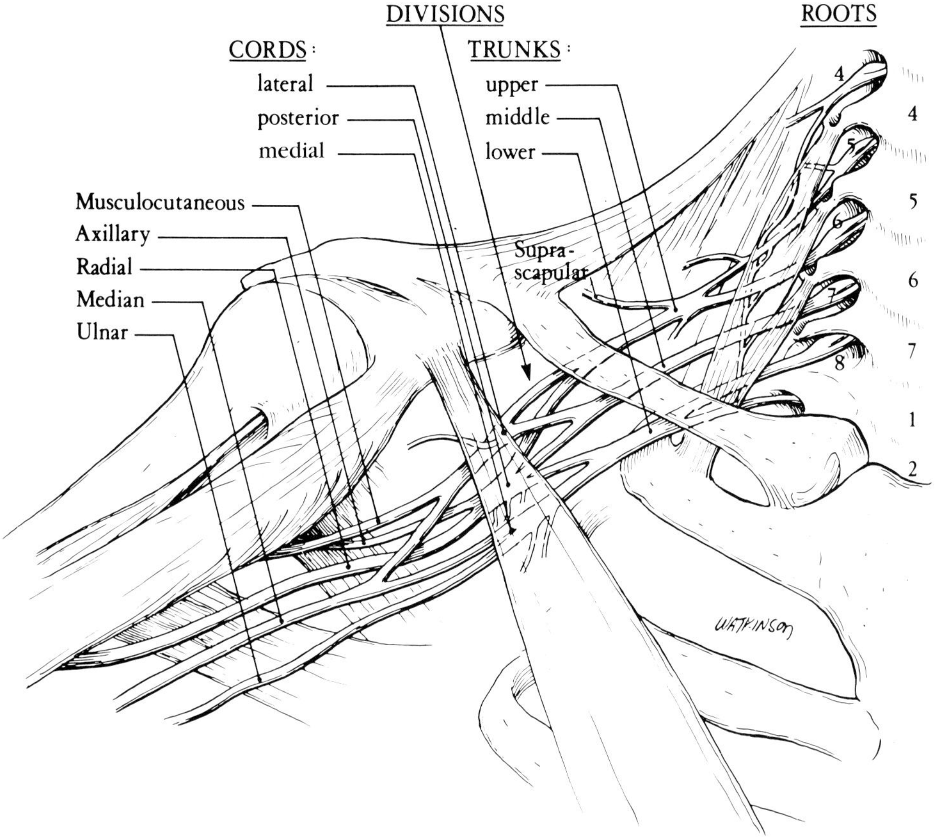

Figure 16-1. The anatomy of the brachial plexus relating the roots, trunks, divisions, and cords to the scalene muscles and clavicle.

nerve originates from the fifth, sixth, and seventh cervical nerve roots and innervates the serratus anterior muscle. The dorsal scapular nerve is a branch of the fifth (and sixth) cervical roots and innervates the levator scapulae and rhomboid muscles. The third branch, the nerve to the subclavius, arising from the fifth and sixth cervical roots innervates the subclavius muscle, and cannot be clinically evaluated. If the muscles innervated by these nerves are not functioning, it suggests a proximal root injury or avulsion of the brachial plexus from the spinal cord. By contrast, if the muscles innervated by these nerves are functioning, even if no other elements are working, it suggests that a living proximal nerve stump can be identified and used to reconstruct the plexus. If the rhomboids and serratus muscles are not functioning, it implies nerve root avulsion with no proximal nerve at that level usable for reconstruction. The presence of a Horner's syndrome suggests root avulsion at the C8, T1 level. Cervical sympathetic fibers (C8 or T1) controlling oculopupillary action accompany the trigeminal nerve to the orbit. The ciliary nerve supplies Mueller's muscle (enophthalmus), tarsal muscles (ptosis), and controls pupillary dilation (myosis). Sweat secretion on the ipsilateral side of the face is also lost with a Horner's syndrome (anhydrosis).

The suprascapular nerve (C5, C6) arises from the upper trunk above the clavicle in the posterior triangle of the neck and innervates the supraspinatus and infraspinatus muscles. It runs deep to the trapezius muscle and through the scapular notch. The nerve can be compressed at the scapular notch and can be decompressed at this level by excision of the ligament that forms the roof of the notch.

The lateral pectoral nerve (C5, C6) is a branch of the lateral cord and innervates the clavicular head of the pectoralis major muscle. Thus, if weakness of the clavicular head of the pectoralis major muscle is present, it implies injury to the lateral cord. The medial pectoral nerve arises from the medial cord and along with the branches from the lateral pectoral nerve innervates the sternocostal head of the pectoralis major muscle. Examination then of the pectoralis major muscle will be critical in localizing injury at the cord level. If the clavicular head is involved, it implies lateral pectoral nerve injury, and, if the sternocostal head is involved, it implies injury to both the lateral and medial pectoralis nerves, that is, both medial and lateral cords.

The musculocutaneous nerve is a continuation of the lateral cord. It enters the coracobrachialis muscle almost immediately, then runs between the biceps and the brachialis muscles. It supplies all three muscles. It continues distally as the lateral antebrachial cutaneous nerve. Where the musculocutaneous nerve enters the coracobrachialis, it is in a relatively tethered position coming off the lateral cord, and, like the axillary nerve, it is, thus, subject to a secondary traction injury at this level in the situation of a brachial plexus stretch palsy.

The posterior cord, after giving off the axillary nerve, also gives off collateral branches to the muscles making up the posterior wall of the axilla. The thoracodorsal nerve (C6,C7,C8) innervates the latissimus dorsi. The subscapular nerve (C5,C6,C7) innervates the subscapularis and teres major muscles.

Intraneural Topography of the Brachial Plexus

The complexity of the intraneural anatomy of the brachial plexus has long been of interest to the anatomist. Abraham Kerr,[37] an anatomist at Johns Hopkins University, reviewed more than 400 brachial plexus dissections done by the medical students between 1895 and 1910. One hundred and seventy-five of these dissections were included in his classic article published in 1918 that described in graphic detail the complexity of the intraneural anatomy of the brachial plexus (Fig. 16-2). Since that time, this anatomy has been well described by many others, including Narakas[38] (Fig. 16-3) and Slingluff et al[39] (Fig. 16-4). These latter investigators stressed that fascicles containing mixed motor and sensory fibers were much more common than either pure motor or pure sensory fascicles. They also noted that the neural to connective tissue ratio was very low in the plexus, for example, percentage of total neural tissue ranged from 1.6% in the axillary (sensory) nerve to

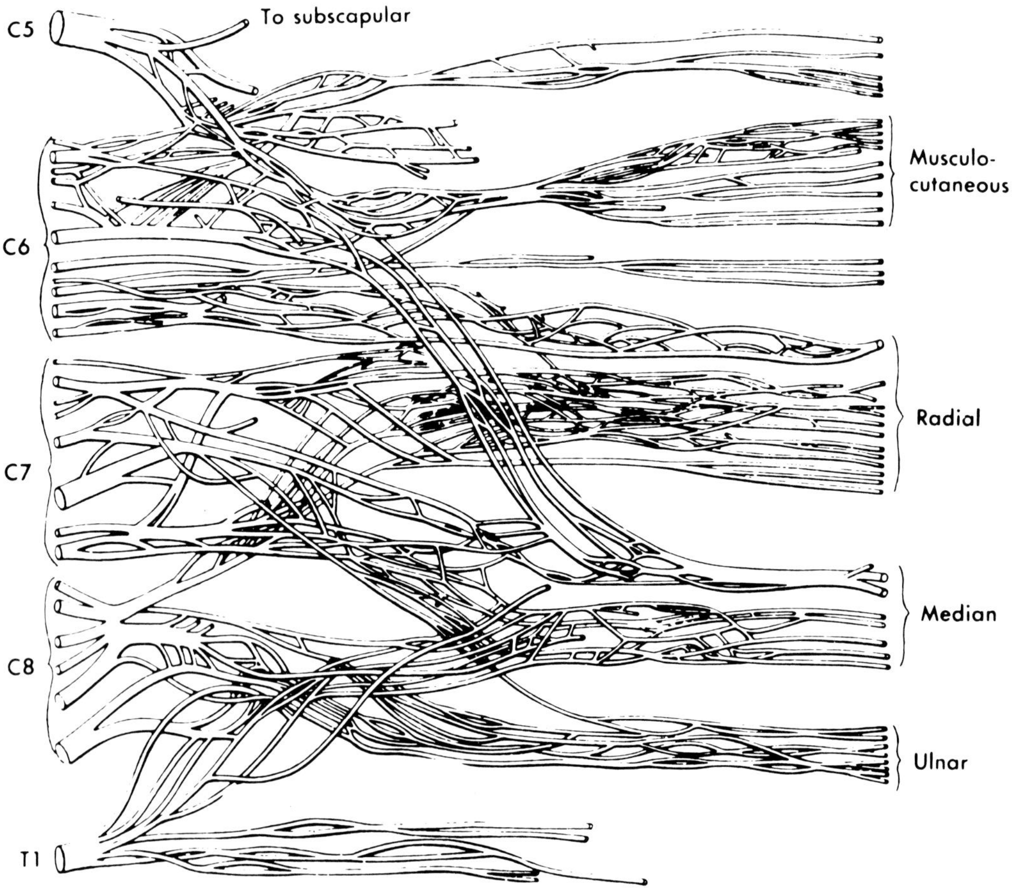

Figure 16-2. Intraneural dissection of the brachial plexus carried out by Kerr demonstrates the tremendous plexus formation. (Reproduced with permission from Kerr.[37])

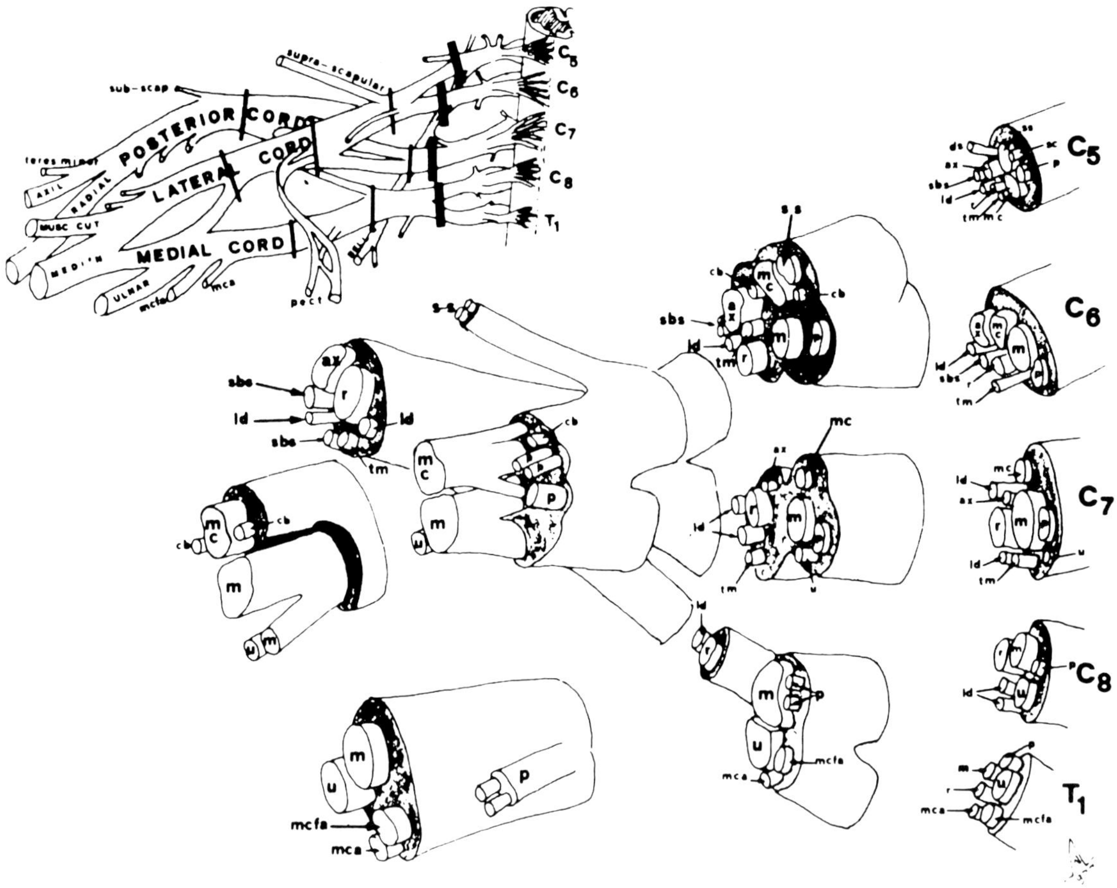

Figure 16-3. Narakas' study of the intraneural topography of the brachial plexus. (Reproduced with permission from Narakas.[27])

8.4% in the musculocutaneous nerve to 24% in C7. They confirmed the presence of marked plexus formation, "rarely, a fascicle will travel over 1 cm. without plexus information," and noted that in the proximal plexus mono- or bifascicularity was the normal finding.

Injury Patterns

The six injury patterns (described in Chapter 2) are, of course, directly applicable to the brachial plexus. In the plexus, injuries can also be classified as three types, root avulsion, nerve interruption, and nerve in-continuity lesions (Fig. 16-5). Millesi[40] reviewed 185 patients with 414 injuries and recorded 226 root avulsions, 127 interruptions, and 61 in-continuity lesions (Table 16-1). Sunderland[41] drew attention to the meningeal-neural relations in the intervertebral foramen with the dura becoming the perineurium as the nerve roots exit from the foramina to become spinal nerves (Figs. 16-6, 16-7).

Clinical Examination

Systematic examination of the patient with a suspected brachial plexus injury is simplified by an understanding of the anatomy of the plexus; as described in the preceding section.

Root Avulsion

Brachial plexus lesions are localized with respect to the location of the dorsal root ganglion (post- or infraganglionic lesions are distal to the dorsal root ganglion, pre- or supraganglionic lesions are proximal to the ganglion) (Fig. 16-8). With both lesions, the patient presents with complete loss of motor and sensory function because the nerve fibers are separated from central structures. With the pre- or supraganglionic lesions, the roots have been avulsed directly from the spinal cord. There is no proximal peripheral nerve tissue and surgical repair is not possible. With a post- or infraganglionic lesion, the

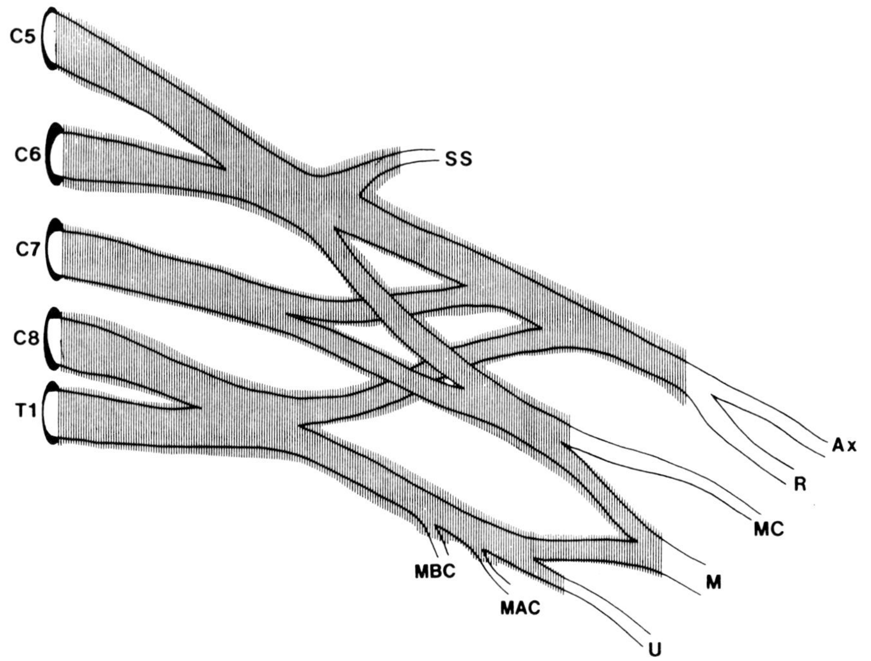

a

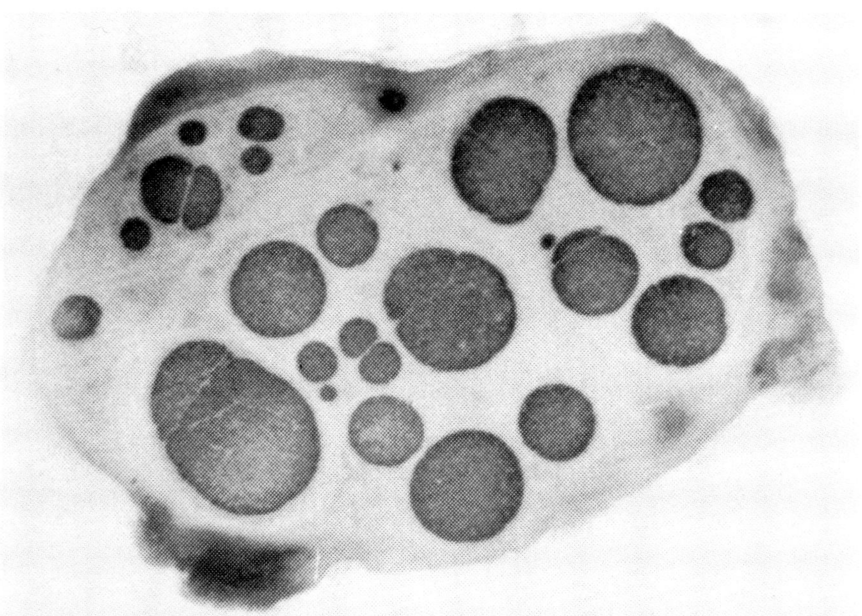

b

Figure 16-4a. Slingluff, et al.[39] carried out a series cross-sections along the entire length of the plexus. This figure demonstrates the multitude of perpendicular sections made through the plexus. Ax: axillary; Median; MAC: medial antebrachial cutaneous; MBC; medial brachial cutaneous; MC: medial cord; R: radial; SS: suprascapular; U: ulnar. **b.** The cross-sections were studied and photographed. This is a representative cross-section from the medial cord (Reproduced with permission from Slingluff, et al.[39])

Table 16-1. Distribution of Avulsions, Interruptions, and Lesions In-Continuity

	C4	*C5*	*C6*	*C7*	*C8*	*T1*	*Total*
Avulsion	1	22	39	68	53	43	226
Interruption	5	57	40	10	6	9	127
Lesion in-continuity	—	3	3	4	23	28	61

Reproduced with permission from Millesi.[40]

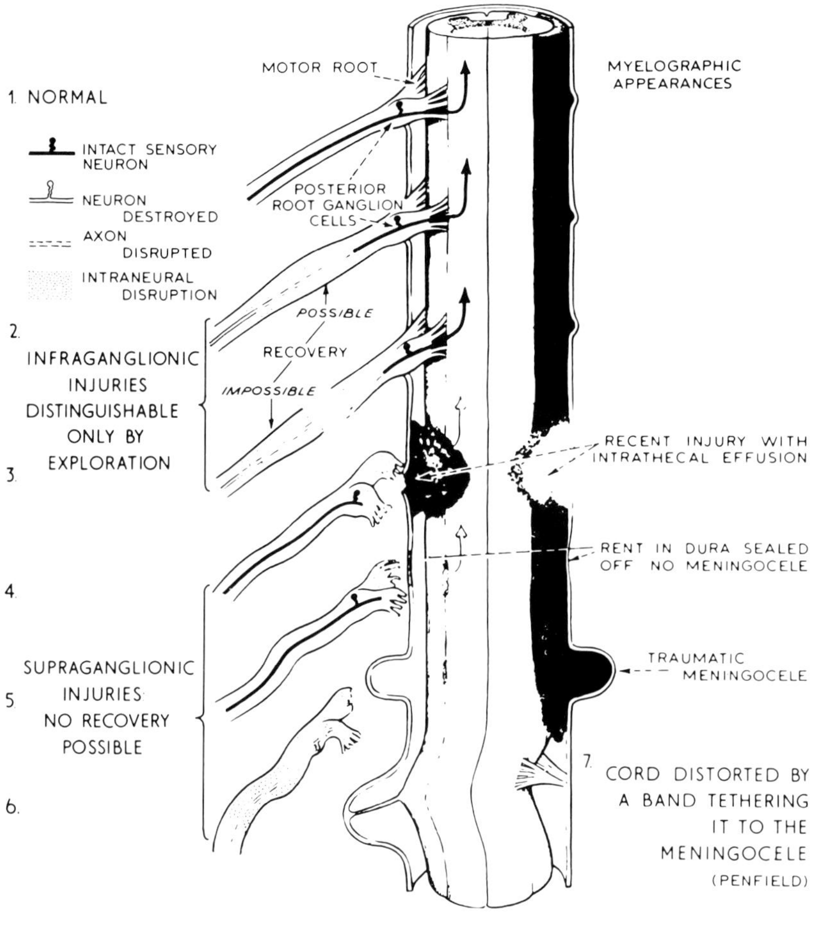

Figure 16-5. Seddon's diagrammatic representation of the types of injury occurring to the roots of the brachial plexus. (Reproduced with permission from Seddon.[68])

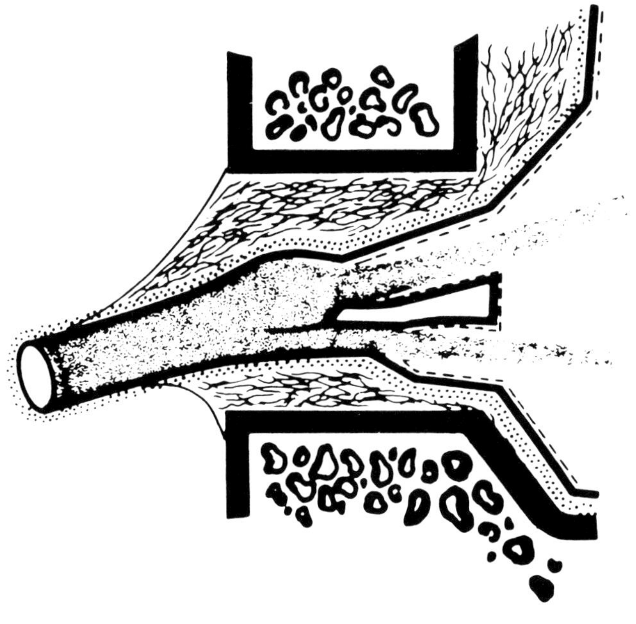

Figure 16-6. Sunderland's classic schema of the nerve root complex between the intervertebral foramen and the meningeal layers that relate to the nerve roots and spinal nerves—dura becoming perineurium; (----) arachnoid; (∴) epidural tissue that is continuous laterally with the epineurial tissue. (Reproduced with permission from Sunderland.[69])

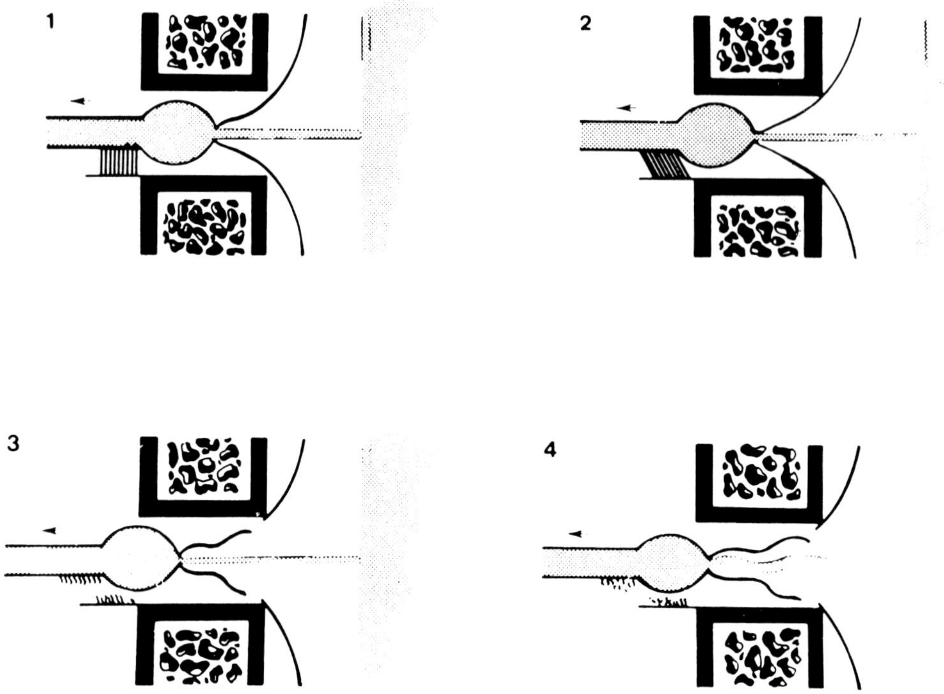

Figure 16-7. Sunderland's classic schema outlining the changes that result in avulsion of the nerve roots secondary to traction on the spinal nerves. The dorsal rootlet is illustrated. (Reproduced with permission from Sunderland.[69])

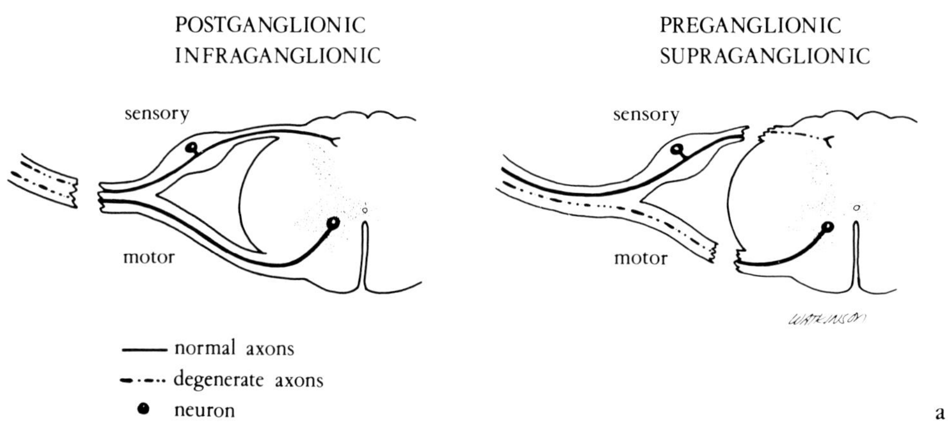

Figure 16-8a. Schematic diagram of post- or infraganglionic lesions that are distal to the dorsal root ganglion and pre- or supraganglionic lesions that are proximal to the ganglion. With postganglionic lesions, Wallerian degeneration occurs in both sensory and motor fibers. With preganglionic lesions, the dorsal root ganglion is in-continuity with the sensory axon. Thus Wallerian degeneration does not occur in the sensory fibers. (*Figure continues.*)

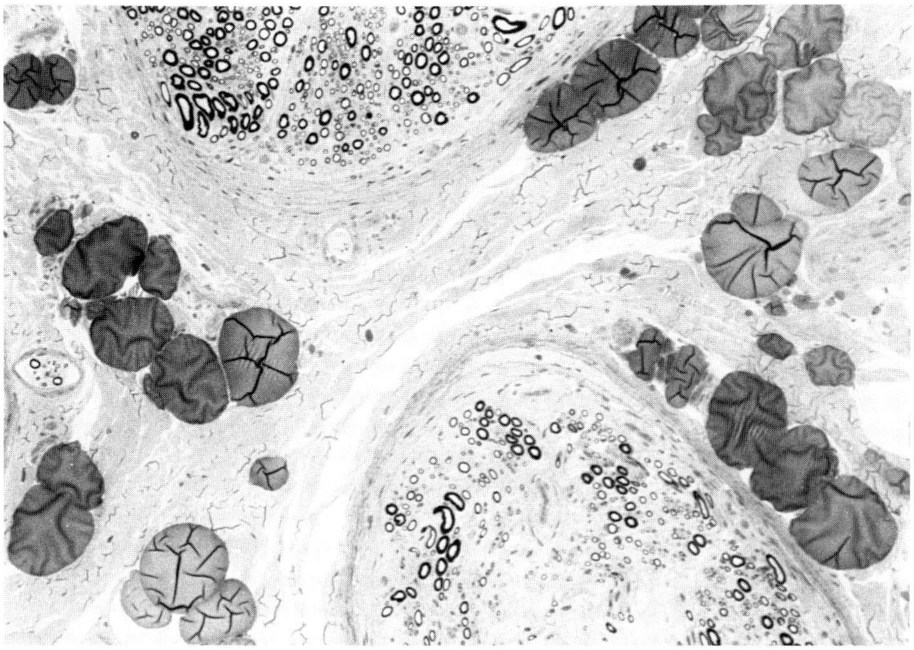

Figure 16-8 (*continued*) **b.** Transverse section of radial nerve, from a patient undergoing a limb amputation after total root avulsion of the brachial plexus (a preganglionic injury site.) Note a population of well-myelinated fibers that are the sensory fibers which are in continuity with their cell body in the dorsal root ganglion. The motor fibers have all degenerated. (Toluidine blue; $\times 368$.)

injury is more distal, normal nerve fibers are present proximal to the lesion and a surgical repair is possible.

With a pre- or supraganglionic lesion, the motor fibers have been separated from the cell bodies in the anterior horn cells, but the sensory fibers are still connected to their neurons in the dorsal root ganglion. Thus, although the patient will have no sensation (because the roots have been avulsed from the cord), there will be no Wallerian degeneration in the sensory fibers and sensory nerve conductions will be normal. Such normal sensory nerve conduction studies combined with the remainder of the clinical examination is helpful in localizing the level of the injury. (For historical purposes it is interesting to note that this also forms the basis for the intact axon flare reflex of Lewis.)

The loss of function of muscles innervated by branches coming directly from the roots of the brachial plexus is highly suggestive of proximal root avulsion injury. The long thoracic nerve, derived from the roots of C5, C6, and C7, innervates the serratus anterior. With serratus anterior paralysis, winging of the scapula is demonstrated (Fig. 16-9). The dorsal scapular nerve, a branch of the C4 and C5 root, innervates the rhomboid muscles (Fig. 16-10). Paralysis of these muscles suggest a very proximal lesion compatible with a root avulsion. If the patient has a Horner's syndrome (myosis, enophthalmos, anhydrosis, and ptosis), it is suggestive of either avulsion of the C-8 or T1 root or traction injury very close to the cord because the preganglionic fibers that mediate this function divide from the spinal nerve immediately after they merge from the T1-T2 intervertebral foramen (Fig. 16-11).

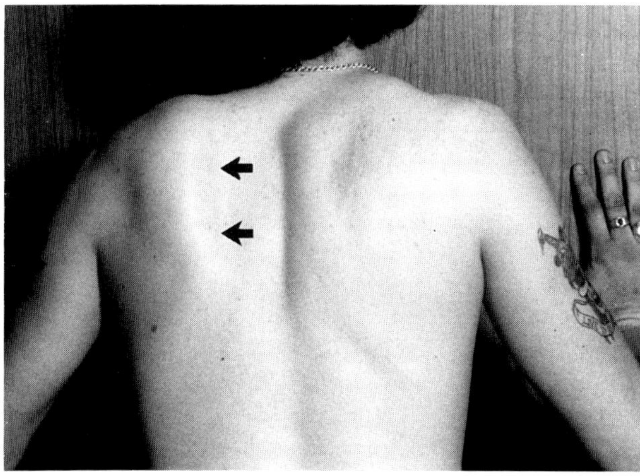

Figure 16-9. Serratus anterior palsy (long thoracic nerve, C5, C6, C7) resulting in winging of the left scapula (arrows).

Trunk Injury

The only branch from the trunk that lends itself to clinical examination is the suprascapular nerve (C5, C6) from the upper trunk. This nerve supplies the supra- and infraspinatus muscles (Fig. 16-12). Wasting of these muscles is readily demonstrated. If the patient with a diffuse plexus injury demonstrates recovery of all mus-

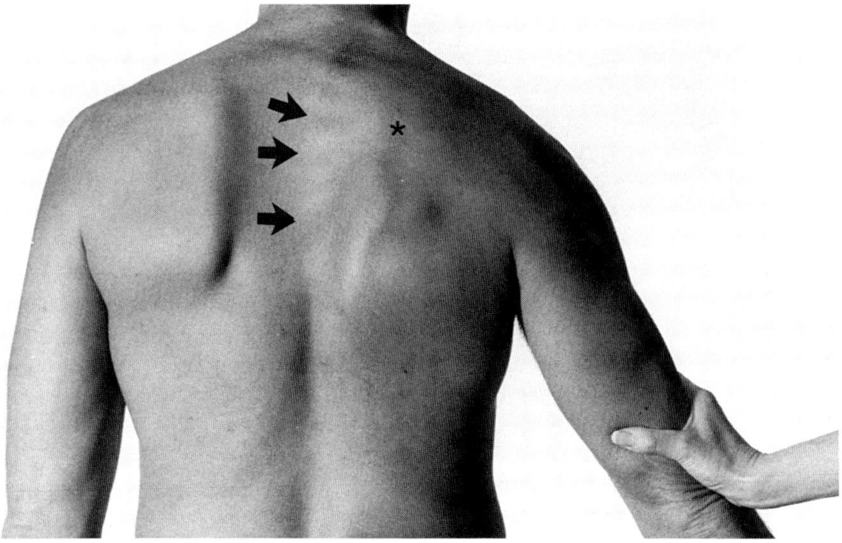

Figure 16-10. The rhomboid muscles (dorsal scapular nerve, C4, C5) can usually be palpated and in this instance are seen (arrows). The muscle belly of the supraspinatus can also be seen and palpated (asterisk).

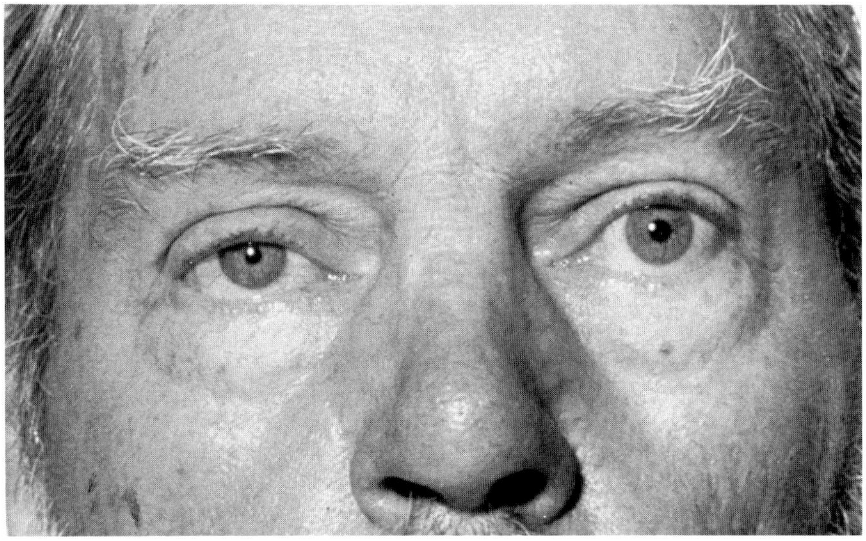

Figure 16-11. Typical appearance of Horner's syndrome with myosis and ptosis of the right eye is apparent. (Photograph courtesy of A.R. Hudson, M.B., Toronto, Canada.)

cle groups except for the infra- and supraspinatus muscles, it suggests superimposed traction injury of the suprascapular nerve in the scapular notch region.

There are no branches arising from the divisions of the brachial plexus.

Lateral Cord

The lateral pectoral nerve innervating both heads of the pectoralis major muscle arises from the lateral cord (Fig. 16-13a). Injury at this level will leave a paralyzed clavicular head of the pectoralis major.

Posterior Cord

From the posterior cord arises the nerves to innervate the muscles of the posterior axilla. The thoracodorsal nerve innervates the latissimus dorsi. The subscapular nerves innervate the subscapularis and the teres major muscles (Figs 16-12, 16-13). Improvement in triceps function but not deltoid may suggest axillary nerve entrapment at the quadrangular space.

Medial Cord

From the medial cord, the medial pectoral nerve innervates the sternocostal head of the pectoralis major muscle and the pectoralis minor. Isolated injury to the nerve is not clinically detectable because of the overlap innervation from the lateral pectoral nerve. The medial cutaneous nerves of the arm and forearm are also branches of the medial cord (Fig. 16-13b).

Terminal Cord Branches

The terminal branches of the cords are the axillary nerve innervating the deltoid muscle and the radial nerve (Fig. 16-14). The ulnar nerve is a terminal branch

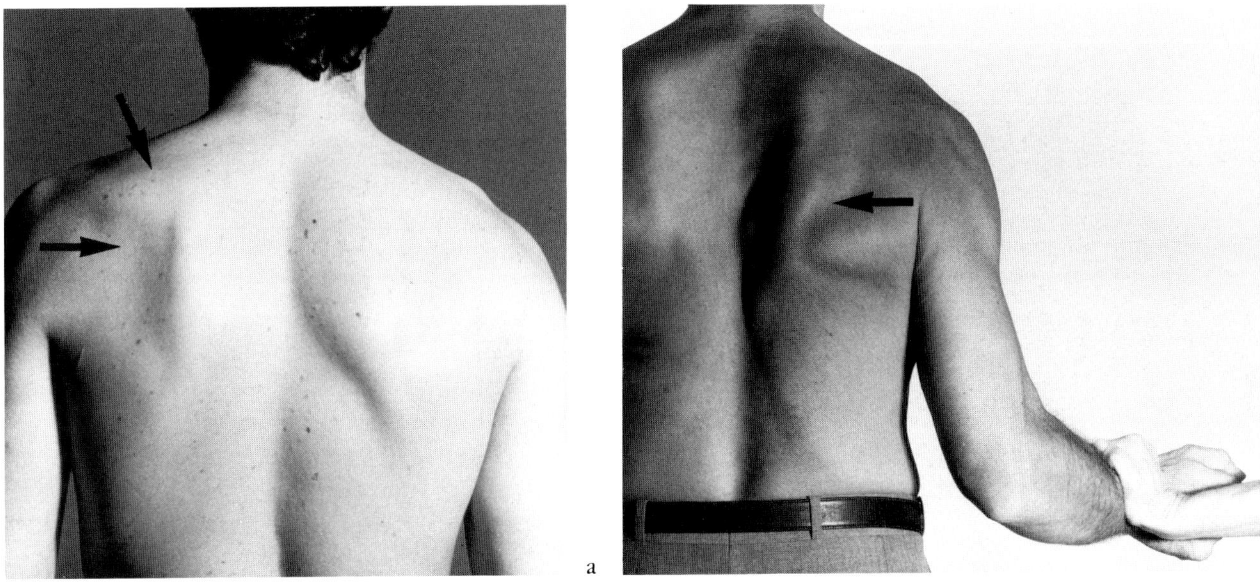

a b

Figure 16-12a. Injury to the suprascapular nerve (C5, C6) with wasting of the left supraspinatus and infraspinatus muscles (arrows). Note, prominence of spine of the scapula on the affected side compared with the normal side. (See operative sequence for this patient Fig. 16-20.) **b.** The infraspinatus muscle is best tested by having the patient externally rotate the arm against resistance (arrow). The supraspinatus muscle is best demonstrated by having the patient abduct the arm against resistance (Fig. 16-10, asterisk). Note that teres major muscle can be seen just below the arrow.

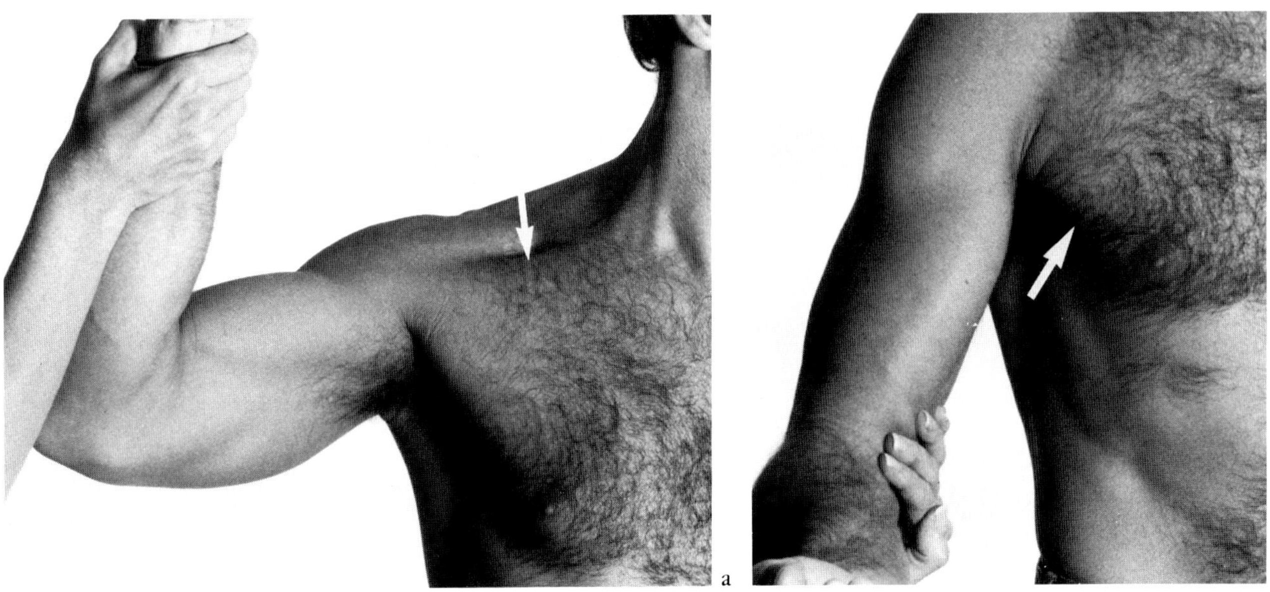

a b

Figure 16-13a. The lateral pectoral nerve (C5, C6) innervates the clavicular head (as well as the sternal head) of the pectoralis major muscle. The clavicular head of the muscle can be demonstrated when the arm is raised above the horizontal and the patient pushes forward against the examiner's hand (arrow, clavicular head). **b.** The medial pectoral nerve innervates only the sternal head of the pectoral major muscle. It does not innervate the clavicular head. The sternal head of the muscle can be demonstrated by having the patient adduct the upper arm against resistance. The sternal head can be seen and palpated (arrow).

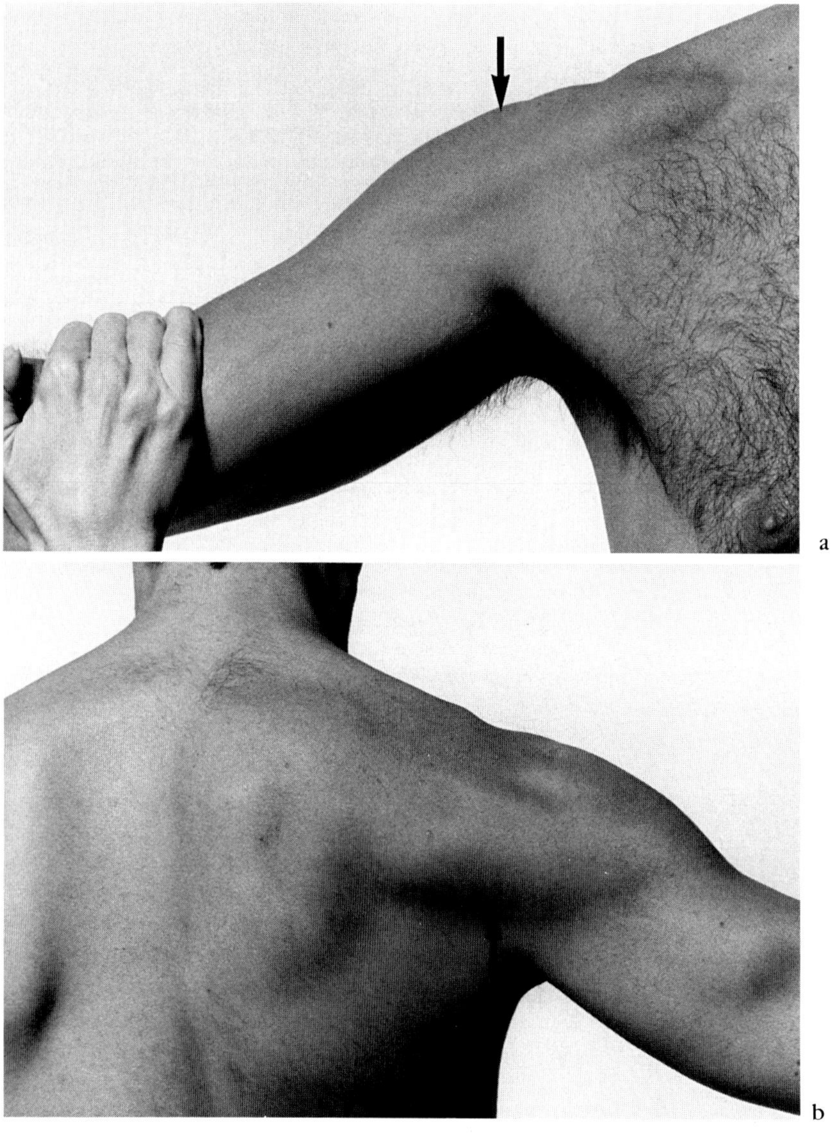

Figure 16-14a. The deltoid muscle (axillary nerve, C5, C6) can be demonstrated by having the patient abduct the upper arm against resistance. The anterior middle fibers are noted (arrow). **b.** The posterior fibers of the deltoid are seen (arrow).

of the medial cord along with the medial cord contributions to the median nerve. The musculocutaneous nerve innervating the coracobrachialis, brachialis, and biceps muscle is the terminal branch of the lateral cord along with the lateral cord contribution of the median nerve. Thus the sensory component of the median nerve comes from the lateral cord while the motor component for the intrinsic muscles comes from the medial cord.

Surgical Treatment of Brachial Plexus Injuries

All of the previous principles discussed in the classification and management of the isolated peripheral nerve injury can be extrapolated to the care of the patient with the brachial plexus injury. These patients will present a major surgical challenge both because of the complexity of the anatomy in the region of the brachial plexus as well as the nature of the injury, which is a proximal injury involving multiple nerves over a variable distance. Management of these patients will be based on a complete understanding of the surgical anatomy of the brachial plexus as well as a clear and realistic reconstructive plan for these patients. It is critical in these cases that both the surgeon and the patient have an understanding of the goals of treatment and be prepared to work together for a prolonged period of time in order to obtain the maximum potential from this devastating injury.

Open Injuries

Traumatic injuries of the brachial plexus only rarely involve open injuries. These injuries should be managed as any injury involving an open wound, that is, early exploration is indicated. The nature of the injury will determine whether or not a primary repair or delayed grafting techniques are used. Clean, sharp lacerations of the brachial plexus will be treated with a primary epineurial repair.

When there has been an actual loss of nerve tissue or an avulsive type injury, the elements of the brachial plexus are explored and identified. With this type of injury, the damage occurs for a variable and unpredictable distance along the length of the nerve. The level

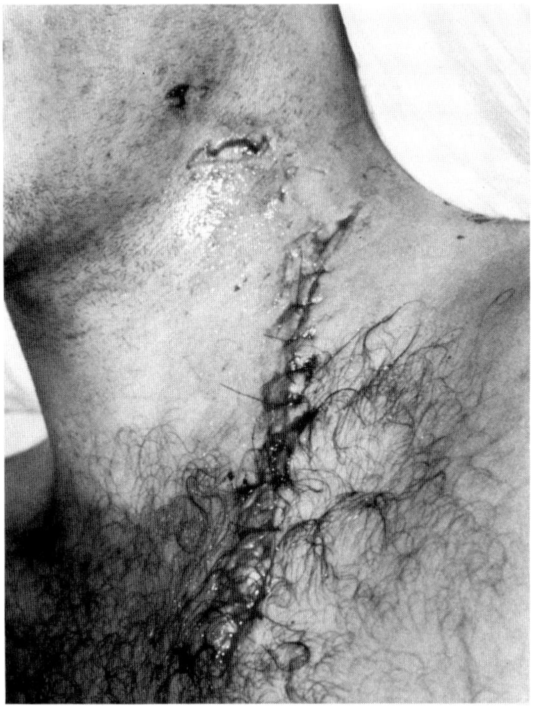

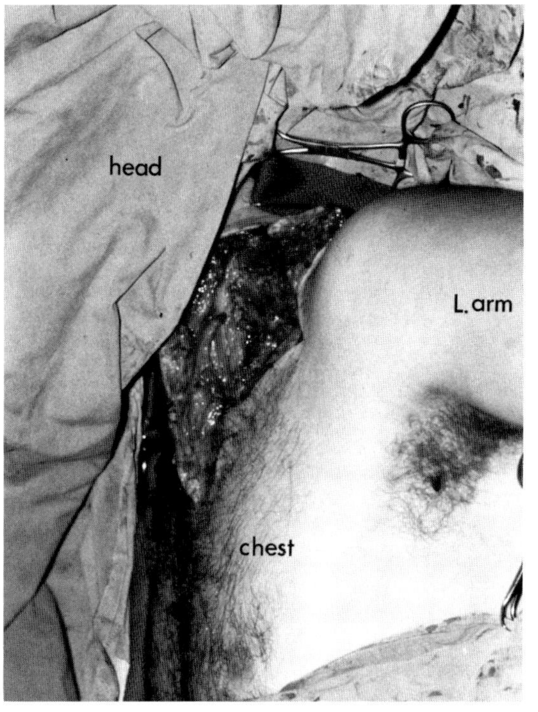

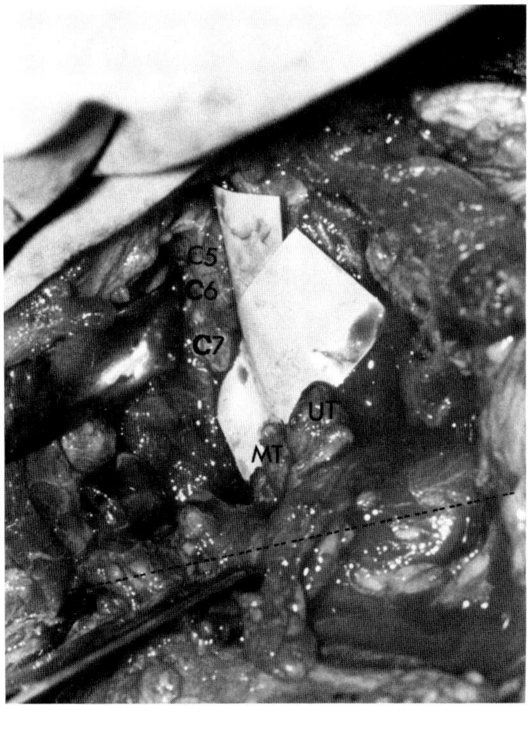

Figure 16-15a. This patient had a chain saw kick-back type of injury to the left supraclavicular brachial plexus. The wound was explored. **b.** The elements of the brachial plexus were identified by extending the laceration along the border of the clavicle. **c.** The patient had divided C5, C6, and C7 with actual loss of nerve tissue of the upper (UT) and middle trunks (MT). The sternomastoid muscle is retracted on the left. The clavicle is represented by the dotted line. (*Figure continues.*)

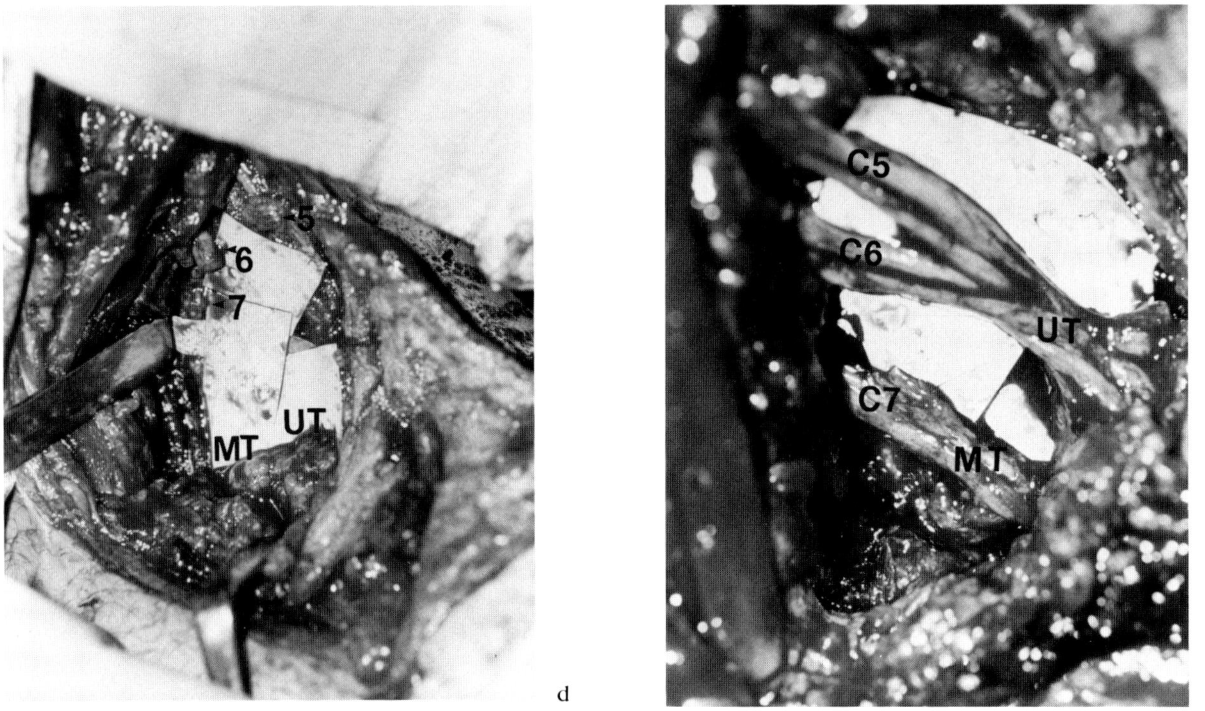

Figure 16-15. (*continued*) **d.** Three weeks after this injury, the wound was reexplored and, with microdissection, scar nerve tissue was excised until a good fascicular pattern was noted both proximally and distally (sternomastoid muscle retracted on the left). **e.** Sural nerve grafts were used to reconstitute the upper and middle trunks.

of the injury cannot be estimated accurately at the time of the initial injury. Thus, delayed repair and grafting is usually indicated. Scaffolding type of sutures may be placed between the appropriate nerve ends in order to facilitate plexus identification at later surgery. By 3 weeks' time, the longitudinal extent of the damage will be defined.[42] At this time, reexploration of the wound with nerve grafting is indicated, as it is still relatively easy to separate the tissue planes because significant soft tissue scarring has not yet developed (Fig. 16-15).

Civilian gunshots to the plexus are usually associated with a significant component of a first-, second-, and third-degree nerve injury.[43] Thus, the surgeon will anticipate that at least the majority of the brachial plexus palsy will improve within the first 3 months after the gunshot wound. Thus, early exploration is not indicated unless there are other associated injuries, i.e., vascular, that necessitate immediate exploration.

Closed Injuries

Closed traction injuries account for the majority of brachial plexus injuries seen in the traumatized patient. These injuries are managed as are all closed nerve injuries. Patient management can be considered in several stages (Table 16-2).

Stage I

In the first 3 months after injury, the patient is treated expectantly and followed both clinically and with electrophysiologic studies. During this stage, a physiotherapist is critical in teaching the patient exercises to ensure maintenance of a full range of passive movement in all joints. The patient is encouraged to feel responsible for his own physiotherapy. Although finger, wrist, and elbow passive movement is easily accomplished by the patient himself, prevention of a shoulder contracture is more difficult. Maintenance of shoulder abduction will require application of a simple overhead pulley system that will allow the patient to pull the arm from the side himself using his normal upper extremity.

In this first stage, the surgeon will outline to the patient both the nature of the injury and the potentially prolonged reconstructive course that he will be undertaking.

Stage II

At the end of the third month, the patient is evaluated clinically, electrophysiologically, and radiographically. As long as the patient demonstrates some return of function that appears to be following an anatomically

Table 16-2. Algorithm for the Management of the Closed Brachial Plexus Injury

First 4–6 weeks			End of 3rd month		4 months and plus
Complete brachial plexus palsy →	NCS* EMG	Clinically complete or partial anatomic recovery →		Monthly electrical and clinical assessments	→ Continued recovery observed; → Failure to recover surgery
		Clinically no recovery →	NCS EMG	Anatomic recovery → Monthly electrical and clinical assessments	
				No or nonanatomic recovery → Myelogram → Surgery	

*NCS: nerve conduction studies; EMG: electromyography.

sequential pattern progressing from proximal to distal, he is followed conservatively. Surgical intervention is indicated if the patient fails to show clinical or electrical evidence of return of function at 3 months or if the patient demonstrates nonanatomic return of function with isolated lack of proximal function in the presence of good distal nerve recovery. The surgeon must not be fooled by this distal recovery pattern in the presence of poor proximal recovery. This would suggest a more severe injury pattern to the nerves innervating the proximal muscles and a much less significant injury to the nerves innervating the distal muscles.

Stage III

If the patient has failed to demonstrate functional return by 3 or 4 months, then surgical exploration is indicated. Adequate surgical exposure is necessary to define the anatomic elements of the plexus. The potential surgical techniques that can be utilized will include primary neurorrhaphy (rarely) and neurolysis and nerve-grafting (frequently). Less often, a nerve transfer or neurotization procedure will be required. Intraoperative direct nerve stimulation is necessary to define the anatomic elements of the plexus. Intraoperative direct nerve stimulation and recording is carried out and excision and nerve grafting of elements of the plexus is indicated if there is no electrical activity across the nerve in an area of injury. If a nerve action potential is recorded, then a simple neurolysis is carried out. In cases involving root avulsion where there is no proximal stump available for nerve grafting, then a neurotization procedure may be considered such as grafting between the intercostal nerves[20,44,46] and the musculocutaneous nerves for elbow flexion and grafting between the cervical sensory plexus and the greater auricular nerve and the ulnar or median nerve for sensory function in the hand. Certainly, in patients with complete brachial plexus palsy, the surgeon must have clearly defined goals at the time of surgery with specific aims to attempt to restore critical function, such as shoulder abduction (axillary nerve),[47] and elbow flexion (musculocutaneous nerve). With regard to restoration of critical sensory function, the territory chosen for reinnervation will be influenced by the possibilities for motor recovery of the wrist and hand. If there is no possibility of restoring movement to thumb and index, then we prefer to reinnervate the medial cord (restoring protective sensation to the small finger and ulnar border of the hand and forearm) than the lateral cord (functional sensation to thumb and index). The traditional concept of restoring thumb and index sensation is not valid in the absence of motor function for these digits (Table 16-3).

Table 16-3. Surgical Priorities in Reconstruction of Complete Plexus Injuries

Restoration of elbow flexion
Restoration of shoulder abduction
Restoration of sensation to medial border of forearm and hand

*Major priorities for reconstruction.

Stage IV

Depending on the nature of the surgery, it will take up to 24 months to realize the extent of the nerve regeneration. During this postbrachial plexus surgery period, the patient is followed periodically by a therapist to maintain joint mobility and is fitted with an appropriate external prosthesis that will provide shoulder stability and static elbow flexion[48] (Fig. 16-16). Although only 25% of our patients use these prostheses, those that do find them very useful. During this stage IV period we use electrical muscle stimulation while awaiting muscle reinnervation (see Chapter 15).

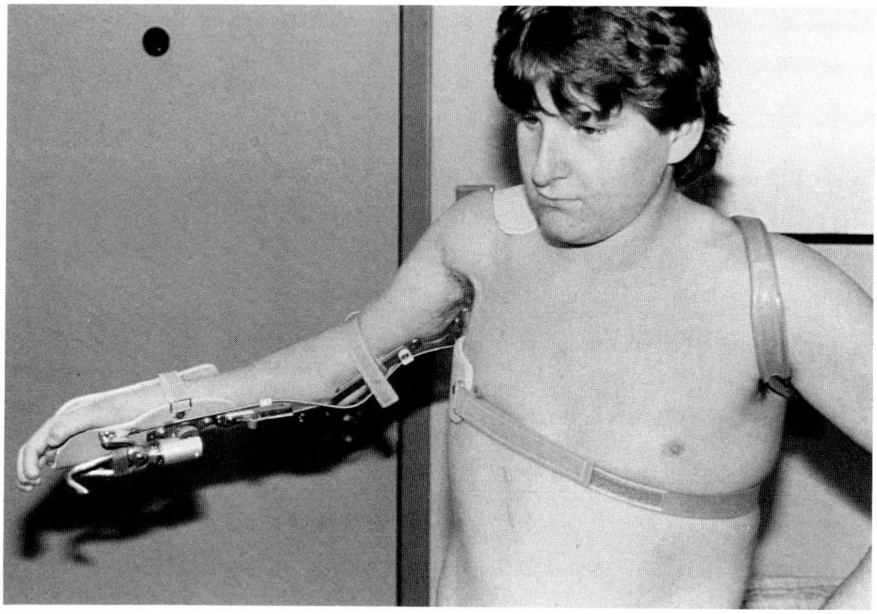

Figure 16-16. While waiting for a neurologic recovery after brachial plexus surgery, the patients are fitted with Stanmore (Wynn-Parry) type prosthesis. (Photograph courtesy of G. Hunter, M.D., Toronto, Canada.)

Stage V

If significant functional return has not occurred after peripheral nerve surgery, then consideration is given to other soft tissue reconstructive procedures such as a muscle or tendon transfer as well as shoulder fusion.[49] Elbow flexion can be restored with transfer of the latissimus dorsi,[50,51] pectoralis major,[52,53] triceps,[54] or forearm flexor muscle units[55–57] (Fig. 16-17). In order for these transfers to give good functional elbow flexion, the muscle transfer should be of close to normal strength before the transfer, since there will be some decrease in muscle strength after the transfer.

Before accepting lack of motor reinnervation after a nerve grafting procedure to the brachial plexus to imply failed nerve regeneration, the surgeon should consider that this failure is due to muscle fibrosis. If this were the situation, then the nerve graft could be used to innervate a free muscle transfer. The principle behind this consideration has developed from experience with cross-facial nerve grafts (Chapter 15). We no longer expect a cross-facial nerve graft to reinnervate denervated facial muscles successfully. We anticipate the need to transfer a free muscle flap to the face after the period of time appropriate for nerve regeneration across the graft has elapsed. It was experience with "failed" cross-facial nerve grafts that prompted us to realize that the failure of this technique was not a failure of nerve regeneration, but a failure of the muscle to respond to reinnervation because of an excessively prolonged period of denervation. This same philosophy can be applied to "failed" brachial plexus surgery. After an appropriate period of time, if the nerve graft has not worked (motor recovery less than M3), the surgeon may consider exploration of the nerve graft involved with intraoperative nerve stimulation. If a nerve action potential is recorded across the nerve graft, then consideration for a free muscle transfer will be entertained. This concept of providing new muscle to "failed" brachial plexus nerve grafts has become a standard philosophy in our unit.

Stage VI

At the end of the third year after injury, after all reconstructive procedures have been completed, the patient must consider his degree of recovery as permanent and either accept the function in his arm or consider amputation and prosthesis. The patient with significant pain after a brachial plexus avulsion injury should at this time be considered for dorsal root entry zone (DREZ) lesion procedure.[58] Certainly amputation should not be considered as a solution for the painful brachial plexus injury but rather for the patient who finds the dead weight of the arm a disability.

Surgical Approach to the Brachial Plexus

The patient is positioned in the supine position with a sand bag under the posterior chest. The neck, thorax, upper extremity, and both lower extremities are prepared and draped. The arm is abducted on an arm board. Preparing the upper extremity will facilitate observation of any muscular contraction during intraoperative nerve stimulation. Both lower extremities are draped in order to facilitate harvesting sural nerve grafts.

The skin incision is marked in order to facilitate

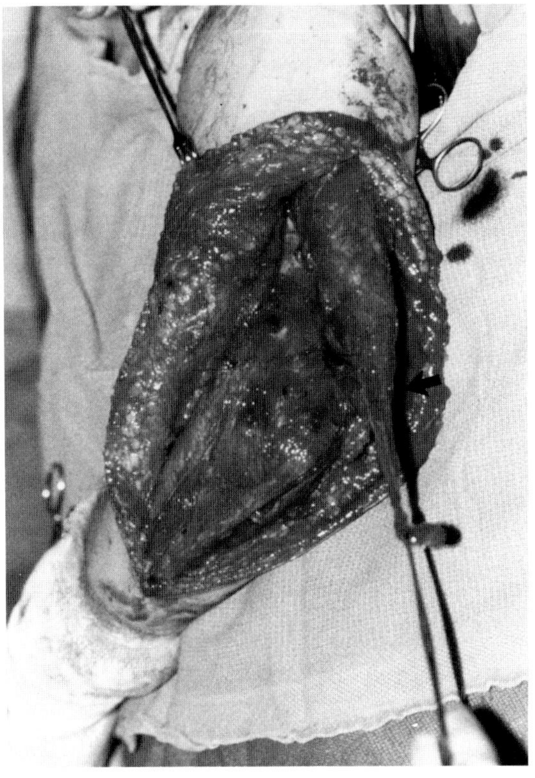

a

Figure 16-17a. This patient recovered good triceps function but had no biceps function. The triceps was transferred anteriorly to restore this function. (retractor on the triceps muscle, arrow, posterior view of left elbow). b. The patient at rest. c. Patient demonstrating elbow flexion with the triceps muscle transfer.

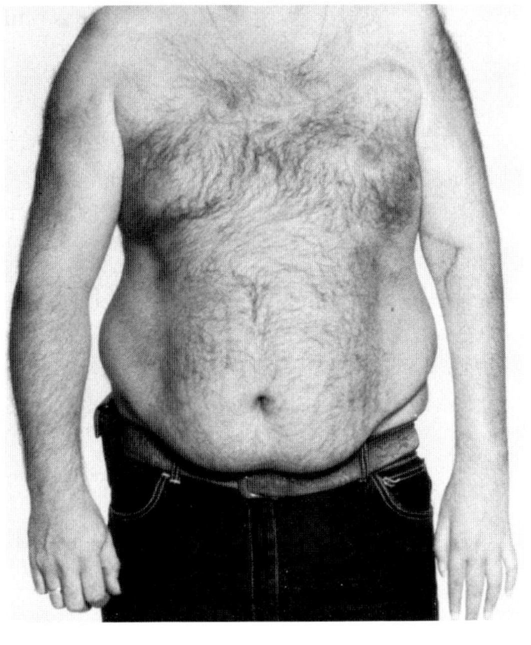

b

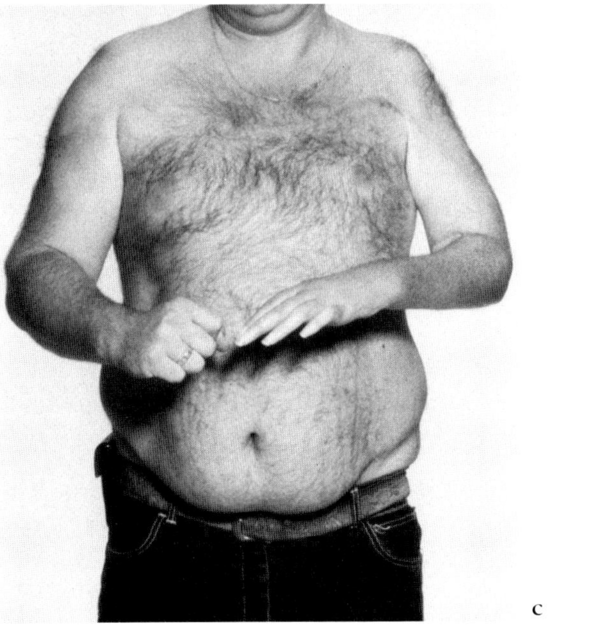

c

exposure of both supra- and infraclavicular portions of the brachial plexus. The superior incision courses along the posterior border of the sternocleidomastoid muscle. At the clavicle, it turns to follow the border of the clavicle until the superior portion of the deltopectoral groove is reached. At this point, the incision is then curved distally to follow the deltopectoral groove (Fig. 16-18a).

The infraclavicular plexus is approached by simply defining the deltopectoral groove. The cephalic vein is reflected and the pectoralis major insertion is identified (Fig. 16-18b). Care is taken to mark the proximal and distal extent of the tendon of the pectoralis major in order that the tendon may be appropriately reinserted at the completion of the procedure (Fig. 16-18c). A cuff of tendon is left on the humerus and marking sutures

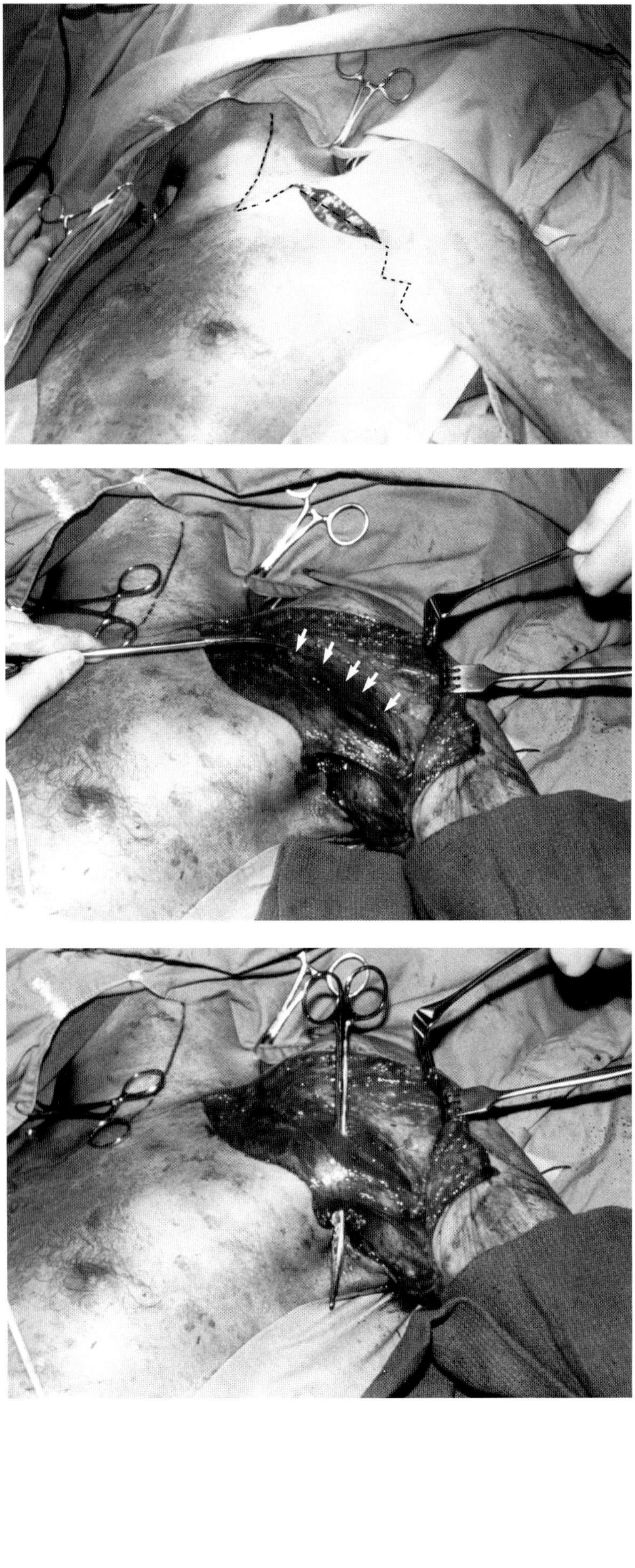

a

b

c

Figure 16-18a. The left arm is abducted. The arm, neck, and chest are prepared. The incision is marked along the posterior border of the sternocleidomastoid continuing along the clavicle and then down along the deltopectoral groove into the axilla. **b.** The cephalic vein in the deltopectoral groove is identified (arrows). **c.** The insertion of the pectoralis major muscle is identified. Note the scissors underneath the pectoralis muscle. (*Figure continues.*)

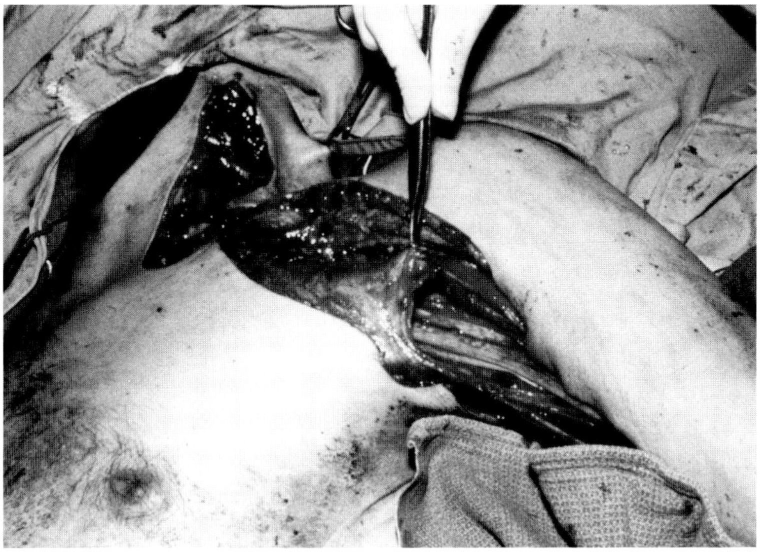

d

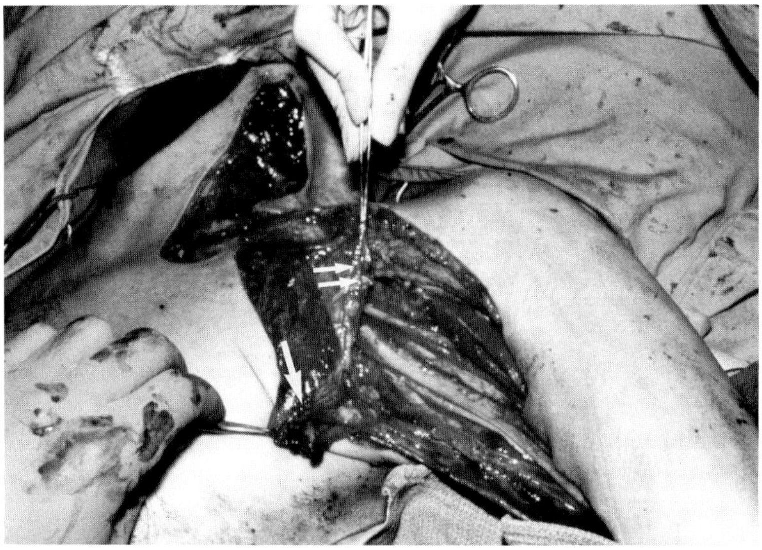

e

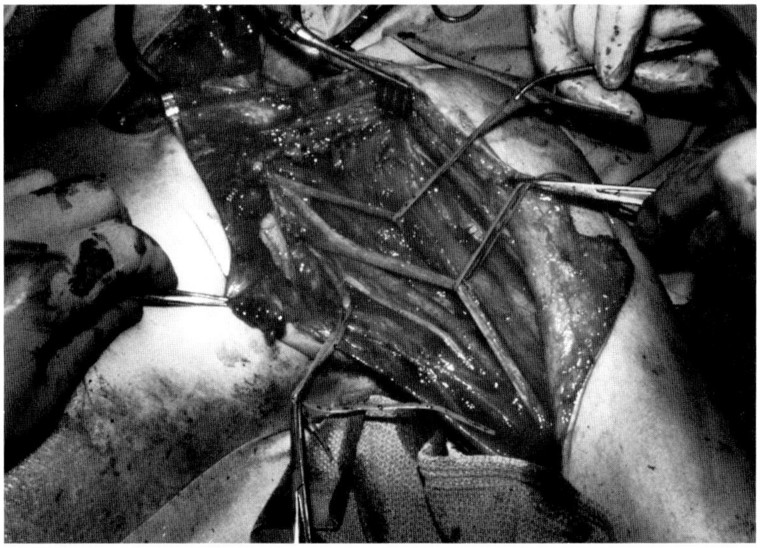

f

Figure 16-18 (*continued*) **d.** The pectoralis muscle insertion is removed. Marking sutures are placed at the insertion in order to allow accurate reinsertion at the conclusion of the procedure. **e.** The pectoralis major is reflected (arrow), as is the pectoralis minor (double arrow). **f.** The brachial plexus is identified. The upper vessel loop is around the musculocutaneous nerve, the middle vessel loop around the median nerve, and the lower vessel loop is around the ulnar nerve. (*Figure continues*)

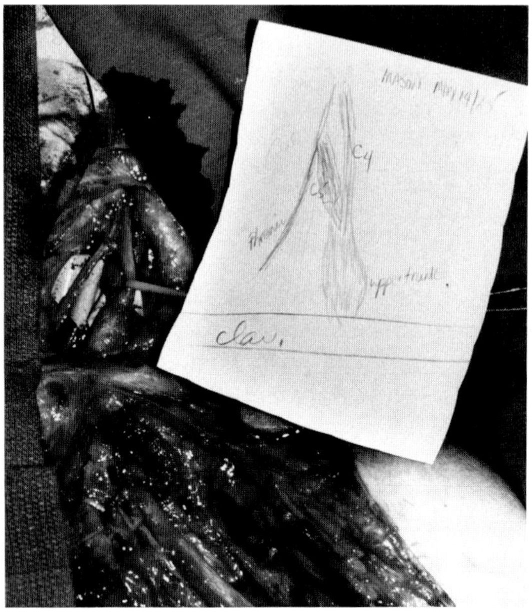

g

Figure 16-18 (*continued*) **g.** The pathologic process involving a large in-continuity neuroma of the upper trunk in this prefixed plexus is diagrammed intraoperatively.

are placed at the proximal and distal ends of the tendon on the humerus. The pectoralis major tendon is tripartate but very short, and meticulous reinsertion of this tendon is imperative (Fig. 16-18d). The pectoralis major is reflected. The pectoralis minor is then identified more proximally. This muscle is reflected and not reinserted (Fig. 16-18e). Just beneath the pectoralis major lies the "M" of the brachial plexus with the terminal divisions of the medial and lateral cord of the plexus. (Fig. 16-18f). In this region as well, the axillary nerve can be identified coursing through the quadrangular space.

The supraclavicular portion of the plexus is identified by dissection along the posterior border of the sternocleidomastoid. With care, the clavicular insertion of the sternocleidomastoid is divided. The subclavian vein lies just behind this muscle. The anterior and middle scalene muscles will be easily palpated and between these muscles lie the roots of the brachial plexus. The anterior scalene muscle may be resected to eliminate it as a potential future site of plexus entrapment. The phrenic nerve crosses this muscle from lateral to medial in a superior to inferior direction. It is preserved on the surface of the anterior scalene muscle. The fifth and sixth cervical roots are easily defined, forming the upper trunk beneath the anterior scalene muscle. Inferior to this lies the seventh cervical root which alone becomes the middle trunk. The eighth cervical root and the first thoracic root are more difficult to expose because they lie in the depths of the exposure behind the clavicle. Downward traction on the arm facilitates their identification.

It has been our practice not to divide the clavicle. We place a gauze around the clavicle and put traction on this gauze in order to elevate the clavicle from the underlying plexus.

Using magnification, the elements of the brachial plexus are identified and the pathologic condition determined. Intraoperative diagrams of the pathologic findings are made (Fig. 16-18g). Intraopoerative nerve stimulation is utilized. A disposable nerve stimulator D current with three settings, 0.5, 1, and 2 mA; (Vari-Stim III, Concept Inc., Clearwater, FL) is used to stimulate the various roots and nerves. If direct stimulation of the elements of the plexus produces any muscle contraction, then only a neurolysis is performed. If stimulation of the plexus does not produce contraction, then interoperative nerve recordings are carried out by stimulating and recording directly from the elements of the plexus (modified evoked potential electromyography unit, GRAS S44 Stimulator with GRAS differential amplifier combined with a NEC personal computer attached to a Datacon A-D board and analyzed with custom software). If no action potential is recorded, the injured area is resected and grafted. Interestingly, we have found an excellent correlation between the simple disposable unit and the costly and elaborate stimulation and recording unit: We have not yet noted any instance whereby a nerve action potential was recorded from a nerve that had not demontrated any functional contraction with the disposable unit.

The sural nerve is routinely used as the donor nerve. Longitudinal incisions are found to be most appropriate because the communicating branch from the common peroneal, the lateral sural, which is present in 80% of cases, can then be carefully preserved. This longitudinal incision allows considerably less trauma to the donor nerves. The sural nerve is normally harvested with the patient in the supine position after the brachial plexus anatomy has been defined. Only on the rare occasion are the nerve grafts harvested with the patient in the prone position at the beginning of the procedure, since the need for the grafts can be determined usually only after the plexus exploration. Other nerves can be used as donor nerves, the medial brachial and medial antebrachial cutaneous nerves provide excellent donor nerves for grafting. The ulnar nerve and radial sensory nerve may also be used, depending upon the overall plan for reconstruction.

On occasion, a posterior approach to the suprascapular or axillary nerves will be required through separate transverse incisions to facilitate grafting. The distal portions of the axillary nerve can be identified in the posterior quadrangular space if through the standard anterior approach good fascicular tissue in the axillary nerve is not defined (Fig. 16-19). Similarly, in patients with injury to the suprascapular nerve, the nerve is frequently decompressed at the level of the suprascapular notch in order to prevent superimposed nerve compression on the suprascapular nerve at this level (Fig. 16-20). The suprascapular notch is easily approached through a trapezius muscle splitting incision. The superior border of the scapula is palpated. The suprascapular vessels are identified on the supraspinatus muscle. The superior transverse ligament is divided in order to decompress the suprascapular nerve at this level.

At the completion of the procedure, the tendon of the pectoralis major is reinserted with nonabsorbable suture. The clavicular head of the sternocleidomastoid muscle is also reinserted. The wounds are closed in layers using subcuticular absorbable suture for skin closure. The arm is positioned at the side with the elbow in a flexed position and held in position with a modified Velpeau dressing. Although passive elbow and hand movement is encouraged, the shoulder is held in the abducted position for 4 weeks in order to allow healing of the tendon of the pectoralis major muscle.

Nerve Repair, Neurolysis, Nerve Graft

Primary nerve repair is only rarely possible in brachial plexus injury. With sharp transection of the plexus, a primary epineurial repair is performed as described in Chapter 4. By comparison, neurolysis is a technique that is utilized in almost every plexus operation. Elements of the plexus that are in-continuity with some clinical or electrical function are neurolysed using the techniques described in Chapter 5.

With magnification and microinstrumentation, the epineurium is opened and dissection is continued until a good fascicular pattern is noted. In these injuries, the epineurial tissue is often very fibrotic and "woody in consistency." With in-continuity lesions that do not conduct any electrical activity, the neurolysis technique is used in order to define good proximal and distal nerve tissue. Neurolysis is started in the area of maximum injury. If only fibrotic tissue is noted, then this area is resected and the resection is continued in a proximal and distal direction until a good fascicular pattern is noted. In the proximal portions of the plexus, the normal fascicular pattern is either mono- or bifascicular, thus, the surgeon will not see the multifascicular pattern typically seen in the distal course of the peripheral nerves. After the surgeon has defined the level of normal proximal and distal nerve tissue, he must reconstitute this defect with nerve grafts. Ideally, the proximal and distal nerve segments will be "synergistic" with respect to nerve fibers. For example, C5 or C6 root would be ideally suited to reinnervate the musculocutaneous nerve for biceps function. Similarly, C8 and T1 roots would ideally be used to innervate ulnar nerve function (Table 16-4). In many instances, the injury to the axillary nerve is very localized just proximal to the quadrangular space and a nerve graft can be used to restore continuity between the proximal and distal axillary nerve. This would be an ideal situation. In some instances, a portion of the posterior cord must be used

Table 16-4. Spinal Root Supply of Critical Nerves for "Synergistic" Muscle Reinnervation

Nerve (Muscle)	*Spinal Root*
Suprascapular	
(infraspinatus, supraspinatus)	*C5*, C6
Axillary	
(deltoid)	*C5*, C6
Musculocutaneous	
(biceps)	C5, C6
Radial	
(triceps)	C6, *C7*, C8
(extensor carpi radialis longus)	C5, *C6*
Ulnar*	
(all muscles)	C8, T1
Median*	
(wrist flexors)	C6, C7
(finger flexors)	C7, *C8*, T1
(pronator)	C6, C7
(intrinsics)	C8, T1

*Successful reinnervation of the distal muscles is unlikely because of proximal nature of injury.

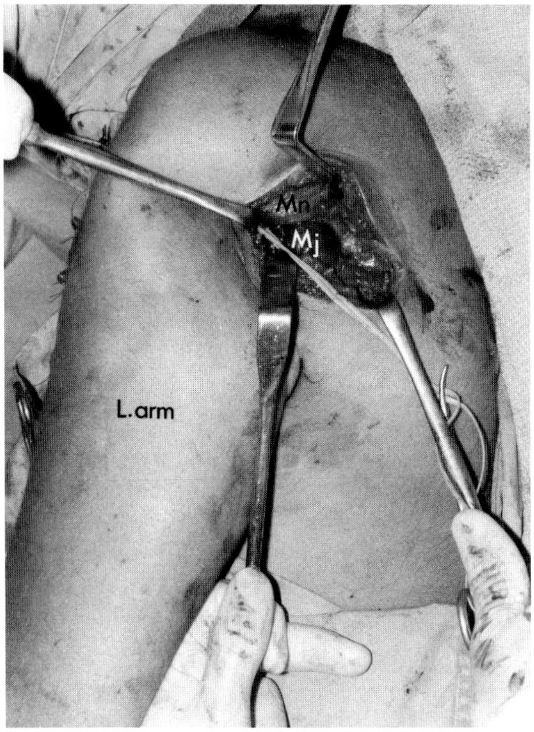

a

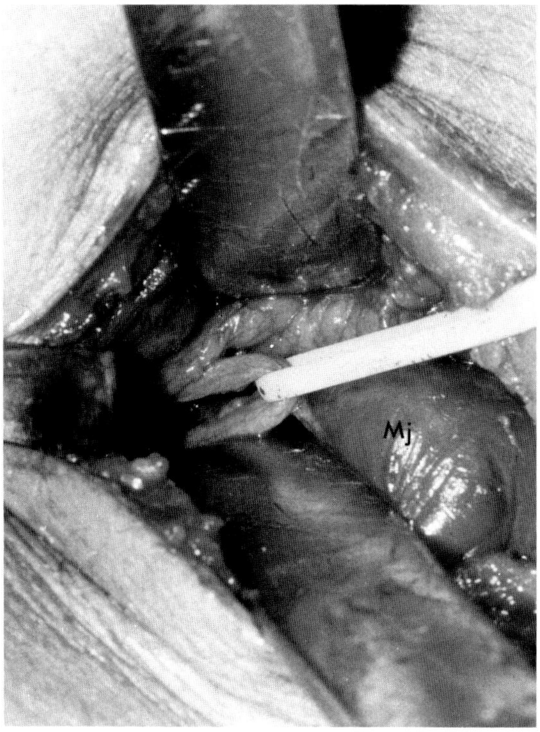

b

Figure 16-19a. On occasion, from an anterior approach, good fascicular pattern in the axillary nerve cannot be identified because the injury extends more distally. The quandrangular space can be explored and the axillary nerve identified in this space between the teres major (Mj) and minor (Mn) muscles, the long head of the triceps and the surgical neck of the humerus (vessel loop around the axillary nerve). **b.** A closer view with the vessel loop around the axillary nerve in the quadrangular space.

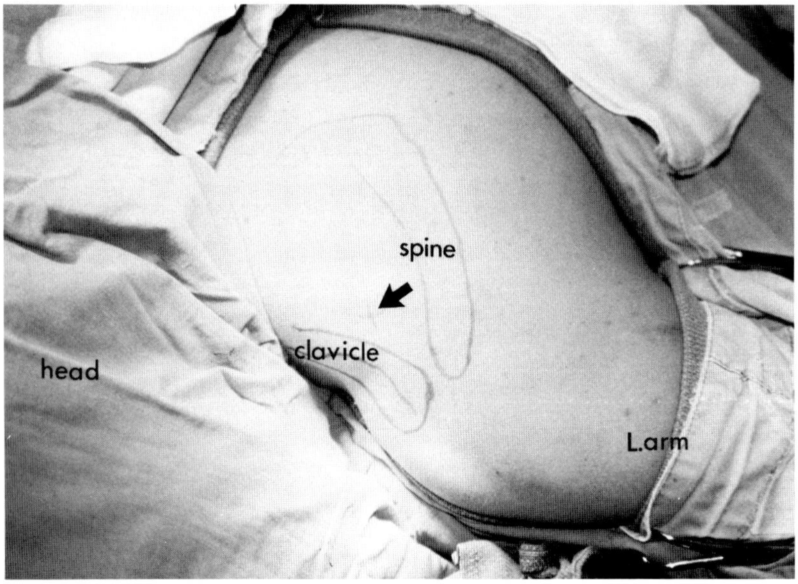

a

Figure 16-20a. The suprascapular nerve was explored, with the patient supine, through a trapezial muscle splitting incision. Arrow points to a point of tenderness. (Tinel) **b.** The suprascapular nerve can be identified through a transverse incision parallel and superior to the spine of the scapula. **Inset:** In the depth of the wound the nerve and ligament are seen.

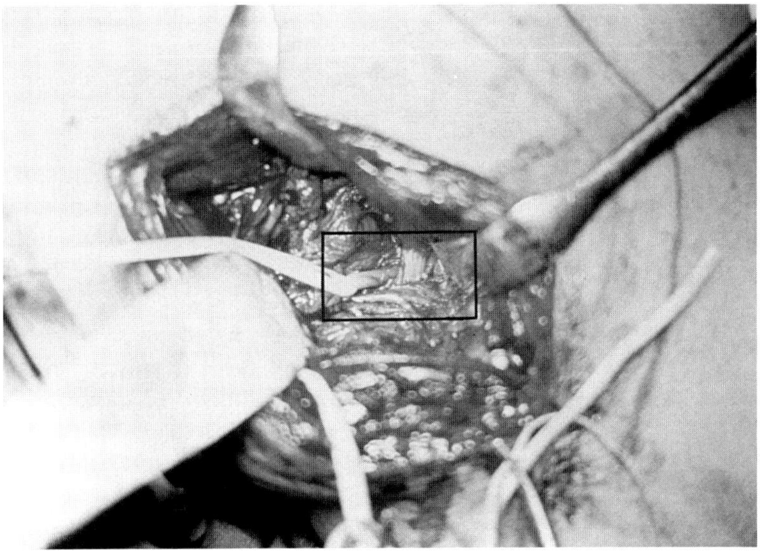

b

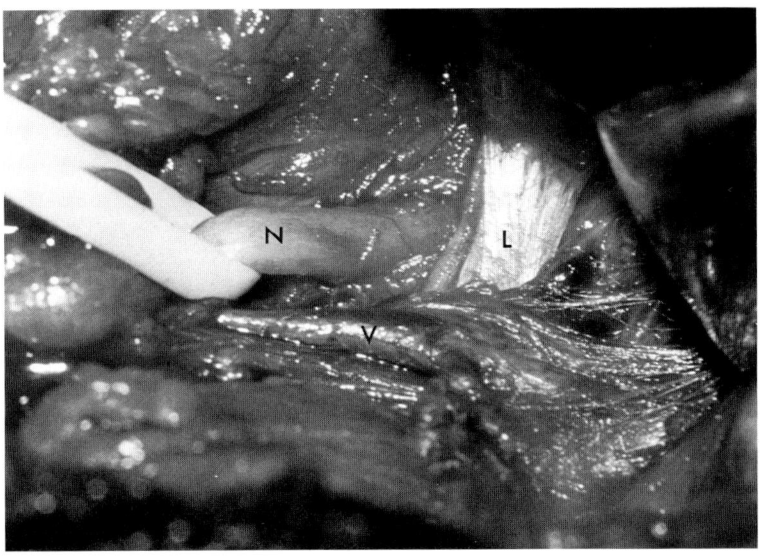

c

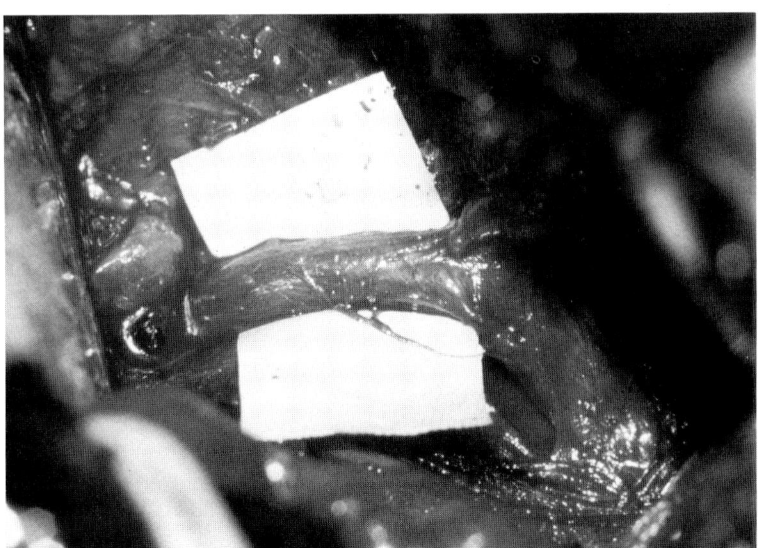

d

Figure 16-20 (*continued*) **c.** The suprascapular vessels (V) lie on the supraspinatous muscle and above the ligament (L). The suprascapular nerve (N) lies beneath the ligament in the suprascapular notch. **d.** The ligament has been excised and the suprascapular nerve will be neurolysed. (Same patient as shown in Figure 16-20a).

to supply proximal nerve fibers to reinnervate the deltoid muscle via the axillary nerve. This is not an ideal situation because the spinal roots C5, C6, C7 and C8 all give significant contributions to the posterior cord and mismatching of motor fibers can occur. If the appropriate proximal nerve tissue is not viable, the surgeon will utilize whatever good proximal nerve is available in order to graft into the axillary and musculocutaneous nerves, preferentially in order to restore some shoulder and elbow function. The nerve grafts are placed under no tension with the head turned to the noninjured side and the shoulder fully abducted to ensure that there is no tension on the proximal or distal repair sites.

Neurotization

With complete root avulsion of the brachial plexus, no proximal functioning nerve is available to restore function to the extremity. In these situations, there are no musculotendinous transfers available for restoration of critical extremity function. It is possible in such instances to transfer a normal nerve as a method of reinnervation of a critical sensory or motor territory. The normal donor nerves are, thus, considered expendable and of less significant functional value than the nerves to which they are being transferred. (Transfer of the hypoglossal nerve to restore facial nerve function in patients with facial nerve palsy is a well-known example of such a neurotization procedure, see Chapter 15) Harris and Low[10] in 1903 are credited with the first neurotization procedure of the brachial plexus transferring a portion of C5 to C6 and C7 in patients with Erb's palsy. Tuttle[11] in 1913 described trànsfer of the spinal accessory nerve as a method of reconstruction of brachial plexus injuries. Neurotization of pectoral nerves to the musculocutaneous or axillary nerves was first described in the 1920s.[59,60]

The transfer of the intercostal nerves to the musculocutaneous nerve is the most common neurotization procedure currently carried out in brachial plexus surgery. In 1963, Seddon[20] reported successful restoration of elbow flexion by transfer of the third and fourth intercostal nerves to the musculocutaneous nerve. The patient, a 17-year-old girl, underwent a below-elbow amputation. The ulnar nerve was used as the interposition nerve graft. In 1968, Tsuyama and Hara[44] described direct suture of the third and fourth intercostal nerves to the musculocutaneous nerve. This transfer did not require the use of a nerve graft. The greatest experience with this technique is from Japan. Takahashi[61] reported the results of this procedure in 72 cases over a 15-year period. In this series, 58% of cases had recovery of muscle strength of grade 4 and another 22% recovered strength to a grade 3 level.

Narakas[38] has had extensive experience with neurotization procedures. Good results were achieved with this technique in 27 of 83 patients (Table 16-5). Based on his experience, Narakas stresses that this technique is still in the developmental stage and that motor transfers are useful in restoration of a single simple function, such as elbow flexion, and that sensory recovery is at best protective.

Our own experience with neurotizing procedures has been limited to transfer of the intercostal nerves using nerve grafts to either the axillary or more commonly to the musculocutaneous nerve. Our results are 50% of patients achieve M3+–M4, and 50% had no function. The cervical sensory plexus as well as the greater auricular nerve have been transferred to the medial cord which has successfully restored protective sensibility to the ulnar border of the forearm and hand in our cases.

In a series of 18 cases, Brunelli[30,62] has reported good results with transfer of the accessory nerve to the musculocutaneous nerve for elbow flexion.

Results of Brachial Plexus Surgery

Problems associated with traumatic injury to the brachial plexus have been recognized for more than 200 years.[3] Surgical correction of these problems has been reported since the early 1900s. Despite this rather lengthy experience, controversy still surrounds brachial plexus surgery. The results of early surgery in the brachial plexus were uniformly poor, which stimulated Seddon[20] to condemn brachial plexus surgery except in upper trunk surgery. The advent of microsurgical technique has resulted in significant improvement of results after plexus surgery. It is, however, difficult to interpret the few end result studies that are available.[43,63–65] There are several reasons for this. It is difficult accurately to stage, quantitate, follow, and report results after brachial plexus injury in view of the fact that the injury patterns are not standardized. Most brachial plexus lesions are combined lesions involving many elements of the plexus with variable degrees of nerve injury. It is standard technique in a given case to use several surgical procedures to reconstruct the plexus, including neurolysis, nerve grafting, and occasionally neurotization procedures. This makes the reporting of end results of brachial plexus surgery extremely difficult and frequently confusing.

Reviewing the results of nerve repair and nerve grafting in Chapter 4, we see that our perception of results after peripheral nerve surgery was greatly influ-

Table 16-5. Neurotizations with Rami of the Cervical Plexus or with Intercostal Nerves (Usually Several from T3 to T7)*

Donors	Receptors	Number of Patients	Available Controls	Results: Good	Results: Doubtful, Poor, or Nil
Long thoracic nerve	C6	1	1	1	0
	Lateral cord	2	2	0	2
	C8	1	1	0	1
Spinal accessory terminal rami to the upper trapezius	Suprascapular nerve	5	2	1	1
Several intercostal nerves	C5 or C6	6	5	1	4
	Lateral cord or musculocutaneous nerve	21	13	9	4
	C7	21	14	7	7
	Posterior cord				
	Axillary nerve	12	8	4	4
	Suprascapular nerve				
	Medial cord C8 or T1				
	Median and/or ulnar nerve	14	9	3 sensory, 1 motor, and sensory result	5

Reproduced with permission from Narakas.[38]

enced by the large experience with war injuries.[17] At that time, these very severe injuries were treated without the modern techniques of microneurosurgery. With the introduction of microsurgical technique, we have seen dramatic improvement in the results of nerve repair and grafting of peripheral nerves. These same techniques recently have been extrapolated to the management of brachial plexus injuries with the anticipated improvement in results.

There have been several reports of long-term results after brachial plexus surgery. Millesi[40] has recently reviewed a large series of patients who underwent surgery to the brachial plexus. In 134 patients with complete brachial plexus lesions, 69% recovered "useful" function after neurolysis, 72%, after nerve grafting, and 50%, after nerve transfer. In 72 patients with injury to the upper brachial plexus, results after surgery were even better, with 95% of patients recovering useful function after neurolysis, 75% recovering useful function after nerve grafting, and 63% recovering useful function after neurotization.

Reviewing 171 patients over a 12-year period with brachial plexus injuries, Kline and Judice[43] noted acceptable results in 65% of nerve repairs and 50% of nerve grafts, with improved results in upper plexus injuries compared with lower plexus injuries. Reviewing 53 patients undergoing neurotization procedures with a follow-up of more than 3 years, Narakas[65] reported good or acceptable results in 54% of patients.

The results of nerve grafting for restoration of motor function when the distance between the proximal nerve and the motor end plate is short (such as for the accesory[66] and axillary nerves[47]) are excellent (Fig. 16-21, 16-22). Our own results have been consistently good for recovery of deltoid function, where the distance between the level of the proximal nerve injury and the deltoid muscle end plate is usually short, and have been 75% to an M4 level. We have seen 50% recovery to level M3+–M4 across very long nerve grafts (>10 cm) for restoration of musculocutaneous function (Fig. 16-23). Because the long distance challenges the time limits of the muscle end-organ response for reinnervation, a free muscle transfer, innervated by the previously placed graft should be considered to improve these results.

Surgery of the brachial plexus is in a continuing state of evolution. The complex nature of the injury pattern combined with the use of multiple surgical techniques in the single case have made the assessment of results after this surgery difficult to quantitate. It is truly remarkable that results after nerve graft and neurotizing procedures are favorable in 50% (or greater) of patients with such proximal and complex injuries. These results should stimulate more centers to consider surgical management of these problems, especially as we begin to extrapolate our understanding of functional free muscle transfers to the management of brachial plexus injuries. We have a new realization that failure of brachial plexus surgery may be related not to a failure of nerve regeneration but an inability of the motor end organ to respond to the nerve regeneration. We would now consider providing a free muscle flap to restore motor function, innervating these muscle flaps with the reinnervated elements of the brachial plexus. We would

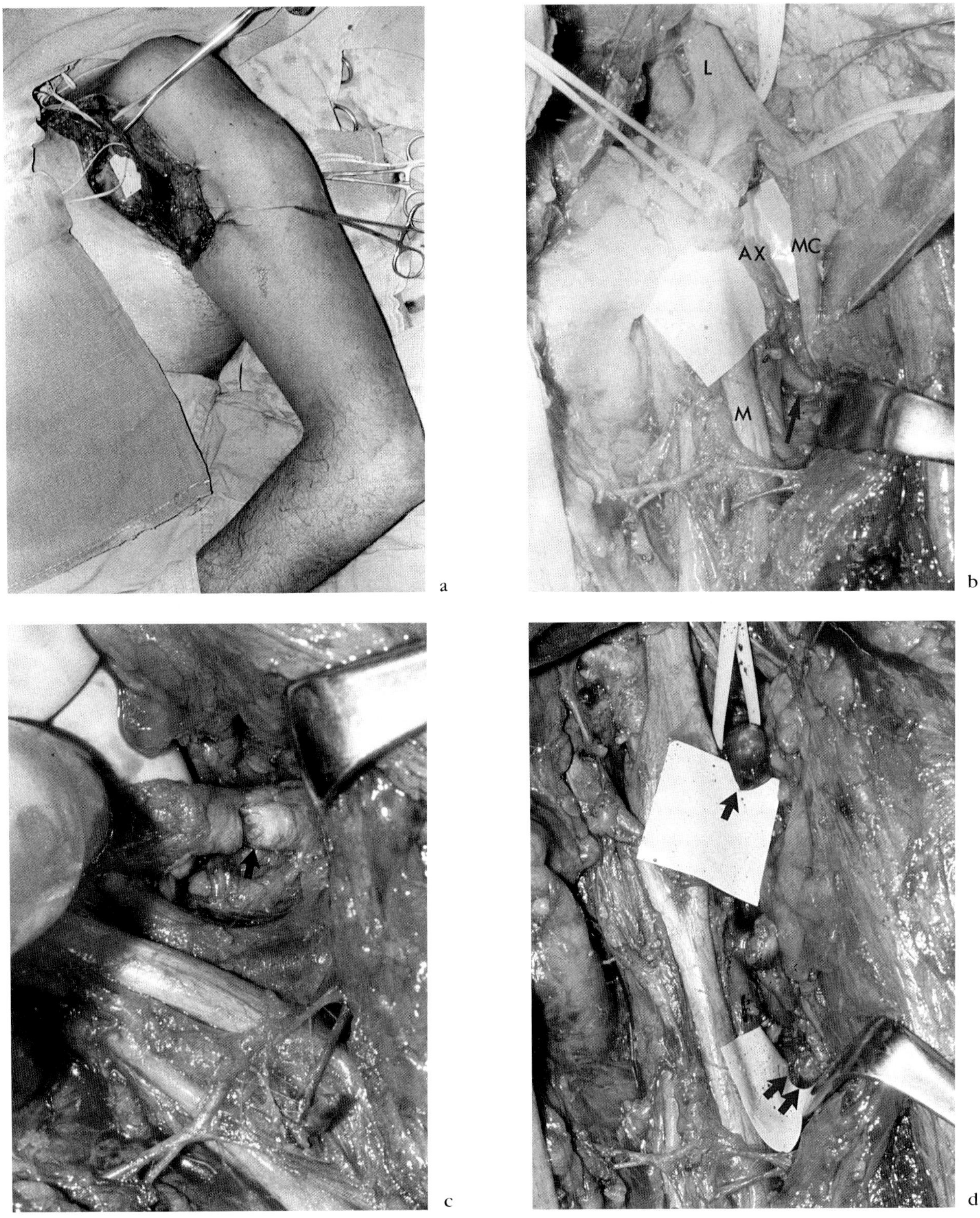

Figure 16-21a. Over a 3-month period, this patient had good recovery of all elements of his plexus injury except for an isolated injury to the axillary nerve. The standard incision was made and the injury was found in the region just proximal to the point where the axillary nerve runs through the quadrangular space. **b.** The axillary artery (arrow) is a good landmark for identifying the axillary nerve in the quadrangular space. The location of the axillary nerve (AX) injury, with respect to the musculocutaneous nerve (MC) and the median nerve (M) and the lateral cord (L), is seen. The axillary nerve demonstrated an in-continuity lesion that did not conduct any electrical activity. **c.** The neuroma in-continuity was transected until a good fascicular pattern was identified proximally and distally. Here, the distal portion of the axillary nerve is beginning to show good fascicular pattern (arrow). **d.** The proximal (single arrow) and distal (double arrows) ends of the axillary nerve are identified. (*Figure continues.*)

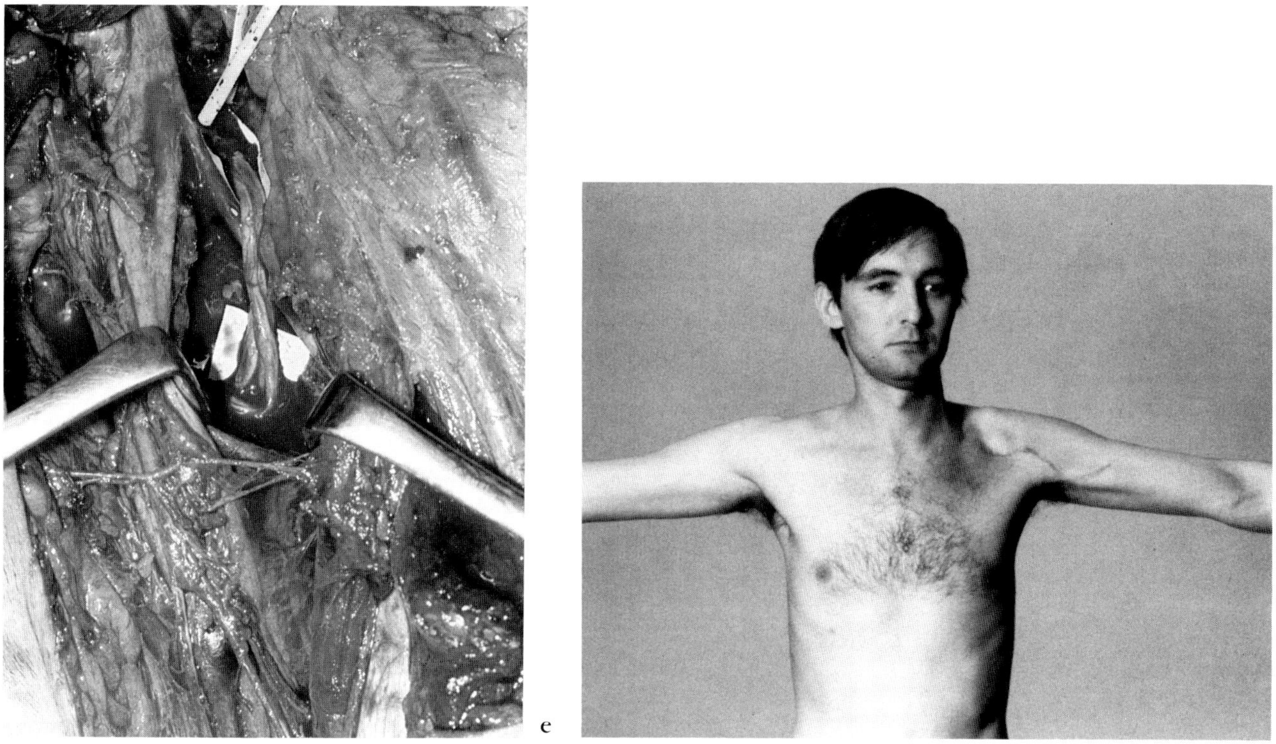

Figure 16-21 (*continued*) **e.** The sural nerve graft is used to restore continuity of this defect. **f.** Eighteen months after this surgery, the patient demonstrates excellent return of deltoid function.

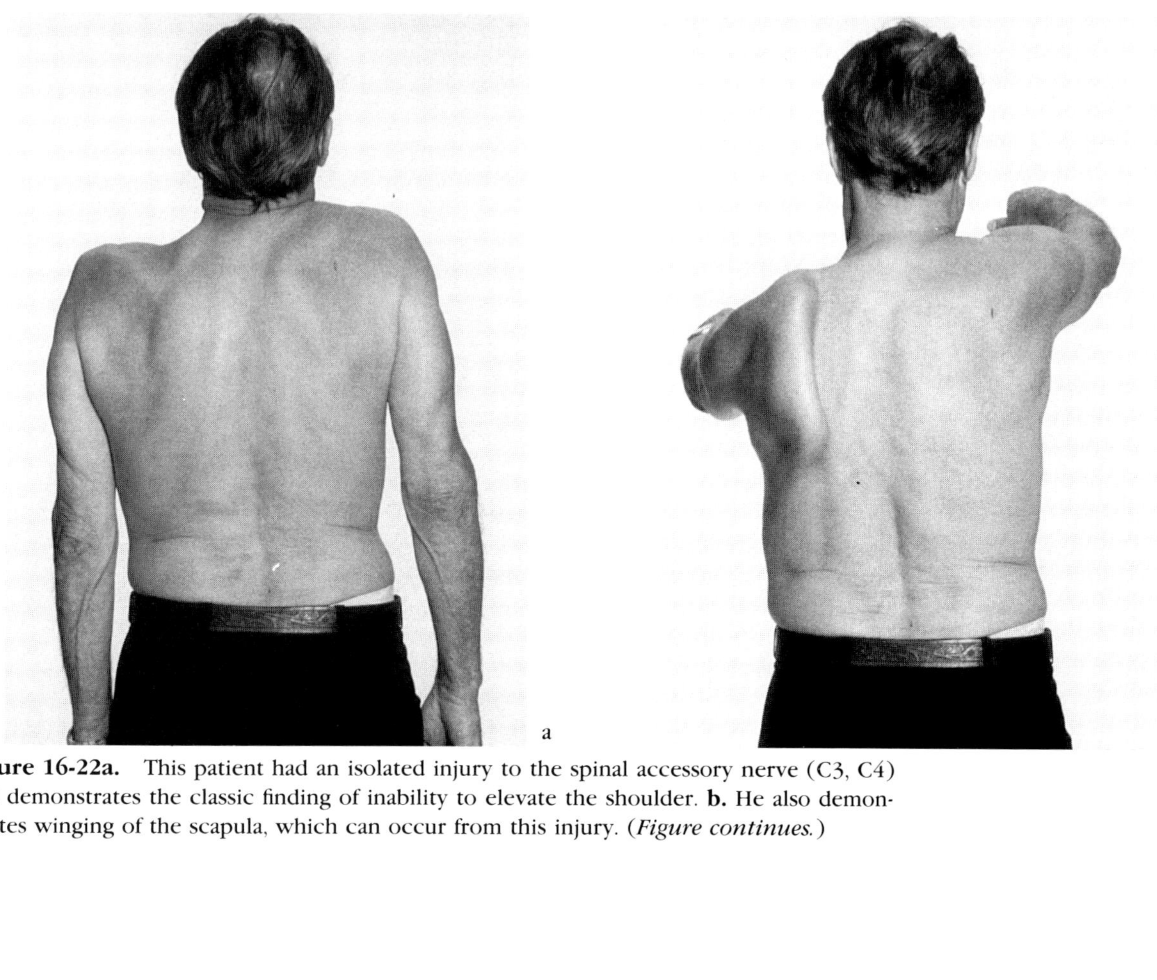

Figure 16-22a. This patient had an isolated injury to the spinal accessory nerve (C3, C4) and demonstrates the classic finding of inability to elevate the shoulder. **b.** He also demonstrates winging of the scapula, which can occur from this injury. (*Figure continues.*)

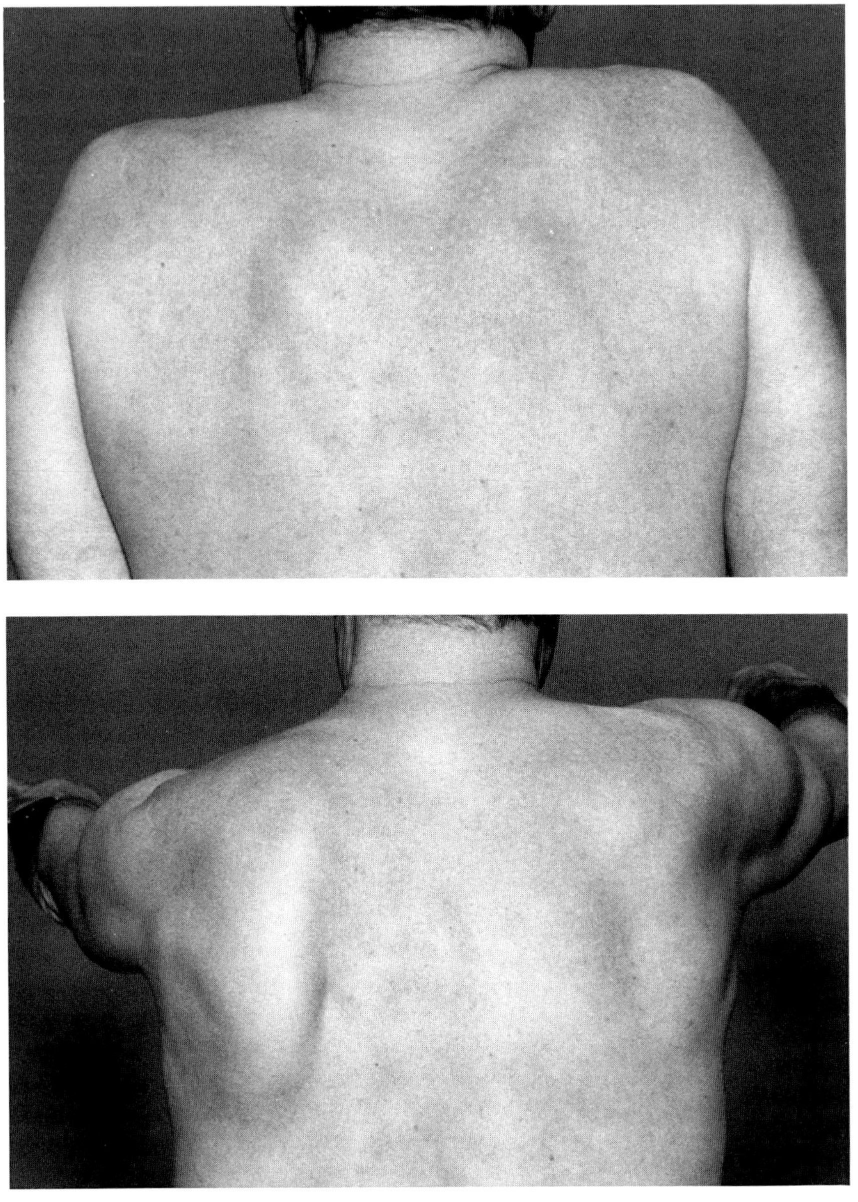

c

d

Figure 16-22 *(continued)* **c.** Two years after a nerve graft to restore continuity in the accessory nerve, he demonstrates excellent recovery of function with ability to elevate his shoulder (c) and significant improvement in the problem of winging of the scapula (d).

not anticipate functional reinnervation of facial muscles by a cross-facial nerve graft alone and would currently plan to provide a free muscle flap for this function after an appropriate period of time to facilitate regeneration of nerve fibers across the cross-facial nerve graft. A similar philosophy extrapolated to the brachial plexus may result in a similar improvement of functional recovery.

Summary—Is It Possible to Make Brachial Plexus Surgery Easy?

While brachial plexus surgery cannot be made easy it can be made far more manageable by adherance to several basic concepts. Treating the brachial plexus patient, the surgeon can use all of the basic techniques of diagnosis of nerve injury (Chapters 2 and 3) and the techniques of nerve repair and grafting (Chapter 4). The anatomy of the brachial plexus is extremely complicated and a thorough understanding of both the anatomy and the surgical exposure is critical before undertaking this surgery. Several cadaver dissections, with an anatomy book close at hand, will allow the surgeon to familiarize himself with this important anatomy. A careful clinical examination, a thorough understanding of the anatomy and surgical competence with both the exposure of the plexus and microneurosurgical techniques are the essential tools the surgeon will require in order to carry out the technical aspects of this surgery.

The decision-making aspects of the surgery are more complicated. There are, however, several basic

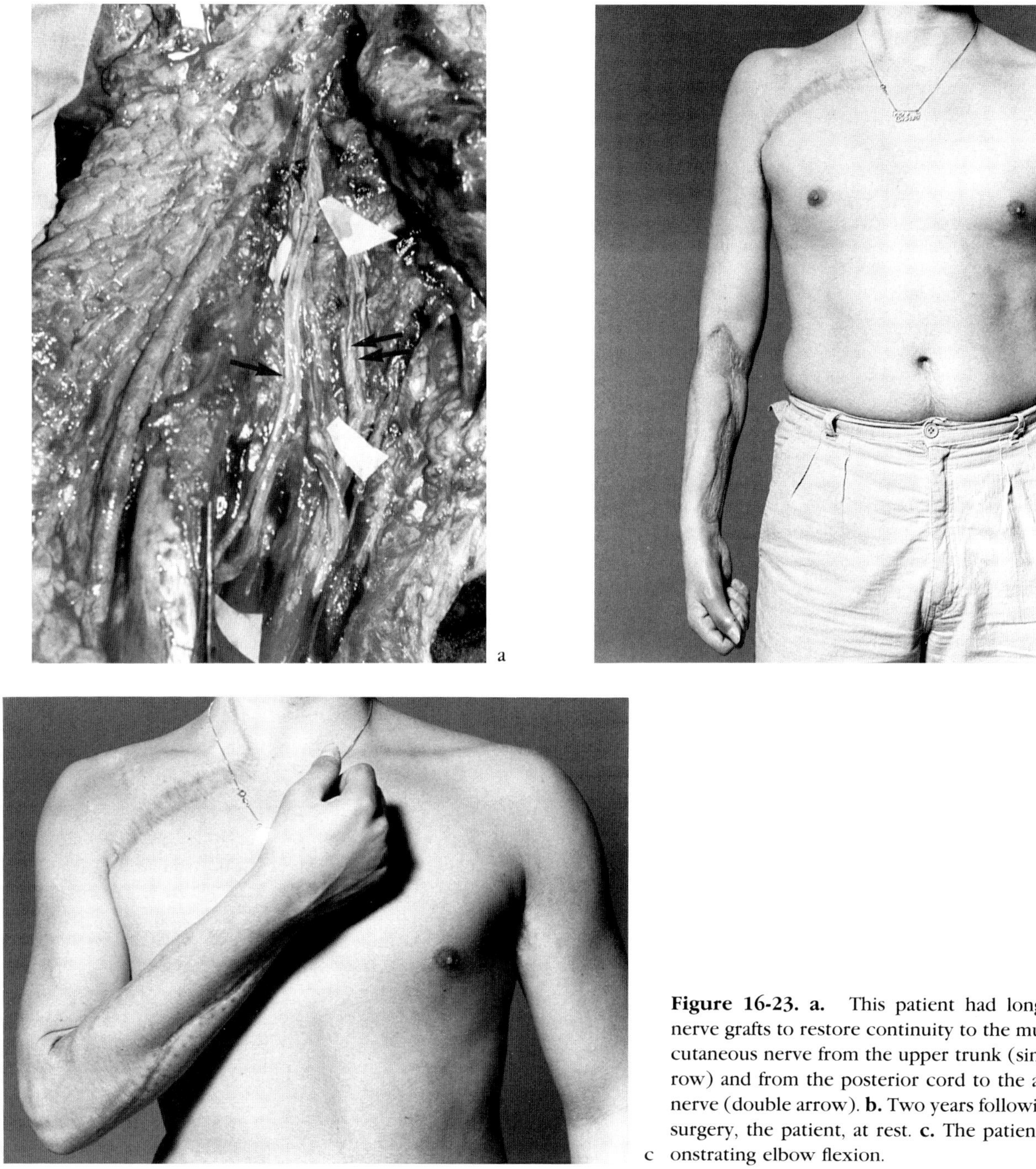

a b c

Figure 16-23. a. This patient had long sural nerve grafts to restore continuity to the musculocutaneous nerve from the upper trunk (single arrow) and from the posterior cord to the axillary nerve (double arrow). **b.** Two years following this surgery, the patient, at rest. **c.** The patient demonstrating elbow flexion.

principles that can be followed in order to simplify the surgical decision-making in dealing with brachial plexus injuries. The reconstructive surgeon has available to him a number of procedures, including nerve, muscle, tendon, and bony reconstructive techniques. He will want to use these techniques at varying times throughout the course of management of this problem in order to restore maximum function to the patient as quickly as possible with the minimum of surgical morbidity.

It is useful to recall the basic principles of tendon transfers because several of these principles can be extrapolated to the patient with brachial plexus injury in order to simplify the decision-making in this problem. Before carrying out a tendon transfer, the surgeon will make a list of the tendons which are available for transfer and the functions that need to be reconstructed. In a similar fashion, preoperatively the surgeon, through clinical examination, determines what function is present in the extremity and prioritize the needs of the extremity for useful function. In outlining the fundamental principles of tendon transfers, Curtis[67] noted that "in choosing the motor muscle one should make a chart and list on one side the needs, on the other side the muscles available should be listed. Then after careful testing and grading of the strength of each muscle, the proper transfers are selected ... it is important when possible to use a synergistic muscle in the transfer."[67] These same principles are used in determining the appropriate organization of the nerve grafts in brachial plexus surgery. Rather than transferring tendons, we are simply transferring nerve fibers from a proximal nerve to a distal nerve using a nerve graft to carry out this transfer (Table 16-4).

The priorities for reconstruction will be shoulder abduction and elbow flexion. (In complete palsy, the distance between the proximal nerve and the motor end organs controlling hand function is too great to anticipate functional recovery.) If possible, shoulder and elbow function should be restored by using a nerve graft that brings appropriate or "synergistic" nerve fibers from the proximal portion of the plexus to the distal nerves (Table 16-4). For example, grafts from the upper trunk (C5, C6) to the musculocutaneous nerve are ideal. Grafts from other portions of the plexus will carry less "synergistic" nerve fibers. With the analogy to tendon surgery, we note that a tendon graft between the proximal and distal ends of an injured tendon is likely to give a superior result than a tendon transfer because no component of relearning or motor re-education is required. Similarly, if a nerve graft can be placed between the proximal and distal ends of the same nerve (such as axillary nerve graft from proximal axillary nerve to distal axillary nerve, then the nerve fibers are far more appropriate than a graft from the proximal portion of the posterior cord to the distal axillary nerve). In some cases, it may not be possible to use the appropriate proximal nerve in order to reinnervate critical muscle units. Wherever possible, however, this should be the goal.

Although many combinations of nerve injuries are frequently seen in trauma to the brachial plexus, there are two patterns that are noted most commonly. The surgical options available to deal with these problems are many; however, we have found that in the decision-making process several patterns emerge for surgical reconstruction. We will see situations in which the entire brachial plexus has been injured and there is no function in the limb. The other frequently seen pattern is that in which there is no shoulder or elbow function but good hand and forearm function. If the entire brachial plexus is involved, the priorities for reconstruction will be shoulder and elbow function via reinnervation of the axillary and musculocutaneous nerves. The surgeon will hope to reinnervate these nerves using "synergistic" fibers from the proximal portion of the plexus. If such fibers are not available, then the surgeon will use other "less synergistic" fibers. If there are no proximal fibers available, then a neurotization procedure is indicated.

In the situation where the patient has good hand and forearm function but lacks elbow flexion and shoulder abduction, the plexus is explored and, if possible, the axillary and the musculocutaneous nerves will be reinnervated. If this is not possible, then the surgeon will consider such musculotendinous reconstructive procedures as a forearm flexorplasty.[55–57] If it is possible to restore continuity to the musculocutaneous nerve, then the patient will be provided with an elbow splint (Fig. 16-16) and the procedure, such as a Steindler flexor plasty, delayed until the results of the nerve grafting procedure can be assessed.

The management of the patient with brachial plexus injury presents the greatest challenge for the upper limb reconstructive surgeon. Knowledge of the complex anatomy of the brachial plexus combined with a clear understanding of all of the techniques available to the reconstructive surgeon will provide the patient with some optimism for eventual useful function of the upper limb.

References

1. Leffert RD: Brachial Plexus Injuries. Churchill Livingstone, New York, 1985.
2. Terzis, JK ed: Microreconstruction of Nerve Injuries. W.B. Saunders, Philadelphia, 1987, pp 285–570.
3. Smellie W: A collection of cases and observations in midwifery, vol 2, 4th ed. London, 1768, p 446.
4. Duchenne GB: De l'electrisation localisee et de son application a la pathologie et a la therapeutique, 3rd ed. Bailliere, Paris, 1872, p 357.
5. Erb W: Uber eine eigenthumliche Localisation von la Hemengen im Plexus brachialis. Verh Naturhist-Med (Heidelberg) 2:130, 1874.
6. Klumpke A: Contribution a l'etude des paralysies radiculaires du plexus brachial. Rev Med 5:591, 1885.
7. Flaubert M: Memoire sur plusiers cas de luxation. Rep Gen Anat Physiol Pathol 3:55, 1827.
8. Thoburn W: Obstetrical paralysis. J Obstet Gynecol Br Emp 3:454, 1903.
9. Kennedy R: Suture of the brachial plexus and birth paralysis of the upper extremity. Br Med J 1:298, 1903.
10. Harris W, Low VW: On the importance of accurate muscular analysis in lesions of the brachial plexus. Br Med J 2:1035–1038, 1903.
11. Tuttle H: Exposure of the brachial plexus with nerve transplantation. JAMA 61:15–17, 1913.
12. Clark LP, Taylor AS, Prout P: Study on brachial birth palsy. Am J Med Sci 130:670, 1905.
13. Taylor AS: Results from the surgical treatment of brachial plexus palsy. JAMA 48:96, 1907.
14. Taylor AS: Conclusions derived from further experience in the surgical treatment of brachial birth palsy. Am J Med Sci 146:836, 1913.

15. Taylor AS: Brachial birth palsy and injuries of similar types in adults. Surg Gynecol Obstet 30:494, 1920.
16. Davis L, Martin J, Perret G: The treatment of injuries of the brachial plexus. Ann Surg 125:647, 1947.
17. Nulsen FE, Slade HW: Peripheral nerve regeneration. In Woodhall, B, Beebe GW, eds: A Follow up Study of 3,656 World War II Injuries. Recovery Following Injury to the Brachial Plexus, Veterans' Administration Medical Myelograph, Washington, DC, 1956, pp 389–408.
18. Tracy JF, Brannon EW: Management of brachial plexus injuries (traction type). J Bone Joint Surg 48:1031, 1958.
19. Bonney G: Prognosis in traction regions of the brachial plexus. J Bone Joint Surg 41B:4–35, 1959.
20. Seddon H: Nerve grafting. J Bone Joint Surg 45:447–461, 1963.
21. Millesi H, Meiszl G, Katzer H: Zur Behandlung der Verletzungen des Plexus brachialis. Vorschlag einer Integrirten Therapie Burns. Beitr Klin Chir 220:429–446, 1973.
22. Millesi H: Surgical management of brachial plexus injuries. J Hand Surg 2:367–379, 1977.
23. Kline DG, Nulsen FE: The neuroma incontinuity—its preoperative and operative management. Surg Clin North Am 52:1189, 1972.
24. Hudson AR, Tamner B: Brachial plexus injuries. In Wilkins RH, Regachary SS eds: Neurosurgery, McGraw Hill, New York 1985, pp 1817–1832.
25. Narakas A: Lesions dans les elongations du plexus brachial. Rev Chir Orthop 63:44–55, 1977.
26. Narakas A: Indications et resultats du traitement chirurgical direct dans les lesions par elongation du plexus brachial. Rev Chir Orthop 63:88, 1977.
27. Narakas A: Surgical treatment of traction injuries of the brachial plexus. Clin Orthop 133:71–90, 1978.
28. Narakas A: Brachial plexus surgery. Orthop Clin North Am 12:303–323, 1981.
29. Gilbert A, Tassin JL: Obstetrical palsy—a clinical pathologic and surgical review. In Terzis JK ed, Microreconstruction of Nerve Injuries. WB Saunders, Philadelphia, 1978, pp 529–553.
30. Brunelli G: Neurotization of avulsed roots of brachial plexus of nerve of cervical plexus. In Oberval, ed: New Techniques in Microsurgery. 1979, pp 145–148.
31. Merle D'Aubigne RN, Deburge A: Etiologie evolution et pronostic des paralysies traumatiques du plexus brachial. Rev Chir Orthop 53:23, 1967.
32. Alnot JY, Jolly A, Rot B: Traitement direct de lesions nerveuses dans les paralysies traumatiques du plexus brachial chez l'adulte. Int Orthop 63:82, 1981.
33. Allieu Y: Exploration et traitement direct des lesions nerveuses dans les paralysies traumatiques par elongation du plexus brachial chez l'adulte. Rev Surg Orthop 63:107–122, 1975.
34. Samii M, Kahl RI: Clinische Resultate der autologen nerven Transplantation. Nelssunger Med Mitteil 46:197–202, 1972.
35. Terzis JK, Liberson WT, Maragh HA: Motorcycle brachial plexopathy. In Microreconstruction of Nerve Injuries. WB Saunders, Terzis JK, ed: Philadelphia, 1987, pp 361–384.
36. Kotani PT, Toshima Y, Matsuda H, et al: Postoperative results of nerve transposition in brachial plexus injury. Orthop Surg (Tokyo) 22:963, 1971.
37. Kerr AT: The brachial plexus of nerves in man—the variations in its formation and its branches. Am J Anat 23:285, 1918.
38. Narakas A: Thoughts on neurotization or nerve transfers in irreparable nerve lesions. In Terzis JK ed: Microreconstruction of Nerve Injuries. WB Saunders, Philadelphia, 1987, pp 447–451.
39. Slingluff CL, Terzis JK, Edgerton MT: The quantitative microanatomy of the brachial plexus in man. Reconstructive relevance. In Terzis JK ed: Microreconstruction of Nerve Injuries. WB Saunders, Philadelphia, 1987, pp 285–324.
40. Millesi H: Brachial plexus injuries: Management and results. In Terzis JK ed: Microreconstruction of Nerve Injuries. WB Saunders, Philadelphia, 1987, pp 347–360.
41. Sunderland L: Nerves and Nerve Injury, 2nd ed. Churchill Livingstone, Edinburgh, 1978.
42. Zachary LS, Dellon AL: Relationship of intraneural damage in the rat sciatic nerve to the method of injury. Microsurgery 8:182–185, 1987.
43. Kline DG, Judice DJ: Operative management of selected brachial plexus lesions. J Neurosurg 58:631–649, 1983.
44. Tsuyama N, Hara T: Reconstructive surgery for traumatic brachial plexus injuries. Clin Orthop Surg 3:675–687, 1968.
45. Minami M, Ishii S: Satisfactory elbow flexion in complete brachial plexus injuries: Produced by suture of third and fourth intercostal nerves to musculocutaneous nerve. J Hand Surg (AM) 12:1114–1118, 1987.
46. Hara T, Tsuyama N: Intercostal nerves anastomosis for brachial plexus injuries with root avulsions. Operation 23:1087–1096, 1969.
47. Petrucci FS, Morelli A, Raimondi PL: Axillary nerve injuries—21 cases treated by nerve graft and neurolysis. J Hand Surg (Am) 7:271–278, 1982.
48. Wynn Parry CB: Rehabilitation of the Hand 4th ed, 1981, pp 157–177.
49. Richards RR, Waddell JP, Hudson AR: Shoulder arthrodesis for the treatment of brachial plexus palsy. Clin Orthop 198:250–258, 1985.
50. Zancolli E, Mitre H: Latissimus dorsi transfer to restore elbow flexion. J Bone Joint Surg 55A:1265–1275, 1973.
51. Axer A, Segal D, Elbson S: Partial transplantation of the latissimus dorsi. J Bone Joint Surg 55A:1259–1264, 1973.
52. Brooks DM, Seddon HJ: Pectoral transplantation for paralysis of the flexions of the elbow a new technique. J Bone Joint Surg 41B:36–50, 1959.
53. Clark JMP: Reconstruction of biceps brachii by pectoralis muscle transplantation. Br J Surg 34:180, 1946.
54. Carroll RE, Kleinman WB: Pectoralis major transplantation to restore elbow flexion to the paralytic limb. J Hand Surg 4:501–507, 1978.
55. Steindler A: Operations on the upper extremity problems in kinetics and results. J Bone Joint Surg 9:404, 1927.
56. Steindler A: Tendon transplantations in the upper extremity. Am J Surg 44:260, 1939.
57. Mayer L, Green W: Experiences with the Steindler flexorplasty at the elbow. J Bone Joint Surg 36A:775–789, 1954.

58. Nashold BS: Current status of the DREZ operation: 1984. Neurosurgery, 15:942–944, 1984.
59. Vulpius O, Stoffel A: Orthopadische Operations-lehre, 2nd ed. Enke, Stuttgart, 1920.
60. Foerster O: Die Therapie der Schuss Verletzungen der peripheren Nerven. In Lewandowski: Handbuch der Neurologie. Ergaenzungsband, Berlin, 1929, pp 1677–1691.
61. Takahashi M: Studies of conversion of motor function in intercostal nerves for complete brachial plexus injuries of root avulsion type. J Jpn Orthop Assoc 57:1799–1807, 1983.
62. Brunelli G: Neurotization of avulsed roots of the brachial plexus by means of anterior nerves of the cervical plexus. In Terzis JK; ed: Microreconstruction of Nerve Injuries. WB Saunders Co, Philadelphia, 1987, pp 435–446.
63. Roraback CH, Harris WR: Factors affecting the prognosis of brachial plexus injuries. J Bone Joint Surg 63B:404–407, 1981.
64. Ransford AO, Hughes SPF: Complete brachial plexus lesions—a ten-year follow-up of twenty cases. J Bone Joint Surg 59B:417–420, 1977.
65. Narakas A: Neurotization or nerve transfer for brachial plexus lesions. Ann Chir Main 1:101–118, 1982.
66. Hudson AR: Personal communication.
67. Curtis RM: Fundamental principles of tendon transfer. Orthop Clin North Am 5:231–242, 1974.
68. Seddon HJ: Surgical Disorders of the Peripheral Nerves. Williams & Wilkins, Baltimore, 1972.

17

Painful Sequelae of Peripheral Nerve Injury

The inevitable consequence of injury to a peripheral nerve is loss of sensory or motor function. Restoration of lost sensibility and muscle strength often presents a formidable task for the reconstructive surgeon. However, the long-term sequelae of nerve injury includes not only this functional loss due to failure of nerve regeneration, but frequently painful sequelae relating to incomplete or abnormal nerve regeneration. Management of these pain problems often provides more of a challenge than does restoration of sensory or motor function. Indeed, patients with pain would often be willing to lose sensory or motor function through nerve division in the hope of achieving pain relief.

It is important to review the basic aspects of nerve regeneration as well as the current thoughts on the neurophysiologic aspects of pain mechanisms. Although some degree of pain follows all nerve injuries, there are several particularly difficult pain problems whose management should be addressed. These problems are:

Painful neuroma
Reflex sympathetic dystrophy, or sympathetic maintained pain syndromes (RSD/SMPS)
The painful neuroma in-continuity
Pain after carpal tunnel surgery

Nerve Regeneration

When a peripheral nerve is divided, Wallerian degeneration occurs distal to the level of the nerve transection. Schwann cells proliferate in the distal nerve and phagocytose myelin and axon debris. In the proximal portion of the nerve, degeneration occurs for a variable distance, and centrally changes in the cell body also occur. An attempt is made by the nerve to regenerate distally in order to restore neural continuity. Nerve fibers in the proximal nerve stump will form regenerating units that contain numerous axon sprouts. If these sprouting fibers make appropriate sensory or motor distal connections, then functional recovery occurs. As the nerve fibers regenerate distally, the patient will experience unpleasant sensations. These are usually more annoying than painful and resolve as the nerve function recovers. If these regenerating fibers do not make appropriate distal connections, then loss of function occurs. Pain may develop at the level of the thwarted regeneration.

The inevitable consequence then of complete division of a peripheral nerve is the formation of a neuroma at the proximal site of the nerve division if the neuron's attempt to regenerate distally is thwarted. Not all of these neuromas will be painful. There is no consensus as to why one neuroma is clinically symptomatic and another is not. If there is partial regeneration at the site of the nerve injury or if partial injury exists, then painful sequelae may develop as a portion of the nerve is transmitting relatively normal impulses and the remainder of the nerve is transmitting abnormal impulses. This problem is particularly relevant in reflex sympathetic dystrophy or sympathetic maintained pain syndromes. One of the first goals in preventing painful neuromas will then be to try to direct appropriate functional regeneration at the level of the nerve injury with meticulous microsurgical technique.

Neurophysiology of Pain

Nerve fibers vary considerably in size. It is the small C-fibers and A-delta fibers that mediate pain responses. These specialized C and A fibers are termed "nociceptors" and mediate the perception of painful stimuli, including the intensity, duration, and frequency of the painful stimuli.

Electrophysiologic assessment of neuromas has been studied in rats.[1–3] When a nerve is severed, there is a brief spontaneous discharge of electrical activity. With time, regeneration in the proximal stump occurs. Using single unit nerve fiber recordings, it is noted that nerve fibers fire spontaneously and send impulses in a central direction from the neuroma.[3] Ephaptic conduction, or "cross-talking," has been demonstrated within the neuroma itself. This concept of ephapses implies that adjacent nerve fibers can induce a neuronal impulse within each other without the occurrence of a true synapse between the nerve fibers. Experimentally, ephapses are demonstrated by stimulating one nerve fiber proximal to a neuroma and recording from a second nerve fiber proximal to the neuroma. After peripheral nerve division, changes also occur centrally in the dorsal ganglion and dorsal horn of the spinal cord as well as in the sympathetic system.[4] Sympathetic afferent fibers may stimulate an injured nerve through norepinephrine release and also influence the release of chemical pain mediators.[5,6] An ephapse between sympathetic (efferent) and pain (afferent) fibers may explain the association between the "neuroma" patient and the patient with reflex sympathetic dystrophy or sympathetic maintained pain syndromes.[4–6]

In 1965, Melzack and Wall[7] described the "gate control theory" of pain to explain some of the neurophysiologic aspects of pain. They noted that small diameter fibers mediate pain. They postulated that large diameter fibers had the ability to "close the gate" to these painful small diameter fibers, thus preventing transmission of pain to the cortex. Since conduction along these larger myelinated touch fibers occurs more quickly than it does along the small unmyelinated or thinly myelinated fibers, stimulation of these large fibers could block or "gate out" the number of pain fiber signals reaching the cortex.

This theory provided the mechanism to explain why stimulation of these large fibers (light touch, pressure) could be used as modalities to treat painful disorders.

A recent study suggests that this theory is somewhat simplistic.[8] A clinical report studied a series of patients with pain after peripheral nerve injury. The effects of a differential block of A-beta fiber (ischemic block) to C-fiber (local anesthetic block) was evaluated. This study demonstrated that hyperalgesia was related to activity in A-beta fibers and not C-fibers because hyperalgesia disappeared when the A-beta fibers were blocked and the C-fiber function was still intact. The hypothesis that hyperalgesia is related to activity in A-beta fibers and not C-fibers is supported by other studies[9,10] and suggests that the previous concept[7] that activity in large caliber afferents block pain signals and that pain after nerve injury reflects a loss of large fiber function is incorrect. Hyperalgesia does not occur because of a decline of large fiber (A-beta) input but is, in fact, mediated by these fibers. Thus, large fibers (A-beta) will normally signal touch, but, after nerve injury when hyperalgesia exists, they will mediate this very painful sensation. In this study,[8] when the large fibers (A-beta) were blocked, the hyperalgesia disappeared but the "neuromatous" pain mediated by the small fibers (A-delta, C-fibers) remained. In summary, then, the traditional "gate control theory" of pain postulated that normally "good" large diameter A-beta fibers "blocked the gate" so that messages from the "bad" pain fibers (C and A-delta) could not reach the cortex. In the patient with pain, it has been shown that large A-beta fibers are not "good" and mediate hyperalgesia. The smaller C and A-delta fibers mediate neuromatous-type pain.

Nomenclature

It is important to define several terms that are related to the painful sequelae of nerve injuries.

Anesthesia: Complete loss of sensation (nonpainful)

Hypesthesia: Decreased nonpainful sensation

Dysesthesia: Abnormal sensation usually described as "pins and needles" or "pricking," an unpleasant and annoying sensation but not particularly painful (synonymous with paresthesia)

Hyperalgesia: Painful sensation so that light tough on the skin produces exquisite and marked pain characterized by a reduced pain threshold with increased pain response to normal stimuli. Hyperalgesia is mediated by large A-beta fibers

Neuromatous pain: A discrete area of tenderness corresponding to a localized injury to a peripheral nerve, percussion at the neuroma produces paresthesia in the distribution of the injured nerve. Neuromatous pain is mediated by C and A-delta fibers

Causalgia: Burning pain and hyperalgesia confined to the distribution of an injured peripheral nerve

Reflex sympathetic dystrophy, or sympathetic maintained pain syndrome: A clinical syndrome of diffuse pain, decreased function, joint stiffness, soft tissue changes, with or without vasomotor instability. This pain syndrome may be instigated by a great number of things but is maintained by an abnormal and prolonged response by the sympathetic nervous system. We prefer the term "sympathetic maintained pain syndrome" (SMPS) to "reflex sympathetic dystrophy" (RSD).

Painful Neuroma

Historical Review

A myriad of techniques suggested for management of the peripheral neuroma attests to the fact that none of these treatment methods reliably prevents the formation of the painful neuroma. Since the earliest description of peripheral neuromas, management of this problem has been associated with controversy, frustration, and failure. It is generally agreed that pain in the region of a scar with altered sensation in the distribution of the peripheral nerve associated with increased pain in the distribution of that nerve when the region of the scar is palpated constitutes the diagnosis of a neuroma. Confronted with this clinical problem, the surgeon traditionally has resected the neuroma, cutting back the nerve to a more proximal level away from the scar. Reportedly, up to 150 methods have been utilized in an attempt to control neuroma formation. Other methods cited for the prevention of neuroma formation have included capping the nerve with various materials, ranging from metal foils to silicone caps and more recently with epineurium.[11–14] Various chemical and physical modalities have been applied to the ends of the proximally cut nerve in an attempt to prevent neuroma formation. These methods have included electrical coagulation, chemical agents (alcohol, phenol, heavy water),[13,15–18] and suture ligation of the transected nerve.[19,20] Recently, experimental work has involved the concept of dipping the proximal ends of the transected nerve in ricin, which is transported retrograde to the cell body and destroys the nerve cell body.[21] This "suicide transport" has not been clinically applicable because the neurotoxic effects of ricin spill over into adjacent normal neurons. Such a technique in the future may have clinical applicability if the "killing" properties of the suicide transport can be made to be more selective.

Critical review of the experimental and clinical literature suggests that the implantation of a transected nerve into muscle may alter classic neuroma formation. Moszkowicz,[22] in 1918, reported that "in two cases, after total resection of the neuroma, the nerve endings were placed into an opening into the muscle. A catgut suture, which grasps also the nerve, closes the opening in the muscle, secures the position of the nerve ending in the muscle." Teneff,[23] writing in Turin, Italy, in 1949, investigated this in an unspecified number of rabbit mixed (sensory and motor) nerves. He reported that the "neurofibrils separate, approach the muscle fibres singly and end upon them firmly attached. Corresponding to these developments, there is no trace of connective tissue proliferation . . . formation of amputation neuroma and the terminal cicatrix is prevented."[23] He reported success with this method in treating one amputation stump neuroma. In 1959, Munro and Mallory,[24] in Boston, reported the successful treatment of an amputation stump recurrent neuroma of the median nerve by a neuroma resection, crush, and ligature of the transected nerve ending and burial of this tied end "in red muscle fibres." Petropoulos and Stefanko[25,26] from Poland in 1961 reported a dog model in which a transected mixed nerve implanted into muscle did not form a neuroma. Our experience with neuroma resection and muscle implantation is reported later.[27–29]

With the realization that the basic biologic process of nerve regeneration and subsequent neuroma formation cannot be prevented has come the concept of moving the neuroma from a region in which the end of the nerve is readily susceptible to injury to a quieter area. This has included transposing the neuromas in the palm to the dorsum of the hand and moving the neuromas from the subcutaneous area into bone or muscle.[30]

In summary, information from the past decade supports the surgical principle of moving the neuroma to an area away from which it is likely to be repeatedly stimulated, with the most recent reports being divided between maintaining the intact mature neuroma during this transposition and resecting the neuroma with or without manipulation of the transected nerve endings. Such an approach appears to give about a 65% satisfactory long-term result.[31–33] Success decreases with repeated surgery on the painful neuroma.

Primate Studies of Neuroma Formation

Rats do not form classic neuromas and the rat has been criticized as a neuroma model because of its inherent superlative regenerative capacity. Thus, electrophysiologic and histologic properties of neuroma formation in the primate must be reviewed. In adult baboons, the radial sensory nerve was transected at the level of the wrist and 2 cm of the distal nerve was excised (Fig. 17-1).[34] At varying times postoperatively, from 1 to 7 months, electrophysiologic studies were carried out. Single unit nerve fiber recordings were used to evaluate the electrical activity originating from the neuroma. Spontaneous activity in both C-fibers and A-delta fibers was noted. These fibers also were exquisitely sensitive to mechanical stimulation (Table 17-1).

Evidence of reinnervation of the previously denervated dorsoradial skin was demonstrated and "cross-talk" activity between nerve fibers at the level of the neuroma was observed. These observations suggested that the neuroma was mechanically sensitive (susceptible to stimulation by touch or by skin, joint, or muscle movement) and was itself a source of pain signals (C-fiber and A-delta fiber activity) through ephaptic conduction and spontaneous fiber activity. These findings supported the concept that the so-called mature neuroma should be resected as part of the surgical treatment of the painful neuroma. The fact that the neuroma is exquisitely mechanically sensitive would suggest that the surgeon can influence the degree of neuroma pain by moving the neuroma to an area that is not mechanically stimulated. The fact that the neuroma is itself spontaneously active with both C and A-delta activity suggests that not all aspects of neuroma pain can be controlled by the surgeon because the neuroma itself without any stimulation will demonstrate spontaneous pain fiber activity.

In a series of cynomolgus monkeys, the three sensory nerves about the wrist, (radial sensory nerve, palmar cutaneous branch of the median nerve, dorsocutaneous branch of ulnar nerve) were transected at the level of the wrist, and 2 cm of the distal nerve was

Table 17-1. Neuroma Properties*

	Neuroma (age in months)			
	1–2	*4*	*7*	*Control*
Number of experiments	4	2	2	3
Number of C-fibers studied	128	73	180	158
Number of A-fibers studied	87	51	70	148
Percent spontaneously active	10	8	18	9
Percent mechanically sensitive	18	17	4	0
Percent apparent cross-talk	0	4	4	2

*Reprinted with permission from Meyer et al.[34]

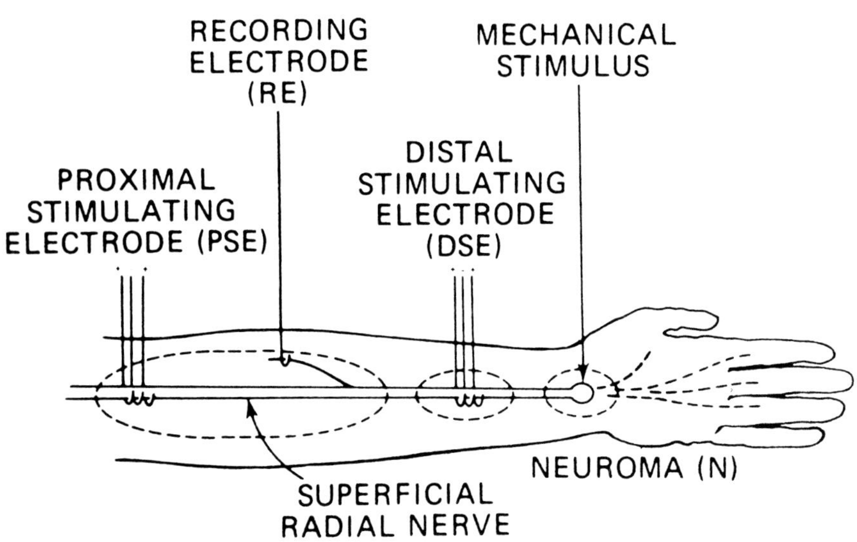

Figure 17-1. Schemata of neuroma experiment. (Reproduced with permission from Meyer et al.[34])

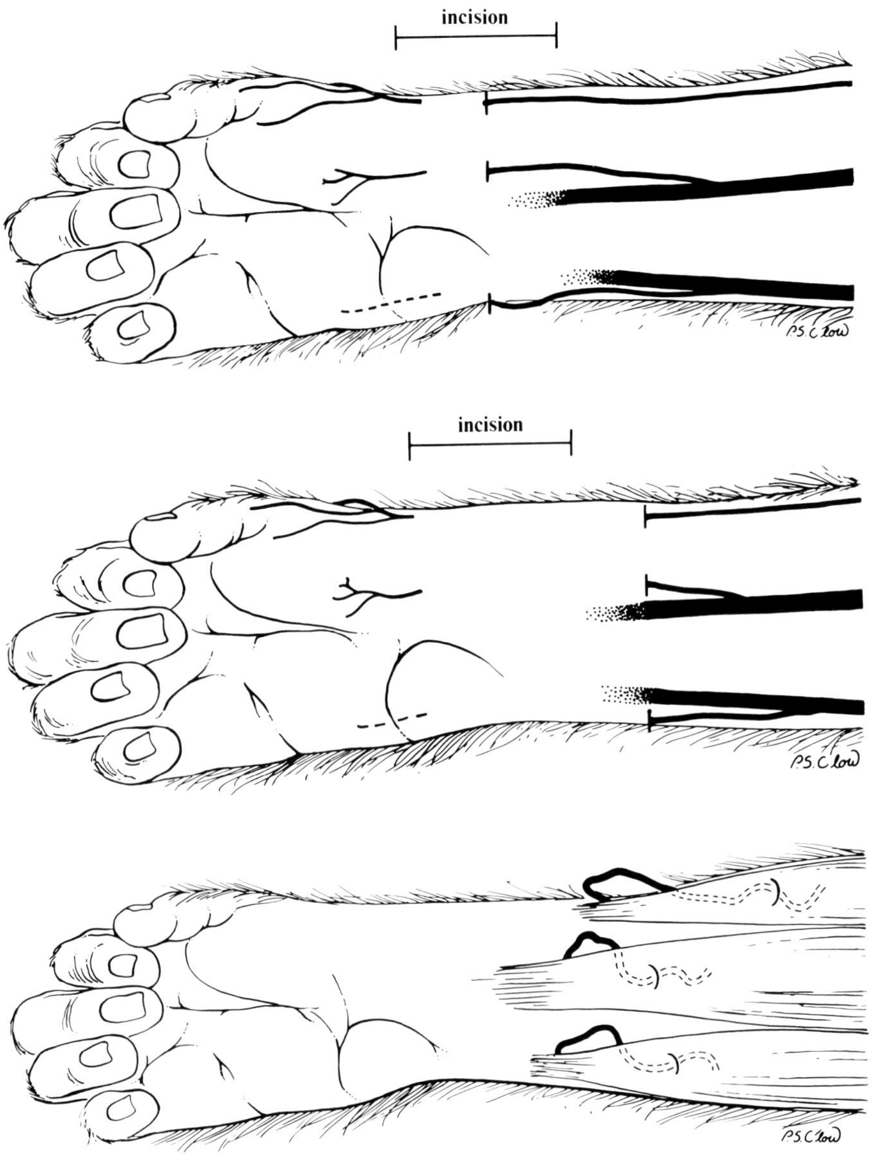

a b c

Figure 17-2. Schematic diagram outlining the experimental technique. In the control group, the transected sensory nerves were left adjacent to the incisional wound at the level of the wrist (**a**). In the proximally cut group, sensory nerves were transected at a level away from the incisional wound and away from the level of the wrist (**b**). In the muscle implantation group, the transected ends of the sensory nerves were implanted into muscle (**c**). (Reproduced with permission from Mackinnon et al.[28])

excised (Fig. 17-2).[28] This group was considered the control "neuroma" group because the freshly cut end of the sensory nerve was left under denervated skin and the incision was in an area subjected to repetitive movement and mechanical stimulation. A second group was treated by proximally cutting these nerves so that the transected end of the sensory nerve was located proximal to the wrist and away from the overlying incision. In the third group of animals, the sensory nerves were implanted into innervated muscles. All nerves were evaluated histologically at 6 months. The control neuromas showed evidence of regeneration into the overlying skin (Fig. 17-3). The neuroma itself was composed of a tangled mass of nerve fibers with regenerating units noted in all orientations. A dense mass of connective tissue was noted between these disorganized fibers. Myofibroblasts were apparent within the neuroma and 80% of the cross-sectional area of the neuroma were made up of collagen and scar tissue (Fig. 17-4).

Histologically, the "proximally cut group" could not be distinguished from the control group except that the neuromas in the proximally cut group failed to reinnervate the overlying skin. This group contained myofibroblasts and 80% of the cross-sectional area of the neuroma were made up of connective tissue.

In marked contrast, the nerves implanted into muscle were found to contain significantly less connective tissue (40%) than the control or proximally cut groups ($p < 0.001$) and showed no evidence of invasion or regeneration into the surrounding innervated muscle (Fig. 17-5). The nerves demonstrated a sharp interface with the muscle and, although a small neuroma did form at the distal end of the transected sensory nerve, the nerve fibers within the neuroma were all arranged in the same direction. Myofibroblasts were not seen and the nerve fibers in the minifascicles were "immature"

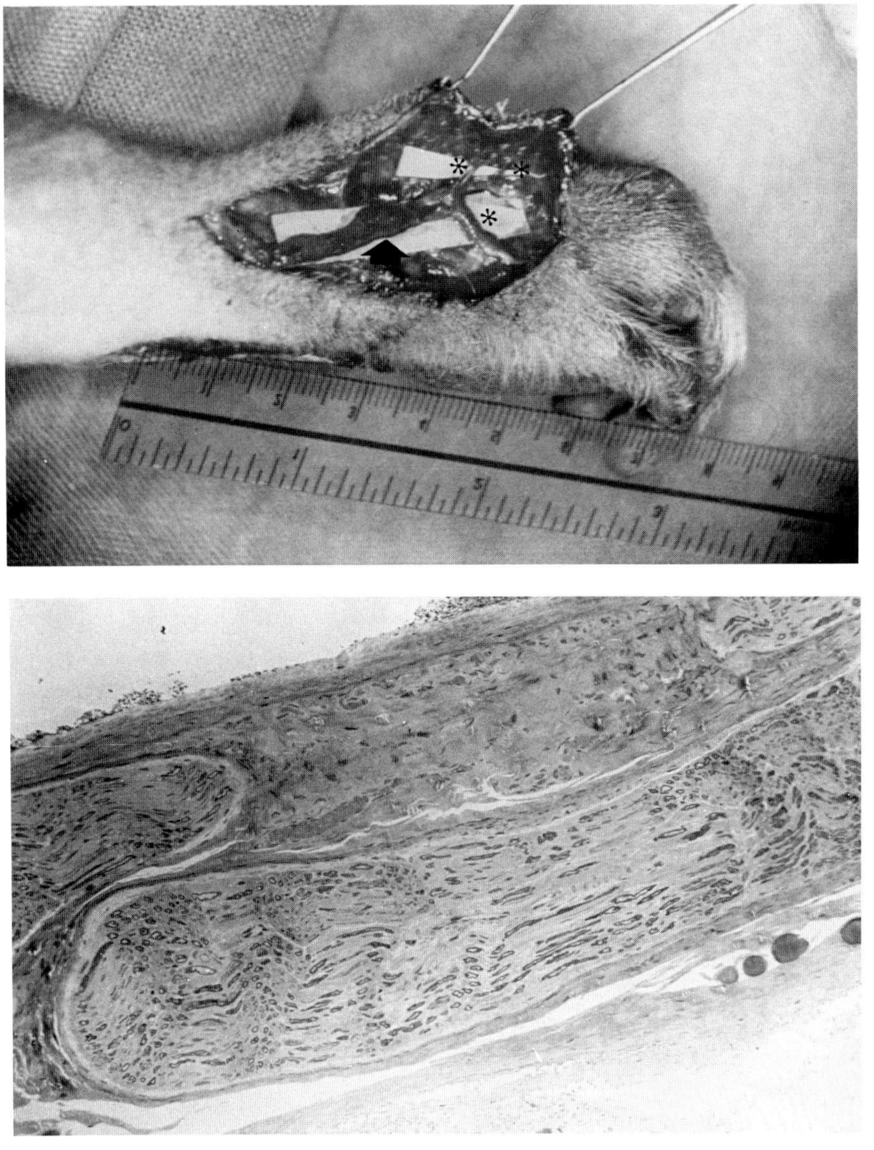

Figure 17-3. The radial sensory nerve has been transected at the level of the wrist (arrow). When reexplored 6 months later, evidence of regeneration into the overlying skin was seen (*; hand toward right; **a**). Longitudinal sections of the regenerating "twigs" identified in a (*). These fibers were identified as nerve tissue (**b**). (Toluidine blue; ×128.) (Reproduced with permission from Mackinnon et al.[28])

and thinly myelinated when compared with the other treatment groups (Table 17-2). It is concluded from this study that, although implantation of the sensory nerve into innervated muscle did not prevent neuroma formation, it did significantly alter neuroma formation, preventing the formation of a classic neuroma. Thus, it is apparent that neuroma formation can be altered by manipulation of the nerve's microenvironment. The implantation of the sensory nerve into muscle theoretically removed the influence of possible neurotrophic factors from the denervated skin and also decreased the effect of wrist movement as a source of tension on the neuroma.

Table 17-2. Morphologic Assessment of Neuroma Formation*

	Treatment Method		
	Control neuroma	*Proximally Cut*	*Muscle Implantation*
Fascicular area, $\mu^2/375{,}000\mu^2$	6268.7 ± 318.00	6558.9 ± 402.80	17764.5 ± 609.81†
Percent neural tissue	20	21	59†
Mean fascicle diameter (μm)	31.7 ± 16.89	30.9 ± 15.51	25.1 ± 9.5‡
Mean fiber diameter (μm)	3.8 ± 0.48	3.6 ± 0.28	2.8 ± 0.30†
Number of fibers/375 μ^2	5.64 ± 1.37	5.00 ± 1.5	3.07 ± 0.83†

*Reprinted with permission from Mackinnon et al.[28]

†$p < 0.001$.

‡$p < 0.05$.

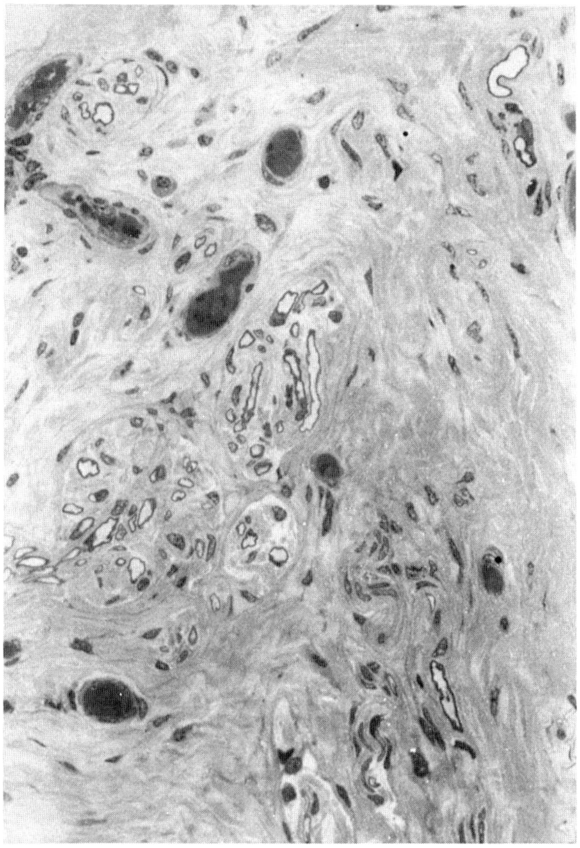

a

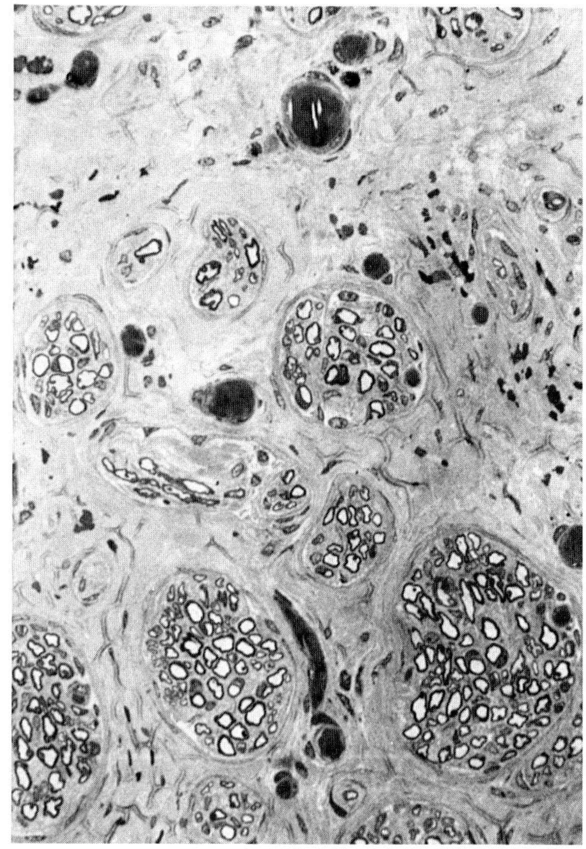

b

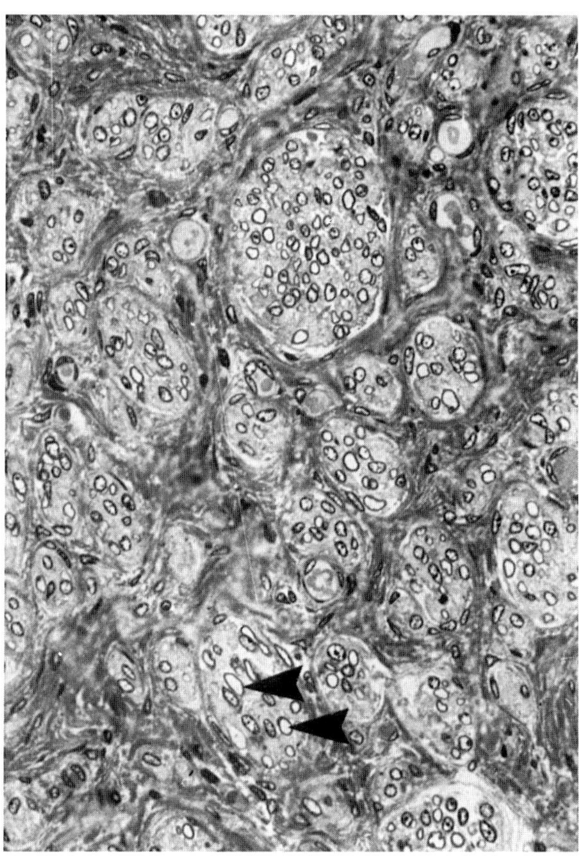

c

Figure 17-4. Transverse section of the neuromas identified in the three experimental groups. In the control group, small nerve fascicles are identified in cross-section and in longitudinal orientation (**a**). In the proximally cut group, fascicles with well-myelinated fibers are identified (**b**). In the muscle implantation group, small minifascicles all oriented in the same direction are noted. Most of the "circular" structures within the regenerating units are Schwann cells and only the occasional myelinated fiber is identified. These minifascicles are densely packed and bounded by perineurium (**c**). (Toluidine blue; ×232.) (Reproduced with permission from Mackinnon et al.[28])

Clinical Studies of Neuroma Treatment with Muscle Implantation Technique

The experimental work just described suggested that implantation of a transected nerve into muscle might alter classic neuroma formation. A recent clinical study evaluated this approach in the management of neuroma problems.[29] The neuroma was excised and the proximal end of the nerve was placed away from denervated skin, scar, and tension and into a well-vascularized muscle environment. Seventy-eight neuromas in 60 patients with a mean follow-up of 31 months (range, 18 to 43) were evaluated (Table 17-3). Sixty-seven percent of these patients involved Workers' Compensation and 57% had had at least one previous operation to treat the pain. The results were good to excellent in 82% of the treated nerves in the entire group. The factors that were predictive of poor outcome were digital neuromas ($p < 0.0005$), Workers' Compensation ($p < 0.01$), and three or more previous operations for pain ($p < 0.01$). Transposition of the nerves into small superficial muscles (such as intrinsic muscles in the hand) or muscles with significant excursion (such as thumb extensors) resulted in treatment failures.

The patients were evaluated pre- and postoperatively using two rating systems (pain and function). The preoperative pain was in each case severe and disabling. Postoperatively, the relief of pain was rated as poor (worse or little improvement), good (not pain-free but significantly improved), and excellent (essentially pain free).

Hand function was graded separately from pain. Many of these patients had other injuries that interfered with their functional performance. Thus, it was noted whether their restriction of hand function was due to residual and unrelieved pain or due to other disabilities (such as decreased tendon or joint function, amputation). Postoperatively, hand function was judged as poor if it was made worse or not improved or if the patient was incapable of activities of daily living only because of residual pain. It was judged good if the patient could work with restriction or do activities of daily living limited by residual deformity but not limited by pain. It was judged as excellent if the patient could work at his or her previous job or was in vocational rehabilitation restricted still by residual deformity.

Table 17-3. Neuromas Treated by Resection and Muscle Implantation*

	Nerves	*Patients in Each Group*
Radial sensory	30	26†
Lateral antebrachial cutaneous	15	15
Palmar cutaneous median	6	6
Digital	7	5
Dorsal cutaneous ulnar	6	5‡
Medial antebrachial cutaneous	9	9
Brachial plexus	3	3
Intercostal	1	1
Sural	1	1
	78	71§

*Reprinted with permission for Dellon and Mackinnon.[29]

†Four patients had the same neuroma reoperated on, transferring it into a different muscle.

‡One patient had the same neuroma reoperated on, implanting it more proximally.

§Eleven patients had more than one neuroma and appear in different categories.

The clinical results relating to specific nerves are noted in Figure 17-6.

Analysis of patients with treated digital neuromas demonstrate that none of the patients enjoyed excellent relief of pain and only 14% had good relief; 86% of patients remained little improved or unchanged.

Analysis of the clinical results related to previous operations demonstrated that the poorer results were obtained in the group of patients with three or more previous operations for pain versus those patients treated for pain for the first time with neuroma resection and muscle implantation ($p < 0.01$) (Fig. 17-7).

In this clinical study, treatment failures were evaluated and it was determined that the choice of muscle was critical in determining treatment outcome. It was thought that 12 patients had little if any relief of pain after the first muscle implantation procedure because of failure to choose an appropriate muscle for implantation. Muscles with large excursions, the abductor pollicis longus or extensor pollicis brevis group, were initially chosen for muscle implantation because of their proximity to the resected radial sensory neuroma. Although good to excellent pain relief was obtained over the dorsoradial aspect of the hand, movement of the thumb and especially forced extension caused significant pain, limiting hand function. All four of these patients who were treated with implantation into these muscles had subsequent operations in which the nerve in the muscle was excised and relocated in the brachioradialis muscle. The brachioradialis, a large muscle with very little excursion, located away from the wrist and the hand, proved to be an excellent muscle in which to implant the dorsoradial sensory nerves.

Implantation of digital nerves into the pronator quadratus muscle or into the small muscles in the hand in no instances produced excellent pain relief. The pronator quadratus implantation site resulted in pain with wrist pronation and supination. The small muscles in the hand were associated with either too much excursion or were small superficial muscles that were subjected to frequent mechanical stimulation with use of the hand.

Another source of treatment failure was not identifying the situation in which more than one cutaneous

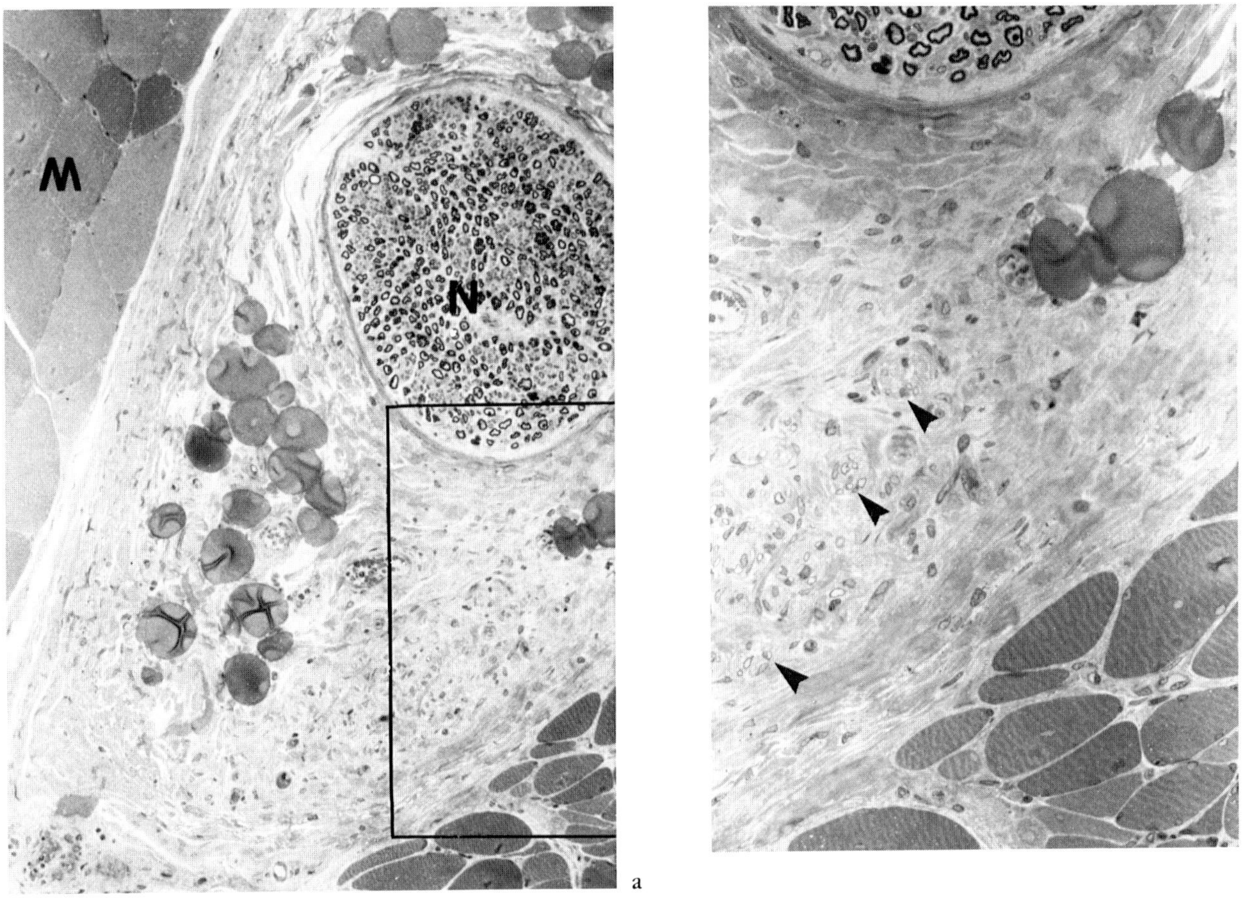

Figure 17-5. Transverse section of sensory nerve implanted into muscle **a.** The original sensory nerve is contained within the muscle. N: nerve; M: muscle. (Toluidine blue; ×82.) **b.** At a higher magnification, clusters of small minifascicles (arrow) can be identified at the interface between the original sensory nerve and the muscle. (Toluidine blue; ×328) (Reproduced with permission from Mackinnon et al.[28])

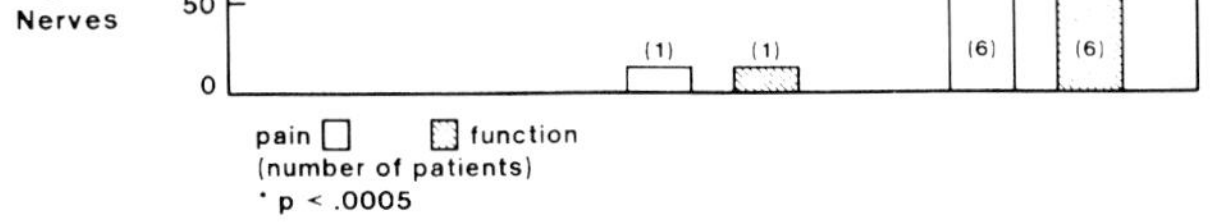

Figure 17-6. Clinical results related to specific nerves. LABC: lateral antibrachial cutaneous; SBR: superficial branch of the radius. (Reproduced with permission from Dellon and Mackinnon.[29])

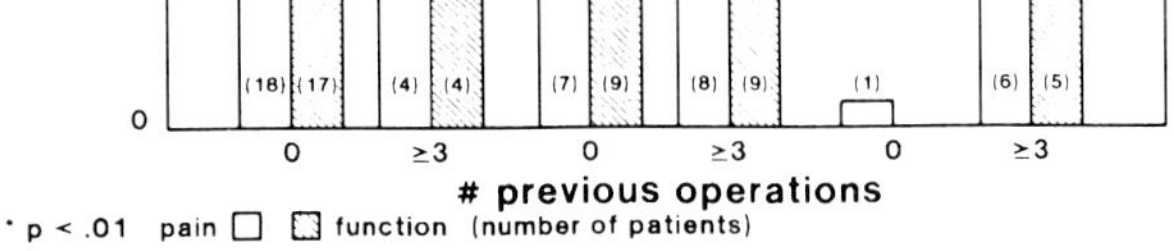

Figure 17-7. Clinical results related to previous operations. (Reproduced with permission from Dellon and Mackinnon.[29])

nerve was involved directly in the neuroma. In particular, the overlap of the lateral antebrachial cutaneous nerve with the radial sensory nerve was not recognized in some of the early patients treated with dorsoradial wrist neuromas. Diagnostic preoperative nerve blocks of the nerves potentially contributing to the pain allowed identification of the various cutaneous nerves innervating the neuromas.

Histopathology of Human Neuromas

The histopathologic examination of a classic neuroma demonstrates regenerating nerve fibers embedded in scar tissue. There is no orientation to the regenerating fibers. The fibers are classically noted to be found in random orientation.

In the clinical evaluation of 68 neuromas previously treated by ourselves with muscle implantation technique, eight clinical specimens were available for histologic evaluation. In all instances, the patients complained of pain at the implantation site. In two cases, this occurred with movement of the muscle. In one of these two cases, the nerve had pulled completely free of the muscle (abductor pollicis longus or extensor pollicis brevis). Histologically, this neuroma demonstrated a pattern of disorganized nerve fibers, which in transverse cuts were noted to be in longitudinal and transverse orientation (Fig. 17-8). In the second case, the nerves had largely pulled out of the muscle (extensor pollicis longus) and only a very small portion of the distal portion of nerve or neuroma remained surrounded by muscle. A classic neuroma of disorganized nerve fibers and dense connective tissue stroma was noted in the proximal sections where the nerve entered the muscle, and in the distal sections of this neuroma, the nerve was seen to be "invading" the muscle (Fig. 17-9). Small nerve fascicles were noted between muscle fibers. The nerve was not bounded and confined by the muscle, as is seen in the subhuman primate studies and in the clinical specimens in which the nerve was found to be completely confined by the muscle.

In the remaining six cases, the patients complained of significant pain with direct palpation of the muscle implantation site. These nerves demonstrated grossly a smoothly tapered mass within the muscle (Fig. 17-10) but were located very superficially in the muscle belly. Serial histologic sections in these six patients demonstrated that the original sensory nerve maintained its orientation well into the muscle bed, and at the distal portion of the nerve only a small neuroma formed. This neuroma was not a classic neuroma. The small fascicles at the distal portion of the nerve were all oriented in the same direction because all fascicles appeared in cross-section. The neuroma did not invade the muscle but was completely confined by the muscle (Fig. 17-10).

Electron microscopic sections demonstrated less connective tissue stroma and a decrease in the number of fibroblasts compared with the case in which the neuroma was not confined by muscle. A similar histologic pattern was seen in all six of these specimens in which the nerve had not pulled out of muscle.

Patient Selection for Surgery

In this chapter, we will not discuss the use of physiotherapy modalities for the management of painful nerve injuries. Desensitization will include many modalities, including those described in Chapter 18 as well as transcutaneous nerve stimulation. All these modalities should be tried before surgical intervention. If the patient has not responded to a 6-month course of such therapy, it is unlikely that he ever will.

The use of pharmacologic agents is only occasionally helpful for these patients. Tricyclic antidepressants may prove useful. Drugs such as amitriptyline and imipramine or amitriptyline and carbamazepine have helped some patients, but their use must be carefully monitored.

Before any surgical procedures for pain secondary to nerve injury, a very critical evaluation of the patient is necessary in order to quantitate the component of the pain complex that is due to functional overlay. We have developed a method of evaluation that has proved

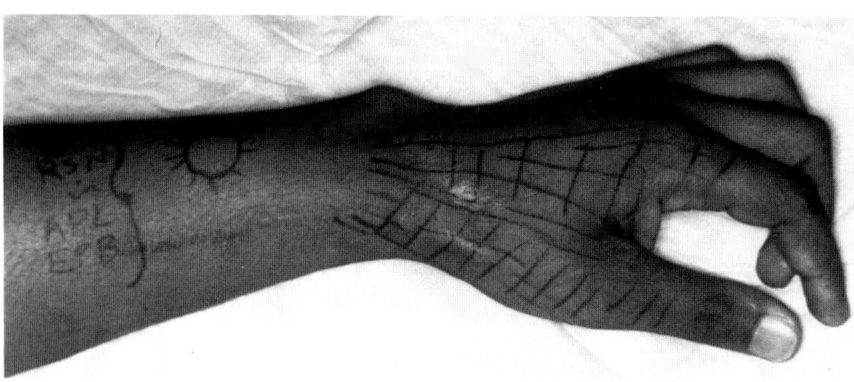

a

Figure 17-8. One year after implantation of the sensory branch of the radial nerve into the abductor pollicis longus and extensor pollicis brevis muscle, the patient continues to have pain in the distribution of the sensory branch of the radial nerve with movement of the thumb (**a**). (*Figure continues.*)

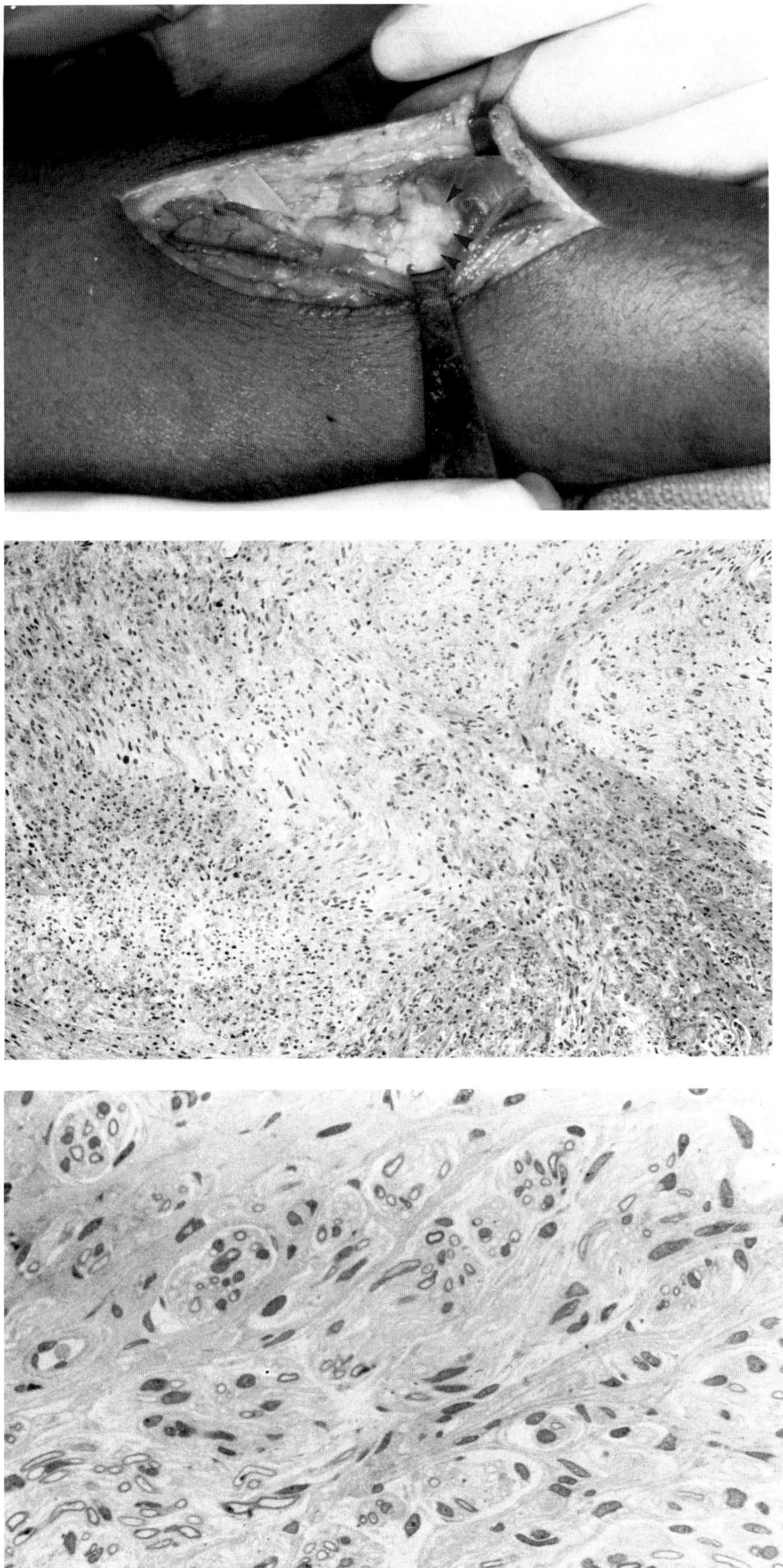

b

c

d

Figure 17-8 (*continued*) **b.** Exploration of the sensory branch of the radial nerve demonstrated that the nerve was no longer completely surrounded by muscle. It had largely pulled free from the muscle and a considerable amount of scarring was noted where the nerve entered the muscle from the previous operative site (arrow) (hand toward right, visibility background beneath the radial nerve) **c.** Histologic changes are representative of a "classic" neuroma. The fibers are seen in longitudinal and in cross-section orientation. (Toluidine blue; ×153.) **d.** At higher magnification, a disorganized pattern of the nerve fibers is embedded in a dense stroma of connective tissue. (Toluidine blue; ×614.) (Reproduced with permission from Dellon and Mackinnon.[29])

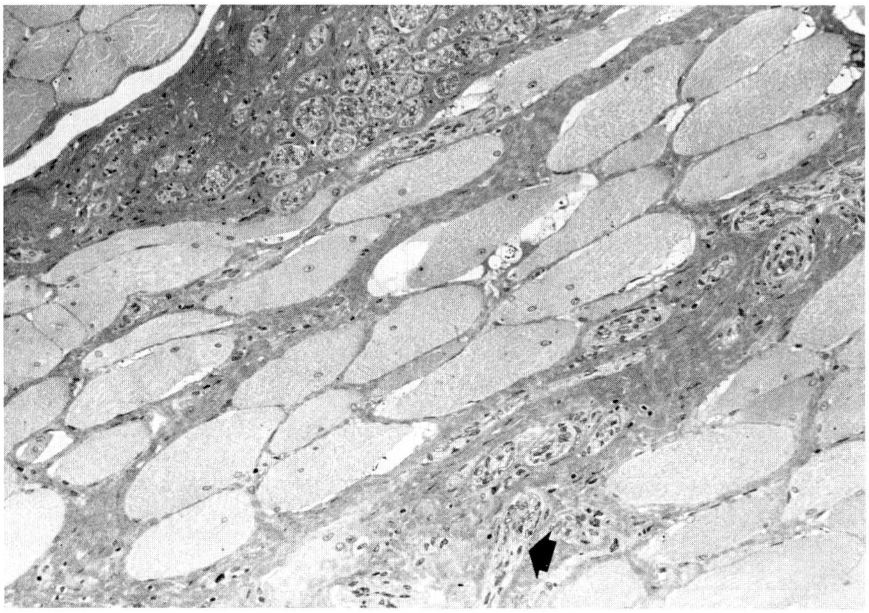

Figure 17-9. Transverse section of the sensory branch of the radial nerve, which had been placed into the adductor pollicis longus and extensor pollicis longus muscles and had partially pulled out of the muscle bed. Nerve fibers are seen to be invading the muscle. They are not confined by the muscle bed but are apparent between muscle fibers (arrow) (Toluidine blue; ×169.) (Reproduced with permission from Dellon and Mackinnon.[29])

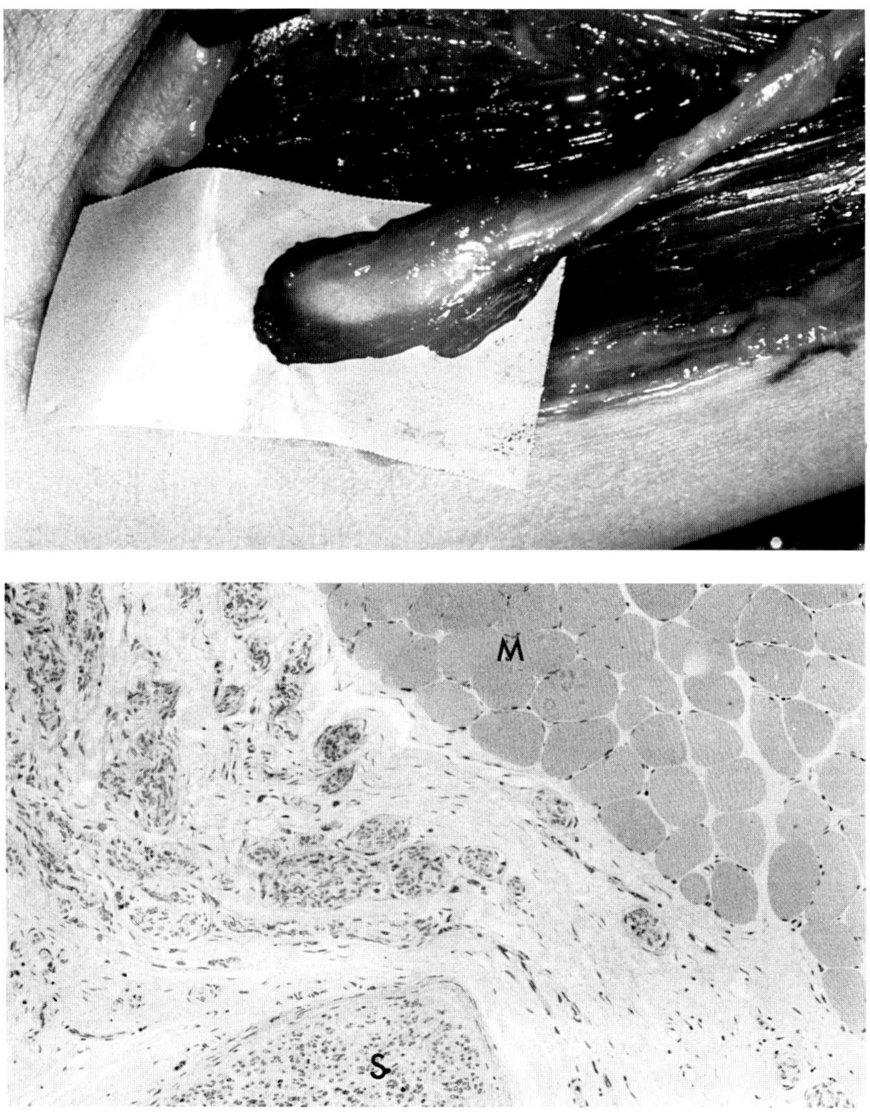

a

b

Figure 17-10. The sensory branch of the radial nerve was biopsied 1 year after implantation into the brachioradialis muscle. **a.** It is tapered smoothly within the muscle and did not appear to extend through the muscle but was surrounded by a cap of muscle tissue. **b.** In the muscle bed, the sensory nerve preserves its normal architecture. A small neuroma not invading the muscle is apparent at the nerve–muscle junction. S: sensory nerve: M: muscle. (Toluidine blue; ×153.) (Reproduced with permission from Dellon and Mackinnon.[29])

helpful in separating the "organic" from the "functional" pain patient. This technique allowed the determination of when there is "too much" functional overlay to allow a good result of the surgical treatment of the problem. Functional overlay may preclude a satisfactory result even if the surgery is done perfectly. Pain is difficult to quantitate and therefore usually repeated assessment of these patients is necessary in order to develop a sense of the magnitude of the pain and the degree of impact on the patient's lifestyle. Consultation with the referring physicians and surgeons is mandatory. If a language barrier exists, the recruitment of an interpretor, preferably a family member, is required. In some cases, when Workers' Compensaton or litigation is not involved and previous surgical procedures directed at the relief of pain have not been attempted, a single preoperative consultation may be all that is required. Otherwise, two or three separate evaluations are recommended. The liberal use of opinions from "respected colleagues" is encouraged.

Pain Rating Scale

A pain rating scale has been modified from Hendler's[35] back pain rating scale to assess patients with extremity pain.[36] The test is given to the patient by the surgeon and takes very little time to administer (Appen-

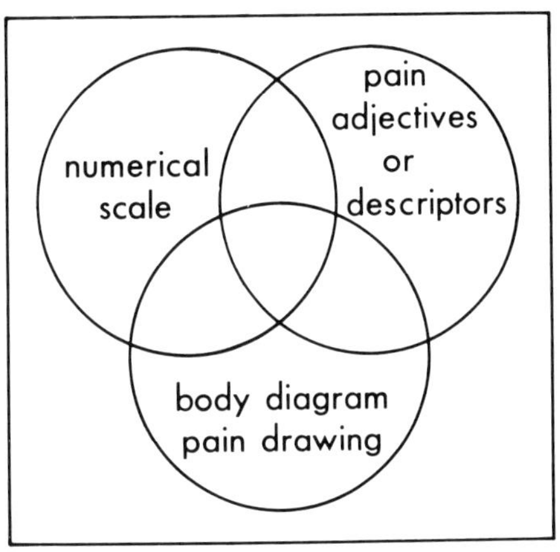

a

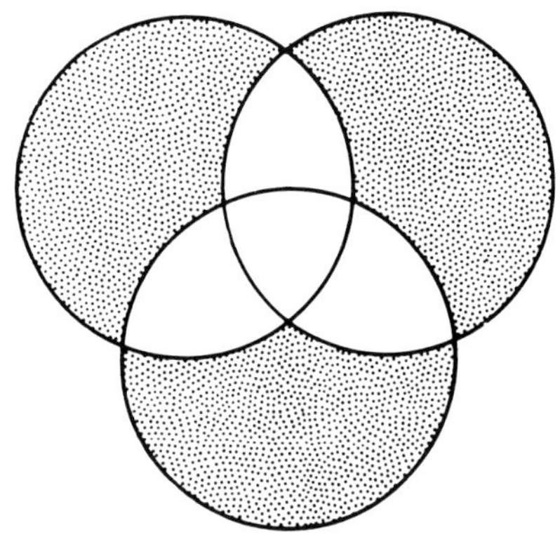
b

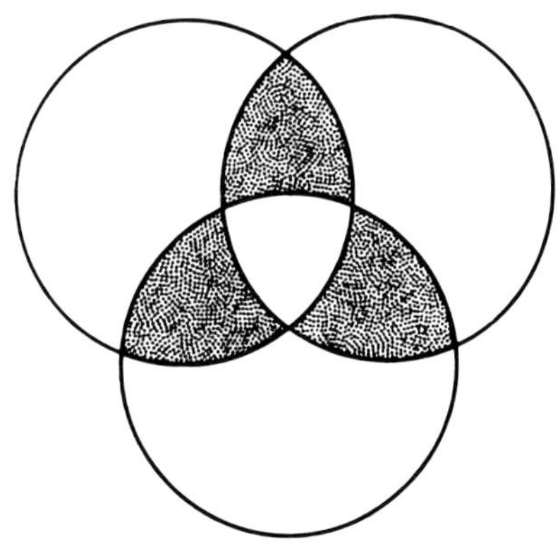
c

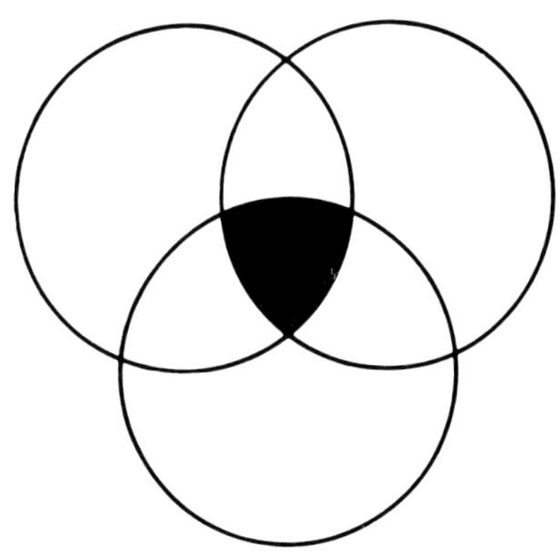
d

Figure 17-11a. Venn construct for pain evaluation rating scale. The patients are evaluated using three broad parameters. A *numerical scale* reflects the answers the patients give to various questions. The *body diagram* pain drawing determines whether or not the pain described by the patient follows any known anatomic pattern. Finally, the *pain descriptors* indicate the number of adjectives the patient uses to describe the pain. **a.** If the patient's scores greater than 14 on the numerical scale, then they fall within the circle outlined for this rating. If they circle more than three adjectives when asked to describe their pain, then they fall within the circle that diagrams the pain adjectives. If the patient describes a location of their pain on the body diagram that does not fit with any known anatomic distribution of pain, then they fall within the circle outlined for the pain drawing. If the patient's grading falls into only one of these circles, the surgeon may proceed with surgery with caution. He will often explain his concern to the patient and solicit psychiatric help at his own discretion. **b.** If the patient's scale falls into one of these three areas, that is, if they are positive for two of the three evaluations, then psychiatric evaluation is always solicited (**c**). If the patient is positive on all three rating scales and falls into the central area, then surgery is contraindicated (**d**).

dix D). It consists of three components (Fig. 17-11a).

The patient is asked to draw on a body diagram the area that corresponds to his pain. The surgeon is looking for a distribution of pain in keeping with some known anatomic distribution. The patient with considerable overlay will draw a wandering pattern of pain that corresponds to no particular anatomic distribution.

The patient is then presented with a list of pain descriptors. He is asked to circle the words that describe his pain. The patient with considerable functional overlay will circle more than three words to describe the pain.

Finally, a series of questions are presented to the patient. Many of these the surgeon will have already covered in his history-taking. The answers to these questions are assigned a numerical grade. A score of 14 or less points suggests that the patient is an objective pain patient. If the patient accumulates greater than 14 points, there is concern that more than just organic disease exists and that the patient is exaggerating the pain.

A Venn diagram is constructed. If the patient scores greater than 14 points on the numerical scale, he is considered to be "within" the circle that describes the numerical scale. If he must use more than three words to describe the pain, he is located within the adjective or descriptor circle. Similarly, if the drawing the patient uses to describe the area involved with pain does not fit a reasonable anatomic pattern, then the patient will score within the circle that represents the drawing portion of the evaluation.

The patient whose scores place him outside of all circles is the "ideal surgical candidate." These scores suggest an objective pain patient reporting a normal response to a painful problem.

The patient who scores positive on just one of the three portions of the test and whose score places him within one circle is likely to be a good surgical candidate but is demonstrating an exaggerated response to his painful problem. The surgeon may want to discuss his concerns regarding the functional component of his pain with the patient preoperatively and may occasionally seek a psychiatric consultation (Fig. 17-11b).

If the patient's scores place him within two circles (Fig. 17-11c), surgery is relatively contraindicated. Psychiatric consultation is always solicited. The surgeon must discuss his concerns with the patient regarding surgery. The patient falling into this category will be seen on several occasions if surgery is seriously considered. Usually, however, they are not considered to be surgical candidates because of the very real concern about the degree of superimposed functional overlay.

Finally, if the patient's scores place him in the situation where all scores are positive (Fig. 17-11d), surgery is absolutely contraindicated.

Tourniquet Test

Several other tests have proven useful in assessing the patient's pain tolerance. In particular, the surgeon will develop a sense of the patient's tolerance for pain by their response to a standard painful stimulus. In the very difficult case, the tourniquet test has been used. (The surgeon must try this test on himself before administering it to a patient.) The pain from tourniquet ischemia is a standard pain stimulus. Patients who cannot tolerate the tourniquet for 5 to 10 minutes without discomfort have a decidedly lowered tolerance to pain.

The use of the tourniquet ischemia to decrease hyperalgesia has been described.[8] After just 4 to 11 minutes of tourniquet time, the hyperalgesia disappears. The area that was previously hyperalgesic can be touched without eliciting pain. This is because the large A-beta fibers mediating hyperalgesia are blocked first by ischemia, probably because they are most sensitive to ischemia because of their size. Certainly after 7 to 11 minutes of tourniquet ischemia, the smaller C-fibers that are responsible for "neuromatous" type pain are still functioning. Thus, light touch to a previously hyper-

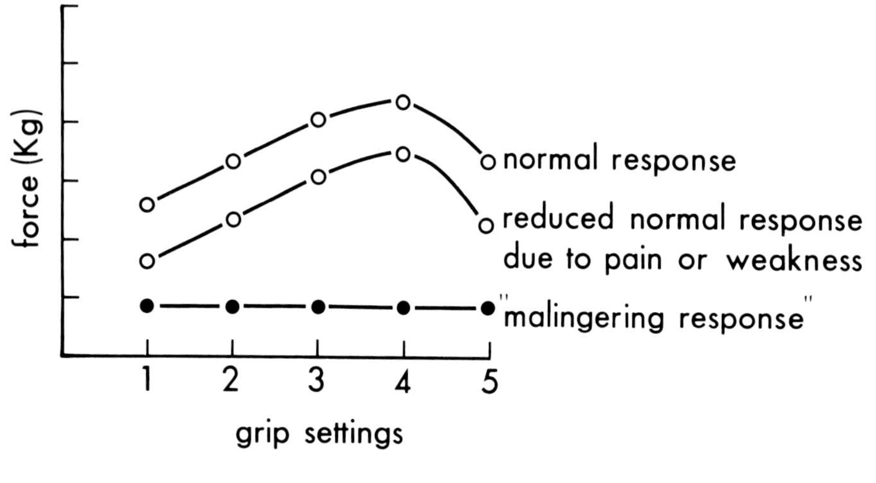

Figure 17-12. When the grip strength is plotted against the various settings available on the grip meter in a normal situation at the extremes of the settings, a weaker grip is noted than in the optimal central settings. A patient who is noncompliant will demonstrate a "flat line" grip strength across all settings.

algesic area is no longer painful but tapping over a neuroma will still elicit pain. This pattern of response to the tourniquet test can also be used to evaluate the reliability of the patient's response.

Jamar Grip Meter

The reliability of the patient's complaints can be assessed using standard assessment of grip measurements.[37] The grip meter has five settings and the grip reading generated will be related to the position or setting of the instrument. In the extremes of the settings, it is difficult to generate much grip force. In the mid ranges, grip strength is maximized. Thus, a normal pattern across the various settings will describe a curve as depicted in Figure 17-12. A malingering patient will present a flat line Jamar grip curve, making no effort to generate a strong grip even when the instrument is set to their advantage (Fig. 17-12).

The rapid exchange grip test has recently been described and has proved useful as another test to evaluate patient reliability.[38] The grip meter is set at the optimum position and baseline grip assessment is made with both hands. The patient is then instructed to move the grip meter back and forth rapidly between both hands. The examiner sits in front of the patient visually reading the level of force generated by each grip. If true disease exists in the hand in question, then the grip readings, during rapid exchange, will be similar to the initial reading. If the readings in the hand in question approach the reading in the normal hand during the rapid exchange testing, then it suggests that the patient is not completely reliable. Although the patient can control the amount of grip strength generated on a single isolated effort when he rapidly exchanges the grip meter, the cortical impulses blend and he can no longer "intellectualize" or control the amount of force in one hand versus another.

Similarly, two grip meters can be used simultaneously, one in each hand, and rapid simultaneous grip recordings carried out. If the patient is asked to do rapid simultaneous grips, he finds it difficult to "intellectualize" his response. Any weakness of grip demonstrated will be "real" during these rapid grip test and not "faked" (Fig. 17-13).

Diagnostic Nerve Blocks

In most patients, diagnostic nerve blocks are an integral part of the evaluation.[39] In a few patients, it is apparent that these blocks cannot be tolerated and an elaborate emotional response is noted with the attempt to give the block or after the blocks. Occasionally, the patient will describe being "so much worse" even a few days after the blocks. Patients who do not tolerate the nerve block are never surgical candidates.

It is recommended that successful nerve blocks can be repeated on more than one occasion to ensure that a positive response with pain relief is not purely due to a placebo effect from the injection.

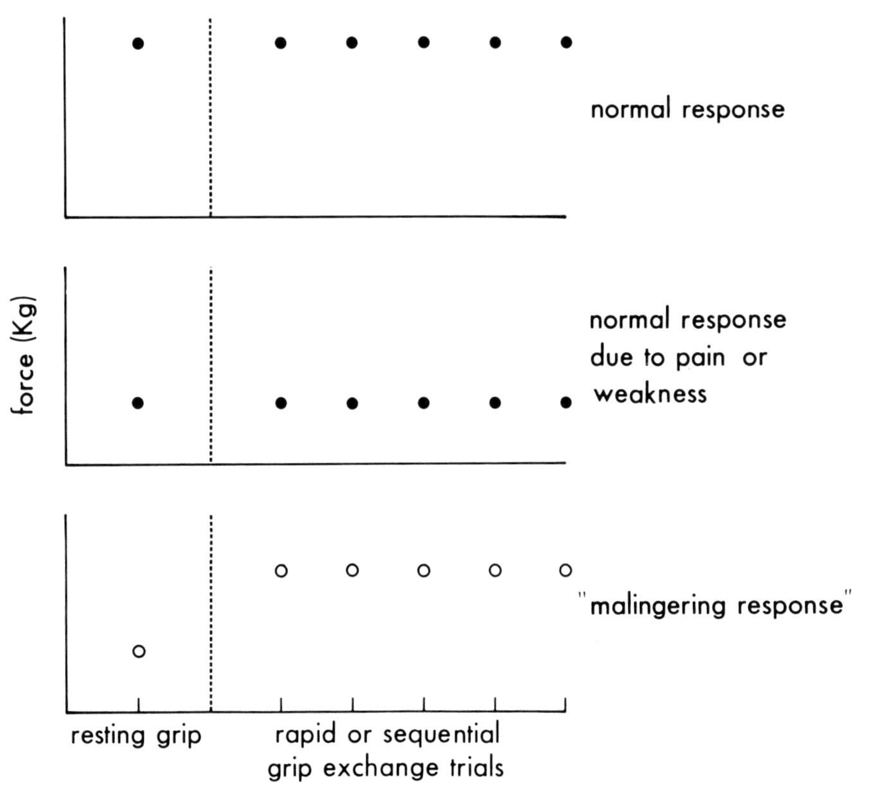

Figure 17-13. Using the rapid exchange grip test, the patient's grip in both hands is tested at the optimum setting. In the isolated, single test, the patient may record a significant difference between the grip strength in the two hands. During rapid exchange grip testing, the strength in the "pathological hand" will approach that in the normal hand if the patient is noncompliant or malingering. Patients with true pathology will not be able to generate a greater strength in the pathologic hand even during the rapid exchange grip test. The points recorded in this figure represent tests from the pathologic hand only, not the normal hand.

Sensory Testing

Sensory testing can also be used to assess the unreliable or "malingering" patient. Several of the tests will be new to the patient and therefore he will not have a rehearsed set of answers or responses.

Using the two-point discriminator (Disk-criminator™), when the examiner nears the patients' limit or actual level of two-point discrimination, the patient will often ask the examiner to push a little harder or the examiner will note that the patient moves his finger up toward the testing instrument to perceive more information from the testing instrument. If the patient makes no such effort, it is suggestive of perhaps less than total compliance on the part of the patient. The 256 cps tuning fork can be used in a similar fashion because frequently the patient has not previously experienced this sensory stimulus. Thus, unlike "light touch" where the patient has prepatterned himself to deny recognition of this touch stimulus the patient will have no such set response to tuning fork stimulation. It is wise to present the first vibration stimulus to the area in question and watch carefully for the patient's response. If the stimulus is presented first to the normal hand, this may be all the "information" the patient needs in order to pattern an "appropriate" response in the other hand. A vibrometer with a consistent frequency and variable amplitude will be extremely helpful in assessing such patients but unfortunately is also expensive (Fig. 17-14).

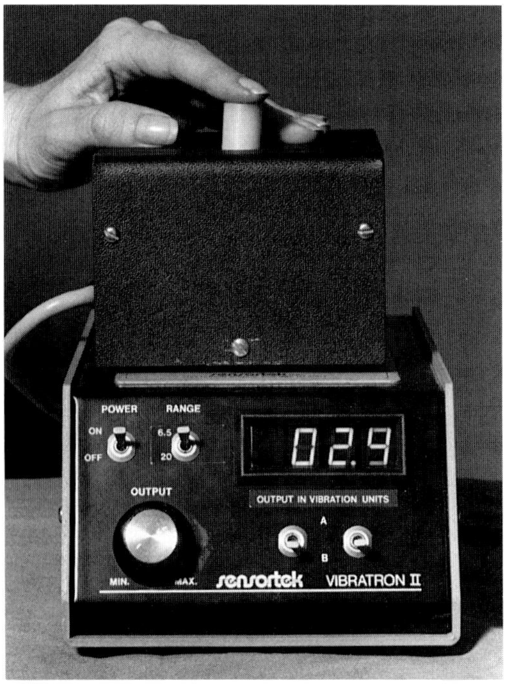

Figure 17-14. A fixed frequency (120 cps) variable amplitude vibrometer with a digital printout is extremely useful in evaluating sensory patterns in all patients, including those who are unreliable or even malingering.

Although the tests described may be time consuming, we have found them extremely helpful in conjunction with the standard assessment (see Chapter 3) in evaluating these very difficult patients. They have been predictive of the surgical result, because, unfortunately, in some patients even the best surgical procedure may be doomed to failure if the patient has a tremendous functional overlay, no pain tolerance, or is outright malingering.

Algorithm for the Management of the Painful Neuroma

Based on clinical and experimental studies, an algorithm for the management of painful neuroma can be described[40] (Table 17-4). The ultimate goal in treating the patient with the painful neuroma will be both to relieve pain and to restore nerve function. Reestablishing continuity in the peripheral nervous system will help to reverse the neuropathologic consequences that occur at various levels in the peripheral nerve spinal cord and central nervous system after nerve injury.

In general, the surgical management of the painful neuroma follows three basic principles:

1. If appropriate distal nerve and sensory receptors are available, a nerve graft can be used to direct the regenerating nerve fibers from the proximal stump distally into normal nerve and sensory receptors. This will reverse the changes that occur along the peripheral nerve and central nervous system subsequent to division of the sensory nerve. At the same time, it will restore sensory function.
2. If a distal nerve is not available and restoration of function in the injured nerve is critical (such as the thumb) innervated free tissue transfers can be used to accept the regenerating nerves from the injured sensory nerve (such as innervated great toe, wrap around flap or innervated full-thickness skin graft, skin flap, or neurovascular island flap).[41,42]
3. If function in the injured nerve is not critical or if the treatment outlined fails, or the distal nerve stump is not available (such as amputation neuroma) or if the tissue bed and local environment are not suitable for a nerve graft (such as sural nerve at the ankle, radial sensory nerve near the wrist),[43] then the neuroma is resected and the proximal stump of the nerve is transposed into an area that is subjected to the least amount of mechanical stimulation.

The management of the painful neuroma throughout the body is based on these three principles. It will be modified only slightly from region to region in the body.

Table 17-4. Surgical Algorithm for Management of Painful Neuroma

- Neuroma resection
  - Arm → Bone
  - Wrist Forearm
    - Critical sensation → Nerve graft
    - Noncritical → Brachioradialis muscle
  - Hand
    - Critical sensation
      - Distal nerve stump Available → Nerve graft → Provide innervated free tissue
      - No distal nerve → Provide innervated free tissue → Bone
    - Noncritical
      - Distal nerve available → Nerve graft → Bone
      - No distal nerve → Bone
  - Lower Extremity
    - Critical sensation → Nerve graft
    - Noncritical
      - Bone
      - Soleus muscle

*Reprinted with permission from Mackinnon and Dellon.[40]

Digital Neuromas

Digital neuromas in *nonamputated digits* are best managed with a nerve graft or a bioabsorbable nerve tube that is used to reestablish continuity of the nervous system (Fig. 17-15). The nerve grafts commonly used are the lateral antebrachial cutaneous nerve or the anterior branch of the medial antebrachial cutaneous nerve. Occasionally, the terminal sensory branch of the posterior interosseous nerve has been used. More recently, nerve tubes have been used to reestablish continuity (see Chapter 20). These nerve tubes are made of polyglycolic acid and being biodegradable are only used to manage the short nerve gap. Nerve tubes are especially useful in the management of digital neuromas in that the patient does not have to experience a new area of sensory loss, a new scar, or potentially a new site of pain from the proximally divided end of the donor nerve. These "neuroma" patients tend to be more susceptible to painful donor site neuromas than patients not complaining postoperatively of painful neuromas.

If a digit is amputated, preoperative evaluation, including anesthetic nerve blocks, may be critical in determining exactly what nerves are involved in the painful neuroma. If a single digital nerve is involved, the painful neuroma is resected and the nerve implanted into bone (Fig. 17-16). If both digital nerves are involved, the amputation is revised with care not to denervate the finger pulp. This will require shortening of the digit so that the digital nerves are skeletonized and

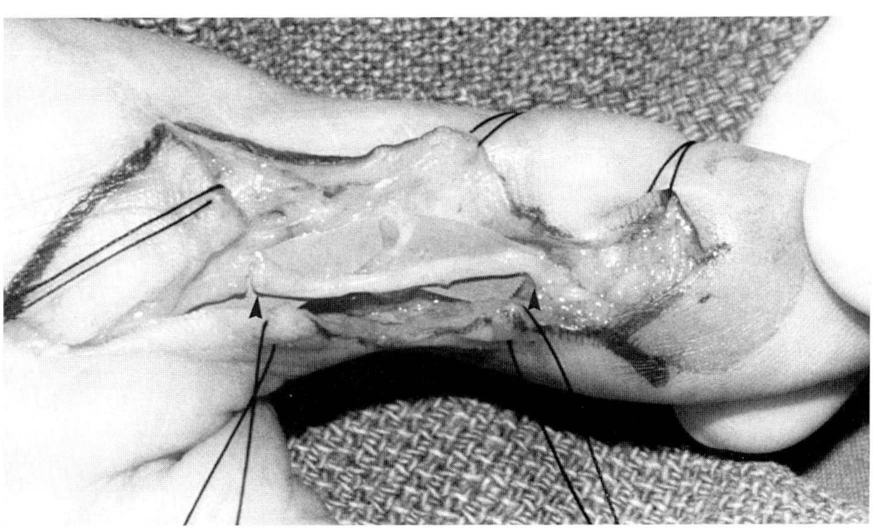

Figure 17-15. A defect in the ulnar digital nerve to the thumb is managed with a nerve graft from the lateral antebrachial cutaneous nerve. (arrows)

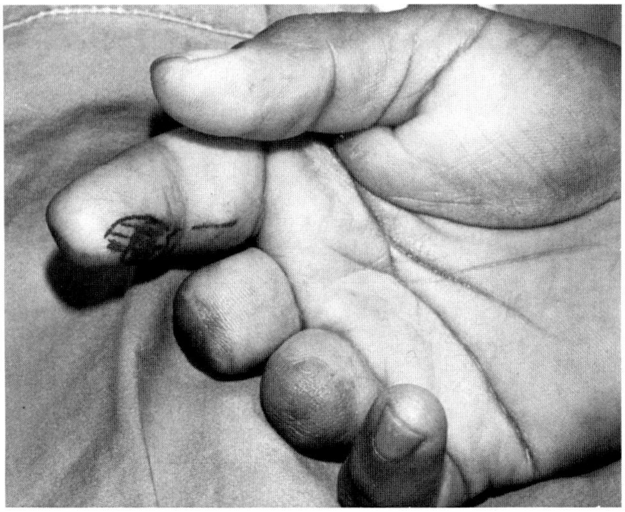
a

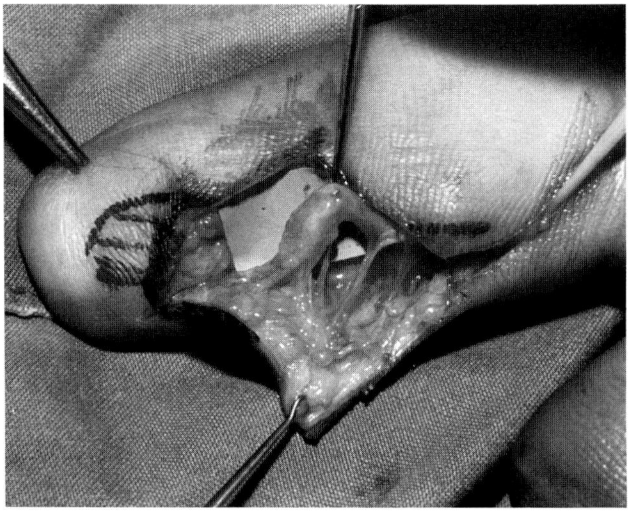
b

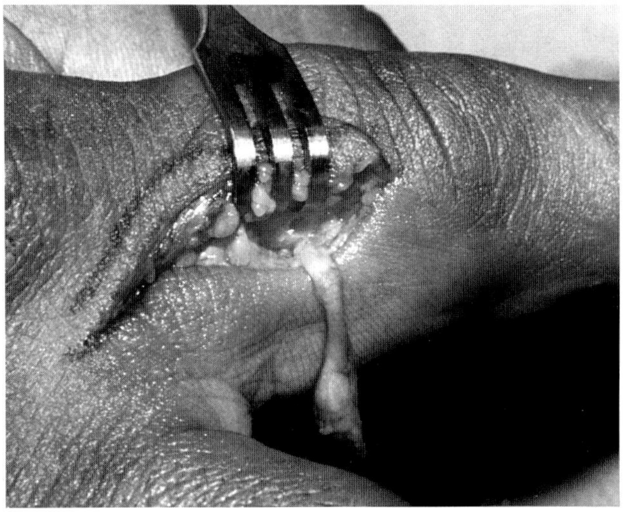
c

Figure 17-16a. The ulnar digital nerve of the index finger was the only nerve with a symptomatic neuroma in this patient with multiple amputations. **b.** Attempted regeneration from the injured digital nerve into the overlying skin is demonstrated. **c.** The neuroma is exposed and the nerve transferred to the dorsum and placed into the ulnar side of the proximal phalanx. (Reproduced with permission from Mackinnon and Dellon.[40])

the skin flaps that are left are not denervated. Denervated sensory receptors will provide a neurotrop(h)ic target for injured sensory nerves in the area and may result in hyperalgesia from abnormal sensory reinnervation of the denervated skin. The terminal branches of the digital nerves are dissected so that remaining skin is innervated. The digital nerves are then transferred into the bone with no tension on the nerves as they enter the phalanx. An epineurial-periosteal nylon suture will hold the nerve in place as it enters the bone. The digit and hand are moved before choosing the appropriate bone implantation site so that there will be no tension on the digital nerve when the hand and fingers are moved. Injured dorsal digital branches may be treated in the same fashion.

Neuromas of the common digital nerves or digital nerves in the palm can be treated with a nerve graft or nerve tube as the initial method of management. If these methods fail, the nerve is exposed in the palm and transferred dorsally away from the palmar contact surface of the hand and implanted into bone, thus sacrificing the cutaneous sensation distribution of the digital nerve involved (Fig. 17-17). We have not found muscle implantation in the hand to be satisfactory because these muscles are small, offering little bulk to pad the neuromas and have significant excursion.

Ray amputations present a very significant problem and a documented high incidence of postoperative painful sequela has been reported after this operation. In reviewing 49 patients with ray amputations, Murray[44] found that 50% of these patients were bothered with significant pain and 10% had pain in the region of the first web space that was totally disabling. In carrying out the primary ray amputation, great care is taken not to denervate the skin flaps by proximally cutting back the nerves. Rather, all terminal sensory nerve entering the digit are identified, dissected, and left long to facilitate transposition into bone. This will usually involve both

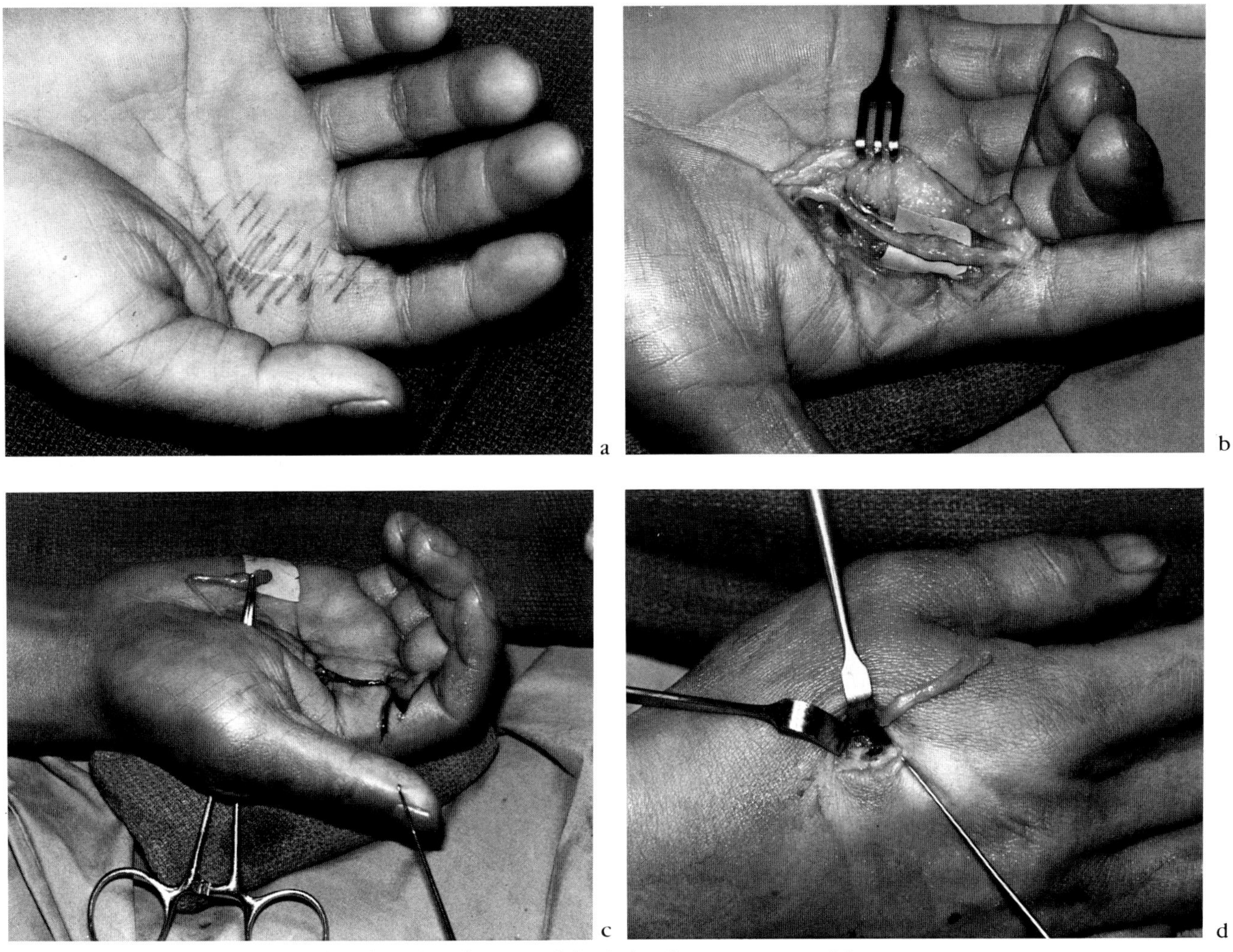

Figure 17-17a. A neuroma of the ulnar digital nerve of the index finger was treated by a short nerve graft. Eighteen months later, the patient still experienced neuromatous type pain in the palm as well as anesthesia in the atonomous zone of the ulnar digital nerve. **b.** The nerve graft was exposed in the palm of the hand and excised. **c.** The digital nerve was transferred to the dorsum of the hand. **d.** The digital nerve was transposed into the second metacarpal with care so that no tension was placed on the nerve as it entered the bone.

dorsal and palmar branches of the digital nerves to the index finger as well as terminal branches of the radial sensory nerves (Fig. 17-18).

For patients with significant pain after ray amputation (which has usually involved just proximally cutting the nerves involved), a very detailed critical examination is necessary. This will involve blocking initially the radial sensory nerve to determine the component of the pain in the web space, which is due to this nerve. In the occasional patient, this will be the only nerve that is giving the patient significant problems. This is best managed by transferring the radial sensory nerve proximally into the brachioradialis muscle. In the majority of instances, the digital nerves to the amputated index finger are the primary cause of the amputation pain. Thus, in most patients, excision of the large neuroma and transposition of the digital nerves involved to the dorsum of the hand and location of these digital nerves in the second metacarpal has proved successful in significantly alleviating pain. (Suturing the two digital nerves to each other [neurocampsis] has not proved effective in our experience.) Through a standard carpal tunnel incision, the affected digital nerves are identified proximally in the wrist and with microneu-

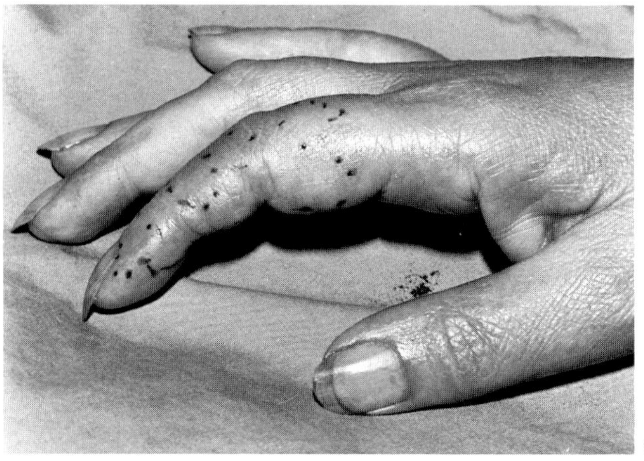

a

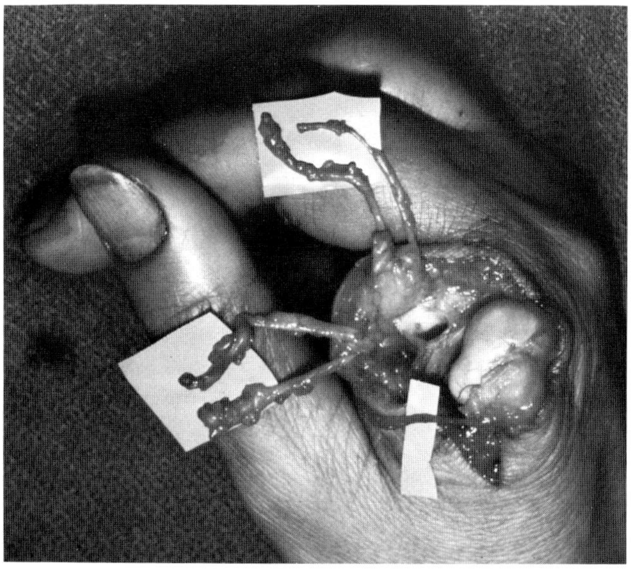

b

Figure 17-18a. After multiple failed procedures, including neurolysis and nerve grafting, this patient continued to have severe pain in the index finger. Subsequently, a ray amputation was performed. **b.** Both digital and dorsal digital nerves as well as a branch of the radial sensory nerve were identified entering the index finger. Care was taken to make sure the skin flaps were left well innervated. The metacarpal was then amputated at a proximal level and the five nerves were placed in the second metacarpal with no tension on the nerves. (Reproduced with permission from Mackinnon and Dellon.[40])

rosurgical technique, the fascicles that are innervating the neuroma can be separated carefully from the main median nerve. The neuroma, which is usually found to be innervating the overlying skin, is excised and the digital nerves are transferred to the dorsum of the hand through the interosseous muscles. Much care must be taken to ensure that the digital nerves in their bone implantation site are placed here in a relaxed, tension-free fashion so that movement of the wrist will not cause tension or any pulling on the nerves. It may be necessary to rotate a small flap of dorsal interosseous muscle and fascia to cover the bone implantation site.

A critical examination of the hand will determine if injury has occurred to the digital nerves to the remaining long finger and thumb. In some patients who have had several operative procedures in order to control the neuromas in the index finger, injury may have occurred to the adjacent nerves of the thumb and long fingers. In these cases, it has been appropriate to use a nerve grafting technique to direct fibers from the amputated index finger and the thumb or long finger into the remaining distal nerves that had had associated digital nerve injury. In these instances, the proximal nerve fibers will greatly outnumber the distal nerve fibers. Care must be taken to divide the nerve fibers proximally at a level so that there is essentially normal nerve architecture because more distally with increasing scar tissue, the size match will be even greater. In these instances, we have used a nerve tube fashioned in a cone shape to allow the discrepancy between the proximal end of the median nerve and the nerve graft to be accommodated (Fig. 17-19) (see Chapter 20).

In patients with significant pain after ray amputation, as a salvage procedure, we have had good success diverting the involved nerves up the forearm into the brachioradialis muscle with long sural nerve grafts.[45] Previously painful digital nerve fibers are, thus, directed along the sural nerve graft and finally into the brachioradialis muscle (Fig. 17-20). In a similar fashion, the involved fascicles have, on occasion, been dissected free from the main median nerve to the mid forearm level (Fig. 17-21). This in some patients is possible because of the lack of plexus formation between the median nerve fascicles in the distal and mid forearm. In these instances, a sural nerve graft was not necessary in order to prolong the nerve and direct the nerves into the brachioradial muscle. Rather the involved fascicles have been "flip flopped" back into the brachioradialis without requiring a nerve graft. These are salvage types of operations to be used in a small select group of patients.

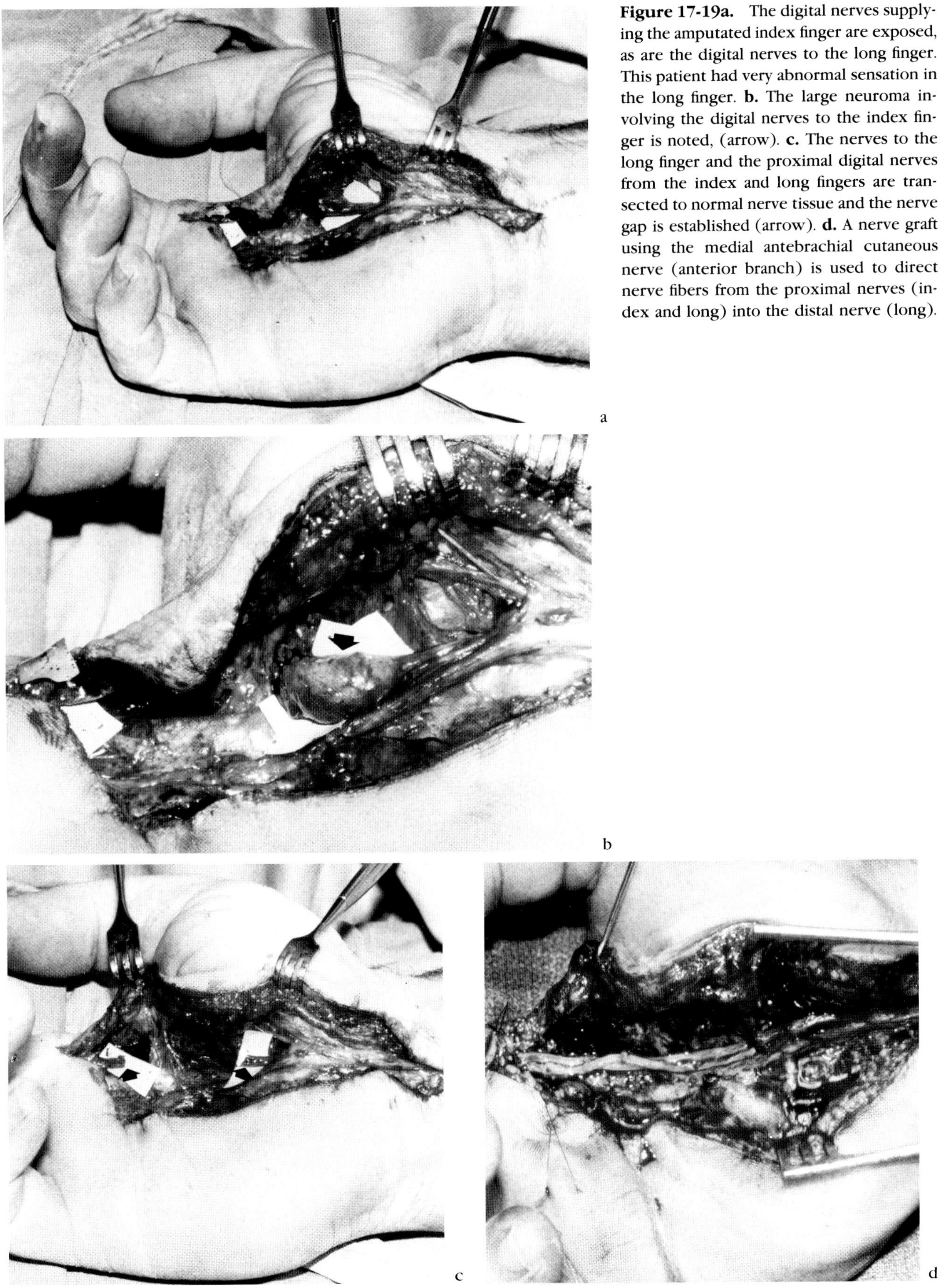

Figure 17-19a. The digital nerves supplying the amputated index finger are exposed, as are the digital nerves to the long finger. This patient had very abnormal sensation in the long finger. **b.** The large neuroma involving the digital nerves to the index finger is noted, (arrow). **c.** The nerves to the long finger and the proximal digital nerves from the index and long fingers are transected to normal nerve tissue and the nerve gap is established (arrow). **d.** A nerve graft using the medial antebrachial cutaneous nerve (anterior branch) is used to direct nerve fibers from the proximal nerves (index and long) into the distal nerve (long).

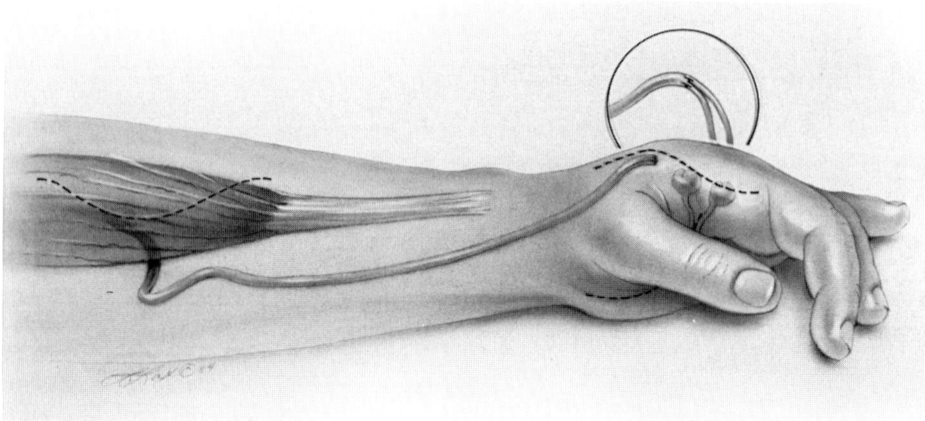

a

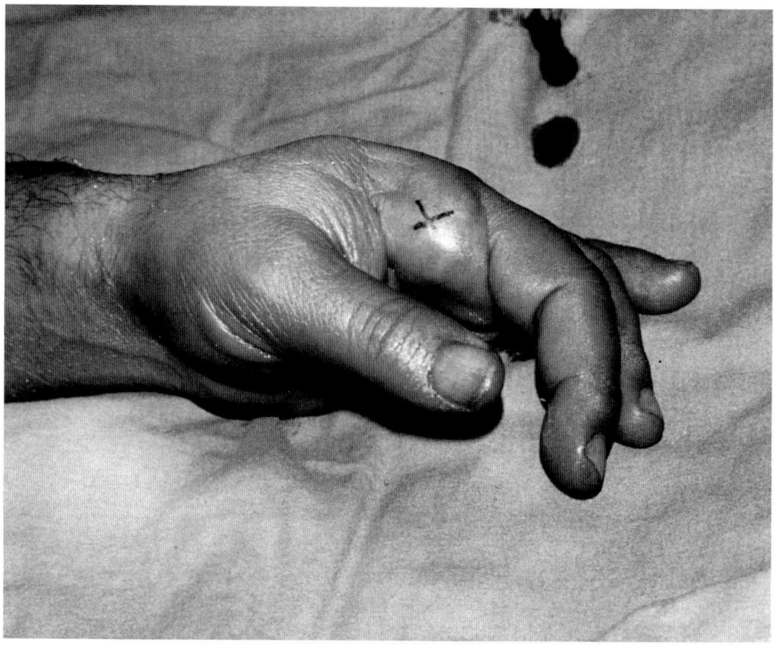

b

Figure 17-20a. The operative procedure is outlined diagrammatically. A standard carpal incision is extended into the hand in order to identify the neuromas to the amputated index finger. A second incision is made on the dorsum in order to carry out the epineural repair between the nerve graft and the dorsally transposed digital nerves. A third incision is made just volar to the region of the muscle belly of the brachioradialis muscle. A sural nerve graft is tunneled subcutaneously underneath the forearm. Incision, broken lines, nerve repair, (inset). **b.** The maximum area of tenderness is marked in the first web space. This was surrounded by an area of shiny erythematous skin and exquisite hyperalgesia. (*Figure continues.*)

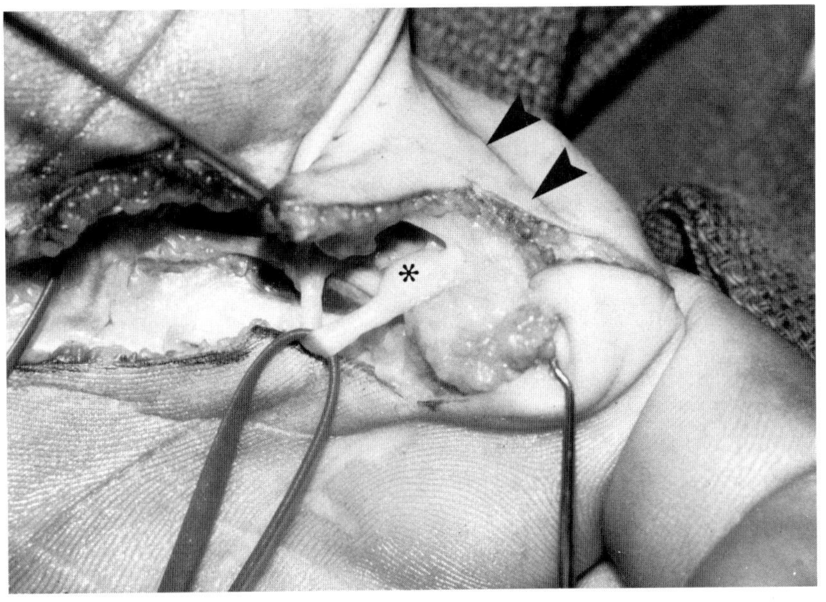

c

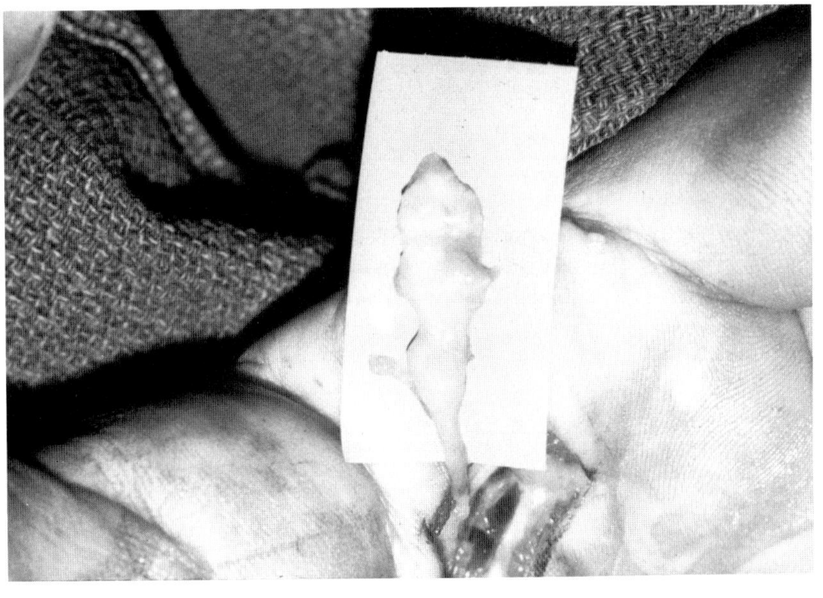

d

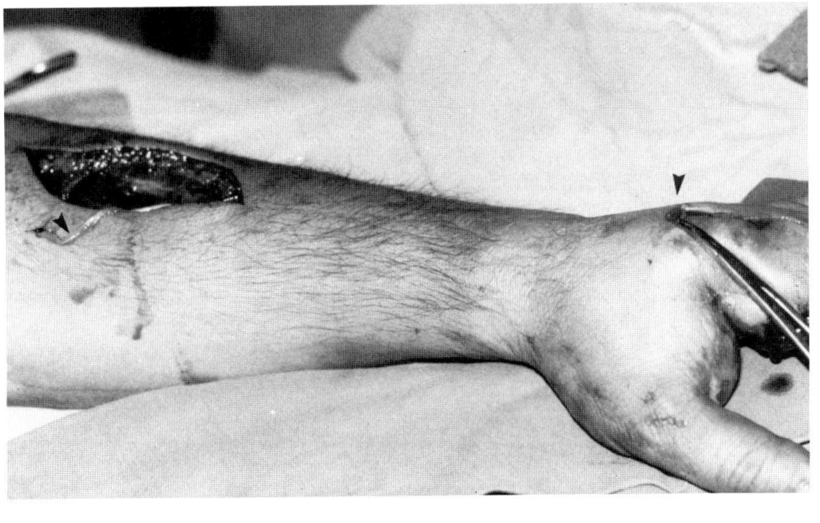

e

Figure 17-20 (*continued*) **c.** A vessel loop is placed about the radial digital nerve to the amputated index finger. A small, smooth neuroma is noted (*). This neuroma is adherent to the scar and dermis in the first web space and traction on this digital nerve causes indrawing of the skin of the first web space (arrow). Thumb top left, long finger to right of photograph. **d.** This neuroma is in-continuity with scar tissue. Long finger to right of photograph. **e.** The digital nerves are transposed dorsally. A sural nerve graft (arrow) is tunneled subcutaneously along the forearm and brought out in the proximal wound near the brachioradialis muscle. (Reproduced with permission from Mackinnon.[45])

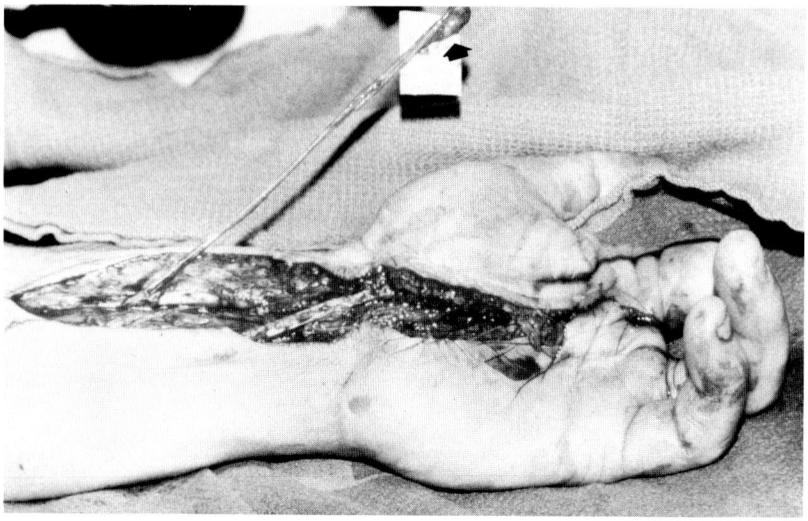

Figure 17-21. Flip-flop operation, the radial digital nerve to the thumb innervates a neuroma (arrow). They are dissected from the median nerve and then transposed proximally and the distal end is buried in the brachioradialis muscle.

The success rate with the latter two procedures is 75%.

Techniques that involve excision of the hyperalgesic skin in the first web space with subsequent resurfacing procedures are to be condemned.[46] With time, the nerve endings will once again reinnervate the skin graft or flap in the web space and usually the pain returns with even more vengeance. We have had success in dealing with some of these problems with use of soft tissue expanders in the hand.[47] The dorsum of the hand is expanded so that the painful skin grafted area can be excised and resurfaced with full-thickness innervated dorsal skin. This limits the neurotrophic effect of the skin graft for the sensory nerves. It will, of course, be critical to deal appropriately with the digital neuromas after the resurfacing procedure has been carried out (Fig. 17-19).

Dorsoradial Wrist Neuromas

At the level of the wrist, the management of the neuroma is influenced by several factors. The significant amount of movement across the wrist and the lack of good local tissues often will dictate against nerve grafting except in the instances of nerves that subserve critical sensation. At the level of the wrist, nerve grafting for management of the painful radial sensory or lateral antebrachial cutaneous neuroma is discouraged. Although it is technically possible to reinnervate the distal territory of these nerves, it is our clinical experience that the range of motion about the wrist puts considerable tension on the nerve repair sites and the relatively poor soft tissue covering at the level of the wrist is often associated with scar formation between the radial sensory nerve graft and the underlying tendons and the overlying skin.[43,48] This may result in successful reinnervation of the dorsoradial aspect of the hand but pain may persist at the level of the nerve graft repair sites. We have described four cases in which a nerve graft of the radial sensory nerve was successful in restoring sensibility to the dorsum of the hand.[43] It failed, however, in controlling pain. When these nerve grafts were reexplored, proximal and distal suture line neuromas were noted at the proximal and distal ends of the nerve graft. Histologic evaluation of the nerve grafts demonstrated excellent regeneration across the nerve grafts and into the distal radial sensory nerve (Table 17-5; Fig. 17-22). The treatment chosen for these patients with pain after this nerve grafting procedure was neuroma resection and implantation of the radial sensory nerve into the brachioradialis muscle.

Table 17-5. Light Morphometric Analysis of SBR Nerve Graft*

	Proximal	*Graft*	*Distal*
Mean fiber diameter (μm) SD	6.9 ± 2.5	4.1 ± 1.7	3.9 ± 1.5
Total number fibers	5639	6417	4698

*Reprinted with permission from Dellon and Mackinnon.[43]

Radial Sensory/Lateral Antebrachial Nerve Overlap

Patients with persistent sensation over the dorsoradial aspect of their hand after resection of the radial sensory nerve demonstrated innervation of this area from the lateral antebrachial cutaneous nerve. Neuromas of the lateral antebrachial cutaneous could be present in addition to or instead of what was assumed to be a neuroma of the radial sensory nerve. This finding stimulated a study of the overlap pattern between the radial sensory nerve and the lateral antebrachial cutaneous nerve.[49]

Ninety-four human upper extremities were dissected to delineate the overlap relationship between

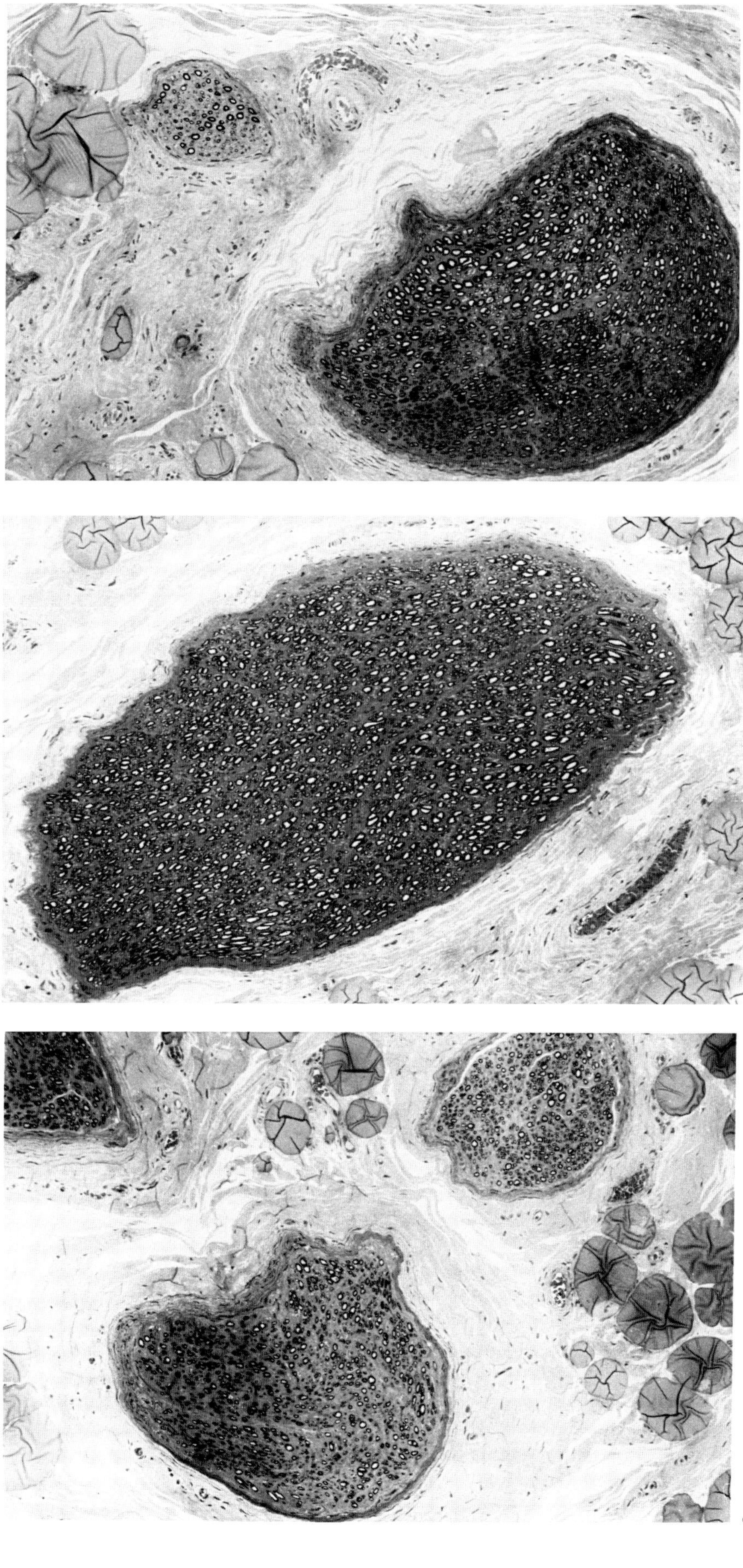

Figure 17-22a. Histologic section demonstrating the radial sensory nerve proximal to the nerve graft. **b.** Section through the center of the nerve graft. **c.** Distal to the area of nerve graft. Note little difference between the proximal and distal section, suggesting that the graft has successfully served as a conduit for nerve regeneration (Toluidine blue; ×120.) (*Figure continues.*)

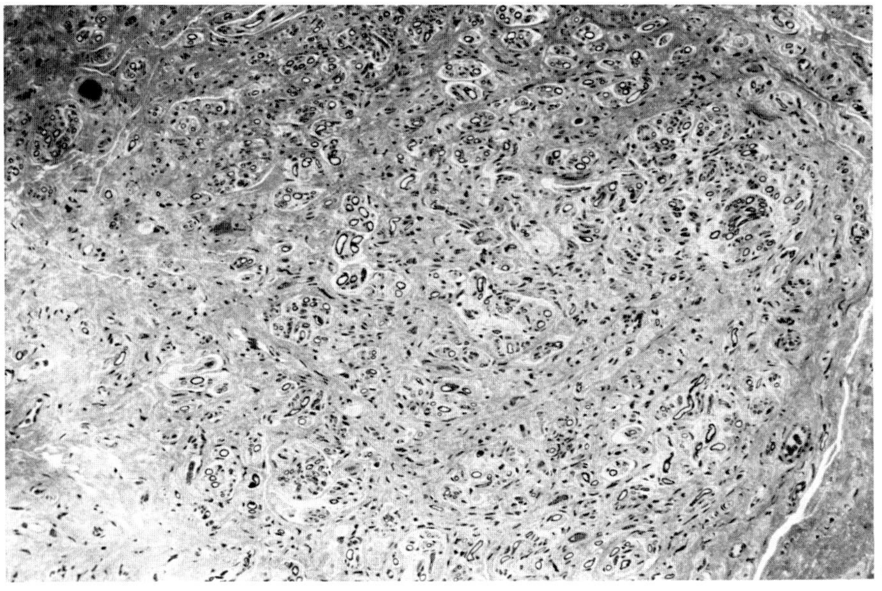

Figure 17-22 (*continued*) **d.** Histologic section through juncture of graft and radial sensory nerve. Appearance is one of a classic neuroma in-continuity. (Toluidine blue; ×120.) (Reproduced with permission from Dellon & Mackinnon.[43])

these two nerves. Of these dissections, 41 were clinical cases explored for neuromas, direct nerve injury, or nerve compression. Fifty-three were carried out in cadaver specimens. This study demonstrated that there was partial or complete overlap of the lateral antebrachial cutaneous nerve on the territory generally presumed to be that of the radial sensory in 75% of the dissected extremities (Fig. 10-2). Invariably, the lateral antebrachial cutaneous nerve had fibers that were thinner and more superficial to those of the radial sensory nerve (Fig. 17-23). From these dissections, it is apparent that occasionally a branch of the posterior cutaneous nerve, the palmar cutaneous nerve, or the dorsocutaneous branch of the ulnar nerve can innervate this dorsoradial area. Thus, it becomes essential in the evaluation and treatment of a neuroma in the dorsoradial aspect of the wrist to be aware of overlap patterns and attempt to distinguish the clinical importance of the nerves in innervating the neuromas preoperatively by serial diagnostic nerve blocks. We have also found the presence of a Tinel sign along the course of the affected nerve proximal to the region of the neuroma helpful in determining which cutaneous nerves are innervating the neuroma. Palpation along the proximal course of a cutaneous nerve that is innervating a neuroma will often produce a Tinel response along the course of the nerve several centimeters proximal to the level of the actual neuroma. This is probably related to the fact that regenerating nerve fibers not only regenerate distally into the overlying skin and scar tissue to form the neuroma itself but may also turn on themselves and regenerate proximally up the injured nerve for a varying distance along the course of the nerve. Regenerating fibers in the neuroma then use the parent nerve as a nerve graft type of material along which to regenerate. This proximal regeneration of fibers from the neuroma would account for the Tinel sign along the proximal course of the nerve. This finding is very useful in determining which cutaneous nerves are innervating the neuroma. This maneuver must always be supplemented with confirmatory diagnostic nerve blocks.

Thus, in the management of the dorsoradial wrist neuroma, we suggest careful and often repeated preoperative examination of the patient. This will be supplemented with diagnostic nerve blocks commencing with the nerve least likely to be involved in the neuroma. Preblock pinch and grip strength and wrist range of motion are measured. The blocks are carried out in the proximal forearm well away from the neuroma itself. The technique of diagnostic nerve blocks is demonstrated in Figure 17-24. The lateral antebrachial cutaneous nerve is adjacent to the cephalic vein. This vein is usually not visible in the proximal forearm but is frequently palpable and lies at the junction between the lateral and middle thirds of the forearm at the medial border of the brachioradialis muscle. The lateral antebrachial cutaneous nerve lies on the muscle fascia. After blocking this nerve, the patient is encouraged to reevaluate the degree of pain at the wrist after 15 to 20 minutes. The strength and range of motion are measured again. The amount of improvement they experience in the pain at the wrist is a good indicator of the amount of involvement of the lateral antebrachial cutaneous nerve in the neuroma formation. The radial sensory nerve is then blocked and the measurements repeated. The posterior cutaneous nerve of the forearm is only occasionally involved in these neuromas and usually when the injury is in a more proximal and a

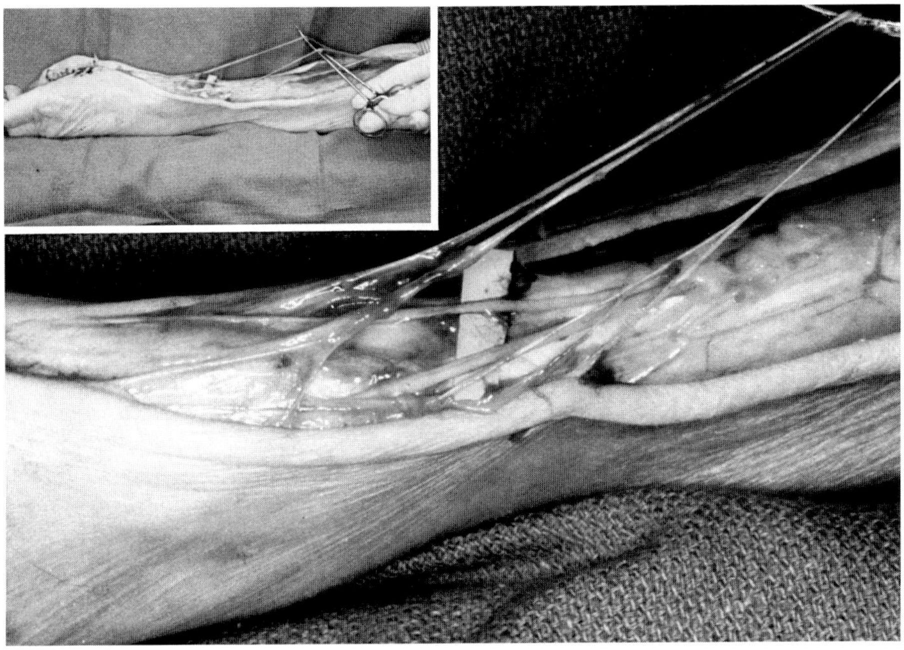

a

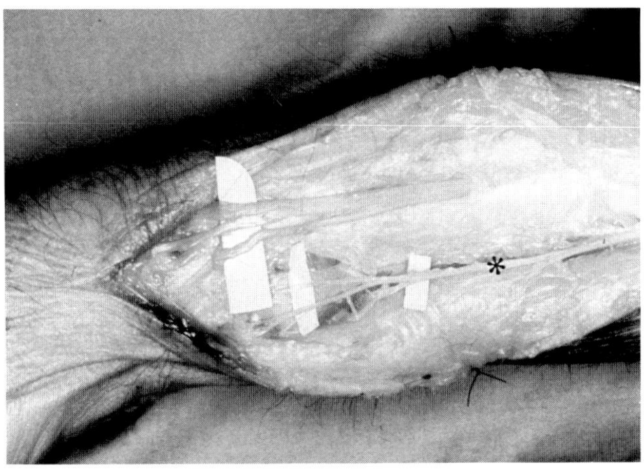

b

Figure 17-23a. Cadaveric dissection of the radial sensory nerve (visibility background) and the lateral antebrachial cutaneous nerve (held on a hemostat) with an overview of the arm (**inset**). The lateral antebrachial cutaneous nerve completely overlaps the territory of the radial sensory nerve and is just superficial to the radial sensory nerve. **b.** The radial sensory and the lateral antebrachial cutaneous (*) demonstrates no overlap. This pattern was found in 25% of dissections. (Reproduced with permission from Mackinnon and Dellon.[49])

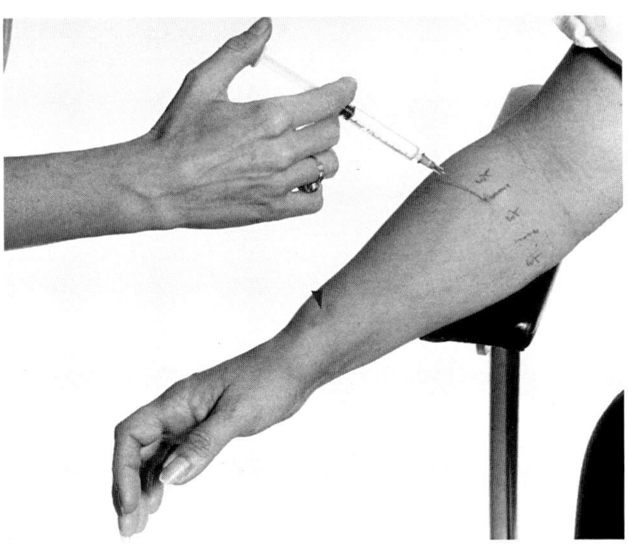

a

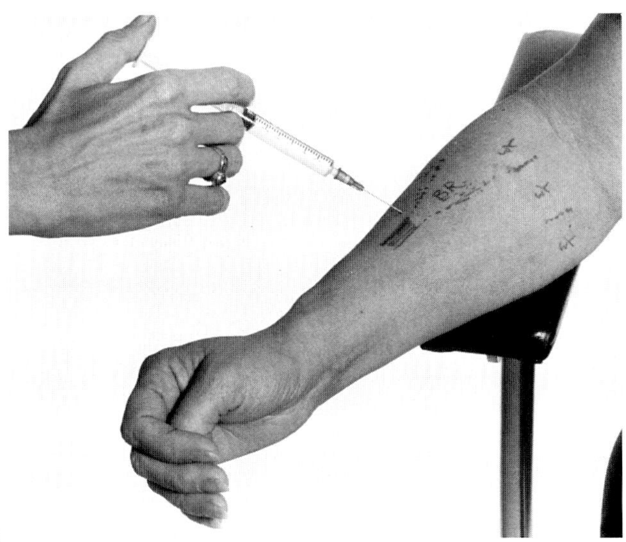

b

Figure 17-24a. The lateral antebrachial cutaneous nerve is blocked in the proximal forearm. The forearm is "divided" longitudinally into thirds. The nerve lies adjacent to the cephalic vein at the junction of the lateral and middle thirds. It lies just medial to the brachioradialis muscle. The patient had pain at the wrist after a previous de Quervain's release (arrow). **b.** The radial sensory nerve lies just dorsal to the musculotendinous junction of the brachioradialis muscle.

more dorsal location. The posterior cutaneous nerve of the forearm is identified on the posterior aspect of the brachioradialis muscle. The radial sensory nerve becomes superficial at the musculotendinous junction of the brachioradialis muscle in the interval between the extensory carpi radialis longus and the brachioradialis tendon. The anatomy of the brachioradialis muscle is critical in determining the location of the nerve blocks with the lateral antebrachial cutaneous lying on the medial border of the brachioradialis muscle and the posterior cutaneous nerve of the forearm lying on the posterior border of the brachioradialis muscle. The radial sensory nerve becomes superficial just at the point where the brachioradialis muscles become tendinous. Thus, a useful maneuver in locating these nerves is to encourage the patient to demonstrate resisted elbow flexion in order to mark out the limits of the brachioradialis muscle. Thus, in the management of the dorsoradial wrist neuromas we suggest careful and often repetitive preoperative examination of the patient with diagnostic nerve blocks.

Surgical Treatment

Our experience in the management of more than 100 patients with dorsoradial neuromas has facilitated a surgical technique that has evolved through the experience in dealing with these patients. The majority of these patients had recurrent dorsoradial neuromas, which had failed to respond to the standard methods of treatment.

Surgery is only considered if, after careful preoperative analysis of the neuroma with diagnostic nerve blocks, satisfactory pain relief is experienced. The patient is taken to the operating room and the procedure carried out under tourniquet control. A lazy S type of incision is made in the region of the proximal forearm just dorsal to the lateral antebrachial cutaneous nerve. The lateral antebrachial cutaneous nerve will be identified at the junction between the lateral and middle thirds of the forearm. With loupe magnification, the branches of the lateral antebrachial cutaneous nerve are identified adjacent to the cephalic vein. The surgeon is encouraged to identify the vein initially and then note the lateral antebrachial cutaneous adjacent to this vein. The vein is an easily identified landmark, and the lateral antebrachial cutaneous nerve will be noted in the soft tissue around the vein. There are usually two branches at this forearm level and these branches of the lateral antebrachial cutaneous nerve are carefully identified and vessel loops placed around the nerve. The radial sensory nerve will be found adjacent to the radial artery and associated veins deep to the brachioradialis muscle. Thus, the brachioradialis muscle is retracted laterally in order to identify the radial sensory nerve. A vessel loop is placed around this nerve. The neuroma, in the more distal forearm, is then identified. Traction on the radial sensory nerve and the lateral antebrachial cutaneous nerve will demonstrate movement of the distal neuroma if these nerves are, indeed, innervating the neuroma. This finding will confirm the findings of the diagnostic nerve blocks. The neuroma is then excised and the nerves innervating the neuroma are divided in the mid forearm and transferred into the proximal incision. The nerves are then directed in the proximal direction into the brachioradialis muscle from the undersurface of the brachioradialis muscle (Fig. 17-25). Several attempts at

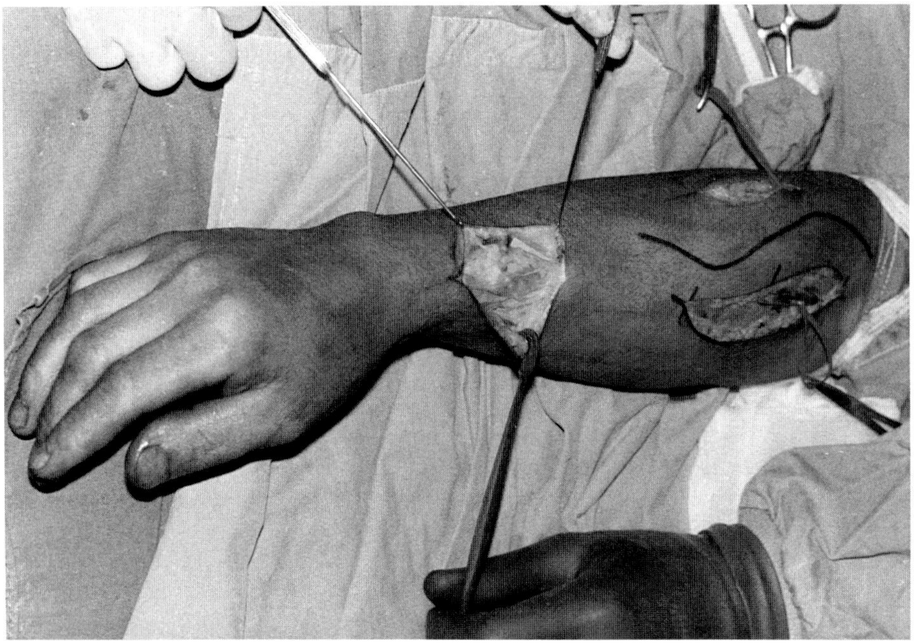

Figure 17-25a. The cutaneous nerves innervating the neuroma are identified proximally. (*Figure continues.*)

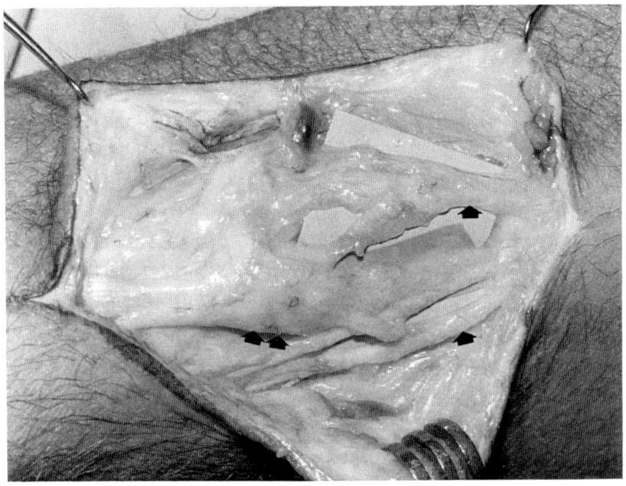

b

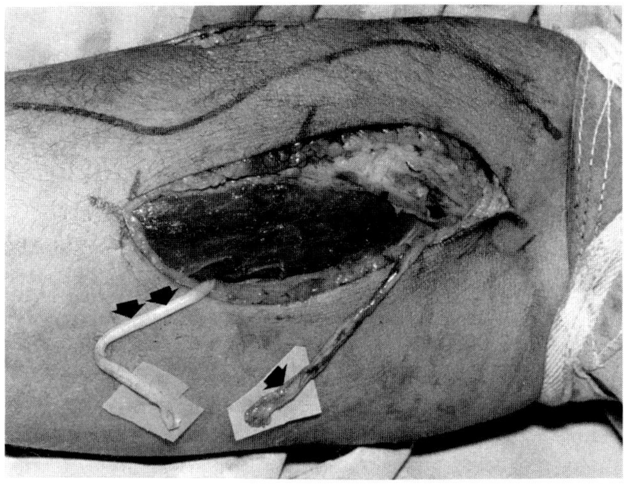

c

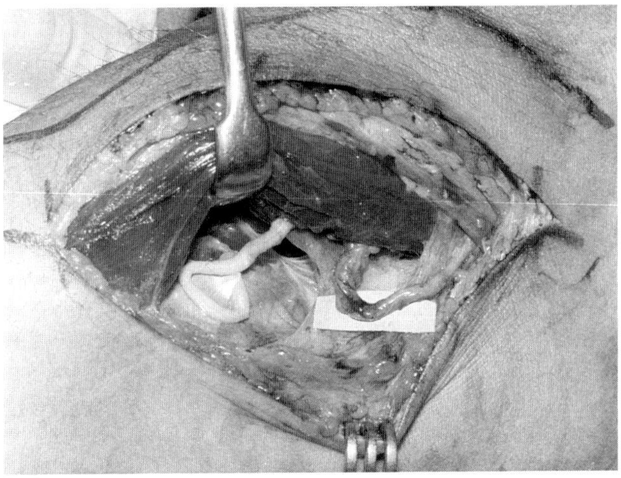

d

Figure 17-25 *(continued)* **b.** The neuroma at the level of the wrist was found to involve the lateral antebrachial cutaneous nerve (arrow) and the sensory branch of the radial nerve (double arrow). Sutures from a previous attempt to repair an injury to the sensory branch of the radial nerve can be seen. The neuroma at the level of the wrist was completely excised. **c.** The lateral antebrachial cutaneous nerve (arrow) and the sensory branch of the radial nerve (double arrow) are divided proximally in the forearm. **d.** These nerves are then implanted into the brachioradialis muscle from the undersurface of the brachioradialis and directed in a proximal direction. Care is taken to place no tension on the nerve as it enters the muscle and the nerves are held in place as they enter the muscle with an epineurial suture. (Reproduced with permission from Dellon and Mackinnon.[29])

positioning these nerves correctly in the mid portion of the muscle belly may be required. The elbow is moved in order to ensure that the nerves do not pull out of the muscle when the elbow is fully extended. An epineurial/muscle suture will hold the nerves in place as they enter the muscle. The nerves will enter the muscle with no tension on the nerves. An intradermal, absorbable, suture is usually used for skin closure. The procedure is schematically outlined in Figure 17-26. The arm is then placed in a well-padded dressing with support for the wrist and elbow. In 7 to 10 days, the patient is allowed gentle elbow movement, recalling that the action of the brachioradialis will involve elbow flexion.

Clinical Evaluation and Results

Analysis of the clinical results of all patients is outlined in Figure 17-27. Analysis of the results as they relate to previous operative procedures directed for pain relief is outlined in Figure 17-28. The patients treated for the first time (primary neuroma) had 60% with excellent and 40% with good pain relief. The patients who had three or more operations for pain relief (subgroup of recurrent neuromas) had 21% with excellent and 35% with good pain relief. The difference between these two groups was statistically significant ($p < 0.05$). In the group of patients for whom this was their second operation, that is, their first treatment of a recurrent neuroma, there was excellent pain relief in 58% and good pain relief in 30%. There was a significant difference in the results of treating this group versus the primary treatment group ($p < 0.05$). The results of all three clinical groups are noted in Table 17-6.

Analysis of the patients as to whether or not Workers' Compensation was involved in the injury is noted in Figure 17-29. The difference between 30% poor result of the Workers' Compensation group and 11% poor results of the non-Workers' Compensation group did not reach clinical significance ($p < 0.08$). However, when Workers' Compensation patients were evaluated as to whether or not they were actually employed or working, it was apparent that those patients who were employed and working achieved better results than those patients who were not ($p < 0.01$). A recent study has suggested that the critical feature of the effect of

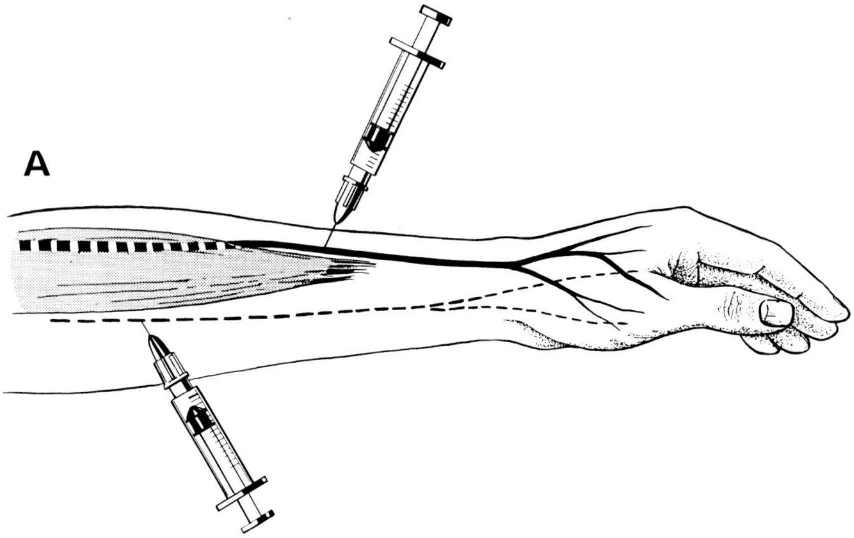

a

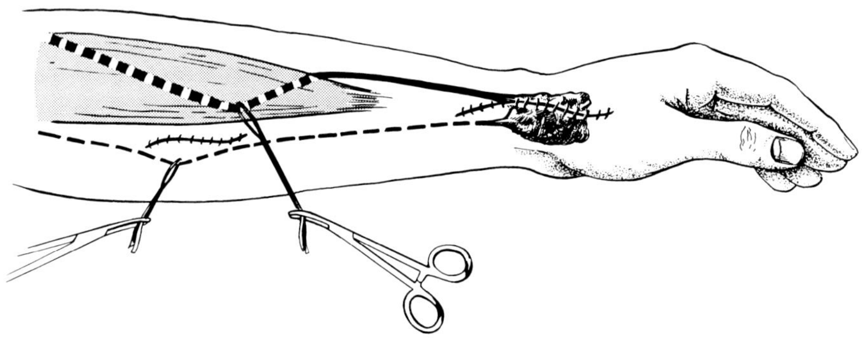

b

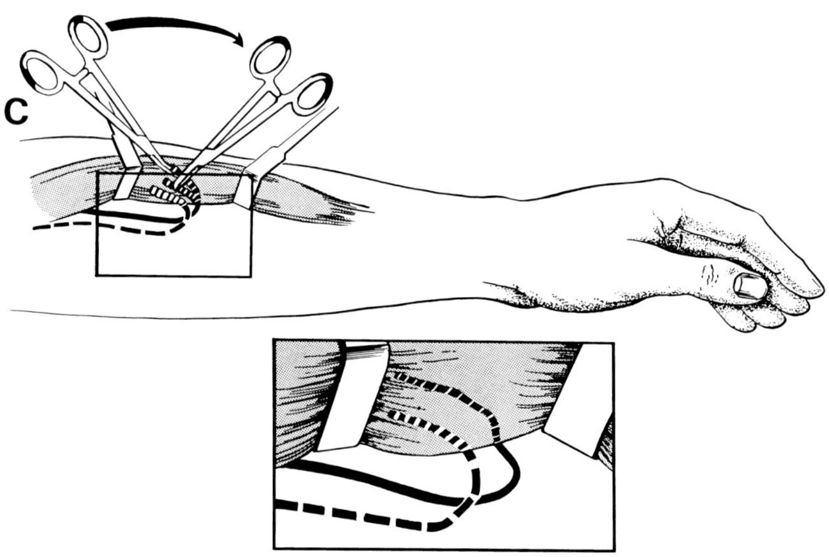

c

Figure 17-26a. Diagnostic nerve blocks are carried out preoperatively. The lateral antebrachial cutaneous nerve is blocked in the proximal forearm adjacent to the cephalic vein. The radial sensory nerve is blocked just dorsal to the muscle tendon junction of the brachioradialis muscle. The nerves are blocked well proximal to the dorsoradial wrist area. **b.** Two separate incisions are used, one over the neuroma and one placed in the proximal forearm. Vessel loops are placed around the lateral antebrachial cutaneous nerve and the radial sensory nerve in order to determine the contribution of these nerves to the neuroma. **c.** The neuroma is excised and the involved nerves are directed from the undersurface of the brachioradialis muscle into the muscle belly in a proximal direction.

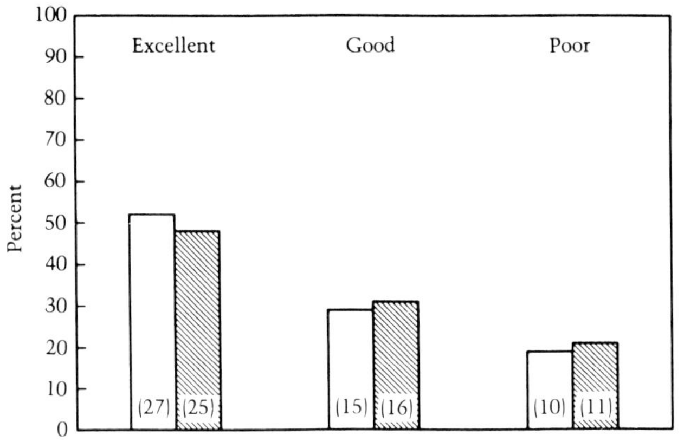

Figure 17-27. Clinical results of dorsoradial nerves. □: pain; □: function (number of patients). (Reproduced with permission from Mackinnon and Dellon.[39])

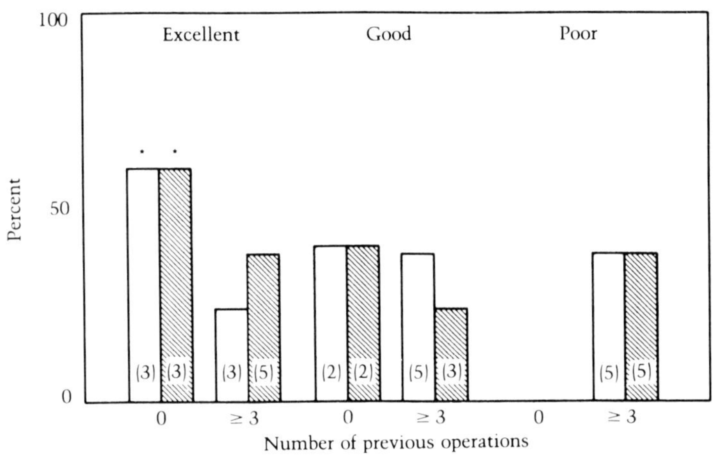

Figure 17-28. Clinical results related to previous operations. □: pain; ▧: function (number of patients): * $p < 0.05$. (Reproduced with permission from Mackinnon and Dellon.[39])

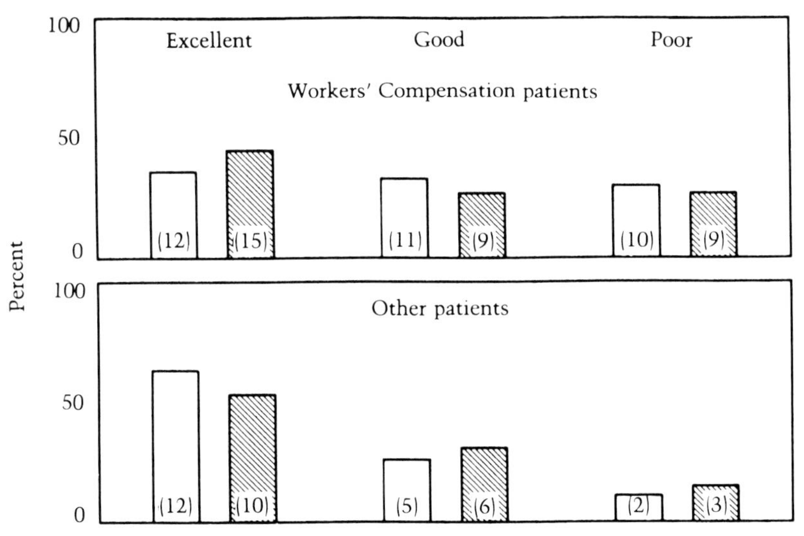

Figure 17-29. Clinical results related to Workers' Compensation. □: pain; ▧: function (number of patients). (Reproduced with permission from Mackinnon and Dellon.[39])

Table 17-6. Results Related to Clinical "Neuroma" Group*

Clinical Group	*No. Previous "Neuroma" Operations*	*No Patients (% of Series)*	*Percentage of Patients with Good or Excellent Pain Relief*
Primary	0	5 (10)	100 (5/5)
First recurrence	1	33 (64)	88 (29/33)
Multiple recurrence	≥3	14 (26)	57 (8/14)

*Reprinted with permission from Mackinnon and Dellon.[39]

Workers' Compensation on the treatment response in chronic pain is not the compensation or litigation but rather actual employment status. In their study, Dworkin et al[50] noted a significantly better response in those patients who were employed or who had a job available for them to return to compared with those patients who were not. This would suggest that attention should be directed away from the "compensation" patient and toward the status of employment in evaluating response to treatment intervention.

The correlation between the duration of pain before definitive neuroma surgery and the surgical outcome demonstrated that the time before surgery in a group of patients with a poor pain relief after surgery was 48 months compared with 24 months for the patients with good or excellent pain relief. Once again, this difference was significant ($p < 0.01$).

The complications associated with this operation can be discussed in terms of donor site morbidity, hyperalgesia in the distribution of the radial sensory nerve, failure to identify all nerves contributing to the neuroma, and the partially injured radial sensory nerve.

All patients had a Tinel-like response with palpation over the brachioradialis muscle at the implantation site for the first 3 months postoperatively. After 1 year, one-third of the patients had a Tinel over the brachioradialis muscle and after 2 years only in one patient was the implantation site in the brachioradialis reexplored because of pain. In this patient, who was treated early in the series, the radial sensory nerve had been placed on the superficial surface of the muscle rather than on the undersurface (Fig. 17-10). Relocation of the neuroma on the undersurface of the muscle resulted in good pain relief. Hyperalgesia did occur but in very few patients in the postoperative period. This seemed to be related to ingrowth into the denervated area by adjacent nerves. This lasted from 6 to 8 weeks and required analgesic support and patient reassurance. In four patients, contribution from the posterior cutaneous nerve of the arm and the medial antebrachial cutaneous nerve was not identified preoperatively. Treatment of these nerves in three of the four patients resulted in a good eventual result.

In five patients, at the time of surgery, it was apparent that only one main branch of the radial sensory nerve had been injured. Using microneural dissection, this branch was dissected away from the injured portion of the nerve preserving one-half of the radial sensory nerve. The injured portion of the nerve was transposed into the brachioradialis in the same fashion. In four of these five patients, pain relief was not obtained and in the second operation transposition of the remainder of the radial sensory nerve into the brachioradialis resulted in good results. This technique of trying to save half of the nerve is not recommended; rather we would suggest that the entire nerve be transposed into the brachioradialis muscle even if a portion of the nerve has not been injured.

Upper Arm

Patients were evaluated using the rating system for pain and function previously described. In each case, the preoperative pain was severe and disabling.

Painful neuromas in the upper arm are less frequent than in the forearm. Small cutaneous nerves (such as posterior cutaneous nerve and medial antebrachial cutaneous nerve) are evaluated preoperatively with diagnostic nerve blocks. No attempt is made to reconstruct these nerves with nerve grafting or nerve tube techniques. After excision of the neuromas involving these nerves, the proximal end of the nerves will be transferred into the depth of the proximal forearm or into bone.

The medial antebrachial cutaneous (MABC) nerve is most commonly injured during ulnar nerve transposition surgery at the elbow. The MACB may be either cut back to lie well proximal to the elbow or be implanted into the triceps muscle after neuroma resection.

Neuromas in amputation stumps are excised and then transferred into bone (Fig. 17-30). Frequently, the main portion of the nerve will be divided more proximally as well and the nerve sutured at this level in an epineurial fashion. This, then, will mean that the distal portion of the nerve (which subsequently enters the bone) will act as a long nerve graft. This technique helps to minimize postoperative recurrence at best and to delay it at least because the nerve fibers must regenerate from the proximal repair site along the length of the nerve. Positioning of the nerve into bone will be influ-

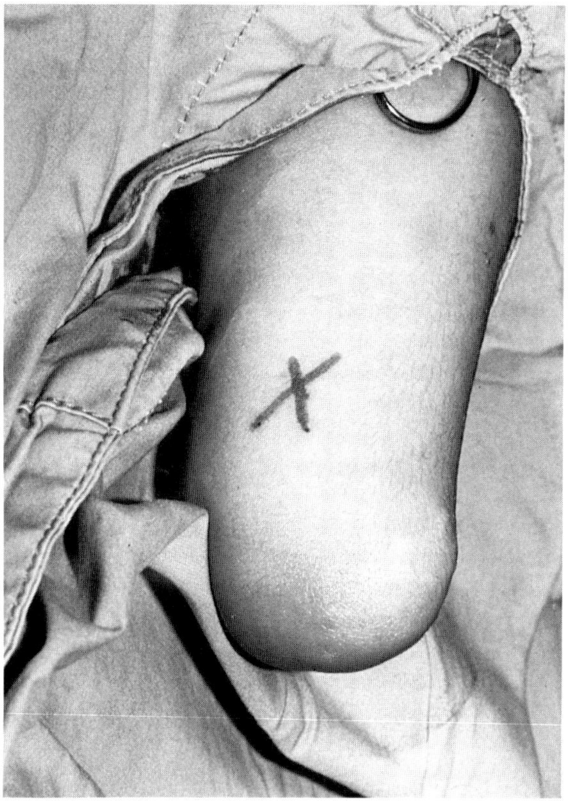

a

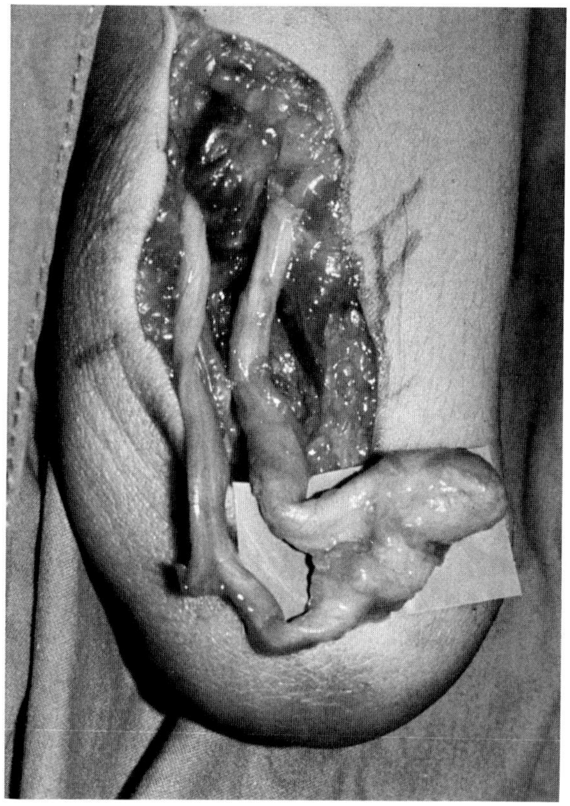

b

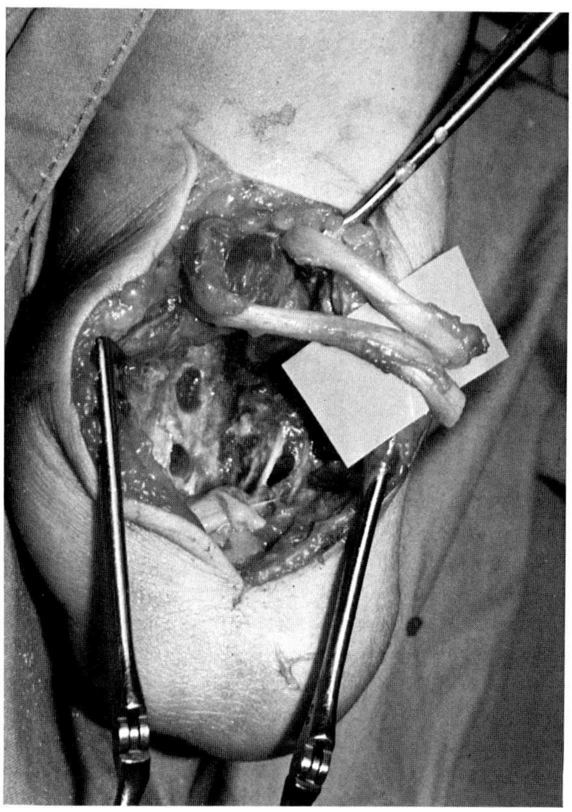

c

Figure 17-30a. This patient had an above-elbow amputation, and neuromatous pain prevented him from wearing his prosthesis. **b.** Exploration of the amputation stump demonstrated large neuromas of the median and ulnar nerves. **c.** These neuromas were excised and the ends of the nerves were transferred into bone.

enced by the nature of the prosthesis that the patient wears. Care is taken to position the nerves well away from any pressure sites or sites that are susceptible to mechanical stimulation with braces or prostheses.

Lower Extremity

A similar approach has been adopted for treatment of neuromas in the lower extremity. If restoration of the injured nerve offers important sensation for the patient (such as posterior tibial nerve) continuity is reestablished with a nerve graft (Fig. 17-31). Neuromas involving less critical nerves (such as sural nerves) are best managed with neuroma resection and muscle implantation. When it is possible, the muscle of choice has been the soleus, since this muscle has minimum excursion and is a large deep muscle well away from the overlying skin (Fig. 17-32). Painful neuromas of the sural nerve may occasionally be seen after harvesting this nerve as nerve graft donor material. This usually occurs in chronic pain patients with preestablished pain patterns (see Chapter 4). Once again, preoperative diagnostic nerve blocks may be critical in identifying the source of the pain and also in letting the patient experience the relationship between pain relief and associated numbness as exemplified with injury to the superficial peroneal nerve (Fig. 17-33). Another commonly encountered lower extremity pain problem is that of heel pain. The common scenario is an operation for a bone spur removal followed by persistent pain, then a tarsal tunnel release without success. Our experience suggests the pathologic processes in these patients combines calcaneal nerve entrapment or neuroma plus inadequate release of the medial and lateral plantar nerves (see Chapter 12 and Fig. 17-34).

Painful Nerve Sequelae Associated with De Quervain's Disease

Traditionally, the surgical management of tenosynovitis of the abductor pollicis longus and extensor pollicis brevis tendons has been a simple procedure with few complications or associated failures. The fallacy of this concept has been recently emphasized and the failure rate, complications, and misdiagnoses have been reviewed.[51] Not mentioned in this report was certain

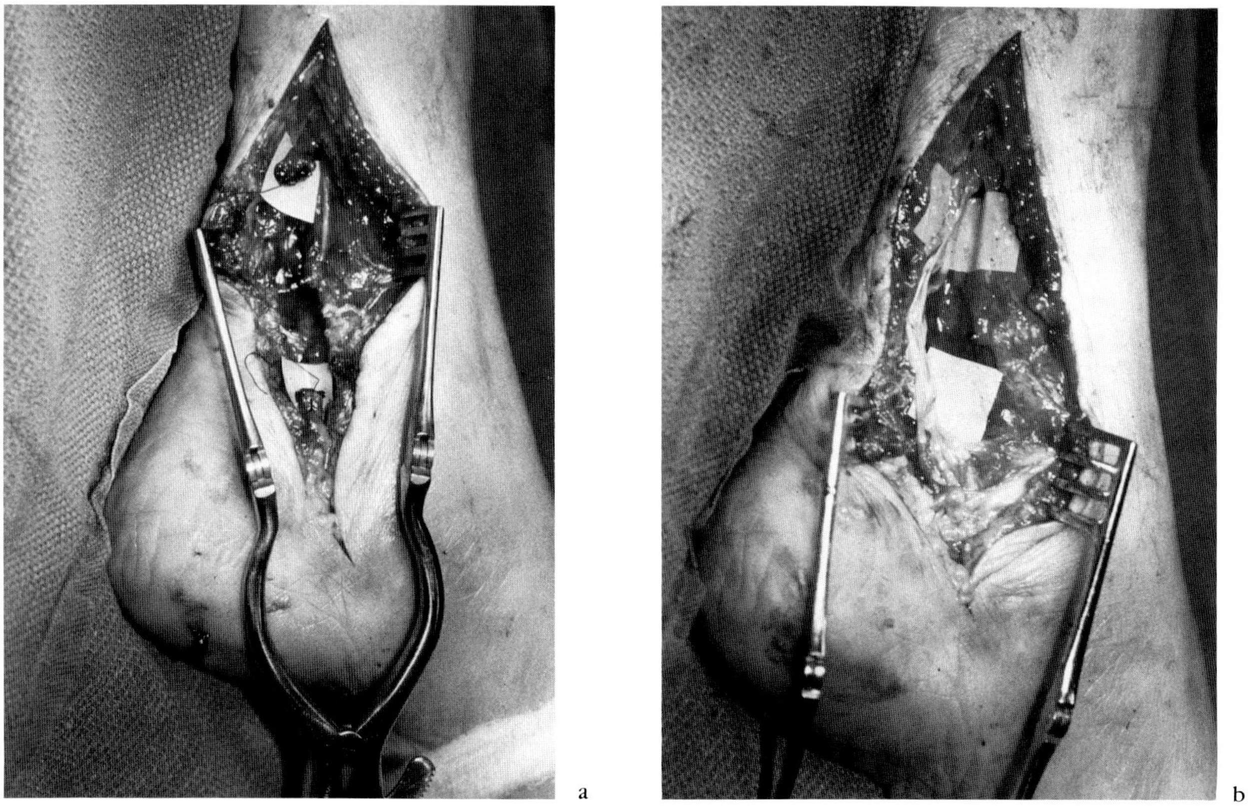

Figure 17-31a. After resection of the posterior tibial nerve for a nerve tumor, this patient has pain in the region of the biopsy and numbness on the sole of the foot. The proximal and distal ends of the nerve lie on the visibility background. **b.** A sural nerve graft is used to reconstruct the nerve gap.

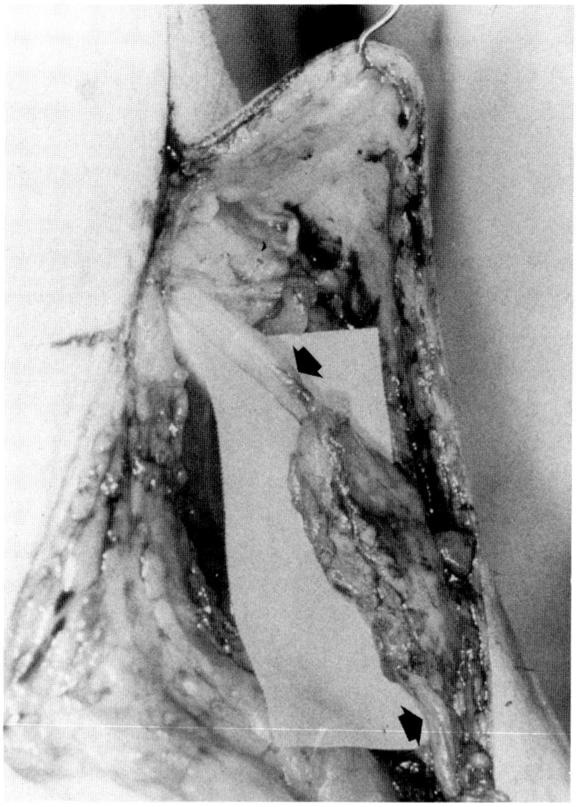
a

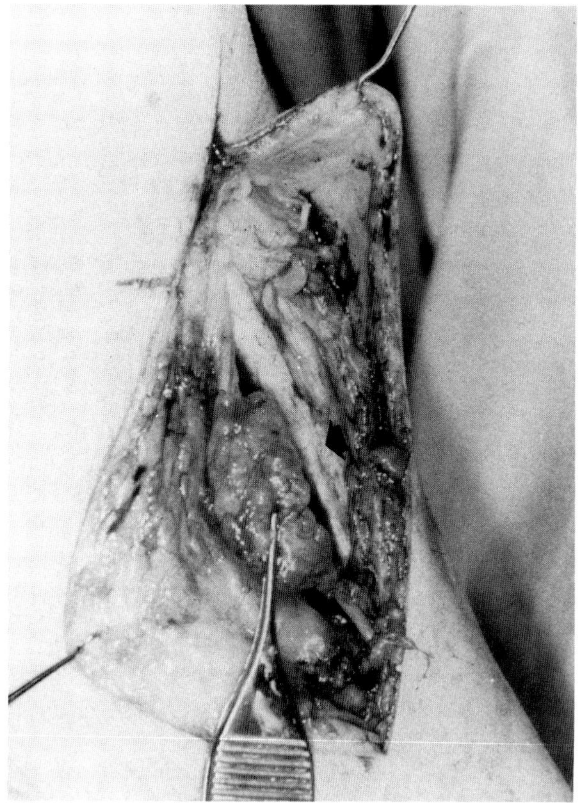
b

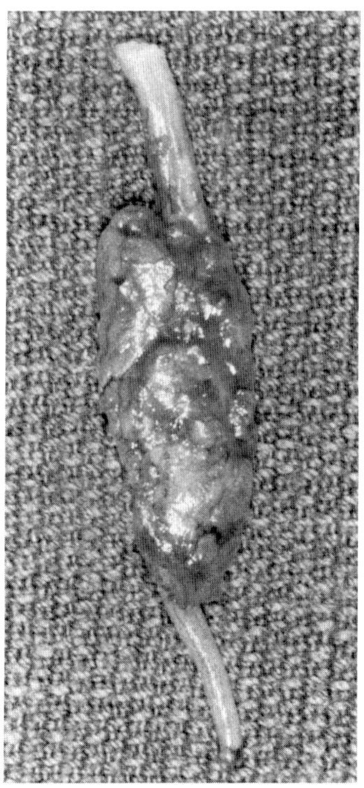
c

Figure 17-32a. After an injury to the sural nerve with a skate blade, a large painful neuroma developed. The sural nerve is seen entering and exiting from the neuroma. **b.** The sural neuroma was adherent to the underlying achilles tendon (arrow). **c.** The neuroma was resected and the proximal end of the sural nerve buried in the soleus muscle.

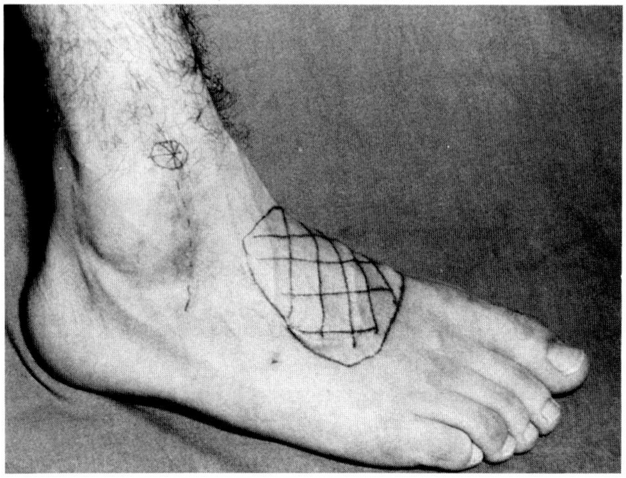

a

Figure 17-33a. This patient with a painful injury to the superficial peroneal nerve had not responded to previous surgical neurolysis. A preoperative anesthetic nerve block convinced the patient that numbness in the distribution of this nerve was significantly more tolerable than pain. **b.** At surgery, a nerve injury is identified (arrow). The neuroma was resected and the proximal portion of the nerve transposed into the deep proximal area in the leg. Foot toward right.

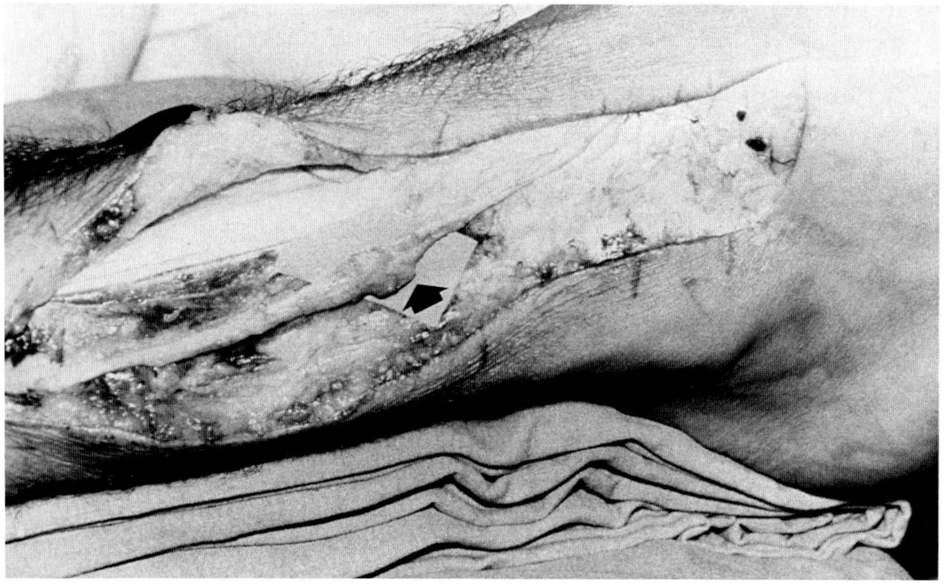

b

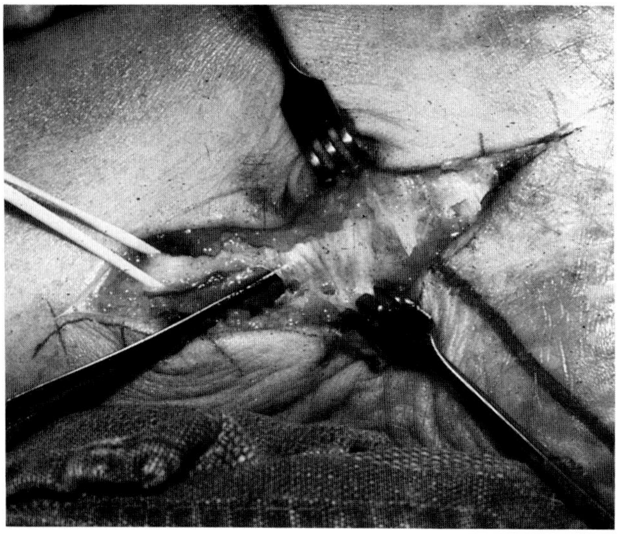

a

Figure 17-34a. This patient with left heel and foot pain had had a previous inadequate release of the left tarsal tunnel. Vessel loop around posterior tibial nerve, elevator under flexor retinaculum. Heel, bottom right of photograph. **b.** The entire tarsal tunnel was released and the medial and lateral plantar nerves are seen (MP, LP). **c.** The neuroma of the calcaneal branch is noted on the visibility background. (*Figure continues.*)

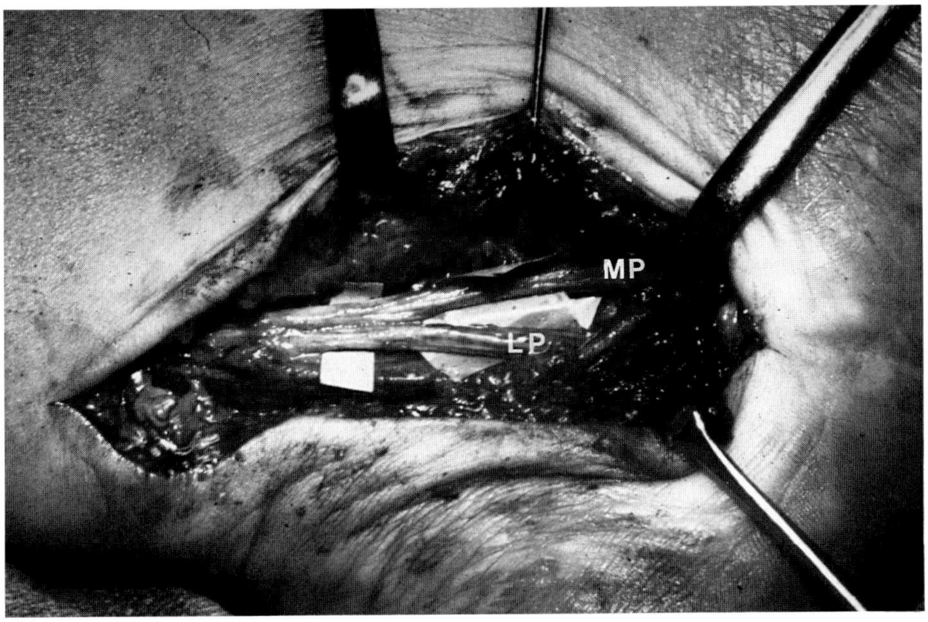

b

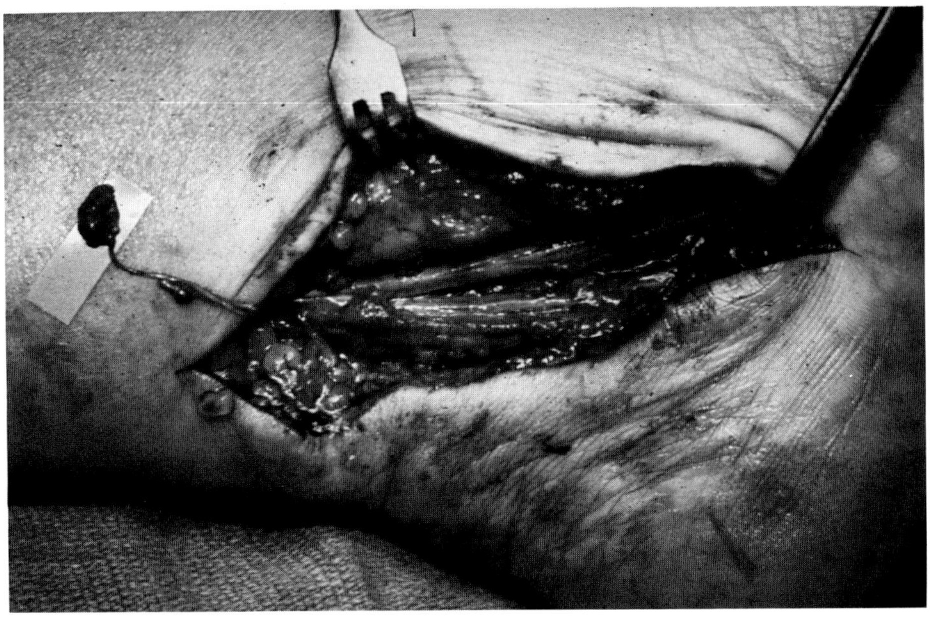

c

Figure 17-34 *(continued)* **b,c.**

pathologic conditions of the dorsoradial sensory nerves. In particular, we would draw attention to the frequent misdiagnosis of radial sensory nerve entrapment as de Quervain's disease. We would also encourage an increased awareness of neuroma formation of the lateral antebrachial cutaneous nerve as well as the radial sensory nerve as a complication of the dorsal compartment release.

Recently, two patient populations have been reviewed[52] (Table 17-7). Seventy-one patients with entrapment of the radial sensory nerve were treated. Seventeen of these patients had been previously diagnosed as having de Quervain's disease. In the same time interval, 82 patients with neuromas of the radial sensory nerve and the lateral antebrachial cutaneous nerve were treated. Twenty-four of these patients had previously been treated for de Quervain's disease (Fig. 17-35). Diagnosis and management of radial sensory nerve entrapment has been described in Chapter 10 and the comparison of symptoms between de Quervain's disease and radial sensory nerve entrapment is outlined in Table 3-8. Patients with radial sensory nerve entrapment will demonstrate sensory abnormalities on the dorsum of the hand that are not apparent in those patients with de Quervain's disease. Sensibility testing will be abnormal in patients with radial sensory nerve entrapment. As well, in the proximal forearm at the junction between the brachioradialis tendon and the tendon

Table 17-7. Clinical Data*

	Radial Sensory Nerve Entrapment	*Dorsoradial Wrist Neuromas*
Patients (no.)	71	82
Male/female	33/38	40/42
Workman's Compensation Board	37	60
Previous trauma	59	55
Diabetes	9	2
Previous diagnosis: de Quervain's disease	17	24
Previous surgery: de Quervain's disease	5	24

*Reprinted with permission from Saplys et al.[52]

of the extensor carpi radialis longus, there will be evidence of entrapment or compression on the radial sensory nerve. Pressure provocative tests at this level will produce sensory abnormalities over the dorsal aspect of the hand. A Tinel sign will often be present at this level as well. Local tenderness over the first extensor compartment will not be present in patients with radial sensory nerve entrapment. Resisted thumb extension or abduction is not painful.

In our experience, the release of the first extensor compartment rarely causes injury to the radial sensory nerve but very frequently causes injury to the lateral antebrachial cutaneous nerve, which is superficial to the radial sensory nerve and of much smaller size at the level of the wrist. Of course, treatment of the radial sensory nerve, with no awareness of the lateral antebrachial cutaneous nerve, will not result in good pain relief for those patients with nerve injury after release of the first extensor compartment.

Unfortunately, radial sensory nerve entrapment is frequently misdiagnosed as de Quervain's disease and surgical treatment of de Quervain's disease is often complicated by injury to the dorsoradial wrist nerves. The diagnosis of neuromas of these nerves is easily made. The scar from the previous injury or surgery is noted. Palpation in this area causes significant pain radiating into the distal distribution of the nerves involved. Patients complain of sensory abnormalities over the dorsum of the hand. Radial sensory nerve and lateral antebrachial cutaneous neuromas can be distinguished by diagnostic nerve blocks.

Dorsoradial wrist pain can be managed reliably given differential diagnosis of de Quervain's tenosynovitis, radial sensory nerve entrapment, and neuromas of the radial sensory and lateral antebrachial cutaneous nerves. A careful history and physical examination is supplemented with diagnostic nerve blocks when indicated.

Reflex Sympathetic Dystrophy or Sympathetic Maintained Pain Syndrome

Although the syndrome to be described was clearly noted in 1864 by Mitchell, et al[53] this syndrome remains a diagnostic and therapeutic dilemma. One of the reasons for this is that the criteria for the diagnosis of reflex sympathetic dystrophy has been extremely lax and often the diagnosis has been applied to patients who most certainly do not have the syndrome. This problem has been compounded by the lengthy and confusing classifications suggested in the past (such as minor and major causalgia, minor and major traumatic dystrophy, and shoulder-hand syndrome).[54] As well, the terms used to describe this syndrome are numerous, and in most reports dealing with reflex sympathetic dystrophy, a myriad of terms are included in the diagnosis: Sudek's atrophy, shoulder, arm, hand syndrome, phantom pain, Leriche's post-traumatic pain syndrome, post-traumatic vasomotor disorders, post-traumatic painful osteoporosis, post-traumatic spreading neuralgia, post-traumatic pain syndrome, minor causalgia, major causalgia, causalgic state, and reflex nervous dystrophy.

The classic description by Silas Weir Mitchell reporting this syndrome secondary to nerve injury involving gunshot wounds during the Civil War is always quoted. Mitchell used the word "causalgia" (meaning burning pain) to describe the pain associated with this

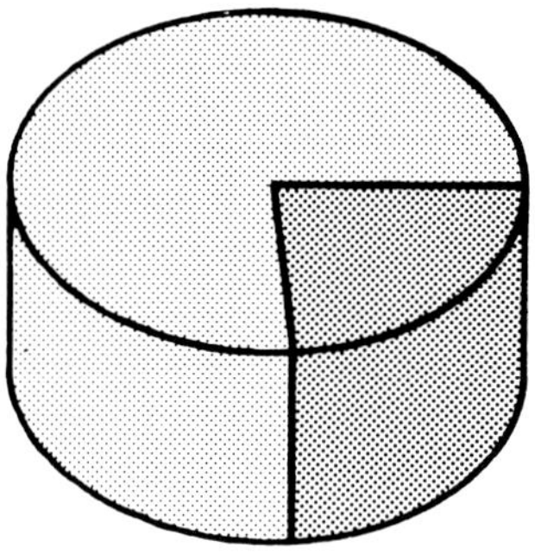
a

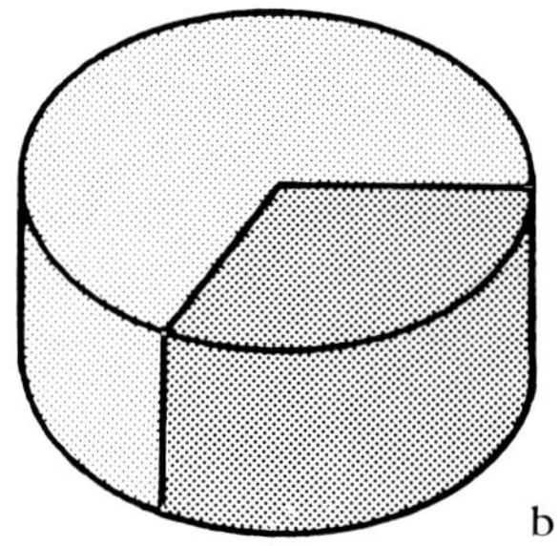
b

Figure 17-35a. Seventeen of 71 patients with a previous misdiagnosis of de Quervain's disease had actual radial sensory nerve entrapment. **b.** Twenty-four of 82 patients with a previous diagnosis and surgical treatment of de Quervain's disease developed dorsal radial wrist neuromas (with permission Saplys et al.[52])

syndrome. Since the time of the Civil War, understanding of the mechanisms behind this causalgia has expanded tremendously. The critical aspects of this understanding have come largely from the advances from the neurophysiologists and not from the clinical surgeons. Unfortunately, during the time that this neurophysiologic neurochemical information was being compiled by the basic scientists, the clinicians from many disciplines were randomly assigning this diagnosis to a very mixed group of patients, ascribing numerous terms to this syndrome and using varying criteria for diagnosis. Although we see many painful sequelae following nerve injury, there is a definite clinical syndrome associated with pain, lack of function, joint stiffness, and soft tissue changes. Most importantly, this pain syndrome is maintained by some abnormality in the sympathetic nervous system. Rather than describe this syndrome as reflex sympathetic dystrophy, we prefer to call it a sympathetic maintained pain syndrome (SMPS). This implies that any number of factors might be the cause of the syndrome but that an abnormality in the response of the sympathetic nervous system to this causative factor is what is maintaining this pain syndrome. A pain syndrome without sympathetic overactivity may be termed "nonsympathetic maintained pain syndrome." Thus pain syndromes may be maintained by many factors other than an abnormality in the sympathetic nervous system. Factors that may maintain pain syndromes include secondary gain (worker's compensation, litigation) functional or psychological problems, joint stiffness due to disuse, injury to other tissue such as bone, soft tissue, or nerves. If we reevaluate the previous classification of RSD[54] we see that "shoulder hand syndrome" is a syndrome maintained by stiffness secondary to disuse; major and minor causalgia is a pain syndrome due to injury to a major or minor peripheral nerve. Major and minor traumatic dystrophy would imply the etiology of a sympathetic dystrophy. Pain syndromes may be maintained by a number of these factors to various degrees. It is important to try to determine what factors are involved in any given patient so that treatment can be directed at whatever factors are felt to be maintaining the pain syndrome in that particular patient. Frequently several factors may be maintaining the pain syndrome to a greater or lesser degree. Some or all of these factors may be ameniable to treatment.

The neurophysiologic events associated with SMPS are not well understood. The theories from the 1930s and 1940s[55–59] of abnormalities in the "internuncial pool" of the spinal cord and peripheral "short circuiting" between somatic "afferent sensory" and autonomic "efferent sympathetic" fibers are still quoted as likely abnormalities in this syndrome.[54,60] Recent advances in our understanding of the neurophysiologic features of the nociceptive "pain" system help to expand these early theories.[61,62] Some of the previously unknown factors in the classic reflex arc or "nociceptive loop"[61] are now well documented. Primary afferent pain impulses are conducted to the spinal cord (spinal thalamic neurons in the dorsal horn) by way of the dorsal root ganglion. Substance P is a neurotransmitter for noxious stimuli at this level.[63–65] It is also located in the sensory terminals in the skin.[62] Substance P has also been shown to induce plasma extravasation in the skin and is a likely candidate for neurogenically induced increased capillary permeability in the skin. This extravasation may result in the release into the tissue of agents that have been shown to facilitate pain (prostaglandins) or to increase the activity in the pain fiber system (bradykinin, histamine).[66] We have observed that localized pain in the hand has frequently been associated with a flushed rubious area that is clearly demarcated and corresponds almost exactly with the subjective area of pain. This finding may well represent local manifestations of this nociceptive system.

The nociceptive loop can be modified by local and encephalon inhibitory systems within the dorsal horn of the medulla.[67] This encephalon system may regulate some aspects of psychogenic pain. Low cerebral fluid levels of these substances has been found in patients believed to have psychogenic rather than somatic pain.[68]

Abnormalities in these nociceptive fiber systems and short circuiting between the somatic and autonomic nervous system at the spinal cord level are possible mechanisms in the pathogenesis of SMPS. Similar mechanisms are believed to be involved in the pathogenesis of pain associated with peripheral nerve injury.[69,70] This may explain why SMPS is often associated with peripheral nerve injury.

The schematic diagram of the nociceptive (pain) system is outlined in Figure 17-36. Skin nociceptors carry afferent information via C-fibers and A-delta fibers and synapse with dorsal horn neurons. These, in turn, convey central information via ascending tracts and also synapse with motor and sympathetic afferents. In SMPS with partial nerve injury or with soft tissue crushing injuries, several components of the nociceptive loop may be influenced. Substances that excite (bradykinin) or sensitize (prostaglandins) skin nociceptors are released in the skin. These same substances also have an effect on the sympathetics and also affect skin capillaries, producing vasodilation and increased capillary permeability.[71–75] In addition, prostaglandins also affect bone metabolism.[76,77] In the case of an injured nerve, the sympathetic nerves may excite the nociceptors, influence the release of various analgesic substances in the skin, and also produce the vasomotor changes typical in SMPS. Short circuiting (ephapsis) between sympathetics and nociceptive afferents has been suggested

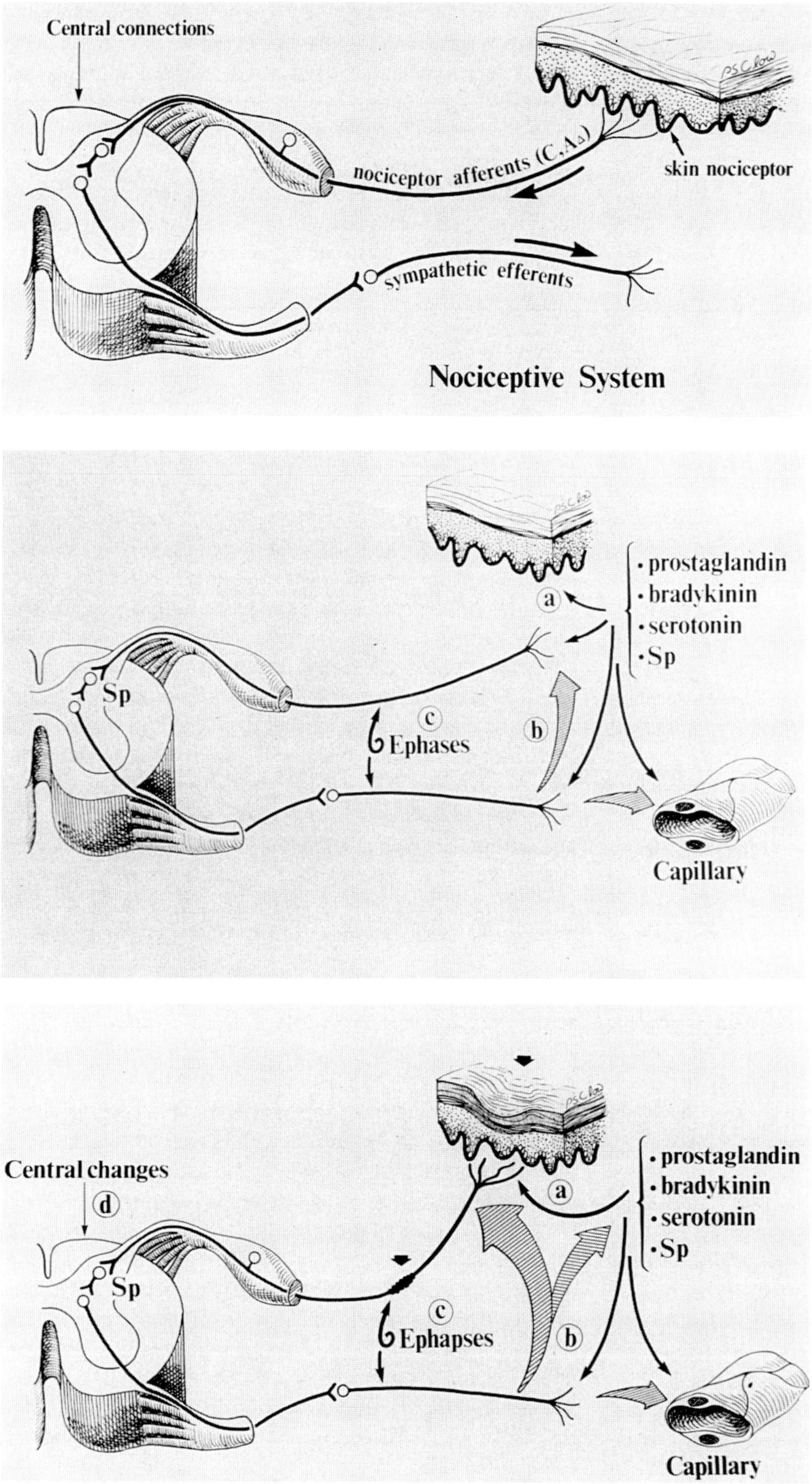

Figure 17-36a. Schematic diagram of the nociceptive (pain) system. Skin nociceptors carry afferent information via C-, A-delta fibers and synapse with dorsal horn neurons. These, in turn, convey central information via ascending tracts and also synapse with motor (not shown) and sympathetic efferents. **b, c.** SMPS with partial nerve injury of soft tissue crush (arrowheads). Several components of the nociceptive loop may be influenced. (a.) (black arrows): Substances that excite (bradykinin) or sensitize (prostaglandins) skin nociceptors are released in the skin. These same substances also have effects on the sympathetics and skin capillaries. In addition, prostaglandins also affect bone metabolism. (b.) (hatched arrows): In the case of any injured nerve, the sympathetic nerves may excite the nociceptors, influence the release of the various algesic substances in the skin, and also produce the vasomotor changes typical in SMPS. (c.) Short circuiting (ephapse) between sympathetics and nociceptive afferents (and also between mechanoreceptors and nociceptors) has been postulated in the clinical situation and documented in experimental animal models.[9] (d.) The peripheral system may have complex influences on the central components of the nociceptive system. (Reproduced with permission from Holder and Mackinnon.[81])

in the clinical situation and has been documented in the experimental animal models. This short circuiting has also been demonstrated between mechanoreceptors and nociceptors. The effects on the complex relationship between the peripheral nervous system and the central nervous system have been well documented.

Diagnosis

The diagnostic criteria for SMPS should be quite strict. Causalgia must and can be distinguished from SMPS. These two entities may exist together, but the unfortunate tendency is to call problems that are purely causalgia, SMPS. Patients with causalgia all have injuries (such as crush, laceration, compression) to a peripheral nerve. These patients demonstrate hyperalgesia in the distribution of that nerve. All the signs and symptoms can be entirely explained by a documented injury to a peripheral nerve. Thus, if the patient has had a median nerve repair or injury and his symptoms are entirely confined to the distribution of the median nerve, the patient has causalgia in the distribution of the median nerve and does not have SMPS. If the remainder of the hand looks normal and good range of movement is noted, then the patient does not have dystrophy from SMPS. Similarly, if the patient has had an injury to the radial sensory nerve at the wrist and demonstrates burning pain in the distribution of the radial sensory nerve with, otherwise, normal hand examination, the patient has causalgia and does not have SMPS. In fact, if it can be demonstrated that the patient has a full range of movement or if the hand looks entirely normal, then the patient does not have SMPS. The number of patients referred with the label of "reflex sympathetic dystrophy" made by otherwise competent physicians is very discouraging.

The recent report by such leading authorities as Kozen et al[78,79] describing reflex sympathetic dystrophy categories as "probable, possible and doubtful" underlines this lack of clear diagnostic criteria in the minds of many clinicians.

A group of surgeons trained in the speciality of surgery of the hand have established diagnostic criteria for SMPS (Table 17-8).[6,80] The patients must complain of pain outside a peripheral nerve distribution. Although the injury itself may have been minor, the pain appears out of proportion to the injury. We have seen two types of SMPS, one involves the hand or even a greater majority of the upper extremity and a second is localized to one or more digits. In no instance can the patient's pain be completely accounted for by an injury to a specific nerve, although injury to a specific nerve may be the causative basis for the more diffuse symptoms. The patient also demonstrates diminished hand function. Several patients have been referred with a diagnosis of SMPS and, on examination, it is quite apparent that, although they may complain of diffuse pain, their hand functions normally with a full range of movement and motor power is demonstrated. These patients, of course do not have SMPS. The patients must also demonstrate some joint stiffness (Fig. 17-37). The skin and soft tissue trophic changes will demonstrate varying amounts of vasomotor instability, depending on the stage of the SMPS (Fig. 17-38).

Table 17-8. Diagnostic Criteria for Sympathetic Maintained Pain Syndrome*

1. Complaint of diffuse pain that does not follow the distribution of a peripheral nerve
2. Diminished (hand) function
3. Joint stiffness
4. Skin and soft-tissue changes with or without vasomotor instability.

*Reprinted with permission from Mackinnon and Holder.[80]

We prefer to describe early, intermediate, and late stages of SMPS. In the *early stages,* vasomotor instability is noted with very dramatic sympathetic overactivity apparent in the hand or digit involved. Instability with changes varying between redness and warmth and cyanosis and sweating are noted in this early stage. Edema is also a classic finding in this early stage. In the *intermediate stage* of SMPS pain is less of a dramatic component and is usually elicited by attempts to move the joints. At rest, the patient may be quite comfortable. The edema and vasomotor changes have settled by this time and the hand has the appearance of a "burned out" dystrophic hand with marked stiffness and atrophy of the soft tissue noted. The normal wrinkles on the dorsum of the hand are no longer apparent. The fingertips may have a tapered appearance. The nail growth is usually more exaggerated than in the normal hand, and the hand is often cool and pale. The intermediate stage will extend over a number of months and is intermediate between the early and late stages. During the *late stage,* all the superimposed problems of disuse atrophy may take effect and during this stage problems with the elbow and shoulder are very common, even though the patient may initially have had just a SMPS involving the hand or a localized problem involving one or more digits. The degree of pain experienced during the late phase is variable and is often the result of disuse and stiffness. SMPS can effect other areas of the body and has been described in the foot, face, and penis.

Three-Phase Radionuclide Bone Scanning

Radionuclide scintigraphy has been demonstrated to be one of the most sensitive tests for describing SMPS. When very strict criteria (as already outlined) are used

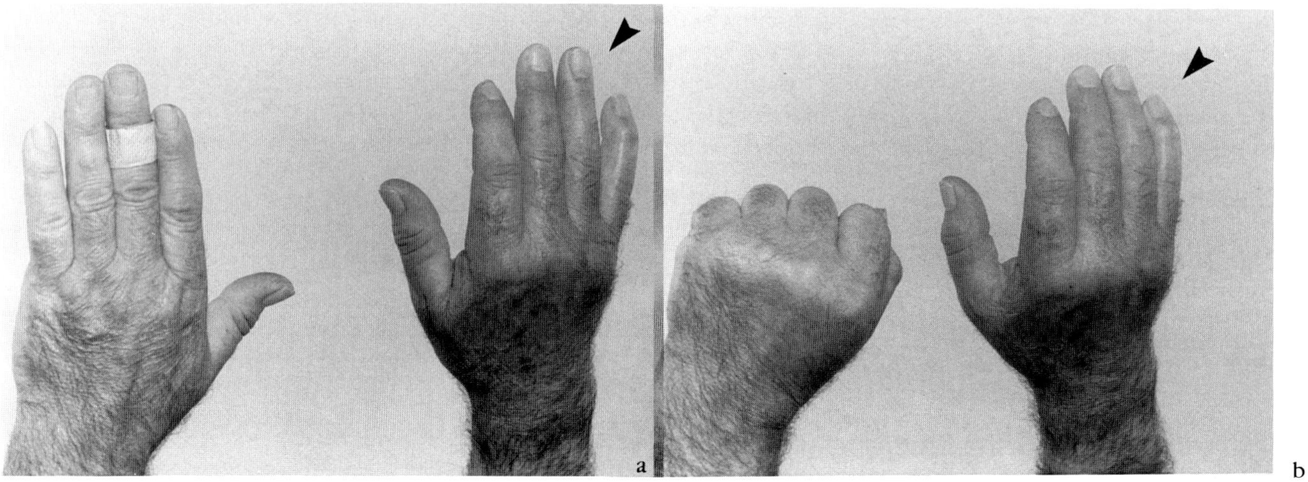

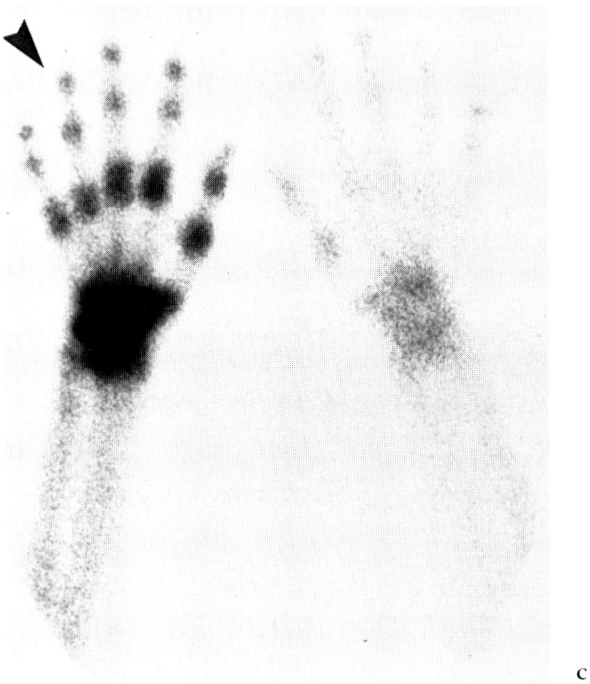

Figure 17-37a. This patient has some trophic skin changes in the right hand (arrow). **b.** He demonstrates marked joint stiffness and is unable to "make a first" (arrow). **c.** His three-phase hand scan demonstrated marked increased uptake in the delayed phase (Posterior view, therefore patient's right hand is on the left side of this scan). (arrow)

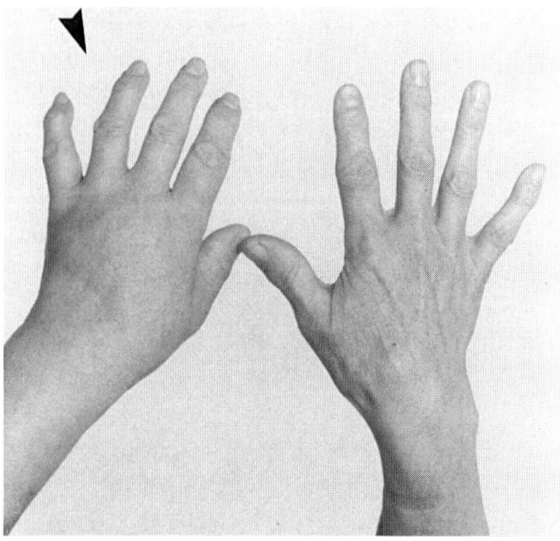

Figure 17-38. Marked swelling and stiffness is noted in this patient with SMPS in the left hand (arrow).

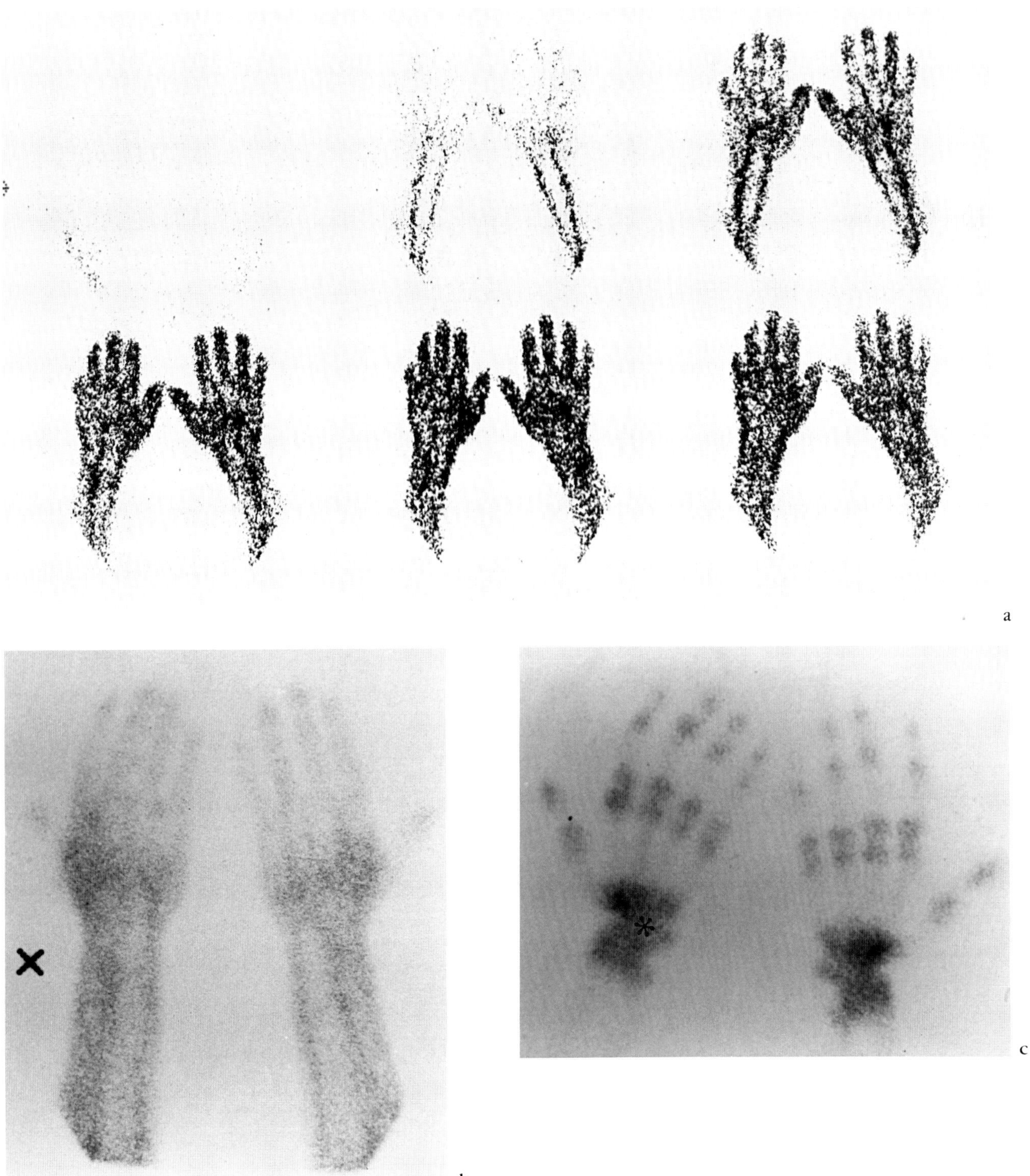

Figure 17-39a. Normal three phase bone scan (RNA), palmar view. Radial and ulnar artery activity on early image (5 to 10 seconds) is followed by activity in the palmar arches (10- to 15-second image) and then in the digits. Activity is represented by black dots on white background. **b.** Blood pool or tissue phase, dorsal view. The relative vascularity of the soft tissue is imaged. The thenar and to a lesser extent the hypothenar musculature is seen. **c.** Delayed image, dorsal view. Activity in the radial carpal, intercarpal, and carpal metacarpal joints is not separable (*). Metacarpal phalangeal and interphalangeal joints are defined by juxta-articular activity two to three times more intense than that in the individual phalanges (clinical diagnosis, dorsal ganglion). (Reproduced with permission from Mackinnon and Holder.[80])

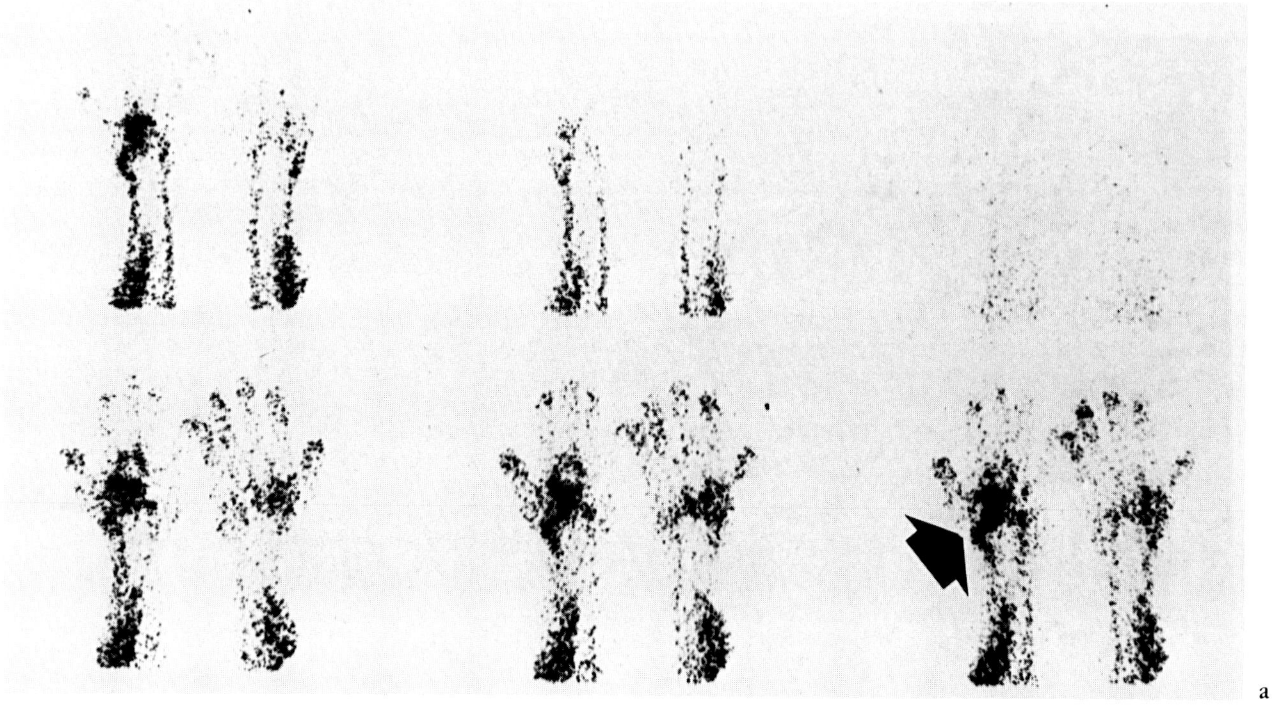

a

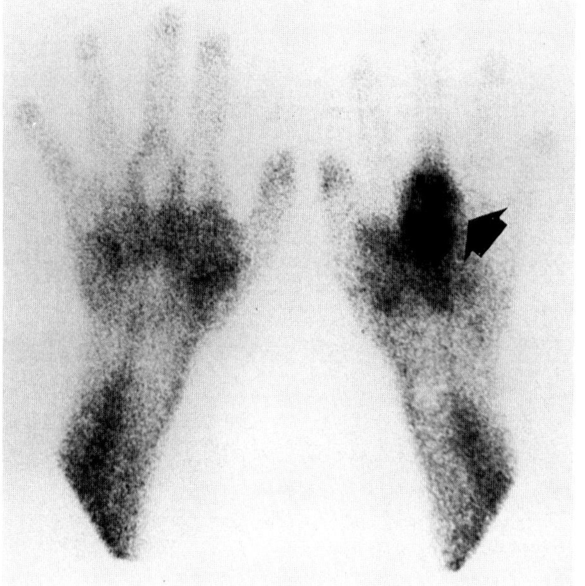

b

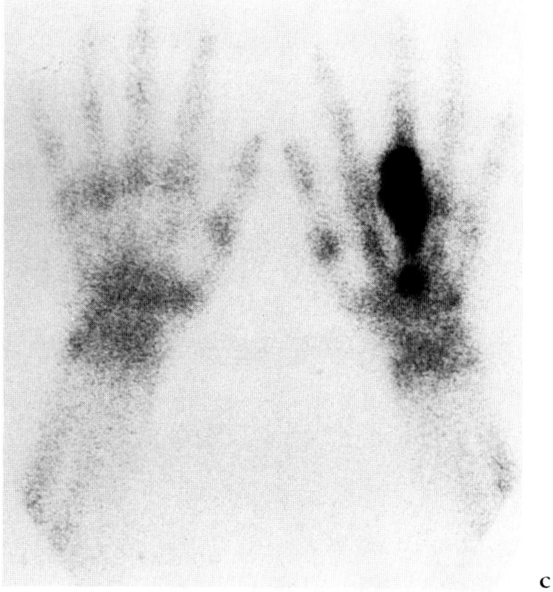

c

Figure 17-40a. Focally abnormal three phase bone scan (RNA), dorsal view. Focal increased perfusion to the area of the third metacarpal phalangeal joint is noted on the left side (arrow). Note the asymmetry of activity of the radial and ulnar arteries and digits when compared with the normal hand. **b.** Blood pool image, palmar view. Poorly marginated increased activity in the area of the head of the third metacarpal and base of the third proximal phalanx is noted (arrow). The thenar and digital vascularity is normal and similar to that in the right hand. **c.** Delayed image, palmar view. More intense abnormal increased tracer accumulation is noted in the distal half of the third metacarpal and proximal half of the third phalanx. Slight increased activity is noted at the base of the third metacarpal. Activity in the wrist and digits is normal and similar to that in the normal hand. Clinical diagnosis: synovitis of the metacarpal phalangeal joint. (Reproduced with permission from Mackinnon and Holder.[80])

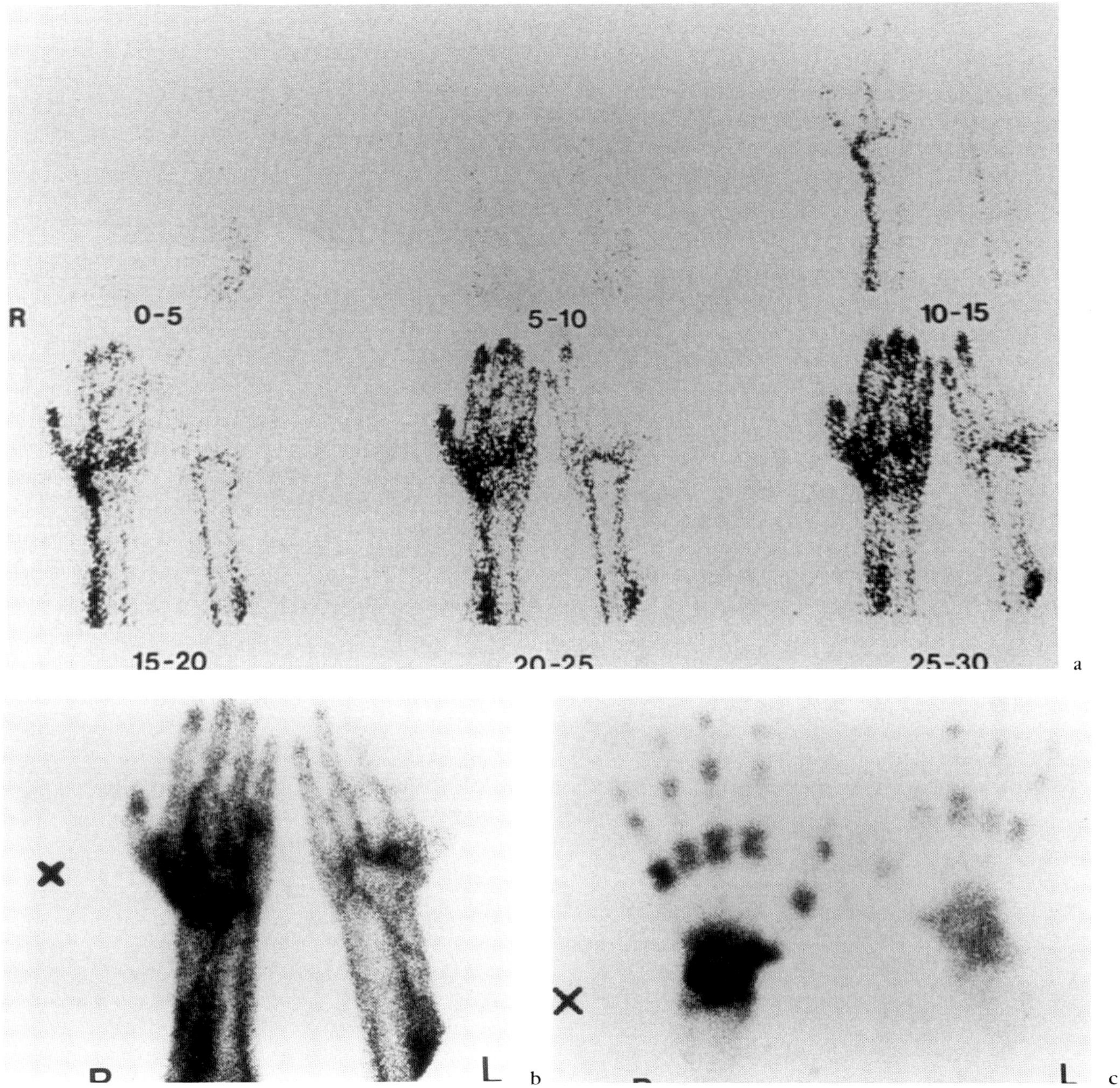

Figure 17-41a. Diffusely abnormal three phase bone scan (RNA), dorsal view. On the right, more perfusion is via the radial artery (arrow). Increased perfusion to the wrist and digits is noted in the right hand compared with the normal left side. Previous traumatic amputation of the digit and parts of the second and third digits is noted on the left hand. **b.** Blood pool image, dorsal view. Diffusely increased relative vascularity involves the wrist and digits when compared with the normal left side. **c.** Delayed image, palmar view. Diffusely increased activity throughout the radial carpal, intercarpal, and carpometacarpal joints is noted. All of the metacarpal phalangeal, and proximal and distal interphalangeal joints show more activity when compared with the normal left hand. Activity in the distal interphalangeal joints on the left is almost imperceptible. As in normal joints, juxta-articular activity is less marked in the more distal joints. Clinical diagnosis: SMPS. (Reproduced with permission from Mackinnon and Holder.[80])

in the diagnosis of SMPS, three phase bone scanning provides an objective marker for SMPS. Hand scans are performed according to the three phase technique. Phase 1 is the radionuclide angiogram (RNA), which consists of sequential 5-second images obtained for 40 seconds with a gamma scintillation camera after rapid bolus injection of 20 mCi of technetium-99m-labeled methylene diphosphonate. Immediately after the RNA, phase-2 (blood pool or tissue phase) images are obtained for 500,000 counts with the high-sensitivity low-energy all-purpose collimator. Phase 3 consists of detailed (metabolic) images obtained with a high-resolution parallel-hole collimator 3 to 4 hours after the injection.

Images can be graded as normal, focally or multifocally abnormal, or diffusely abnormal. To be considered diffusely positive, RNA perfusion has to be increased in all portions of the wrist and hand. Phase 2 blood pool and phase 3 delayed images have to demonstrate increased activity in the areas of the radial and ulnar carpal, intercarpal, carpometacarpal, metacarpal phalangeal, and the juxta-articular digits to be considered diffusely positive. A normal scan is demonstrated in Figure 17-39. A focally abnormal scan is demonstrated in Figure 17-40. A diffusely abnormal three phase bone scan that is diagnostic of SMPS is demonstrated in Figure 17-41.

The specificity and sensitivity of the three phase bone scan was determined evaluating 145 scans. Using the strict diagnostic criteria already outlined, four clinical groups were determined (Table 17-9). The hand scan findings are outlined in Table 17-10. The analysis of the results is presented in Table 17-11 and diagrammatically depicted in Figure 17-42. It is apparent that *the diffuse increased tracer uptake in the delayed image (phase three) is diagnostic for SMPS.* The sensitivity is 96% and the specificity is 98%. The strictly interpreted delayed radionuclide image is extremely sensitive in the diagnosis of SMPS. Changes in the delayed image can be graded in Figure 17-43.

Table 17-9. Clinical Groups*

Clinical Group	*No. Patients*
I. Definite RSD/SMPS	23
II. Diffuse hand pain (not RSD/SMPS)	26
III. Focal pain	51
IV. Other	45
Total	145

*Reprinted with permission from Mackinnon and Holder.[80]

Table 17-10. Findings on Delayed Image of Three Phase Bone Scan of the Hands*

	Hand-Scan Findings		
Clinical Groups	*Normal*	*Focal Changes*	*Diffuse RSD/SMPS Pattern*
1. RSD/SMPS	1/23	6/23	22/23
2. Diffuse pain	13/26	12/26	1/26
3. Focal pain	20/51	29/51	2/51
4. Other	16/45	24/45	0/45†

*Reprinted with permission from Mackinnon and Holder.[80]

†Two patients with vascular lesions had diffusely decreased scan activity; delayed scanning was not performed in three patients.

Table 17-11. Correlation Between the Clinical and RNA Diagnosis of RSD/SMPS*†

	Clinical	
Scan	*SMPS Negative*	*SMPS Positive*
RSD/SMPS negative	119	1
RSD/SMPS positive	3	22

*Reprinted with permission from Mackinnon and Holder.[80]

†Sensitivity $\frac{22}{22+1}$ = 96%; specificity $\frac{119}{119+3}$ = 98%; positive predictive value $\frac{22}{22+3}$ = 88%; negative predictive value $\frac{119}{119+1}$ = 99%.

We have found the diffuse abnormal uptake in the third phase of the three phase bone scan to be diagnostic of SMPS. We have found that the same criteria can be used to evaluate SMPS localized to one or more digits in the hand (Fig. 17-44).

Treatment

No treatment has proved to be completely satisfactory for this problem; however, it is generally recognized that early diagnosis and aggressive treatment is important in patient management.

We have found in the very late stages of this syndrome that no treatment is particularly useful. In the early and intermediate stages, careful physical examination will be necessary in order to rule out any underlying surgical problem that may have caused the syndrome. It has been previously suggested that the presence of SMPS is a contraindication to surgery. Although this may occasionally be true, frequently, we have found, in the early and intermediate stages, some surgical problem that most likely caused the syndrome in the first place and which is likely to continue to mitigate against a resolution of SMPS until it is treated. Neuromas of the radial sensory nerve, partial injuries to the larger nerves, or crush injuries with subsequent significant nerve compression have all been found to be causative factors of the pain syndrome. Treatment of these underlying problems may facilitate successful treatment of the superimposed SMPS. Surgery is carried out in conjunction with indwelling brachial plexus catheters for long-term anesthetic block.[81]

Therapy, including desensitization and range of movement exercises, are utilized. Frequently, nerve blocks, often with indwelling continuous infusion of local anesthetic adjacent to major nerves, are utilized.

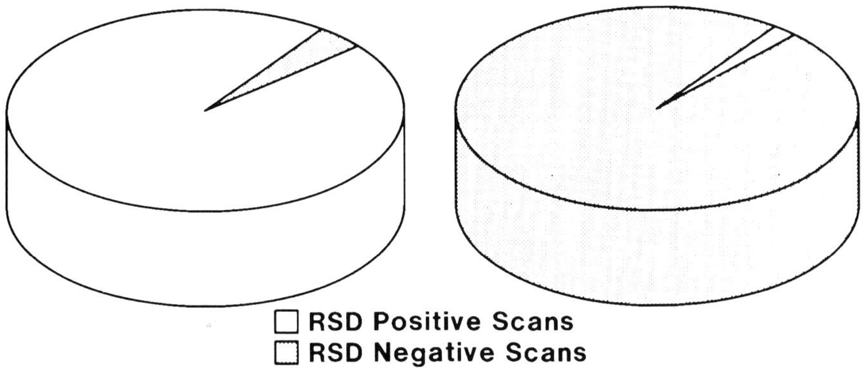

Figure 17-42. In those patients with clinically positive and clinically negative SMPS (RSD), delayed scans that were positive and negative for SMPS are depicted to demonstrate diagrammatically the sensitivity and specificity of the test.

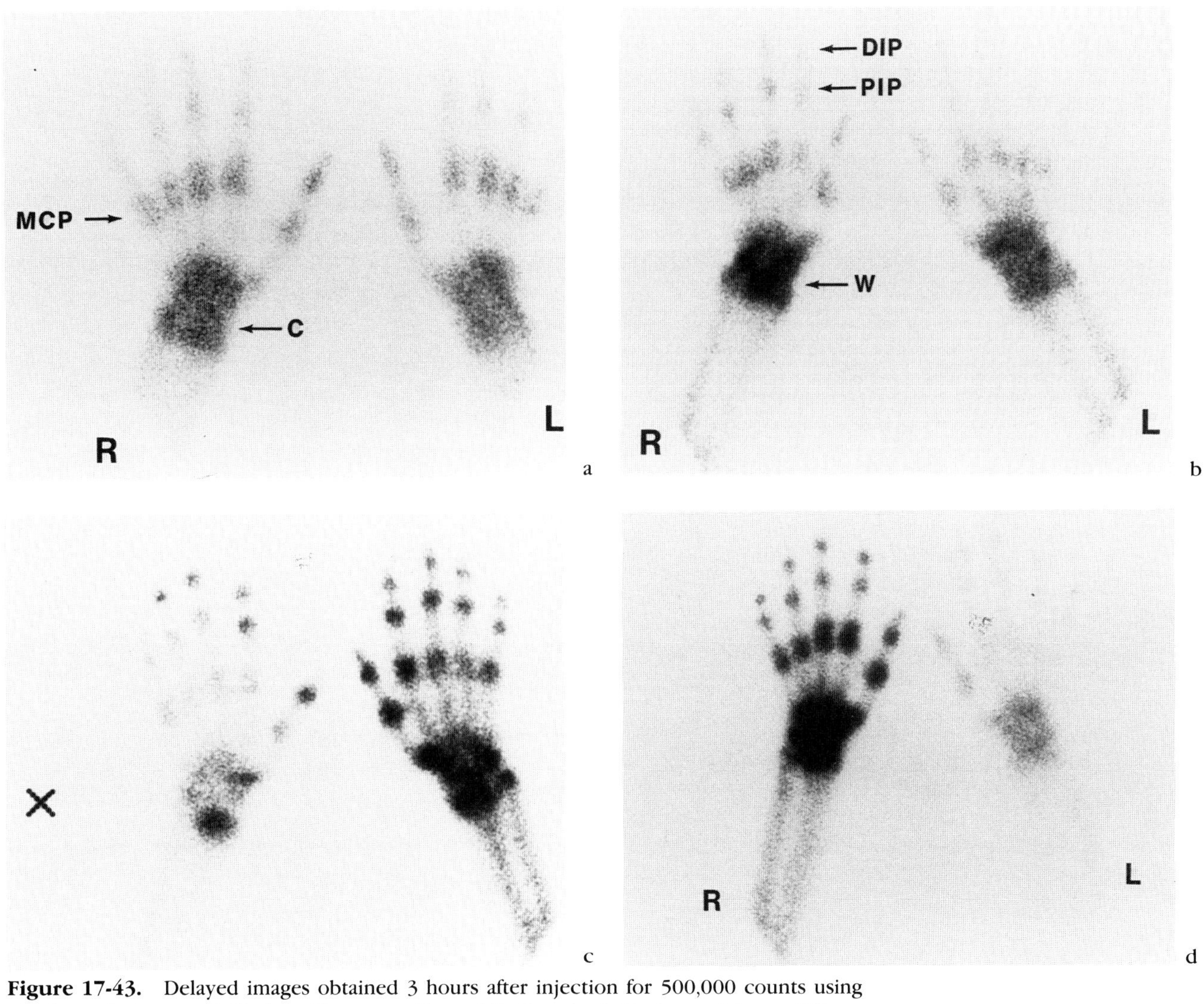

Figure 17-43. Delayed images obtained 3 hours after injection for 500,000 counts using a high resolution parallel hole collimator. **a.** Normal findings. Individual carpal bones (C) are not defined. Metacarpophalangeal (MCP) joints are defined with 0.5 to 2 times more activity than the metacarpal or phalangeal shafts. **b.** Grade 1/3 diffusely positive. Minimal increased activity in abnormal right hand, most easily appreciated in the wrist (W), and, for example, when comparing activity in proximal and distal interphalangeal (PIP and DIP) joints. **c.** Grade 2/3 diffusely positive. Easily seen differences in the abnormal left hand. A few areas of non-inflammatory arthritis in the right hand contrast with the increased juxta-articular activity in all the joints of the left hand. **d.** Grade 3/3 diffusely positive. Very intense activity throughout the abnormal right hand. The rapid acquisition of counts from the right hand results in a decreased contribution to the 500,000 total from the normal left hand, and its washed-out appearance compared with what is expected in a normal hand (Fig. 17-3A). (Reproduced with permission from Holder and Mackinnon.[6])

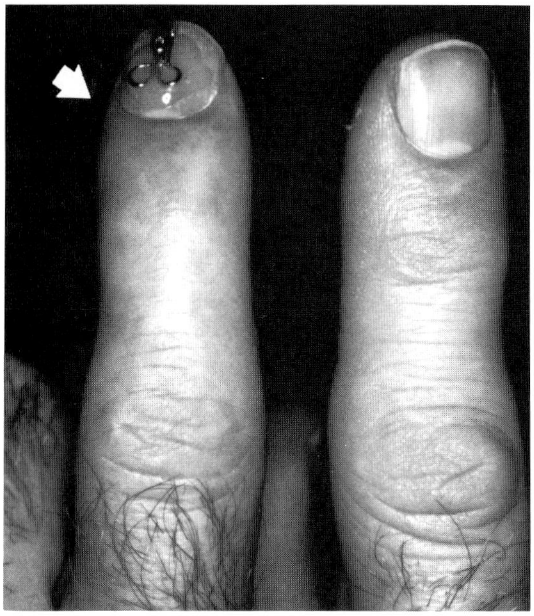

a

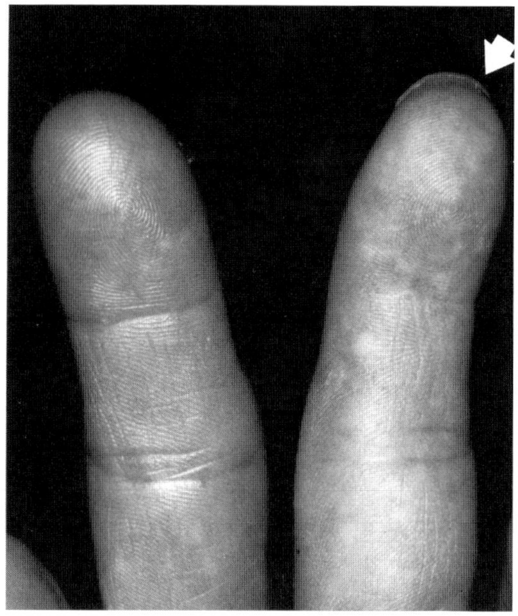

b

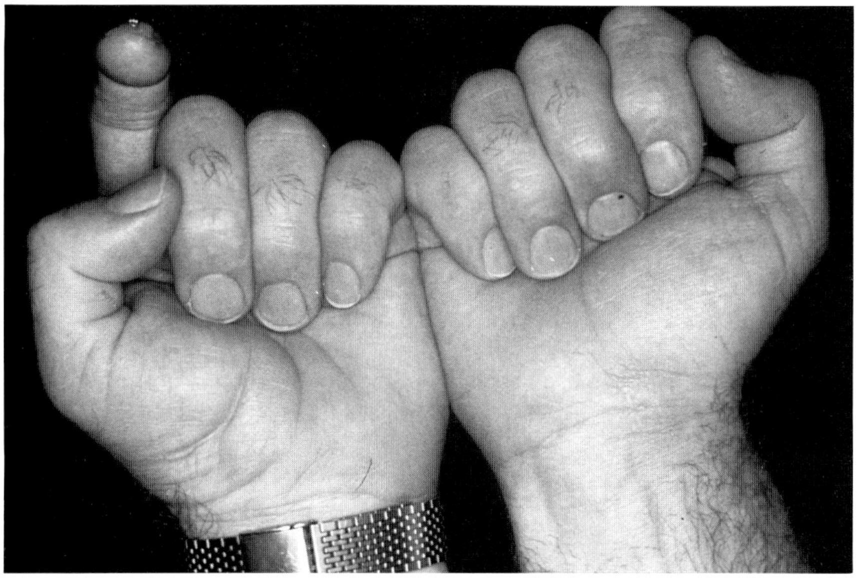

c

Figure 17-44a, b. After a minor injury to the left index finger, this patient developed localized SMPS. The trophic skin changes are noted both on the dorsal and volar aspect of the left index finger (arrow). **c.** The digit demonstrated stiffness. (*Figure continues.*)

Controlled physiotherapy is carried out during the period of the nerve blocks. Sympathetic blocks have been utilized in a similar fashion. A series of sympathetic blocks will help to break the pain cycle, allow the patient to move the extremity without pain, and demonstrate to the patient that it is, indeed, possible to break the pain cycle. A series of blocks over 5 to 6 consecutive days is recommended.

Permanent surgical sympathectomy is only considered when the clinical problem persists despite a full conservative course of therapy and repeated blocks and after underlying surgical problems have been treated. Of course, the patient must have demonstrated a consistent positive response to sympathetic blocks if permanent surgical sympathectomy is to be considered.

The use of an intravenous regional sympathetic block with chemical agents has been popularized by Hannington-Kiff.[82] In our hands, the use of reserpine and guanethidine has not offered significant improvement over stellate ganglion blocks.

In the late stages of this syndrome, we have found considerable success using intravenous regional anesthetic Bier blocks with 80 mg of methylprednisolone sodium succinate added to the intravenous anesthetic solution. With the Bier block in place, the surgeon will gently manipulate the stiff joints (Fig. 17-45). Its role is largely in the later stages of the syndrome when pain is not as important a characteristic as stiffness. This steroid block has been useful in improving the range of motion in the late stages of the dystrophy phase and is a useful

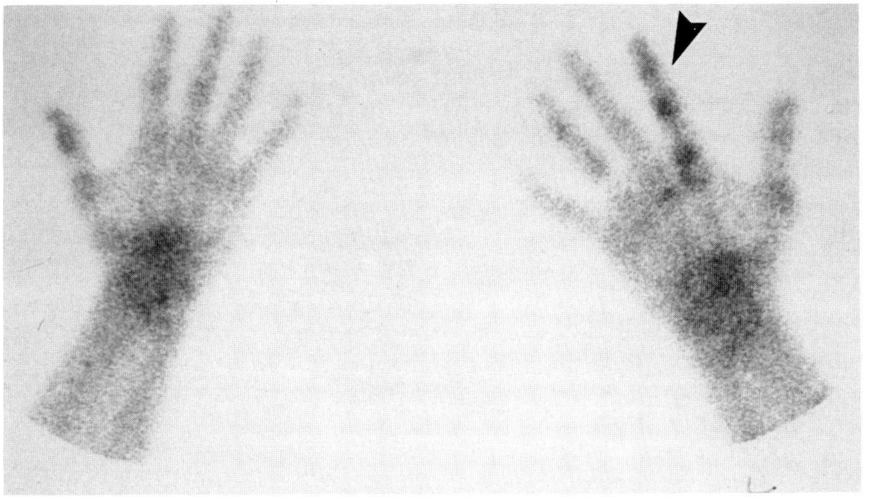

d

Figure 17-44 (*continued*) **d.** The delayed phase of the hand scan was positive for RSD (SMPS) localized to the left index finger (arrow). (Photography courtesy of Dr. J.F. Murray Toronto Canada.)

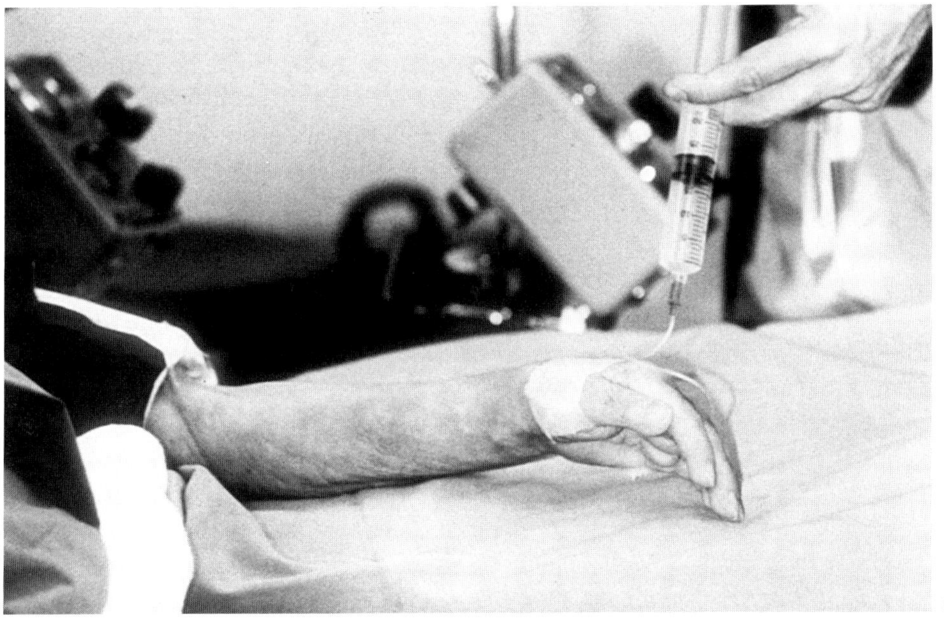

a

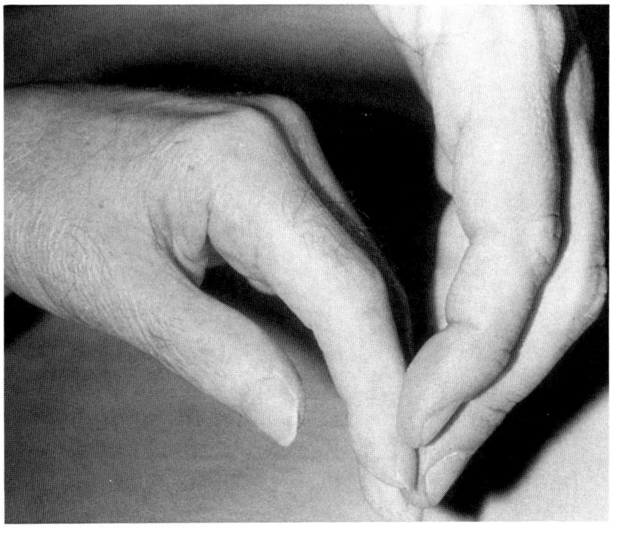

b

Figure 17-45a. This patient with SMPS is being treated with a steroid Bier block. **b.** Gentle manipulation of the digits is done under the influence of the steroid block.

modality for treating stiffness but will not necessarily improve any pain associated with the dystrophy unless the pain is due to joint stiffness and disuse.

After the manipulation, under the steroid block, the use of continuous passive movement has maintained the range of movement obtained during the steroid block. Once again, a series of steroid blocks over several days is recommended. Oral steroid, using a tapering regimen over 2 to 3 weeks, is used in conjunction with these blocks.

Painful Neuroma Sixth Degree Injury In-Continuity

The prototype of the painful nerve injury is the partial nerve injury. This is seen after traumatic injury to a major nerve with partial recovery of nerve function after repair and very frequently after iatrogenic nerve injury. The technique for dealing with this type of pain problem follows the basic principles previously described and rests firmly on a detailed clinical examination of the peripheral nerve involved. The surgeon is dealing with a mixed or sixth degree injury (Chapter 2). He will evaluate the patient and make a detailed clinical assessment of function in each fascicle or groups of fascicles of the nerve in question. With this clinical examination, he will be making a mental picture of the injury pattern within the nerve, separating, with his clinical examination, those components of the nerve that are functioning appropriately from those that are not. When no sensation (or motor function) exists, the surgeon will be dealing with a fourth or fifth degree injury. This portion of the nerve will require reconstitution with nerve grafting or nerve tube techniques (see Chapter 4 and 20). Evaluation of the type of sensibility testing in the remainder of the nerve will influence the surgeon's surgical management. If diminished and nonpainful light touch exists, preoperatively, the surgeon will plan to simply neurolyse the fascicles involved. If, however, the light touch that exists is exquisitely painful so that hyperalgesia is present, the surgeon will be influenced toward a nerve-grafting technique. On several occasions, however, in the face of exquisite hyperalgesia in the hand, exploration of the nerve demonstrates only marked scarring around the nerve and after a detailed neurolysis has been carried out the fascicles themselves look normal. In these cases, neurolysis would be all that was required. Thus, preoperatively, the surgeon, through a very detailed examination involving his entire battery of sensory testing instruments and electrophysiologic diagnosis, distinguishes the parts of the nerve that have no function and require nerve grafting, from those parts of the nerve that have diminished but present nonpainful sensory function and require only neurolysis. Those fascicles that mediate hyperalgesia may not require nerve grafting technique, depending on the findings at surgery. The smaller cutaneous nerves in the region of the major nerve injury that mediate nonfunctional sensation will be evaluated in the identical fashion to the major nerve injury. With the smaller cutaneous nerves (such as palmar cutaneous branch median nerve), the surgeon will not be planning nerve grafting techniques but either neurolysis or resection of the nerve and transposition in a more proximal soft tissue location.

Surgical Technique

Under tourniquet control with magnification, the nerve involved is exposed proximal and distal to the area of the injury in-continuity. The normal proximal and distal architecture of the nerve will be displayed before exploring the in-continuity lesion itself. When the injury is in the distal forearm, as it is frequently, it is possible to identify the various fascicles entering the main portion of the nerve through identification of distal nerve branches. These distal fascicles are then traced back proximally to the major nerve injury. Magnification and microneurosurgical technique will be required to separate the neuroma in-continuity into its various components (Fig. 6-7 and Fig. 4-7). The techniques of internal neurolysis (Chapter 5) will be required. Fascicles mediating no function will be replaced with a nerve graft or nerve tube. All fascicles will be neurolysed and those fascicles that on clinical examination had been noted to have poor sensation and significant hyperalgesia will be reconstructed with nerve grafts or a nerve tube.

If nerve grafts are required for the management of this nerve injury, all that is usually needed is a portion of the lateral antebrachial cutaneous nerve (5 to 6 cm) or the anterior branch of the medial antebrachial cutaneous nerve (6 to 12 cm). The nerve tube technique is described in Chapter 20.

Local Muscle Flaps

In those patients who have significant injury to the major nerves at the wrist, two local muscle flaps have been used with good success, the abductor digiti quinti muscle[83] and the pronator quadratus muscle.[84] These flaps are indicated for those patients who have significant pain and hyperalgesia in the skin over the volar aspect of the wrist. The patients usually have had several operative procedures in the past and have a very significant painful nerve injury. Transposition of these local muscle flaps over the injured nerve will act as a target for any stray sensory nerve fibers. Because these muscle flaps remain innervated, they will inhibit neuroma formation and certainly prevent reinnervation of the overlying scarred and denervated skin. This will markedly diminish the possibility of the redevelopment of hyperalgesia in the skin. It is very important to realize that transposition of these muscle flaps is not the panacea for nerve injury. These muscle flaps must only be transferred over nerve injuries that have been completely and appropriately treated with microneurosurgical techniques, as already described. Transposition of these flaps over an in-continuity neuroma that has not been appropriately managed with neurolysis and nerve grafting technique will not adequately treat the patient's pain. The abductor muscle flap can be used to cover injuries distal to the proximal wrist crease. The pronator quadratus flap can be used to cover injuries more proximal to this level. The techniques of elevation of these flaps is described below.

Abductor Digiti Quinti Muscle Flap

The standard carpal tunnel incision is used as well as a hypothenar incision, which is based along the border of the glabrous and hairy skin extending from the pisiform to the abductor tendon insertion. The abductor digiti minimi muscle is identified and any cutaneous branches of the dorsocutaneous branch of the ulnar nerve are preserved. These branches rarely cross the site of this incision. The muscle is dissected at the subfascial level, protecting the digital nerve to the little finger, which is superficial to the muscle fascia. The tendon of the abductor muscle is identified distally and this makes the separation of the abductor muscle from the other hypothenar muscles much easier. A portion of the tendon is taken with the muscle flap and serves as a good point of traction. The neurovascular bundle coming into the abductor muscle is noted at the very proximal base of the muscle, 1 cm lateral and 1 cm distal to the pisiform. The bundle is carefully preserved. A tunnel then is made connecting the two incisions. Care is taken to protect the ulnar vessels and nerve. There are usually several thin fascial bands extending from the hypothenar muscles to the overlying skin that need to be divided in order to allow the transposition of the muscle. A portion of the proximal origin of the muscle from the pisiform can be divided in order to allow the muscle to rotate easily into the carpal tunnel incision. The fascia over the muscle can be incised in order to allow the abductor flap to fan out over the nerve injury in a proximal distal direction. This muscle transfer can never be used both to pad the nerve injury and as an opponensplasty because it must be directed in a proximal distal direction in the region of the carpal tunnel to pad the nerve, and to serve as an opposition tendon transfer it must be directed toward the metacarpophalangeal joint of the thumb (Fig. 17-46). Volar radial skin may require elevation to permit ease of skin closure.

The transposition of this flap is easily carried out with an additional 30 minutes of tourniquet time. A volar splint maintaining the wrist in neutral is applied for 8 days. The patient will begin massage of the incisions at about the 10th postoperative day. In only one patient have we had any problem with the hypothenar donor site. This involved an abduction contracture of the little finger that was difficult to explain and proved impossible to treat. It did not, however, interfere with the patient's hand function. Importantly, these donor sites have never been painful and the loss of the muscle has not been a disability to the patient.

Pronator Quadratus Muscle

This flap is extremely useful for painful nerve injuries in the distal forearm. The muscle will cover an area directly above its anatomic location (Fig. 17-47). It cannot be transferred more distally than its own in situ position even though it is elevated on a neurovascular island flap. The technique of elevation is much more demanding than elevation of the abductor digiti quinti muscle flap and adds an additional 45 to 60 minutes of tourniquet time to the operative procedure. In the postoperative period, the patients will experience considerable pain at the operative site and for several weeks postoperative pronation and supination may be painful for them. The long-term results for pain relief are, however, excellent. The functional loss of the pronator quadratus is nonexistent and no long-term sequelae from the use of this muscle has been noted. The details of the surgical technique are outlined next.

The flap is used in conjunction with surgery to the injured nerve. Any preexisting palmar wrist or distal forearm scar can be used. The incision must be extended approximately 12 cm from the wrist crease in order to identify the neurovascular pedicle to the pronator quadratus muscle. Whatever procedures need to be carried out on the painful nerve can be done before elevating the muscle, but the delicate techniques of nerve grafting or the use of a nerve tube should be left until the flap has been elevated.

With the tourniquet inflated, the muscle flap is approached by identifying the pronator muscle between the flexor profundus and flexor pollicis longus muscle tendons (Fig. 17-48). The distal edge of the muscle is divided sharply from the radius and ulna and the terminal branches of the anterior interosseous nerve and

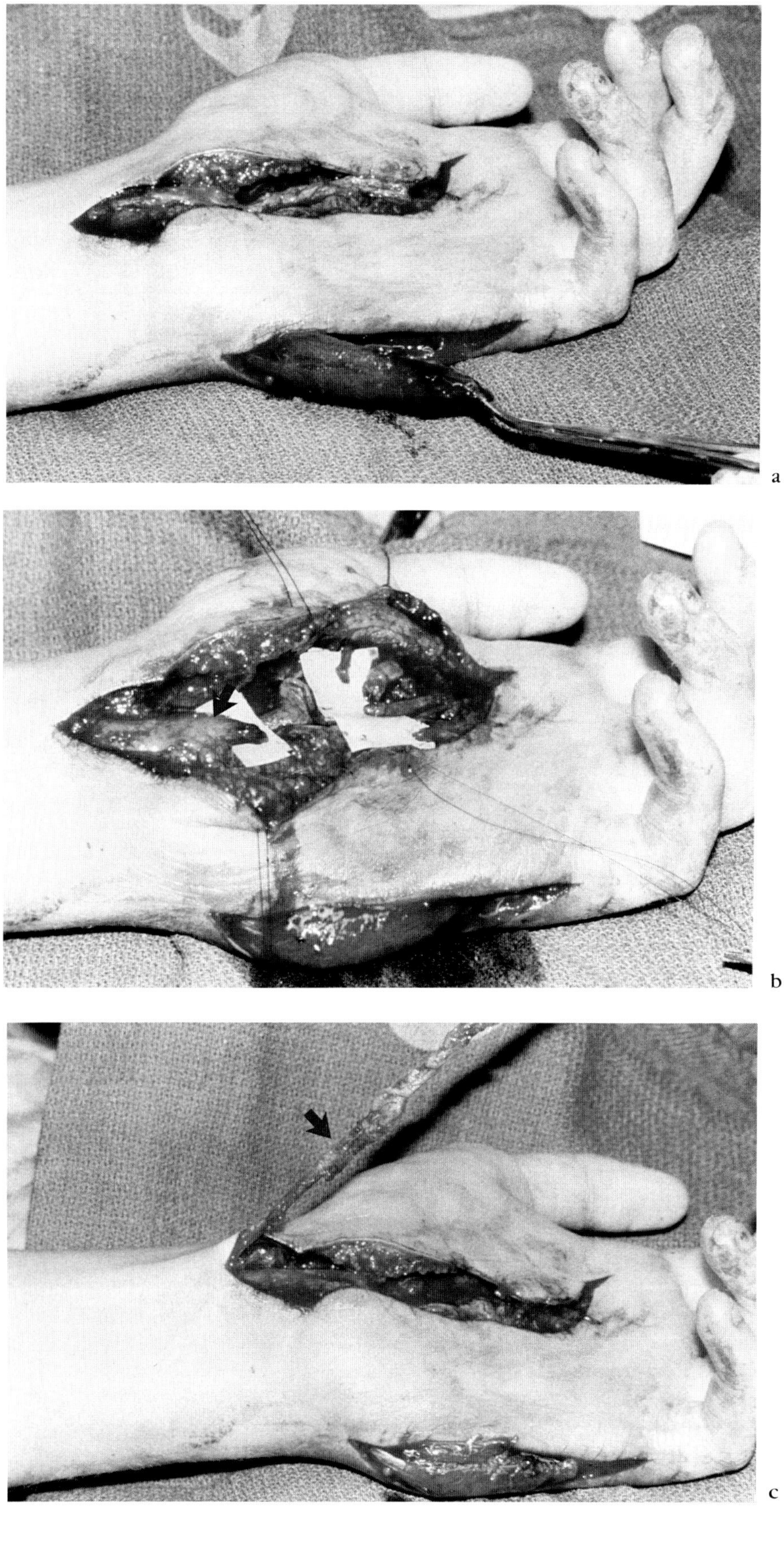

Figure 17-46a. Using an incision along the medial border of the hand,the abductor digiti quinti muscle is identified and isolated on its proximal attachment and the neurovascular bundle. **b.** In this patient with a painful median nerve injury, the proximal median nerve neuroma is noted (arrow). The distal digital and common digital nerves are identified. **c.** A tendon transfer (prolonged palmaris longus) is used to restore opposition of the thumb (arrow). (*Figure continues.*)

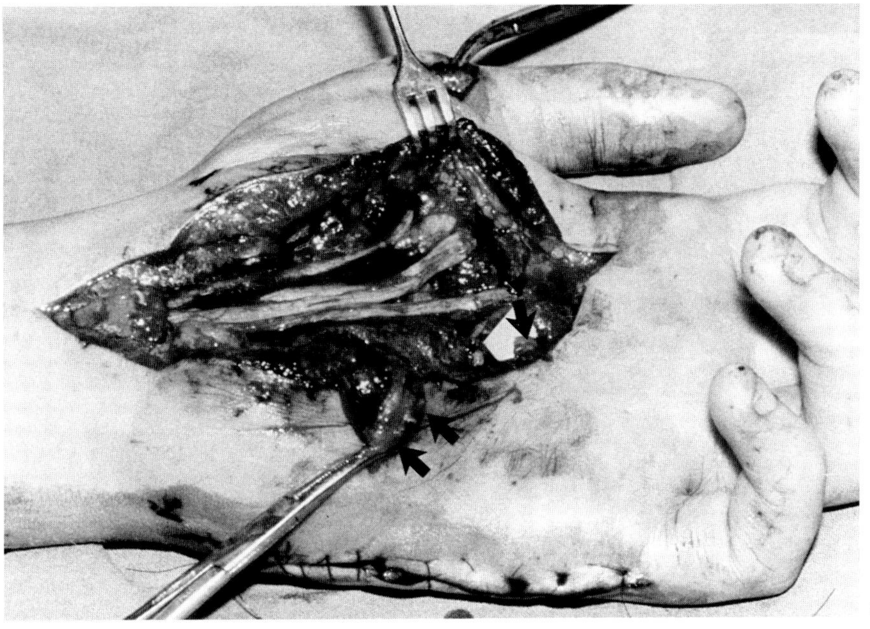

d

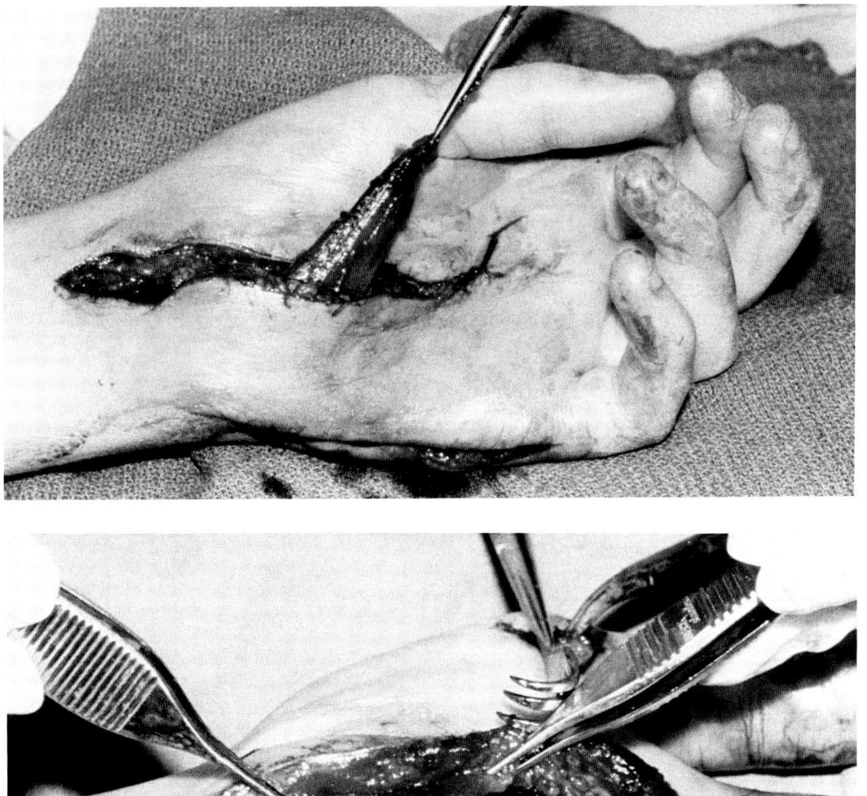

e

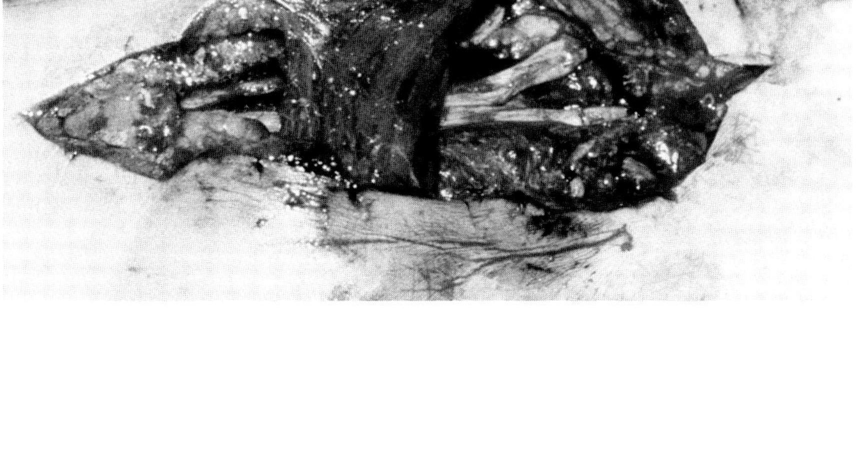

f

Figure 17-46 (*continued*) **d.** Sural nerve grafts are used to reconstruct the median nerve injury. Note the common digital nerve to the long and ring fingers has not been reconstructed because enough proximal nerve tissue was not available (arrow). Thus, the nerve grafts were oriented to maximize regeneration into the thumb and index fingers. Note the abductor flap has been transfered into the extended carpal tunnel incision before the nerve grafting is performed (double arrow). **e.** The abductor flap can be advanced toward the thumb (as for a tendon transfer). **f.** In this case, the flap is spread out over the nerve graft and directed in a proximal and distal direction. Thus, it cannot be used both as a tendon transfer and to provide good nerve coverage in the same case.

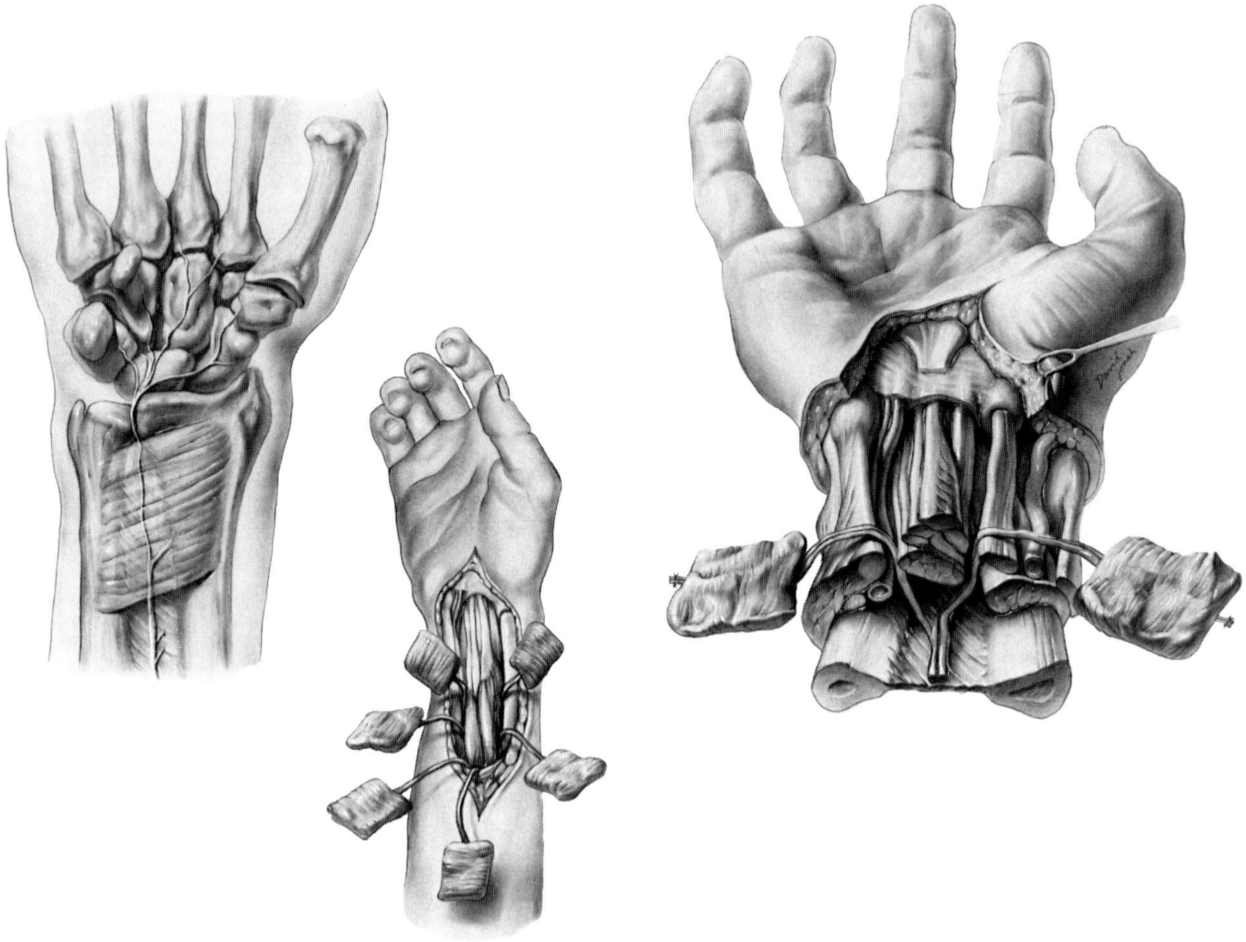

Figure 17-47. The pronator quadratus muscle is shown schematically supplied by the anterior interosseous neurovascular bundle with vessels perforating the interosseous membrane. Center, the arc of rotation of the pronator quadratus muscle flap allows coverage of the medial and lateral aspects of the forearm and distally to the proximal wrist crease. Right, the flap may be extended superficially by either a radial or ulnar route. (Reproduced with permission from Dellon and Mackinnon.[84])

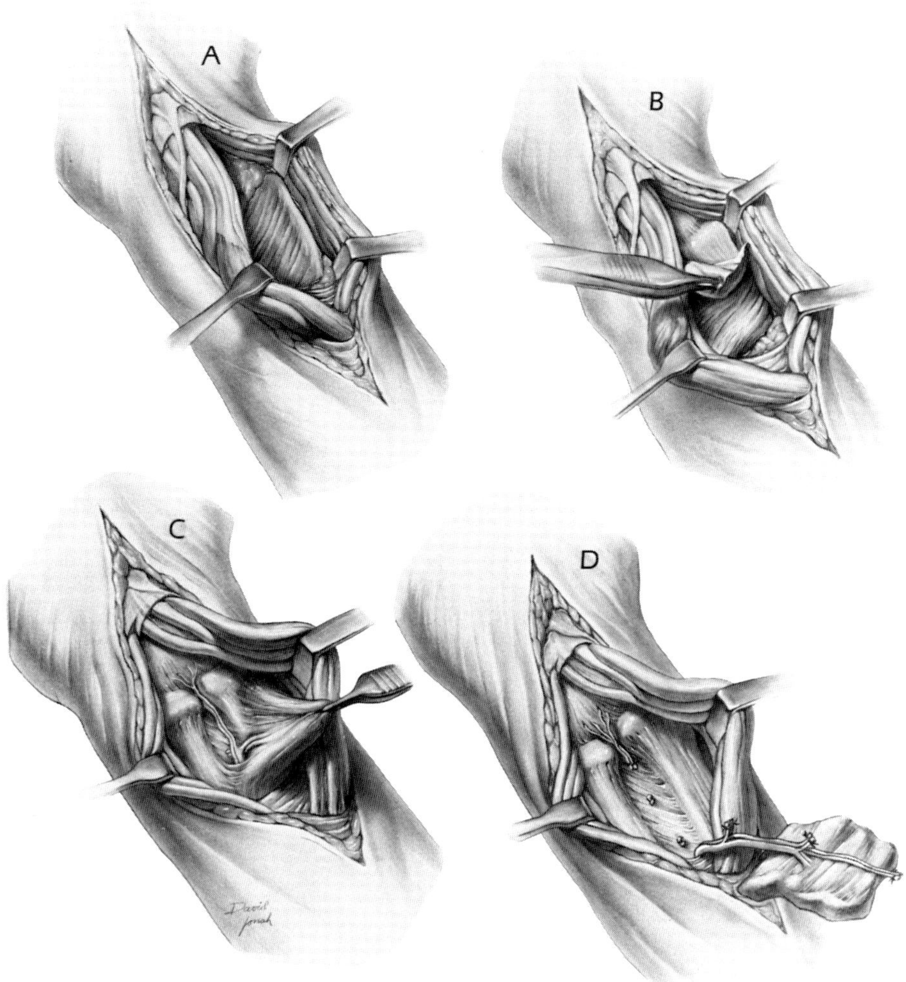

Figure 17-48. The technique of pronator quadratus muscle flap elevation is noted with exposure of the muscle in **a,** elevation of the muscle from the radius and ulna in **b** and **c,** with elevation of the muscle in the neurovascular pedicle in D. (Reproduced with permission from Dellon and Mackinnon.[84])

artery are divided. The muscle is then elevated by sharply dissecting the muscle first from the radius and then the ulna. The anterior interosseous neurovascular bundle is identified proximally and a vessel loop placed around it. The muscle is then lifted beginning distally and with gentle traction is elevated from the interosseous membrane. Perforating branches from the neurovascular bundle will be ligated and the flap can be elevated on its neurovascular bundle. After elevation of the flap, the tourniquet is deflated in order to allow the flap to perfuse and to obtain hemostasis. Any procedures still required to treat the nerve injury are carried out before rotating the flap into its final position (Fig. 17-49).

Pain after Carpal Tunnel Surgery

With the incidence of carpal tunnel syndrome on the rise and with a new awareness of this problem, surgery for median nerve compression at the wrist and the complications related to this surgery have also increased. Unfortunately, after failed carpal tunnel surgery, the patient frequently complains more of pain than loss of sensory or motor function.[85] The treatment of these painful sequelae is difficult.

Cause of Painful Complications

Fortunately, there is no longer widespread use of the transverse wrist incision for the release of the carpal tunnel (Fig. 17-50). This incision is to be soundly condemned. Should a complication arise after surgery carried out through such a transverse incision, there can be no basis for medicolegal defense. The recommended incision has been discussed in detail in Chapter 6. It is located in line with the long axis of the fourth digit in order to avoid injury to the palmar cutaneous branch of the median nerve and any ulnar cutaneous branches that are occasionally in this area. If the incision crosses the wrist crease, it will be necessary to use some "zig-zagging" technique. In our experience, if there ever is

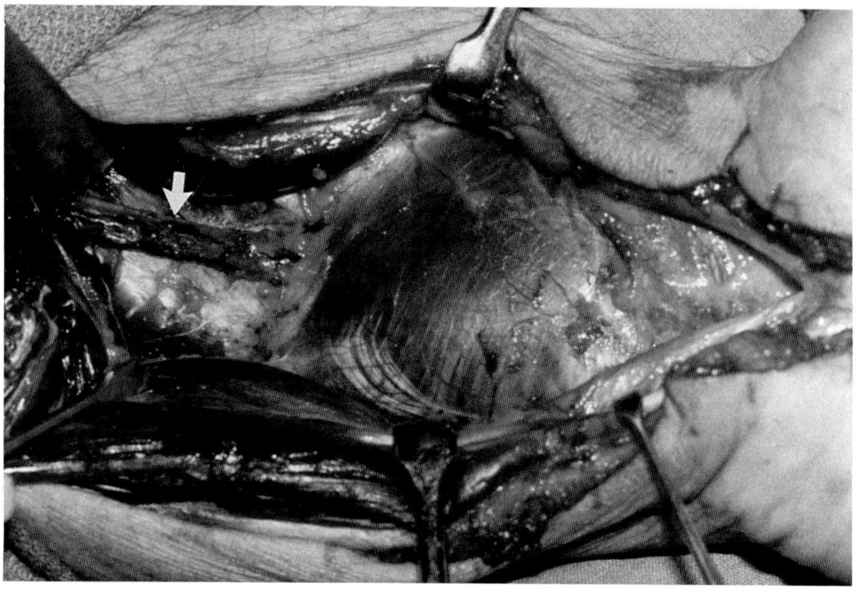

a

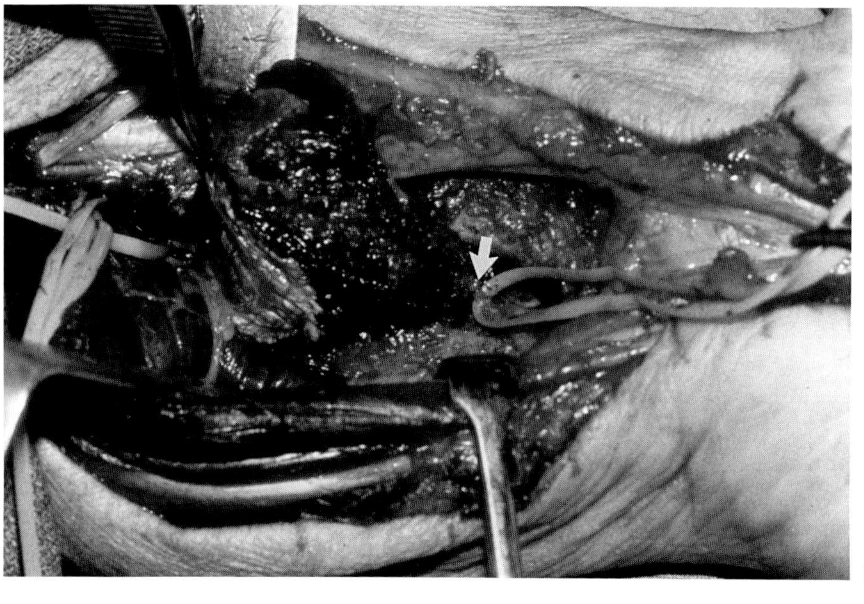

b

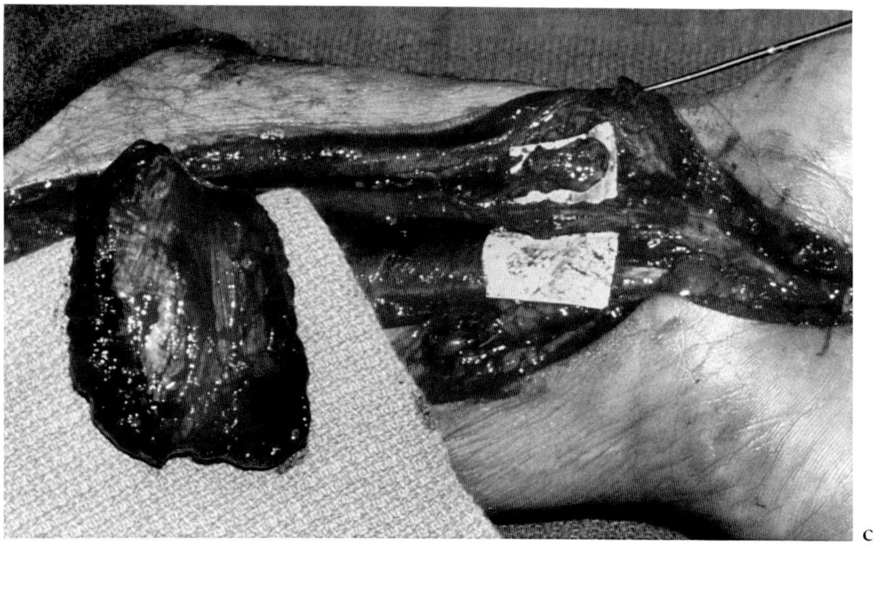

c

Figure 17-49. Intraoperative views (hand toward right). **a.** Pronator quadratus muscle exposed. Note proximal neurovascular bundle (left) (arrow). **b.** Pronator quadratus muscle elevated to show neurovascular bundle entering its deep side (vessel loop to the right). (arrow) **c.** Pronator quadratus muscle elevated. Note neurolysed median nerve and palmar cutaneous neuroma (overlying background). (*Figure continues.*)

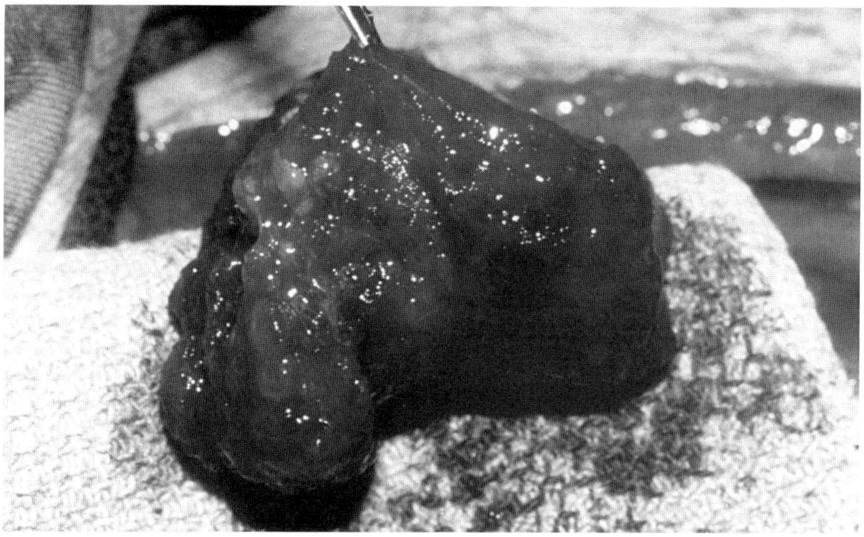

d

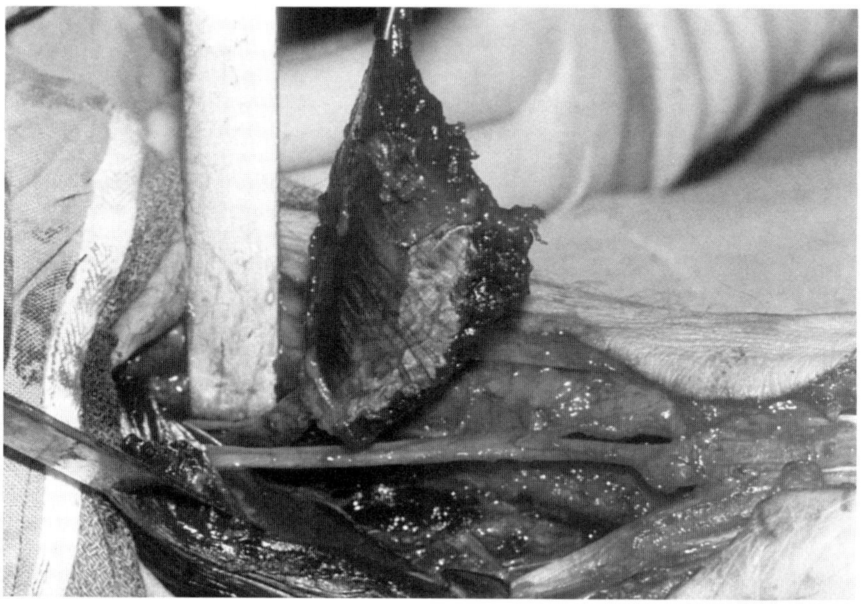

e

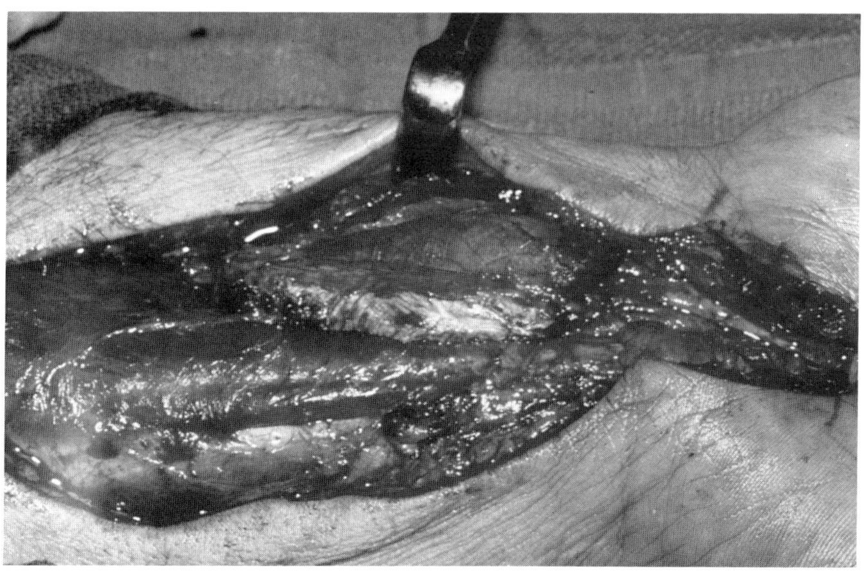

f

Figure 17-49 (*continued*) **d.** Tourniquet let down. Note bleeding from edges of flap. **e.** Muscle flap being interposed between skin and neurolysed median nerve. **f.** Flap in place. Palmar cutaneous neuroma has been resected and nerve end implanted into the muscle. (Reproduced with permission from Dellon and Mackinnon.[84])

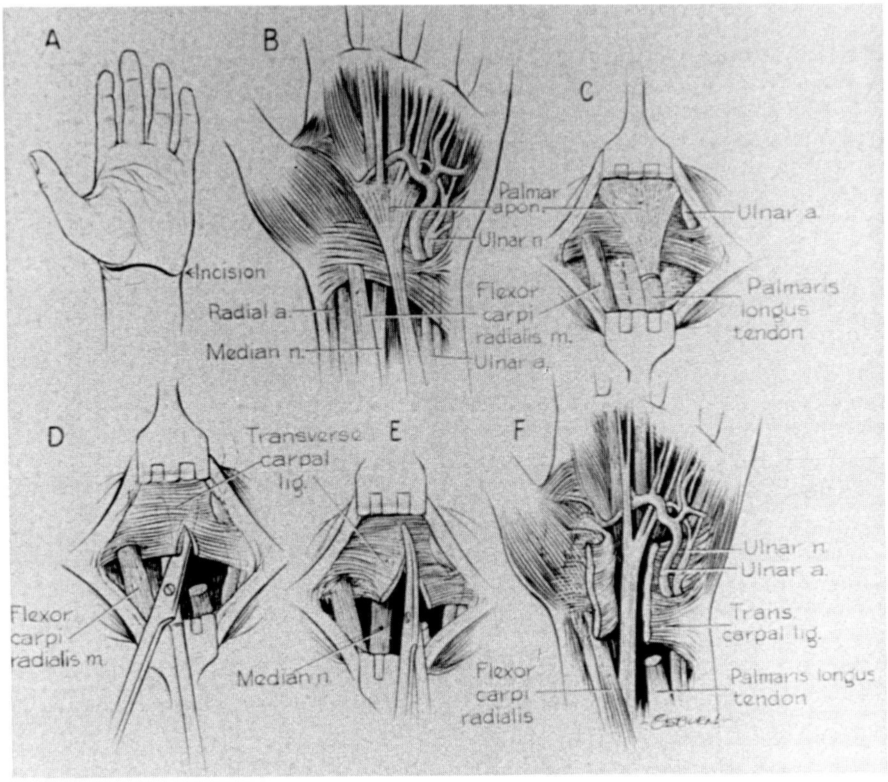

Figure 17-50. The technique for release of the carpal tunnel through a transverse wrist incision is to be condemned. (Reproduced with permission from Poppen[88].)

a painful area of local tenderness along the scar from carpal tunnel release, it is in the region of the wrist. Thus, if a neurolysis is not necessary, the incision may well stop short of crossing the wrist. Of course, the distal portion of the antebrachial fascia must be released through direct visualization underneath the distal forearm skin.

Twenty percent of the patients referred for consideration for repeat carpal tunnel release had associated inappropriate incisions used at the initial surgery.

Table 17-12 outlines the findings on physical examination and at surgery to account for the patient's pain problems. Table 17-13 outlines the procedures done to treat these problems.

Entrapment of the palmar cutaneous nerve has mimicked a neuroma. In these cases, only release of the palmar cutaneous branch was required (Fig. 17-51).

Table 17-12. Cause of Painful Symptoms in Patients After Carpal Tunnel Release

Incomplete first operation
Pathologic scar, reformation of flexor retinaculum, entrapment palmar cutaneous branch
Surgical misadventure (lacerated, median, palmar cutaneous branch)
Neuroma formation
Proximal entrapment of median nerve

Table 17-13. Surgical Procedures Performed on Patients with Persistent Symptoms After Carpal Tunnel Release

Surgery
Nerve grafting (lateral antebrachial cutaneous nerve to median)
Muscle flap (Abductor digiti minimi muscle flap)
Excision or burying neuroma (palmar cutaneous nerve)
Neurolysis
Internal
External
Excision of reformed ligament
Simple incision of carpal ligament
Removal of foreign body
Release of median nerve forearm
Release of palmar cutaneous nerve entrapment

Frequently, all that is required is a detailed neurolysis (Fig. 17-52). Occasionally, nerve grafting will be required.

It is concluded, from review of these patients, that careful examination coupled with careful surgery will result in relief of symptoms in most of these patients. In patients who have carpal tunnel syndrome after major forearm crush or injury, the incision should be extended well across the wrist and into the distal forearm. The distal forearm fascia in these instances will constitute a significant component of the cause of the entrapment neuropathy (Fig. 17-53).

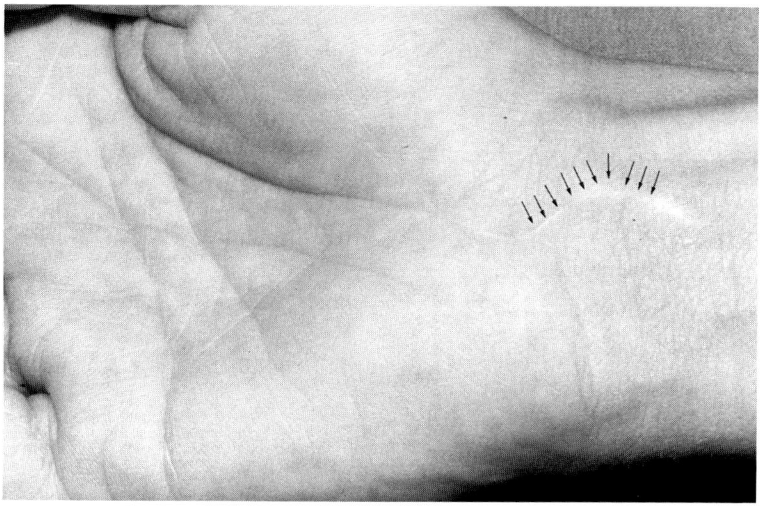

a

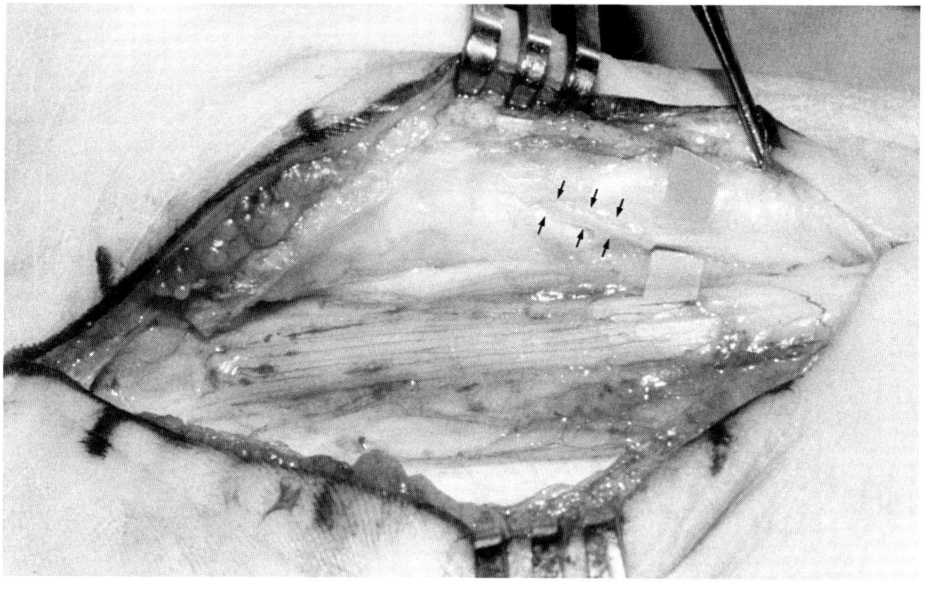

b

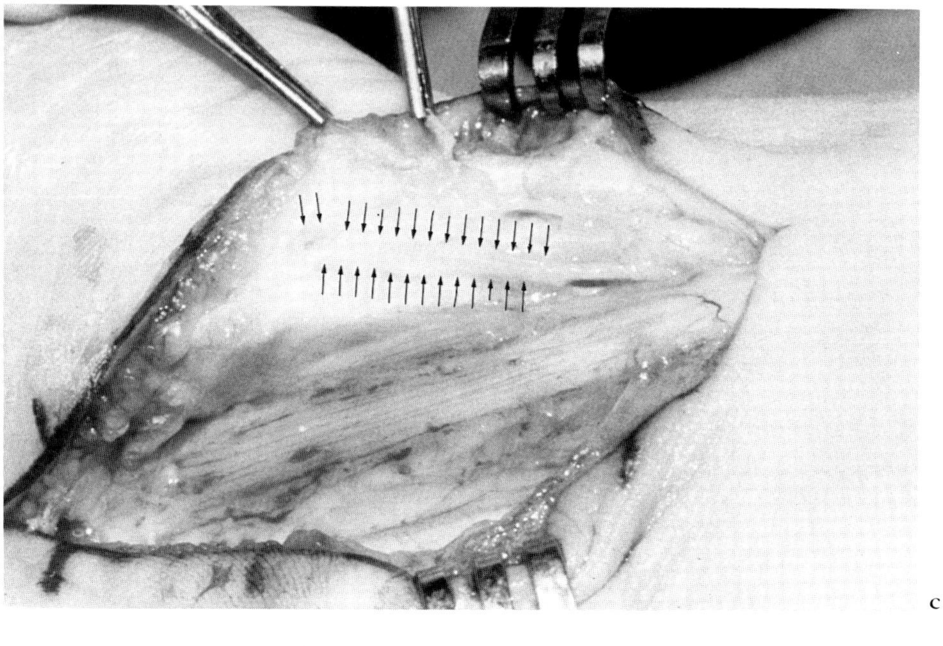

c

Figure 17-51a. The previous carpal tunnel incision passes over the course of the palmar cutaneous branch of the median nerve. The patient had symptoms of a neuroma of the palmar cutaneous nerve. **b.** At exploration, the palmar cutaneous nerve was not divided but was compressed and entrapped in its own separate tunnel. **c.** It was subsequently decompressed well into the carpal region. Note neurolysis of median nerve.

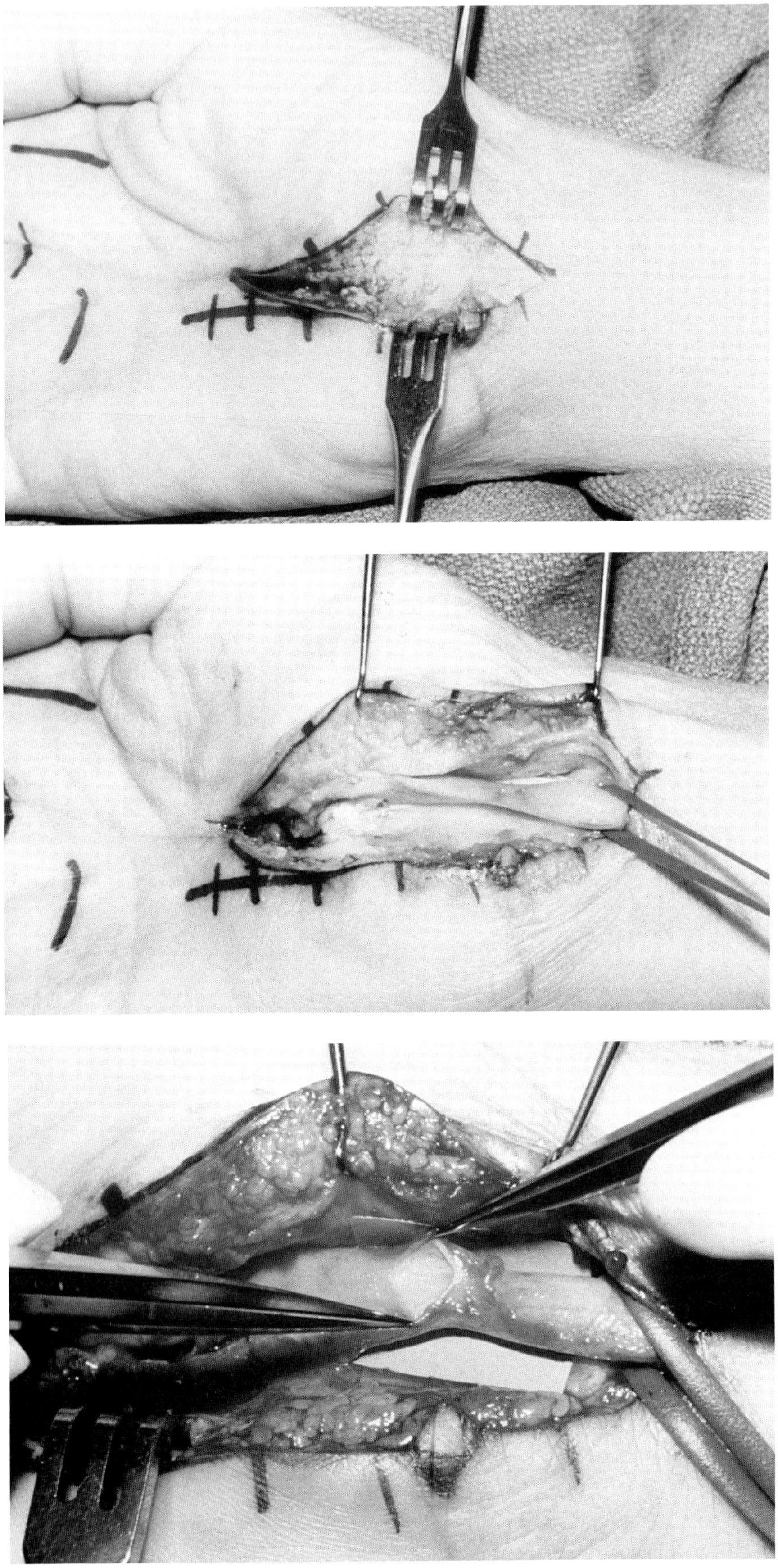

a

b

c

Figure 17-52a. This diabetic patient lost all median nerve function after a carpal tunnel release. At the time of her repeat carpal tunnel surgery, a "new" transverse arch had formed. **b.** The median nerve was adherent to the carpal ligament and very scarred and narrowed. **c.** An epineurotomy was carried out. (*Figure continues.*)

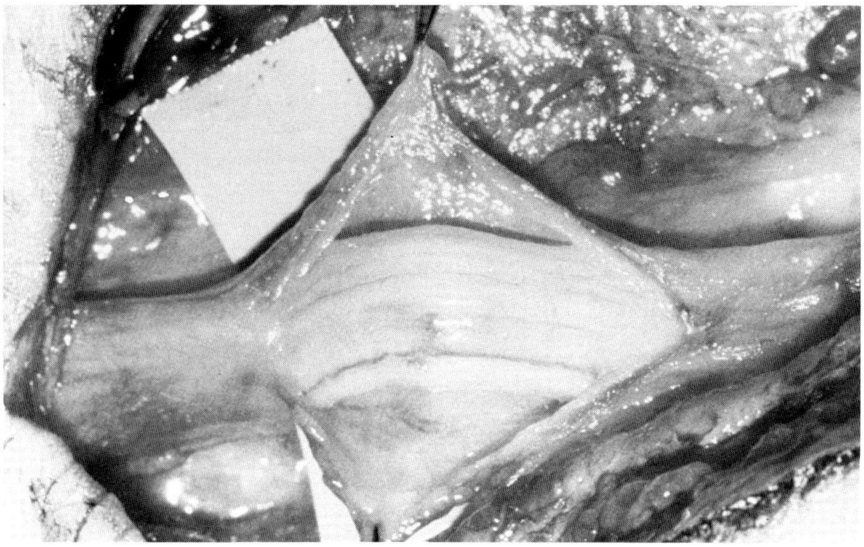

d

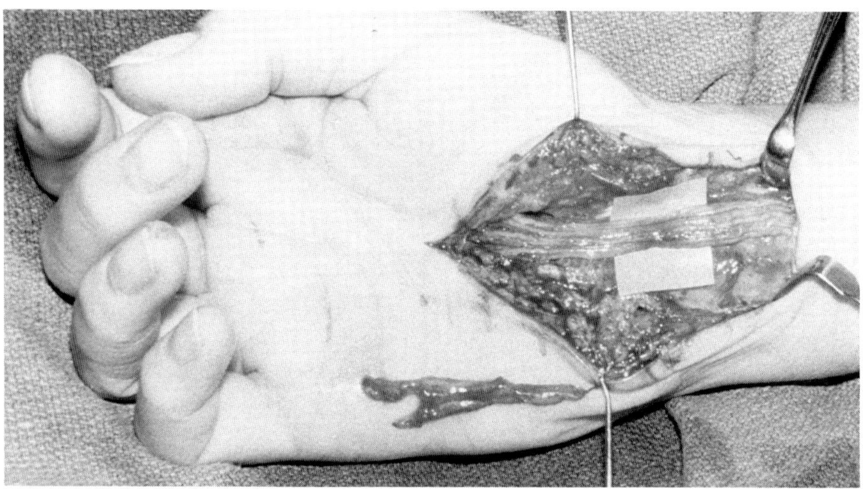

e

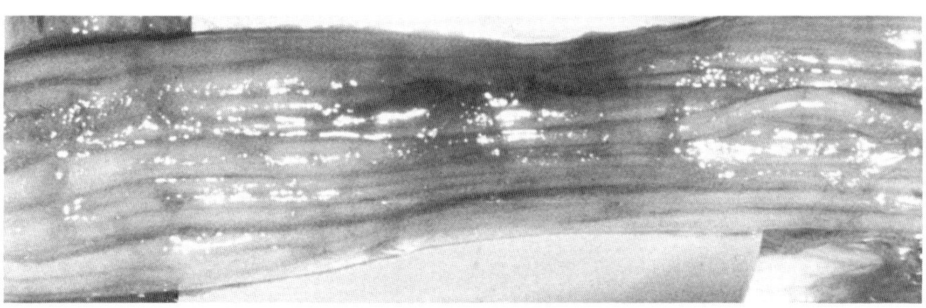

f

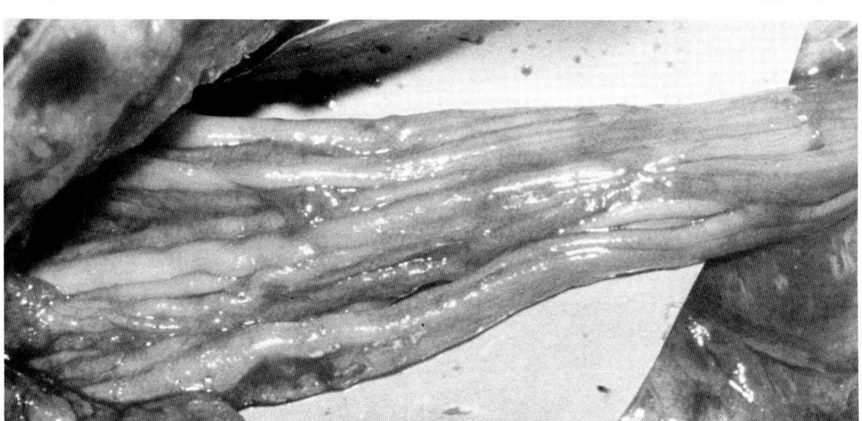

g

Figure 17-52 (*continued*) **d.** The normal fascicular pattern is noted after the epinerium is opened. **e.** After detailed microneurosurgical internal neurolysis, an improved fascicular pattern is seen, the epineurium excised is noted on the hypothenar eminence. **f.** A closer view of the portion of the nerve under the visibility background shows some hyperemia. **g.** In the median nerve distal to the compression,the fascicles are tortuous and distended because of the backup in the axonal transport due to the proximal nerve compression. Excellent return of function occurred after this procedure, but it returned slowly over the following 10 months.

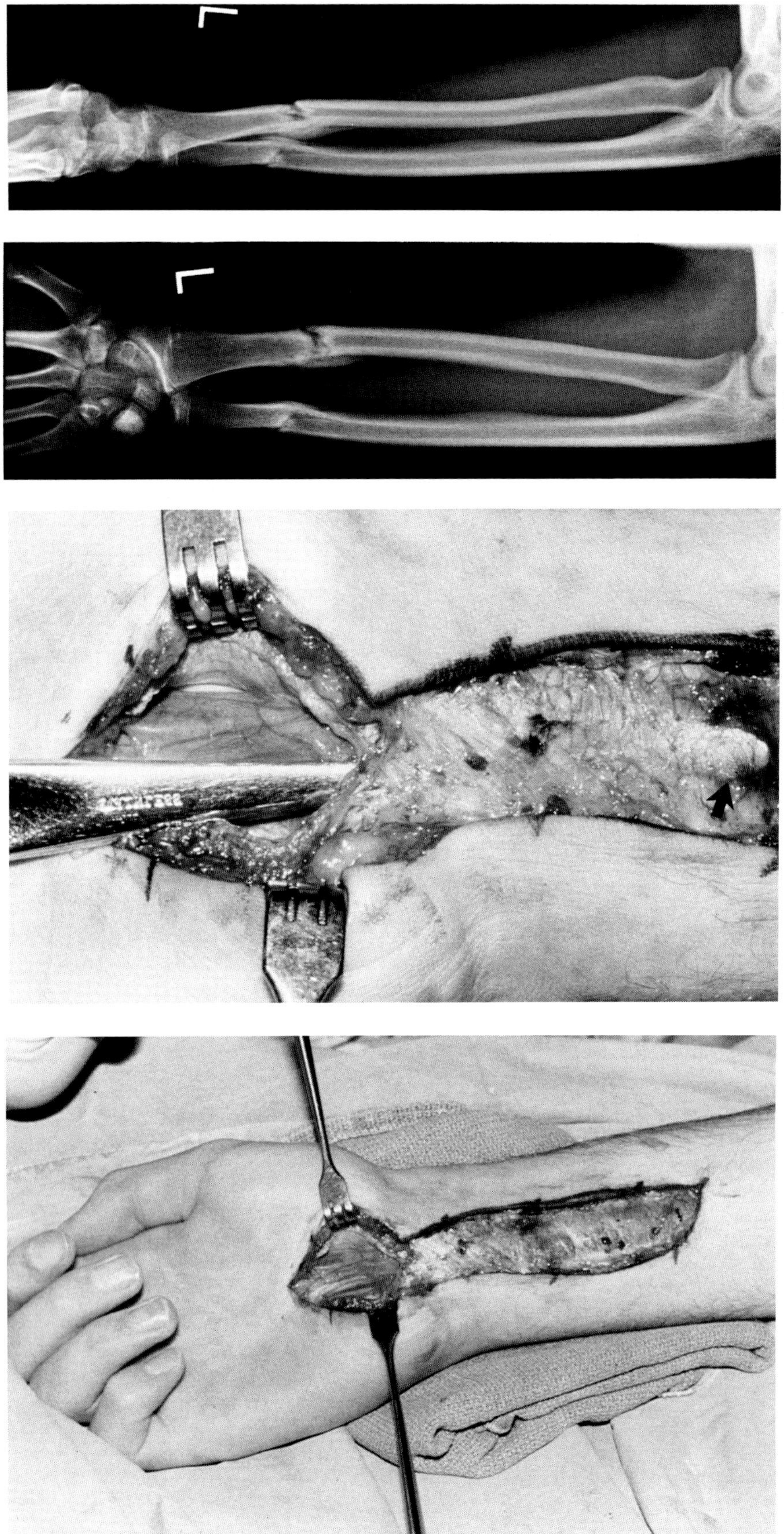

a

b

c

Figure 17-53a. After fractures of both bones of the forearm, this patient developed pain and diminished in the median nerve distribution. **b.** The median nerve was released at the carpal tunnel. The fascia of the forearm was also compressing the nerve. The elevator is visualized only at the far right of this photograph (arrow). **c.** The incision was extended proximally and the entire median nerve decompressed. (*Figure continues.*)

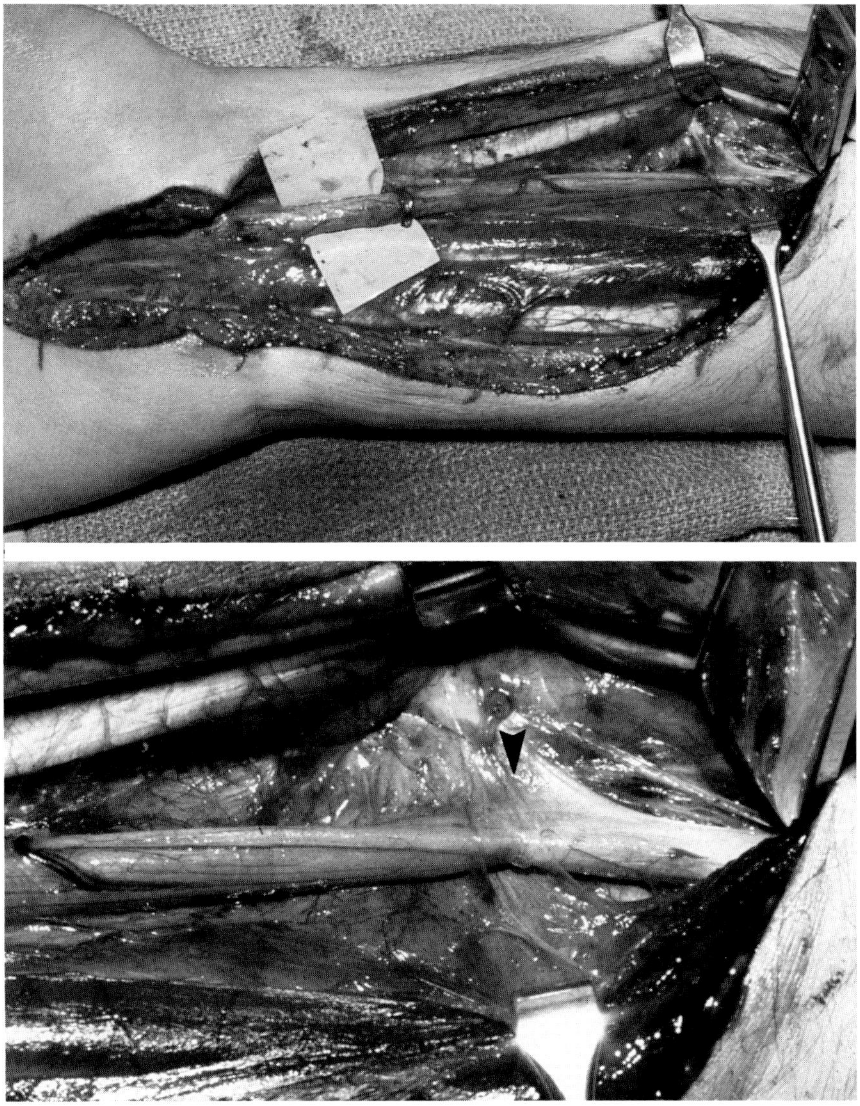

d

e

Figure 17-53 *(continued)* **d.** An area of nerve compression and scarring was found at the level of the fracture at the proximal extent of this incision **e.** Close-up view of the injury (arrow).

Wrist Pain

The perception of pain arising in the wrist can be either of joint origin or from injury to the terminal portions of the anterior and posterior interosseous nerves that innervate these joints. Discussion of the diagnosis and management of pathologic conditions within the wrist joint is beyond the scope of this chapter. Diagnosis of wrist pain amenable to treatment by partial wrist denervation can be made by appropriate local anesthetic blocks of these nerves. If pain is relieved and function is judged by increased grip strength and range of motion is improved, either a partial volar or partial dorsal wrist denervation procedure can be done.[86,87]

References

1. Seltzer Z, Devor M: Ephaptic transmission in chronically damaged peripheral nerves. Neurology (Minneap) 29: 1061–1064, 1974.
2. Wall PD, Devor M: Sensory afferent impulses originate from dorsal root ganglia as well as from the periphery in normal and nerve injured rats. Pain 17:321, 325, 1983.
3. Wall PD, Gutnick M: Properties of afferent nerve impulses originating from a neuroma. Nature 248:740, 742, 1974.
4. Wall PD: Alterations in the central nervous system after deafferentation connectivity control. Adv Pain Res Ther 5:677–689, 1983.
5. Bonica JJ: Causalgia and other reflex sympathetic dystrophies. In Bonica JJ, Liebskind JC, Alke-Fessaid DG eds: Adv. Pain Res Ther 3:141–166, 1979.
6. Holder LE, Mackinnon SE: Reflex sympathetic dystrophy in the hands: Clinical and scintigraphic criteria. Radiology 152:517–522, 1984.
7. Melzak R, Wall PD: Pain mechanisms—a new theory. Science 150:971, 1965.

8. Campbell JN, Raja SN, Meyer RA, Mackinnon SE: Myelinated fibres in peripheral nerves signal hyperalgesia that follows nerve injury. Pain 32:89–94, 1988.
9. Lindbloom U, Verillo RT: Sensory functions in chronic neuralgia. Neurol Neurosurg Psychiatry 42:422–435, 1979.
10. Wallin G, Torebjork E, Hallin R: The preliminary observations on the pathophysiology of hyperalgesia in the causalgic pain syndrome. In Zotterman Y, ed: Sensory Functions of the Skin in Primates. Pergamon Press, Elmsford, NY, 1976, 489–499.
11. Battista AF, Cravioto HM, Budzilovich GN: Painful neuroma: Changes produced in peripheral nerve after fascicle ligation. Neurosurgery 9:589–600, 1981.
12. Frackelton WH, Teasley JL, Tauras A: Neuromas in the hand treated by nerve transposition and silicone capping. J Bone Joint Surg 53A:813, 1971.
13. Munro D: Prevention of amputation neuromas. Consultant 12:26, 1972.
14. Swanson AB, Boeve NR, Biddulph SL: Silicone-rubber capping of amputation neuromas. Investigational and clinical experience. Interclin Info Bull 11:1, 1972.
15. Guttman L, Medawar PB: The chemical inhibition of fiber regeneration and neuroma formation in peripheral nerves. J Neurol Neurosurg Psychiatry 5:130, 1942.
16. Huber GC, Lewis D: Amputation neuromas. Their development and prevention. Arch Surg 1:85–113, 1920.
17. Poth EJ, Bravo-Fernandez E, Dreager GA: Prevention of formation of end-bulb neuromata. Proc Soc Exp Biol Med 60:200–207, 1945.
18. Snyder CC, Knowles RP: Traumatic neuromas. J Bone Joint Surg 47A:641–648, 1965.
19. Evans LE, Campbell JB, Pinner-Poole B, Jenny J: Preventation of painful neuromas in horses. Am Vet Med Assoc 153:313, 1968.
20. Farley HH: Treatment of painful stump neuroma. Minn Med 48:347, 1950.
21. Wiley RG, Blessing WW, Reis DJ: Suicide transport: Destruction of neurons by retrograde transport of ricin abrin and modeccin. Science 216:889, 1982.
22. Moszkowicz LP: Zur Behandlung der schmerzhaften neuroma. Zentralbl Chir 45:547, 1918.
23. Teneff S: Prevention of amputation neuroma. J Int Coll Surg 12:16, 1949.
24. Munro D, Mallory GK: Elimination of the so called amputation neuromas of derivative peripheral nerves. J Med 260:358, 1959.
25. Petropoulos PC, Stefanko S: Experimental studies of post-traumatic neuroma under various physiologic conditions. J Surg Res 1:235, 1961.
26. Petropoulos PC, Stefanko S: Experimental observations on the prevention of neuroma formation. J Surg Res 1:241, 1961.
27. Dellon AL, Mackinnon SE, Pestronk A: Implantation of sensory nerve into muscle: Preliminary, clinical and experimental observations on neuroma formation. Ann Plast Surg 12:30–40, 1984.
28. Mackinnon SE, Dellon AL, Hudson AR, Hunter DA: Alteration of neuroma formation produced by manipulation of neural environment in primates. Plast Reconstr Surg 76: 345–352, 1985.
29. Dellon AL, Mackinnon SE: Treatment of the painful neuroma by neuroma resection and muscle implantation. Plast Reconstr Surg 77:427–436, 1986.
30. Boldney E: Amputation neuroma in nerves implanted in bone. Ann Surg 118:1052–1057, 1943.
31. Herndon JH, Eaton RG, Littler JW: Management of painful neuromas in the hand. J Bone Joint Surg 58A:369–373, 1976.
32. Laborde KG, Kalisman M, Tsai T: Results of surgical treatment of painful neuromas of the hand. J Hand Surg 7:190–193, 1982.
33. Tupper JW, Booth DM: Treatment of painful neuromas of sensory nerves in the hand: A comparison of traditional and newer methods. J Hand Surg 1:144–151, 1976.
34. Meyer RA, Raja SN, Campbell JN, Mackinnon SE, Dellon AL: Neural activity originating from a neuroma in the baboon. Brain Res 325:255–260, 1985.
35. Hendler N: Hendler ten minute screening test for chronic back pain patients. Psychosomatics 20:806–808, 1979.
36. Mackinnon SE, Dellon AL: Screening test for evaluation of patients with hand pain. In preparation. 1990.
37. Stokes HM: The seriously uninjured hand—weakness of grip. J Occup Med 25:683–684, 1983.
38. Hildreth D: The Jamar Dynamometer. Presented at the 41st Annual Meeting of the American Society for Surgery of the Hand, New Orleans, February 19, 1986.
39. Mackinnon SE, Dellon AL: Results of treatment of recurrent dorsal radial wrist neuromas. Ann Plast Surg 19:54–61, 1987.
40. Mackinnon SE, Dellon AL: Algorithm for management of painful neuroma. Contemp Orhtop 13:15–27, 1986.
41. Tada K, Nakashima H, Yoshida T, Kitano K: A new treatment of painful amputation neuroma: A preliminary report. J Hand Surg [Br] 12:273–276, 1987.
42. Berger A, Meissl G: Innervated skin grafts and flaps for restoration of sensation to anesthetic areas. Chir Plast 3:33–37, 1975.
43. Dellon AL, Mackinnon SE: Pain after radial sensory nerve grafting. J Hand Surg [Br] 11:341–346, 1986.
44. Murray JF, Carman W, Mackenzie JK: Transmetacarpal amputation of the index finger and clinical assessment of hand strength and complications. J Hand Surg 2:471–481, 1977.
45. Mackinnon SE: The wandering nerve graft technique for the management of the recalcitrant painful neuroma in the hand. Microsurgery 9:46—51, 1988.
46. Brown H, Flynn JE: Abdominal pedicle flap for hand neuromas and entrapped nerves. J Bone Joint Surg 55A:875, 1973.
47. Mackinnon SE, Dellon AL: The use of soft tissue expansion in the hand. J Hand Surg [Br] 12:73–77, 1987.
48. Dellon AL, Mackinnon SE: Susceptibility of the superficial sensory branch of the radial nerve to form painful neuromas. J Hand Surg [Br] 9:42–45, 1984.
49. Mackinnon SE, Dellon AL: The overlap pattern of the lateral antebrachial cutaneous nerve and the superficial branch of the radial nerve. J Hand Surg [Am] 10:522–526, 1985.
50. Dworkin RH, Handlin DS, Richlin DM: Unravelling the effects of compensation, litigation and employment on the treatment response in chronic pain. Pain 23:49, 1985.

51. Arons MS: deQuervain's release in working women: A report of failures, complications and associated diagnoses. J Hand Surg [Am] 12:40–44, 1987.
52. Saplys R, Mackinnon SE, Dellon AL: The relationship between nerve entrapment versus neuroma complications and the misdiagnosis of deQuervain's disease. Contemp Orthop 15:51–57, 1987.
53. Mitchell SW, Morehouse GR, Keen WW: In gunshot wounds and other injuries of nerves. JB Lippincott, Philadelphia, 1864.
54. Lankford LL: Reflex sympathetic dystrophy. In Omer GE, Spinner M, eds: Management of Peripheral Nerve Problems. WB Saunders, Philadelphia, 1980. 216–244.
55. Doupe J, Cullen CH, Chance GQ: Posttraumatic pain and causalgia syndrome. J Neurol Neurosurg Psychiatry 7:332–348, 1944.
56. Livingston WK: In Livingston WK, ed. Pain Mechanisms of Physiological Interpretation of Causalgia and its Related States. Plenum Publishing, New York, 1943.
57. Lorento DE, No R: Analysis of the activity of the chains of enternuncial neurons. J Neurophysiol 1:207–244, 1938.
58. Lewis T: Experiments relating to cutaneous hyperalgesia and its spread through somatic nerves. Clin Sci 2:373–423, 1936.
59. Lewis T: The nocifensor system of nerves and its reactions. Br Med J 1:431–435, 1937.
60. Lankford LL: Reflex sympathetic dystrophy. In Green DP ed: Operative Hand Surgery, Churchill Livingstone, New York, 1982, pp 539–562.
61. Wilson PR: Neurologic mechanisms of pain. In Cousins MJ, Bridenbaugh POD eds: Neural Blockade in Clinical Assessment and Management of Pain. JB Lippincott, Philadelphia, 1982, pp 557–585.
62. Yaksh TL, Hammond DL: Peripheral and central substrates involved in the rostrad transmission of nociceptive information. Pain 13:1–85, 1982.
63. Cuello AC, Delfiacco MD, Paxinos G: The central and peripheral ends of substance P contaning sensory neurons in the rat trigeminal system. Brain Res 152:499–500, 1978.
64. Jessell TM, Iversen LL, Guello AC: Capsaician-induced depletion of substance P from primary sensory neurons. Brain Res 152:183–188, 1978.
65. Henry JL: Effects of substance P on functionally identified units in cat spinal cord. Brain Res 114:439–451, 1976.
66. Szolcsanyi J: A pharmacological approach to lucidation of the role of different nerve fibres and receptor endings in mediation of pain. J Physiol (Paris) 73:251–259, 1977.
67. Almay BGL, Johansson F, von Knorring L: Endorphins in chronic pain—differences in CSF endorphin levels between organic and psychogenic pain syndromes. Pain 5: 153–162, 1978.
68. von Knorring L, Almay BGL, Johansson F: Pain perception and endorphin levels in cerebrospinal fluid. Pain 5:359–365, 1978.
69. Wall PD: In Seigfried J, Zimmerman M, eds: Phantom and Stump Pain. Springer-Verlag, New York, 1981, pp 2–14.
70. Blumpber H, Janig W: In Seigfried J, Zimmerman M, eds: Phantom and Stump Pain. Springer-Verlag, Berlin, 1981, pp 15–31.
71. Vane JR: Prostaglandin Thromboxane Res 2:791–801, 1976.
72. Higgs GA, Higgs EA, Salmon JA: Prostacyclin in inflammation. In Vane JR, Bergstrom S, eds: Prostacyclin. Raven Press, New York, 1979, pp 187–193.
73. Kaley G, Weiner R: Prostaglandin E_1: A potential mediator of the inflammatory response. Ann NY Acad Sci 180:338–350, 1971.
74. Ferreira SH, Mondcada S, Vane JR: In Robinson JH, Vane JR, eds: Prostaglandins and Signs and Symptoms of Inflammation. Raven Press, New York, 1974.
75. Bennett A: In Turner PW, Syhand DG, eds: Prostaglandins. Churchill Livingstone, Edinburgh, 1979, pp 17–30.
76. Dekel S, Lenthall G, Francis MJO: Release of prostaglandins from bone and muscle after tibial fracture: An experimental study in rabbits. J Bone Joint Surg 63B:185–189, 1981.
77. Bennett A, Harvey W: Prostaglandins in orthopedics. J Bone Joint Surg 63B:152–154, 1981.
78. Kozin F, Soin JS, Ryan LM: Bone scintigraphy in reflex sympathetic dystrophy syndrome. Radiology 138:437–443, 1981.
79. Kozin F, Ryan LM, Carerra GF: Reflex sympathetic dystrophy syndrome, Part III. Am J Med 70:23–30, 1981.
80. Mackinnon SE, Holder LE: The use of three-phase radionuclide bone scanning in the diagnosis of reflex sympathetic dystrophy. J Hand Surg [Am] 9:556–563, 1984.
81. Hobelmann CJ, Dellon AL: The use of prolonged sympathetic blockade as an adjunct to surgery in the patient with sympathetic maintained pain. Miscrosurg 10:151—153, 1989.
82. Hannington-Kiff JG: Pharmocological target blocks in hand surgery and rehabilization. J Hand Surg [Br] 9:29–36, 1984.
83. Reisman N, Dellon AL: The abductor digiti minimi muscle flap—a salvage technique for palmar wrist pain. Plast Reconstr Surg 72:859–863, 1983.
84. Dellon AL, Mackinnon SE: The pronator quadratus muscle flap. J Hand Surg [Am] 9:423–427, 1984.
85. Rutka J, Mackinnon SE: Results of treatment of recurrent carpal tunnel syndrome. J Hand Surg 1988. In press.
86. Dellon AL: Partial dorsal wrist denervation: Resection of posterior interosseous nerve. J Hand Surg [Am] 10:527–533, 1985.
87. Dellon AL, Mackinnon SE: Terminal branch of anterior interosseous nerve as source of volar wrist pain. J Hand Surg 9B:316—322, 1984.
88. Poppen JL: Atlas of Neurosurgical Techniques. WB Saunders, Philadelphia, 1960.

18

Sensory Rehabilitation After Nerve Injury

Physicians interested in rehabilitation after nerve injury have emphasized electrodiagnostic studies and restoration of motor function through physical modalities. Excellent texts on this approach exist.[1–5] Rehabilitation of sensory function has been neglected. The earliest attempts to rehabilitate sensation began in patients following cerebrovascular accidents. These studies devised various objects that the stroke patients could manipulate, emphasized the performance of activities of daily living and adaptive objects, such as forks and knives with larger handles, and resulted in some research studies that, in fact, demonstrated that patients with better recovery of sensation after stroke had a quicker discharge from the hospital and quicker return to activities of their daily lives.[6–9]

As surgeons became increasingly interested and able to operate on the peripheral nervous system, they, as well as the rehabilitation team, became interested in measuring the results of these attempts to restore sensation to the hand. In the 1960s, the physiatrist, Wynn Parry in England began to rehabilitate patients after peripheral nerve surgery and was the first to use the term "re-education of sensation."[10] His attempt focused on utilizing large objects and smaller shaped objects and recording the time it took for the patient to recognize these objects. The same series of test objects were utilized from the beginning of sensory recovery. The patient could use his time improvements as a guide to his rehabilitation. In subsequent reports, Wynn Parry's team has demonstrated that sensory re-education has been useful to them for patients with repair of the median nerve at the wrist.[11,12]

In 1968, Dellon became interested in evaluating sensibility based on the correlation of histologic and neurophysiologic concepts of slowly and quickly adapting fibers. This type of sensory evaluation was applied to patients recovering from peripheral nerve repairs and a consistent pattern of sensory recovery was noted.[13] This pattern was that the thinly myelinated and unmyelinated fibers recovered first, restoring perception of pain and temperature and these recovered at approximately the same time as pseudomotor function. Later, the touch perception recovered and could be subdivided into the following: the first to recover was the perception of 30 cps vibratory stimulus; the next was the perception of moving touch; the third was perception of constant touch; the last was the perception of 256 cps vibratory stimulus. Utilizing this type of sensibility evaluation protocol, this pattern of recovery was also found by Gelberman et al[14] in their studies of sensory recovery after digital replantation. Most recently, investigators under the directorship of Professor Tajima in Niigata, and reported at the 28th Meeting of the Japanese Society for Surgery of the Hand by Tachikawa, have made similar confirmatory observations of this pattern of recovery.[15]

Rehabilitation specialists have long been aware of the early frustrations of patients when required to perform motor tasks beyond their ability in the early stages of recovery. This same possibility for frustration exists in the sensory recovery process. To avoid this frustration, the most appropriate approach to re-education of sensation is to apply specific sensory exercises at the appropriate time in the sensory recovery. The timing for this exercise schedule is determined by the pattern of sensory recovery. Such an attempt at sensory re-education was reported by Dellon to the Johns Hopkins Medical Society in 1970 and before The American Society for Surgery of the Hand in 1971.[16,17]

What Is Sensory Re-education?

Sensory re-education is a method in which the patient learns to interpret the pattern of abnormal sensory impulses generated after an intervention in the peripheral nervous system.[18] Sensory re-education is required when the pattern of sensory impulses that is transmitted to the central nervous system from the peripheral nervous system is different for a given stimulus than it was before the injury. For example, after a nerve repair, we know that the transmission of neural impulses centrally will be different because: (1) less than the normal number of axons than before injury will have regenerated distally after the nerve repair; (2) misdirection of axons exists after nerve repair (axons that formerly carried messages from the index finger may now carry messages from the thumb or middle finger after median nerve repair); (3) possibility for incorrect reinnervation of peripheral receptors by regenerating axons (a slowly adapting fiber that previously had innervated a Merkel cell-neurite complex, coding for constant touch and pressure, may reinnervate a former quickly adapting receptor, such as a Meissner corpuscle, formerly coding for moving touch and vibration). Thus, after a nerve repair, the profile of transmitted neural impulses is altered for sensory perception in quantity, location of the message, and mechanical transduction potential. When this altered profile of sensory impulses reaches the somatosensory cortex, it must be interpreted. This interpretation is our conscious perception of neural impulses and what is most appropriately termed "sensation." (Sensibility refers most appropriately to the neural events occurring at the periphery. Thus, we evaluate sensibility and re-educate sensation.)

When we attempt to interpret, at a conscious level, this altered profile of neural impulses, we, in some way, must match the current profile to our memories of those profiles stored in some "association" cortex elsewhere in the brain. If no match is made, then either the altered profile of sensory impulses are ignored or the patient, when asked what he has just felt in his fingertip, says: "I do not know." If, in fact, he was asked whether he felt one or two points, he might answer incorrectly, when he had received sufficient sensory information to make that discrimination. Thus, sensory re-education is an attempt to give the patient a new set of matching profiles. Sensory re-education is an attempt to place an old familiar name on a new unfamiliar sensory message. This concept must be explained to the patient at the start of the re-education process so that he may understand that it is as if someone has repainted his house or apartment in which he has lived for many years and is now asking him to give the same old name to the new colors.

Who Does Sensory Re-education?

Sensory re-education is begun by the operating surgeon at the time the patient is first tested in his office. The surgeon is the first to introduce the concept to the patient in terms of its need and importance. The surgeon explains that sensory reeducation will be used at the same time as motor rehabilitation. Sensory re-education is done by the surgeon each time the patient is seen simply by the surgeon examining the patient, reviewing neural regeneration, mislocalization, progressing Tinel's sign, and going over the moving and static two-point discrimination testing procedures. The surgeon does these tests and records them in the chart as part of the follow-up and checks whether the patient is carrying out the exercises as directed by the therapist.

The therapist sees the patient on referral from the physician, and in the early phase of sensory re-education will see the patient at least every 3 to 4 weeks. In the later phases of sensory re-education, the patient will be monitored by the therapist at 4- to 6-week intervals.

The patient will do sensory re-education for 5 to 10 minutes, three to four times a day at home on his own until he has returned to his normal activities of daily living and household or job requirements.[18]

Techniques of Sensory Re-education

There is no one technique for sensory re-education. Any technique that forces the patient to focus on the altered profile of sensory impulses he is receiving and learning to identify them properly is an appropriate technique for sensory re-education. In this concept, "desensitization," as will be discussed later, is a form of sensory re-education. It will be fruitless in the future for anyone to attempt to define their particular program as the "best" program for sensory re-education. Techniques from the different hand center programs can be shared and, indeed, should be modified for the patient's basic needs, future job requirements, and hand potential (there may be restrictions in hand function due to loss of digits, permanent paralysis of muscles, contractures).

Early phase re-education is directed to that point in recovery of sensation when just moving and constant touch, but not two-point discrimination, are present. After a median nerve repair at the wrist, it can be begun when moving or constant touch is perceived over the thenar eminence and palm. It is directed at having the patient learn to identify correctly the difference between the function of the slowly and quickly adapting fiber receptor systems. Thus, the patient is to learn to discriminate between a constant and a moving touch. Early phase re-education also is directed at correcting mislocalization. Thus, when the patient is touched over the thenar eminence and believes the fingertip is being touched, he must learn to localize correctly this stimulus to the thenar eminence. A form of re-education technique here is the specific sensory exercise appropriate to this stage of recovery. Thus, the patient needs only to take the eraser end of a pencil and move it over the thenar eminence while directly observing this to perceive what is actually happening, and then to shut his eyes and think about what the stimulus feels like. He then opens his eyes and sees again that, no matter what his consciousness says is occurring, in fact what is happening is that an eraser is moving over the thenar eminence. He now shuts his eyes again and says to himself that he is feeling moving touch over the thenar eminence. The same sequence is repeated for constant-touch using different degrees of pressure (Fig. 18-1). The patient says to himself that he is perceiving constant touch that is either light or heavy over the thenar eminence. The patient may simply use his fingertip to carry out this exercise and the therapist in testing him repeats the same type of test procedures.

During this visit, the therapist will use the 30 and 256 cps vibratory stimuli and draw out the pattern of

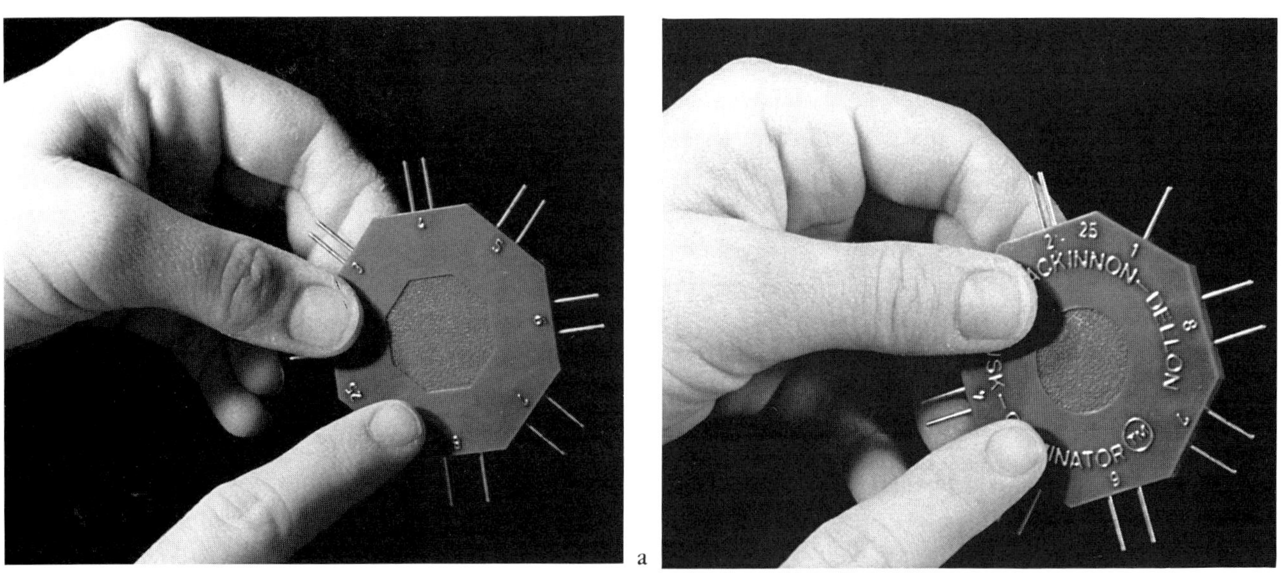

a b

Figure 18-1a, b. Early phase re-education: Correction of mislocalization and relearning moving from constant touch (quickly from slowly adapting fiber receptor systems). Observe the stimulus. Turn head, close eyes and concentrate on stimulus. Observe stimulus again to reinforce the perception. Here the Disk-Criminator™ is utilized by moving or pressing the fingers against its smooth, rough, or raised surfaces.

sensory recovery on a map of the hand, moving and static two-point discrimination are not tested, since there can be no ability to do two-point discrimination until moving and constant touch have returned to the tips of the fingers. It is inefficient to do any more sensibility evaluation at this stage than the perception of the tuning fork stimuli and moving and constant touch from proximal to distal until the 256 cps vibratory stimuli is perceived at the tip of the finger. When the 256 cps vibratory perception is perceived at the tip of the finger, then all the nerve fibers for touch perception have been recovered at the tip of the finger. The end of early phase sensory re-education occurs when moving and constant touch are perceived at the tip of the finger. At that point, the first moving and static two-point discrimination test measurements can be obtained and the patient moves on to the next phase of sensory re-education.[18]

Late Phase Sensory Re-education

Late phase re-education is designed to improve the patient's sensory discrimination capacity. For late phase sensory re-education, exercises are designed to emphasize dynamic activity of the hand. These exercises require the patient to move objects with his fingers and attempt to identify the objects. The series of objects is begun by first maximizing differences in size and shape and texture and materials. Objects are chosen that may be familiar to the patient for ease of identification. Thus, small jars, scissors, spool of thread, a pencil and a pen, a paperclip, and safety pin may be utilized in one series, going from large to small. Other series of objects that may be used are materials of different textures, from coarse to fine weave, from materials with heavy pile to those with fine pile, wool to silk. The objects may be in small garment remnants or may be wrapped around blocks of the same size. A similar technique may use sandpaper of different grades from rough to smooth (Fig. 18-2). The patient is periodically measured in moving and static two-point discrimination.

Over a period of time, the patient will improve in his ability to identify these objects, and more difficult combinations are then introduced, which will require increased ability to discriminate. Thus, small nuts or bolts of finer size may be used. Nuts that have six sides versus those that have four sides may be used. Coins that have rough edges (50 yen) versus those with smooth edges (10 yen) or coins that are solid (100 yen) versus those that have a hole in the center (50 yen, 10 yen) may be used. Difficult combinations, such as the difference between a paperclip and safety pin, may be used. If a patient's discrimination improves, finer degrees or distinctions between test pairs may be utilized (Fig. 18-3).

Other forms of re-education may be introduced as a type of game. A large bowl may contain beans or rice or small lightweight stones or Styrofoam pieces. Then objects, such as a matchbook or small eraser, a marble, a paperclip, money, are introduced into this medium. The patient must use his fingers searching through the beans or Styrofoam pieces in an attempt to find the different objects within and identify them before they are pulled out (Fig. 18-4). A large bag may have objects placed within it. The patient has to reach in and grab something and identify it before it is pulled out. This leads to the type of exercises the patient can do at home. The patient can take small buttons or coins or nuts or paperclip and safety pin combinations and carry them in a pocket or purse. At various times during the

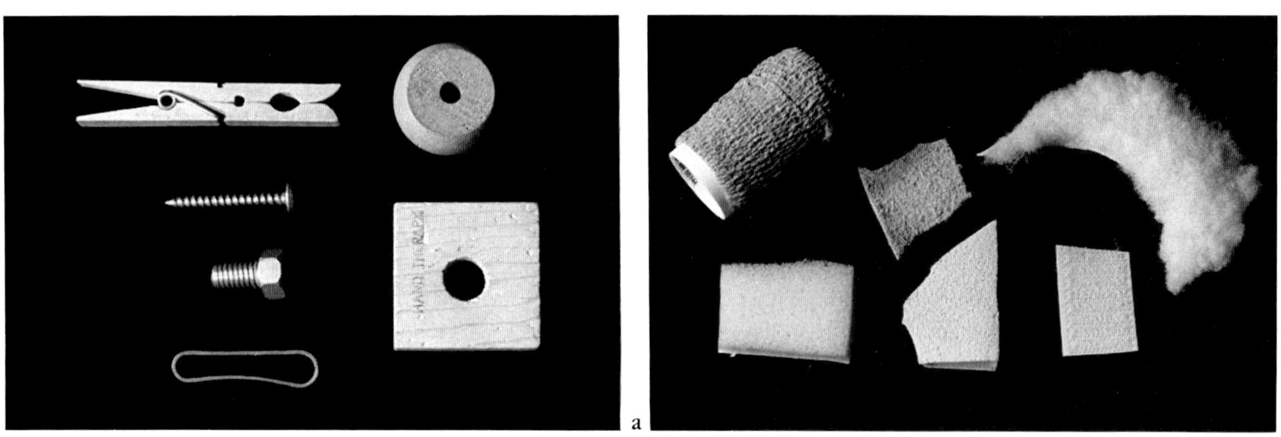

a b

Figure 18-2. Late phase re-education: Object recognition by shape (**a**) and texture (**b**). Begin with large objects, varying in as many attributes as possible (temperature, texture, shape). Go through sequences with each object similar to those sequences described in Figure 18-1.

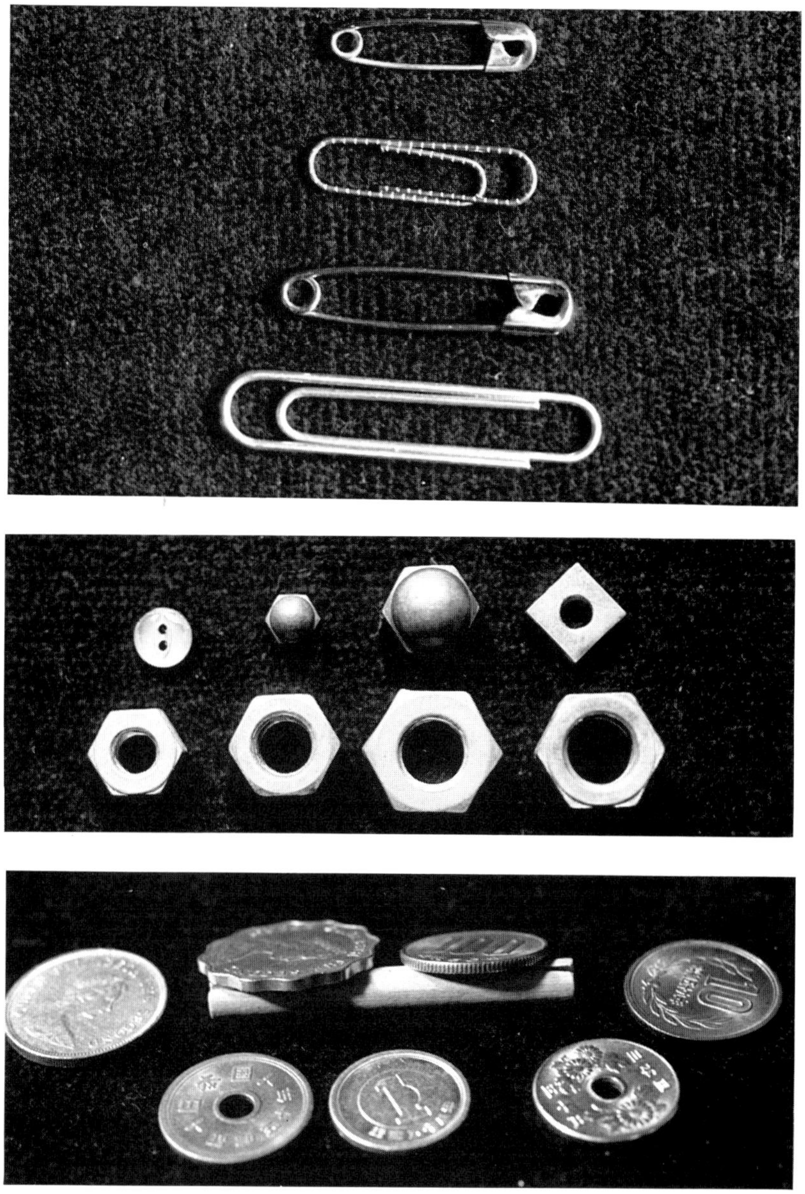

a

b

c

Figure 18-3. Late phase re-education: Object recognition is possible as two-point discrimination recovers. Utilize object pairs with only a few attribute differences: paper clip versus safety pin (a). Smaller 4 to 6 sided bolts, hex nuts, and buttons (b). Coins with differences in edges (serrated versus nonserrated), center open versus center solid (c).

day, the patient may then have these objects available for practice of fine sensory discrimination in the late phase sensory re-education program.

It is possible to use very different forms of sensory stimuli, such as vibrations. A vibrometer can stimulate the patient with vibrations of different frequencies, and the patient can attempt to tell which frequency is being utilized, or differences in intensity at the same frequency.

It is emphasized again that there is no one correct method for this sensory re-education and the techniques are limited only by the therapist's imagination.

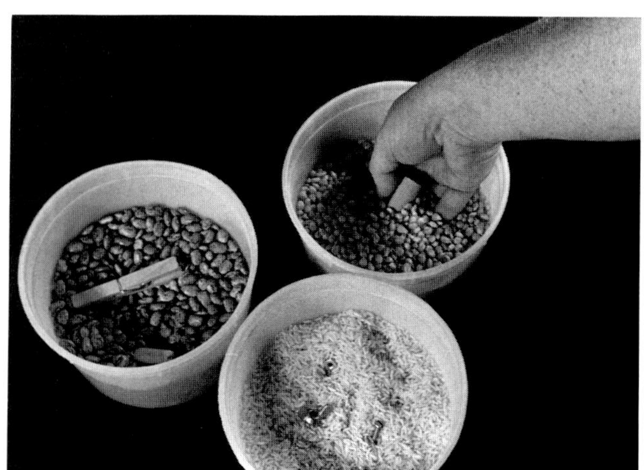

Figure 18-4. Objects hidden in media; such as matchbook in rice, marbles in coffee beans. See text. The fingers move through the media and attempt to identify the object.

A protocol for sensory re-education for the Union Memorial Hospital (which uses objects such as those in Figures 18-1 through 18-4) is given in Appendix E. Sensory re-education works by the patient trying to learn the name of the stimulus and coordinating this with what is perceived.

Examples of specific sensory re-education programs and protocols are: the Disk-Criminator (Fig. 18-5); kit developed by Royce Lewis, Lubbock, Texas, see Appendix E (Fig. 18-6); kit developed by Susan Mackinnon and Louise Kelly, Toronto, Ontario, Appendix E (Fig. 18-7); and Dewey Disc kit developed by Linda Shultis Kiernan, North Palm Beach, Florida, Appendix D (Fig. 18-8).

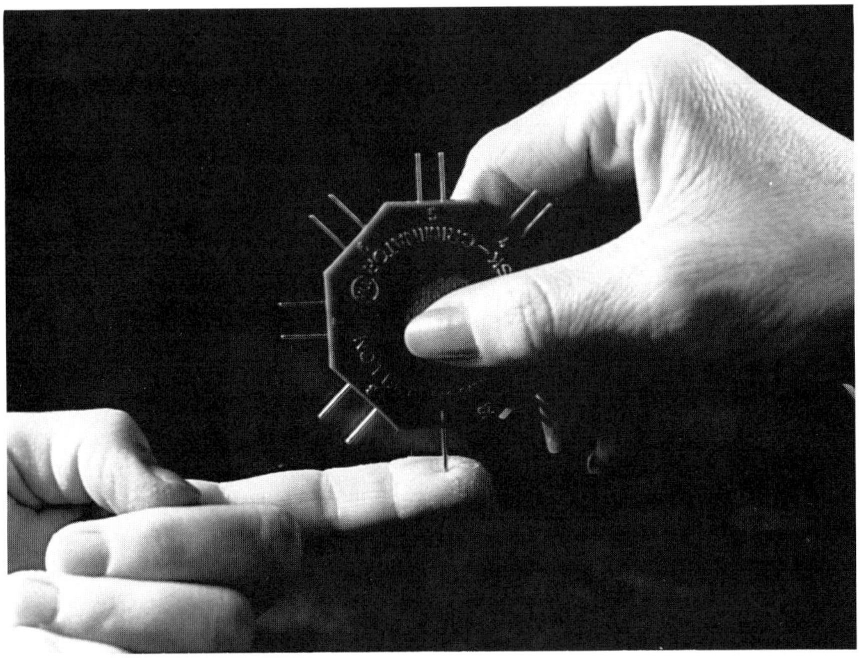

a

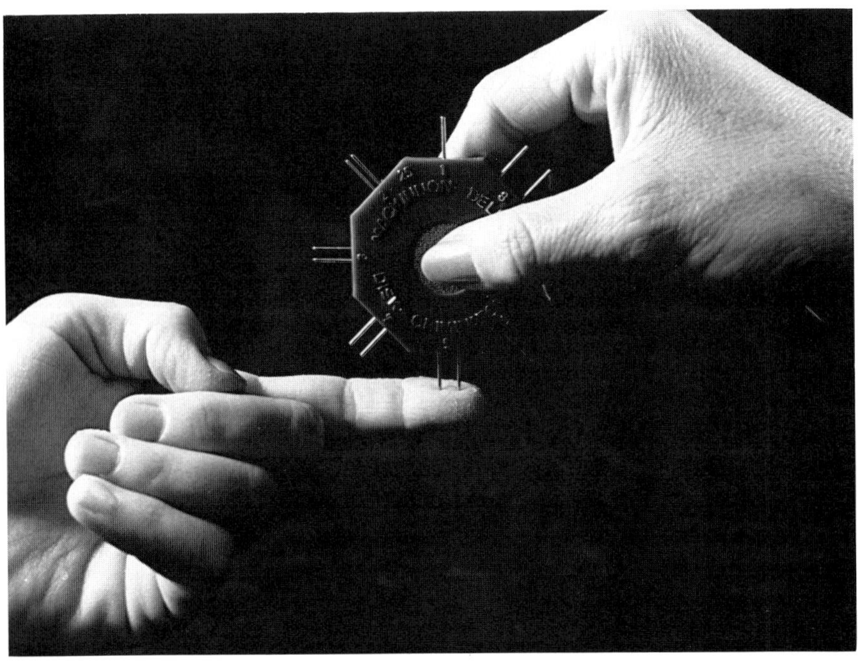

b

Figure 18-5. The Disk-Criminator™ for sensory re-education. In early phase, the fingertip moves across the surface of the Disk-Criminator™; with the patient attempting to perceive the rough from the smooth surfaces and the surface with the raised letters, as in Figure 18-1. The side with the octagon rough center can be distinguished from the side with circular rough center, also. In late phase, the patient learns to make finer and finer determinations of one versus two points (**a**, **b**). A friend or relative can test him, and he can record his progress. One disk has a range of 2 to 8 mm, the other from 9 to 22 mm.

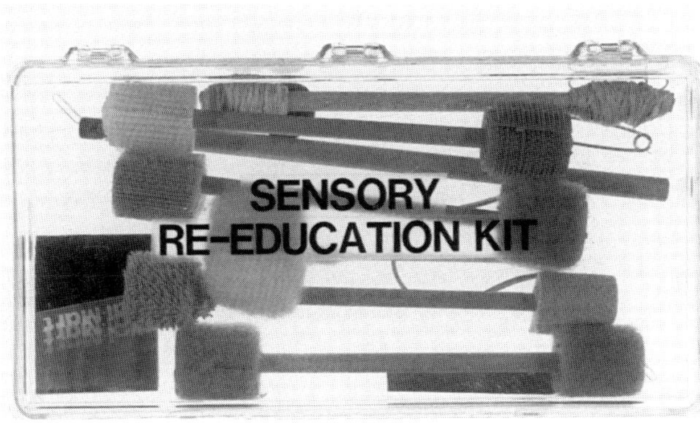

a

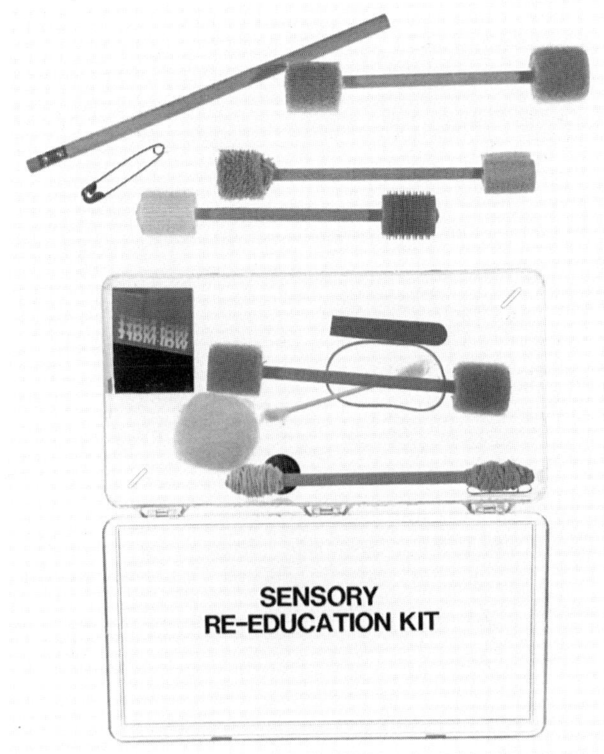

b

Figure 18-6a, b. The Royce Lewis Sensory Re-education Kit, Lubbock, Texas. See description in Appendix E.

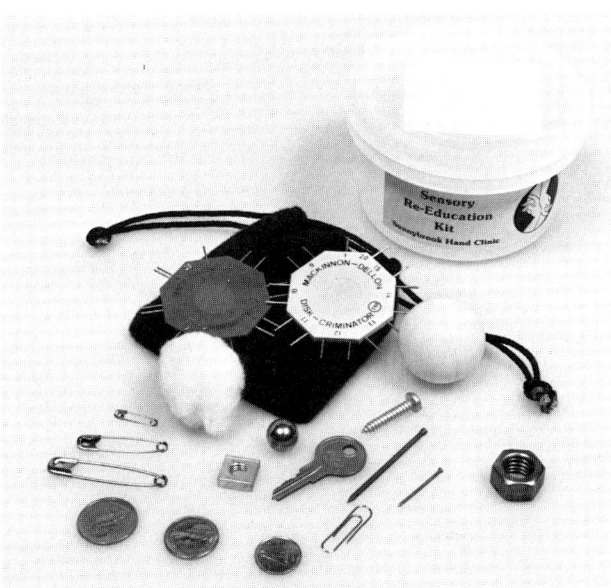

a

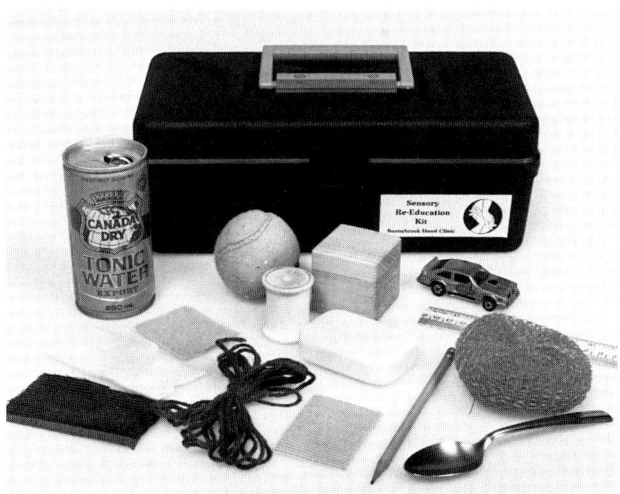

b

Figure 18-7. The Mackinnon/Kelly Sensory Re-education Kit, Sunnybrook Medical Center Hand Services, University of Toronto, Ontario, Canada (**a** for late phase, **b** for early phase). See description in Appendix C.

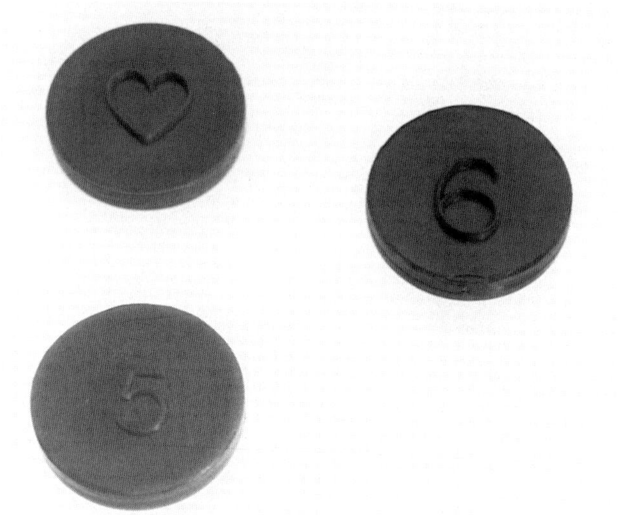

Figure 18-8. The Dewey Disc Sensory Re-education Kit, North Palm Beach, Florida, developed by Linda Shultis Kiernan. See description in Appendix D.

Results of Sensory Re-education

In order to determine whether sensory re-education techniques are effective, it is important to appreciate the level of sensory recovery without sensory re-education. Measurements were determined by static two-point discrimination classified according to the British system, so that their classification of S4, representing normal, would be equivalent to 6 mm or less static two-point discrimination, and category S3+ would be equivalent to "some" discrimination, 7 to 15 mm. A review of the published articles for median and ulnar repairs to the wrist and digital nerve repairs has been compiled.[18] That review demonstrated that less than 1 in 100 adults recovered to a level of S4 even by 5 years after repair of the median or ulnar nerve at the wrist and less than 11% of adults recovered to a level of S4 after a digital nerve repair. It should be noted that those digital nerve repair series reviewed in general did not include an anesthetic block of the intact functioning digital nerves, and there were some children included in the digital nerve repair series that could not be excluded from the calculations, so that the actual results of digital nerve repair are probably worse than was reported.

Dellon's series of patients who had sensory re-education achieved, for the median nerve, 54% to the level of S4, and for the ulnar nerve, 80% to the level of S4 by 2 years after nerve repair at the wrist. Eighty-two percent of the patients with digital nerve repair recovered to the level of S4 by 2 years after nerve repair and in this series the intact and functioning digital nerve was blocked with lidocaine before carrying out the sensory testing.[18] Thus, from comparison of Dellon's re-educated peripheral nerve patients with the historical series, sensory re-education significantly improved the degree of sensory recovery and shortened the time required for that recovery over patients who were repaired and did not receive sensory re-education techniques.

Another way to evaluate the results of sensory re-education after nerve repair is to adopt a suggestion by Erik Moberg:[19] "Recognize that no studies in the future will accrue enough patients to permit a randomized prospective study design, matching nerve lesions for type of injury and location of injury and patient age and recognize that patient's age is the main factor in the degree of sensation recovered. Then to evaluate your results, the individual patient should be plotted by his age versus degree of static two-point discrimination recovered." This plot can be compared with "Önne's line." In 1962, Önne[20] evaluated Professor Moberg's primary nerve repairs at 5 years after the time of repair and found essentially that the degree of static two-point discrimination recovered was equal to the patient's age in years. Thus, Moberg suggested that if a line were drawn on a graph in which age equaled static-two point discrimination in millimeters, that line would represent the results of an ideal nerve repair. The patients are plotted as a single dot on that chart and if this dot falls below the diagonal Önne's line, so that the two-point discrimination was less in millimeters than the patient's age in years, then the results of whatever technique was done for the nerve repair or rehabilitation would represent an improvement over the traditional techniques. Dellon's series of median and ulnar nerve repairs at the wrist and digital nerve repairs were plotted as Moberg suggested. All the points fell well below Önne's line (Fig. 18-9). This was at 2 years' follow-up compared with the traditional time for determination of results, 5 years. Thus, with sensory re-education, adults can achieve static two-point discrimination in the normal range.

There remains no series of patients reported for whom moving two-point discrimination with sensory re-education has been reported. We, in particular, wished to report static two-point discrimination in our re-education patients so that the results could be compared with the historic controls. There are no historic controls for moving two-point discrimination in patients who have not been re-educated.

At the 28th Meeting of the Japanese Society for Surgery of the Hand, Imai, under the direction of Tajima, reported[21] a series of patients with median nerve repair at the wrist. In that series of patients, the most recently operated group received sensory re-education and were

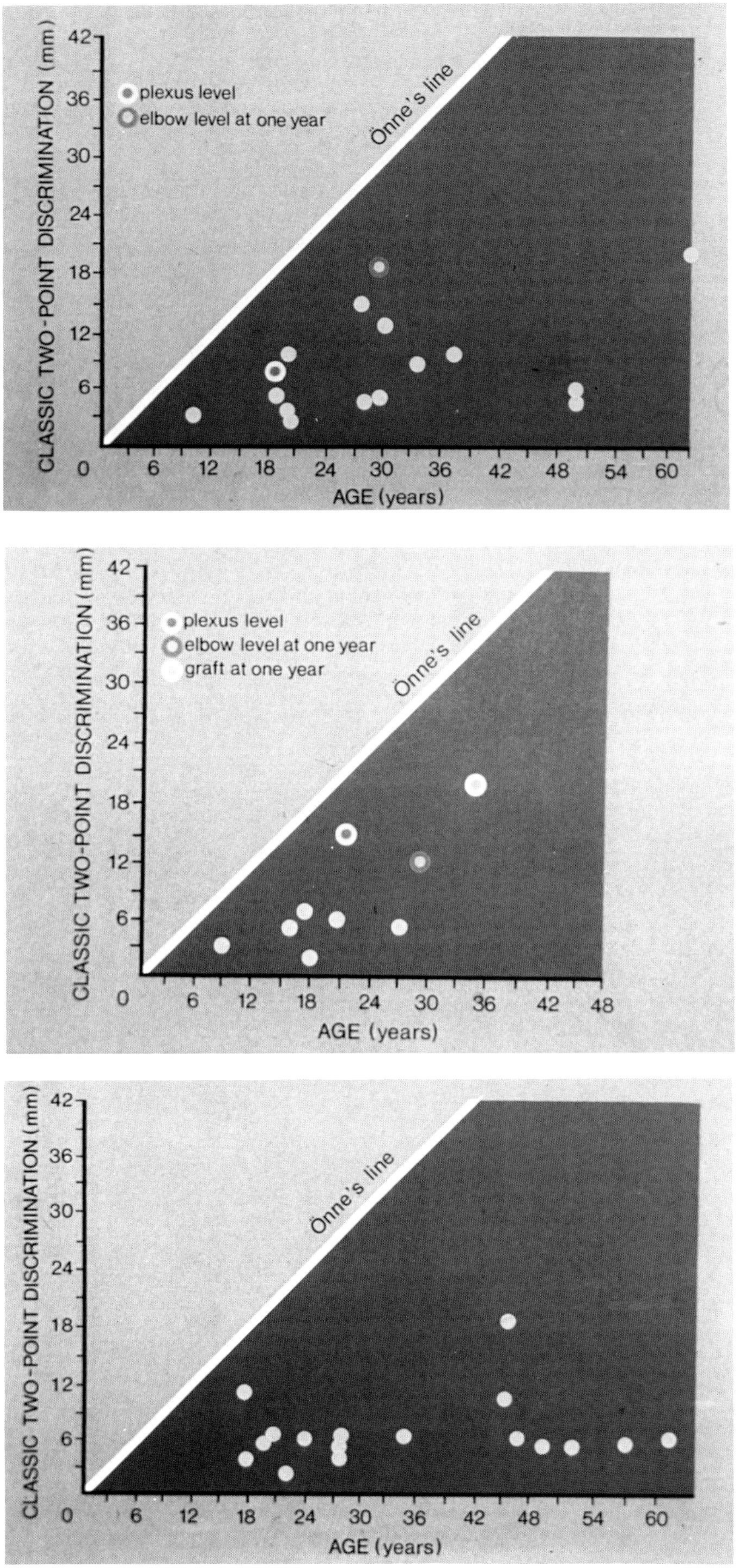

a

b

c

Figure 18-9. Dellon's results of median nerve (a), ulnar nerve (b), and digital nerve (c) sensory re-education plotted by patient age. Each patient's dot is below Önne's line, the expected result for a repair without re-education. Thus, sensory re-education improved the patients results over that expected without it.

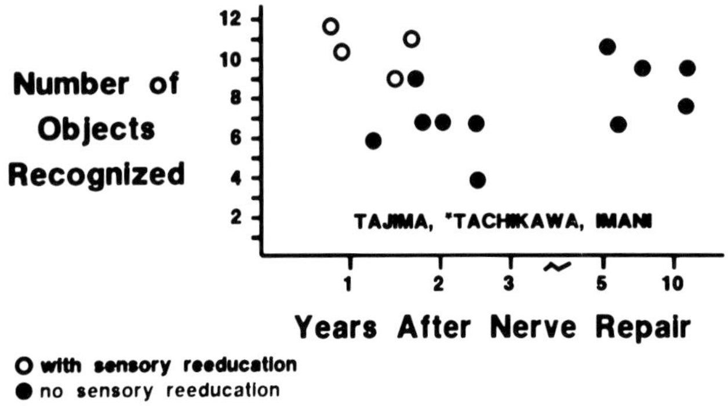

Figure 18-10. Tajima's results with sensory re-education enabled patients after median nerve repair to identify 9 to 12 objects by 1 to 1½ years after repair, whereas those patients without sensory re-education did not obtain this ability even 5 years or more after repair.

evaluated at times up to 1½ years after nerve repair. The level of static and moving two-point discrimination recovered in this group of patients was better than that in a group of patients repaired by the same operative technique between 3 and 5 years after surgery who had not been re-educated. The results in the re-educated group were also better than the group of patients who had not received re-education and who had been operated on between 5 and 10 years previously (Fig. 18-10). This latter group demonstrated some improvement over time from the group operated on 3 to 5 years previously. This improvement may be considered to have occurred as the patients "re-educated themselves" during their activities of daily living and normal work routine. It is this type of slow improvement with time up to and, indeed, after 5 years that led earlier surgeons to suggest that patients with nerve repairs not be evaluated until 5 years after their surgery to determine the final results. It was this philosophy of "wait and see" that left the gap that the present sensory re-education can fill.

Our present concept is that each operation gives the patient a certain potential for ultimate sensory recovery. Without sensory re-education, the patient achieves some level but only sensory re-education enables the patient to fulfill the potential given to him at surgery and in a shorter time period than he would be able to achieve without rehabilitation techniques.

Sensory re-education results can also be judged by a review of patients reported to have had replantation of digits and those reported to have had reconstruction by toe-to-thumb transfers. The literature on this subject has been recently reviewed.[22] In summary, those centers not using sensory re-education techniques have reported sensory recovery in replanted digits that averages 15 mm static two-point discrimination. Those centers using sensory re-education routinely after digital replantation have reported results of sensory recovery that, in general, are better than those centers reporting replantation results without re-education techniques. Groups who have replanted digits followed by sensory re-education have a significant number of their patients who have been reported to have recovered static two-point discrimination in the normal range. The same trend may be observed between those centers carrying out toe-to-thumb transfers without sensory re-education techniques, where the average reported sensation recovered in the big or second toe has averaged 15 mm static two-point discrimination in contrast to those that have used sensory re-education, where a significant number of patients have recovered static two-point discrimination in the normal range.[22]

In a recent report from Minami in Sapporo,[23] patients were evaluated by both moving and static two-point discrimination so that each of these results can be correlated. These patients did have sensory re-education. In their patients with thumb reconstruction by a variety of techniques, moving two-point discrimination always recovered to a more normal degree than did static two-point discrimination. In their toe-to-thumb transfers, for example, static two-point discrimination was 6.7 mm and moving two-point discrimination was 2.7 mm.

Thus, in summary, from the reports of sensory re-education that are available for review, we may conclude that sensory re-education appears to allow the patient to achieve a better level of functional sensation and to achieve this level sooner than he would if he did not receive sensory rehabilitation techniques.

Theoretical Mechanism of Sensory Re-education

What is the mechanism by which the results of sensory re-education work? We can say for certain that re-education does not work by causing increased regeneration in the peripheral nervous system. Sensory re-education does not make axons grow faster or cause receptors to form. Most likely, the site of sensory re-education is in the central nervous system. The mechanism for this in the central nervous system is generally considered under the category of plasticity, the ability of central sensory mechanisms to reorganize in some way. It is possible that this reorganization includes the growth of new nerve fibers or terminals; however, this is most unlikely. More likely, plasticity represents an "uncovering" of existing terminals, which are allowed to come into functional use when previously existing ones no longer function.

Evidence is becoming available on the plasticity in the somatosensory cortex. For example, if a digit is amputated and mapping carried out of the hand area in the sensory cortex, with time a new sensory map appears in that area, so that, for example, if the middle finger were amputated, the area occupied by the index and ring fingers might expand to cover the previous middle finger area. Another example would be that for the median nerve divided at the wrist, the area formerly occupied by the pulp aspect of the thumb would become occupied by the sensory portion of the radial nerve and that by the pulp of the middle and ulnar half of the ring finger by the area previously related centrally to the ulnar nerve.[24–26]

The most compelling evidence for central mechanisms existing in sensory re-education comes from a recent abstract reported by Merzenich in which a normal monkey was trained to receive his food and drink by manipulating a wheel in his cage with the pulps of several fingers without being able to use his other fingers. The centrally recorded map from this hand area demonstrated, over time, an increase in size of the sensory map devoted to the fingers used daily by the monkey to manipulate his environment and the shrinkage of those areas where fingers were not required for this use.[27]

Table 1. Desensitization* Protocol of the Raymond M. Curtis Hand Center, Union Memorial Hospital, Baltimore, Maryland

Indications
1. Neuromas
2. Sensitive amputation tips (stumps)
3. Hypersensitive scars and surrounding areas
4. Nerve injuries with dysesthesia (a painful and persistent sensation induced by a gentle touch of the skin)

Contraindications
1. Diffuse pain will not be helped with this technique
2. Do not use desensitization in areas with open wounds
3. Desensitization has greatest effect on hyperalgesic skin
   Deep pain is not remediated with desensitization

Desensitization program
1. Desensitization should be done for a standard amount of therapy time, approximately 5 minutes up to 30 minutes. Treatment time varies for each patient. Treatment session is stopped at the point when stimulus becomes unbearable, noxious, or irritating.
2. Patients find that moving touch is most bothersome
3. Do not touch patient, demonstrate on self
4. Sometimes a protective splint with a bubble is needed for comfort. Also, a cuff of lambswool is useful for protection of an area
5. The last step of each material should feel comfortable before advancing to the next texture.

*Desensitization is a modality to decrease hypersensitivity of skin to tactile stimulation. Several techniques are used, including stimulation with non-irritating media progressing to various textures or weights of objects used for stimulation.

Desensitization (Re-education of Unpleasant Sensations)

Sensory re-education cannot be applied to the painful, stiff, or swollen extremity. During the first phases of rehabilitation after injury, efforts to reduce edema by wrapping, elevation, massage, and intermittent compression are begun. With edema reduction, range of motion exercises are instituted. Together, these activities restore an extremity to one that is soft, pliable, and ready to be reeducated. These activities and early phase sensory re-education may need to be stopped temporarily for the onset of unpleasant sensations as the nerves regenerate into the previously anesthetic area. This unpleasant sensation is best termed "dysesthesia."[28] Although often termed a "hypersensitive" area, for which desensitization is the indicated treatment, hypersensitivity should imply a more than normal response to a normally nonpainful stimuli. Patients with true hyperalgesia do not respond well to densensitization. Patients with long standing neuromatous pain also do not respond well to desensitization programs (see Chapter 17).

The treatment techniques described as "desensitization"[29–33] are effective in treating dysesthesia. Like sensory re-education techniques, a variety of desensitization techniques have developed that use the application of a series of graded stimuli, from soft to harsh, for example, cotton wisps through sandpaper, or gentle finger stroking through vibrator stimulation. These gradually increase the patient's tolerance for touch to the area and permit the reinstitution of sensory re-education techniques.

Desensitization techniques are identical in concept to sensory re-education (Table 18-1), and indeed they may work through the same mechanism of cerebral plasticity.[34] Instead of the patient learning to associate an old name with a new pattern or altered profile of transmitted impulses so that he can identify an object he is touching, the patient is learning to filter out the unpleasant sensations to permit perception of the underlying meaningful sensory input. The analogy is given to the patient of listening to a song on a radio channel that has a lot of static. At first, the song is only poorly heard. As one listens, however, the mind can "filter out" the static and the melody can be discerned. So, too, with the dysesthetic hand. Through desensitization techniques, the brain learns to discount the unpleasant signals, and the patient can focus on the sensory messages that convey useful information. In essence, this is re-education of the pain sensation, instead of re-education of the touch sensation. Vibration units are useful for desensitization.

To aid in desensitization, the transcutaneous nerve stimulators are also often helpful. Still, there will be patients in whom those units are ineffective. Physiologically, the electrical stimulation of these units elicits a response in both large and small fibers and both quickly and slowly adapting fibers. We have found that many of these nonresponding patients will be helped by continued mild pressure on their hand, such as obtained by wearing a regular glove, an elastic glove, or gently wrapping their extremity with an elastic bandage. This technique stimulates selectively the slowly adapting fiber or receptor group, as opposed to the entire range of nerve fibers. Although it is unclear why this treatment adjunct should be effective, it is recommended during this stage when sensory (touch) re-education must be suspended. The use of a drug "to calm the nerve endings," such as hydroxyzine (Vistaril, Atarax), instead of a narcotic has been helpful also during this time. The drug is prescribed as 25 mg orally three times a day and 50 mg at bedtime, increasing to 75 mg three times a day and 100 mg at bedtime over a period of 2 weeks if needed. It is possible that as the balance of small to large fibers is restored at the periphery and as the fiber-receptor connections "mature," restoring normal stimulus thresholds, these desensitization techniques will be effective therapeutically, permitting institution of late-phase sensory re-education.

Sensory Re-education: Future Areas for Investigation

Every type of sensory impairment may benefit from sensory re-education. Currently, sensory re-education techniques using the type of evaluation procedures outlined and similar re-education techniques are being applied to stroke patients by Naomi Aoki in Tokyo.[35] Furthermore, under her direction, re-education techniques and moving two-point discrimination values are being studied in blind patients with diabetic neuropathy and in patients with leprosy.[36] In the brachial plexus region, Shiina[37] is studying the evaluation of sensibility and re-education utilizing the protocols already described, also in patients in Tokyo. We look forward to the results of these investigations because the potential for sensibility in these patients has not been well-documented and their potential for re-education is unknown.

The current use of microsurgery to carry out free tissue transfers with flaps that can be innervated remains an area for future investigation with these techniques. For example, the areas that can be transferred represent those that are not daily used for sensory function. Their actual moving and static two-point discrimination values have not been determined. Their potential in the normal site for sensation is not determined. Thus, it remains for each of these potential sites to have sensory re-education normally so that we know what the potential for each site truly is. For example, what is the true sensory potential of the pulp of the big toe and the second toe and the region of the web space dorsally between the first and second toes?

When we find that a second toe can be transferred for a thumb and that the sensibility recovered in that second toe is better than the normal contralateral intact second toe, and almost as good as the patient's normal thumb, should we be surprised? The toes have Meissner corpuscles present in very significant density. The actual axon counts in the plantar digital nerves of the second and big toes, we are finding, are less than those present in digital nerves (500 to 800 axons per plantar nerve in contrast to 2500 for thumb digital nerves).[38] How does this relate to the Meissner corpuscles' normal innervation with between three to nine separate fibers? How does this relate to the capacity for sensory re-education to maximize the patient's potential? Each of these separate factors is suitable for investigation. A simple approach would be to take, for example, the dorsoradial aspect of the hand, the web space between the first and second toes, and the pulp of the first and second toes in normal patients and subject them to a period of sensory re-education and then measure moving and static two-point discrimination. In this way, the full potential for these tissues might be better appreciated.

New techniques for re-education will almost certainly be developed. Brunelli's "gnostic" rings may be an ideal postoperative rehabilitation tool. The patient could gradually increase his ability to discriminate the shapes and textures on the big ring, then progress to the smallest ring of figures as his recovery progresses.[40,41]

References

1. Umphred DA: Neurological Rehabilitation. CV Mosby, St. Louis, 1985.
2. Sahs AL, Hartman EC, Aronson SM, eds: Stroke: Cause, Prevention, Treatment and Rehabilitation. Castle House Publications, London, 1979.
3. Van Hoff MW, Mohn G, eds: Functional Recovery from Brain Damage. Elsevier/North Holland Biomedical Press, Amsterdam, 1981.
4. Basmajian JE: Biofeedback—Principles of Practice for Clinicians. Williams & Wilkins, Baltimore, 1979.
5. Hunter JM, Snyder LH, Mackin EJ, Callahan AD, eds: Rehabilitation of the Hand. CV Mosby, St. Louis, 1984.
6. Ruch TC, Fulton JF, German WJ: Sensory discrimination in monkey, chimpanzee and man after lesions of parietal lobe. Arch Neurol Psychiatry 39:919–938, 1938.

7. VanBuskirk C, Webster C: Prognostic value of sensory defect in rehabilitation of hemiplegics. Neurology (Minneap) 5:407–411, 1955.
8. Forster FM, Shields CD: Cortical sensory defects causing disability. Arch Phys Med Rehabil 40:56–61, 1959.
9. Vinograd A, Taylor E, Grossman S: Sensory retraining of the hemiplegic hand. Am J Occup Ther 5:246–250, 1962.
10. Wynn Parry CB: Rehabilitation of the Hand, 2nd ed. Butterworths, London, 1966, pp 19, 107–108.
11. Wynn Parry CB, Salter M: Sensory re-education after median nerve lesion. Hand 8:250–257, 1976.
12. Wynn Parry CB: Rehabilitation of the Hand, 4th ed. Butterworths, London, 1984.
13. Dellon AL, Curtis RM, Edgerton MT: Evaluating recovery of sensation in the hand following nerve injury. Johns Hopkins Med J 130:235–243, 1972.
14. Gelberman RH, Urbaniak JR, Bright DS, et al: Digital sensibility following replantation. J Hand Surg 3:313–319, 1978.
15. Tachikawa K, Tajima T: Investigation of recovering process of sensation following peripheral nerve repair. Presented at 28th Meeting of the Japan Society of Surgery of the Hand, Kobe, May, 1985.
16. Dellon AL, Curtis RM, Edgerton MT: Re-education of sensation in the hand following nerve injury. (Abstr.) J Bone Joint Surg 53A:813, 1971.
17. Dellon AL, Curtis RM, Edgerton MT: Re-education of sensation in the hand following nerve injury. Plast Reconstr Surg 53:297–305, 1974.
18. Dellon AL: Evaluation of Sensibility and Re-education of sensation in the Hand. Williams & Wilkins, Baltimore, 1981.
19. Moberg E: Future hopes for the surgical management of peripheral nerve lesions. In Michon J, Moberg E, eds: Traumatic Nerve Lesions. Churchill Livingstone, New York, 1975.
20. Önne L: Recovery of sensibility and sudomotor activity in the hand after nerve suture. Acta Chir Scand [Suppl] 300:1–70, 1962.
21. Imai H, Tajima T: Sensory re-education in patients following median nerve repair. Presented at 28th Meeting of the Japan Society of Surgery of the Hand, Kobe, May, 1985.
22. Dellon AL: Sensory recovery following digital replantation and toe-to-thumb transfer. J Reconstr Microsurg, 2:123, 1986.
23. Minami A, Masamichi V, Hiroyuki K, Seiichi J: Thumb reconstruction by free sensory flaps from the foot using microsurgical techniques. J Hand Surg [Br] 9:239–244, 1984.
24. Merzenich MM, Nelson RJ, Stryker MP, Cynader MS, Schoppmann A, Zok JUM: Somatosensory cortical map changes following digital amputation in adult monkey. J Comp Neurol 224:591–605, 1984.
25. Dykes RW: Central consequences of peripheral nerve injuries. Ann Plast Surg 13:412–422, 1984.
26. Kang R, Herman D, MacGillis M, Zarecki P: Convergence of sensory inputs in somatosensory cortex: Interactions from separate afferent sources: Exp Brain Res 57:211–278, 1985.
27. Jenkins WM, Merzenich MM, Ochs MT: Behaviorally controlled differential use of restricted hand surfaces induce changes in the cortical representation of the hand in areas 3b of adult owl monkeys. (Abstr.) Soc Neuroscience 10: 665, 1984.
28. Dellon AL, Seiler WA, Schneider RA: Dysesthesia. Unpublished observations, 1987.
29. Wolpe J: Systematic desensitization. J. Nerv Ment Dis 132:198, 1961.
30. Wilson RL: Management of pain following peripheral nerve injuries. Orthop Clin North Am 12:343–359, 1981.
31. Hardy MA, Moran CA, Merritt H: Desensitization of the traumatized hand. Va Med 109:134–137, 1982.
32. Yerxa EJ, Barber LM, Diaz O, Black W, Azens P: Development of hand sensitivity test for use in desensitization when it presents in the hand. Am J Occup Ther 37:176–181, 1983.
33. Barber LM: Desensitization of the traumatized hand. In Hunter, JM, Schneider LH, Mackin EJ, Callahan AD, eds: Rehabilitation of the Hand. CV Mosby Co., St. Louis, 1984, pp 493–502.
35. Sawa S, Iwosak T, Aoki N: Correlation of sensibility evaluation and object recognition in stroke patients. Am J Rehabil Med. In preparation. 1988.
36. Aoki N: Personal communication, May 11, 1985.
37. Shiina K: Personal communication, May 11, 1985.
38. Mackinnon SE, Dellon AL: Unpublished observations.
39. Dellon AL: Mechanism of sensory re-education: Cerebral Plasticity. In Evaluation of Sensibility and Re-education of Sensation in the Hand, 2nd edition. Dellon Publishing, Baltimore, 1988.
40. Brunelli G, Stefani G: Nuovi anelli di gnosia per la volutazione della ripresa dello sensibilata lattile dopo interventi riparatori. Riv Di Chir delle Mano 17:187–189, 1980.
41. Brunelli G: Gnostic rings for quantifying sensitive regeneration. In Gorio A, et al., eds. Post-traumatic Peripheral Nerve Regeneration: Experimental Basis and Clinical Implication. Raven Press, New York, 1981, pp 611.

19

Tumors of the Peripheral Nerve

Peripheral nerve tumors will be encountered only infrequently, even in practices devoted primarily to the management of surgical problems of the peripheral nerve. These tumors comprise less than 5% of tumors of the hand and upper extremity.[1–5] Peripheral nerve tumors may be considered of neurogenic or non-neurogenic origin, neoplastic or non-neoplastic. We have modified the classification by Harkin and Reed[3] (Table 19-1). The classification of neural sheath tumors has been somewhat controversial. Stout[6] introduced the term "neurilemmoma" in 1935. This term was replaced by the more appropriate term "schwannoma" by Ehrlich and Martin in 1943.[7] It is believed that "neurilemmoma," which refers to the neuroectodermal origin of the tumor, is not as specific as "schwannoma," which refers to the cell type involved in the tumor.[8]

Fisher and Vusevski[9] have demonstrated the unique "double basement membrane" of the Schwann cell. This double basement membrane distinguishes a fibroblast from a Schwann cell. This distinction can only be made by elecron microscopy. Although the epineurium is made up of fibroblasts, the perineurium is composed of perineural fibroblasts, which have a similar basement membrane to Schwann cells. These perineural cells are more primative and are considered to be non-myelin-producing Schwann cells. It is suggested that these cells give origin to the more invasive neurofibromas and the Schwann cells to the less invasive schwannomas.[10]

Table 19-1. Classification of Peripheral Nerve Tumors

- I. Neoplasms of nerve sheath origin
  - A. Benign primary nerve sheath tumors
    - 1. Schwannoma
    - 2. Neurofibroma
  - B. Malignant primary nerve sheath tumors
    - 1. Malignant schwannoma
    - 2. Nerve sheath fibrosarcoma
- II. Neoplasms of nerve cell origin*
  - 1. Neuroblastoma
  - 2. Ganglioneuroma
  - 3. Pheochromocytoma
- III. Tumors metastatic to peripheral nerves
- IV. Neoplasms of non-neural origin
  - 1. Lipofibromatosis of the median nerve
  - 2. Intraneural lipoma, hemangioma, ganglion
- V. Non-neoplasms
  - 1. Traumatic neuroma†
  - 2. Compressive "neuroma"‡ (Morton's neuroma, Bowler's thumb)

*Not discussed.
†Chapter 17.
‡Chapter 13.

The peripheral nerve tumors with which the peripheral nerve surgeon must be familiar are the schwannoma, neurofibroma, fatty infiltration of the median nerve, lipofibroma, intraneural lipoma, intraneural ganglion, and intraneural hemangioma. Malignant variations of the nerve sheath cell tumors are fortunately rarely encountered.

This chapter will discuss neurofibromatosis, since tumors of neural origin are frequently seen associated with this disease. Cutaneous neurofibromas and plexiform neurofibromas are frequently encountered in neurofibromatosis. Schwannomas are encountered although much less frequently. In this disease, malignant degeneration occurs with an incidence reported up to 10%,[11] nerve sheath cell sarcoma occurring much more frequently than malignant schwannoma. Thus, it is important for the surgeon dealing with nerve problems to have some knowledge of this interesting and puzzling disease.

Neoplasms of Nerve Sheath Origin

Schwannoma (Neurilemoma)

Schwannomas arise from the nerve sheath and can occur anywhere that a nerve has a Schwann cell sheath. The eighth cranial nerve is involved more than all other cranial nerves (acoustic neuroma). Schwannomas tend to be solitary but can be multiple, and multiple schwannomas along a single nerve have been described. Rarely, they are associated with neurofibromatosis.

The patient is frequently asymptomatic, noticing only the localized small tumor mass. Occasionally, there may be some sensory symptoms, and palpation of the tumor often produces a Tinel-like response. On physical examination, the tumor is mobile from side to side but not along the long axis of the nerve. Clinically, they may mimic a ganglion or a lipoma.

Nerve fibers are not found in the schwannoma. Of surgical significance, the schwannomas tend to displace the fascicles of the nerve. Grossly, the fascicles of the nerve will appear stretched out over the schwannoma.

Peripheral nerve schwannomas can be completely excised without injury to the nerve (Fig. 19-1). Microscopic magnification is indicated so that no damage is done to the peripheral nerve. The tumor can be enucleated from the nerve without damage to any of the fascicles. Excision of the nerve in order to remove the tumor is unacceptable treatment. Solitary schwannomas that are enucleated rarely recur. Malignant change in a solitary schwannoma is very rare.[12]

In contrast to the peripheral nerve, it is occasionally not possible to excise a VIIIth nerve schwannoma without causing damage to a segment of the nerve. This relates to the anatomical relationships especially the rigid bony anatomy and the fact that the nerve is monofascicular at this level. The vestibular component is frequently injured without significant clinical consequence. The cochlear component of the (vestibulocochlear VIII) nerve is usually not harmed. Associated VIIth nerve damage is rare (5%) and once again relates to the intricate anatomy of this area and probably direct injury to the VIIth nerve.

On gross examination, the tumor is encapsulated and on cut section may be either solid or cystic. Histologically, there are two types of schwannomas, Antoni A and Antoni B. Both types may be found in the same tumor. An Antoni A pattern is characteristically cellular, made up of spindle-shaped cells that often align themselves into a palisade formation (Verocay bodies) (Fig. 19-2a). Collagen fibers, produced by the Schwann cell,

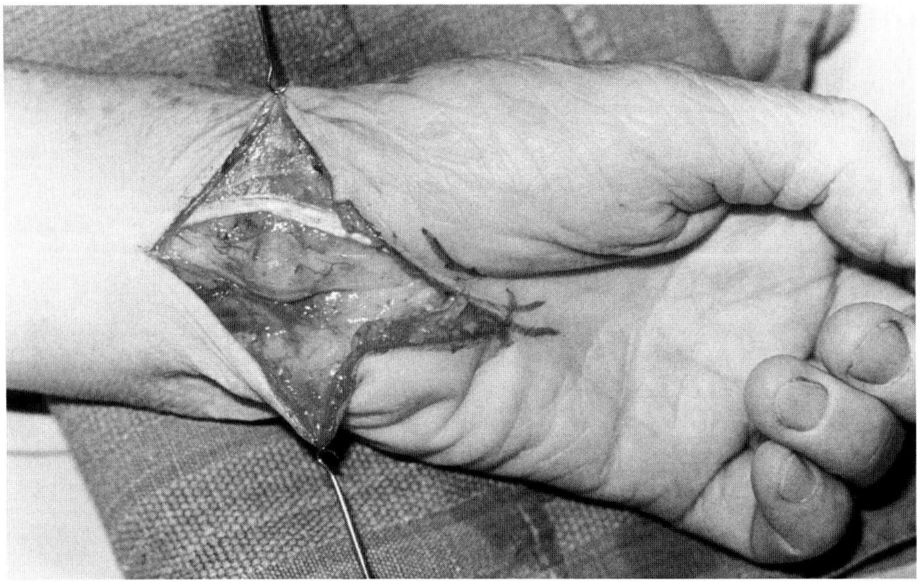

a

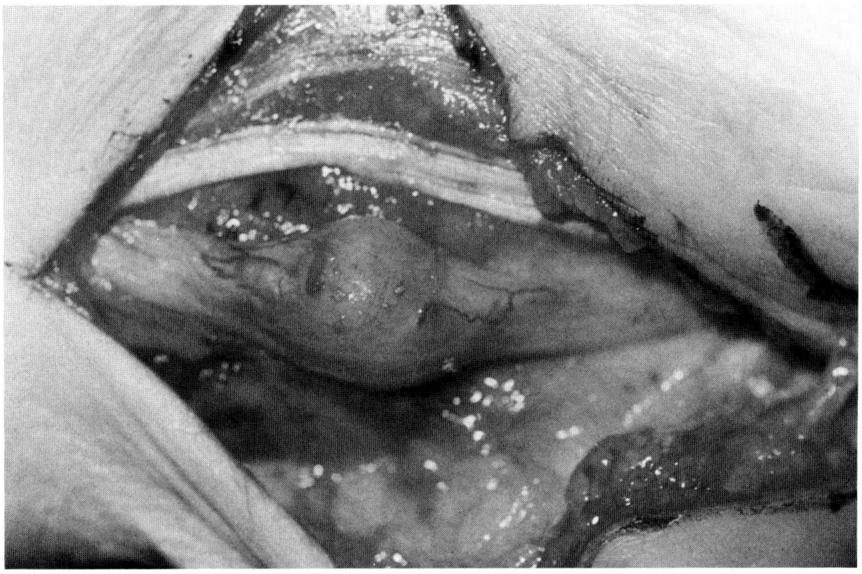

b

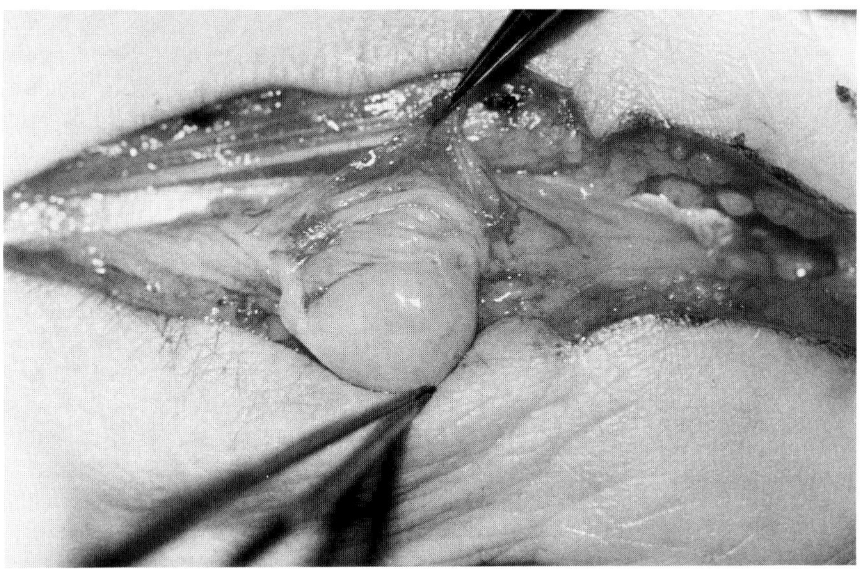

c

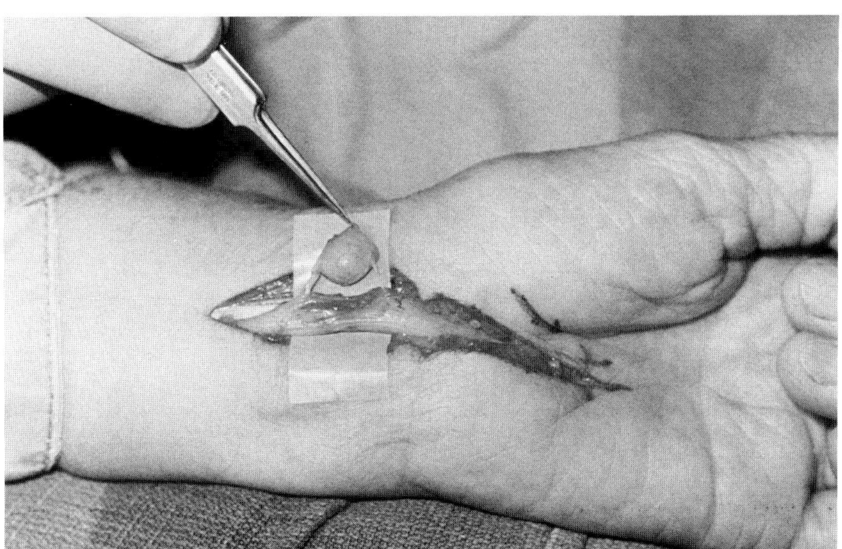

d

Figure 19-1a. This woman presented with a mass in the distal forearm. Percussion of the mass produced paresthesia into the distribution of the median nerve. At exploration, a mass is noted in the median nerve. **b.** The palmaris longus tendon is noted above the median nerve. The fascicles of the median nerve are displaced around the tumor mass. **c.** With magnification, the normal fascicles are dissection from the median nerve. **d.** The parent fascicle is seen to enter and exit from this schwannoma. The size difference between the larger proximal fascicle and the smaller exiting fascicle is noted.

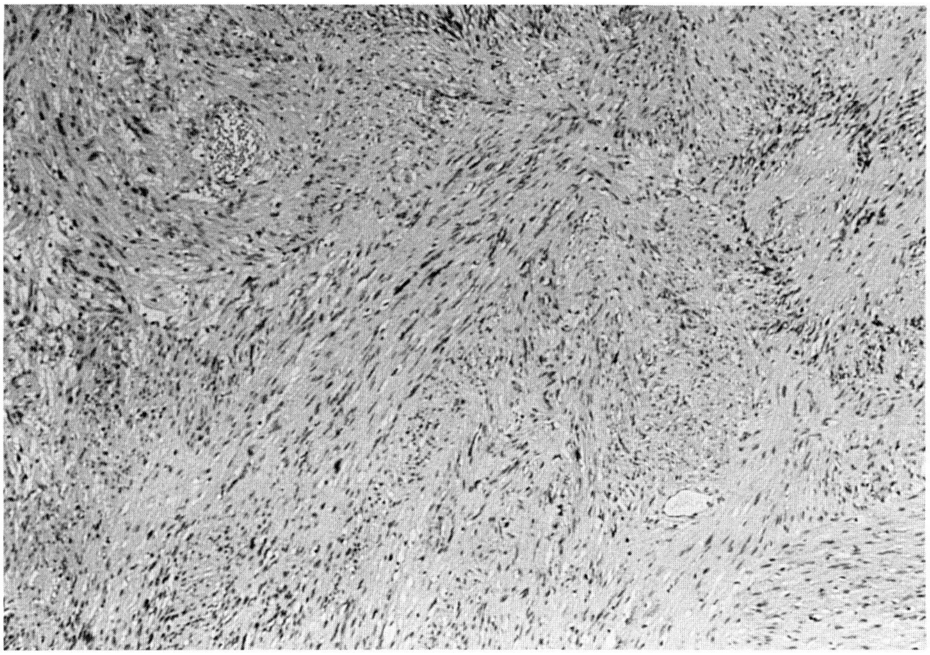

a

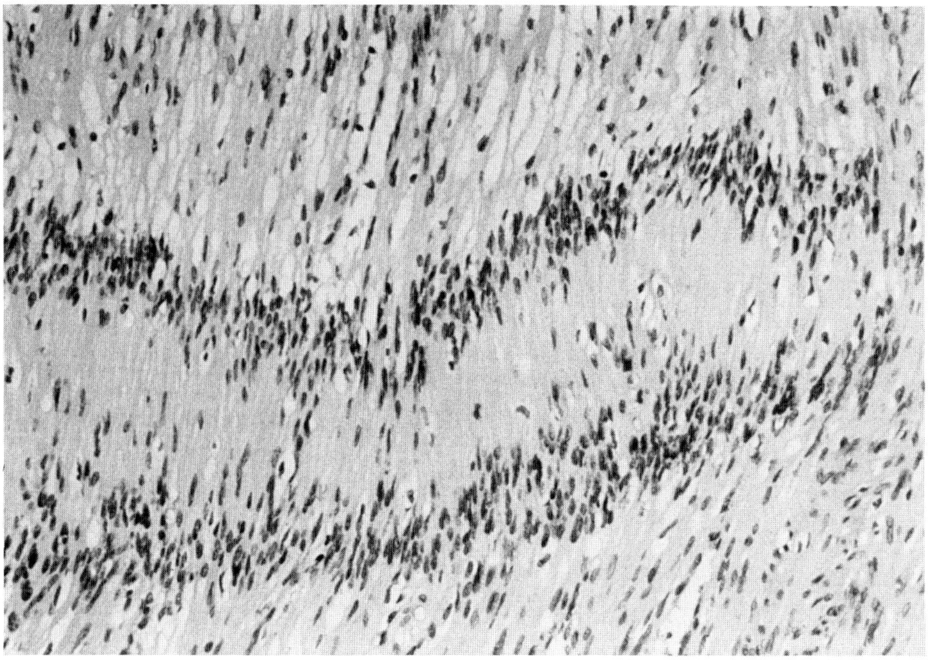

b

Figure 19-2a. Antoni type A tissue is composed of compactly arranged spindle cells (H&E × 80). **b.** A Verocay body is seen as the nuclei of the cells arrange themselves in a pattern of palisades. (H&E; × 240.) (*Figure continues*)

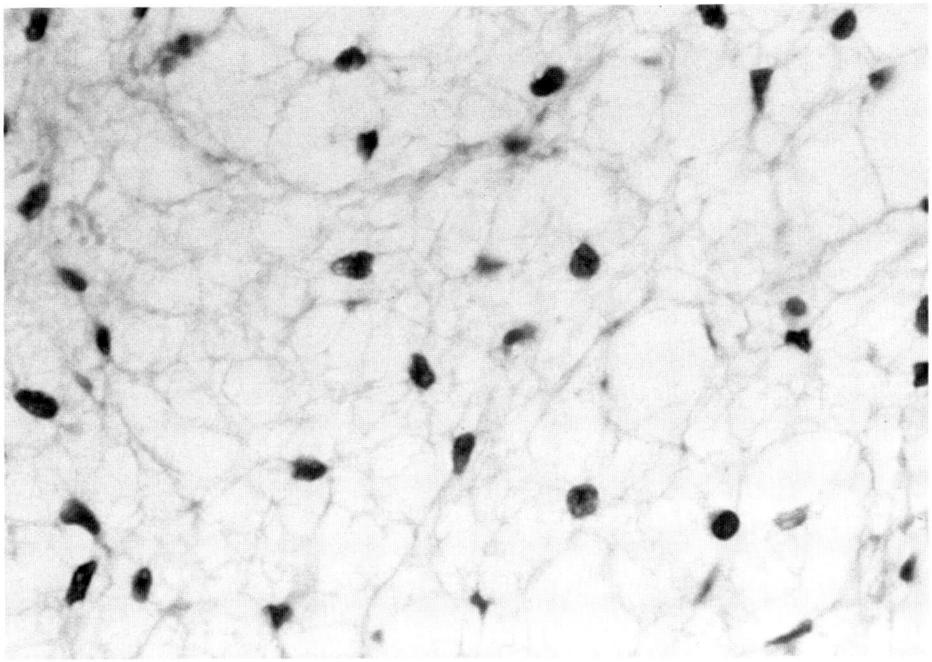

c

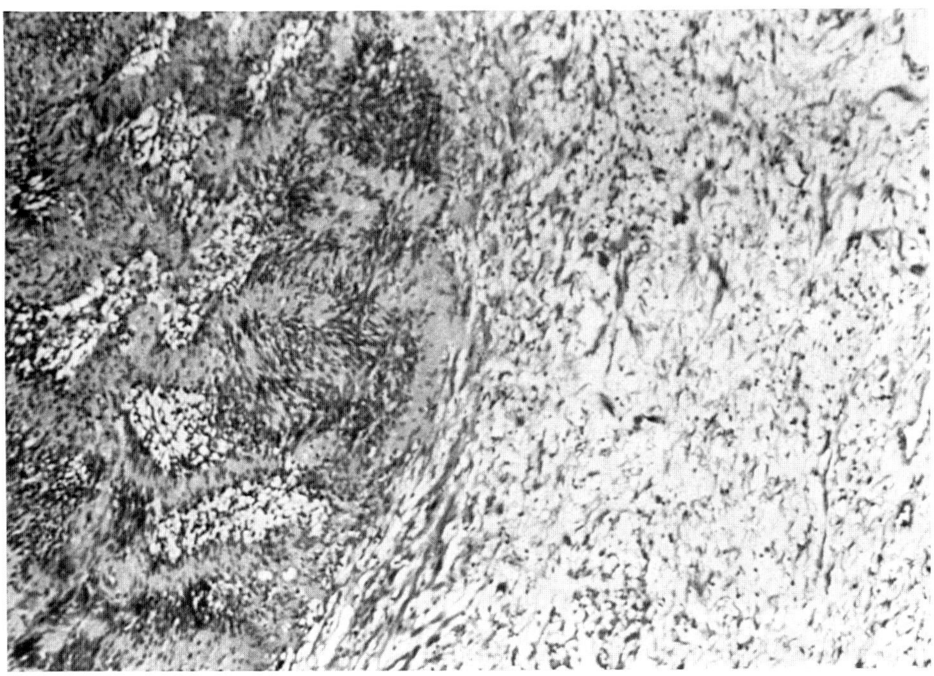

d

Figure 19-2 (*continued*) **c.** Antoni type B tissue in this schwannoma demonstrates less cellularity with loosely arranged cells in a watery matrix. (H&E, ×420.) Figure 19-2a, 19-2b, 19-2c courtesy of J. Rutka, M.D., Toronto) **d.** This tumor displayed areas of a neurofibroma (right) and schwannoma (left). Verocay bodies are noted in the left of the field, typical of a schwannoma. Collagen and Schwann cells are present in the left field in a mucinous matrix, typical of a neurofibroma. (Histologic findings of the tumor displayed in Figure 19-5.) (H&E; ×80.) (*Figure continues.*)

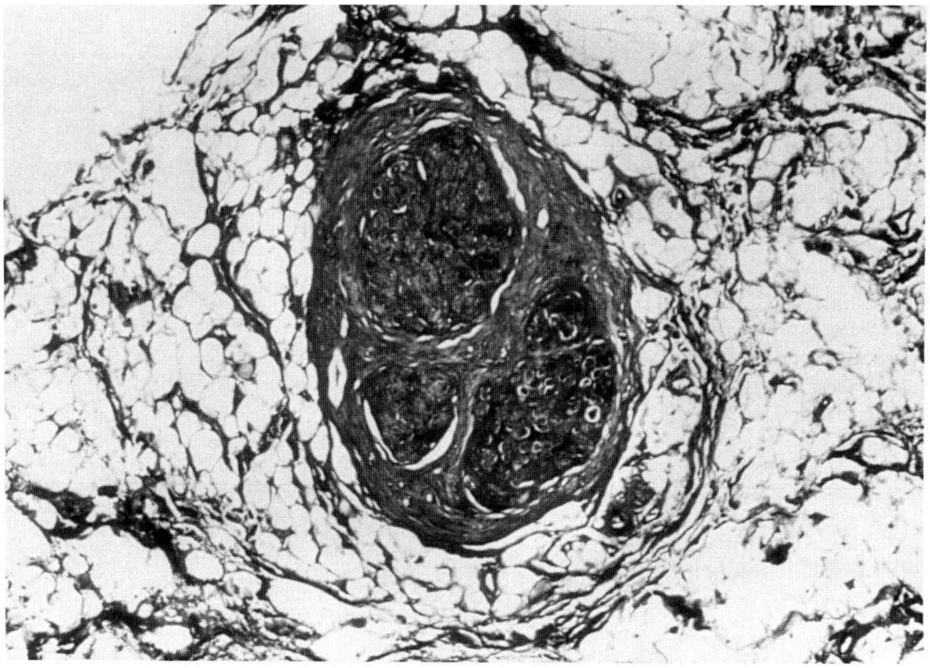

e

Figure 19-2 (*continued*) **e.** Cross-section of digital nerve involved with lipofibromatosis of the median nerve (see Fig. 19-7). The digital nerve in the center of the field has a marked increased thickness of the internal and external epineurium. This may represent chronic compression of the nerve by the tumor. A fibrofatty mass surrounds the digital nerve. Note that the fatty tumor is outside, not inside, the perineurium. (Masson; $\times$ 10.)

may be found in this highly cellular tumor (Fig. 19-2b).

The Antoni B pattern is much less cellular, with a loose arrangement of spindle cells in a clear, watery, mucinous matrix (Fig. 19-2c). This histologic distinction has no known clinical significance, although mucopolysaccharide staining might in the future prove to be a test to differentiate the poorly staining Antoni B pattern from the prominent mucopolysaccharide staining of the neurofibroma.

Cellular Schwannoma

Attention has been drawn to the differentiation between a benign cellular schwannoma and a malignant schwannoma. Woodruff et al[13] have reported that some cases previously described as malignant schwannomas are, in fact, benign cellular schwannomas. Cellular schwannomas are a rare variant of the benign schwannoma that demonstrate hypercellularity and nuclear atypia. The differentiation between a benign cellular and a malignant schwannoma is that in the former tumor no more than six mytotic figures per 40 high-powered fields are noted and no areas of frank necrosis are seen. Necrosis is not present in the cellular schwannomas, as it is in the malignant schwannoma. Ultrastructural examination has been recommended for the differentiation of these two tumors. Woodruff's work highlights the necessity of making a histologic diagnosis of the nature of a peripheral nerve tumor with careful permanent section evaluation. Prognosis of a benign, cellular schwannoma is no different from that of other benign schwannomas.

Neurofibroma

Neurofibromas may occur as a solitary nerve tumor, not associated with the disease of neurofibromatosis. Clinically, this tumor usually presents as a solitary mass in the subcutaneous tissue. It may occur as a solitary mass along the course of the peripheral nerve.

The neurofibroma arises from the nerve sheath, as does the schwannoma. Both the schwannoma and the neurofibroma arise from a cell with a double basement membrane characteristic of the Schwann cell. The neurofibroma can also arise from a perineural fibrocyte that is embryologically more primative than the Schwann cell. Unlike the schwannoma, the neurofibroma is intimately associated with the nerve fibers running through the tumor (Fig. 19-3). This relative "invasiveness" within the nerve may relate to the more primative cell of origin. Thus, unlike the schwannoma, which is basically intraneural but separate from the nerve tissue, nerve fibers are found within the neurofibroma. Thus, the patient with a neurofibroma may complain of neurologic abnormality. Although the degree of nerve dysfunction is usually not great, excision of the tumor, if it involves a peripheral nerve, will result in loss of nerve

Schwannoma

Neurofibroma

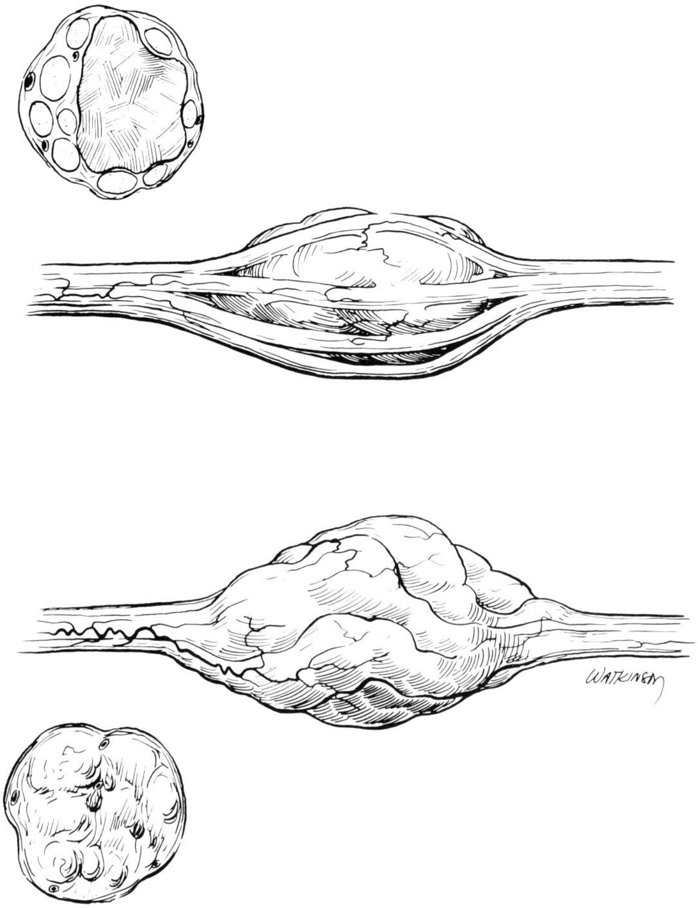

Figure 19-3. Schematic drawing to demonstrate the difference between a Schwannoma and a neurofibroma.

function. A neurofibroma in the skin or subcutaneous tissue may be completely excised without consequence, but a neurofibroma encountered within the nerve should be biopsied only for tissue diagnosis. Excision of the neurofibroma will only be indicated in rare instances. In these cases, neural continuity will usually be restored with a nerve repair or nerve graft.

Although the schwannoma is composed almost entirely of Schwann cells, the neurofibroma is of a more mixed composition. Histologically, the tumor cells are fusiform and present in a mucoid matrix with numerous collagen fibers present. Unlike the schwannoma, the nerve is involved in the tumor and nerve fibers will be present within the tumor.

The majority of neurofibromas found in the skin will be solitary and not associated with neurofibromatosis. Neurofibromas at other sites are usually associated with neurofibromatosis. Plexiform neurofibromas are only seen in patients with neurofibromatosis and not as isolated entities not associated with neurofibromatosis. All patients with a solitary neurofibroma should be examined for evidence of neurofibromatosis.

Neurofibromatosis

Neurofibromatosis is a puzzling disease that has diverse clinical presentation extending from a few subcutaneous nodules of no clinical significance to a devastating disease involving many organs in the body with a tendency toward malignancy. It is difficult to explain the myriad of clinical presentations of neurofibromatosis. Neurofibromatosis is a disorder of neural crest-derived cells.[14] The genetic disorder involves an autosomal dominant mutant gene that has full penetrance but variable expression. This variable expression of a gene or genes that is involved in influencing the behavior of cells from neural crest origin helps to explain the very diverse clinical presentations of this disease.[14,15] A basic feature of neurofibromatosis is a tendency for neoplasia and dysplasia with malignant transformation in multiple tissues.[11] Cardinal features of neurofibromatosis are the café-au-lait spots of the skin and neurofibromas in peripheral, autonomic, and central nervous systems. The cells involved in the neoplastic process are all derived from neural crest origin. Skeletal, vascular, and organ abnormalities can be associated with this disease. The presence of six or more café-au-lait spots, greater than 1.5 cm, is considered pathognomonic of neurofibromatosis.[14] These spots usually occur in early childhood before the appearance of cutaneous neurofibromas. Various classifications of neurofibromatosis have been proposed in order to understand this bizarre disease better.[16,17] Four types of neurofibromatosis have been described; central, peripheral, and visceral and a forme fruste of the disease:[3]

Central neurofibromatosis is characterized by tumors of the central nervous system, including gliomas, meningiomas, schwannomas, and neurofibromas.

Peripheral neurofibromatosis is characterized by multiple cutaneous tumors and plexiform neuromas.

Visceral neurofibromatosis is characterized by neurofibromas and ganglioneuromas of the visceral, or autonomic, nervous system.

The formes frustes involve a limited number of café-au-lait spots and cutaneous neurofibromas of a given region of the body.

Riccardi and Mulvihill[17] have recently described eight types of neurofibromatosis that point to the complexity of this disease.

The incidence of this disease is quoted as 1 in 3000 births.[11] Many of those with the disease will have trivial manifestations. However, the tendency toward malignancy, the complexity of presentations, and the relative high incidence of this problem make neurofibromatosis a disease entity of importance for the surgeon dealing with peripheral nerve problems.

Historical Review

The first description of the cutaneous manifestations of neurofibromatosis was by Akenside in 1768.[18,19] In 1849, Smith described two cases of multiple neurofibromatosis.[20] It was, von Recklinghausen, in 1882, who describing two patients, emphasized the relationship between tumors of nerves and skin, thus, justifying the name neurofibromatosis.[21,22] Frederick Treves, in 1884, met John Merrik who was severely affected by the disease. Treves' presentation of the "elephant man" dramatically emphasized the devastating nature of this disease.[23]

The hereditary nature of the disorder was suggested by Thomson in 1900.[24] In 1910, Verocay[25] suggested that the tumors arose from Schwann cells. Recently, it has been recognized as a neurocristopathy.[14] Nerve growth factor has been implicated in the pathogenesis of neurofibromatosis.[17] The importance of the genetic transmission of this disease has been clarified. The disease phenotype is dependent on a mutant gene, and although the penetrance is complete, the expression of the mutation is very variable. The actual mechanism by which the mutant gene or genes act to result in such variety of the phenotypic presentations of this disease is not known.[17]

Clinical Data

The clinical presentation will depend on the type of neurofibromatosis. Neurofibromatosis type 1, essentially the disorder described by von Recklinghausen, comprises the majority of all neurofibromatosis cases (90%). This is the peripheral type of neurofibromatosis with cutaneous and subcutaneous neurofibromas associated with café-au-lait spots. The presence of plexiform neurofibromas in the involved nerves may produce flabby redundant tissue (Fig. 19-4). There may be hypertrophy of peripheral nerve trunks (Fig. 19-5, 19-2d) or even gigantism of a limb.[26]

Malignant degeneration can occur in lesions of neurofibromatosis. An incidence of 3 to 10% has been described if the tumor involves the major nerve trunks. Malignant degeneration of the cutaneous neurofibromas is reported much less frequently. A rapid growth of tumor size or pain and loss of nerve function signals malignant change in a preexistent neurofibroma.[11] (Fig. 19-6). Reviewing 902 patients with peripheral nerve tumors between 1920 and 1970, Ghosh et al[12] reported

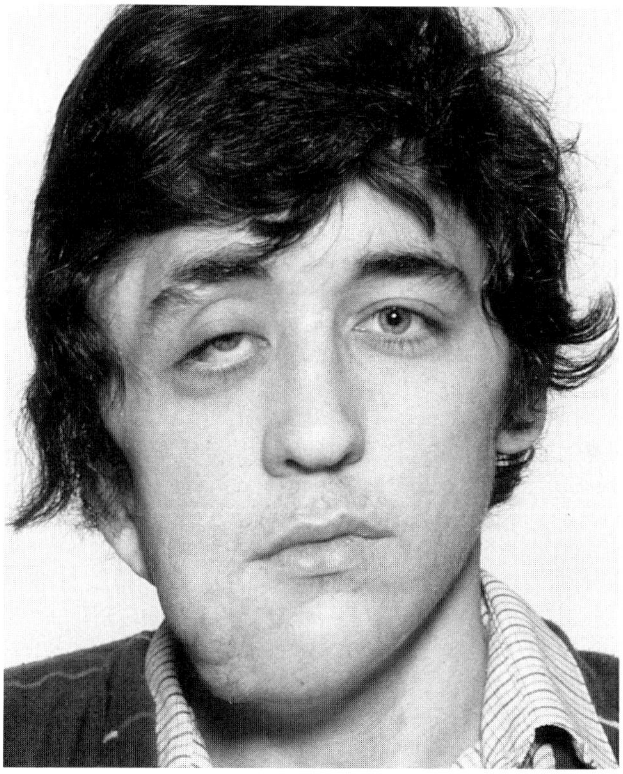

Figure 19-4. A patient with neurofibromatosis of the right facial nerve demonstrates overgrowth of the tissues on the right side of his face.

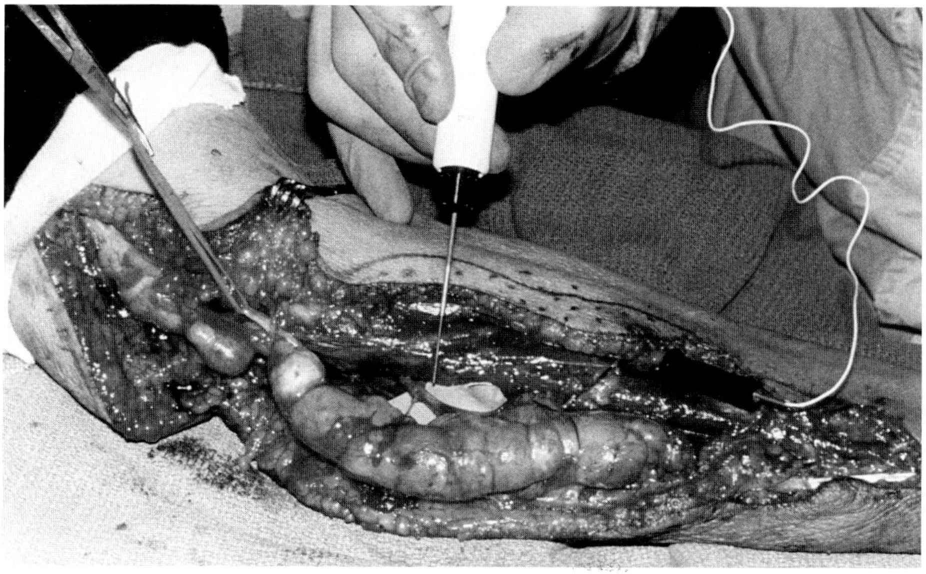

a

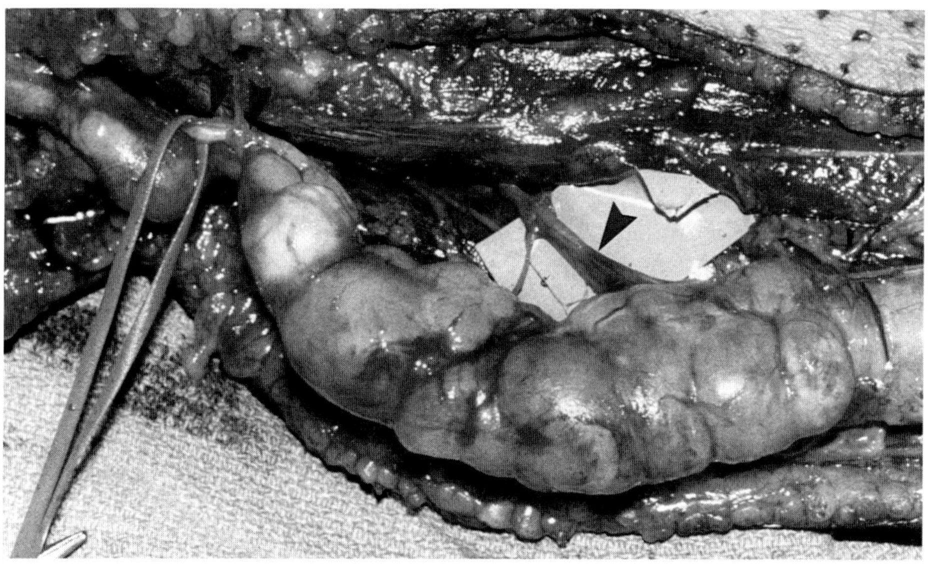

b

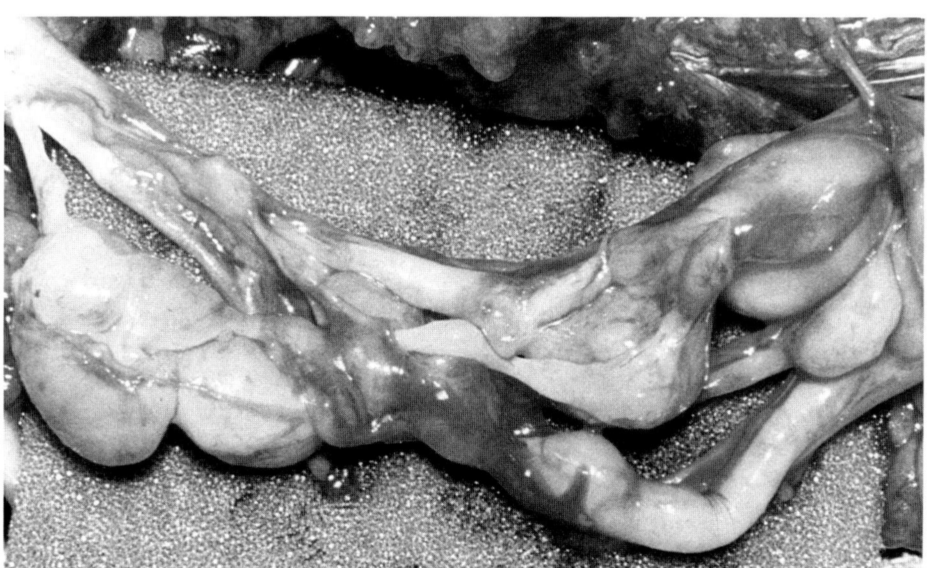

c

Figure 19-5a. This patient had severe pain and no sensation in the ulnar nerve distribution of the left hand. She had diminished ulnar nerve function of the intrinsic muscles. The ulnar nerve was exposed from above the elbow to the wrist (hand toward right, axilla toward left). A Martin-Gruber anastomosis was noted between the median and ulnar nerves (visibility background). Stimulation of this anastomosis produced movement of the intrinsic muscles in the hand. **b.** A closer view of the Martin-Gruber anastomosis (visibility background, arrow); a band of tissue compressed the ulnar nerve in the region of the cubital tunnel and narrowing of the tumor in this region is noted (double arrow, vessel loop). **c.** A close view of the tumor in the distal arm and proximal forearm demonstrates the plexiform nature of the tumor. The tumor was excised, preserving the Martin-Gruber anastomosis. The pathologic condition is demonstrated in Figure 19-2d. No evidence of malignancy was noted.

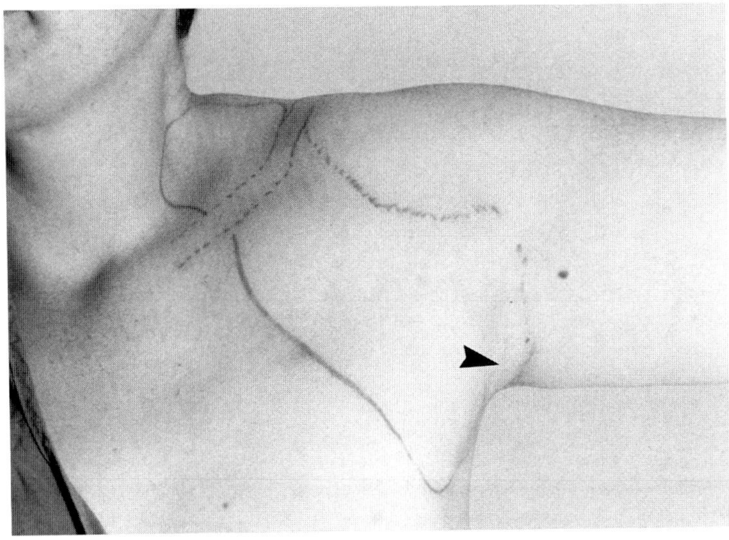

a

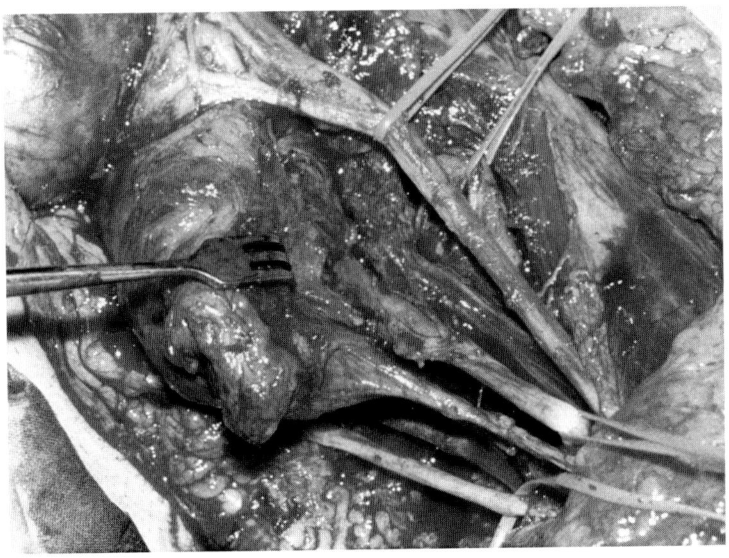

b

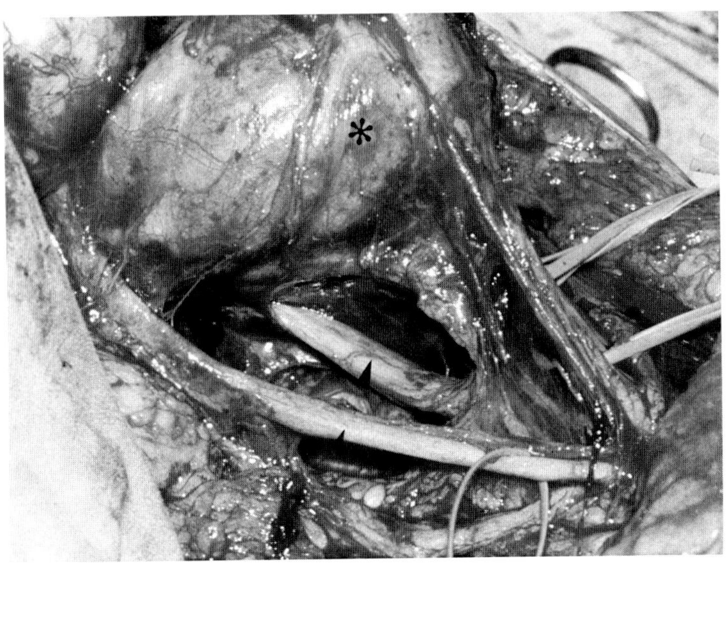

c

Figure 19-6a. This young woman had ignored a slowly growing mass in the left axilla. The mass was palpable above and below the clavicle. An initial biopsy, by the referring surgeon (arrow), revealed only a benign schwannoma. **b.** At the time of formal brachial plexus exploration, a large tumor mass involving the entire brachial plexus was noted. The various elements of the brachial plexus are seen to be entering the large tumor mass, which is retracted by the small retractor. The tumor was debulked, permanent sections demonstrated a malignant schwannoma. The patient declined the recommended forequarter amputation. The patient is alive with persistent local disease at 3 years post surgery.

that 115 of these cases fulfilled the clinical diagnosis of malignant schwannoma. They noted that, when associated with neurofibromatosis, the prognosis was poor. Thus, malignant degeneration in a patient with neurofibromatosis is associated with a higher mortality rate than a similar change in an isolated neurofibroma. In their study, 74% of patients had solitary malignant schwannomas and 26% of these patients had associated neurofibromatosis. The 5-year survival in those patients with a solitary malignant schwannoma was 75% and only 30% in the patients with neurofibromatosis. These investigators suggested that radical, local excision controlled small tumors but muscle group resection or major amputation was indicated in the management of large, malignant schwannomas or after recurrence after a local excision. Lymphatic invasion and lymph node involvement was not observed. Therefore, lymph node dissection was not recommended. The association between neurofibromatosis and other malignancies has been stressed.

Histology

The histologic picture of the cutaneous multiple neurofibromas is the same as that seen in the solitary neurofibromas. Bundles of Schwann cells and axons are noted in the connective tissue matrix.[3] Nerve fibers are seen throughout the tumor (a feature not seen in a schwannoma).

Plexiform neurofibromas are clinically recognized as a mass of redundant soft tissue. The thickened nerves can sometimes be palpated through the skin. Grossly, these plexiform neurofibromas appear as tortuous swellings and nodules along the nerve. It may be difficult at the time of surgery to determine whether the tumor is malignant or benign because the plexiform neurofibromas have the same fusiform oval tumors along the course of the nerve trunk as do the malignant schwannomas (Fig. 19-5, 19-6). The cut section of the malignant tumors often shows areas of hemorrhage or necrosis and the microscopic appearance of these malignant tumors shows aggressive mitotic activity (1 mitosis per high-powered field).

The common site for the plexiform neuromas are the extremities, trunk, and head and neck. Histologically, these lesions may show elements of a normal nerve associated with a disorderly arrangement of Schwann cells, axons, and collagen.

Malignant degeneration can occur as noted previously. These tumors will have an anaplastic appearance similar to a fibrosarcoma.

Clinical Management

The management of the cutaneous neurofibroma is symptomatic. Isolated, painful cutaneous lesions can be excised. Large pendulous masses associated with plexiform neurofibromas can be excised in order to debulk the tumor mass. Management of an isolated plexiform neuroma involving a major nerve is initially that of tissue diagnosis. Excision of the lesion will result in loss of nerve function. As long as there is no concern for malignancy, the patient can be managed conservatively. The incidence of malignant degeneration (up to 10%) is usually heralded by a loss of neurologic function or the presence of pain. In these instances, a high rate of local recurrence is frequently noted after inadequate local resection, and radial local excision will give the best chance of cure. Once again, spread is not by lymphatics. Intraneural extension over a significant distance has been noted. The tumors are notoriously radioresistant.

Schwannomas are uncommonly seen with neurofibromatosis. Once excised, they are more likely to recur in patients with neurofibromatosis, although they rarely undergo malignant transformation.

Malignant Nerve Sheath Tumors

Malignant nerve sheath tumors are very rare and usually are associated with neurofibromatosis. The two types of malignant primary nerve sheath tumors are the malignant schwannoma and the nerve sheath fibrosarcoma. The latter is the most common type of malignant neuroplasm found associated with neurofibromatosis.[27] The tumor cell appears to be a fibroblast. These tumors are usually associated with a plexiform neurofibroma and are highly malignant, with a tendency toward local recurrence and metastasis. Recommended treatment is usually amputation.

Although malignant schwannomas can appear sporadically, they are usually found in patients with neurofibromatosis. The malignant schwannoma does not develop from a benign schwannoma but usually from a plexiform neurofibroma. Histologically, necrosis and numerous mitoses are noted and malignant schwannomas should be treated with wide local excision and reconstitution of nerve function with nerve grafting techniques.

It is difficult to differentiate between a malignant schwannoma and a nerve sheath fibrosarcoma or neurogenic sarcoma. Malignant nerve sheath tumor is probably the better and more accurate term.[10]

Harkin and Reed[3] have emphasized that an erroneous diagnosis of malignant schwannoma is frequently made. A benign schwannoma is mistakenly called a malignant schwannoma. A leiomyosarcoma or fibrosarcoma may be mistakenly called a malignant schwannoma. This confusion points to the necessity of careful evaluation of permanent histologic sections.

Neoplasms of Non-Neural Origin

Lipofibromatosis of the Median Nerve

Several names have been given to this tumor, including intraneural lipoma, lipofibroma, fibrofatty infiltration, lipomatous or lipofibromatous hamartoma.[28–37] This tumor has been described largely involving the median nerve. Macrodactyly has been reported associated with this tumor. These tumors present usually as a soft mass in the palm in childhood or early adulthood. The symptoms are usually slowly progressive. Carpal tunnel syndrome frequently arises secondary to the tumor mass. The tumor may spread to involve digital nerves. Patients will usually eventually complain of pain and sensory abnormalities as well as motor weakness in the median nerve distribution. Carpal tunnel release usually gives only temporary relief. Extensive microsurgical neurolysis is possible because the fibrofatty tumor is present circumferentially around the nerve (Fig. 19-2e). Removal of large amounts of fibrofatty tissue preserving nerve function is possible. Occasionally, the tumor will need to be excised in order to control pain symptoms. In these instances, nerve grafting can successfully restore functional sensibility to the hand (Fig. 19-7).

In the differential diagnosis is Dejerine-Sottas disease, which has a familial pattern of inheritance and is called hereditary hypertrophic interstitial neuritis.[38] It is a rare disease that presents as local swelling of a peripheral nerve caused by this hypertrophic interstitial neuropathy. Unlike lipofibromatosis of the median nerve, the histologic picture of Dejerine-Sottas disease is one of Schwann cell proliferation and myelin sheath

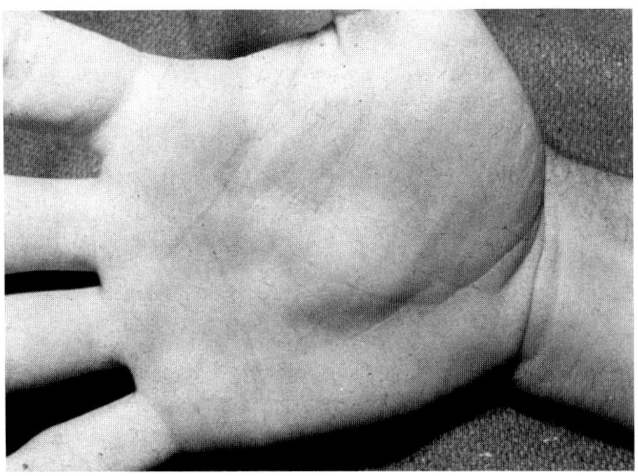

a

Figure 19-7a. This man presented with a carpal tunnel syndrome and a mass in the palm. **b.** Exploration of the median nerve demonstrated the typical appearance of lipofatty infiltration of the median nerve and common digital nerves. After several unsuccessful neurolyses, the median nerve was excised because of pain. (Photograph courtesy of W.R.N. Lindsay, M.D.) **c.** The same patient was referred to us many years later because of problems with lack of sensation in the median nerve distribution. The divided median nerve was found in the proximal forearm (arrow). The digital nerves to the thumb, index, and long fingers were identified in the hand. (*Figure continues.*).

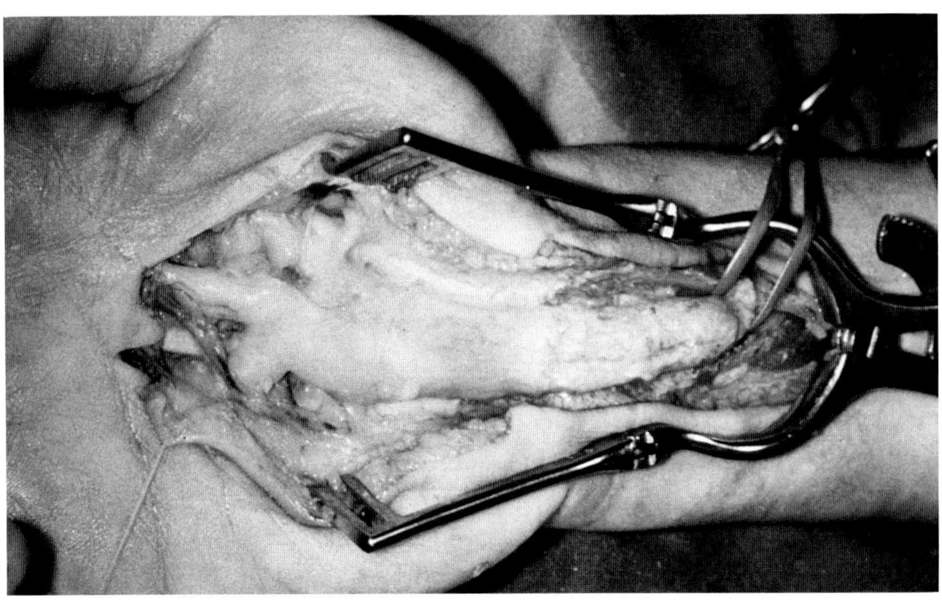

b

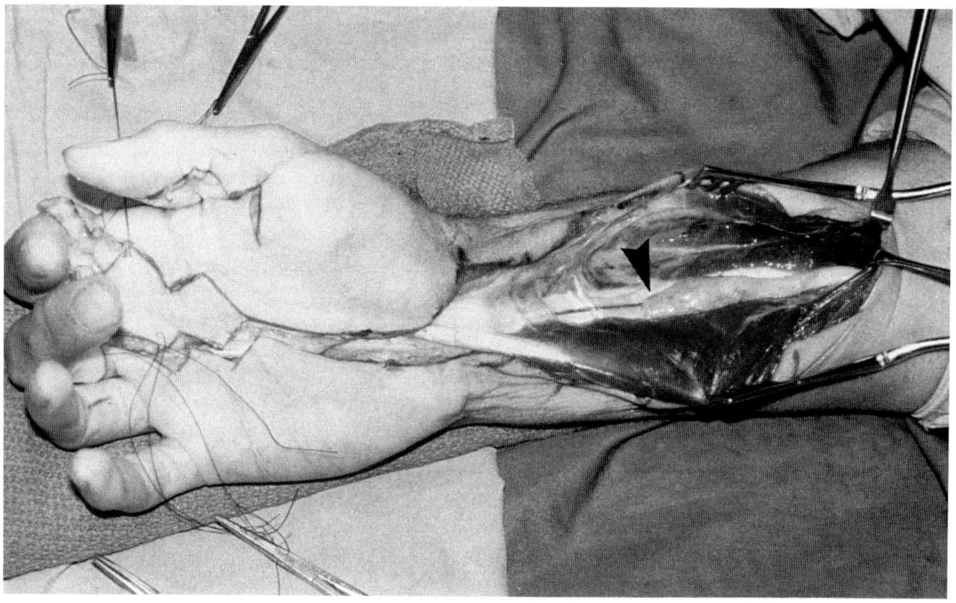

c

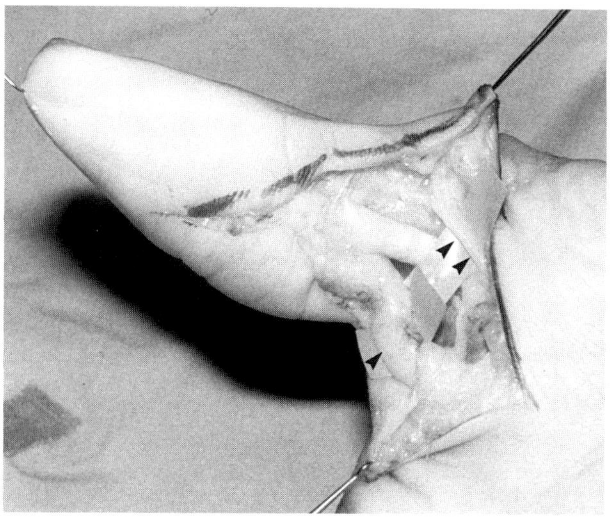

d

Figure 19-7 (*continued*) **d.** Some of the digital nerves were involved with tumor (arrow) and others were not (double arrow). **e.** Long sural nerve grafts were used to reconstitute the nerve gap. The abductor digiti minimi muscle flap was used as a apponensplasty. The patient developed protective sensation in the median nerve distribution.

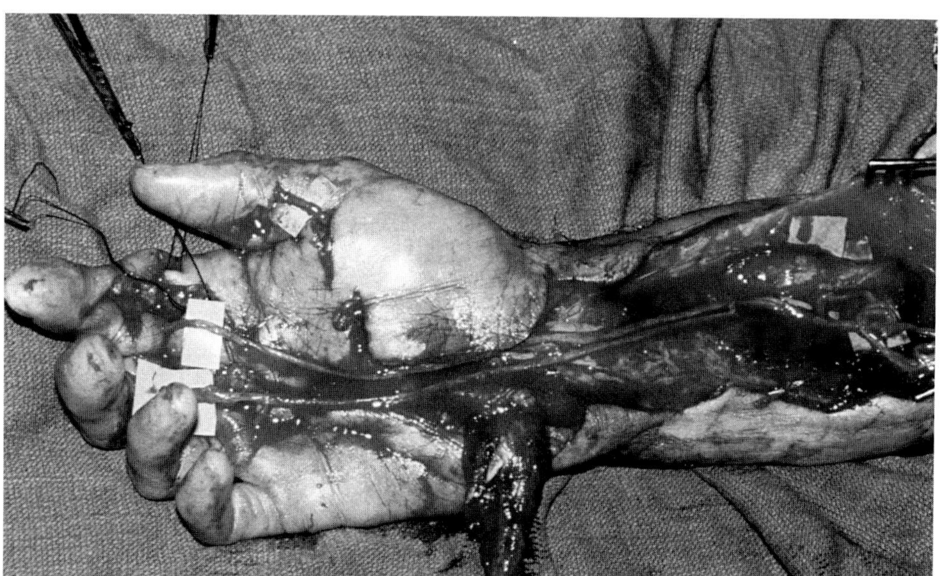

e

degeneration without fatty infiltration of the nerve. The tumor involves the nerve directly and, thus, excision of the tumor will result in loss of nerve function. Macrodactyly has also been described associated with this disease process.

Intraneural Lipoma, Hemangioma, Ganglion

Intraneural lipomas,[39,40] hemangiomas[41–43] and ganglions[44] have been described. These usually present with a mass or neurologic symptoms, or both. Surgical removal, using microneurosurgical technique, should result in no loss of neurologic function.

Tumors of the Brachial Plexus

In 1886, Courvoisier[45] described the first surgical excision of a brachial plexus schwannoma. In 1952, Godwin[46] described 11 benign Schwannomas involving the brachial plexus. In 1970, Dart et al[47] described 27 cases of brachial plexus tumors. In 1983, Kline and Judice reported 23 tumors of the brachial plexus, and in 1978 Lusk and Kline[10] reported 57 tumors involving the brachial plexus. Their article constitutes the largest clinical series of these tumors (Table 19-2). In their series, the 40 neural sheath tumors included 26 neurofibromas, 8 schwannomas, 4 malignant neural sheath tumors, 1 fibrosarcoma, and 1 meningioma. The 17 other tumors were not of neural sheath origin. Seven of these non-neural sheath tumors were benign and ten were metastatic malignant tumors. The benign neurofibromas and the malignant sheath tumors usually presented with pain or a functional neural deficit, and the solitary schwannomas usually presented with a palpable mass and no other symptoms. The investigators utilized intraoperative nerve action potential recordings in order to protect functional elements in the brachial plexus. Forequarter amputation was advised for malignant tumors if the tumor was located distally enough in the plexus in order to facilitate the interscapulothoracic amputation.

Table 19-2. Tumors of the Brachial Plexus (1968–1985)*

Tumor Type	*No.*
Neural sheath-associated tumors	
Neurofibromas	
With VRD†	9
Without VRD	15
Lengthy solitary plexiform (regionalized VRD)‡	2
Total	26
Schwannomas	
With VRD	0
Without VRD	8
Total	8
Malignant sheath tumors	
Malignant schwannoma	
With VRD	1
Without VRD	2
Lengthy solitary plexiform (regionalized VRD)	1
Fibrosarcoma	1
Total	5
Meningioma	1
Total	40
Non-neural sheath type tumors	
Benign tumors	
Desmoid	1
Myoblastoma	1
Lymphangioma	1
Lipoma	2
Myositis ossificans with lipoma	1
Brachial cleft cyst	1
Total	7
Malignant secondary tumors§	
Breast cancer infiltration	5
Lung extension (Pancoast)	3
Melanoma	1
Malignant thymoma	1
Total	10
Total all tumors (40 + 17)	57
No. patients	56

*Reprinted with permission from Lusk et al.[10]

†VRD: von Recklinghausen's disease.

‡One patient with a benign lengthy plexiform tumor subsequently developed a malignant tumor at the same site.

§Does not include 14 operated cases of radiation fibrosis involving plexus, but without evidence of active cancer.

References

1. Butler ED, Hamill JP, Seipel RS, et al: Tumours of the hand. Am J Surg 100:293–303, 1960.
2. Stack HG: Tumours of the hand. Br Med J 1:919–922, 1960.
3. Harkin JC, Reed RJ: Tumours of the Peripheral Nervous System. Armed Forces Institute of Pathology, Washington, D.C., 1968.
4. Mason ML: Tumours of the hand. Surg Gynecol Obstet 64:129–148, 1937.
5. Stout AP, Laidlaw GF, Haagensen DC: Tumours of the Peripheral Nerve. Williams & Wilkins, Baltimore, 1937.
6. Stout AP: The peripheral manifestations of the specific nerve sheath tumour (neurilemmoma). Am J Cancer 24: 751–796, 1935.
7. Ehrlich H, Martin H: Schwannomas (neurilemmomas) in the head and neck. Surg Gynecol Obstet 76:577–583, 1943.
8. Russell DS, Rubinstein LJ: Pathology of Tumors of the Nervous System, 4th ed. Williams & Wilkins, Baltimore, 1977, pp 293–297.
9. Fisher ER, Vusevski VD: Cytogenesis of Schwannomas (neurilemmomas) neurofibromas, dermatofibromas, and dermatofibrosarcomas as revealed by electron microscopy. Am J Clin Pathol 49:941–954, 1968.
10. Lusk MD, Kline DG, Garcia CA: Tumors of the brachial plexus. Neurosurgery 21:439–453, 1987.
11. Hope DG, Mulvihill JJ: Malignancy in neurofibromatosis. Adv Neurol 29:33–54, 1981.
12. Ghosh BC, Ghosh L, Huvos AG, Fortner JG: Malignant schwannoma. Cancer 31:184–190, 1973.
13. Woodruff JM, Godwin TA, Erlandson RA, et al: Cellular schwannoma. Am J Surg Pathol 5:733–744, 1981.
14. Bolande RP: Neurofibromatosis—the quintessential neurocristopathy. Adv Neurol 29:67–75, 1981.
15. Lott IT, Richardson EP: Neuropathological findings in the biology of neurofibromatosis. Adv Neurol 29:23–32, 1981.
16. Riccardi VM: von Recklinghausen's neurofibromatosis. N Engl J Med 305:1617–1627, 1981.
17. Riccardi VM, Mulvihill JJ: Neurofibromatosis (von Recklinghausen's disease). Adv Neurol 29:1–282, 1981.
18. Akenside M: Observations on cancers. Med Trans Coll Physicians Lond 1:64, 1768.
19. Ober WB: Mark Akenside, M.D. (1721–1770). Physician and philosophic poet. New York State J Med 68:3116, 1968.
20. Stay EJ, Vawter G: Relationship between nephroblastoma and neurofibromatosis. Cancer 39:2550–2555, 1977.
21. Recklinghausen VF: Ueber die multiplen Fibrome der Haut und ihre Beziehung zu den multiplen Neuromen. Verleg v. A. Hirschwald, Berlin, 1882.
22. Warkany J: Friedrich von Recklinghausen and his times. Adv Neurol 29:251–257, 1981.
23. Massey JM, Massey WE: Dr. Trevelyan and Mr. Treves, Sherlock Holmes and the elephant man. South Med J 78:854, 1985.
24. Thomson A: A Neuroma and Neurofibromatosis. Turnball and Speers, Edinburgh, 1900.
25. Verocay J: Zur Kenntnis der Neurofibrome. Beitr Pathol Anat 48:1–68, 1910.
26. Tsuge K, Ikuta Y: Macrodactyly and fibrofatty proliferation of the median nerve. Hiroshima J Med Sci 22:83–101, 1973.
27. Ducatman BS, Scheithauer BW, Piepgras DG, et al: Malignant peripheral nerve tumours. Cancer 57:2006–2021, 1986.
28. Johnson RJ, Bonfiglio M: Lipofibromatous hamartoma of the median nerve. J Bone Joint Surg 51A:984–990, 1969.
29. Lewis DS, Dick HM: Ossifying lipofibroma of the median nerve. J Bone Joint Surg 55A:1082–1084, 1973.
30. Rowland SA: Lipofibroma of the median nerve in the palm. J Bone Joint Surg 49A:1309–1313, 1967.
31. Pulvertaft RG: Unusual tumours of the median nerve. J Bone Joint Surg 46B:731–733, 1964.
32. Emmett AJJ: Lipomatous hamartoma of the median nerve in the palm. Br J Plast Surg 18:208–213, 1965.
33. Strickland JW, Steichen JB: Nerve tumours of the hand and forearm. J Hand Surg 2:285–291, 1977.
34. Lewis DS, Hankin FM, Greene TL, et al: Lipofibromas of the median nerve. Long term follow-up of four cases. J Hand Surg [Am] 10:403–407, 1985.
35. Rowlan SA: Case report—ten year follow-up of lipofibroma of the median nerve in the palm. J Hand Surg 2:316–317, 1977.
36. Yoman PM: Fatty infiltration of the median nerve. J Bone Joint Surg 46:737–739, 1964.
37. Abu Jamra FN, Rebeiz JJ: Lipofibroma of the median nerve. J Hand Surg 4:160–163, 1979.
38. Edmonson AS, Crenshaw AH: Campbell's Operative Orthopedics. CV Mosby, St. Louis, 1980, p 383.
39. Morley GH: Intraneural lipoma of the median nerve in the carpal tunnel. J Bone Joint Surg 46B:734–735, 1964.
40. Mikhail IK: Median nerve lipoma in the hand. J Bone Joint Surg 46B:726–730, 1964.
41. Kojima T, Yoshita I, Marumo E, et al: Hemangioma of the median nerve causing carpal tunnel. Hand 8:62–65, 1976.
42. Losli EJ: Intrinsic hemangiomas of the peripheral nerves. Arch Pathol 53:226–232, 1952.
43. Purcell FH, Gurdjian ES: Hemangiomata of peripheral nerves. Am J Surg 30:541, 1935.
44. Barrett R, Cramer F: Tumours of the peripheral nerves and socalled ganglia of the peroneal nerve. Clin Orthop 27:135–146, 1963.
45. Courvoisier LG: Die Neurome. Eine klinische Monographie. B. Schwode, Basel, 1886.
46. Godwin JT: Encapsulated neurilemmoma (Schwannoma) of the brachial plexus. Report of 11 cases. Cancer 5:708–720, 1952.
47. Dart L, MacCarty CS, Love JG, et al: Neoplasms of the brachial plexus. Minn Med 53:959–964, 1970.
48. Kline DG, Judice DJ: Operative management of selected brachial plexus lesions. J Neurosurg 58:631–649, 1983.

Future Directions in Peripheral Nerve Surgery

20

Recent advances in our understanding of nerve regeneration provide encouragement for a new optimism in the surgical treatment of peripheral nerve injury. Over the last half century, technical achievements have been utilized by people interested in the peripheral nerve to provide a foundation for our current management of injuries to these vital structures. World War II provided a large volume of nerve injuries, the treatment of which provided important information for surgeons interested in the management of nerve-injured patients.[1] Although the functional results of these early nerve repairs were generally poor,[2] the clinical material and surgical techniques used at that time provided the important reference point from which our current surgical management has developed. Anatomic studies by Sunderland,[3] the concept of tension-free nerve repair by Millesi,[4] and efforts by Moberg[5] and ourselves,[6–8] to quantitate the clinical assessment of sensory function have significantly influenced our understanding of nerve injury and repair. The emergence of surgeons dedicating the majority of their practice to the management of surgery of the injured nerve, has aroused a new critical awareness and sophistication not previously expended toward these problems. Important advances in the field of microsurgery have provided us with the technical skills required to deal with these injuries, and although the importance of all aspects of careful surgical technique cannot be overemphasized, we believe that it is unlikely that improved clinical results will come from further refinements in microsurgical techniques. We are now limited by a working knowledge and understanding of the details of the neurobiology and the neurochemistry of nerve regeneration.

It has been the responsibility of the surgeon to align correctly fascicles of the peripheral nerve in such a fashion as to permit appropriate motor and sensory nerve regeneration. Both experimental and clinical experience has demonstrated that nerve repair without tension[9–11] and with proper fascicular alignment will minimize scar formation at the repair site and maximize the appropriate direction of axons. Although adherence to these principles has improved functional results after nerve repair, normal function is almost never restored and the average result is still far from excellent.

Neuroscientists have recently studied the cell biology of neural regeneration:[12] the interaction of the Schwann cell and the axon,[13] the dynamics of axoplasmic transport[14] and the neurophysiology of sensory receptor,[15] and motor end-plate function.[16] The efforts of these researchers has until recently had no real effect on the clinical management of nerve injury. As the peripheral nerve surgeon becomes more knowledgeable in the writings of the basic scientists and involved in his own basic science research, it becomes more apparent that improved clinical results are likely to be realized from a greater understanding of the neurobiology of nerve repair. Of particular importance for the nerve surgeon is the concept of neurotrop(h)ism and contact guidance in determining regeneration across a nerve gap.[47] Neurotrophism implies an ability to influence *maturation* of the nerve, neurotropism to influence *direction* of nerve regeneration). We coin the term, "neurotrop(h)ism" to suggest influences that both facilitate nerve maturation and appropriate directional regeneration.[42]

Neurotropism, Neurotrophism, and Contact Guidance

In 1880, Gluck[17] used the central canal of a decalcified bone to provide a pathway between the divided ends of two nerves. In 1898, a Swedish bacteriologist, Forssman[18] observed that regeneration across small gaps could occur after peripheral nerve transection. He introduced nerves into straw tubes and noted regeneration toward nerve tissue. Forssman attributed this influence to neurotropism. This concept was popularized by the Spanish biologist, Ramon y Cajal[19] (Figs. 20-1, 20-2), who postulated that chemical agents (myelin or Schwann cells) from the distal nerve stump could attract nerve sprouts from the proximal stump.

Many years later this concept of neurotropism was questioned by the Americans Weiss and Taylor.[20] They conceded that "continuity is restored between severed nerve stumps even when the latter has been separated and brought out of line" but proposed that "this connection is affected not by attraction but by the influence of the stump and their surroundings" so that surrounding tissue preferentially guides fibers toward the distal stump.[20,21] In a series of multiple choice experiments using Y-shaped arteries (abdominal aorta with the iliac bifurcation), Weiss and Taylor[20] showed that "in no cases were the regenerating nerve fibers attracted to-

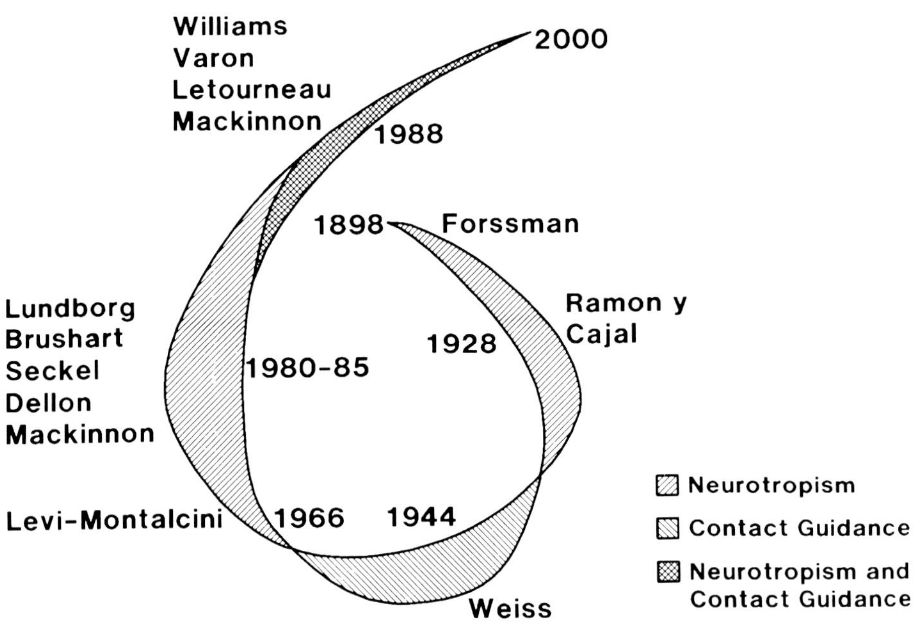

Figure 20-1. The concepts of neurotropism and contact guidance have evolved considerably in the 20th century. In the early part of the century, Forssman and Ramón y Cajal spoke in favor of neurotropism. In the 1940s the concept of neurotropism was strongly opposed by Weiss. In 1966, Levi-Montalcini described a nerve growth factor (two decades later, she was awarded the Nobel Prize for this work). In the 1980s the pendulum swung again toward neurotropism and against contact guidance as target-specific neurotropism was demonstrated at many levels of specificity. In the late 1980s we see that neural regeneration is influenced by both contact guidance and neurotropism. We recognize that both concepts can be utilized to influence nerve regeneration.

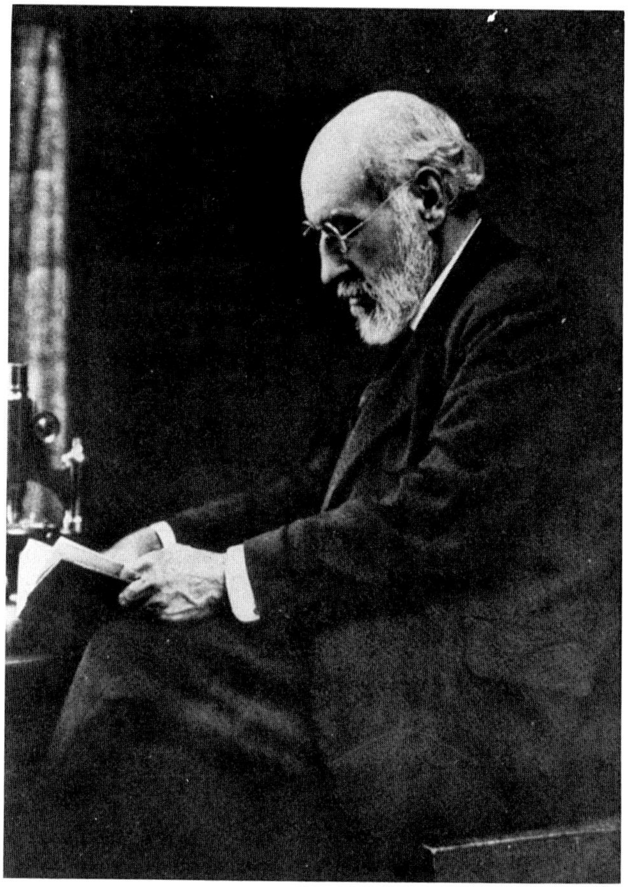

a

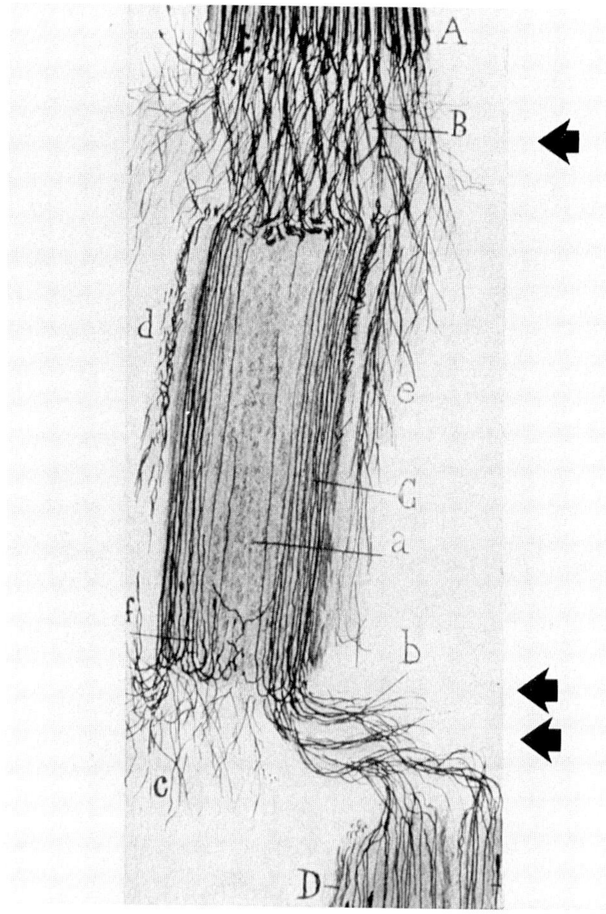

b

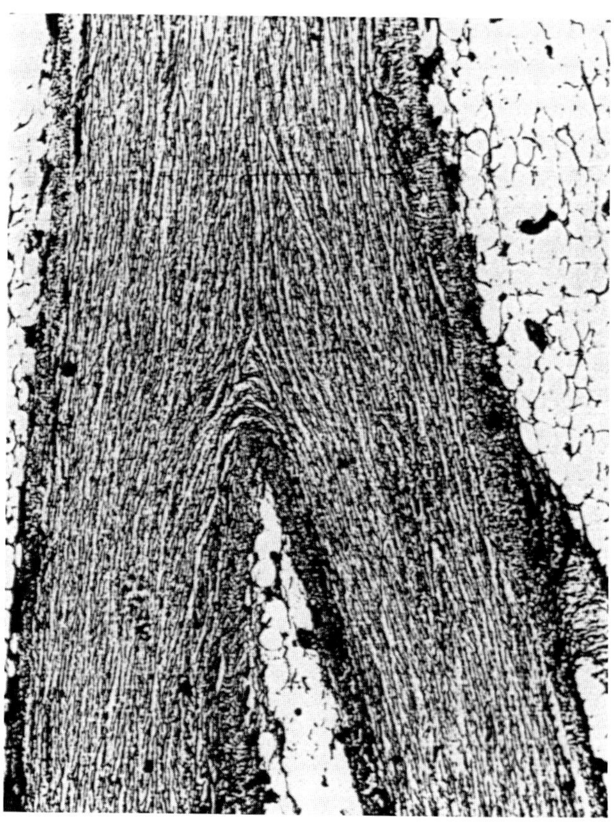

c

Figure 20-2a. Ramón y Cajal supported the concept of neurotropism. **b.** Cajal reconstructed this drawing to show that when the nerve ends were separated the nerve sprouts would grow to the distal nerve (arrow) even when the nerve ends were brought out of line (double arrow). **c.** Weiss' classic Y experiment demonstrated that nerve regeneration occurred independent of the distal target and supported the concept of nerve growth by contact guidance. Note that the fibers grow in equal numbers into each distal limb.

ward the peripheral nerve fragment but the fiber stream divided itself more or less evenly regardless of the kind of destination awaiting them". This work was used to support the concept of "contact guidance" rather than neurotropism. It is important to note that the silver stain used to assess nerve regeneration did not facilitate either quantitation or ultrastructural assessment. The presence of neurotropism in Weiss and Taylor's models may well have been obscured because of an immunologic response directed toward the aortic homografts that were used as the "Y" channels in their experimental model.

Weiss suggested that contact guidance was important in determining nerve regeneration as axons elongated and oriented themselves along strands of fibrin clot.

From the 1940s until the mid 1980s, this controversy between contact guidance and neurotropism existed. In the 1980s, a series of experiments combined to refute Weiss' theory in favor again of Forssman's concept of neurotropism.

As we will see, very recent work shows us that neurotropism and contact guidance are both important in determining nerve regeneration and both properties can be utilized to our advantage to improve the results of nerve repair (Figs. 20-1, 20-2).

Recent in vitro and in vivo studies have demonstrated a basis for the concept of neurotropism. These studies have demonstrated not only that neurotropism exists but also that there is a high degree of specificity associated with this neurotropism. Target-specific nerve regeneration has been documented at various levels of specificity. Tissue specificity,[22,23] fascicular specificity,[24] and end-organ specificity[25] have all been demonstrated (Chapter 1).

Experimental Evidence

In eight adult cynomolgus monkeys, the sensory component of the femoral nerve was sectioned and introduced into the proximal channel of a silicone "Y" chamber.[23] The proximal stump was given distal choices of various tissues that were inserted into the remaining arms of the chamber. The targets presented were combinations of tendon, muscle, intact distal nerve, distal nerve graft, or an empty silicone channel. After 6 weeks, ultrastructural analysis confirmed axonal growth toward distal nerve tissue and minimal or no nerve regeneration toward tendon, muscle, or empty silicone channels (Fig. 20-3). These results showed that either a distal nerve stump or a nerve graft would act as a specific target to the regenerating primate proximal nerve stump. No axonal growth was directed toward tendon, muscle, or empty chambers and ultrastructural assessment showed regeneration into the distal nerve segments (both distal nerve intact and nerve graft). A comparison of nerve regeneration into the limb with the nerve graft versus the nerve intact demonstrated that the degree of regeneration directed toward the intact nerve was greater than that directed toward the nerve graft, suggesting that the presence of an intact end organ might influence eventual maturation of nerve regeneration (Fig. 20-4). We have recently completed a similar study in which regeneration through the Y chamber was followed to 6 months. The distal targets were a nerve graft and a distal nerve intact to distal sensory receptors. Improved regeneration was seen directed towards the nerve intact to distal receptors (total nerve fibers 1277 ± 656) versus the nerve graft (516 ± 624 nerve fibers) $p < .005$.

Another study evaluated the effect of the distal nerve in influencing nerve regeneration across a long nerve graft. Cross-facial nerve grafts were carried out in the cynomolgus monkey. In one group, the distal end of the nerve graft was coapted to the distal end of the opposite facial nerve that had been transected but had distal motor end-plate connections intact. In the second group, the distal end of the graft was left in the subcutaneous tissue, remote from any muscle. At the conclusion of the experiment (12 months) improved regeneration was noted in the group with motor end-plate connection (Fig. 15-10).

Seckel et al[24] have demonstrated that when the peroneal nerve is placed in the proximal limb of a Y chamber, it will grow preferentially by a ratio of 2 to 1 to the appropriate distal peroneal nerve fascicle when presented with the distal nerve choice of peroneal and posterior tibial nerve. In another study by Brushart[25] investigating end-organ specificity, a proximal motor nerve was given distal choices of sensory and motor fascicles. When a very short distance (2 mm) was present between the proximal and distal nerve stumps, axonal behavior was "independent of the nature of the distal stump." With a longer gap (5 mm), neurotropism

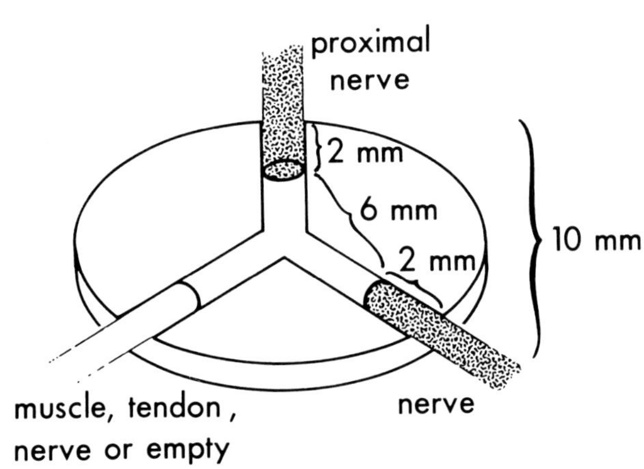

Figure 20-3 Experimental design. The proximal end of the nerve was inserted 2 mm into the silicone Y chamber and distal choices were presented, including nerve intact, nerve graft, muscle, tendon, and empty chamber.

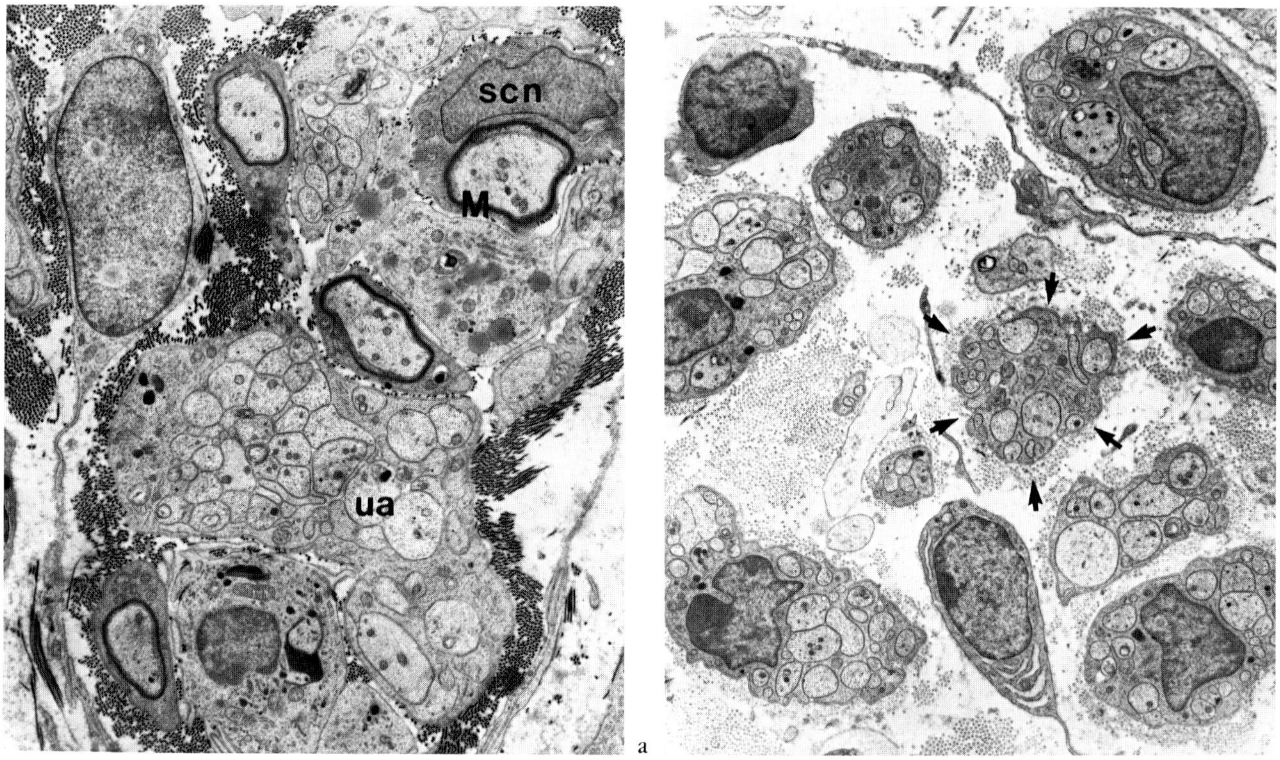

Figure 20-4. Histology from Y-tube experiment where proximal nerve is given choice of a distal nerve graft of its own distal (intact) nerve end. Transverse section. **a.** distal channel (nerve intact), large regenerating units with large unmyelinated fibers and a few myelinated fibers are noted. **b.** distal channel (nerve graft) smaller regenerating units spaced farther apart with smaller unmyelinated fibers seen. No myelinated fibers are noted. Arrow: regenerating units; ua: unmyelinated fibers; M: myelinated fibers; scn: Schwann cell nucleus. (Uranyl lead acetate stain; ×6160.) (Reproduced with permission from Mackinnon, et al.[23])

was demonstrated with evidence of preferential growth of the motor nerve toward the distal motor nerve (Fig. 20-5).

It has been demonstrated that regenerating motor axons will preferentially reinnervate a distal motor branch versus a distal sensory branch. Brushart has further explored this specificity of motor reinnervation in a study presented to the American Society for Surgery of the Hand at their annual meeting in 1988. The femoral nerve in the rat was divided at a level where the sensory and motor axons are diffusely mixed and the proximal and distal nerve stumps were separated by 5 mm within a silicone tube. Brushart used 2 retrograde tracers, horseradish peroxidase (HRP) and Fluoro Gold. HRP was applied to one femoral branch of each femoral nerve and Fluoro Gold to the other. These tracers were then transported proximally to the spinal cord. The cords were then examined to determine the number of motor neurons which projected axons into the sensory and motor branches of each femoral nerve as well as the number of motor projecting axons into both branches (double-labeled neurons). These evaluations were made at 2, 6 and 8 weeks. This study demonstrated, at 2 weeks, that the motor neurons projected axons into both the motor and sensory nerve stumps. Thus, at 2 weeks, the motor axons did not selectively reinnervate distal motor branches. This finding supports the concept of neurotrophism versus neurotropism. At 6 and 8 weeks, however, there was statistically significant increased labelling in the distal motor branch to confirm selective reinnervation of the distal motor stump. This study suggests that it is neurotrophism which is influential in determining the preferential motor reinnervation and that there is a selective "pruning" of inappropriate motor-sensory reinnervation with time. One would hypothesize that initially the motor nerve will regenerate equally towards motor and sensory nerves but once end organ contact has been reestablished, the trophic interaction between the motor axons and the distal muscle end organ supports appropriate motor axonal regeneration at the expense of inappropriate motor to sensory regeneration.

Thus, the properties of neurotropism will direct nerve regeneration toward nerve versus other tissue. This study would suggest that it is the property of neurotrophism that influences preferential motor regeneration toward distal motor nerve.

Recent work has demonstrated that contact guid-

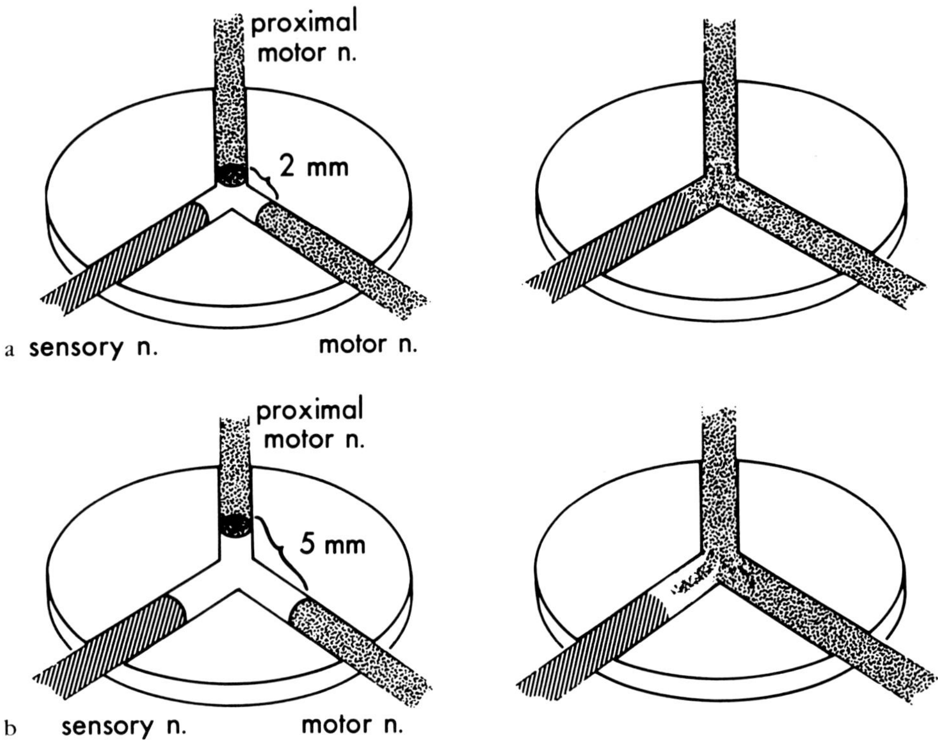

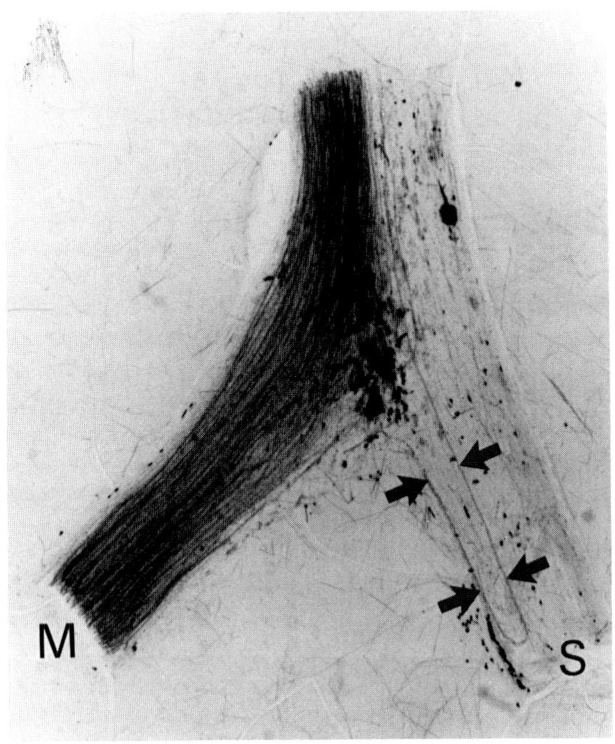

c

Figure 20-5. Schematic diagram of Brushart's study (see text). When the distance between the proximal and distal nerves was only 2 mm, evidence of neurotropism was not apparent **a.** When the gap distance was increased to 5 mm, the proximal motor nerve regenerated preferentially toward the distal motor nerve **b.** Horseradish peroxidase staining of longitudinal section of the 2 mm Y tubes demonstrating ability of this staining technique to track nerve fibers. M: motor; S: sensory. **c.** The horseradish peroxidase labelling techniques used by Brushart to demonstrate specificity of nerve regeneration. (Courtesy T.M. Brushart, Baltimore.)

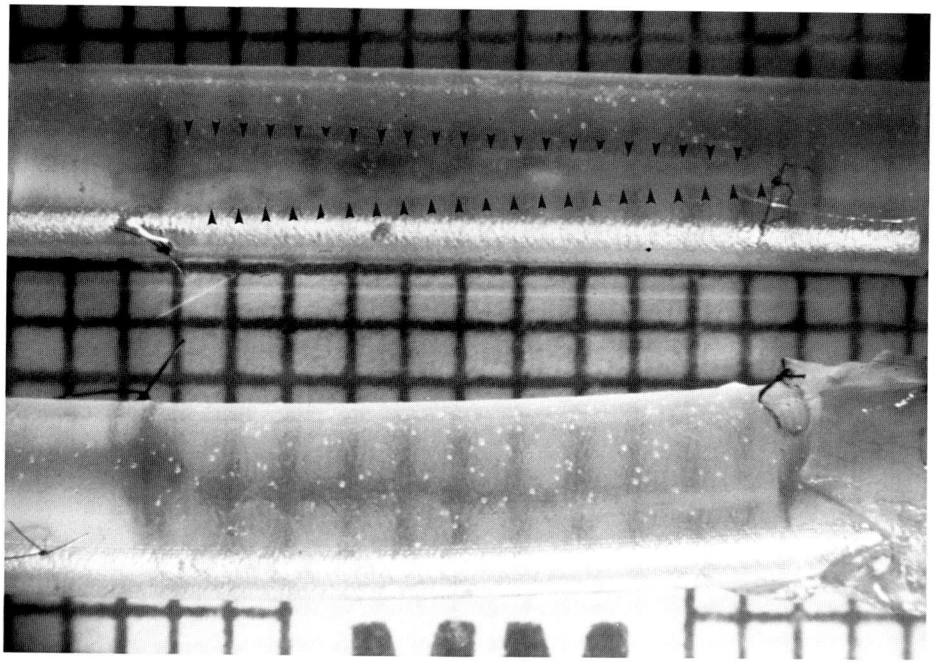

Figure 20-6. The two ends of the divided sciatic nerve were inserted into a silicone chamber that was prefilled with heparinized saline. Four weeks after this procedure, the nerve had regenerated across the gap (above; arrows). When the chamber was left empty, at 4 weeks there was no evidence of nerve regeneration (below).

ance is also extremely important in influencing early axonal elongation. Williams[26] has emphasized the importance of a longitudinal fibrin matrix within a nerve conduit. In an isolated chamber model of nerve regeneration, the proximal and distal nerve was separated 1.5 cm and each end of the nerve inserted into a silicone tube. If axons are allowed to elongate into an empty chamber, they will not do so until fluid has either been placed in the chamber or enough time has passed to allow the nerve itself to fill the chamber completely as fluid moves from the severed ends of the nerve. Thus, if fluid is placed in the chamber, axonal elongation will be enhanced, and if the fluid in the chamber forms a linear fibrin matrix, then axons will elongate in a linear fashion along this matrix and will cross the nerve gap more rapidly than if the axons must elongate along a random, disorganized matrix pattern. If a longitudinal fibrin matrix (such as serum or heparinized saline) exists within the environment of the chamber, axonal regeneration is enhanced. When a disorganized randomly oriented matrix pattern existed (clot) within the chamber or when the chamber was left completely empty, axonal elongation was inhibited. In the empty chambers, axonal elongation did not occur until the chamber became filled with fluid that came from the severed ends of the cut nerves. In this model, it took several weeks for the fluid to collect before axonal elongation could finally occur. In a similar experiment, we have investigated the ability of chamber contents to influence nerve regeneration and have demonstrated that when a disorganized blood clot or an empty chamber was the environment for regeneration, axonal elongation was retarded. When a chamber was prefilled with a matrix that supported longitudinal elongation of the nerve fibers, regeneration was enhanced (Fig. 20-6).

In 1915, Kirk and Lewis[27] studied nerve regeneration in the dog across tubes made of fascia lata. It is interesting to note their concern regarding blood products was the same then as ours is now. "Hemorrhage from the ends of the nerve must be controlled, for blood within the tube will prevent the axis cylinders (axons) passing downward. The tubes in cases in which hemorrhage occurred into them were almost occluded by scar tissue."[27]

It is concluded that axons will elongate along a fibrin matrix, thus, although certainly neurotrop(h)ic effects can be utilized to influence nerve regeneration, contact guidance is also important in directing axonal elongation. The long-standing Weiss-Cajal controversy of contact guidance versus neurotropism is perhaps artificial. It would appear that nerve regeneration can be influenced by neurotropic and neurotrophic factors as well as contact guidance.

With a standard nerve grafting or nerve repair technique, it is the surgeon who determines the topography of the proximal and distal nerve fascicles. It is the surgeon who directs nerve regeneration as his experience and wisdom deems most appropriate. It is possible

Table 20-1. Primate Neural Regeneration in Pseudosheath: Light Microscopic Assessment of Fiber Diameter and Density*

Months	*Proximal*	*Mid Sheath*	*Distal*
Mean Fiber Diameter (μm)			
3	6.1		
5	5.5	3.4	2.5
7	6.0	3.6	2.8
9	5.1	4.2	3.9
Percent neural tissue			
3	35	0.2	
5	35	5	2
7	40	5	7
9	32	7	20

*Reprinted with permission from Mackinnon et al.[35]

that the fascicular alignment he chooses may not be appropriate. The ideal nerve repair should maximize neurotrop(h)ic effects.

This work would suggest that a short nerve gap between the nerve ends may even be desirable as long as fascicular alignment can be ensured, perhaps, with some type of nerve conduit or guide. When tight end-to-end suture coaptation is utilized, as in current neurorrhaphy technique, the benefits to be gained from neurotropic effects may be overcome by the regenerative drive of the proximal stump.

The awareness of the tremendous potential benefits of neurotrop(h)ism in directing appropriate nerve regeneration led us to the investigation of nerve regeneration across a controlled surgical gap. The problems to investigate were the possibility of directing nerve regeneration across a nerve gap in primates and the identification of an ideal nerve conduit to direct such regeneration.

The Nerve Gap

It has been recognized since the late 1800s that peripheral nerves will cross small gaps when guided through various preformed tissue spaces. More recently, in the rat model, regeneration across distances of up to 15 mm has been demonstrated.[28–30] Lundborg et al[31–33] developed an experimental model using preformed pseudosynovial tubes to investigate regeneration of peripheral nerve tissue. Although these experiments have been of considerable neurobiologic significance, there was considerable doubt that these experiments in lower animals would have any practical significance in the human situation. Recognizing the rat's excellent regenerative capacities,[34] a primate model was developed to investigate nerve regeneration across 3 cm gaps.[35] It was believed that a primate nerve separated by as much as a 3 cm gap would merely form a proximal and distal end-bulb neuroma. Thus, when the experimental situation was developed to separate a divided ulnar nerve by a 3 cm gap to study regeneration through a pseudosynovial sheath, we were surprised to note that histologic evaluation at 3, 5, 7, and 9 months demonstrated evidence of nerve regeneration across this gap. Nerve fiber diameter and density assessment demonstrated a maturation of the nerve fiber pattern with time (Table 20-1, 20-2; Fig. 20-7). The overall morphologic pattern of the regenerating nerve within the pseudosheath was that of multiple small fascicles, each within its own perineurial compartment, these are classical regenerating units. This type of regeneration across the conduit should not be called "neuromatous neurotization." Thus, contrary to our hypothesis that a primate nerve separated by a 3 cm gap would not regenerate across this distance, we did see histologic evidence of regeneration with maturation of nerve fibers in the distal ulnar nerve apparent over the 3- to 9-month period of the study. Since regeneration was not anticipated in this primate model, a control experimental group to assess regeneration across a classic nerve graft had not been included in the first study. A second study was designed to compare the quality of regeneration across a vascularized pseudosheath and a classic sural nerve graft in a primate model using histologic and electrophysiologic parameters.[36] The experimental design is noted in Figure 20-8. A 3 cm gap in the ulnar nerve of a primate was reconstructed with either a sural nerve graft or a preformed pseudosynovial sheath. Histologic and electrophysiologic evaluation was made 1 year after the initial procedures. Histologic evaluation demonstrated comparable regeneration across both the pseudosheath and the sural nerve graft (Fig. 20-9). Electrophysiologic evaluation demonstrated similar findings (Fig. 20-10).

This study then confirmed regeneration across a 3 cm gap in a primate model through a vascularized

Table 20-2. Primate Neural Regeneration in Pseudosheath: Characteristics of "Mini" Fascicles in Midsheath*

Months	*Mean Fascicular Diameter (μm)*	*% Neural Tissue/ Fascicle*	*No. Fibers/Fascicle*	*Mean Fiber Diameter (μm)*
5	38 ± 16	8.5	6 ± 1	3.46 ± 1.03
7	42 ± 18	15.3	45 ± 7	3.64 ± 1.13
9	33 ± 14	16.0	56 ± 18	4.21 ± 1.20

*Reprinted with permission from Mackinnon et al.[35]

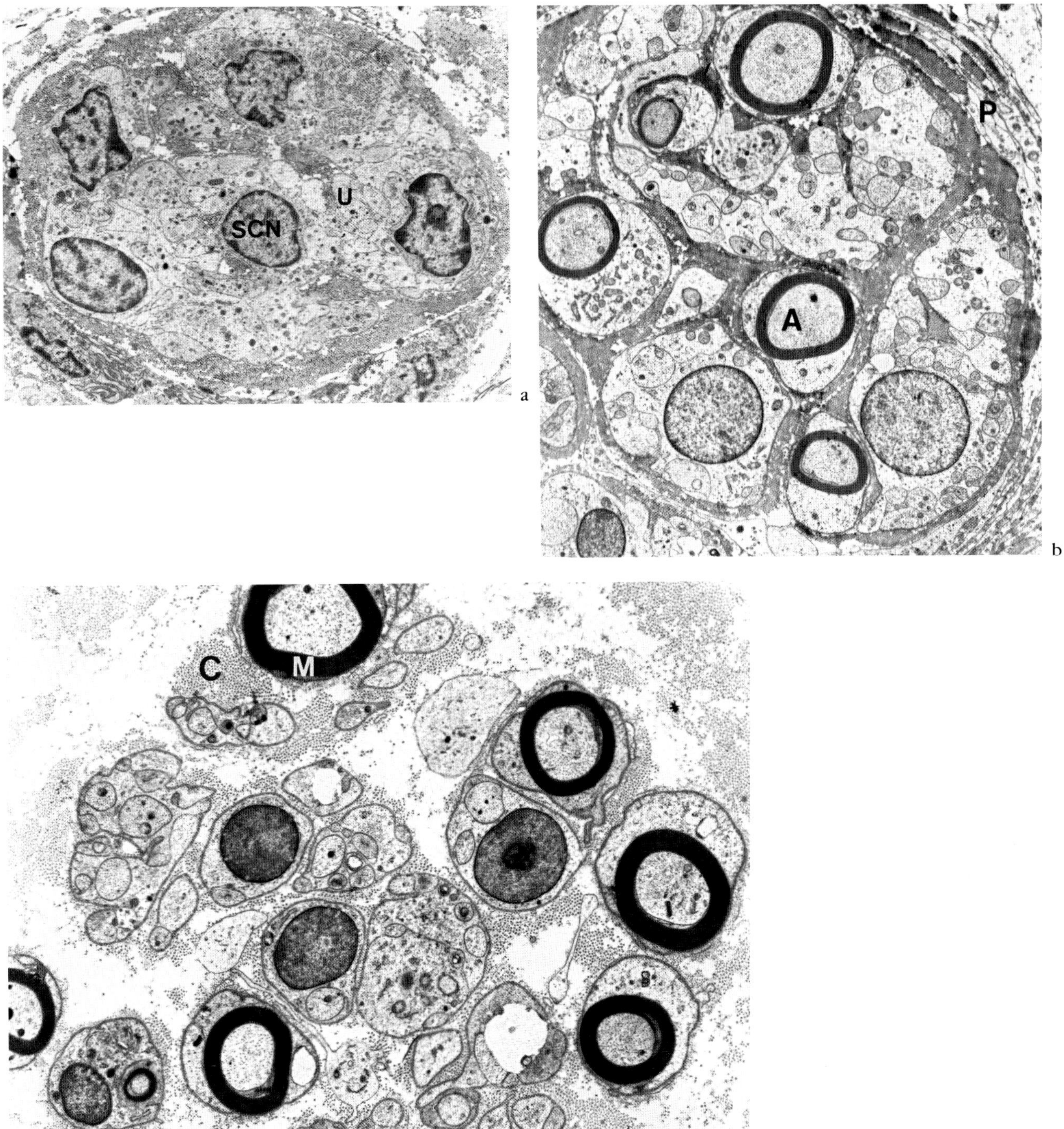

a b c

Figure 20-7a. Primate neural regeneration in pseudosheath. Cross-section through the mid-sheath area at 3 months demonstrates numerous unmyelinated fibers (x3876) **b.** Cross-section through the mid sheath at 5 months demonstrates five myelinated fibers and numerous unmyelinated axons. (×3876.) **c.** Cross-section at nine months demonstrates six well-myelinated fibers. (×4560.) A: axon; M: myelin sheath; U: unmyelinated axon; SCN: Schwann cell nucleus; C: collagen; P: perineurium. (Reproduced with permission from Mackinnon et al.[35])

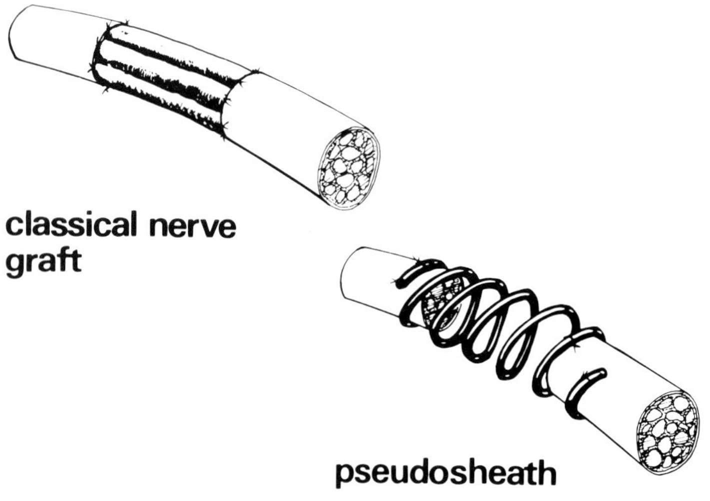

Figure 20-8. Experimental design of a study to compare nerve regeneration across a pseudosynovial sheath and a sural nerve graft. (Reproduced with permission from Mackinnon et al.)[36]

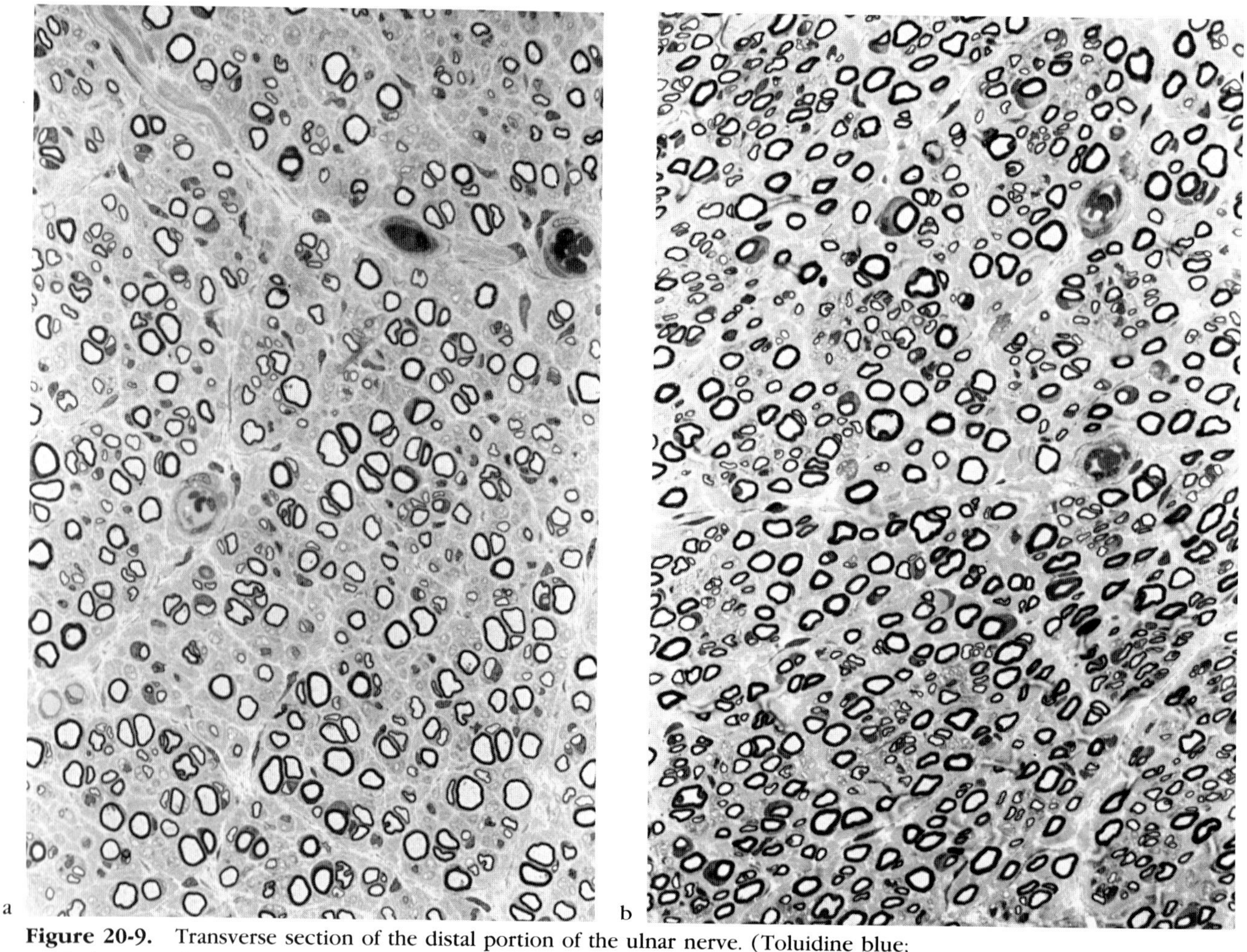

Figure 20-9. Transverse section of the distal portion of the ulnar nerve. (Toluidine blue; ×563.) **a.** Distal to the sural nerve graft. **b.** Distal to the pseudosheath. (Reproduced with permission from Mackinnon et al.)[36]

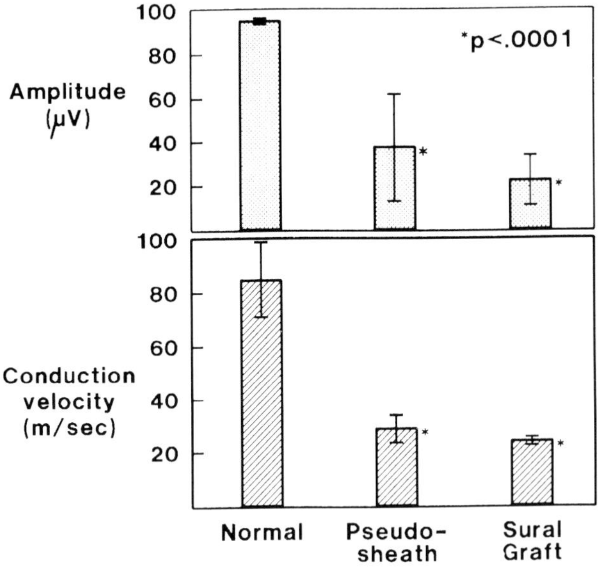

Figure 20-10. Electrophysiologic data demonstrated no significant difference between the two experimental groups. (Reproduced with permission from Mackinnon et al.)[36]

pseudosynovial sheath. The formation of the pseudosheath, however, required two operations staged approximately 6 weeks apart. A readily available, biodegradable conduit would be especially attractive for the management of the short nerve gap. Theoretically, such a conduit could utilize potential benefits of neurotropism in directing nerve regeneration and neurotrophism in supporting nerve fiber maturation. It would also importantly obviate the morbidity associated with harvesting a nerve graft. The problem then would be to define the ideal nerve conduit. It has been demonstrated recently in a number of animal models that nerves will regenerate across a nerve gap through various tubes and conduits.[37–44] Autogenous conduits, such as vein and pseudosynovial sheaths of the kind used in this study, have been used as well as nonabsorbable and bioabsorbable nerve tubes.

The characteristics of the ideal nerve conduit would include availability, biodegradability, and low antigenicity. Such conduits would be readily vascularized and porous enough to facilitate oxygen transport. The presence of a circular nondegradable structure around a peripheral nerve would most likely with time produce changes of chronic nerve compression (Chapter 2). This is a major criticism for the silicone nerve wrap recently presented for clinical use.

A number of investigators are currently exploring the use of collagen as a nerve conduit.[44,45] By necessity, this collagen is either allogenic or zenogenic in origin and, thus, will stimulate an immune response that may inhibit nerve regeneration. Conduits that are antigenic are likely to interfere with nerve regeneration because of a cellular or humoral response directed toward the immunologically foreign material. Similarly, if any substances are to be added to the contents of the conduits they must not be antigenic.

A study was designed to compare nerve regeneration across conduits of polyglycolic acid[46] (Dexon,™ PGA supplied by Davis & Geck Division of American Cyanamid). The experimental design is noted in Figure 20-11. Regeneration across a three cm gap in the ulnar nerve, through both rigid PGA and meshed PGA tubes, was compared with regeneration across a three cm sural nerve graft. One year after surgery, histologic and electrophysiologic studies were carried out. Regeneration similar to that across the sural nerve graft was noted in the experimental situations in which PGA tubes were used. Such a readily available, biodegradable nerve tube would be especially attractive for the management of short nerve gap where the problems of harvesting a donor nerve with associated donor site morbidity (loss of sensation, scar, potential painful neuromas) are emphasized for both the patient and the surgeon.

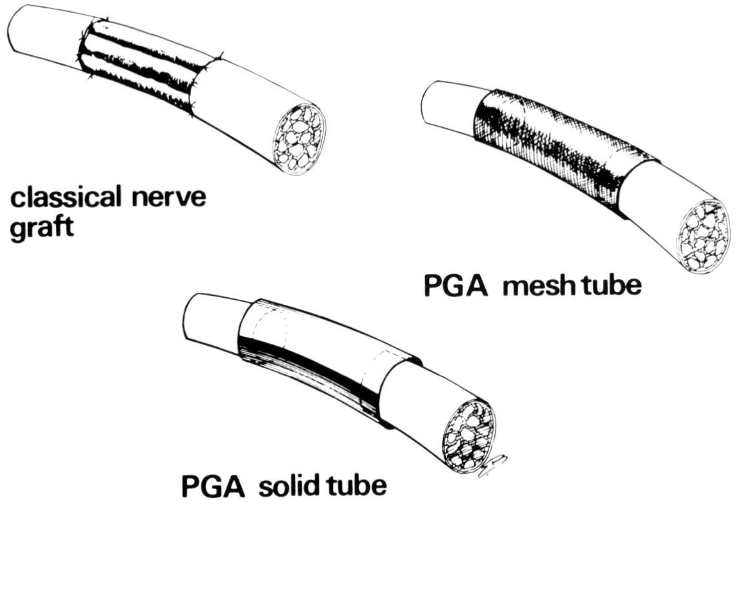

Figure 20-11 Experimental design of a study to compare regeneration across a sural nerve graft and nerve conduits of polyglycolic acid. (Reproduced with permission from Dellon and Mackinnon.)[46]

Table 20-3. Clinical Data—PGA Nerve Conduit Patients*

Number of patients	33
Number of neurotubes	45
Workers' Compensation patients	21
Male/female	23/10
Mean follow-up (months)	25 ± 6

*Reprinted with permission from Mackinnon and Dellon.[48]

Table 20-4. Clinical Date—PGA Conduit Patients*

Nerve	*Number Patients*	*Number Tubes*
Digital	17	21
Median	11	18
Ulnar	2	3
Facial	2	2
Radial	1	1
	33	45

*Reprinted with permission from Mackinnon and Dellon.[48]

Table 20-5. Clinical Results of PGA Nerve Conduit Reconstructions*,**

	Median Nerve $n = 4$ (%)	*Digital Nerve* $n = 16$ (%)
Excellent m2PD ≤ 3 mm s2PD ≤ 6 mm	75	81
Good m2PD 4-7 mm s2PD 7-15 mm		6
Poor m2PD ≥ 8 mm s2PD ≥ 16 mm	25	13
Worse		

*Reprinted with permission from Mackinnon and Dellon.[48]
**Patients routinely had sensory re-education postoperatively.

Clinical Study of the PGA Tube

Millesi has demonstrated the problems associated with tension at the neurorrhaphy and has made the once controversial peripheral nerve grafting technique a reliable method of management of surgical nerve gap (see Chapter 4). Thus, a technique that was controversial only two decades ago is now the "gold standard" for the management of the peripheral nerve gap. In the situation in which only a very short nerve gap exists, the morbidity of harvesting the short nerve graft becomes a concern for both the patient and the surgeon. It is in these latter cases that an alternative to the standard nerve graft for the management of the short nerve gap would be especially useful. Between December 1985 and December 1987, PGA tubes were used in 33 patients to reconstruct 37 nerves in these patients. Table 20-3 presents the clinical data and Table 20-4 presents the various nerves that were repaired using this technique. The general uses of the PGA tube are outlined in Table 20-5. The nerve gaps treated varied between 1.0 and 3.0 cm.

Clinical Uses of PGA Tubes

Failed Nerve Repair

A PGA tube was used for secondary reconstruction after nine failed major nerve repairs and nineteen failed digital nerve repairs. In these cases, a primary repair had been done one to four years previously (mean, 2.8 years) without any recovery of nerve function. Seventeen of the 19 digital nerve patients complained of significant pain at the level of the nerve repair and numbness in the distribution of the digital nerve involved. In ten of these cases, the hand pain prevented the patients from working. In all patients, the pain was significantly disabling (Fig. 20-12). After excision of the fourth degree injury (neuroma in-continuity) at the level of the nerve repair, the median length of the gap between the proximal and distal nerve ends was 2.4 cm for the major nerves and 1.7 cm for the digital nerves (Figs. 20-13, 20-14).

Iatrogenic Nerve Injury

In four cases, major nerves had been injured after operative procedures for other conditions. In these cases, the use of PGA obviated the need for a donor nerve graft (Fig. 20-15).

Acute Injuries

In four instances, a PGA tube was used at the time of the acute nerve injury (Fig. 20-16). In these cases, the nature of the injury was such that a primary repair was not possible due to the severity of the injury with loss of nerve tissue. The use of a primary nerve graft is relatively contraindicated because it is difficult to determine the exact longitudinal extent of the nerve injury. It is inappropriate in these cases to sacrifice a donor nerve for a nerve graft unless the surgeon can be absolutely certain of the longitudinal extent of the injury. In these four cases, it was elected to reconstitute the nerve gap with PGA tubes in order to facilitate some approximation of the nerve ends and obviate the use of the nerve graft.

Size Mismatch

In four cases, the proximal and distal ends of the nerve to be repaired at the site of the nerve graft were mismatched in terms of size. A PGA tube was fashioned in a cone shape to facilitate the incongruity in the size of the nerves to be approximated (Fig. 20-17).

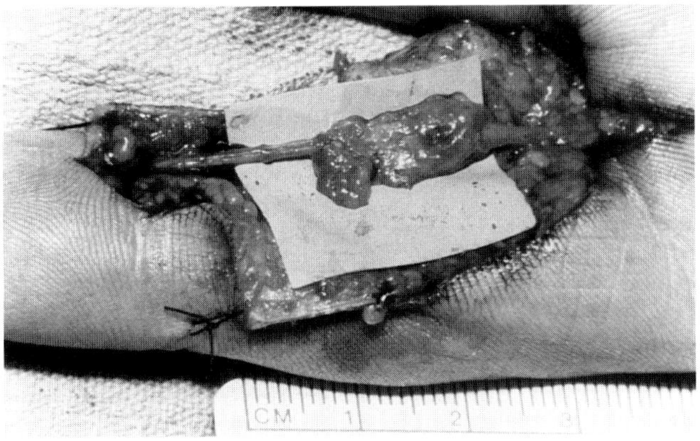

a

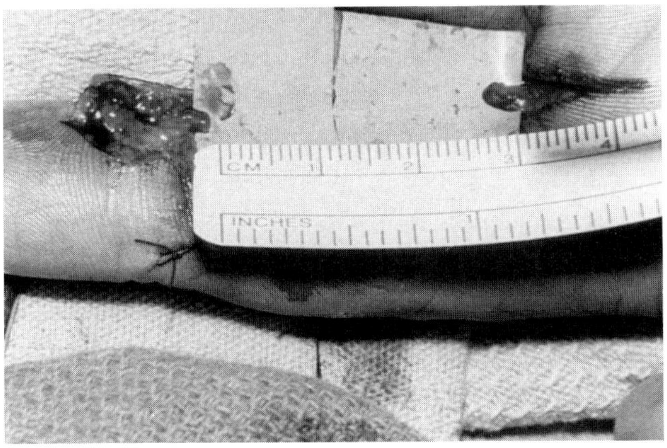

b

Figure 20-12a. The ulnar digital nerve had been previously injured and not repaired. A large painful neuroma developed. **b.** The neuroma was excised. The nerve gap was 2.5 cm. **c, d.** Nerve was reconstructed with a PGA tube. (Reproduced with permission from Mackinnon and Dellon.)[48]

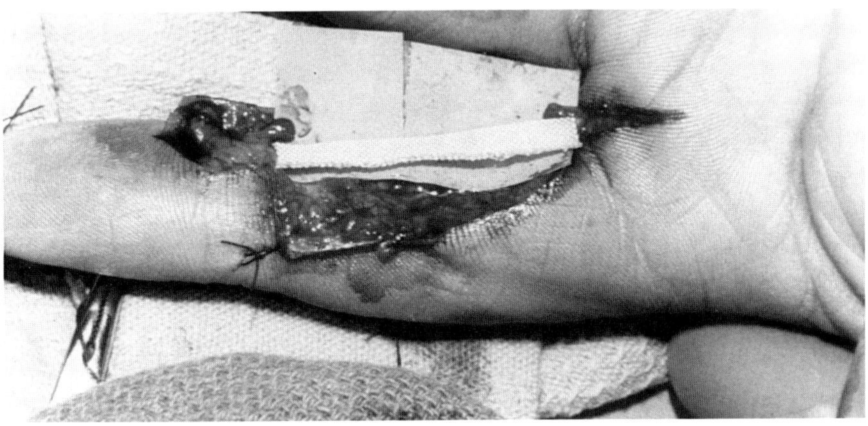

c

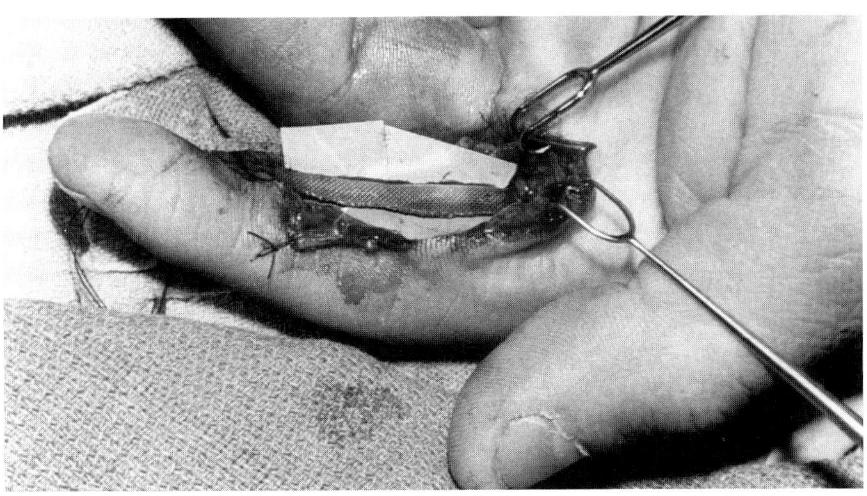

d

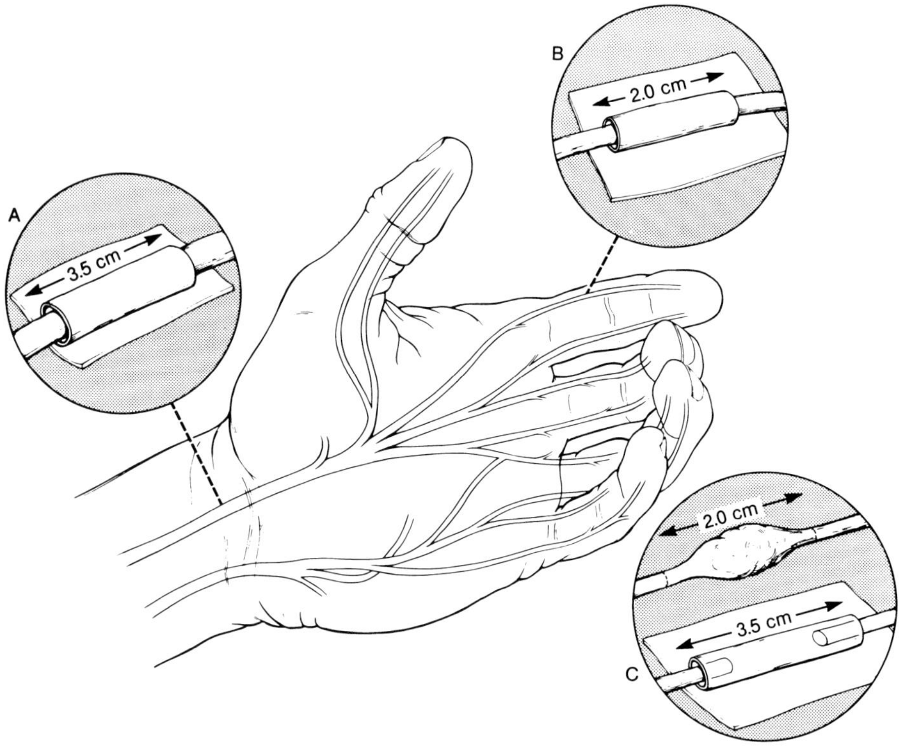

Figure 20-13. The PGA tube has been used largely for short nerve gaps in the digital nerves and to redo failed primary repairs of major nerves at the wrist level.

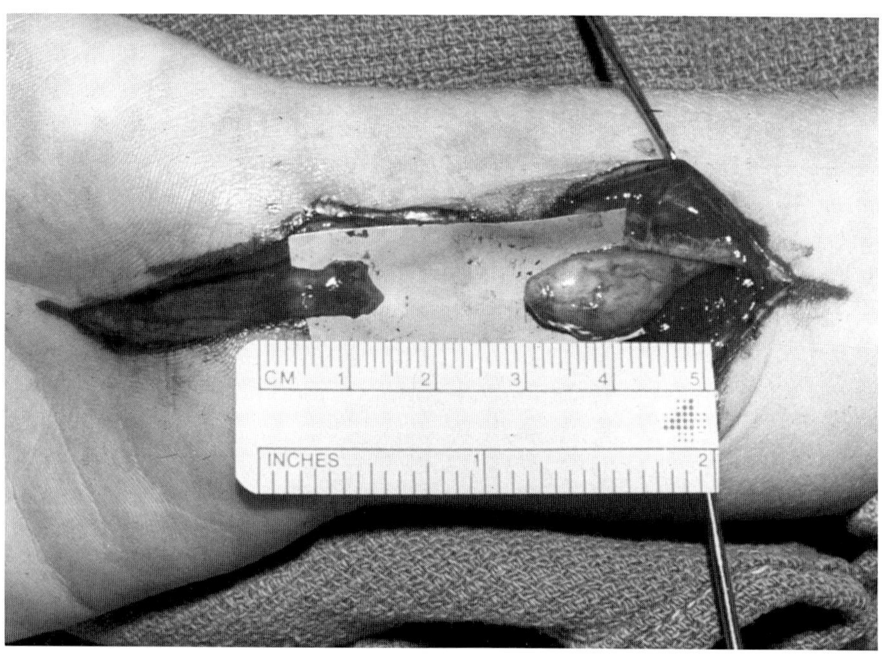

a

Figure 20-14a. This median nerve was injured and not repaired. When explored 1 year later, a large proximal neuroma was seen. **b.** The neuroma was cut back until a good fascicular pattern was seen. **c.** The nerve tube was filled with the patient's own serum. (*Figure continues.*)

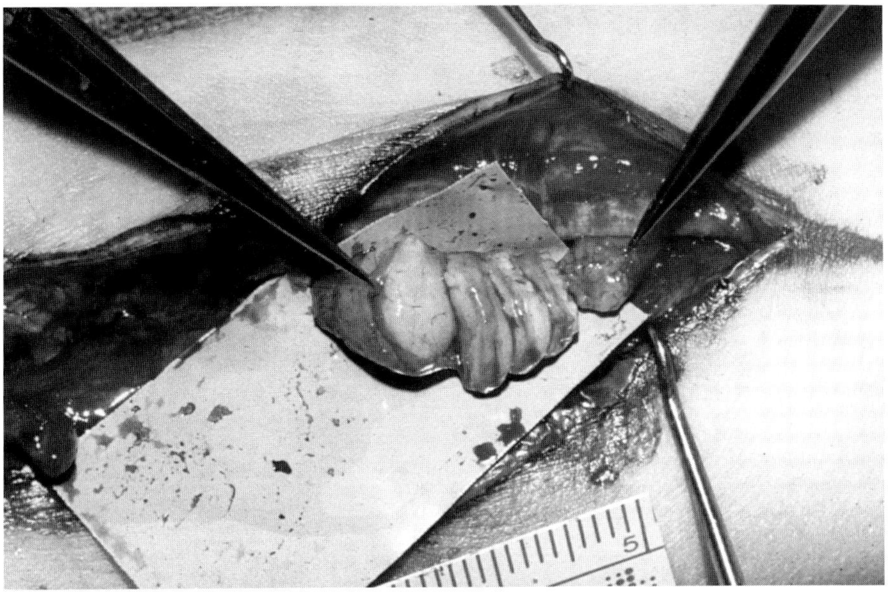

b

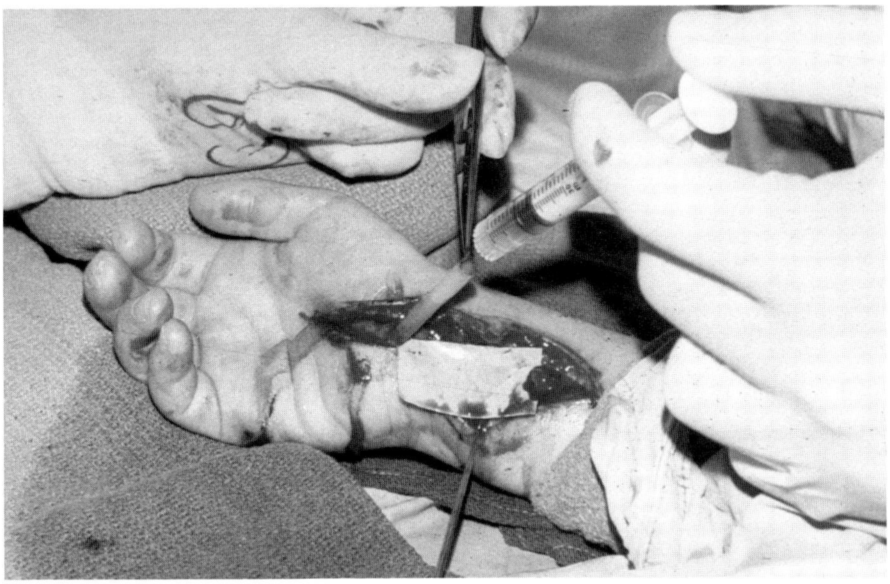

c

Surgical Technique for Clinical PGA Tube Reconstruction

Various techniques were initially used to fashion the PGA tubes from sheets of mesh PGA. Initially, the tubes were sutured together with PGA sutures. This was unsatisfactory for several reasons. In particular, if the length of the tube had to be changed, the tubes unraveled when cut. Disposable cautery units were then used to "heat weld" the edges of the PGA tubes. This proved to be a very satisfactory technique in that the cautery could be used to heat seal the proximal and distal ends of the tube in a circular configuration to prevent collapse of the tube. Also, if the length of the tube was found to be too long, it could be easily shortened without the concern of the tube unraveling. Most importantly, the heat welding technique could be used to fabricate the cone-shaped tubes to accommodate the instances in which the proximal and distal nerves were of dissimilar sizes.

The evolution of the use of PGA tubes stimulated

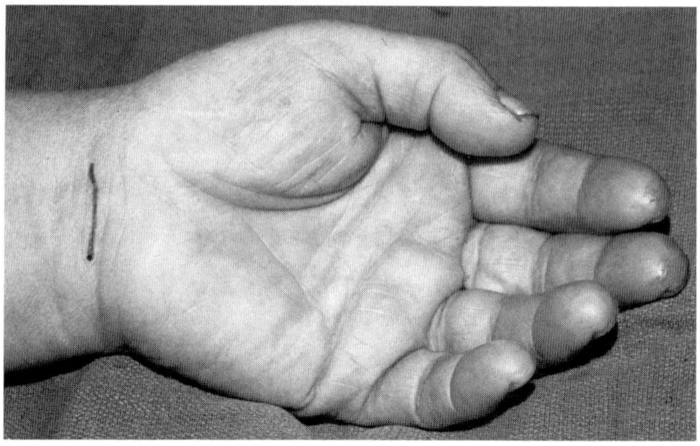

a

Figure 20-15a. This patient had had several previous procedures to remove ganglions in the wrist area and had developed median nerve loss following these procedures. **b.** At exploration, the median nerve was found to be iatrogenically injured at two levels. PGA tubes were fashioned to reconstitute the median nerve and covered with an abductor digiti quinti muscle flap. Due to chronic thenar muscle denervation, no attempt was made to reinnervate the motor branch. (*Figure continues.*)

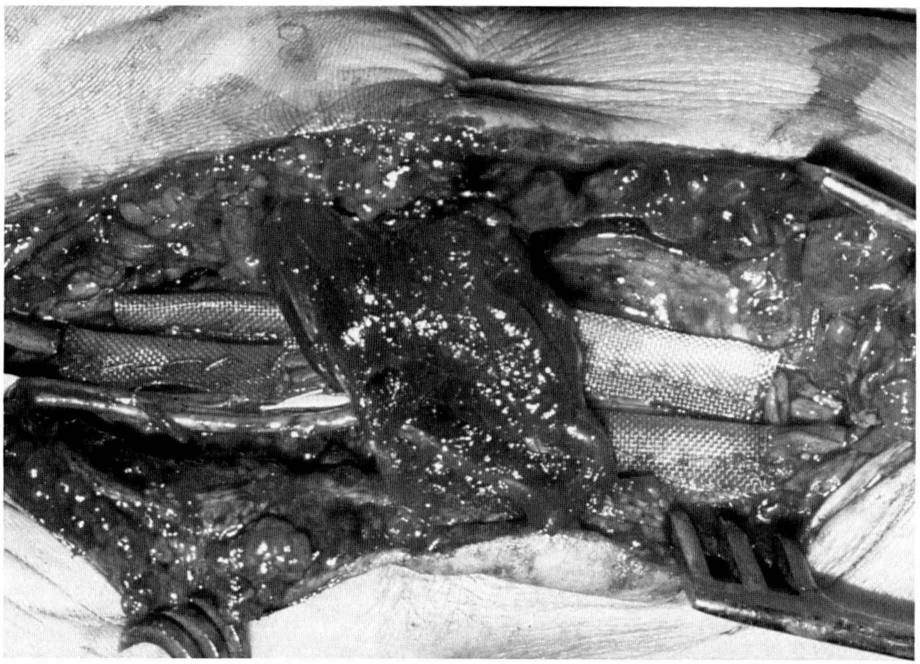

b

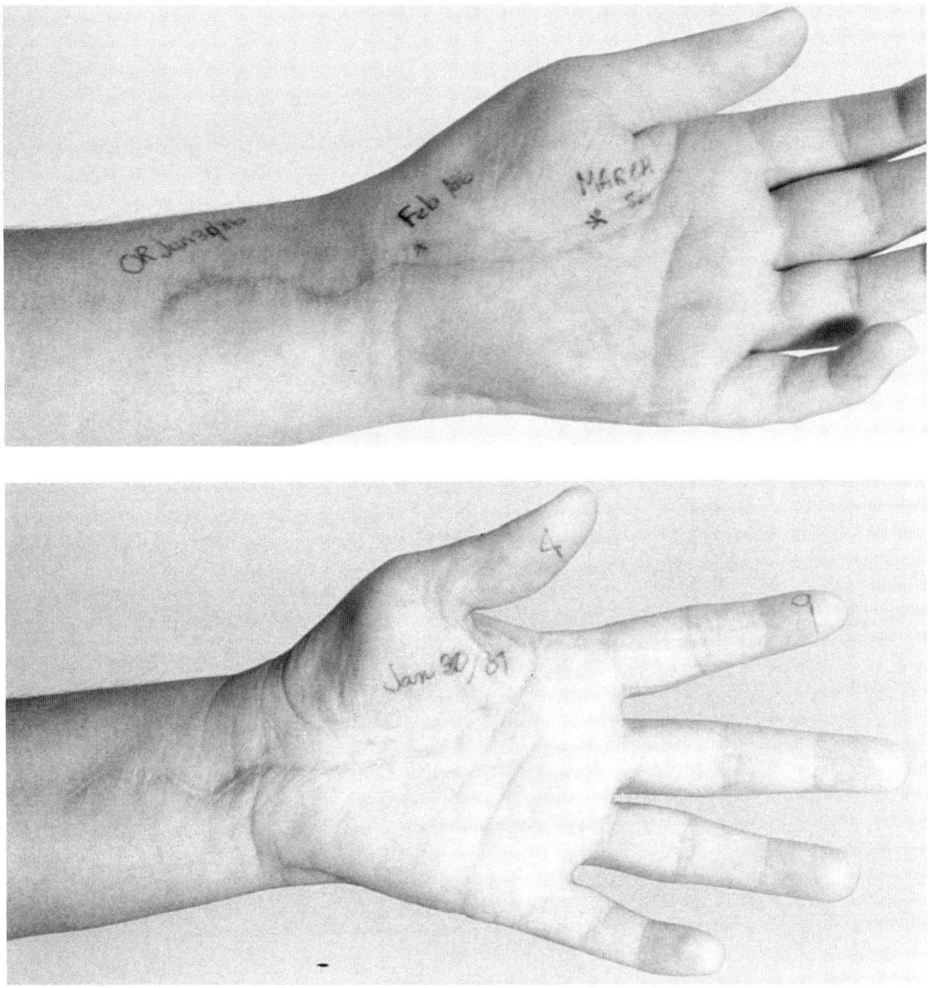

c

d

Figure 20-15 (*continued*) **c.** The Tinel sign advanced appropriately. **d.** One year after surgery, the patient demonstrated light touch perception in the median nerve distribution, and point discrimination had returned to the distribution of the median nerve.

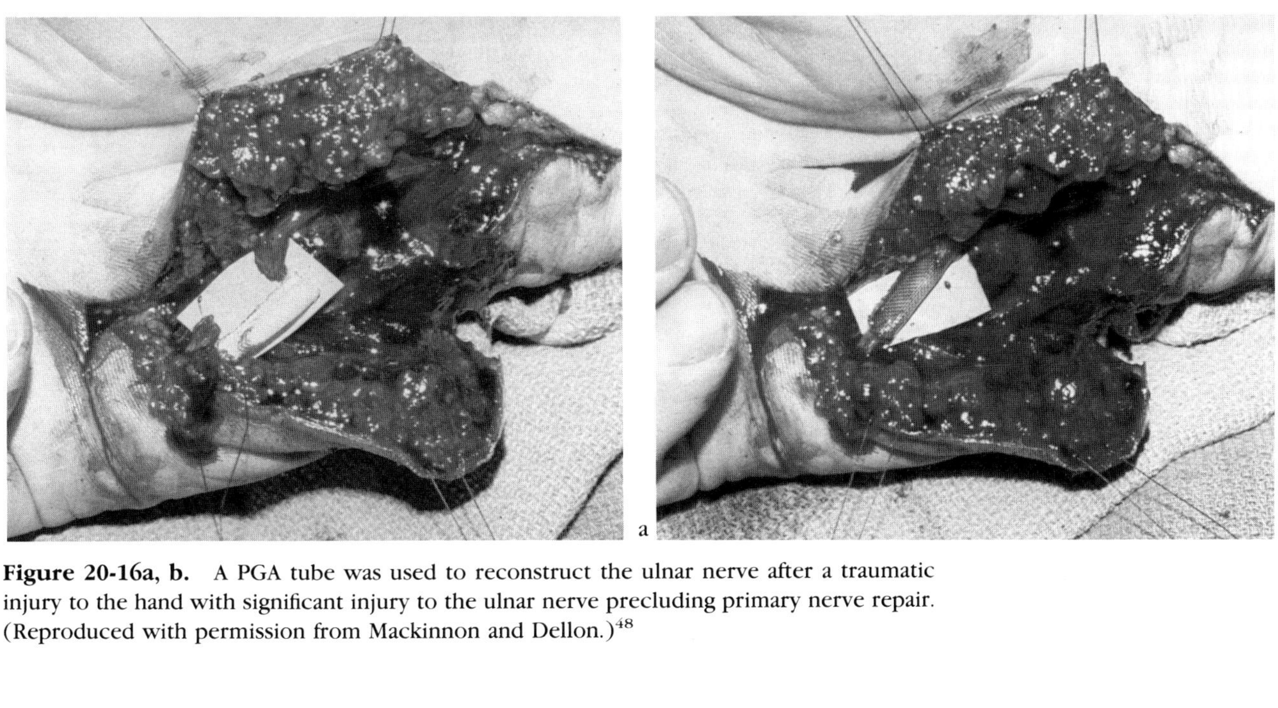

a b

Figure 20-16a, b. A PGA tube was used to reconstruct the ulnar nerve after a traumatic injury to the hand with significant injury to the ulnar nerve precluding primary nerve repair. (Reproduced with permission from Mackinnon and Dellon.)[48]

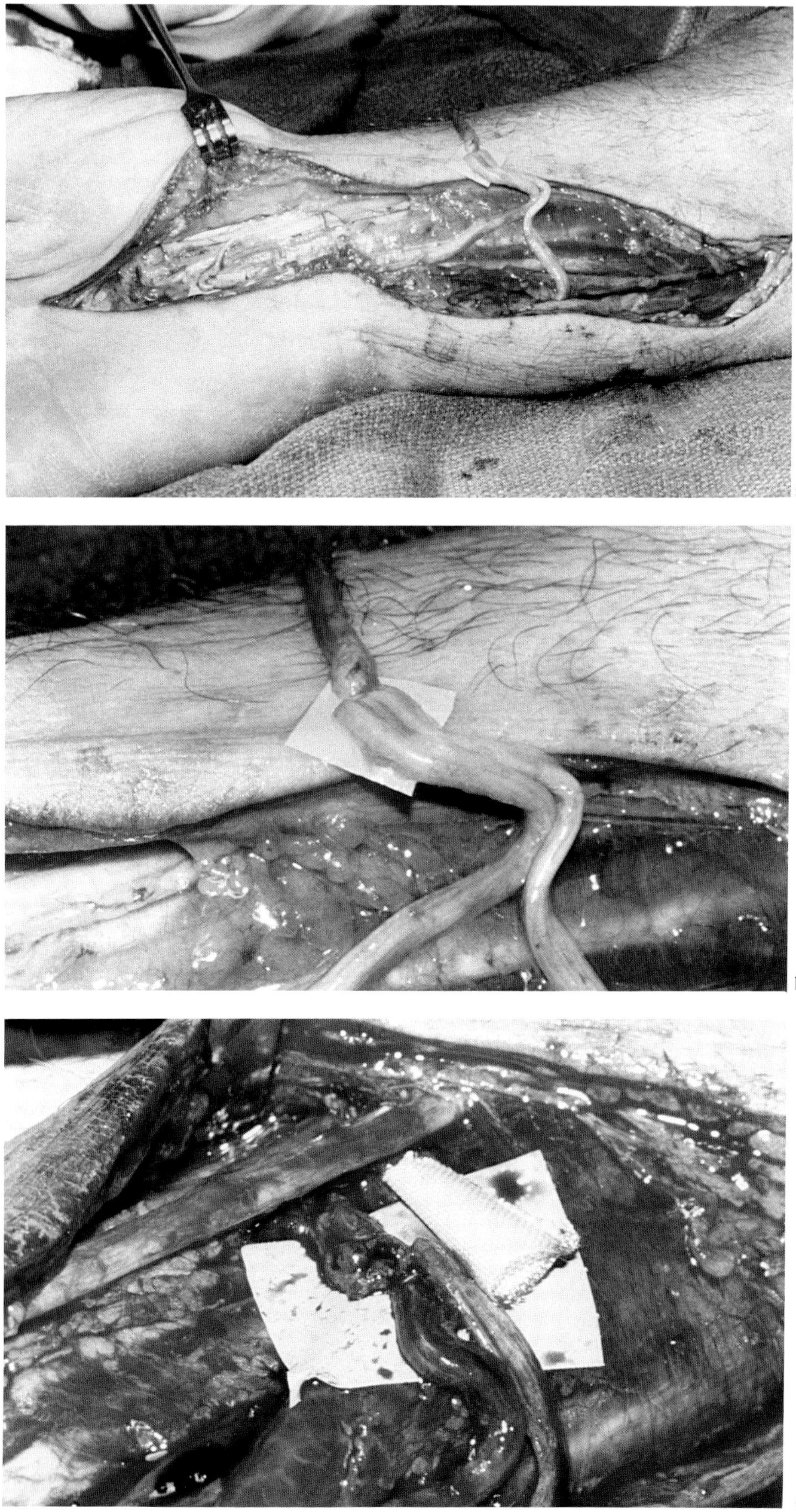

Figure 20-17. **a**. Patient with an irreparable ulnar nerve injury in the proximal arm. The radial sensory nerve was neurotized to the distal sensory ulnar fascicles. **b**. A size discrepancy is apparent between the radial sensory and ulnar nerve. **c**. A PGA tube was fashioned in the shape of a cone to facilitate the incongruity in the size of the proximal and distal nerves.

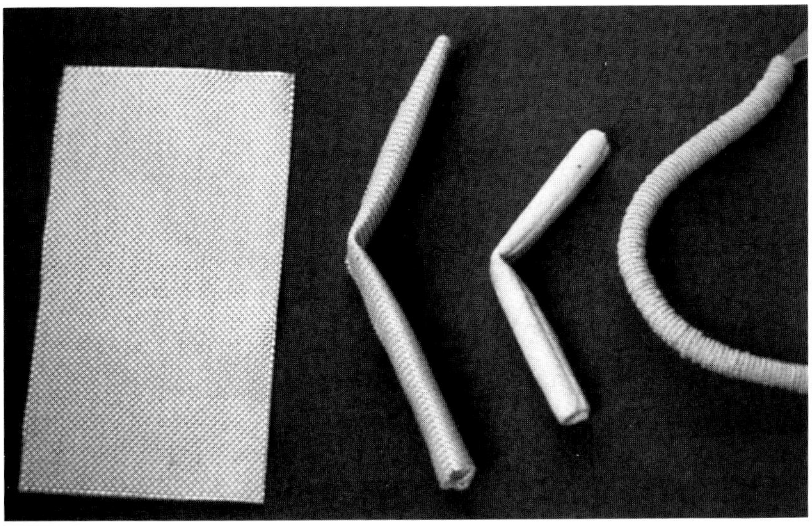

Figure 20-18. Initially, sheets of polyglycolic acid mesh were rolled and sutured together to form tubes. A cautery was subsequently used to heat weld the edges of the tube together to prevent unraveling. In order to prevent "kinking" of the tube, a corrugated tube was fashioned that would allow significant bend before kinking of the tube. On the left, a flat sheet of polyglycolic acid could be rolled and heat welded to make a tube. These tubes were, however, subject to kinking (center) and a corrugated tube would tolerate some degree of bending before kinking (right).

the development of a series of tubes with varying internal diameters that were smooth on the inside and crimped or corrugated on the outside. This was done to prevent kinking or collapse of the tube (Fig. 20-18). This design was inspired in the operating room. Observation of the anesthetist's corrugated tubes stimulated the development of these prefabricated PGA tubes (Davis & Geck Division of American Cyanamid). The technique for insertion of the nerve ends and the use of the patient's serum or heparinized Ringer's remains the same. In some instances, these prefabricated PGA tubes have been used to accommodate size mismatch although it has been necessary to make made-to-measure cone-shaped PGA tubes using the heat welding technique (Figs. 20-17c, 20-19).

The proximal and distal end of the nerves are inserted approximately 0.5 cm into the tube using horizontal mattress technique. Usually one suture is all that is necessary; in some instances, two sutures have been used. Magnification and 9-0 nylon microsuture with microinstruments are used to facilitate this maneuver (Fig. 20-20). Care is taken to ensure that the PGA tubes are positioned so that no tension is present on either the proximal or distal end of the nerve when the joints are moved. The tubes are always placed with the extremity in an extended position without flexing the joints.

If the operative procedure is done under tourniquet control, which is usually the case, the tourniquet is released and hemostasis is obtained before inserting the nerve ends into the tube. This is done to prevent the deleterious effects that blood can have on nerve regeneration.[26,27] Either the patient's serum or heparinized Ringer's solution is inserted into the PGA tube with a micro blunt-tipped needle and syringe.

Postoperative Care

The nerve reconstruction site is kept in protective splinting for three to four weeks and then any joints crossed by the PGA tube are gently mobilized by the therapist. At the appropriate time in the recovery of sensation, sensory re-education is introduced (see Chapter 18).

Complications of Clinical PGA Tube Reconstructions

Complications occurred in our early experience with this technique. There were six complications among 45 tubes (13.3%): two extrusions and one kinking, leading to a failure rate of 6.7%, and three cases of pain at the repair site associated with functional sensation (6.7%) not requiring further treatment. In one patient, a tenolysis of the flexor pollicis longus tendon with pulley reconstruction was carried out at the same time as two PGA tubes were inserted for nerve injury of both thumb digital nerves. In the very early postoperative period, the thumb was mobilized to prevent tendon adhesions. Unfortunately, during this first postoperative week, this early movement resulted in extrusion of both PGA tubes. This patient was later successfully reconstructed using the anterior branch of the medial antebrachial cutaneous nerve as a nerve graft. A second patient, early in the series, extruded a portion of the PGA tube at four weeks. Fortunately, in this short tube, neural regeneration had been completed and this did not compromise his long-term satisfactory result. In a third patient, two PGA tubes were used to reconstruct the sensation to

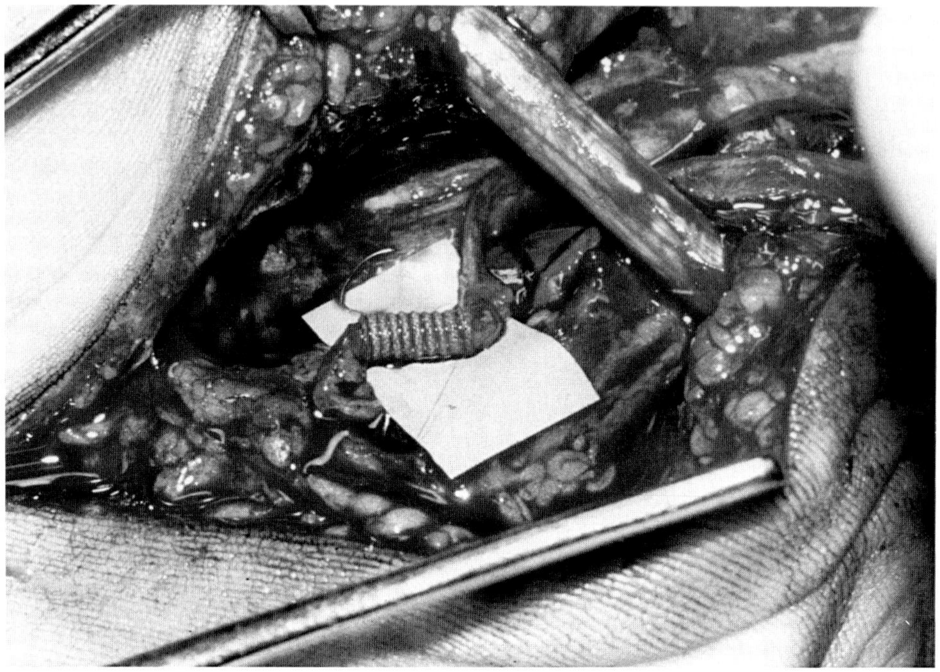

Figure 20-19. A corrugated PGA tube is used to carry out this nerve repair of a 2.0 cm nerve gap in the palm.

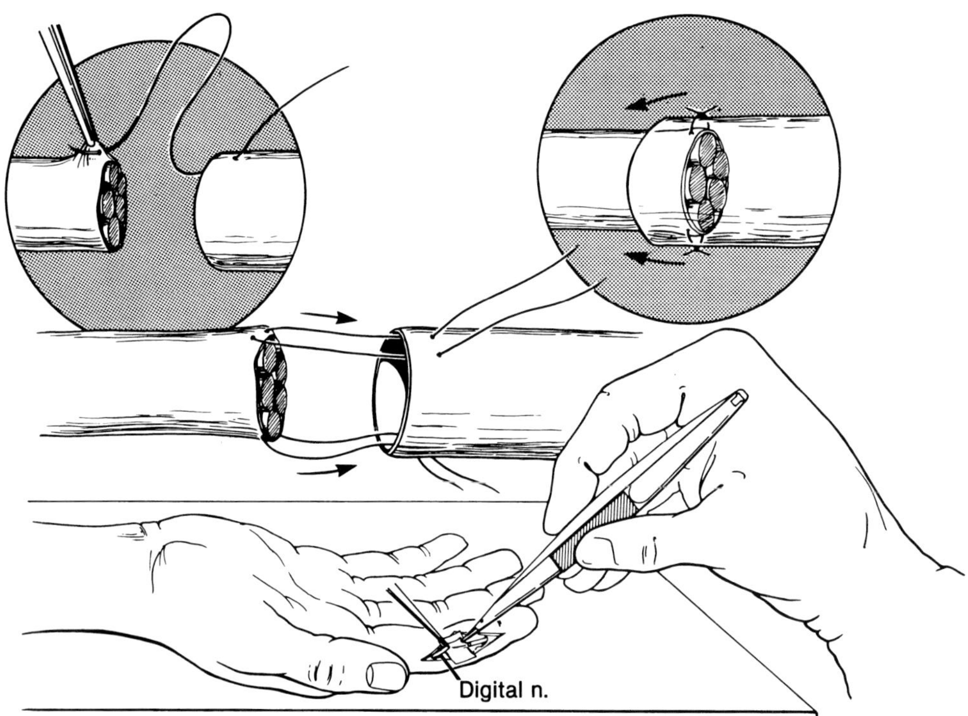

Figure 20-20. Technique of inserting the nerve into the PGA tube. (Reproduced with permission from Mackinnon and Dellon.)[48]

the thumb and radial side of the index finger. These non-crimped tubes to the thumb were placed in position of considerable angulation around the thenar musculature. Regeneration did not occur past this angulation point at which the tube must have kinked. The patient subsequently went on to be salvaged with the classic nerve graft procedure. Three other patients, after use of the PGA tubes in the digits, have persistent discomfort at the location of the tube despite the fact that satisfactory nerve regeneration has occurred across the tube and into the distribution of the digital nerve. None of these patients has agreed to reexploration and either secondary nerve grafting or relocation of the digital nerve to the dorsum of the hand.

Clinical Results of PGA Tube Reconstruction

The results using this PGA tube technique have been excellent and in general superior to the use of a nerve graft. The progress of nerve regeneration across the PGA tube appeared to be faster than across a classic nerve graft or a nerve repair. The localization of sensory recovery after regeneration across the PGA tubes that were used for reconstruction of median nerve injuries was appropriate demonstrating little mislocalization.

Patient acceptance of this technique has been excellent. It is explained to all patients that if the PGA tube technique fails, then the recourse would be to carry out a standard nerve graft. When given the option preoperatively of a nerve graft or a PGA tube reconstruction, all except one patient selected the tube technique. This one patient did not want to consider having a second procedure, a nerve graft, if the PGA tube failed and was treated with a nerve graft.

Results of the PGA tube reconstructions were evaluated in February 1988 for those patients with more than a one year follow-up (Table 20-5).[48] An excellent result was defined as recovery of either three mm. or less moving two-point discrimination (m2PD) or six mm or less static two-point discrimination (s2PD). Sixteen of the 21 digital nerve reconstructions were available for follow-up of greater than 1 year (mean, 15.6 months, range 9 to 25 months) and four of the eleven median nerve reconstructions (mean, 20 months, range 18 to 25 months). Of the 16 digital nerve follow-up evaluations, eleven included a local anesthetic block of that finger's normal intact digital nerve. In only one of those fingers blocked did the measured two-point discrimination in the autonomous zone of the reconstructed nerve change by one mm. and this did not affect the end result classification. Thirteen of the 16 digital nerves (81%) and three of the four median nerves (75%) achieved excellent recovery of sensation. These results may be compared with historical reports (see Chapter 4) where through 1981 the literature reported that only about ten percent of digital nerve repairs and one percent of median nerve repairs gave such excellent results even with a follow-up of five years.

The results among the other nerves reconstructed (Table 20-3) are encouraging as well. Where the PGA tube was utilized to adjust for mismatching of nerve diameter, as in the facial nerve reconstructions, satisfactory regeneration has occurred such that facial reanimation has been possible (see Chapter 15). Motor functional results are not available yet as the high median nerve reconstructions are not sufficiently long postoperatively. The one radial nerve reconstructed was done acutely for a severely damaged nerve and will require secondary tendon transfers and the delayed repair of the low median nerve injuries all had severe thenar wasting at the time of reconstruction, so the median motor branch was not reconstructed.

While the role of the nerve tube for the reconstruction of digital nerve injuries appears established, the role for reconstruction of major large nerves is not yet clear and a much larger follow-up will be necessary.

The Future and the Lifeboat

The future of microneurosurgery, predictable in the logical progression of ideas from basic research to clinical reality, is that neurobiology will be an integral part of nerve reconstruction, including primary nerve repair. The future will most likely witness the use of a bioabsorbable conduit to reconstruct short nerve gaps of three cm or less. If a more slowly absorbable conduit is developed, and if subhuman primate neural regeneration can be demonstrated to occur across longer gaps, then the techniques developed in this investigation will be extended to reconstruct longer nerve gaps. With the realization that neurotrop(h)ic forces may result in more functionally appropriate reinnervation of target tissues than will increasing manual (surgeon's) micromanipulation of the fascicles, will come the use of bioabsorbable nerve conduits for primary nerve repair. Frequently the appropriate fascicular matching of motor and sensory fascicles of the proximal and distal nerve stumps is not clear to the surgeon. For these future "repairs", where topography is uncertain a very small, perhaps three to five mm , gap may deliberately be created between the two ends of the nerve.

The lifeboat, as Sir Harold Gilles cautioned us,[49] must always be available. The results of our clinical use of PGA for nerve reconstruction demonstrated a majority of excellent results, but there were complications which required salvage of the nerve reconstruction. Where the indication for the conduit will be restoration of function, the lifeboat will be the classic interposition nerve graft (see Chapter 4). Where the indication for a conduit is a painful neuroma with a distal nerve available, the lifeboat may again be a nerve graft, or resection of the neuroma with implantation of the proximal stump into an appropriate muscle or bone (see Chapter 17).

The Future Role of Immunology in Nerve Regeneration

Albert performed the first human nerve allograft in 1878, no followup was reported for this patient.[50] Subsequently, many investigators have reported the use of clinical nerve allografts.[51-56] While some authors have reported functional[57] recovery, others have reported little functional recovery.[52-53]

With a greater understanding of transplantation immunology we were encouraged to investigate the nerve allograft response in a rat model. The nerve allograft response was investigated:

1. Regeneration across an allogeneic nerve graft from a donor with only minor histocompatibility disparity from the recipient was shown to be superior to that across one from a donor with major histocompatibility disparity.[58,59]
2. Pretreatment of the donor nerve grafts with high dose irradiation (35,000 rads) or lyophilization (freeze drying) demonstrated significantly decreased immunological responsiveness to these pretreated nerve allografts.[60]
3. Regeneration across these irradiated and lyophilized pretreated grafts was inferior to that which occurred across a standard nerve autograft.[61]
4. Host immunosuppression with azathioprine and steroids improves regeneration across the nerve allograft. This immunosuppression was required only for the period of time required for host axons to traverse the nerve allograft.[62]
5. We have shown that the nerve allograft is not particularly immunogeneic. Only very low dosages of Cyclosporin A (5 mg/kg) is necessary in order to suppress the nerve allograft response.[63]
6. In the rat immunosuppressed with Cyclosporin A, regeneration across the nerve allograft is equal to that seen across the autograft.[64]
7. Only a short course of Cyclosporin A is necessary in order to allow host axons to traverse the nerve allograft. The allograft is thus necessary only to provide a structural and not a functional support system for axonal elongation. Immunosuppression treatment can be stopped once host axons have traversed the allograft.[65]
8. In a primate model, it has been shown that nerve regeneration across the nerve allograft in the host immunosuppressed with Cyclosporin A is comparable to that which occurs across the autograft. Immunosuppression is only required for the time necessary to support axonal regeneration across the nerve allograft.[68]

These experimental studies will facilitate the logical extension of the use of the nerve allograft in the clinical situation in which a large amount of nerve graft material is required. The use of the nerve allograft for large nerve gaps and the nerve conduit for short nerve gaps will facilitate surgical repair of nerve injuries.

The conclusion is that the future shows promise for improved nerve reconstruction of all types, as we move from basic research to clinical reality.

References

1. Omer GE: Injuries to nerves of the upper extremity. J Bone Joint Surg, 56A:1615–1624, 1974.
2. Seddon HJ: Surgical Disorder of the Peripheral Nerves. Williams & Wilkins, Baltimore, 1972.
3. Sunderland S: Nerves and Nerve Injuries, 2nd ed. Churchill Livingstone, Edinburgh, 1978.
4. Millesi H: Nerve grafting. Clin Plast Surg 11:105–120, 1984.
5. Moberg E: Methods for examining sensibility in the hand. In Flynn JE ed: Hand Surgery. Williams & Wilkins, Baltimore, 1966, pp 435–439.
6. Dellon AL: Evaluation of Sensibility and Re-education of Sensation in the Hand. Williams & Wilkins, Baltimore, 1981.
7. Antonyshyn O, Kesarwani A, Mackinnon SE, Kelly L, Novaks C: Evaluation of facial sensation in the normal and posttraumatic patient. Ann Plast Surg, 1988. In press.
8. Mackinnon SE, Dellon AL: Two-point discrimination tester. J Hand Surg [Am] 10:906–908, 1985.
9. Terzis J, Faibisoff BA, Williams BH: The nerve gap: Suture under tension versus graft. Plast Reconstr Surg 56:166, 1975.
10. Miyamoto Y, Tsuge K: Effects of tension on intraneural microcirculation and end to end neurorrhaphy. In Gorio A, Millesi H, Mingrino S, eds: Posttraumatic Peripheral Nerve Regeneration. Raven Press, New York, 1981, pp 81–91.
11. Millesi H, Meissl G: Consequences of tension at the suture site. In Gorio A, Millesi H, Mingrino S, eds: Posttraumatic Peripheral Nerve Regeneration. Raven Press, New York, 1981, pp 277–279.
12. Hammarback JA, Palm SL, Furct LT, Letourneau PC: Guidance of neurite growth by pathways of substra absorbed laminin. J Neurosci Res 13:213–222, 1985.
13. Weinberg HJ, Spencer PS: The fate of Schwann cells isolated from axonal contact. J Neurocytol 7:555–569, 1968.
14. Smith BH, Kornblith PL: Axonoplasmic transport and neurological surgery. Neurosurgery 10:268–276, 1982.

15. Horch K: Guidance of regrowing sensory axons after cutaneous nerve lesions in the cat. J Neurophysiol 42:1437–1449, 1979.
16. Aguayo AJ, Karpati G: Current topics in nerve and muscle research. In Aguayo AJ, Carpati G, eds: Excerpta Medica, Amsterdam, 1979.
17. Gluck T: Ueber Neuroplastik aut dem Wege der Transplantation. Arch Klin Chir 25:606–616, 1880.
18. Forssman J: Ueber de Ursachen, welche die Wachstumstrichtung der peripheren Nervenfasern bei der Regeneration bestimmen. Beitr Pathol Anat 24:55, 1898.
19. Ramón y Cajal SR: Mechanismo de la degeneracion y regeneration de nervos. Trab Lab Inbest Biol, Madrid 4:119, 1905.
20. Weiss P, Taylor AC: Further experimental evidence against (neurotropism) in nerve regeneration. J Exp Zoo 95:233–257, 1944.
21. Weiss P: The technology of nerve regeneration: A review of sutureless tubulation and related methods of nerve repair. J Neurosurg 1:400, 1944.
22. Lundborg G, Danielson N, Dahlin LB, Nachensson A, Polloryd P: Tissue specificity in nerve regeneration. Scand J Plast Surg. 1988. In press.
23. Mackinnon SE, Dellon AL, Lundborg G, Hudson AR: A study of neurotropism in the primate model. J Hand Surg [Am] 11:888–894, 1986, and manuscript in preparation.
24. Seckel BR, Ryan SE, Gagne RJ, Tin Ho Chiu CST, Watkins E: Target specific nerve regeneration through a nerve guide in the rat. Plast Reconstr Surg 78:793–798, 1986.
25. Brushart TM, Seiler WA IV: Selective reinnervation of distal motor stumps by peripheral motor axons. Exp Neurol 97:289–300, 1987.
26. Williams LR: Exogenous fibrin matrix precursors stimulate the temporal progress of nerve regeneration within a silicone chamber. Neurochem Res. 1988. In press.
27. Kirk EG, Lewis D: Fascial tubulization in the repair of nerve defects. JAMA 65:486–492, 1915.
28. Lundborg G, Dahlin L, Danielson N, et al: Nerve regeneration across an extended gap. J Hand Surg 7:580–587, 1982.
29. Chiu DTW, Janecka I, Krizek TJ, et al: Autogenous vein graft as a conduit for nerve regeneration. Surgery 91:226, 1982.
30. Spencer PS, Politis MJ: Guidance of nerve fibers during regeneration. Presented at Sunderland Society, Third Annual Meeting, New Mexico, May, 1983.
31. Lundborg G, Dahlin L, Danielsen MP, Hansson HA, Larsson K: Reorganization and orientation of regenerating nerve fibres, perineurium and epineurium in preformed mesothelial tubes. An experimental study in the sciatic nerve of rats. J Neurosci Res 6:265–281, 1981.
32. Lungborg G, Hansson HA: Regeneration of peripheral nerve through a preformed tissue space, preliminary observations on the reorganization of regenerating nerve fibres and perineurium. Brain Res 178:573–576, 1979.
33. Lundborg G, Hansson HA: Nerve regeneration through preformed pseudosynovial tubes. A preliminary report of a new experimental model for studying regeneration and reorganization of peripheral nerve tissue. J Hand Surg 5:35, 1980.
34. Mackinnon SE, Hudson AR, Hunter DA: Histologic assessment of nerve regeneration in the rat. Plast Reconstr Surg 75:384–388, 1985.
35. Mackinnon SE, Dellon AL, Hudson AR, Hunter DA: Nerve regeneration through a pseudosynovial sheath in a primate model. Plast Reconstr Surg 75:833–839, 1985.
36. Mackinnon SE, Dellon AL, Hudson AR, Hunter DA: Comparison of regeneration across a sural graft in a vascularized pseudosheath. J Hand Surg. November, 1988. In press.
37. Politis MJ, Ederle K, Spencer PS: Trophism in nerve regeneration. In vivo attraction of regenerating axons by diffusable factors derived from cells in distal nerve stumps of transected peripheral nerve. Brain Res 253:1–12, 1982.
38. Lundborg G, Longo FM, Varon S: Nerve regeneration model in trophic factors in vivo. Brain Res 232:157–162, 1982.
39. Lundborg G, Gelberman R, Longo FM, Powell H, Varon S: In vivo regeneration of cut nerve encased in silicone chambers. Growth across a 6 mm gap. J Neuropathol Exp Neurol 41:412–422, 1982.
40. Uzman BG, Villegas GM: Mouse sciatic nerve regeneration through semipermeable tubes. A quantitative model. J Neurosci Res 9:325, 1983.
41. Seckel BR, Chiu TH, Nyilas E, Sidman RL: Nerve regeneration through synthetic biodegradable nerve guides: Regulation by the target organ. Plast Reconstr Surg 74:173–181, 1984.
42. Molander H, Olsson Y, Engkvist O, Bowald S, Eriksson I: Regeneration of peripheral nerve through a polyglactin tube. Muscle Nerve 5:54–57, 1982.
43. Cuadros CL: Nerve regeneration through a synthetic microporous tube (expanded polytetrafluoroethylene) experimental study in sciatic nerve of the rabbit. Microsurgery 8:41–46, 1987.
44. Collin W, Donoff RB: Nerve regeneration through collagen tubes. J Dent Res 63:987–993, 1984.
45. Madison R, daSilva CF, Dikes P, Sidman RL, Chiu TH: Increased rate of peripheral nerve regeneration using bioabsorbable nerve guides and a laminin containing gel. Exp Neurol 88:767–772, 1985.
46. Dellon AL, Mackinnon SE: An alternative to the management of the short nerve gap. Plast Reconstr Surg 82:849—856, 1988.
47. Mackinnon SE, Dellon AL: Reply to Thomas Brushart's Letter to the Editor on "Neurotropism versus neurotrophism." J Hand Surg 12A:809, 1987.
48. Mackinnon SE, Dellon AL: Clinical nerve reconstruction with bioabsorbable polyglycolic acid tube. Plast Reconstr Surg 1990. In press.
49. Gilles HD, Millard DR Jr: Principles and Art of Plastic Surgery. Little Brown Co., Boston, 1957.
50. Albert E: Berichte des Naturwissenschaftlich-Medizinischen in Innsbruck. Innsbruck, vol 9, p 97, 1878.
51 Davis L, Ruge D: Functional recovery following the use of homogenous nerve grafts. Surgery 27:102–114, 1950.
52. Delageniere H: A contribution to the study of the surgical repair of peripheral nerves. Surg Gynecol Obstet 37:543–553, 1924.
53. Hoen TI: The repair of peripheral nerve lesions. Am J Surg 72:489–495, 1946.

54. Ingebrigtsen R: A contribution to the biology of peripheral nerves in transplantation. J Exp Med 22:418–428, 1915.
55. Jacoby VW, Fahlbusch R, Mackert B, Braun B, Rolle J, Schnell J: Uberbruckung peripherer nervendefekte mit lyophilisierten und desantigenisierten homologen transplanten. Munch Med Wschr 112:586–589, 1970.
56. Jacoby W, et al: Fortschritte in der Behandlung peripherer Nervenverletzungen. Forschr Med 89:181–223, 1971.
57. Singh R, de Lange SA: Experience with homologous lyophilized nerve grafts in the treatment of peripheral nerve injuries. Acta Neurochirurgica 32:125–130, 1975.
58. Mackinnon SE, Hudson AR, Falk R, Bilbao J, Hunter DA, Kline D: Nerve allograft response: A quantitative immunological study. Neurosurg 10:61–69, 1982.
59. Mackinnon SE, Hudson AR, Falk RE, Hunger DA: The nerve allograft response—an experimental model in the rat. Ann Plast Surg 14:334–339, 1985.
60. Mackinnon SE, Hudson AR, Falk RE, Kline D, Hunter DA: Peripheral nerve allograft: an immunological assessment of pretreatment methods. Neurosurg 14:167–171, 1984.
61. Mackinnon SE, Hudson AR, Hunter DA: Peripheral nerve allograft: an assessment of regeneration across pretreated nerve allografts. Neurosurg 15:690–696, 1984.
62. Mackinnon SE, Hudson AR, Bain JR, Falk RE, Hunter DA: The peripheral nerve allograft: an assessment of regeneration in the immunosuppressed host. Plast Reconstr Surg 79:436–444, 1987.
63. Bain JR, Mackinnon SE, Hudson AR, Falk RE, Hunter DA: The nerve allograft response with rat immunosuppressed with Cyclosporin A. Plast Reconstr Surg 82:447-455, 1988.
64. Bain JR, Mackinnon SE, Hudson AR, Falk RE, Falk J, Hunter DA: Evaluation of functional recovery across the nerve allograft in the rat immunosuppressed with Cyclosporin A. Plast Reconstr Surg 82:1052—1064, 1988.
65. Bain JR, Mackinnon SE, Hudson AR. The nerve allograft response in the primate immunosuppressed with Cyclosporin A. Transplantation Proceedings 21:695-697, 1989.

Appendices: Adjuncts for Patient Care

Appendix A
Carpal Tunnel Syndrome
Information for the Patient Having Surgery for a Pinched Nerve at the Wrist

The Problem

The problem you have is called a carpal tunnel syndrome. This means the symptoms you are experiencing and the problems you are having are due to a nerve at your wrist, called the median nerve, which is being pressed upon in a tunnel called the carpal tunnel. This is commonly called a pinched nerve at the wrist. The tunnel is made up of the wrist bones, which are close to the skin over the back of the hand as well as on the thumb and little finger sides of the hand. Over the palm of the hand, there is a strong ligament connecting these bones. This creates a tunnel between the ligament and the bones. Through the tunnel go the nine tendons, which bend your fingers, and one nerve, the median nerve. This is a big nerve, the size of a pencil or pen. This nerve contains thousands of small individual nerve fibers. Some of these make the muscles to the thumb work: lift the thumb up and out from your hand and allow the thumb to turn and touch the other fingertips when pinching. The rest of the nerve fibers give feeling to the tip of the thumb, index, middle, and part of the ring fingers.

Pressure on this nerve usually comes from a thickened amount of the lining tissue that surrounds the nine tendons that move the fingers. There are many other reasons that can cause increased pressure in this carpal tunnel. When the pressure builds up, the blood flow in the nerve decreases. When the nerve does not get enough oxygen, it begins to give you the numbness and tingling feelings that you experience in your fingers. When the wrist bends down, which it does when you are asleep at night, the nerve gets pressed harder against the ligament. This further decreases the blood flow to the nerve and causes you to awaken at night with the feeling that you hand is "asleep." The splinting that is often done to treat this problem before surgery places the wrist in a straight or neutral position, attempting to take pressure off the nerve. This is especially useful at night. When you reach the stage where the splinting no longer is helpful, then another form of treatment becomes necessary.

Combined with the splinting will be any medical treatment that has been used to prevent the swelling in these tissues, like the medicines that are used to treat different forms of arthritis or medicines used to treat some overall disease that your body has, such as the treatment for diabetes or thyroid problems. Changing the activities that you do with your hand every day, such as taking time off from work or changing your hobbies, for example, doing less sewing or less knitting or playing less tennis or golf, also may be helpful in decreasing the swelling in this tunnel. When all that can be done by either medicines or changing your activities or by splinting prove to be ineffective in relieving your symptoms, the last possible technique to help you is an operation to relieve the pressure in this carpal tunnel. If an operation is not done and the problem with pressure on the nerve continues, all the feeling in the thumb, index and middle fingers, and part of the ring finger can become lost so that you do not feel hot or cold or pain. Thus, the fingers are more likely to be injured. Additionally, the thumb will lose the ability to lift out from the palm of the hand, because some of the thumb muscles become paralyzed.

The Operation

The operation consists of cutting the ligament that forms the roof of the tunnel (Fig. 1). When the ligament is released, the pressure on the nerve is released. Additional parts to the operation can be performed. The swollen tissue in the tunnel or anything else present in the tunnel that is pressing on the nerve, such as a cyst from the joint or a fatty tumor, can be removed. When the nerve has been compressed for a long time, scar tissue builds inside the nerve. When this has happened, usually the fingers remain numb all the time and you lose the ability to tell whether one or two objects are being pressed against or moved along the surface of the finger at the same time. The muscles that lift the thumb out from the hand may also have become partly paralyzed. When this amount of scar tissue is present, an addition to the ligament release operative procedure can be done, called an internal neurolysis. In this procedure, using magnification, the outer wrapping of the nerve is opened and the scar tissue is removed from within the nerve.

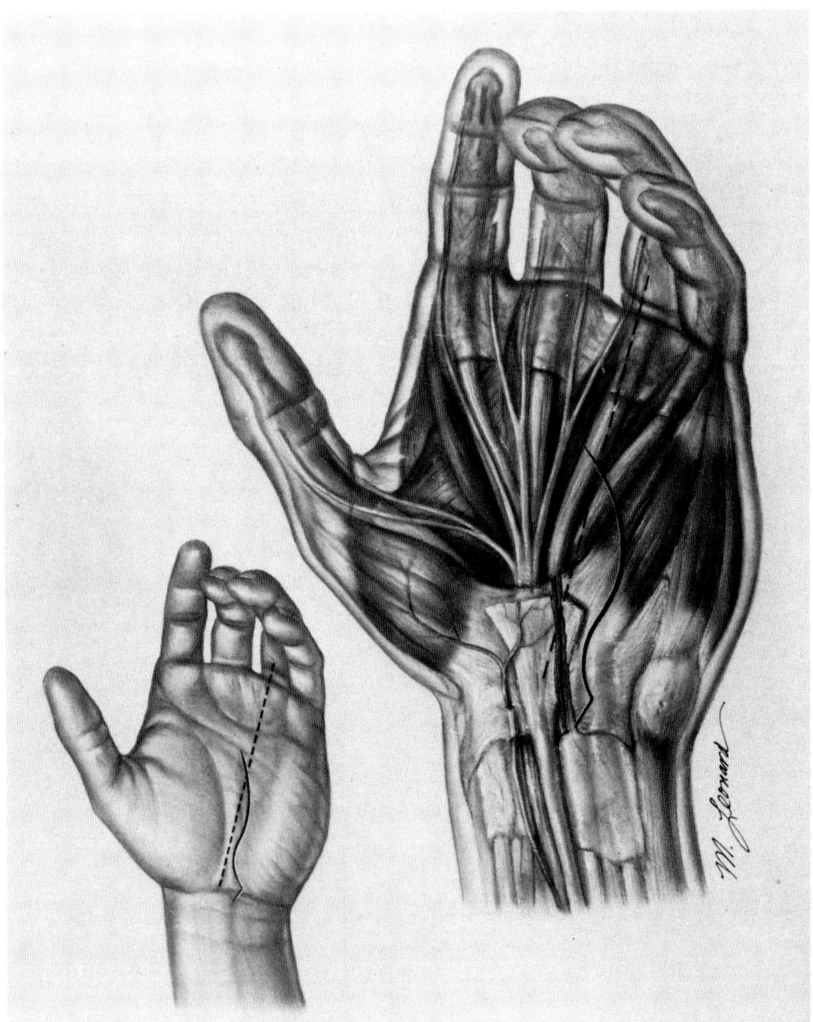

Figure 1.

Complications

The risks and complications from the operation include a scar that will always be present, a scar that may become painful, bleeding, which may be serious enough to require a return visit to the operating room to stop the bleeding, infection, and pain in the fingers after surgery. The pain in the fingers after surgery may last for only a brief period or may last for a few weeks. This pain is usually from the nerve growing back, or regenerating, into the fingers. The pain may be such that the fingers feel extremely sensitive to normal touch, heat, or cold. These problems are not the only ones that may occur. Rarely, the main nerve, itself, or one of its branches, may be injured or pain and swelling and stiffness may persist.

Postoperative

After surgery, the hand is placed in a splint for 1 week. Then the dressing is removed. The sutures are removed at 1 to 2 weeks. Sometimes the dressing and sutures will remain longer, based on the type of healing that is occurring or if it is expected that the healing process may take longer than usual. This occurs if you are taking cortisone for different types of arthritis, have diabetes, or have some other types of wound-healing problems. When the stitches are removed, the palm of the hand and the place where the sutures are remains swollen for a period of 3 to 8 weeks. During this time, gentle heat and massage of the scar with some type of hand lotion or mild cream is helpful in aiding to decrease the swelling. Opening and closing the fingers a few times each hour is helpful in keeping the tendons that move the fingers from becoming stuck to the surrounding tissues by scar. This movement is also helpful in causing the nerve that has been operated upon to slide through the tissues so that it does not become stuck down to the area that was operated upon. After 3 to 6 weeks, if the scar remains thick and pink, it may be necessary to apply a cortisone-containing cream to the scar to help soften it. A resting wrist splint may be used for a week or two in the postoperative period, especially if early return to work is necessary.

Physical therapy occasionally is needed to help the hand regain its softness, movement, and strength, but usually the exercises can be taught to you and you can carry them out yourself at home. If the activities you are doing at home cause the hand to swell more or the numbness to return, then you are doing too much activity and this must be stopped. Good examples are the numbness and swelling coming back after doing excessive housecleaning, waxing the floor, washing the car, or cutting the lawn in the period of time that is between 6 weeks and 3 months after the surgical procedure. Those whose job activities require frequent gripping, pushing, and pulling motions or excessive hand use may find that they cannot return to work until at least 6 to 8 weeks after the operative procedure.

Recovery Phase

The recovery process occurs generally in two stages. The operation, itself, causes release of pressure on the nerve and blood flow improves in the nerve immediately after the operative procedure. By the time the sutures are removed, you may have observed that the numbness and tingling is either gone or greatly diminished from your hand and the nighttime awakening no longer occurs. The parts of your symptoms due to scarring inside the nerve or from actual death or degeneration in the nerve fibers, such as muscle wasting or inability to discriminate fine points with the ends of the fingers, do not recover this quickly. The nerve fibers must regenerate from the site of the nerve injury, the wrist, to the muscles or fingertips. Thus, over a period of 6 months to a year, there will be continued improvement in muscle strength and ability to discriminate with the tips of the fingers. There is no way to hurry this neural regeneration process. This process may be associated with pain, similar to that experienced when your leg and foot "come back to life" after falling asleep. Such pain may last six weeks and require additional pain medication, massage, and prolonged postoperative care.

This information can be reviewed by you with your doctor and any information not understood discussed with him. It is hoped that this information may make you better aware of the operation, the potential benefits, risks, and complications, and help you in the recovery period following surgery.

Appendix B
Cubital Tunnel Syndrome
Information for the Patient Having Surgery for a "Pinched Nerve" at the Elbow

The Problem

The problem you have is called a cubital tunnel syndrome. This means that your symptoms and the problems you are experiencing are due to pressure on a nerve, the ulnar nerve, in a bony tunnel called the bubital tunnel. This is the area where a bump to the elbow gives a tingling in the little and ring fingers, and people frequently say they have "hit their funny bone." This familiar expression takes origin in the fact that one of the bones that contributes to this bony tunnel is the bone in the upper arm called the humerus. However, when this nerve in the cubital tunnel becomes compressed, the situation is not humorous.

The tunnel has a bone on either side and a bony groove at its base with a ligament crossing the nerve from the top of one bone to the other. The ulnar nerve, which is the size of a pen or pencil, controls the muscles for grip strength, primarily in the little, ring, and often the middle fingers. It controls the muscles for most of the pinch strength and it controls all of the small muscles in the hand that coordinate fine movements in the hand, with the exception of two muscles that lift the thumb up and out from the palm and turn the thumb for pinching. This ulnar nerve also controls the feeling in the little and ring fingers on both the palm and back side of the hand. The complaints that you have when this nerve becomes compressed may result from either sensory or motor (muscle) causes. For example, the complaints may primarily involve numbness and tingling in the little and ring fingers, the side of the hand and the back of the hand. These complaints worsen or are brought on when the elbow is bent, such as in holding a telephone in the hand or resting the head on the hand or with the arms crossed over the chest or during the night when the arm is curled beneath the body when asleep. You may notice that the hand becomes cold when it is on top of a steering wheel. The other group of symptoms involve motor functions of the nerve and you may be aware that the hand has become weaker, so that you have trouble opening jars. Frequently, you find that you drop things or that the hand cannot be made to do things quite as easily as it did before, for example, playing the violin, guitar, or piano or typing may cause problems with coordination of the fingers, especially when this activity is carried out for a long period of time. In many people, there are both sensory and motor symptoms present. Many times we do not know the cause of this problem. Often, the patient has experienced some injury to the region of the elbow, either with a fracture or dislocation about the elbow, a fall on the elbow, a twisting of the elbow, a sudden forceful flexion and extension of the elbow, as may occur in arms when the hands are on the wheel of a car and it is hit from the back in an automobile accident. Occupations requiring significant elbow flexion throughout the day, such as typing, computer data, or assembly line work may be contributory Problems with pressure on this nerve are more common in people with arthritis, diabetes, thyroid problems, and those who consume a great deal of alcohol.

Nonoperative Treatment

When the elbow is bent, the nerve becomes pulled up between the bones into the bony groove, causing increased pressure on the nerve. Every time the elbow is bent the nerve is tightened and the blood supply to the nerve is reduced (Fig. 1). The main nonoperative method for relieving pressure on the ulnar nerve at the elbow is therefore to keep the elbow straight as much as possible. It is clear that this cannot be done throughout the day because we need to bend our elbow to do many tasks. Regular daily activities must be altered, however, to avoid crossing the arms across the chest, keeping the elbow bent when talking on the telephone (people who need to use the telephone a lot may wish to get a cradle attachment or headset), changing the sleeping position by lying on your back when asleep with the arm at the side, changing the chair and desk angle and position so that when working at a typewriter or a computer keyboard, the elbow is flexed no more than 30° and the wrist is in a neutral position, or obtaining a nightstand for bedtime reading so that the book is not always held with the elbow bent. Most of these changes are common sense and require you to pay attention to your daily activities. A splint can be provided to keep the elbow straight or just slightly (30°) flexed. We often suggest that you fabricate your own elbow extension splint with soft toweling or use hockey elbow pads, which prevent elbow flexion. An additional aspect of the treatment before any operative procedure is to treat any underlying medical problem, such as arthritis or diabetes.

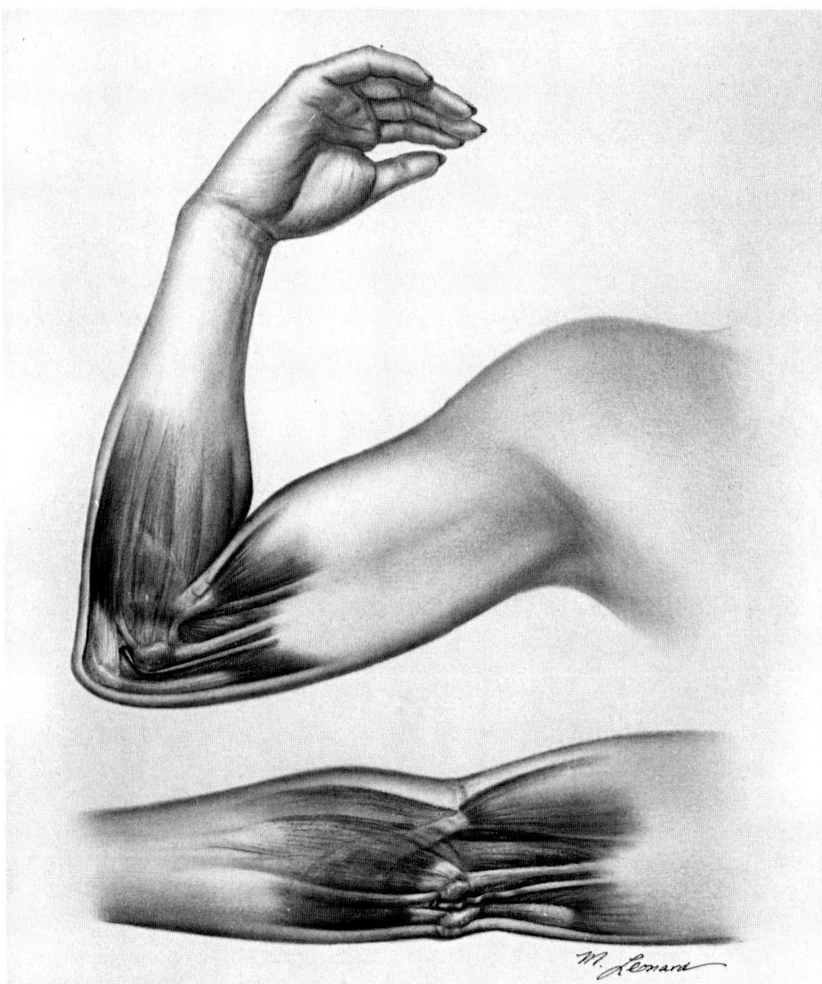

Figure 1.

The Operation

The operation is designed not only to take pressure off the nerve, but also to move the nerve to a place where it no longer will be pressed on by the common activities of daily living. There are many approaches to the treatment of compression of the ulnar nerve at the elbow. The one that will be described, as well as the postoperative care, is an operation that will move the nerve from its location behind the elbow to a location in front of the elbow. Thereafter, when the elbow is bent, the nerve will no longer be pulled into the bony groove, causing pressure on it. The location in which the nerve will be placed in front of the elbow will be one that lies beneath a muscle layer. Placement in this location is designed to prevent the nerve from slipping back into the bony groove behind the elbow, while at the same time providing a source of increased blood supply to help the nerve with healing. The placement of the nerve in this position, beneath the muscle, will protect it from injury (Fig. 2). Because the nerve must be moved from

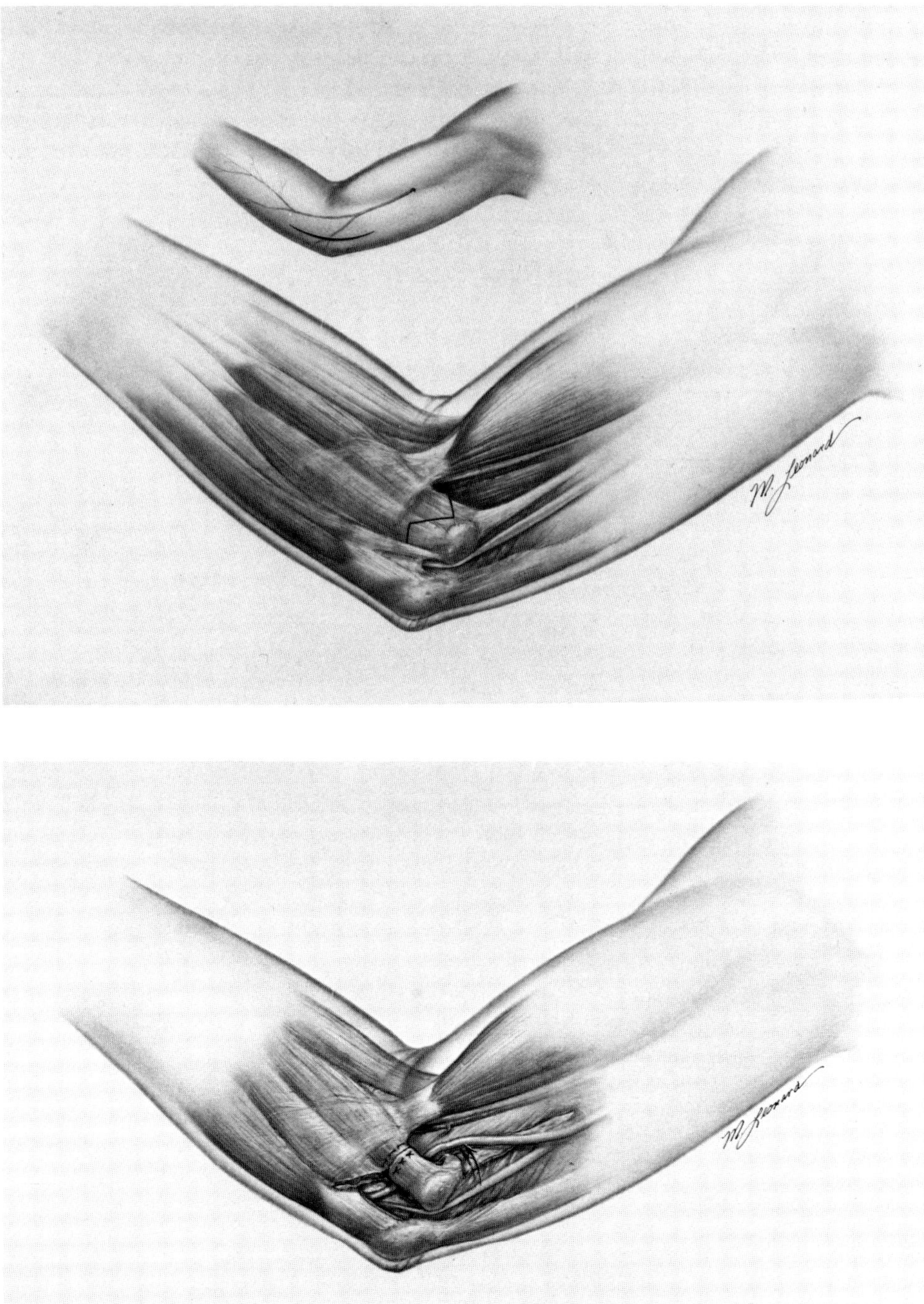

a

b **Figure 2.**

one location to another, there is the possibility that the nerve can become compressed or pinched in its new location by new areas of the anatomy that the nerve must pass along. The operation that will be described is designed to remove these potential sites for future nerve compression and thereby minimize the chance of the nerve compression occurring again. In its "new" position in front of the elbow, elbow flexion will no longer pinch, stretch, or decrease blood supply to the nerve.

The operation is called an anterior submuscular transposition of the ulnar nerve. The incision is made behind the elbow. The length of the incision varies, depending on the thickness of the arm, the size of the arm, the amount of fat tissue present, and the presence of any unusual anatomic arrangements that may require lengthening the incision in order to be sure the surgeon can see everything he is doing and do it safely. A nerve crosses the area of the incision. This is a small nerve that supplies the skin behind the elbow and in part of the forearm. This nerve may become injured during the operative procedure even though great care is taken to avoid injury to this nerve. After surgery, pain in the scar or loss of sensation in areas about the elbow are possible despite the care that the surgeon takes in attempting to identify this nerve at the time of surgery. Magnifying glasses (operating microscope or loupes) are worn during the operation to minimize the chances of this occurring. The main nerve to be operated on, the ulnar nerve, is identified in the bony tunnel and the bands causing pressure on it are released. The muscles that go from the inside of the elbow across the forearm and are related to turning the forearm, bending the wrist, and bending some of the fingers, are lifted from the bone. This mass of muscle is called the flexor-pronator muscle mass. In order to be sure that the place in which the nerve will be newly positioned does not cause compression on the nerve, the strong tissues that cover this muscle mass are lengthened, so that when the muscle mass is reattached to the bone, no tightness is placed on the nerve. The areas above and below the elbow that the nerve passes through are checked so that any places that might cause future compression of the nerve are also treated. Patients who have numbness in the little and ring fingers, which is present all the time, or who have severe weakness in the muscles of gripping or pinching, or who have wasting of the muscles, may have scar tissue built up inside the nerve. In these cases, an additional operative procedure is done called a microsurgical internal neurolysis. The operation is performed with magnifying glasses. In this situation, the outer wrapping of the nerve is opened and the scar tissue within the nerve is removed. Care is taken not to injure any of the small connections between the nerve fibers.

Postoperative Management

After surgery, the dressing is placed so that the elbow is flexed and the wrist is kept straight. This is done by means of plaster placed in the dressing. The forearm may be placed in a sling. The sling can be worn for 2 weeks to allow the muscle to heal back to the bone, but the heavy plaster dressing is removed at approximately the eighth day after surgery, at which time any sutures are also removed. A lighter plastic splint may be made at this time for use for another 7 to 10 days. The timing of these aspects of the postoperative care may vary and may be lengthened if it is anticipated that there will be wound-healing problems, such as occurs if you are taking cortisone for arthritis or if you have diabetes or some other type of wound-healing problem. Movement of the fingers is encouraged early on in the postoperative period.

During the second week after surgery, when the arm is out of its dressing but still in a sling or light splint, the fingers are moved, the wrist is moved and the elbow may be flexed and extended slightly to allow the nerve to slip and slide through the area in which the operation was done. In the third week after surgery, which is the week after which the sling or splint is no longer worn, the elbow may begin to be extended. This is done by placing a warm cloth on the incision or gently massaging the incision for 5 minutes, utilizing some type of hand cream or lotion, and then gently letting gravity, itself, attempt to extend the elbow when the arm is held at the side. When the arm begins to ache, the arm can be placed back into a flexed position and the person may sit down. This should be repeated several times throughout the day with the expectation that at some time during the third or fourth week after surgery, the elbow will become straight again. In terms of exercising the hand to regain strength, it will be found that it takes approximately 3 months for the strength that was present before surgery to return. This may happen sooner in some people or later in others. Exercise may be begun in the third week, preferably by squeezing Play-Doh™ or exercise putty. This should be done just until swelling or aching occurs in the hand or forearm. Until the muscles are healed and the nerve has grown back into the muscles that were becoming paralyzed, it will not be possible to increase strength simply by forcing the arm and hand through these periods of swelling and discomfort. It is better to do the exercise for shorter periods of time and repeat the series more frequently. Pinching and rolling out the Play-Doh™ into small pieces strengthens the small muscles of the hand. If recovery of two-point discrimination is slow, you may use a Disk-Criminator™ for a home sensory re-education program.

Recovery Phase

The recovery process occurs generally in two phases. The symptoms that are due to pressure on the nerve with decreased blood flow to the nerve and therefore decreased oxygen to the nerve fibers are those that may cause muscle weakness and numbness and tingling. Frequently, by the time the sutures are removed, you will note some improvement in the numbness and tingling in the fingers. Especially considering that before surgery bending the elbow for just 1 or 2 minutes would cause numbness and tingling to occur, you now will have had the arm flexed for 8 days and the numbness and tingling may be improving. However, when the muscle weakness, muscle wasting or loss of ability to discriminate one or two points on the tips of the fingers is present, or when the numbness in the little and ring fingers has been present all the time throughout the day for a considerable period of time before surgery, actual degeneration or death of the nerve fibers has occurred. In this instance, recovery can only occur when the nerve regrows into the muscles. This takes approximately 4 to 5 months for this to occur for the gripping muscles. It takes approximately 1 to 1½ years for this to occur for the small muscles in the hand. It may take the same amount of time for sensation to improve in the little and ring fingers. Thus, recovery can extend up to 1½ years and may extend to 2 years if you are over the age of 50 years. In some patients with a very severe degree of nerve compression recovery may be incomplete.

If the scar becomes painful in the period after surgery, this may be helped by massage with a cortisone-containing cream. If there are areas of sensory loss about the elbow or forearm after the operative procedure due to injury to the small nerves that cross this area, as already discussed, these areas frequently diminish in size over a period of time, but they may remain permanent in nature. The process of neural regeneration may be associated with pain, similar to that experienced when your leg and foot "come back to life" after falling asleep. Such pain may last for 6 to 12 weeks going down the side of the forearm to the wrist and finally into the little finger. This may require prolonged postoperative medication, massage, and therapy.

The potential complications and risks from the operation, in addition to the painful scar and loss of sensation behind the elbow that have been mentioned already, are the scar itself. Bleeding or bruising may occur, occasionally severe enough to require a return to surgery to stop the bleeding. Infection may occur requiring antibiotic treatment. Persistent numbness in the little and ring fingers and tingling down the forearm, usually due to regeneration of the sensory nerve fibers, may occur and may become permanent. In a few people, the symptoms may either not be improved or may recur eventually.

This information should be reviewed with your doctor and any information not understood brought up and discussed with him. It is hoped that this information may make you better aware of the operation, its potential benefits, risks, and complications and help you in the recovery period after surgery.

Appendix C
Multiple Crush Syndrome

The problem you have concerns more than one reason why your nerve(s) are not functioning normally. The approach taken to correct this problem is to begin one at a time with the causes of nerve compression that are giving you your symptoms. For example, numbness in the little finger may be caused by pressure upon the nerves as they leave the spine (the discs in the neck), pass under the collarbone (thoracic outlet syndrome or brachial plexus compression), cross behind the elbow (cubital tunnel syndrome), and enter the hand through a tunnel (Guyon's Canal) at the wrist. A similar situation exists when a disease, such as diabetes, alcoholism, thyroid dysfunction, or arthritis makes all the nerves in the body more sensitive (susceptible) to pressure at a normal area of anatomic tightness (like those mentioned above). The surgical approach may require release of pressure at just the worst site of compression.

An everyday experience found useful in describing the multiple crush syndrome is a garden hose used to water the lawn or flowers. When the hose is turned on with more than enough water necessary to keep the plants watered or the grass green, someone may come along and step on the hose, partially compressing it. There will be some decrease in water flowing through the hose, similar to the way the first site of compression of a peripheral nerve causes a decrease in axoplasmic flow, but enough water may still come out the end to keep the grass or flowers nourished and green. A second person may come by and step on the hose somewhat closer to the nozzle and further decrease the amount of water flowing through the hose and decrease the amount of water coming out the nozzle, although there may still be enough water to keep the flowers or grass alive. However, if an additional person steps on the hose, it may narrow the opening in the hose sufficient that only a small trickle of water will come out and this may keep the flowers going for a while but people observing the flowers or the grass will notice that they are beginning to wilt. This is similar to the symptoms being produced, the symptoms calling the patient's and physician's attention to the problem.

At this point, it may only be necessary to remove any one of the three areas in which the hose is being pressed on to increase the flow enough that, although the flow is not as much as possible, it is still enough to keep the flowers or grass alive. If, however, no one noticed that the flowers were wilting or the grass dying, or no one paid attention to the sign, and the decreased flow continued at a very low trickle, then the flowers or grass would become brown and at some point they would be unable, even with additional water, to come back to life. Thus, serial constraints on flow, each summates to contribute to decreased flow and at some point this flow will be sufficiently decreased to cause some functional change. If the flow is returned at an appropriate time, no permanent damage may occur, but if a sufficient length of time elapses, then it may not be possible, even if the flow could be increased, to permit a return to normal functioning.

Appendix D
Pain Questionnaire: Pain Rating Scale*

*adapted from the McGill Pain Scale Questionnaire and Hendler's Chronic Back Pain Scale

PREOPERATIVE ASSESSMENT OF PATIENTS WITH HAND PAIN

NAME: ______________________ HISTORY # ____________ DATE: ____________

A. Pain Descriptors

Is your pain like: (circle as many as you wish)						
	BURNING	THROBBING	ACHING	STABBING	TINGLING	DULL
	TWISTING	CRAMPING	CUTTING	SHOOTING	NUMBING	VAGUE
	STINGING	SQUEEZING	PULLING	SMARTING	PRESSURE	COLDNESS
	INDESCRIBABLE		OTHER: ____________			

How is your pain now? (mark on any part of the line below)

No Pain |————————————————————————| Severe Pain

How is your mood now? (Mark on any part of the line below)

Worse Mood |————————————————————————| Best Mood

B. Body Diagram

Where is your pain? (Please indicate on the diagram, may use color pen)

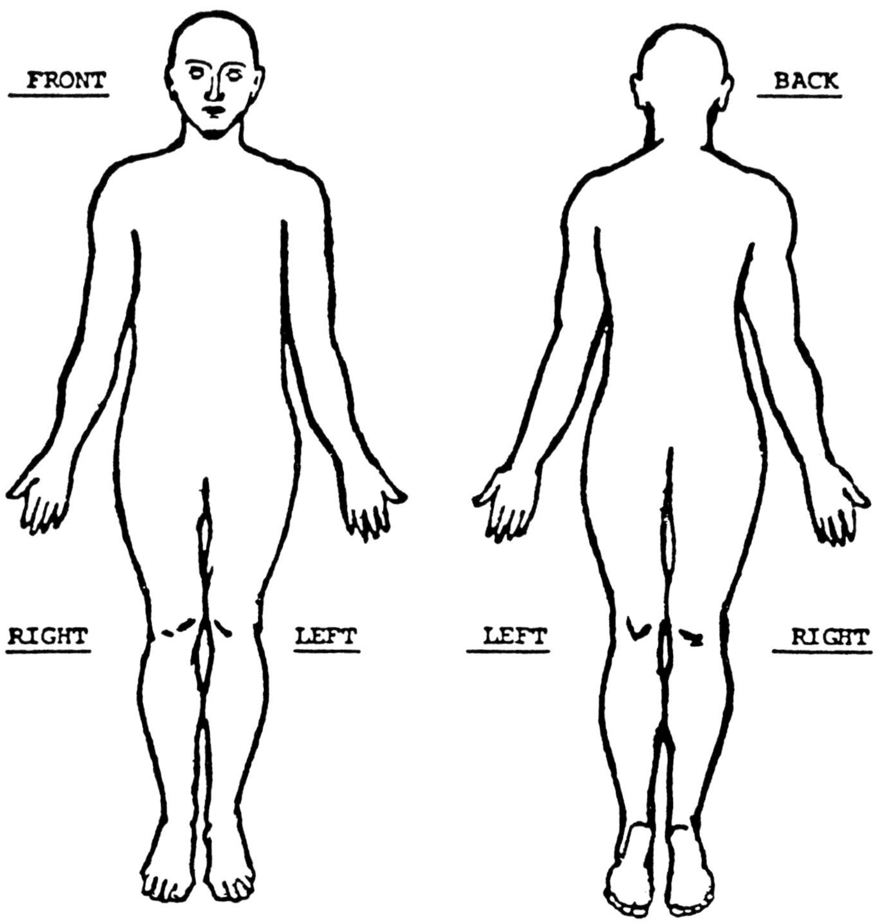

C. Numerical Scale

Instructions Each question is asked by an examiner and the patient is given points according to the appropriate response. Number of points to be awarded for the various responses is circled in the column at the right, and at the end of the test, the examiner calculates the total number of points.

Age ______ sex ____________
Workman's Compensation Board Yes ______ No ______
Nature of Complaint:

Duration of Complaint:
Nature of Surgical Procedures Performed:

If the patient has had surgery by the evaluating surgeon, please document the patients response to that surgery.
If the patient has had a psychiatric evaluation, please document that report.
In the examining surgeons evaluation, is the pain due to:
a. Arthritis
b. Vascular disorder
c. Bony or ligamentous injury
d. Sympathetic maintained pain syndrome
e. Nerve injury, neuromatous type pain hyperalgesia or neuroma incontinuity

1. How did the pain that you are now experiencing occur?
   a. Sudden onset with accident or definable event. 0
   b. Slow progressive onset. 0
   c. Slow progressive onset with acute exacerbation without an accident or definable event. 3
   d. A sudden onset without an accident or definable event. 4
2. Where do you experience the pain?
   a. One site, specific, well-defined consistent with anatomical distribution. 0
   b. Two sites each with well-defined and consistent with an anatomical distribution. 0
   c. One site inconsistent with anatomical considerations or not well defined. 2
   d. Greater than two sites but each well anatomically defined. 2
   e. Vague description, more than one site, of which one is inconsistent with anatomical considerations or not well-defined or anatomically explainable. 3
3. Do you ever have trouble falling asleep at night or are you ever awakened from sleep? If the answer is no, score 3 points and go on to question 4. If the answer is yes, proceed.

3A. What keeps you from falling asleep or what awakens you from sleep?
   a. Trouble falling asleep every night due to pain. 0
   b. Trouble falling asleep due to pain most nights of the week. 1
   c. Occasionally during the week having difficulty falling asleep due to pain. 2
   d. No trouble falling asleep due to pain. 3
   e. Trouble falling asleep which is not related to pain. 4

3B. a. Awakened by pain every night. 0
   b. Awakened from sleep by pain most nights. 1
   c. Not usually awakened from sleep by pain. 3
   d. Restless sleep, or early morning awakening with or without being able to return to sleep, both unrelated to pain. 4

4. Does weather have any effect on your pain?
   a. The pain is usually worse with damp weather or the cold weather. 0
   b. The pain is occasionally worse with damp or cold weather. 2
   c. The weather has no effect on the pain. 3

5. How would you describe the type of pain that you have?
   a. Any of the adjectives, burning, sharp shooting, pins and needles, coldness, numbness, dull aching, with occasional sharp shooting pains or the patient is experiencing hyperalgesia. 0
   b. The patient describes the pain as; spasm type or tension type pain or nagging or bothersome pain. 3
   c. The patient describes the pain as excruciating, overwhelming or unbearable pain or bringing them to tears. 4
6. Does movement or position have any effect on the pain?
   a. The pain is worsened by use or movement. 0
   b. The pain is usually worsened by use and movement. 2
   c. The pain is not altered by the use of the hand. 5
7. What medications have you used in the past month?
   a. No medications or nonnarcotic pain relievers. 0
   b. Valium. 2
   c. Frequent narcotic use. 3
   d. Psychotrophic or antidepressant drugs 4
8. Have you ever thought of suicide?
   a. No. 0
   b. Yes. 2
   c. History of suicide attempt. 5
9. Are you presently receiving psychiatric treatment?
   a. Yes. 4
   b. No. 0
10. Have you ever received psychiatric treatment?
    a. Yes. 2
    b. No. 0
11. How many surgical procedures have been carried out on your hand *in order to try to eliminate the cause of the pain?*
    a. None or one. 0
    b. Two surgical procedures. 2
    c. Three or four surgical procedures. 3
    d. Greater than four surgical procedures. 4
12. Do you still participate in the hobbies that you enjoyed prior to the development of the painful hand?
    a. Reduced number of hobbies or activities relating to a hobby. 0
    b. Unable to participate in any hobbies that were formally enjoyed. 1
    c. Still able to participate in hobbies but with some discomfort. 2
    d. Participates in hobbies as before without any restrictions. 3
13. Are you still working or doing your household chores?
    a. Works every day at the same prepain job or same level of household duties. 0
    b. Works every day but the job is not the same as the prepain job with reduced responsibility or physical activity. 0
    c. Works sporadically or does a reduced amount of household chores. 2
    d. Not at work or most household chores are now performed by others. 3
14. If you had three wishes for anything in the world, what would you wish for?
    a. Get rid of the pain is the only wish. 0
    b. Get rid of the pain is one of the three wishes. 1
    c. Doesn't mention getting rid of the pain but has specific wishes usually of a personal nature such as for more money, better relationship with spouse or children, etc. 2
    d. Does not mention pain and the wishes are nonpersonal for such things as world peace, etc. 3
15. Is the patient involved in any litigation process regarding their physical complaint?
    a. No. 0
    b. Yes. 3
16. Is this a Workers' Compensation Board case?
    a. No. 0
    b. Yes. 2

Total Point Score ______________

Summary

A. Pain Descriptors: positive/negative (> 3 adjectives considered positive)
B. Body Diagram: positive/negative (nonanatomical pain distribution considered positive)
C. Numerical Scale: positive/negative (> 14 considered positive)

Note: See Chapter 17, Dellon AL, Mackinnon SE: Surgery of the Peripheral Nerve. Thieme, New York, 1988.

Interpretation

If A, B, C are all positive this is an absolute contraindication for surgery. If two of the assessment parameters are positive this is a relative contraindication and the patient is referred for psychiatric evaluation. If one of the assessment factors is positive, then the surgeon explains his concern to the patient and uses his own discretion regarding the appropriateness of a psychiatric consultation. If all of the three parameters are negative then the patient should be a valid pain patient, reporting a normal response to organic pain without a significant functional or psychogenic component to his perception of pain.

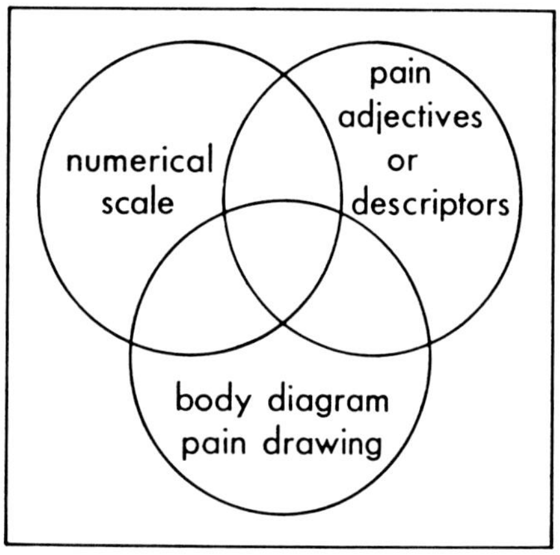

a

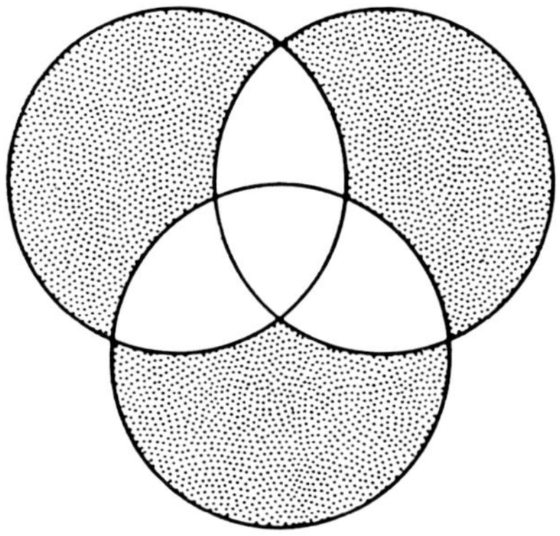

b

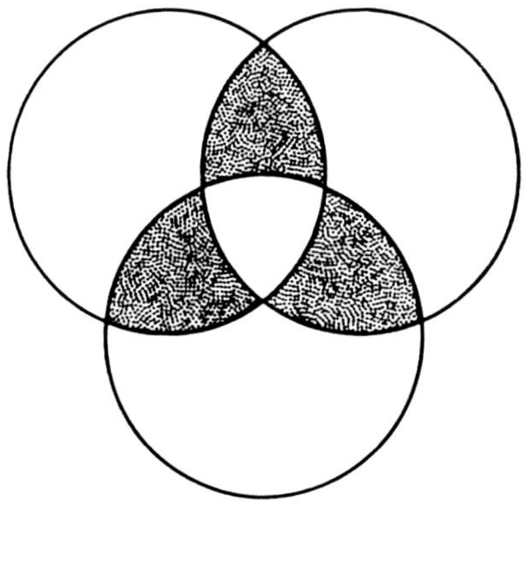

c

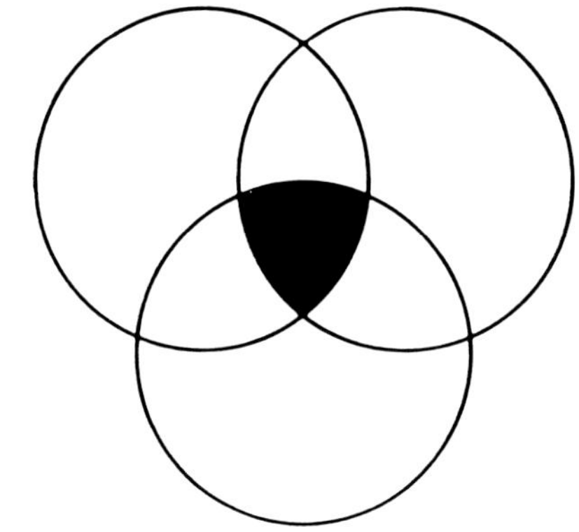

d

Figure 17-11a. Venn construct for pain evaluation rating scale. The patients are evaluated using three broad parameters. A *numerical scale* reflects the answers the patients give to various questions. The *body diagram* pain drawing determines whether or not the pain described by the patient follows any known anatomic pattern. Finally, the *pain descriptors* indicate the number of adjectives the patient uses to describe the pain. **a.** If the patient's scores greater than 14 on the numerical scale, then they fall within the circle outlined for this rating. If they circle more than three adjectives when asked to describe their pain, then they fall within the circle that diagrams the pain adjectives. If the patient describes a location of their pain on the body diagram that does not fit with any known anatomic distribution of pain, then they fall within the circle outlined for the pain drawing. If the patient's grading falls into only one of these circles, the surgeon may proceed with surgery with caution. He will often explain his concern to the patient and solicit psychiatric help at his own discretion. **b.** If the patient's scale falls into one of these three areas, that is, if they are positive for two of the three evaluations, then psychiatric evaluation is always solicited (**c**). If the patient is positive on all three rating scales and falls into the central area, then surgery is contraindicated (**d**).

Appendix E Sensory Education Protocol Re-education

*Raymond M. Curtis Hand Center, Union Memorial Hospital, Baltimore, Maryland 21218

Techniques of Sensory Re-education

Sensory re-education is a method or combination of techniques that help the patient with a sensory impairment learn to reinterpret the altered profile of neural impulses reaching his conscious level after his injured hand has been stimulated. In the normal state, stimulation of the hand by contact with the external environment stimulates the sensory receptors and a profile of neural impulses is elicited. These impact on the sensory cortex, associate with previous memory or experiences, and ultimately become a recognized perception. After a nerve division and nerve repair, the same contact with the external world, the same stimulus, now elicits a different or an altered profile of neural impulses. When these reach the sensory cortex, they may find no match in the association cortex. Thus, the sensation is new, cannot be named, and may even pass unnoticed.

This is the basic philosophy for sensory re-education treatment after nerve laceration or compression. Unless these neural impulses are trained, sensation will be nonfunctional.

Early Phase Sensory Re-education

When 30 cps and moving touch have returned to an area, for example, the palm, early phase re-education may begin. It is most critical to begin by the time recovery has reached the proximal phalanges.

Goals at this Stage

1. To re-educate specific perceptions, movements versus constant touch and pressure
2. To re-educate misdirection or incorrect localization

The exercise is for the patient to use a soft instrument, like a pencil eraser, or someone else may use their fingertip to stroke up and down the length of the area being re-educated. The patient observes what is happening, shuts his eyes, and concentrates on what he is perceiving and then opens his eyes to confirm again what is really happening. He should verbalize to himself what he is perceiving as specifically as he can (example: "I feel something moving up (down) my index finger near the palm" [may draw numbers].

When the patient can perceive constant touch, the same type of early phase re-education is done for this touch submodality (example: the eraser is pressed down into one spot on the palm or finger within the area of recovered constant touch perception and the patient first directly observes what is occurring, then shuts his eyes and repeats the stimulus, verbalizes to himself what he is perceiving, opens his eyes and reaffirms the stimulus and perception. Again, he should be saying, "I feel something pressing (hard or soft) on my index finger near my palm."

How hard should the stimulus be pressed into the finger? The newly reunited fiber or receptor system is "immature," its threshold is therefore high and early in the recovery of sensation more stimulus intensity must be used for perception to occur. Press the moving or stationary eraser as hard as necessary for the patient to perceive constant touch or movement. (Stimulus intensity should never evoke perception of pain. We are not re-educating pain perception.)

The patient should not stimulate one hand directly with the other. The patient's right index finger should not be used to stroke or press on the patient's left palm or left thumb. If this were to occur, the patient would be receiving two sets of sensory information, one from each hand. At this early point in re-education, this only confuses the distorted sensory picture.

Who Performs Early Phase Sensory Re-education?

The surgeon, whenever he examines the patient, will be doing these exercises to ascertain for his own records the degree of recovery. This may be about once a month and should reinforce the whole motivational and emotional systems and the need for re-education.

The therapist should be seeing the patient in a quiet, distraction-free room, two to three times a week, if possible, for approximately 10 to 15 minutes, to reinforce the goals, check the progress, and provide reassurance.

The patient should be encouraged to practice early phase sensory re-education three to four times a day, even if just for 5 minutes a day, in a quiet, distraction-free room.

Any interested person (spouse, mother, sister, boyfriend) can be shown the sensory re-education techniques and be "pressed" into service.

Early phase sensory re-education should be introduced to the fingertip 4 to 6 months after a median or ulnar nerve repair at wrist level.

Late Phase Sensory Re-education

Late phase sensory re-education should begin as soon as moving touch and constant touch can be perceived at the fingertip with good localization. This can be as early as 6 to 8 months after median or ulnar nerve repair at the wrist. It is important at the beginning of this phase that the patient be told that he will continue slow improvement in his ability to recognize objects. He will not be able to differentiate the smallest objects until 10 to 12 months after nerve repair at the wrist.

Goal at This Stage

To guide the patient to recovery of tactilegnosis (object identification)

Sensory re-education cannot induce axonal regeneration. Sensory re-education can only help the patient achieve the fullest potential provided by the nerve repair.

Since the goal of late phase sensory re-education is recovery of functional sensation, the specific exercises should involve object identification.

Tactile discrimination recovers progressively over time as measured by both static and moving two-point discrimination. At any given time in the recovery process that moving two-point discrimination has recovered to a greater degree than static two-point discrimination, the object recognition tasks should incorporate movement.

The exercises should be graded, beginning with the discrimination of larger objects, with greater differences among them in size, shape, and texture, if possible, and progressing to more subtle differences.

Late phase sensory re-education is begun with a set of familiar household objects, differing widely in shape, size, and texture. Again, the sequence of object grasp with eyes open and shut with concentration of perception, eyes open for reinforcement, is utilized. After the patient has practiced with the object, the therapist may test him and record either the number of objects identified correctly or the time required (in seconds with a stop watch) for object identification. A record such as this provides evidence to the patient, therapist, and referring physician that progress is occurring. It gives the patient a goal "to beat" next time. It assists patient motivation.

Late phase sensory re-education is continued by progressing to objects differing largely in texture and then to objects that are smaller, differing in size and shape, but not in texture and requiring subtle discrimination. At this stage, the patient will be clinically recovering, static two-point discrimination will be less than 7 mm. As moving two-point discrimination drops below 5 mm, patients will be able to identify the smallest objects correctly, although the objects may fall from the patient's grasp because the slowly adapting fiber and receptor system has not regenerated and matured sufficiently. A Disk-Criminator™* can be given to the patient for continuation of late phase re-education at home.

Late phase sensory re-education also provides motor education. Activities that duplicate or incorporate

*P.O. Box 16392, Baltimore, Maryland 21210.

work motions or activities should be included in the patient's therapy. It is ideal to have the patient attend the workshop, working on work simulator, to practice specific sensory grips before the patient is ready to try the actual tool at his job.

Who Performs Late Phase Sensory Re-education?

The surgeon, whenever he examines the patient, should test moving and static two-point discrimination and object recognition. In so doing, praise, reinforcement, reassurance, and motivation are provided to sustain the patient and back-up what the therapist has been doing. At this point, the surgeon should be seeing the patient every 3 months.

The therapist should be seeing the patient weekly, progressing to biweekly and perhaps monthly, between the start of late phase re-education (6 to 9 months after repair) and the patient's return to work. The therapist should be working through the exercises, testing and recording the results of object recognition, encouraging and reinforcing the patient. At each session, both static and moving two-point discrimination should be recorded.

The patient should be practicing at home three to four times a day, 5 to 10 minutes each time. Frequent short sessions are more productive than longer, less frequent sessions. Late phase exercises can be modified, depending on the nerve involved.

Median Nerve

All of the exercises described are applicable and essentially involve three-jaw chuck pinch or gripping of objects between thumb, index and middle fingers and manipulating the object. A glove may be cut and modified to cover the ulnar digits leaving the thumb, index, and long fingers exposed. This will facilitate mobility of the hand but decrease sensory input from the ulnar nerve.

Ulnar Nerve or Digital Nerve Injuries

A second person's presence during exercise is helpful. That person can place objects for recognition onto the surface of the fingertip being re-educated. Less precise, but still helpful, is for the patient to manipulate an object between the thumb and the fingertip being reeducated. Here, the patient must try to concentrate on the perceptions being transmitted via the injured finger instead of those coming from the thumb.

Other Techniques of Re-education

Bilateral exercises are useful by having the patient differentiate between various textures of material and grades of sandpaper with vision and then feel with vision eliminated.

Sand, rice, or bean media can be used for sensory reeducation. Patients, without visual clues, must identify objects within a pile of sand, rice, or beans.

How long should sensory re-education be continued once the patient has recovered functional sensation? The program should be followed for a long time. If the patient returns to work, or resumes housekeeping, or is a child, the re-education is continued at this level and no formal program is required.

If patient discontinues sensory re-education exercises and active daily use of the hand, the effect of the re-education program is lost by the time the patient is next tested. This is "early on." If re-education exercises are resumed, function is quickly recovered. After recovery has proceeded for some time, the patient becomes increasingly able to maintain his re-educated status.

This re-education program must be designed and modified on an individual basis.

Sunnybrook Medical Center Hand Service, University of Toronto, Toronto, Ontario, Canada

Sensory Re-education Home Program

Purpose: To *concentrate* on sensations until your brain learns the correct responses.

Procedure: Choose a quiet area with few distractions.
Complete the exercises three times each day.

Sequence: Follow an *eyes open, eyes closed, eyes open* sequence for each exercise

Early Phase

Localization

1. Light touch or pressure
   a. Use a pencil eraser. Place it on the area indicated and hold for 1 second, then release. Notice where you placed it
   b. Close eyes and repeat. Try to describe where the eraser was felt
   c. Repeat entire *sequence* five times. Move to another area
2. Disk-Criminator™
   a. Use the point of the Disk-Criminator™. Follow the same directions as for no. 1 above. Ask yourself. "Does this feel sharp or dull?"
   b. Repeat the *sequence* five times. Move to another area.

Discrimination

1. Two-point discrimination
   a. Use device provided.* Set points 1 cm apart (use ruler to guide). Place points on area indicated and hold for 1 second, then release. Do you feel one point or two points?
   b. Repeat the *sequence* (eyes open, eyes closed, eyes open) five times, asking this question each time. Move to another area
   c. The points can be moved closer together, 1 mm at a time, only when you can correctly feel two points in seven of ten tries in one area
2. Moving two-point discrimination
   a. Use device provided. Follow the directions as for no. 1 above, *moving* the points slowly within the area indicated. Do you feel one point or two points?
   b. Repeat the *sequence* five times. Move to another area
   c. The points can be moved closer together, 1 mm at a time, only when you can correctly feel two points seven of ten tries in one area.
3. Texture discrimination
   a. Use the dowels provided
   b. Move the two ends of each dowel in the area indicated. After rubbing with both ends, ask yourself:
      Are the textures the same or different?
      How are they different?
      Describe to yourself the texture felt at each end
   c. Repeat the *sequence* five times with each dowel. Move to another area

*P.O. Box 16392, Baltimore, Maryland 21210.

Lubbock Orthopedic Surgery Clinic and Hand Surgery Service, Department of Orthopedic Surgery, Texas Tech University School of Medicine, Lubbock, Texas

Sensory Re-education Program

Guidelines for Persons with Decreased Sensation

1. Avoid exposing your hand to sharp, hot, or very cold objects.
2. To keep skin soft and smooth, follow a daily routine of skin care, including soaking in warm water and massaging with NIVEA creme.
3. If blisters, cuts, or other wounds occur, treat them with the utmost care to avoid further injury and possible infection. If you are uncertain about an injury, please call the office.
4. When gripping an object, do not apply more force than is necessary.
5. Avoid work that requires use of one tool for a long period of time. (Especially if the hand is unable to change its manner of grip.)
6. Change tools or objects you use frequently to rest tissue and skin.
7. Watch the skin for signs of stress: redness, swelling, warmth. Rest the hand if these signs occur.
8. Begin sensory reeducation program as soon as the doctor or therapist advises you to do so.

Sensory Re-education Home Program

For the early phase see the protocol for the Sunnybrook Medical Center Hand Service.

Late Phase

Stereognosis: The ability to recognize common objects by touch alone.

1. Good motor function
   a. Place objects provided in a bowl in front of you. Pick out one object at a time and manipulate it with eyes open. Describe its shape.
   b. Close your eyes and manipulate the object. Describe the object.
   c. Open your eyes and repeat. Do this *sequence* with each object.
   d. Replace all objects in bowl.
   e. With eyes closed, pick out one object at a time and try to identify it.
   f. Open your eyes and see if you were correct.
   g. Repeat this with each object until all are removed from the bowl.
2. Poor motor function
   a. Using your other hand (or with assistance), place one object at a time into your affected hand and move it around. Describe its shape.
   b. Close your eyes and move the object around in your palm. Describe its shape.
   c. Open your eyes and repeat. Do this *sequence* with each object.
   d. Follow the same directions as for d, e, f, and g above.

Note: When you are able to identify correctly all the objects provided with eyes open and closed, gather your own set of ten household items and repeat the exercises. Try to find objects that are similar in shape.

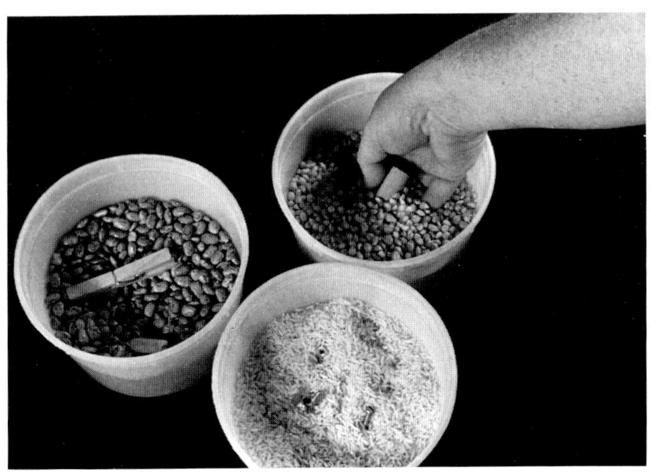

North Palm Beach Hand Rehabilitation, North Palm Beach, Florida

Dewey Disc Sensory Re-education System

As hand therapists, we instruct patients in various methods and techniques to re-educate their damaged cutaneous sensory nerves. There are a few home programs, such as the Dellon program utilized at the Curtis Hand Center, that are simple to use and cost effective for the patient to perform on a repetitive basis at home.

The Dewey Disc program has 3 cm plastic discs with a 1/16 and 1/32 inch raised number (1.5 cm width) from 0 to 9. Once the 1/16 numbers can be correctly identified by the affected digit with vision occluded, the patient progresses to the 1/32 inch raised numbers at 1.5 cm width and then possibly to smaller numbers as sensation improves. The discs are small and can easily be carried during the day for frequent manipulation. They can be held flat on a table for single digit manipulation, or held against the thumb for manipulation.

We suggest this program for patients with more advanced cutaneous sensibility, because we have found that static two-point discrimination must be present at the digit pulp for success with identification of the 1/32 inch raised numbers. We anticipate that identification of geometric shapes with 1/16 inch rise will be easier to identify.

We issue the patient with nerve-injured digits three or four discs to begin a sensory reeducation program. We request that he begin by manipulating the discs with his involved digits by looking and feeling first, and then by feeling without looking. We ask that the patient carry the discs in his pocket and manipulate them constantly throughout the day, or that he work on this reeducation program for 15 to 20 minutes at least four times a day. We initially give patients unlike numbers, such as 1, 3, and 7, and when they have mastered identification of unlike numbers, exchange their discs for like numbers, such as 3, 8, and 9. We record progress on a weekly or bimonthly basis by asking the patient to identify the discs in the clinic with vision occluded. We give the patient ten trials and record the number of correct responses.

The discs are packaged as a complete sensory re-education kit, including three geometric shapes and numbers 1 through 8. The number 6 can also be correctly identified as a 9, and the number 0 can also be used as the circle in the geometric shapes.

Combined Bibliography

1. Aasar YH: A peculiar relation of the femoral head of the bicep femoris to the common peroneal nerve. J Anat 72:305, 1938.
2. Abbott LC, Saunders JB: Injuries of the median nerve in fractures of the lower end of radius. Surg Gynecol Obstet 57:507, 1933.
3. Abu Jamra FN, Rebeiz JJ: Lipofibroma of the median nerve. J Hand Surg 4:160–163, 1979.
4. Adams CWM, Grant RT, Davis OB: Cholinesterases in peripheral nervous system. 1. mixed, motor and sensory trunks. Brain Res 5:366–367, 1967.
5. Adelaar RS, Foster WC, McDowell C: The Treatment of Cubital Tunnel Syndrome. J Hand Surg [Am] 9:90–95, 1984.
6. Adeymo O, Wyburn GN: Innervation of skin grafts. Trans Bull 4:152–153, 1957.
7. Adson AW: Surgical treatment of progressive ulnar paralysis. Minn Med 1:455–460, 1918.
8. Adson AW: Surgical treatment for symptoms produced by cervical ribs in the scalene anticus muscle. Surg Gynec Obstet 85:687–696, 1947.
9. Adson AW, Coffey JR: Cervical rib—a method of anterior approach for relief of symptoms by division of the scalenus anterior. Ann Surg 85:839–844, 1927.
10. Aegineta: The seven books translated by F. Adams. Vol. 2. Sydenham Society, London, 1844–1847.
11. Akenside M: Observations on cancers. Med Trans Coll Physicians Lond 1:64, 1768.
12. Albert E: Einige Operationen an Nerven. Wien Med 26:1285, 1885.
13. Allieu Y: Exploration et traitement direct des lesions nerveuses dans les paralysies traumatiques par elongation du plexus brachial chez l'adulte. Rev Surg Orthop 63:107–122, 1975.
14. Almay BGL, Johansson F, von Knorring L: Endorphins in chronic pain—differences in CSF endorphin levels between organic and psychogenic pain syndromes. Pain 5:153–162, 1978.
15. Alnot JY, Jolly A, Rot B: Traitement direct de lesions nerveuses dans les paralysies traumatiques du plexus brachial chez l'adulte. Int Orthop 63:82, 1981.
16. Althaus B, Maillard GF: Spatrsultate nach chirurgis cher behandlung fon fifty karpaltunnel syndromen unter anwendung der mikrochirurgis chen endoneurolyse. Helv Chir Acta 48:89–93, 1981.
17. Alvine FG, Schurrer ME: Postoperative ulnar nerve palsy. J Bone Joint Surg 62A:255–259, 1987.
18. Amadio PC: Pyridoxine as an adjunct in the treatment of carpal tunnel syndrome. J Hand Surg [Am] 10:237–241, 1985.
19. Amadio PC, Beckenbaugh RD: Entrapment of the ulnar nerve by the deep flexor-pronator aponeurosis. J Hand Surg [Am] 11:83–87, 1986.
20. Ametewee K, Harris A, Samuel M: Acute carpal tunnel syndrome produced by anomalous flexor digitorum superficialis indicis muscle. J Hand Surg [Br] 10:83–84, 1985.
21. Anatomical Society of Great Britain and Ireland: Report of Committee of Collective Investigation on the Distribution of Cutaneous Nerves on the Dorsum of the Foot. J Anat Physiol 26:89–90, 1892.
22. Anderl H: Reconstruction of the face through cross-face nerve transplantation in facial paralysis. In Converse JM: Reconstructive Plastic Surgery, 2nd ed. WB Saunders, Philadelphia, 1977, pp 1848–1862.
23. Andrae H: Uber traumatische Luxation des Nervus ulnaris am Ellenbogen. Inaugural dissertation: Greifswald, 1889.

24. Apfel E: The effect of thumb interphalangeal joint position on strength of key pinch. J Hand Surg [Am] 11: 47–51, 1986.
25. Apfelberg DB, Larson SJ: Dynamic anatomy of the ulnar nerve at the elbow. Plast Reconstr Surg 51:76–81, 1973.
26. Aguayo AJ, Karpati G: Current topics in nerve and muscle research. In Aguayo AJ, Carpati G, eds: Excerpta Medica, Amsterdam, 1979.
27. Arnason BGW: Idiopathic polyneuritis and experimental allergic neuritis in comparison. In Rowland LP, ed: Immunological Disorders of the Nervous System, Vol. 49. Williams & Wilkins, Baltimore, 1971.
28. Arons MS: deQuervain's release in working women: A report of failures, complications and associated diagnoses. J Hand Surg [Am] 12:40–44, 1987.
29. Asbury AK: Renaut bodies—a forgotten endoneurial structure. J Neuropathol Exp Neurol 32:334–343, 1973.
30. Asbury AK, Aldredge H, Hirshberg R, Fisher CM: Oculomotor palsy in diabetes mellitus: A clinicopathological study. Brain 93:555–560, 1970.
31. Asbury AK, Brown MJ: The evolution of structural changes in distal axonopathies. In Spencer PS, Schaumberg HH, (eds) Experimental and Clinical Neurotoxicology. Williams & Wilkins, Baltimore, 1980, p 179.
32. Ash EN, Hurst EM: Anatomical factors in etiology of ulnar neuropathy. Can Med Assoc J 87:159–163, 1962.
33. Assaky G: Du la suture des nerfs a distence. Arch Gen Med 17:529–553, 1886.
34. Auger RG, Piepgras DG, Laws ER, Miller RH: Microvascular decompression of the facial nerve for hemifacial spasm. Clinical and electrophysiological observations. Neurology (NY) 31:346–350, 1981.
35. Axer A, Segal D, Elbson S: Partial transplantation of the latissimus dorsi. J Bone Joint Surg [Am] 55:1259–1264, 1973.
36. Babcock WW: A standard technique for operations on peripheral nerves, with a special reference to the closure of large gaps. Surg Gynecol Obstet 45:364–378, 1927.
37. Babcock WW: Nerve disassociation; a new method for the surgical release of certain painful or paralytic afflictions of nerve trunks. Ann Surg 46:686–693, 1907.
38. Backhouse KM, Church-Davidson D: Anomalous palmaris longus muscle producing carpal tunnel-like compression. Hand 7:22–24, 1975.
39. Baird DB, Fredenberg ZB: Delayed ulnar nerve palsy following a fracture of the hamate. J Bone Joint Surg 50A:570, 1968.
40. Baker DC, Conley J: Facial nerve grafting: A thirty year retrospective review. Clin Plast Surg 6:343–360, 1979.
41. Bakke JL, Wolff HG: Occupational pressure neuritis of the deep palmar branch of the ulnar nerve. Arch Neurol Psychiatry 60:549–555, 1948.
42. Barba GE: Burning foot syndrome: Bilateral occurrence with radical cure. Med J Aust 1:764–65, 1965.
43. Barber LM: Desensitization of the traumatized hand. In Hunter, JM, Schneider LH, Mackin EJ, Callahan AD, eds: Rehabilitation of the Hand. CV Mosby Co., St. Louis, 1984, pp 493–502.
44. Bardosi A, Goebel HH, Stennert E: The ultrastructure of normal and denervated human facial muscle. Plast Reconstr Surg 79:171–176, 1987.
45. Barfred T, Hojlund AP, Bertheussen K: Median artery in carpal tunnel syndrome. J Hand Surg [Am] 10:864–867, 1985.
46. Barker NW, Hines ES Jr: Arterial occlusion in the hands and fingers associated with occupational trauma. Proc Staff Meet Mayo Clinic 19:345–349, 1944.
47. Barnard LB, McCoy SM: The supercondyloid process of the humerus. J Bone Joint Surg 28:845–850, 1946.
48. Barrett R, Cramer F: Tumours of the peripheral nerves and socalled ganglia of the peroneal nerve. Clin Orthop 27:135–146, 1963.
49. Bartlett SP, May JW Jr, Yaremchuk MJ: The latissimus dorsi muscle: A free cadaver study of the primary neurovascular pedicle. Plast Reconstr Surg 67:631, 1981.
50. Barton NJ: Radial nerve lesions. Hand 5:200–208, 1973.
51. Basmajian JE: Biofeedback—Principles of Practice for Clinicians. Williams & Wilkins, Baltimore, 1979.
52. Batt M, Griffet JE, Scotti LE, Bas P: Thoracic outlet syndrome: Report of 112 cases toward a more defined tactical approach (translation from French) J Chir (Paris) 120:687–691, 1983.
53. Battista AF, Cravioto HM, Budzilovich GN: Painful neuroma: Changes produced in peripheral nerve after fascicle ligation. Neurosurgery 9:589–600, 1981.
54. Beazley WC, Milek MA, Reiss BH: Results of nerve grafting in severe soft tissue injuries. Clin Orthop 188:208–212, 1984.
55. Behan PO, Currie S: In Behan PO, Currie S, eds: Clinical Neuroimmunology. WB Saunders, London, 1978.
56. Bell C: On the nerves giving an account of some experiments on their structure and functions, which leads to a new arrangement of the system. Trans Soc Lond 3:398, 1821.
57. Bell GE Jr, Goldner JL: Compression neuropathy of the median nerve. South Med J 49:966–972, 1956.
58. Bennett A: In Turner PW, Syhand DG, eds: Prostaglangins. Churchill Livingstone, Edinburgh, 1979, pp 17–30.
59. Bennett A, Harvey W: Prostaglandins in orthopedics. J Bone Joint Surg 63:152–154, 1981.
60. Bennett JB, Crouch CC: Compression syndrome of the recurrent branch of the median nerve. J Hand Surg 7:407–409, 1982.
61. Benoit BG, Preston DN, Atack DM, Da Silva VF: Neurolysis combined with the application of a Silastic envelope for ulnar nerve entrapment at the elbow. Neurosurgery 20:594–598, 1987.
62. Berger A, Meissl G: Innervated skin grafts and flaps for restoration of sensation to anesthetic areas. Chir Plast 3:33–37, 1975.
63. Bergouignan FX, Vital C: Occurrence of Renaut bodies in a peripheral nerve. Arch Pathol Lab Med 108:230–233, 1984.
64. Berry H, Richardson PM: Common peroneal nerve palsy: A clinical and electrophysiological review. J Neurol Neurosurg Psychiatry 39:1162–1171, 1962.
65. Betts LO: Morton's metatarsalgia: Neuritis of the fourth digital nerve. Med J Aust 1:514–515, 1940.

66. Bierman HR: Nerve compression due to a tight watch band. N Engl J Med 261:237–238, 1959.
67. Bisby MA, Keen P: The effect of a conditioning lesion on the regeneration rate of peripheral nerve axons containing substance P. Brain Res 336:201–206, 1985.
68. Biom S, Dahlback LO: Nerve injuries in dislocations of the shoulder joint and fractures of the neck of the humerus. A clinical and electromyographical study. Acta Chir Scand 136:461–466, 1970.
69. Black IB: Growth and development of cholinergic and adronergic neurons in a sympathetic ganglion. In Fuxe K, Olson L, Zotterman Y, eds: Dynamics of Degeneration in Growth in Neurons. Proceedings of the International Symposium, Stockholm, May, 1973. Pergamon Press, New York, 1974, pp 455–467.
70. Bland JH, Nakano KK: Neck Pain. In Edgar S, Kelly WN, Harris ED, Ruddy S, Sledge CCB, Textbook of Rheumatology. WB Saunders, Philadelphia, 1981, pp 411–446.
71. Bleecker ML, Bohlman M, Moreland R, Tipton A: Carpal tunnel syndrome: Role of carpal canal size. Neurology (Cleve) 35:1599–1604, 1985.
72. Blumpber H, Janig W: In Seigfried J, Simmerman M, eds: Phantom and Stump Pain. Springer-Verlag, Berlin, 1981, pp 15–31.
73. Blunder R: Neuritis of the deep branch of the ulnar nerve. J Bone Joint Surg 40B:354, (Abstr.) 1958.
74. Blunt MJ: The vascular anatomy of the median nerve in the forearm and hand. J Anat 93:15–22, 1959.
75. Bodian D, Howe HA: Experimental studies of intraneural spread of poliomyelitis virus. Bull Johns Hopkins Hosp 68:248–267, 1941.
76. Bodian D, Howe HA: The rate of progression of poliomyelitis virus in nerve. Bull Johns Hopkins Hosp 69: 79–85, 1941.
77. Bolande RP: Neurofibromatosis—the quintessential neurocristopathy. Adv Neurol 29:67–75, 1981.
78. Boldney E: Amputation neuroma in nerves implanted in bone. Ann Surg 118:1052–1057, 1943.
79. Bolton CF, MacFarland RM: Human pneumatic tourniquet paralysis. Neurology (NY) 28:787–793, 1978.
80. Bonica JJ, Liebskind JC, Alke-Fessaid DG, eds: Adv Pain Res Ther 3: 1979.
81. Bonney, G: Prognosis in traction regions of the brachial plexus. J Bone Joint Surg 41B:4–35, 1959.
82. Bonney G, Birch R, Jamieson AM, Eames RA: Experience with vascularized nerve grafts. In Terzis JK, ed: Microreconstruction of Nerve Injuries. W B Saunders, Philadelphia, 1986, pp 403–414.
83. Bora FW: Peripheral nerve repair in cats. The fascicular stitch. J Bone Joint Surg 49A:659–666, 1967.
84. Bora FW, Brown MJ, Summer AJ: Prosthetic nerve grafts. The use of a resorbable tube as an alternative to autogenous nerve grafting. Presented at the 41st Annual Meeting of the American Society for Surgery of the Hand, New Orleans, September, 1986.
85. Bora FW, Pleasure DE, Didizian NA: A study of nerve regeneration and neuroma formation after nerve suture by various techniques. J Hand Surg 1:138–143, 1976.
86. Borges LF, Hallett M, Selkoe DJ, Welch K: The anterior tarsal tunnel syndrome. J Neurosurg 54:89–92, 1981.
87. Boswick JA, Schneewind J, Stromberg W: Evaluation of peripheral nerve repairs above the elbow. Arch Surg 90:50–51, 1965.
88. Bowen TL, Stone KH: Posterior interosseous nerve paralysis caused by a ganglion at the elbow. J Bone Joint Surg 48B:774–776, 1966.
89. Boyes JH: On The Shoulder of Giants: Notable Names in Hand Surgery. JB Lippincott, Philadelphia, 1976, pp 103–105.
90. Braidwood AS: Superficial radial neuropathy. J Bone Joint Surg 57B:380–383, 1975.
91. Bramwell E: Lesion of the first dorsal nerve root. Rev Neurol Psychiatr 1:299, 1903.
92. Braun R: Comparative studies of neurorrhaphy and sutureless peripheral nerve repair. Surg Gynecol Obstet 120:15, 1966.
93. Braun RM, Newman J, Thatcher B: Injury to the brachial plexus as a result of diagnostic arteriography. J Hand Surg 3:90–94, 1978.
94. Breidenbach WC, Terzis JK: The blood supply of vascularized nerve grafts. J Reconstr Microsurg 3:43–56, 1986.
95. Breidenbach W, Tsai T, Manstein C: Ipsilateral pronator teres and carpal tunnel compression of the median nerve. (Abstr.) J Hand Surg [Am] 10:432, (Proc, Abstr), 1985.
96. Brismar T, Tegner R: Experimental uremic neuropathy. Part II (Sodium permeability decrease and inactivation in potential clamped nerve fibers). J Neurol Sci 65:37–45, 1984.
97. Broadbent TR, Odom GL, Woodhall B: Peripheral nerve injuries in the administration of penicillin. Report of four clinical cases. JAMA 140:1008–1010, 1949.
98. Broca A, Mouchet A: Complications nervuses des fractures de l'extermite inferieure de l'humerus. Rev Chir (Paris) 19:701, 1899.
99. Brock AJ: Greek Medicine. JM Dent & Sons, New York, 1929.
100. Brones MF, Wilgis EFS: Anatomical variations of the palmaris longus, causing carpal tunnel syndrome. Plast Reconstr Surg 62:798–800, 1978.
101. Brooks D: The place of nerve grafting in orthopedic surgery. J Bone Joint Surg 37A:299–326, 1955.
102. Brook DM: Editorial. J Bone Joint Surg 32B:291–292, 1950.
103. Brooks DM: Nerve compression by simple ganglia. J Bone Joint Surg 34B:391–400, 1952.
104. Brooks DM, Seddon HJ: Pectoral transplantation for paralysis of the flexions of the elbow a new technique. J Bone Jt Surg [Br] 41:36–50, 1959.
105. Broudy AS, Leffert RD, Smith RJ: Technical problems with ulnar nerve transposition at the elbow: findings and results of reoperation. J Hand Surg 3:85–89, 1978.
106. Brown DM, Nahai F, Wolf S, Basmajian JV: Electromyographic biofeedback in the re-education of facial palsy. Am J Phys Med 57:183–190, 1978.
107. Brown HA: Internal neurolysis in the treatment of peripheral nerve injuries. Clin Neurosurg 17:99–107, 1970.
108. Brown H, Flynn JE: Abdominal pedicle flap for hand neuromas and entrapped nerves. J Bone Joint Surg 55A: 875, 1973.

109. Brown MJ, Somner AJ, Greene DA, Diamond SM, Asbury AK: Distal neuropathy in experimental diabetes mellitus. Ann Neurol 8:168–178, 1980.
110. Brown PW: The time factor in surgery of upper extremity peripheral nerve injury. Clin Orthop 68:14, 1970.
111. Brown WF, Ferguson GG, Jones MW, Yates SK: The location of conduction abnormalities on human entrapment neuropathies. J Can Sci Neurol 3:111–114, 1976.
112. Brown WF, Yates SK: Percutaneous localization of conduction abnormalities in human extremities. Can J Neurol Sci 9:391–400, 1982.
113. Brunelli, G: Neurotization of avulsed roots of brachial plexus of nerve of cervical plexus. Oberval Ed, New Techniques in Microsurgery, 1979, pp 145–148.
114. Brunelli G: Neurotization of avulsed roots of the brachial plexus by means of anterior nerves of the cervical plexus. In Microreconstruction of Nerve Injuries, WB Saunders, Philadelphia, 1987, pp 435–446.
115. Brushart TM: The central course of primate digital nerve axons. American Society for Surgery of the Hand, Scientific Session, 1985.
116. Brushart TM, Seiler WA: Selective reinnervation of distal motor stumps by peripheral motor axons. Exp Neurol 97:289–300, 1987.
117. Brushart TM, Henry EW, Mesulam M: Reorganization of muscle afferent projections accompanies peripheral nerve regeneration. Neuroscience 6:2053–2061, 1981.
118. Brushart TM, Mesulam MM: Alteration in connections between muscle and anterior horn motoneurons after peripheral nerve repair. Science 208:603–605, 1980.
119. Brushart TM, Tarlov E, Mesulam MM: A comparison of motor neuron pool organization after epineurial and perineurial repair of the rat sciatic nerve. Orthop Trans 4:19–20, 1980.
120. Brushart TM: Experiments on the mechanism of preferential motor reinnervation. American Society for Surgery of the Hand, Scientific Session 1988.
121. Bryan FS, Miller LS, Panijaganond P: Spontaneous paralysis of the posterior interosseous nerve. A case report and review of the literature. Clin Orthop 80:9–12, 1971.
122. Bryce TH: The long muscular branch of the musculocutaneous nerve of the leg. J Anat 31:5–12, 1896.
123. Buchthal F, Rosenthalk A, Trojaborg W: Electrophysiological findings in entrapment of the median nerve at the wrist and elbow. J Neurol Neurosurg Psychiatry 37:340–360, 1974.
124. Buncke HJ: Digital nerve repairs. Surg Clin North Am 52:1267–1285, 1972.
125. Bunnell S: Surgery of the nerves of the hand. Surg Gynecol Obstet 44:145–152, 1927.
126. Bunnell S: Suture of the facial nerve within the temporal bone with a report of the first successful case. Surg Gynecol Obstet 45:7–12, 1927.
127. Bunnell S: Repair of nerves and tendons of the hand. J Bone Joint Surg 10:1–16, 1928.
128. Bunnell S, Boyes JH: Nerve grafts. Am J Surg 44:64–75, 1939.
129. Burkhardt FL, Daly JW: Sciatic and peroneal nerve injury: A complication of vaginal operations. Obstet Gynecol 28:99–101, 1966.
130. Butler ED, Hamill JP, Seipel RS, et al: Tumours of the hand. Am J Surg 100:293–303, 1960.
131. Byers CM, Delisa JA, Frankel DL, Kraft GH: Pyridoxine metabolism in carpal tunnel syndrome with and without peripheral neuropathy. Arch Phys Med Rehabil 65: 712–716, 1984.
132. Byrd JW, Ricciardi JM, Jun BI: Regional migratory osteoporosis in tarsal tunnel syndrome. Clin Orthop 157: 164–169, 1981.
133. Calder FWG: Effects of a division of the ulnar nerve. Lancet 1:489–490, 1833.
134. Campbell JB, Bassett CA, Girado JM, et al: Application of monomolecular filter tubes in bridging gaps in peripheral nerves and for prevention of neuroma formation. A preliminary report. J Neurosurg 13:635, 1956.
135. Campbell JB, Post KD, Marantz RA: A technique for relief of motor and sensory deficits occurring after anterior ulnar transposition. J Neurosurg 40:405–409, 1974.
136. Campbell JN, Raja SN, Meyer RA, Mackinnon SE: Myelinated fibres in peripheral nerves signal hyperalgesia that follows nerve injury. Pain, 32:89–94, 1988.
137. Cancilla PA: General reactions of muscle to injury. In Heffner RR, ed: Muscle Pathology. Contemporary Issues in Surgical Pathology. Churchill Livingstone, New York, 1984, pp 15–30.
138. Cannieu JMA: Recherches sur une anastomse. Entra la branche profnude du cubitale et le median. Bull Soc Anat Physiol Bordeaux 18:339–340, 1897.
139. Cannon BW, Love JG: Tardy median nerve palsy: median neuritis amenable to surgery. Surgery 20:210–216, 1946.
140. Capener N: Posterior interosseous nerve lesions. Proceedings of the Second Hand Club. J Bone Joint Surg 46B:361, 1964.
141. Capener N: The vulnerability of the posterior interosseous nerve of the forearm. J Bone Joint Surg 48B: 770–773, 1966.
142. Carayon A: Investigations on physiopathology of the nerve in leprosy. Int J Leprosy 81:278–294, 1971.
143. Carlton JM, Goldberg N: Quantitating integrated muscle function following reinnervation. Surg Forum 37:611–612, 1986.
144. Carroll RE, Hurst LC: The relationship of thoracic outlet syndrome and carpal tunnel syndrome. Clin Orthop Rel Res 164:149–153, 1982.
145. Carroll RE, Kleinman WB: Pectoralis major transplantation to restore elbow flexion to the paralytic limb. J Hand Surg 4:501–507, 1978.
146. Cavanagh JB: The dying back process. A common denominator in many naturally occurring and toxic neuropathies. Arch Pathol Lab Med 103:659–664, 1979.
147. Cavanagh JB: The significance of the "dying back" process in experimental and human neurologic disease. Int Rev Exp Pathol 3:219–267, 1964.
148. Chabaud HE, Rodkey WG, McCarroll HR, et al: Epineurial and perineurial fascicular nerve repairs. A critical comparison. J Hand Surg 1:131–137, 1976.

149. Chabaud HE, Rodkey WG, McCarrol HR: Peripheral nerve injuries. Studies in higher nonhuman primates. J Hand Surg 5:201–206, 1980.
150. Chaise F, Roger B: Neurolysis of the common peroneal nerve in leprosy. J Bone Joint Surg 67B:426–429, 1985.
151. Chan RC, Paine KW, Varughese G: Ulnar nerve at the elbow: Comparison of subcutaneous decompression and anterior transposition. Neurosurgery 7:545–550, 1980.
152. Chang KSF, Low WD, Chan ST: Enlargement of the ulnar nerve behind the medial humeral epicondyle. Anat Rec 145:149–153, 1963.
153. Chapman DR, Bennett JB, Bryan WJ, Tullos HS: Complications of distal radial fractures: Pins and plaster treatment. J Hand Surg 7:509–512, 1982.
154. Guy de Chauliac on wounds and fractures (translated by W.A. Brennan), W.A. Brennan, Chicago, 1923.
155. Checkles NS, Russakov AD, Pareo DL: Ulnar nerve conduction velocity: Effect of elbow position on the measurement. Arch Phys Med Rehabil 52:362–365, 1971.
156. Chen ZW, Yu HL: Lower limb replantation. In Urbaniak JR, ed: Microsurgery for Major Limb Reconstruction. CV Mosby, Co, St. Louis, pp 67–73, 1987.
157. Childress HM: Recurrent ulnar nerve dislocation at the elbow. J Bone Joint Surg 38A:978–984, 1956.
158. Chisholm CD, Clark DE: Effect of pneumatic antishock garment on intramuscular pressure. Ann Emerg Med 13:8, 1984.
159. Chiu DTW, Janecka I, Krizek TJ, et al: Autogenous vein graft as a conduit for nerve regeneration. Surgery 91: 226, 1982.
160. Chow JA, Sunderland S, Van Beek AL: Surgical significance of the motor fascicular group of the ulnar nerve in the forearm. J Hand Surg [Am] 9:605, 1985.
161. Chusid JG: Yoga foot drop. JAMA 217:827–828, 1971.
162. Creuz KA, Thomas JE, Lambert EH, Love JG, Lipscomb PR: Long-term results of operation for carpal tunnel syndrome. Mayo Clin Proc 41:232–241, 1966.
163. Clagett OT: Presidential Address: Amer Thorac Surg, Research and Prosearch. J Thorac Cardiovasc Surg 44: 153–166, 1962.
164. Clark AW, Griffin JW, Price DL: The axonal pathology in chronic IDPN intoxification. J Neuropath Exp Neurol 39:42–55, 1980.
165. Clark CB: Cubital tunnel syndrome. JAMA 241:801–802, 1979.
166. Clark JMP: Reconstruction of biceps brachii by pectoralis muscle transplantation. Br J Surg 34:180, 1946.
167. Clark K, Williams PE Jr, Willis W, McGavran WL III: Injection injury of the sciatic nerve. Clin Neurosurg 8:17:111–125, 1970.
168. Clark LP, Taylor AS, Prout P: Study on brachial birth palsy. Am J Med Sci 130:670, 1905.
169. Clarke SA, Allard T, Jenkins WM, Merzenich MM: Receptive fields in the body-surface map in adult cortex defined by temporally correlated inputs. Nature 332:444, 1988.
170. Clarke E, Bearn JG: The spiral bands of Fontana. Brain 95:1, 1972.
171. Clawson DK, Seddon HJ: The late consequences of sciatic nerve injury. J Bone Joint Surg 42B:213, 1960.
172. Clawson DK, Seddon HJ: The results of repair of the sciatic nerve. J Bone Joint Surg 42B:205, 1960.
173. Clayburgh RH, Beckenbaugh RD, Dobyns JH: Carpal tunnel release in patients with diffuse peripheral neuropathy. J Hand Surg [Am] 12A:380–383, 1987.
174. Clodius L, Uhlshmid G, Hess K: Irradiation plexitis of the brachial plexus. Clin Plast Surg 11:161–165, 1984.
175. Cohen DJ, Loertscher R, Rubin MF, Tilney NL, Carpenter CB, Strom TB: Cyclosporine: A new immunosuppressive agent for organ transplantation. Ann Intern Med 101:677–682, 1984.
176. Collin W, Donoff RB: Nerve regeneration through collagen tubes. J Dent Res 63:987–993, 1984.
177. Converse JM: In Kazanjian and Converse JM, eds Surgical Treatment of Facial Injuries, 3rd ed, Williams & Wilkins, Baltimore, 1974, pp 1235–1288.
178. Coote H: Pressure on the axillary vessels and nerve by an exostosis from a cervical rib: interference with the circulation of the arm. Removal of rib and exostosis: recovery. Med Times Gaz 2:108, 1861.
179. Cornblath DR, Dellon AL, Mackinnon SE: Electrodiagnostic evaluation of peripheral nerves in Type I diabetic primate. Muscle or Nerve, 1988. In press.
180. Corradi M, Mandrioli R, Rinaldi E, Ugolotti U: La sindrome dell "uncinato. Riv Chir Mano 20:445–449, 1983.
181. Cosh JA: Studies on the nature of vibration sense. Clin Sci 12:131, 1953.
182. Costigan DG, Riley JM, Coy FE: Thrombofibrosis of the ulnar artery in the palm. J Bone Joint Surg 41A:702–704, 1959.
183. Courvoisier LG: Dei Neurome. Eine klinische Monographie. B. Schwode, Basel, 1886.
184. Couse WP: Epicondylitis (Franke) or tennis elbow. Boston Med Surg J 170:461, 1914.
185. Cragg C: Isolated paralysis of the flexor pollicis muscle. An unusual variation of the anterior interosseous nerve syndrome. Case report. Scand J Plast Reconstr Surg 8: 250–252, 1974.
186. Craven RR, Green DP: Cubital tunnel syndrome: Treatment by medial epicondylectomy. J Bone Joint Surg 62A:986–990, 1980.
187. Crow RS: Treatment of the carpal tunnel syndrome. Br Med J 1:1611–1615, 1960.
188. Crumley R: Spatial anatomy of facial nerve fibers—a preliminary report. Laryngoscope 90:274, 1980.
189. Cseuze KA, Thomas JE, Lambert EH, Love JG, Lipscomb PR: Long-term results of operation for carpal tunnel syndrome. Mayo Clin Proc 41:232–241, 1966.
190. Cuadros CL: Nerve regeneration through a synthetic microporous tube (expanded polytetrafluoroethylene) experimental study in sciatic nerve of the rabbit. Microsurgery 8:41–46, 1987.
191. Cuello AC, Delfiacco MD, Paxinos G: The central and peripheral ends of substance P containing sensory neurons in the rat trigeminal system. Brain Res 152:499–500, 1978.
192. Culver JE: Compression neuropathy at the elbow treated by medial humeral epicondylectomy. Long term follow-up. J Bone Joint Surg. In press.

193. Curtis BF: Traumatic ulnar neuritis—transplantation of the nerve. J Nerv Ment Dis 25:480–481, 1898.
194. Curtis RM: Fundamental principles of tendon transfer. Orthop. Clinics N Amer 5:231–242, 1974.
195. Curtis RM, Eversmann WW Jr: Internal neurolysis as an adjunct to the treatment of the carpal tunnel syndrome. J Bone Joint Surg 55A:733–740, 1973.
196. Dahlin LB, Meiri KF, McEan WG, Rydevik B, Sjostind J: Effects of nerve compression on fast axonal transport and Streptozotocin-induced diabetes mellitus. Diabetologia 29:181–185, 1986.
197. Dart L, MacCarty CS, Love JG, et al: Neoplasms of the brachial plexus. Minn Med 53:959–964, 1970.
198. Das SK, Brown GH: In search of complications in carpal tunnel decompression. Hand 8:243–249, 1976.
199. Davidson AJ, Horowitz MT: Late or tardy ulnar paralysis. J Bone Joint Surg 17:844–856, 1935.
200. Davidson JK, ed: Clinical Diabetes Mellitus. NY, Thieme, New York, 1986, p xvii.
201. Davidson MB: Diabetes Mellitus: Diagnosis and Treatment, 2nd ed. NY, John Wiley & Sons, 1986, p x.
202. Davies F, Laird M: The supinator muscle in the deep radial (posterior interosseous) nerve. Anat Rec 101: 243–250, 1948.
203. Davis L: The return of sensation to transplanted skin. Surg Gynecol Obstet 59:533–543, 1934.
204. Davis L, Cleveland DA: Experimental studies in nerve transplants. Ann Surg 99:271–283, 1934.
205. Davis L, Martin J, Perret G.: The treatment of injuries of the brachial plexus. Ann Surg 125:647, 1947.
206. Davis RA, Anson BJ, Puddinger JM, Kurth RE: Surgical anatomy of the facial nerve and parotid gland based upon study of 350 cervical facial halves. Surg Gynecol Obstet 102:385–412, 1956.
207. Merle D'Aubigne RN, Deburge A: Etiologie evolution et pronostic des paralysies traumatiques du plexus brachial. Rev Chir Orthop 53:23, 1967.
208. Dawson DM, Hallett M, Millender LH: Entrapment Neuropathies. Little, Brown & Co, Boston, 1983.
209. DeAndrade Jr, Casagrende PA: Ulnar nerve entrapment in rheumatoid arthritis. Arthritis Rheum 8:294–301, 1965.
210. De Jesus PV, Stiner JC: Spontaneous recovery of ulnar neuropathy at the elbow. Electromyogr Clin Neurophysiol 16:239–248, 1976.
211. Dekel S, Lenthall G, Francis MJO: Release of prostaglandins from bone and muscle after tibial fracture: An experimental study in rabbits. J Bone Joint Surg (Br) 63B:185–189, 1981.
212. Delageniere H: A contribution to the study of the surgical repair of peripheral nerves based on 375 cases. Surg Gynecol Obstet 39:543–553, 1924.
213. Delagi EF: Electrodiagnosis in peripheral lesions. Ch 3 in Omer GE Jr, Spinner M, eds: Management of Peripheral Nerve Problems. WB Saunders, Co, Philadelphia, 1980.
214. Dell PC: Compression of the ulnar nerve at the wrist secondary to rheumatoid synovial cyst: Case report and review of literature. J Hand Surg 4:468–473, 1979.
215. Dellon AL: A cause for optimism in diabetic neuropathy. Ann Plast Surg 20:103–105, 1988.
216. Dellon AL: Clinical use of vibratory stimuli to evaluate peripheral nerve injury and compression neuropathy. Plast Reconstr Surg 65:466–476, 1980.
217. Dellon AL: Evaluation of Sensibility and Re-education of Sensation in the Hand. Williams & Wilkins, Co, Baltimore, 1981.
218. Dellon AL: Interruption of nerve function. In Current Therapy in Plastic and Reconstructive Surgery. (ed) Marsh J, BC Becker Inc, Toronto, 1988.
219. Dellon AL: Musculotendinous variations about the medial humeral epicondyle. J Hand Surg [Br] 11:175–181, 1986.
220. Dellon AL: Operative technique for submuscular transposition of the ulnar nerve. Contemp Orthop. 16:17—24, 1988.
221. Dellon AL: Partial dorsal wrist denervation: Resection of posterior interosseous nerve. J Hand Surg [Am] 10: 527–533, 1985.
222. Dellon AL: Peripheral New Injuries. In Surgical Emergencies, eds Gardner B, Shaftan GW, eds: JB Lippincott, Philadelphia, 1986, pp 533–537.
223. Dellon AL: Reinnervation of denervated Meissner corpuscles. A sequential histological study in primates following interfascicular nerve repair. J Hand Surg [Am] 1:98–109, 1976.
224. Dellon AL: Sensory recovery in replanted digits and transplanted toes. A review. J Reconstr Microsurg 2: 123—129, 1986.
225. Dellon AL: The moving two-point discrimination test; clinical evaluation of the quickly-adapting fiber receptor system. J Hand Surg 3:474–481, 1978.
226. Dellon AL: Tinel or not Tinel? J Hand Surg [Br] 9:216, 1984.
227. Dellon AL: The Vibrometer. Plast Reconstr Surg 71:427–431, 1983.
228. Dellon AL, Curtis RM, Edgerton MT: Evaluating recovery of sensation in the hand following nerve injury. Johns Hopkins Med J 130:235–243, 1972.
229. Dellon AL, Curtis RM, Edgerton MT: Re-education of sensation in the hand following nerve injury. (Abstr.) J Bone Joint Surg 53A:813, 1971.
230. Dellon AL, Curtis RM, Edgerton MT: Re-education of sensation in the hand following nerve injury. Plast Reconstr Surg 53:297–305, 1974.
231. Dellon AL, Hendler N, Hopkins JET, Karas AC, Campbell JN: Team management of patients with diffuse upper extremity complaints. Md Med J 35:849–852, 1986.
232. Dellon AL, Kallman CM: Evaluation of functional sensation in the hand. J Hand Surg 8:865–870, 1983.
233. Dellon AL, Mackinnon SE: Anatomic investigations of nerves at the wrist: II. Instance of fibrous arch overlying the motor branch of the ulnar nerve. Ann Plast Surg. 21:36–37, 1988.
234. Dellon AL, Mackinnon SE: Terminal branches of anterior interosseous nerve as source of volar wrist pain. J Hand Surg 9B:316—322, 1984.
235. Dellon AL, Mackinnon SE: Basic scientific and clinical applications of peipheral nerve regeneration. In Nyhus LM, ed: Surgery Annual. Appleton, Lange, Norwich, Conn., pp 81–83, 1988.
236. Dellon AL, Mackinnon SE: Evaluation of musculoten-

dinous variations about the median nerve in forearm. J Hand Surg (Br) 12A:359–365, 1987.
237. Dellon AL, Mackinnon SE: Gentle passage of nerve grafts. J Hand Surg 8:108–109, 1983.
238. Dellon AL, Mackinnon SE: Human ulnar nerve compression at the elbow: Clinical, histologic and electrodiagnostic correlations. J Reconstr Microsurg, 4:179–187, 1988.
239. Dellon AL, Mackinnon SE: Injury to the medial antebrachial cutaneous nerve during cubital tunnel surgery. J Hand Surg [Br] 10:33–36, 1985.
240. Dellon AL, Mackinnon SE: Musculoaponeurotic variations along the course of the median nerve in the proximal forearm. J Hand Surg [Br] 12:359–363, 1987.
241. Dellon AL, Mackinnon SE: Pain after radial sensory nerve grafting. J Hand Surg [Br] 11:341–346, 1986.
242. Dellon AL, Mackinnon SE: Radial sensory nerve entrapment. Arch Neurol 43:833–837, 1986.
243. Dellon AL, Mackinnon SE: Radial-sensory nerve entrapment in the forearm. J Hand Surg 11A:199–205, 1986.
244. Dellon AL, Mackinnon SE: Segmentally innervated latissimus dorsi muscle: Microsurgical transfer for facial reanimation. J Reconstr Microsurg 2:7–12, 1985.
245. Dellon AL, Mackinnon SE: Susceptibility of the superficial sensory branch of the radial nerve to form painful neuromas. J Hand Surg [Br] 9:42–45, 1984.
246. Dellon AL, Mackinnon SE: The pronator quadratus muscle flap. J Hand Surg [Am] 9:423–427, 1984.
247. Dellon AL, Mackinnon SE: Tibial nerve branching in the tarsal tunnel. Arch Neurol 41:645–646, 1984.
248. Dellon AL, Mackinnon SE: Treatment of the painful neuroma by neuroma resection and muscle implantation. Plast Reconstr Surg 77:427–436, 1986.
249. Dellon AL, Mackinnon SE, Crosby PM: Reliability of two-point discrimination measurements. J Hand Surg, 12A:693–696, 1987.
250. Dellon AL, Mackinnon SE, Daneshvar A: Terminal branch of anterior interosseous nerve as source of wrist pain. J Hand Surg [Br] 9:316–322, 1984.
251. Dellon AL, Mackinnon SE, Hudson AR, Hunter DA: Effect of submuscular versus intramuscular placement of the ulnar nerve: An experimental model in the primate. J Hand Surg 11B:117–119, 1986.
252. Dellon AL, Mackinnon SE, Pestronk A: Implantation of sensory nerve into muscle: Preliminary, clinical and experimental observations on neuroma formation. Ann Plast Surg 12:30–40, 1984.
253. Dellon AL, Mackinnon SE, Schlegel R: Validity of electrodiagnostic studies following anterior transposition of the ulnar nerve. J Hand Surg 12A:700–703, 1987.
254. Dellon AL, Mackinnon SE, Seiler WA: Models for peripheral nerve research. In Adams RJ, Swindle MM, eds: Induced Animal Models of Human Disease. Williams & Wilkins, Baltimore, 1988.
255. Dellon AL, Mackinnon SE, Seiler WA IV: Susceptibility of diabetic nerve to chronic compression. Ann Plast Surg, 20:117–119, 1988.
256. Dellon AL, Schlegel RW, Mackinnon SE: Validity of nerve conduction velocity studies following anterior transposition of the ulnar nerve. J Hand Surg, 12A:700–703, 1987.
257. Dellon AL, Schneider R, Burke R: Effect of acute compartmental changes upon response to vibratory stimuli. Plast Reconstr Surg 72:208–216, 1983.
258. Dellon AL, Seiff SS: Neuroma of the posterior interosseous nerve simulating a recurrent ganglion: A case report and anatomical dissections relating the posterior interosseous nerve to the carpus. Etiology of dorsal ganglion pain. J Hand Surg 3:326–332, 1978.
259. Dellon AL, Witebsky FG, Terrill RE: The denervated Meissner corpuscle. A sequential histologic study following nerve division in the Rhesus monkey. Plast Reconstr Surg 56:182–193, 1975.
260. de Medinaceli L, Freed WJ, Wyatt RJ: An index of the functional condition of rat sciatic nerve based on measurements made from walking tracks. Exp Neurol 77:634–643, 1982.
261. Denny-Brown D, Brenner C: Division in peripheral nerve resulting from compression by a spring clip. Arch Neurol Psychiatry 52:1, 1944.
262. Denny-Brown D, Brenner C: Paralysis of nerve induced by direct pressure and by tourniquet. Arch Neurol Psychol 51:119, 1944.
263. deMaura W, Gilliert A: Surgical anatomy of the sural nerve. J Reconstr Microsurg 1:31–39, 1984.
264. Destot M: Paralaysie cebritale par l'usage de la bicyclette. Gaz Anaphitaux 69:1176–1177, 1896.
265. Dharapak C, Minberg GA: Posterior interosseous nerve compression. Report of a case caused by traumatic aneurysm. Clin Orthop 101:225–228, 1974.
266. Dhuner KG: Nerve injuries following operations: A survey of cases occurring during a six-year period. Anesthesiology 11:289–293, 1950.
267. Diamond C: Facial nerve. Hofstra University Press, New York, 1979.
268. Diamond ML, Lister GD: Cubital tunnel syndrome treated by long-arm splintage. (Abstr.) J Hand Surg [Am] 10:430, 1985.
269. Donoso RS, Ballantyne JP, Hansen S: Regeneration of sutured human peripheral nerves. An electrophysiological study. J Neurol Neurosurg Psychiatry 42:97–106, 1979.
270. Dorfman LJ, Jayram AR: Handcuff neuropathy. JAMA 239:957, 1978.
271. Doupe J, Cullen CH, Chance GQ: Posttraumatic pain and causalgia syndrome. J Neurol Neurosurg Psychiatry 7:332–348, 1944.
272. Dreyfus D, Kessler J: Snapping elbow due to dislocation of the medial head of the triceps. J Bone Joint Surg 60B:56–58, 1978.
273. Droz B, Leblond CP: Axonal migration of proteins in the central nervous system and peripheral nerves as shown by radio autography. J Comp Neurol 121:325, 1963.
274. Droz B, Leblond CP: Migration of proteins along the axons of the sciatic nerve. Science 137:1047, 1962.
275. Droz B, Rambourg A, Koenig HL: The smooth endoplastmic reticulum. Structure and role in the renewal of axonal membrane and synaptic vesicles by fast axonal transport. Brain Res 93:1–13, 1975.
276. Ducatman BS, Scheithauer BW, Piepgras DG, et al:

Malignant peripheral nerve tumours. Cancer 57:2006–2021, 1986.

277. Duchenne, GB: De l'electrisation localisee et de son application a la pathologie et a la therapeutique. 3rd ed, pp 357 Baillie re, Paris, 1872.

278. Ducker PB: The central cell body in axonal regeneration. In Gorio A, Millesi H, Mingrino S, eds: Posttraumatic Peripheral Nerve Regeneration. Raven Press, New York, 1981, pp 7–11.

279. Ducker TB: Pathophysiology of peripheral nerve trauma. In Omer GE, Spinner M, eds: Management of Peripheral Nerve Problems. WB Saunders, Philadelphia, 1980, p 476.

280. Dunn WA: Fractures and dislocations of the carpus. Surg Clin North Am 52:1513, 1972.

281. Dupont C, Cloutler GE, Prevost Y, Dion MA: Ulnar-tunnel syndrome at the wrist. J Bone Joint Surg 47A:757–761, 1965.

282. Dworkin RH, Handlin DS, Richlin DM: Unravelling the effects of compensation, litigation and employment on the treatment response in chronic pain. Pain 23:49, 1985.

283. Dyck PJ, Lais AC, Karnes JL, Sparks MS, Hunder H, Low PA, Windbank AG: Permanent axotomy, a model of axonal atrophy in secondary segmental demyelination and remyelination. Ann Neurol 9:575–583, 1981.

284. Dyck PJ, Thomas PK, Asbury AK, Winegrad AI, Porte D Jr: Diabetic Neuropathy. WB Saunders, Philadelphia, 1987, p 171.

285. Dyck PJ, Thomas PK, Lambert EH, Bunge R: Peripheral Neuropathy, Vol. 1 & 2: 2nd ed. WB Saunders, Philadelphia, 1984.

286. Dykes RW: Central consequences of peripheral nerve injuries. Ann Plast Surg 13:412–422, 1984.

287. Eames RA, Lange LS: Clinical and pathological study of ischemic neuropathy. J Neurol Neurosurg Psychiatry 30:215–226, 1967.

288. Earl CJ, Fullerton PM, Wakefield GS, Shutta HD: Hereditary neuropathy with liability to pressure palsies. QJ Med 33:41–98, 1964.

289. Earle H: Cases and observations illustrating the influence of the nervous system in regulating animal heat. Med Chir Trans 7:173–185, 1816.

290. Eaton RG, Crowe JF, Parkes JC III: Anterior transposition of the ulnar nerve with a non-compressing fasciodermal sling. J Bone Joint Surg 62A:820–825, 1980.

291. Eaton RP: The collagen hydration hypothesis: A new paradym for the secondary complications of diabetes mellitus. J Chron Dis 39:763–766, 1986.

292. Ebeling P, Gilliatt RW, Thomas DK: A clinical and electrical study of ulnar nerve lesions in the hand. J Neurol Neurosurg Psychiatry 23:1–9, 1960.

293. Eckhoff NL: Tourniquet paralysis: A plea for the extended use of the pneumatic tourniquet. Lancet 2:343–345, 1931.

294. Eckman PB, Pearlstein G, Altorcchi PH: Ulnar neuropathy in bicycle riders. Arch Neurol 32:130–131, 1975.

295. Eden KC: The vascular complications of cervical ribs in first thoracic rib abnormalities. Br J Surg 27:111–139, 1939–40.

296. Edmonson AS, Crenshaw AH: Campbell's Operative Orthopedics. CV Mosby, St. Louis, 1980, p 383.

297. Edsage S: Peripheral nerve suture. A technique for improved intraneural topography. Acta Chir Scand (Suppl) 331:1–104, 1964.

298. Edstrom A, Hanson M: Retrograde axonal transport of proteins in vitro in frog sciatic nerves. Brain Res 61:311–320, 1973.

299. Edwards WG, Lincoln R, Bassett FH, Goldner JL: Tarsal tunnel syndrome. JAMA 207:716–720, 1969.

300. Ehrlich W, Dellon AL, Mackinnon SE: Cheiralgia paresthetica (entrapment of the radial sensory nerve). J Hand Surg [Am] 11:196–198, 1986.

301. Ehrlich H, Martin H: Schwannomas (neurilemmomas) in the head and neck. Surg Gynecol Obstet 76:577–583, 1943.

302. Eicken O, Carstam N, Eddland A: Anomalous distal branching of the median nerve. Scand J Plast Reconstr Surg 5:149–152, 1971.

303. Eisen A: Early diagnosis of ulnar nerve palsy: An electrophysiologic study. Neurology (Minneap) 24:256–262, 1974.

304. Eisen A, Dannen J: The mild cubital tunnel syndrome. Neurology (Minneap) 24:608–613, 1974.

305. Ekerot L: Post-anesthetic ulnar neuropathy at the elbow. Scand J Plast Reconstr Surg 11:225–229, 1977.

306. Ellis J, Folkers K, Levy M, Takemura K, Shizukuishi S, Ulrich R, Harrison P: Therapy with vitamin B_6 with and without surgery for treatment of patients having the idiopathic carpal tunnel syndrome. Res Commun Chem Pathol Pharmacol 33:331–344, 1981.

307. Ellis JM, Folkers K, Levy M, Shizukuishi S, Lewandowski J, Nishii S, Schubert HA, Ulrich R: Response of vitamin B-6 deficiency and the carpal tunnel syndrome to pyridoxine. Proc Natl Acad Sci USA 79:7494–7498, 1982.

308. El-Sharkawai AH, Fattah HA: Treatment of displaced supracondylar fractures of the humerus in children on full extension and supination. J Bone Joint Surg 47B:273–276, 1965.

309. Emery SE, Gifford JF: One hundred years of tennis elbow. Contemp Orthop 12:53–58, 1986.

310. Emmett AJJ: Lipomatous harmartoma of the median nerve in the palm. Br J Plast Surg 18:208–213, 1965.

311. Engel J, Ganel A, Melamed R, et al: Choline acetyltransferase for differentiation between human, motor and sensory nerve fibres. Ann Plast Surg 4:367–380, 1979.

312. Erb W: Uber eine eigenthumliche localisation von la hemengen im plexus brachialis verhandl. naturhist-med (Hiedelberg) 2:130, 1874.

313. Erdman WJ II: Electromyography and electrical testing in hand rehabilitation. In Hunter DA, Schneider R, Mackinnon SE: Rehabilitation of Hands. CV Mosby, St. Louis, 1984.

314. Evans JA: Reflex sympathetic dystrophy: Report on 57 cases. Ann Intern Med 26:417–426, 1947.

315. Evans LE, Campbell JB, Pinner-Poole B, Jenny J: Prevention of painful neuromas in horses. J Am Vet Med Assoc 153:313, 1968.

316. Eversmann WW Jr: Entrapment and Compression Neuropathies. In Green DP, ed: Operative Hand Surgery,

2nd ed, Churchill Livingston, Inc., New York, 1988, pp 1423–1478.
317. Eversmann WW Jr, Retsick JA: Intraoperative changes in motor nerve conduction latency in carpal tunnel syndrome. J Hand Surg 3:77–81, 1978.
318. Fachinelli A, Masquelet A, Restrepo J, Gilbert A: A vascularized sural nerve. Int J Microsurg 3:157, 1981.
319. Fahrer M, Millroy PJ: Ulnar compression neuropathy due to an anomalous abductor digiti minimi: Clinical and anatomic study. J Hand Surg 6:266, 1981.
320. Falconer MA, Weddell G: Costoclavicular compression of the subclavian artery and vein in relations to the scalenus anticus syndrome. Lancet 2:539–544, 1943.
321. Fannin TF: Local decompression in the treatment of ulnar nerve entrapment at the elbow. J R Col Surg Edinb 123:362–366, 1978.
322. Farber JS, Bryan RS: The anterior interosseous nerve syndrome. J Bone Joint Surg 58:521–523, 1968.
323. Farley HH: Treatment of painful stump neuroma. Minn Med 48:347, 1950.
324. Fasching MC, VanBeek AL: Monitoring muscle viability using M Waves. Plast Reconstr Surg 75:217–272, 1985.
325. Fatah MF: Palmaris profundus of Frohse and Frankel in association with carpal tunnel syndrome. J Hand Surg [Br] 9:142–144, 1984.
326. Fearn CB, D'a Goodfellow JW: Anterior interosseous nerve palsy. J Bone Joint Surg 47B:91–93, 1965.
327. Feindel W, Stratford J: The role of the cubital tunnel in tardy ulnar palsy. Can J Surg 1:287–300, 1958.
328. Fennay JB: Deep ulnar nerve paralysis resulting from an anatomical abnormality. J Bone Joint Surg 47A:1381, 1965.
329. Ferguson JA, Allen L: Complete medial dislocation of the knee joint with division of the common peroneal nerve. J Bone Joint Surg 21:1012–1014, 1939.
330. Ferrara G: Nuova Selva di Cirurgia Divisia in tre Parti Venice. S Combi. 1608.
331. Ferreira MC, Marchese AT, Spinno Y: Injectos transfacia les des nervios en al tratamiento de le paralysis facial observaciones iniciales. Chir Plat Ibero Lat Am 3:301, 1977.
332. Ferreira SH, Mondcada S, Vane JR: In Robinson JH, Vane JR, eds: Prostaglandins and Signs and Symptoms of Inflammation. Raven Press, New York, 1974.
333. Fierro B, Modica A, D'Arpa A, Santangelo R, Raimondo D: Analysis of F wave in metabolic neuropathies: A comparison study in uremic and diabetic patients. Acta Neurol Scand 75:179–185, 1987.
334. Fine EJ, Wongjirad C: The ulnar flexion maneuver. Muscle Nerve. 8:612 (Abstr) 1985.
335. Finkelstein H: Stenosing tendovaginitis at the radial styloid process. J Bone Joint Surg 12A:509–539, 1930.
336. Fisch U: Extracranial surgery for facial hyperkinesis. In May M, ed: The Facial Nerve. Thieme, New York, 1986, pp 509–523.
337. Fisher ER, Vusevski VD: Cytogenesis of Schwannomas (neurilemmomas) neurofibromas, dermatofibromas, and dermatofibrosarcomas as revealed by electron microscopy. Am J Clin Pathol 49:941–954, 1968.
338. Fissette J, Onkelinx A: Treatment of carpal tunnel syndrome. Comparative study with and without epineurolysis. Hand 11:206–210, 1979.
339. Flaubert, M: Memoire sur plusiers cas de luxation. Rep Gen Anat Physiol Pathol 3:55, 1827.
340. Flourens P: Experiences sur la reunion ou cicatrisation des plaies de la moelle epiniere et des nerfs. Ann Sci Nat 13:113–122, 1828.
341. Flynn JE, Flynn WF: Median and ulnar nerve injuries. Ann Surg 156:1002–1009, 1962.
342. Foerster O: Die therapie der Schuss Verletzungen der peripheren Nerven. In Lewandowski: Handbuch der Neurologie. Ergaenzungsband, Berlin, 1929, pp 1677–1691.
343. Fontana F: Taite sur le venin de la vipere sur la poisons, Americains, vol 2. Florence, 1798.
344. Forman DS, Wood DK, Desilva S: The rate of regeneration of sensory axons in transected rat sciatic nerve repaired with epineurial sutures. J Neurol Sci 44:55–59, 1979.
345. Forssman J: Ueber de Ursachen, welche die Wachstumstrichtung der peripheren Nervenfasern bei der Regeneration bestimmen. Beitr Pathol Anat 24:55, 1898.
346. Forster FM, Shields CD: Cortical sensory defects causing disability. Arch Phys Med Rehabil 40:56–61, 1959.
347. Foster RJ, Edshage S: Factors related to the outcome of surgically managed compressive ulnar neuropathy at the elbow level. J Hand Surg 6:181–192, 1981.
348. Foucher G, Schuind F, Merle M, Brunelli F: Fractures of the hook of the hamate. J Hand Surg [Br] 10:205–210, 1985.
349. Frackelton WH, Teasley JL, Tauras A: Neuromas in the hand treated by nerve transposition and silicone capping. J Bone Joint Surg 53A:813, 1971.
350. Frank DH, Robson MD: Unusual occurrence of chronic nerve compression syndromes at the wrists of thermally injured patients. Orthop Rev 8:180, 1979.
351. Frazier DM, Campbell IW, Ewing DJ, Clark BF: Mononeuropathy in diabetes mellitus. Diabetes 28:96–101, 1979.
352. Freeman BS: Facial Palsy. In Converse JM, ed: Reconstructive Plastic Surgery, 2nd ed. WB Saunders, Philadelphia, 1977, pp 1774–1868.
353. French JH: Post-injection sciatic nerve palsies in infants and children. J Pediatr 58:195–204, 1961.
354. Freshwater MF, Arons MS: The effects of various adjuncts on the surgical treatment of carpal tunnel syndrome secondary to chronic tenosynovitis. Plast Reconstr Surg 61:93–96, 1978.
355. Frey M, Gruber H, Havel M, Sterner E, Freilinger G: Experimental free-muscle transplantation with microneurovascular anastomoses. Plast Reconstr Surg 71:689, 1983.
356. Fröhse F, Frankel M: Die Muskeln des Menschlichen Armes. Bardeleben's Hendbuch der Anatomie des Menschlchen. Fisher, Jena, 1908.
357. Froment MJ: La paralysie de l'adductur du pouce et le signe de la prahnsion. Rev Neurol (Paris) 28:1236–1240, 1915.
358. Froimson AI, Zahraw IF: Treatment of compression neuropathy of the ulnar nerve at the elbow by epicon-

dylectomy and neurolysis. J Hand Surg 5:391–395, 1980.

359. Frykman G: Fracture of the distal radius including sequelae—shoulder-hand syndrome, disturbance of the distal radioulnar joint and impairment of nerve function. A clinical and experimental study. Acta Orthop Scand [Suppl] 108:1, 1967.
360. Fullerton PM, Gilliatt RW: Pressure neuropathy in the hind foot of the guinea pig. J Neurol Neurosurg Psychiatry 30:18–25, 1967.
361. Fu R, DeLiso JA, Kraft GH: Motor nerve latencies through the tarsal tunnel in normal adult subjects. Arch Phys Med Rehabil 61:243–248, 1980.
362. Gabbay KH, Snider JJ: Nerve conduction defect in galactose-fed rats. Diabetes 21:295–300, 1972.
363. Ganel A, Engel J, Raymond S: Intraoperative identification of peripheral nerve fascicle: Use of a new rapid biochemical assay technique. Orthop Rev 15:85–88, 1986.
364. Garcia A Jr, Maeck BH: Radial nerve injuries and fractures of the shaft of the humerus. Am J Surg 99:625–627, 1960.
365. Gardner-Thorpe C: Anterior interosseous nerve palsy: Spontaneous recovery in two patients. J Neurol Neurosurg Psychiatry 37:1146–1150, 1974.
366. Garfin S, Mubarak SJ, Owen CA: Excertional anterolateral compartment syndrome. Case report with a fascial defect, muscle herniation and superficial peroneal nerve entrapment. J Bone Joint Surg 59A:404–405, 1977.
367. Gartsman GM, Kovach JC, Crouch CC, Noble PC, Bennett JB: Carpal arch alteration after carpal tunnel release. J Hand Surg [Am] 11:372–374, 1986.
368. Gassman N, Stegmuller G, Stanisic M: Das karpaltunnel Syndrom. Indikation, Technik und Resultate nach epineuraler und inter aszikularer Neurolyse. Handchirurgie 9:137–142, 1977.
369. Gauthier G: Thomas Morton's disease: A nerve entrapment syndrome. Clin Orthop 142:90–92, 1979.
370. Gay J, Love J: Diagnosis and treatment of tardy paralysis of the ulnar nerve. J Bone Joint Surg 29B:1087–1097, 1947.
371. Gaul JS: Electrical fascicle identification as an adjunct to nerve repair. Hand Clin 2:709–722, 1986.
372. Gelberman RH, Urbaniak JR, Bright DS, et al: Digital sensibility following replantation. J Hand Surg 3:313–319, 1978.
373. Gelberman RH, Aronson D, Weisman MH: Carpal tunnel syndrome. Results of a prospective trial of steroid injection and splinting. J Bone Joint Surg 62A:1181–1184, 1980.
374. Gelberman RH, Pfeffer GB, Galbraith RT, Szabo RM, Rydevik B, Dimik M: Results of treatment of severe carpal tunnel syndrome without internal neurolysis of the median nerve. J Bone Joint Surg 69A:896–903, 1987.
375. Gentili F, Hudson AR, Hunter D, et al: Nerve injection injury with local anesthetic agents: A light and electron microscopic, fluorescent microscopic and horseradish peroxidase study. Neurosurgery 6:263–272, 1980.
376. Gentili F, Hudson AR, Kline DG, Hunter D: Morphological and physiological alterations following internal neurolysis of normal rat sciatic nerve. In Gorio A, et al, ed: Post-traumatic Peripheral Nerve Regeneration: Experimental Basis and Clinical Implications. Raven Press, New York, 1981, pp 183–210.
377. Gentili F, Hudson AR, Kline D, et al: Peripheral nerve injection injury. Neurosurgery 4:244, 1979.
378. Gerl A, Thorwith V: Ergebnisse der Ulnarisver Lagering. Acta Neurochir (Wien) 30:227–246, 1974.
379. Gessini L, Jandols B, Pietrangeli A: The anterior tarsal tunnel syndrome. J Bone Joint Surg 66A:786–787, 1984.
380. Gessini L, Jandolo B, Pietrangeli A: Entrapment neuropathies of the median nerve at and above the elbow. Surg Neurol 19:112–116, 1983.
381. Ghosh BC, Ghosh L, Huvos AG, Fortner JG: Malignant schwannoma. Cancer 31:184–190, 1973.
382. Gilbert A, Tassin JL: Obstetrical palsy—a clinical pathologic and surgical review. In Microreconstruction of Nerve injuries, ed, Terzis, W.B. Saunders Co, Philadelphia, 1978, pp 529–553.
383. Gilliatt RW, Thomas PK: Changes in nerve conduction with ulnar lesions at the elbow. J Neurol Neurosurg Psychiatry 23:312—320, 1960.
384. Gilliatt RW, Wilson TG: A pneumatic tourniquet test in the carpal tunnel syndrome. Lancet 2:595–597, 1953.
385. Gilliatt RW, Wilson RG: Peripheral nerve conduction in diabetic neuropathy. J Neurol Neurosurg Psychiatry 25:11–16, 1962.
386. Gloobe H, Picket P: An anomalous muscle in the canal of Guyon. Anat Anz 133:477, 1973.
387. Gluck T: Ueber Neuroplastik aut dem Wege der Transplantation. Arch Klin Chir 25:606–616, 1880.
388. Godwin JT: Encapsulated neurilemmoma (Schwannoma) of the brachial plexus. Report of 11 cases. Cancer 5:708–720, 1952.
389. Goldie I: Epicondylitis lateralis humeri. Acta Chir Scand (Suppl) 339:7, 1964.
390. Goldman S, Honet JC, Sobel R, Goldstein AS: Posterior interosseous-nerve palsy in the absence of trauma. Arch Neurol 21:435–441, 1969.
391. Goodgold J, Koeppel HP, Sprelholz NI: The tarsal tunnel syndrome: Objective diagnostic criteria. N Engl J Med 173:742–745, 1965.
392. Gore D, Larson S: Medial epicondylectomy for subluxing ulnar nerve. Am J Surg 111:851–853, 1966.
393. Gorio A, Carmignoto G: Reformation, maturation and stabilization of neuromuscular junctions in peripheral nerve regeneration. In Gorio A, Millesi H, Mingrino S, eds: Posttraumatic Peripheral Nerve Regeneration. Raven Press, New York, 1981, pp 481–492.
394. Grabb WC, Bement SL, Kaepke GH, et al: Comparison of methods of peripheral nerve suturing in monkeys. Plast Reconstr Surg 46:31–38, 1970.
395. Grablis M, Puentes J, Lidski M: Tarsal tunnel syndrome in rheumatoid arthritis. Arch Phys Med Rehabil 62:401–403, 1981.
396. Graham RA: Carpal tunnel syndrome: A statistical analysis of 214 cases. Orthopedics 6:1283–1287, 1985.

397. Grantham SA: Ulnar compression in the loge de Guyon. JAMA 197:229–230, 1966.
398. Gray's Anatomy, 36th British ed, WB Saunders, Philadelphia, 1977, p. 1068.
399. Gregg EC: Absolute measurements of the vibratory threshold. Arch Neurol 66:403, 1951.
400. Green DP: Diagnostic and therapeutic value of carpal tunnel injection. J Hand Surg (Am) 9:850–854, 1984.
401. Green MD, House WF: Disorders of the Facial Nerve; Anatomy, Diagnosis and Management. Raven Press, New York, 1980.
402. Greene MH, Hadied AM: Bipartite hamulus with ulnar tunnel syndrome—case report and literature review. J Hand Surg 6:605, 1981.
403. Grigoresco D, Iordanesco G: Une cas rare de paralysie partielle du nerf radial. Rev Neurol (Paris) 12:102–104, 1937.
404. Gross MS, Gelberman RH: Anatomy of the distal ulnar tunnel. Clin Orthop 196:238–247, 1985.
405. Grossman LA, Kaplan HJ, Ownby FD, Grossman M: Carpal tunnel syndrome—initial manifestation of systems disease. JAMA 176:259–261, 1961.
406. Gruber W: Ueber die Verbindung des Nervus Medianus mit dem Nervus ulnaris am Unterarme des Menschen und der Sangethiete. Arch Neurol Physiol 37:501–522, 1870.
407. Grundberg AB: Carpal tunnel decompression in spite of normal electromyography. J Hand Surg 8:348–349, 1983.
408. Gu Y, Zheng Y, Li H, Zu Y: Arterialized venous free sural nerve grafting. J Plast Surg 15:332, 1985.
409. Guiloff RJ, Sagratt RM: Sensory conduction in medial plantar nerve. J Neurol Neurosurg Psychiatry 40:1168–1181, 1977.
410. Gullain G, Courtellemont R: L'action du muscle court supinator dans la paralysie du nerf radial. Presse Med 13:50–52, 1905.
411. Gutmann E: Factors effecting recovery of motor function after nerve lesions. J Neurol Neurosurg Psychiatry 5:81–95, 1942.
412. Gutmann L: Atypical deep peroneal neuropathy in the presence of accessory deep peroneal nerve. J Neurol Neurosurg Psychiatry 33:453–456, 1970.
413. Guttman L, Medawar PB: The chemical inhibition of fiber regeneration and neuroma formation in peripheral nerves. J Neurol Neurosurg Psychiatry 5:130, 1942.
414. Guyon F: Note sur une disposition anatomique propre a la face anterieure de la region du poignet et non encore decrite par le docteur. Bull Soc Anat Paris 6:184–186, 1861.
415. Hagstrom P: Ulnar nerve compression at the elbow. Scand J Plast Reconstr Surg 11:59–62, 1977.
416. Hakstian RW: Funicular orientation by direct stimulation: An aid to peripheral nerve repair. J Bone Joint Surg 50:1178–1186, 1968.
417. Hakstian RW: Perineurial neurorrhaphy. Orthop Clin North Am 4:945–956, 1973.
418. Hall HH, Mackinnon SE, Gilbert RW: An approach to the posterior interosseous nerve. Plast Reconstr Surg 74:435–437, 1984.
419. Hallett J: Entrapment of the median nerve after dislocation of the elbow: A case report. J Bone Joint Surg 63B:408–412, 1981.
420. Hallett J, Tandon D, Berardelli A: Treatment of peripheral neuropathies. J Neurol Neurosurg Psychiatry 48:1193–1207, 1985.
421. Halsted WS: An experimental study of circumscribed dilation of an artery immediately distal to a partially occluding band, and its bearing on dilation of the subclavian artery observed in certain cases of cervical rib. J Exp Med 24:271–290, 1916.
422. Halsted WS: As to the cause of the dilatation of the subclavian artery observed in some cases of cervical rib: A clinical and experimental study. Trans Am Surg Assoc 34:272–288, 1916.
423. Hammarback JA, Palm SL, Furct LT, Letourneau PC: Guidance of neurite growth by pathways of substra absorbed lamini. J Neurosci Res 13:213–222, 1985.
424. Hannington-Kiff JG: Pharmocological target blocks in hand surgery and rehabilitation. J Hand Surg [Br] 9:29–36, 1984.
425. Hara T, Tsuyama N: Intercostal nerves anastomosis for brachial plexus injuries with root avulsions. Operation 23:1087–1096, 1969.
426. Hardy MA, Moran CA, Merritt H: Desensitization of the traumatized hand. Va Med 109:134–137, 1982.
427. Hargens AR, Romine JS, Sipe JC, et al: Peripheral nerve conduction block by high muscle-compartment pressure. J Bone Joint Surg 61A:192, 1979.
428. Harii K, Ohmori K, Toru S: Free gracilis muscle transplantation with microneurovascular anastomoses for treatment of facial paralysis. Plast Reconstr Surg 57:133, 1976.
429. Harkin JC, Reed RJ: Tumours of the Peripheral Nervous System. Armed Forces Institute of Pathology, Washington, D.C., 1968.
430. Harris W, Low, VW: On the importance of accurate muscular analysis in lesions of the brachial plexus. Br Med J 2:1035–1038, 1903.
431. Harris WD: Topography of the facial nerve. Arch Otolaryngol 82:264, 1968.
432. Harrison DH: The pectoralis minor vascularized muscle graft for the treatment of unilateral facial palsy. Plast Reconstr Surg 75:206–213, 1985.
433. Harrison MJG, Nurick S: Results of anterior transposition of ulnar nereve for ulnar neuritis. Br Med J 1:27–29, 1970.
434. Hart UL: Two unusual injuries of the wrists. J Bone Joint Surg 23:948–949, 1941.
435. Hartel R: Munch Med Wochenschr 113:1580–1582, 1971.
436. Hartz CR, Linscheid RL, Gramser RR, et al: The pronator teres syndrome. Compressive neuropathy of the median nerve. J Bone Joint Surg 63A:885–890, 1981.
437. Hayashi Y, Kojima T, Kohno T: Case of cubital tunnel syndrome caused by the snapping of the medial head of the triceps brachii muscle. J Hand Surg [Am] 9:96–99, 1984.
438. Hayes JR, Mulholland RC, O'Connor BT: Compression of the deep palmar branch of the ulnar nerve. J Bone Joint Surg 51B:469–472, 1969.

439. Heinenmann O: Ueber Schlussverletzungen der peripheren Nerven. Arch Klin Chir 108:107, 1916.
440. Heininger K, Liebert UG, Toyka KV, Hanivoll FT, et al: Chronic inflammatory polyneuropathy: Reduction of nerve conduction velocities in monkeys by systemic passive transfer of Immunoglobulin G. J Neurol Sci 66: 1–14, 1984.
441. Hendler N: Hendler ten minute screening test for chronic back pain patients. Psychosomatics 20:806–808, 1979.
442. Hendler N, Biernstein M, Gucer RP, Long D: A preoperative screening test for chronic back pain patients. J Acad Psychosom Med 20:801–808, 1979.
443. Hendler N, Fink H, Long D: Myofascial syndrome: response to trigger point injections. J Acad Psychosom Med 24:990–999, 1983.
444. Hendler N, Uematesu S, Long D: Thermographic validation of physical complaints in psychogenic "pain" patients. J Acad Psychosom Med 23:4–9, 1982.
445. Henrickson B: Supracondylar fractures of the humerus in children. Acta Chir Scand [Suppl] 369:1, 1966.
446. Henry JL: Effects of substance P on functionally identified units in cat spinal cord. Brain Res 114:439–451, 1976.
447. Hempel GK, Rusher, AH Jr, Wheeler CG, Hunt DG, Bukhari HI: Supraclavicular resection of the first rib for thoracic outlet syndrome. Am J Surg 141:213–215, 1981.
448. Herndon JH, Eaton RG, Littler JW: Management of painful neuromas in the hand. J Bone Joint Surg 58A:369–373, 1976.
449. Higgs GA, Higgs EA, Salmon JA: Prostacyclin in inflammation. In Vene JR, Bergstrom S eds: Prostacyclin. Raven Press, New York, 1979, pp 187–193.
450. Highet WB, Sanders FK: The effects of stretching nerves after suture. Br J Surg 30:355, 1943.
451. Hill NA, Howard FM, Huffer BR: The incomplete anterior interosseous nerve syndrome. J Hand Surg [Am] 10:4–16, 1985.
452. Hildreth D: The Jamar Dynamometer. Presented at the 41st Annual Meeting of the American Society for Surgery of the Hand. New Orleans, February 19, 1986.
453. Hillbom M, Wennberg A: Prognosis of alcoholic peripheral neuropathy. J Neurol Neurosurg Psychiatry 47:699–703, 1984.
454. Hirasawa Y, Marmor L: The protective effect of radiation combined with sheathing methods on experimental nerve heterografts. Silastic, autogenous veins and heterogenous arteries. J Neurol 27:401, 1967.
455. Hirasawa Y, Sawamura H, Sakakida K: Entrapment neuropathy due to bilateral epitrochleoanconeus muscles: A case report. J Hand Surg 4:181–184, 1979.
456. Hirschel G: Erfahrungen uber Schussverletzungen der Nerven. Munch Med Wochenschr 62:159, 1915.
457. Ho KC, Marmor L: Entrapment of the ulnar nerve at the elbow. Am J Surg 121:355–356, 1971.
458. Ho PK, Dellon AL, Wilgis EFS: True aneurysms of the hand resulting from athletic injury: Report of two cases. Am J Sports Med 13:136–138, 1985.
459. Hoase J, Bjerre P, Simesen K: Median and ulnar nerve transections treated with microsurgical interfascicular cable grafting with autogenous sural nerve. J Neurosurg 53:73–84, 1980.
460. Hobhouse N, Heald CB: A case of posterior interosseous paralysis. Br Med J 1:841, 1936.
461. Hoehn JG: Neurolysis in the treatment of carpal tunnel syndrome. A preliminary report. Orthop Rev 9:103–107, 1980.
462. Hoen TI, Brachett CE: Peripheral nerve lengthening. 1. Experimental. J Neurosurg 13:43, 1956. 22. Garriety RW: The use of plastic and rubber tubing in the management of irreparable nerve injuries. Surg Forum 6:517, 1955.
463. Hoffert MJ, Greenberg RP, Walshee PJ, Gracely RH, Werdzeh PR, Vinayakom K, Dubner R: Abnormal collateral innervations of sympathetic and peripheral sensory fields associated with causalgia. Pain 20:1–12, 1984.
464. Holder LE, Mackinnon SE: Reflex sympathetic dystrophy in the hands: Clinical and scintigraphic criteria. Radiology 152:517–522, 1984.
465. Holmes JC, Skolnick MD, Hall JE: Untreated median nerve entrapment in bone after fracture of the distal end of the humerus: Postmortem findings after 47 years. J Bone Joint Surg 61A:309–310, 1979.
466. Honner R, Fragiadakis FG, Lamb DW: An investigation of factors affecting the results of digital nerve division. Hand 2:21–31, 1970.
467. Hope DG, Mulvihill JJ: Malignancy in neurofibromatosis. Adv Neurol 29:33–54, 1981.
468. Horch K: Central responses of cutaneous sensory neurons to peripheral nerve crush in the cat. Brain Res 151:581–586, 1978.
469. Horch K: Guidance of regrowing sensory axons after cutaneous nerve lesions in the cat. J Neurophysiol 42:1437–1449, 1979.
470. Horowitz MT: Normal anatomy and variations with the peripheral nerves of the leg and foot. Arch Surg 36:626–636, 1938.
471. House JW: Facial nerve grading system. Laryngology 93:1056–1069, 1983.
472. Howard FM: Ulnar nerve palsy in wrist fractures. J Bone Joint Surg 43A:1197, 1961.
473. Hoyt CS: Ulnar neuropathy in bicycle riders. Arch Neurol 33:372, 1976.
474. Huber GC: A study of the operative treatment for loss of nerve substance in peripheral nerves. J Morphol 11:629, 1895.
475. Huber GC, Lewis D: Amputation neuromas. Their development and prevention. Arch Surg 1:85–113, 1920.
476. Hudson AR, Kline D, Gentili F: Peripheral nerve injection injury. In Omer G, Spinner M, eds: Management of Peripheral Nerve Problems. WB Saunders, Philadelphia, 1980, pp 639–653.
477. Hudson AR, Tamner B: Brachial plexus injuries. In Neurosurgery, RH Wilkins, SS Regachary, eds. McGraw Hill, pp 1817–1832, 1985.
478. Huffman JD: Electrodiagnostic techniques for and con-

servative treatment of thoracic outlet syndrome. Clin Orthop 207:21–23, 1986.

479. Hunt JR: Neural atrophy of the muscles of the hand without sensory disturbances. Rev Neurol Psychiatr 12:137, 1914.

480. Hunt JR: Occupational neuritis of the deep palmar branch of the ulnar nerve. J Nerv Ment Dis 35:676–689, 1908.

481. Hunt JR: Thenar and hypothenar types of neural atrophy of the hand. Am J Med Sci 141:224, 1911.

482. Hunt JR: Thenar and hypothenar types of neural atrophy of the hand. Br Med J 2:642, 1930.

483. Hunter JM, Snyder LH, Mackin EJ, Callahan AD, eds: Rehabilitation of the Hand. CV Mosby, St. Louis, 1984.

484. Hurst LC, Weissberg D, Carroll RE: The relationship of the double crush to carpal tunnel syndrome (an analysis of 1,000 cases of carpal tunnel syndrome). J Hand Surg 10B:202–204, 1985.

485. Ijkelenstam PA: Compression of the posterior tibial nerve (the tarsal tunnel syndrome). Arch Chir Neeland 20:1–6, 1968.

486. Inserra A, Spinner M: An anatomic factor significant in transposition of the ulnar nerve. J Hand Surg (Am) 11A:80–82, 1986.

487. Iwakuma T, Matsumoto A, Nakamura N: Hemifacial spasm: Comparison of three different operative procedures in 110 patients. J Neurosurg 57:753–756, 1982.

488. Jabaley M: Personal observations on the role of the lumbrical muscles in carpal tunnel syndrome. J Hand Surg 3:82–84, 1978.

489. Jabaley ME, Wallace WH, Heckler FR: Internal topography of major nerves in the forearm and hand. A current view. J Hand Surg 5:119, 1980.

490. Jaboulay. 1899, as cited by Kirtley JA, Riddell DH, Stoney WS, Wright JK: Cervicothoracic sympathectomy in neurovascular abnormalities of the upper extremities: Experience in 76 patients with 104 sympathectomies. Ann Surg 165:869–879, 1967.

491. Jackson JP: Traumatic thrombosis of the ulnar artery in the palm. J Bone Joint Surg 36B:438, 1954.

492. Jacoby W, Fahlbusch R, Mackert B, et al: Transplantation lyophilisierter Homoioplasticher Nerven sur Uberbrukung peripherer Nervendefekte beim Menschen. Fortschr Med 88:183, 1970.

493. Jaeger SH, Read R, Smullens SN, Breme P: Thoracic outlet syndrome: Diagnosis and treatment. In Hunter JM, Schneider LH, Macken EJ, Callahan AD eds: Rehabilitation of the Hand, 2nd ed. St Louis, CV Mosby Co, 1984, pp 378–389.

494. Jakobsen J: Axonal dwindling in early experimental diabetes. II. A study of isolated nerve fibers. Diabetologia 12:547–553, 1976.

495. Jakobsen J: Peripheral nerves in early experimental diabetes. Expansion of the endoneurial space as a cause of increased water content. Diabetologia 14:113–119, 1978.

496. Jakobsen J, Malgrin L, Olsson Y: Permeability of blood-nerve barrier in the Streptozotocin diabetic rat. Exp Neurol 60:277–285, 1978.

497. Jakobsen J, Sidenius P: Decreased axonal flux of retrogradally transported glycoproteins in early experimental diabetes. J Neurochem 33:1055–1060, 1979.

498. Jakobsen J, Sidenius P: Decreased axonal transport of structural proteins in Streptozotocin diabetic rats. J Clin Invest 66:292–296, 1980.

499. Janeka IV, Conley J: Primary neoplasms of the facial nerve. Plast Reconstr Surg 79:177–185, 1987.

500. Janetta PJ: Arterial compression of the trigeminal nerve and the pons in patients with trigeminal neuralgia. J Neurosurg 26:159–162, 1967.

501. Janetta PJ: Microsurgical approach to the trigeminal nerve for tic douloureux. Prog Neurol Surg 7:180–200, 1976.

502. Janetta PJ: Microsurgical exploration and decompression of the facial nerve in hemifacial spasm. Curr Top Surg Res 2:217–220, 1970.

503. Janetta PJ: Microvascular decompression for hemifacial spasm. In May M, ed: The Facial Nerve. Thieme, New York, 1986, pp 499–508.

504. Janetta PJ: Neurovascular compression in cranial nerve and systemic disease. Ann Surg 192:518–525, 1980.

505. Janetta PJ, Abbosy M, Maroon JC, et al: Etiology and definitive microsurgical treatment of hemifacial spasm. Operative technique and results in 47 patients. J Neurosurg 47:321–328, 1977.

506. Jefferson D, Eames RA: Subclinical entrapment of the lateral femoral cutaneous nerve: An autopsy study. Muscle Nerve 2:145–154, 1979.

507. Jefferson D, Neary D, Eames RA: Renaut body distribution at sites of human peripheral nerve entrapment. J Neurol Sci 49:19–29, 1981.

508. Jeffrey AK: Compression of the deep palmar branch of the ulnar nerve by an anomalous muscle. J Bone Joint Surg 53B:718, 1971.

509. Jenkins SA: Osteoarthritis of the pisiform-triquetral joint. J Bone Joint Surg 33B:532–534, 1957.

510. Jenkins SA: Solitary tumors of peripheral nerve trunks. J Bone Joint Surg 34B:401–411, 1952.

511. Jenkins WM, Merzenich MM: Reorganization of neocortical representations after brain surgery. Brain Res 71:249–266, 1987.

512. Jenkins WM, Merzenich MM, Ochs MT: A behaviorally controlled differential use of restricted hand surfaces induces changes in the cortical representation of the hand in areas 3b of adult owl monkeys. Soc. Neurosci Abstr 10:665, 1984.

513. Jessell TM, Iversen LL, Guello AC: Capsaician-induced depletion of substance P from primary sensory neurons. Brain Res 152:183–188, 1978.

514. Jhee WH, Oryshkevich RS, Wilcox R: Severe carpal tunnel syndrome with sparing of sensory fibers. Orthop Rev 15:93–96, 1986.

515. Johnson EW, Ortez PR: Electrodiagnosis of tarsal tunnel syndrome. Arch Phys Med Rehabil 47:776–780, 1966.

516. Johnson RJ, Bonfiglio M: Lipofibromatous hamartoma

of the median nerve. J Bone Joint Surg 51A:984–990, 1969.

517. Johnson RK, Shrewbury MM: Anatomical course of the thenar branch of the median nerve—usually in a separate tunnel through the transverse carpal ligament. J Bone Joint Surg 52A:269–273, 1970.
518. Johnson RK, Spinner M, Shrewsbury MM: Median nerve entrapment syndrome in the proximal forearm. J Hand Surg 4:48–51, 1979.
519. Jones ET, Louis DS: Median nerve injuries associated with supercondylar fracture of the humerus in children. Clin Orthop 150:181–186, 1980.
520. Jones RE, Gauntt C: Medial epicondylectomy for ulnar nerve compression syndrome at the elbow. Clin Orthop 139:174–178, 1979.
521. Joplin RJ; The proper digital nerve, vitallium stem arthroplasty and some thoughts about foot surgery in general. Clin Orthop 76:199–212, 1971.
522. Kaley G, Weiner R: Prostaglandin E_1: A potential mediator of the inflammatory response. Ann NY Acad Sci 180:338–350, 1971.
523. Kalisman M, Laborde K, Wolff TW: Ulnar nerve compression secondary to ulnar artery false aneurysm at the Guyon's canal. J Hand Surg 7:137–139, 1982.
524. Kameda Y: An anomalous muscle (accessory scapularis-tres-latissimus muscle) in the axilla penetrating the brachial plexus in man. Acta Anat 96:513–533, 1976.
525. Kane E, Kaplan EB, Spinner M: Observations on the course of the ulnar nerve in the arm. Ann Chir 27:470–496, 1973.
526. Kang R, Herman D, MacGillis M, Zarecki P: Convergence of sensory inputs in somatosensory cortex: Interactions from separate afferent sources. Exp Brain Res 57:211–278, 1985.
527. Kaplan EB: Correction of a disabling flexion contraction of the thumb. Bull Hosp Joint Dis 3:51–54, 1942.
528. Kaplan EB: Functional and Surgical Anatomy of the Hand, 2nd ed, JB Lippincott, Philadelphia, 1965.
529. Kaplan EB: Variation of the ulnar nerve at the wrist. Bull Hosp Joint Dis 24:85–88, 1963.
530. Kaplan EB, Spinner M: Normal and anomalous innervation patterns in the upper extremity. In Omer G, Spinner M, eds: Management of Peripheral Nerve Problems. WB Saunders, Philadelphia, 1980.
531. Kaplan PE, Kernahan WT: Tarsal tunnel syndrome: An electrodiagnostic and surgical correlation. J Bone Joint Surg 63A:96–99, 1981.
532. Karpati G, Carpenter S, Sharron L: Experimental reinnervation attempts of skeletal muscle cells by nonmotor nerves. In Gorio A, Millesi H, Mingrino S, eds: Posttraumatic Peripheral Nerve Regeneration. Raven Press. New York, 1981, pp 495–506.
533. Katims JJ, Naviasky EH, Rendell MS, Ng LKY, Bleeker ML: Constant current sine wave transcutaneous nerve stimulation for the evaluation of peripheral neuropathy. Arch Phys Med Rehabil 68:210–213, 1987.
534. Keck C: The tarsal-tunnel syndrome. J Bone Joint Surg 44A:180–182, 1962.
535. Kelly MJ, Jackson BT: Compression of median nerve at the elbow. Br Med J 2:283–286, 1976.
536. Kempe LF: Topical organization of the distal portion of the facial nerve. J Neurosurg 52:671, 1980.
537. Kendall D: Aetiology, diagnosis and treatment of paraesthesiae in the hands. Br Med J 2:1633–1640, 1960.
538. Kendall HO, Kendall FP: Muscles: Testing and Function. Williams & Wilkins Company Baltimore, 1949.
539. Kennedy R: Suture of the brachial plexus and birth paralysis of the upper extremity. Br Med J 1:298, 1903.
540. Kenzora JE: Symptomatic incisional neuromas on the dorsum of the foot. Foot Ankle 5:2–15, 1984.
541. Kerr AT: The brachial plexus of nerves in man—The variations in its formation and its branches. Am J Anat 23:285, 1918.
542. Kessel L, Wang M: Supercondylar spur of the humerus. J Bone Joint Surg 48B:765–769, 1966.
543. Kiloh LG, Nevin S: Isolated neuritis of the anterior interosseous nerve. Br Med J 1:850–851, 1952.
544. Kim LYS: Compression neuropathy of the radial nerve due to pentazocine-induced fibrous myopathy. Arch Phys Med Rehabil 68:49–50, 1987.
545. Kimura J: Electrodiagnosis in diseases of nerve and muscle. FA Davis, Philadelphia, 1983.
546. King LSL: Note on the pathology of Morton's metatarsalgia. Am J Clin Pathol 16:124–128, 1946.
547. King T, Morgan FP: Later results of removing the medial humeral epicondyle for traumatic ulnar neuritis. J Bone Joint Surg 41B:51–55, 1959.
548. King T, Morgan FP: Treatment of traumatic ulnar neuritis. Aust NZ J Surg 20:33–42, 1950.
549. King TS, Orahilly RM: Palmaris accessorius and duplication of the M. palmaris longus. Acta Anat [Suppl] 10:327–331, 1950.
550. Kirk EG, Lewis D: Fascial tubulization in the repair of nerve defects. JAMA, 65:486–492, 1915.
551. Kirklin JW, Murphy F, Berkson J: Suture of peripheral nerves: Factors affecting prognosis. Surg Gynecol Obstet 88:719–730, 1949.
552. Kishi H, Kishi T, William RH, Folkers K: Human deficiencies of vitamin B_6. I. Studies on parameters of the assay of the glutamic oxaloacetic transaminase by the CAS principle. Res Commun Chem Pathol Pharmacol 12:557–569, 1975.
553. Kitayamo Y, Tsukasass, Kurokawa M: High division of the median nerve: Unusual anatomical variations. Ann Plast Surg 14:74–76, 1985.
554. Kleinert HE, Boliantis GJ: Thrombosis of the palmar arterial arch and its tributaries: Etiology and newer concepts in treatment. Trauma 5:447–457, 1965.
555. Kleinert HE, Hayes JE: Ulnar tunnel syndrome. Plast Reconstr Surg 47:21–24, 1971.
556. Kline DG: Comments on "Neurolysis combined with the application of a Silastic envelope for ulnar nerve entrapment at the elbow." Neurosurgery 20:597–598, 1987.
557. Kline DG: Operative experience with major lower extremity nerve lesions including the lumbosacral plexus and the sciatic nerve. In Omer G, Spinner M, eds: Management of Peripheral Nerve Problems. WB Saunders, Philadelphia, 1980, pp 607–625.
558. Kline DG, Hackett ER: Value of electrophysiologic tests

for peripheral nerve neuromas. J Surg Oncol 2:299–310, 1970.

559. Kline DG, Hackett ER, Davis GD, Myers MB: Microcirculation of peripheral nerves. J Neurosurg 42:114, 1975.
560. Kline DG, Hackett ER, May PF: Evaluation of nerve injuries by evoked potentials and electromyography. J Neurosurg 31:136–138, 1969.
561. Kline DG, Hudson AR, Bratton BR: Experimental study of fascicular nerve repair with and without epineurial closure. J Neurosurg 54:513–520, 1981.
562. Kline, DG, Judice DJ: Operative management of selected brachial plexus lesions. J Neurosurg 58:631–649, 1983.
563. Kline DG, Nulsen FP: The neuroma-in-continuity: Its preoperative and operative management. Surg Clin North Am 52:1189–1209, 1972.
564. Klumpke A: Contribution a l'etude des paralysies radiculaires du plexus brachial. Rev Med 5:591, 1885.
565. Kojima T, Harase M, Ietsune T: Pronator syndrome: Report of six cases. Orthop Surg (Jpn) 19:1147–1148, 1968.
566. Kojima T, Yoshita I, Marumo E, et al: Hemangioma of the median nerve causing carpal tunnel. Hand 8:62–65, 1976.
567. Kopell HP: Carpal tunnel compression median neuropathy treated nonsurgically. NY State J Med 58:744–745, 1958.
568. Kopell HP: Lower extremity lesions. In Omer GE Jr, Spinner M: Management of Peripheral Nerve Problems. WB Saunders, Philadelphia, 1980.
569. Kopell HP, Thompson WAL: Peripheral entrapment neuropathy of the lower extremity. N Engl J Med 262:56–60, 1960.
570. Kopell HP, Thompson WAL: Peripheral Entrapment Neuropathies. Williams & Wilkins, Baltimore, 1963.
571. Kopell HP, Thompson WAL: Pronator syndrome. N Engl J Med 259:713–715, 1958.
572. Kornberg M, Aulicino PL, Dupuy TE: Laceration of the ulnar nerve with a closed fracture of the distal radius and ulna. Orthopedics 6:729–731, 1983.
573. Kosinski C: The course, mutual relations and distribution of the cutaneous nerves of the metatarsal region of the leg and foot. J Anat 60:274–297, 1926.
574. Kotani PT, Toshima Y, Matsuda H, et al: Postoperative results of nerve transposition in brachial plexus injury. Ortho Surg (Tokyo) 22:963, 1971.
575. Kozin F, Ryan LM, Carerra GF: Reflex sympathetic dystrophy syndrome, Part III. Am J Med 70:23–30, 1981.
576. Kozin F, Soin JS, Ryan LM: Bone scintigraphy in reflex sympathetic dystrophy syndrome. Radiology 138:437–443, 1981.
577. Krause KH, Witt T, Ross A: The anterior tarsal tunnel syndrome. J Neurol 217:67–74, 1977.
578. Kredel FE, Evans JP: Recovery of sensation in denervated pedicles and free skin grafts. J Neurol Neurosurg Psychiatry 19:1203–1221, 1933.
579. Kristensson K: Retrograde signalling of nerve cell body response to trauma. In Gorio A, Millesi H, Mingrino S, eds: Posttraumatic Peripheral Nerve Regeneration. Raven Press, New York, 1981, pp 27–34.
580. Kristensson K: Retrograde signalling of nerve cell body response to trauma. In Gorio A, Millesi H, Mingrino S, eds: Posttraumatic Peripheral Nerve Regeneration. Raven Press, New York, 1981, pp 115–128.
581. Gruber H, Zenker W: Acetylcholinesterase: Histochemical differentiation between motor and sensory nerve fibres. Brain Res 51:207–214, 1973.
582. Kruse F, Jr: Paralysis of the dorsal interosseous nerve not due to direct trauma. A case showing spontaneous recovery. Neurology (Minneap) 8:307–308, 1958.
583. Kuhlendahl H, Mumenthaler M, Penzholz H, et al: The treatment of peripheral nerve injuries with homologous nerve grafts. Acta Neurochir (Wien) 26:339, 1972.
584. Kulick MI, Gordillo G, Javidi T, Kilgore ES, Newmeyer WL III: Long-term analysis of patients having surgical treatment for carpal tunnel syndrome. J Hand Surg (Am) 11:59–66, 1986.
585. Kuncl RW, Duncan G, Watson D, Alderson K, Rogawaski MK, Peper M: Colchicine myopathy and neuropathy. N Engl J Med 316:1562–1568, 1987.
586. Kunzel KH, Fischer C, Ander H: The ulnar nerve of the vascularized transplant. J Reconstr Microsurg 2:175, 1986.
587. Kurihara K, Cohen M, Schultz RC: Nerve staining with leucomethylene blue: An experimental study. Plast Reconstr Surg 73:960–964, 1984.
588. Kutz JE, Shealy G, Lubbers L: Interfascicular nerve repair. Orthop Clin North Am 12:277–286, 1981.
589. Laborde KG, Kalisman M, Tsai T: Results of surgical treatment of painful neuromas of the hand. J Hand Surg 7:190–193, 1982.
590. Laha RK, Panchal PD: Surgical treatment of ulnar neuropathy. Surg Neurol 11:393–398, 1979.
591. Lahey MD, Aulicino PL: Anomalous muscles associated with compression neuropathies. Orthop Rev 40:19–28, 1986.
592. Laitung JKG, Peck F: Shoulder function following the loss of the latissimus dorsi muscle. Br J Plast Surg 38:375, 1985.
593. Lam SJS: A tarsal-tunnel syndrome. Lancet 2:1354–1355, 1962.
594. Lam SJS: Tarsal-tunnel syndrome. J Bone Joint Surg 49B:878–892, 1967.
595. Lamb D: Ulnar nerve compression lesions at the wrist and hand. Hand 2:17–18, 1970.
596. Lambert EH: The accessory deep peroneal nerve: A common variation in innervation of the extensor digitorum brevis. Neurology (Minneap) 19:1169–1176, 1969.
597. Langloh ND, Linscheid RL: Recurrent and unrelieved carpal-tunnel syndrome. Clin Orthop 83:41–47, 1972.
598. Lankford LL: In Green DP ed: Operative Hand Surgery, Churchill Livingstone, New York, 1982, pp 539–562.
599. Lankford LL: In Omer GE, Spinner M eds: Management of Peripheral Nerve Problems. WB Saunders, Philadelphia, 1980, 216–244.
600. Lansen RD, Posch JL: Nerve injuries in the upper extremity. Arch Surg 77:469–482, 1958.

601. Lanz V: Anatomic variations of the median nerve in the carpal tunnel. J Hand Surg 2:44–53, 1977.
602. Larsen RD, Posch JL: Nerve injuries in the upper extremity. Arch Surg 77:469–482, 1958.
603. Larson DL, Rodin AE, Robertson DK, O'Steen WK, Rapperport AS, Lewis SR: Perineural lymphatics: Myth or fact. Am J Surg 12:488, 1966.
604. Lasek JR, Shelanski ML, Brinkely BR, Condeelis JS, Ellisman MH, Goldman RD, Solomon F, Taylor EW: Cytoskeletons and the architecture of nervous systems. Neurosci Res Program Bull 19:1–153, 1981.
605. Lasek RJ, McQuarrie IG, Wujek JR: The central nervous system regeneration problem. Neuron and environment. In Gorio A, Millesi H, Miringo S, eds: Posttraumatic Peripheral Nerve Regeneration. Raven Press, New York, 1981, pp 59–70.
606. Lass R, Shrewsbury MM: Variation in the path of the deep motor branch of the ulnar nerve at the wrist. J Bone Joint Surg 57A:990–991, 1975.
607. Lassman G, Lassman H, Stockinger L: Morton's metatarsalgia: Light and electron microscopic observations and their relation to entrapment neuropathies. Virchow's Arch [A] 370:307–321, 1976.
608. Learmonth JR: Technique for transplanting the ulnar nerve. Surg Gyn Obst 75:792–793, 1942.
609. Learmonth JR: A variation in the distribution of the radial branch of the musculospiral nerve. J Anat 53:371–372, 1919.
610. Leffert, RD: Anterior submuscular transposition of the ulnar nerves by the Learmonth technique. J Hand Surg 7:147–155, 1982.
611. Leffert, RD: Brachial Plexus Injuries. Churchill Livingstone, New York, 1985.
612. Lehar K, Dujobny M, deCastro SC: Entrapment of median nerve by supercondylar process of the humerus. J Neurosurg 46:252–255, 1977.
613. Lehmann W: Foester O, et al, eds: In Allgemeine Therapie. Springer-Verlag, Berlin, 1936, pp 165, 205.
614. Lenman JAR, Ritchie AE: Clinical electromyograph. Pitman Publishing, London, 1983. 3rd ed.
615. Lenz U: Lahmung des Tiefen Hohlhandastes des Nervus Ulnaris, bedingt durch eine Anatomsche Variante. Handchirwigin 6:83–86, 1974.
616. Letievant JJE: Traite des sections nerveuses. JB Bailliereetfils, Paris, 1873.
617. Letourneau PC: Cell-to-substratum adhesion and guidance of axonal elongation. Dev Biol 44:92–101, 1975.
618. Letourneau PC: Cell-substratum adhesion of neurite growth cones and its role in neurite elongation. Exp Cell Res 124:127–138, 1979.
619. Letourneau PC: Chemotactic response of nerve fibre elongation to nerve growth factor. Dev Biol 66:183–196, 1978.
620. Letourneau PC: Distribution of Laminin in the Developing nervous system of the chick. Dev Biol 98:212, 1986.
621. Letourneau PC: Neurite extension by peripheral and central nervous system neurons in response to substratum bound fibronectin and laminin. Dev Biol 98: 212, 1983.
622. Letourneau PC, Wessels MK: Migratory cell locomotion versus nerve axon elongation. J Cell Biol 44:92–101, 1974.
623. Levi-Montalcini R, Hamburger V: Selective growth stimulating effects of sarcoma on sensory and sympathetic nervous system of the chick embryo. J Exp Zool 116:321, 1951.
624. Levin ME: Pathophysiology of diabetic foot lesions. Ch 29, In Clinical Diabetes Mellitus. Davidson JK, ed. Thieme, New York, 1986, pp 381–383
625. Levinthal R, Brown WJ, Rand RW: Comparison of fascicular, interfascicular and epineural suture techniques in the repair of simple nerve lacerations. J Neurosurg 47:744–750, 1977.
626. Levy DM, Apfelberg DB: Results of anterior transposition for ulnar neuropathy at the elbow. Am J Surg 123:304–308, 1972.
627. Lewis DS, Dick HM: Ossifying lipofibroma of the median nerve. J Bone Joint Surg 55A:1082–1084, 1973.
628. Lewis DS, Hankin FM, Greene TL, et al: Lipofibromas of the median nerve. Long term follow-up of four cases. J Hand Surg [Am] 10:403–407, 1985.
629. Lewis T: Experiments relating to cutaneous hyperalgesia and its spread through somatic nerves. Clin Sci 2:373–423, 1936.
630. Lewis T, Pickering G: Observations upon maladies in which the blood supply to the digits ceases intermittently or permanently. Clin Sci 1:327–366, 1934.
631. Lewis T: The nocifensor system of nerves and its reactions. Br Med J 1:431–435, 1937.
632. Lichtman DM, Florio RL, Mack GR: Carpal tunnel release under local anesthesia: Evaluation of the outpatient procedure. J Hand Surg 4:545–546, 1979.
633. Lidstrum A: Fractures of distal end of radius. A clinical and statistical study of end result. Acta Orthop Scand [Suppl] 41:1, 1959.
634. Lieber CS, DeCarli LM: Feeding of alcohol and liquid diets: Two decades of applications. A 1982 update. Alcoholism (NY) 6:523–531, 1982.
635. Lieber CS, Jones DP, Mendlison J, DeCarli LM: Fatty liver, hyperlipemia and hyperuricemia produced by prolonged alcohol consumption despite adequate dietary intake. Trans Assn Am Physic 76:289–300, 1963.
636. Lilla JA, Phelps DB, Boswick JA: Microsurgical repair of peripheral nerve injuries in the upper extremity. Ann Plast Surg 2:24–31, 1979.
637. Lilly CJ, Magnell TD: Severance of the thenar branch of the median nerve as a complication of carpal tunnel release. J Hand Surg [Am] 10:399–402, 1985.
638. Lind R, Wood MB: Comparison of the patterns of early revascularization of conventional versus vascularized nerve grafts in the canine. J Reconstr Microsurg 2:229, 1986.
639. Lindbloom U, Verillo RT: Sensory functions in chronic neuralgia. Neurol Neurosurg Psychiatry 42:422–435, 1979.
640. Ling CM, Loong SC: Injection injury of the radial nerve. Injury 8:60–62, 1976.

641. Linscheid RL: Injuries to radial nerve at the wrist. Arch Surg 91:942–946, 1965.
642. Linscheid RL, Burton RC, Fredericks EJ: Tarsal tunnel syndrome. South Med J 63:313–316, 1970.
643. Lipscomb PR: Duplication of hypothenar muscles simulating soft tissue tumor of the hand. J Bone Joint Surg 42A:1058–1060, 1960.
644. Lipscomb PR, Burleson RJ: Vascular and neural complications in supercondylar fractures of the humerus in children. J Bone Joint Surg 37A:487–492, 1955.
645. Lister G: The Hand: Diagnosis and Indications. Churchill Livingstone, Edinburgh, 1977.
646. Lister GD, Belsole RB, Kleinert HE: The radial tunnel syndrome. J Hand Surg 4:52–59, 1979.
647. Liveson JA, Renschoff J, Goodgold J: Electromyographic studies in the case of foramen magnum meningioma. J Neurol Neurosurg Psychiatry 36:561–564, 1973.
648. Liveson JA, Spielholz NI: Peripheral Neurology (Philadelphia,) FA Davis, Co, 1979, p 20.
649. Livingston WK: In Livingston WK, ed. Pain Mechanisms of Physiological Interpretation of Causalgia and its Related States. Plenum Publishing, New York, 1943.
650. Lloyd K, Agarwal A: Tarsel tunnel syndrome, a presenting feature of rheumatic arthritis. Br Med J 3:32, 1970.
651. Lluch AL: Ulnar nerve entrapment after anterior transposition at the elbow. NY Stat J Med 75:75–76, 1975.
652. Lord JW Jr: Surgical management of shoulder girdle syndromes. Arch Surg 66:69–83, 1953.
653. Lorento DE, No R: Analysis of the activity of the chains of enternuncial neurons. J Neurophysiol 1:207–244, 1938.
654. Losli EJ: Intrinsic hemangiomas of the peripheral nerves. Arch Pathol 53:226–232, 1952.
655. Lotem M, Fried A, Levy M, Solzi P, Najenson T, Nathan H: Radial palsy following muscular effort: A nerve compression syndrome possibly related to a fibrous arch of the lateral head of the triceps. J Bone Joint Surg 53B:500–506, 1971.
656. Lott IT, Richardson EP: Neuropathological findings in the biology of neurofibromatosis. Adv Neurol 29:23–32, 1981.
657. Louie G, Mackinnon SE, Dellon AL, Patterson GA, Hunter DA: Medial antebrachial cutaneous—lateral femoral cutaneous neurotization in restoration of sensation to pressure bearing areas in a paraplegic. Ann Plast Surg 19:572–576, 1987.
658. Louis DS, Hankin FM: Symptomatic relief following carpal tunnel decompression with normal electroneuromyographic studies. Orthopedics 10:434–436, 1987.
659. Lowndes HE, Baker T: Toxic site of action in distal axonopathies. In Spencer PH, Schaumberg HH eds: Experimental and Clinical Neurotoxicology. Williams & Wilkins, Baltimore, 1980, pp 193–205.
660. Lubinska L, Niemierko S: Velocity and intensity in bidirectional migration of acetylcholinesterase in transected nerves. Brain Res 27:329–342, 1971.
661. Luce EA, Futrell JW, Wilgis EF, Hoopes JE: Compression neuropathy following brachial arterial puncture in anticoagulated patients. J Trauma 16:717–721, 1976.
662. Lugnegard H, Waldheim G, Wenberg G: Operative treatment of ulnar nerve neuropathy in the elbow region. Acta Orthop Scand 48:168–176, 1977.
663. Lundborg G: A method for long term *in vivo* studies on the microcirculation of a peripheral nerve. Adv Microcirc 3:91, 1970.
664. Lundborg G: Intrinsic vascularization of human peripheral nerves: Structural and functional aspects. J Hand Surg 4:34–41, 1979.
665. Lundborg G: Mechanical effects on circulation and nerve function. In Gorio A, Mellesi H, Mingerino S, eds: Posttraumatic Nerve Regeneration. Raven Press, New York, 1981, pp 157–158.
666. Lundborg G: Structure and function of the intraneural microvessels as related to trauma, edema formation and nerve function. J Bone Joint Surg 57A:938–948, 1975.
667. Lundborg G: The theory of the double crush syndrome. Correspondence Newsletter #9, 1986. Am Soc Surg Hand, dated Oct 24, 1985.
668. Lundborg G, Branemark PI: Microvascular structure and function of peripheral nerves. Vital microscopic studies of the tibial nerve in the rabbit. Adv Microcirc 1:66, 1968.
669. Lundborg G, Dahlin L, Danielson N, et al: Nerve regeneration across an extended gap. J Hand Surg 7:580–587, 1982.
670. Lundborg G, Dahlin L, Danielsen MP, Hansson HA, Larsson K: Reorganization and orientation of regenerating nerve fibres, perineurium and epineurium in preformed mesothelial tubes. An experimental study in the sciatic nerve of rats. J Neurosci Res 6:265–281. 1981.
671. Lundborg G, Gelberman R, Longo FM, Powell H, Varon S: In vivo regeneration of cut nerve encased in silicone chambers. Growth across a 6 mm gap. J Neuropathol Exp Neurol 41:412–422, 1982.
672. Lundborg G, Gelberman RH, Minteer-Convery M, Lee YF, Hargens AR: Median nerve compression in the carpal tunnel—functional response to experimentally induced controlled pressure. J Hand Surg 7:252, 1982.
673. Lundborg G, Hansson HA: Nerve regeneration through preformed pseudosynovial tubes. A preliminary report of a new experimental model for studying regeneration and reorganization of peripheral nerve tissue. J Hand Surg 5:35, 1980.
674. Lundborg G, Hansson HA: Regeneration of peripheral nerve through a preformed tissue space, preliminary observations on the reorganization of regenerating nerve fibres and perineurium. Brain Res 178:573–576, 1979.
675. Lundborg G, Longo FM, Varon S: Nerve regeneration model in trophic factors in vivo. Brain Res 232:157–162, 1982.
676. Lundborg G, Rydevik B: Effects of stretching the tibial nerve of the rabbit. A preliminary study of the intraneural circulation and the barrier function of the perineurium. J Bone Joint Surg 55B:390, 1973.
677. Lusk MD, Kline DG, Garcia CA: Tumors of the brachial plexus. Neurosurgery 21:439–453, 1987.
678. Lusskin R, Campbell JB, Thompson WAL: Posttraumatic lesions of the brachial plexus: Treatment by

transclavicular exploration and neurolysis or autograft reconstruction. J Bone Joint Surg 55A:1159–1176, 1973.

679. Lux P, BreidenbachW, Firrell J: Determination of temporal changes in blood flow in vascularized and nonvascularized nerve grafts in the dog. Plast Reconstr Surg 82:133–142, 1988.
680. Lyle HHM: Traumatic luxation of the head of the fibula. Ann Surg 82:635–639, 1925.
681. Lynch AC, Lipscomb PR: The carpal tunnel syndrome and Colles' fracture. JAMA 185–363, 1963.
682. MacCarty CS: Two stage autograft for repair of extensive damage to the sciatic nerve. J Neurosurg 8:319, 1951.
683. MacDonald RI, Lichtman DM, Hanlon JJ, Wilson JN: Complications of surgical release for carpal tunnel syndrome. J Hand Surg 3:70–76, 1978.
684. Mackenzie JAJ: Resection of the sciatic nerve, neuroplasty, end results. Surg Gynecol Obstet 9:30–44, 1909.
685. Mackey D, Colbert DS, Chater EH; Musculocutaneous nerve entrapment. Ir J Med Sci 146:100–102, 1977.
686. Mackinnon SE: A surgical algorithm for the management of facial palsy. Microsurgery 9:30–35, 1988.
687. Mackinnon SE, Dellon AL: Anatomic investigation of nerves at the wrist I. Orientation of the motor fascicle in the carpal tunnel. Ann Plast Surg 21:32–35, 1988.
688. Mackinnon SE, Dellon AL: A histologic assessment of the effects of the distal nerve in determining regeneration across a nerve gap. Microsurgery 9:46–51, 1988.
689. Mackinnon SE, Dellon AL: Algorithm for management of painful neuroma. Contemp Orthop 13:15–27, 1986.
690. Mackinnon SE, Dellon AL: Evaluation of microsurgical internal neurolysis in a primate median nerve model of chronic nerve compression. J Hand Surg 13A: 54–61, 1988.
691. Mackinnon SE, Dellon AL: Homologies between the tarsal and carpal tunnels: Implications for surgical treatment in the tarsal tunnel syndrome. Contemp Orthop 14:75–78, 1987.
692. Mackinnon SE, Dellon AL: Overlap of lateral antebrachial cutaneous nerve and superficial sensory branch of the radial nerve. J Hand Surg [Am] 10:522–526, 1985.
693. Mackinnon SE, Dellon AL: Pain after radial sensory nerve grafting. J Hand Surg [Br] 11:341–34, 1986.
694. Mackinnon SE, Dellon AL: Reply to T. Brushart's letter on the stury of neurotrophism in a primate model. J Hand Surg 12A:809, 1987.
695. Mackinnon SE, Dellon AL: Results of treatment of recurrent dorsoradial wrist neuromas. Ann Plast Surg 19:54–61, 1987.
696. Mackinnon SE, Dellon AL: The use of soft tissue expansion in the hand. J Hand Surg [Br] 12:73–77, 1987.
697. Mackinnon SE, Dellon AL: Two-point discrimination testor. J Hand Surg [Am] 10:906–907, 1985.
698. Mackinnon SE, Dellon AL, Daneshvar A: Histopathology of the tarsal tunnel syndrome: Examination of a human posterior tibial nerve. Contemp Orthop 9:43–48, 1984.
699. Mackinnon SE, Dellon AL, Daneshvar A: Tarsal tunnel syndrome: Histopathological examination of a human posterior tibial nerve. Contemp Orthop 9:43–47, 1984.
700. Mackinnon SE, Dellon AL: The latissimus dorsi muscle flap—a segmentally innervated muscle transfer for facial examination. Technical considerations. Microsurg 9:36–45, 1988.
701. Mackinnon SE, Dellon AL, Hudson AR, Hunter DA: Alteration of neuroma formation by manipulation of neural environment. Plast Reconstr Surg 76:345, 1985.
702. Mackinnon SE, Dellon AL, Hudson AR, Hunter DA: A primate model for chronic nerve compression. J Reconstr Microsurg 1:185–194, 1985.
703. Mackinnon SE, Dellon AL, Hudson AR, Hunter D: Chronic nerve compression—experimental model in the rat. Ann Plast Surg 13:112–120, 1984.
704. Mackinnon SE, Dellon AL, Hudson AR, Hunter DA: Histopathology of compression of the superficial radial nerve in the forearm. J Hand Surg [Am] 11:206–209, 1986.
705. Mackinnon SE, Dellon AL, Hudson AR, Hunter DA: Nerve regeneration through a pseudosynovial sheath in a primate model. Plast Reconstr Surg 75:833–839, 1985.
706. Mackinnon SE, Dellon AL, Hudson AR, Hunter DA: Histopathology of chronic human nerve compression. Neuropathol Appl Neurobiol 12:547–565, 1986.
707. Mackinnon SE, Dellon AL, Lundborg G, Hudson AR: A study of neurotropism in the primate model. J Hand Surg [Am] 11:888–894, 1986.
708. Mackinnon SE, Holder LE: Use of three-phase radionuclide bone scanning in the diagnosis of reflex sympathetic dystrophy. J Hand Surg [Am] 9:556–563, 1984.
709. Mackinnon SE, Hudson AR, Hunter DA: Histologic assessment of nerve regeneration in the rat. Plast Reconstr Surg 75:384–388, 1985.
710. Mackinnon SE, Hudson AR, Llamas F, Dellon AL, Kline DG, Hunter DA: Peripheral nerve injury by chymopapain injection. J Neurosurg 61:1–8, 1984.
711. Mackinnon SE, Hudson AR, Bojanowski V, Hunter DA, Maraghi E: Peripheral nerve injury with purified bovine collagen—an experimental model in the rat. Ann Plast Surg 14:428–436, 1985.
712. Mackinnon SE, Hudson AR, Gentili F, et al: Peripheral nerve injection study with steroid agents. Plast Reconstr Surg 69:482–490, 1982.
713. Mackinnon SE, Hudson AR, Trued S, Hunter DA: Nerve regeneration in the rat model. Peripheral Nerve Repair Regeneration. 1:41–48, 1986.
714. Mackinnon SE, O'Brien JP, Dellon AL, McLean AR, Hudson AR, Hunter DA: A model of chronic nerve compression in the rat model. Ann Plast Surg, 19:430–435, 1987.
715. Mackinnon SE, O'Brien JP, Dellon AL, MacLean AR, Hudson AR, Hunter DA: An assessment of the effects of internal neurolysis, on a chronically compressed rat sciatic nerve. Plast Reconstr Surg, 81:251–256, 1988.

716. MacNichol MF: Results of operations for ulnar neuritis. J Bone Joint Surg 61B:159–164, 1979.
717. McCarroll HR: Nerve injuries associated with wrist trauma. Orthop Clin North Am 15:279–287, 1984.
718. McEwan LE: Median and ulnar nerve injuries. Aust NZ J Surg 32:89–104, 1962.
719. McFarlane RM, Moyer JR: Digital nerve grafts with the lateral antebrachial cutaneous nerve. J Hand Surg 1:169–173, 1976.
720. McFarlane RM, Mayer JR, Hugill JV: Further observations on the anatomy of the ulnar nerve at the wrist. Hand 8:115, 1976.
721. McGowan AJ: Results of transposition of the ulnar nerve for traumatic ulnar neuritis. J Bone Joint Surg 32B:293–301, 1950.
722. McLellan B, Phillips JM, Hunter GA: Bilateral lower extremity amputation after prolonged application of pneumatic antishock garment. Can J Surg 30:55–56, 1987.
723. McNamara MJ, Garrett WE, Seaber AV, et al: Neurorrhaphy nerve grafting and neurotization: A functional comparison of nerve reconstruction techniques. J Hand Surg [Am] 12:354–361, 1987.
724. McQuarrie IG: Acceleration of axonal regeneration in rat somatic motor neurons by using a conditioning lesion. In Gorio A, Millesi H, Mingrino S, eds: Posttraumatic Nerve Regeneration. Raven Press, New York, 1981, pp 49–58.
725. McQuarrie IG, Grafstein B, Gershon MD: Axonal regeneration in rat sciatic nerve. Effect of a conditioning lesion and of dcb-AMP. Brain Res 132:443–453, 1977.
726. McQuarrie IG, Graftstein B: Axon outgrowth enhanced by a pervious nerve injury. Arch Neurol 29:53–55, 1973.
727. Madison R, daSilva CF, Dikes P, Sidman RL, Chiu TH: Increased rate of peripheral nerve regeneration using bioabsorbable nerve guides and a laminin containing gel. Exp Neurol 88:767–772, 1985.
728. Mallet BL, Zilkha KJ: Compression of the ulnar nerve at the wrist by the ganglion. Lancet 1:890, 1955.
729. Mandruzzato F: Patholgeia e chirurgia del processo sopraepitrocleare del'omero. Chir Organi Mov 24:123–132, 1938.
730. Mangini U: Flexor pollicis longus muscle. Its morphology and clinical significance. J Bone Joint Surg 42A:467–470, 1960.
731. Manktelow RF, McKee NH, Veltese T: Anatomical study of pectoralis major muscle as related to functioning free muscle transplantation. Plast Reconstr Surg 65:610, 1980.
732. Manktelow RT, Zuker RM: Muscle transplantation by fascicular territory. Plast Reconstr Surg 73:751, 1984.
733. Manktelow RT, Zuker RM, McKee NH: Functioning free muscle transplantation. J Hand Surg 9A:32, 1984.
734. Manktelow RT: Free muscle transplantation for facial paralysis. In Terzis JK, ed: Microreconstruction of Nerve Injuries. WB Saunders, Philadelphia, 1987, pp 607–615.
735. Mann RA: Tarsal tunnel syndrome. Orthop Clin North Am 5:109–115, 1971.
736. Mannerfelt L: Evaluation of functional sensation of skin grafts in the hand area. Br J Plast Surg 15:136–154, 1962.
737. Mannerfelt L: Studies on the hand in ulnar nerve paralysis. A clinical-experimental investigation in normal and anomalous innervation. Acta Orthop Scand [Suppl] 87:1, 1966.
738. Mannerfelt L, Norman O: Attrition ruptures of flexor tendons in rheumatoid arthritis caused by bony spurs in the carpal tunnel. J Bone Joint Surg 51B:270–277, 1969.
739. Manske PR: Compression of the radial nerve by the triceps muscle. A case report. J Bone Joint Surg 59A:835–836, 1977.
740. Marie P, Foix C: Atrophie isolee de l'eminence thenar d'origine nevritique. Role du ligament annulaiare anterieus du carpe dans la pathoogenie de la lesion. Rev Neurol (Paris) 26:647–648, 1913.
741. Marie P, Meige H, Patrikios R: Paralysie radiale dissociee simulant une griffe cubitale. Rev Neurol (Paris) 24:123–124, 1917.
742. Marinacci AA: Applied Electromyography Lea & Febiger, Philadelphia, 1968.
743. Marinacci AA: Neurological syndromes of the tarsal tunnels. Bull Los Angeles Neurol Soc 33:90–100, 1968.
744. Markoe TM: Secondary nerve suture. Ann Surg 2:181, 1885.
745. Marmor L, Lawrence JF, Dubois E: Posterior interosseous nerve paralysis due to rheumatoid arthritis. J Bone Joint Surg 49A:381–383, 1967.
746. Marshall CF: Tennis elbow. Br Med J 1:559, 1907.
747. Marshall SC, Murray WR: Deep radial nerve palsy associated with rheumatoid arthritis. Clin Orthop 103:157–162, 1974.
748. Martens V, Bugden C: Thoracic outlet syndrome: A review of 67 cases. Canad J Surg 23:357–358, 1980.
749. Martin R: Tal om Nervus allmanna Egenskaper i Mannsikans Krobp. Stockholm, Lars Salvius, 1763.
750. Martin J, Gaspar DJ, Johnston PW, Kohl RD, Jr, Dietrick W: Vascular manifestations of the thoracic outlet syndrome and surgical urgency. Arch Surg 111:779–782, 1976.
751. Martinelli P, Gabollini AS, Poppi N, et al: Pronator syndrome due to thickened bicipital aponeurosis. J Neurol Neurosurg Psychiatry 45:181–182, 1982.
752. Mason ML: Tumours of the hand. Surg Gynecol Obstet 64:129–148, 1937.
753. Massey EW, Pleet AB: Handcuffs and cheiralgia paresthetica. Neurology (NY) 28:1312–1313, 1978.
754. Massey EW, Riley TL, Pleet AB: Co-existent carpal tunnel syndrome and cervical radiculopathy (double crush syndrome). South Med J 74:957–959, 1981.
755. Massey JM, Massey WE: Dr. Trevelyan and Mr. Treves, Sherlock Holmes and the elephant man. South Med J 78:854, 1985.
756. Matev I: A radiologic sign of entrapment of the median

nerve in the elbow joint after posterior dislocation. J Bone Joint Surg 58B:353–355, 1976.
757. Mathiowetz V, Weber K, Volland G, et al: Reliability and validity of grip and pinch strength evaluations. J Hand Surg [Am] 9:222–226, 1984.
758. Matsen FA III: Compartmental Syndromes. Grune & Stratton, New York, 1980.
759. Matsen FA, Crugmire RB: Compartmental syndromes. Surg Gynecol Obstet 147:943, 1978.
760. Matson DD: Early neurolysis in treatment of injury to the peripheral nerves due to faulty injection of antibiotics. N Engl J Med 242:973–975, 1950.
761. Matzdorf P: Zivei seltene Falle von Peripherer Sensibler Lahmung. Klin Wochenschr 5:1187, 1926.
762. Mayer L, Green W: Experiences with the Steindler flexorplasty at the elbow. J Bone Surg [Am] 36:775–789, 1954.
763. May M: Anatomy of the facial nerve (spatial orientation of fibers in the temporal bone). Laryngoscope 83:1311, 1973.
764. May M: The Facial Nerve. Thieme, New York, 1986.
765. May M: Muscle transposition for facial reanimation. Arch Otol 110:184–189, 1984.
766. May JW, Lukash FN, Galico GG, Sterrat CR: Removable thermocouple probe microvascular patency monitor: An experimental and clinical study. Plast Reconstr Surg 72:366, 1983.
767. May JW, Rosen H: Division of sensory ramus communicans between the ulnar and median nerves: A complication following carpal tunnel release: Case report. J Bone Joint Surg 63A:836–838, 1981.
768. Mayo-Robson AW: Nerve grafting as a means of restoring function in limbs paralysed by gunshot or other injuries. Br Med J 1:117, 1917.
769. Mayou BJ, Watson JS, Harison DH, Wynn Parry CB: Free microvascular and microneural transfer of the extensor digitorum brevis muscle for the treatment of unilateral facial palsy. Br J Plast Surg 34:362, 1981.
770. Meals RA: Peroneal nerve palsy complicating ankle sprain. J Bone Joint Surg 59A:966–968, 1977.
771. Meissl G, Millesi H: Nerve suture and grafting to restore extratemporal facial nerve. Clin Plast Surg 6:335, 1979.
772. Melzak R, Wall PD: Pain mechanisms—a new theory. Science 1950:971, 1965.
773. Merle M, Amend P, Cour C, Foucher G, Michon S: Microsurgical repair of peripheral nerve lesions: A study of 150 injuries of the median and ulnar nerves. Peripheral Nerve Repair Regeneration 2:17–26, 1986.
774. Merzenich MM: Alteration in cortical map following preferential digital stimulation in the adult monkey. (Abstr.) Neuroscience 10:1984.
775. Merzenich MM, Nelson RJ, Stryker MP, Cynader MS, Schoppmann A, Zok JUM: Somatosensory cortical map changes following digital amputation in adult monkey. J Comp Neurol 224:591–605, 1984.
776. Metzler J, Marks PS: Functional changes in cat somatosensory-motor cortex during short term reversible epidural blocks. Brain Res 177:379–383, 1979.
777. Meyers RR, Powell HC: Galactose neuropathy: Impact of chronic endoneurial edema on nerve-blood flow. Ann Neurol 16:587–594, 1984.
778. Meyer RA, Raja SN, Campbell JN, Mackinnon SE, Dellon AL: Neural activity originating from a neuroma in the baboon. Brain Res 325:255–260, 1985.
779. Miani N: Proximal-distal movement along the axon of protein perikaryon of regenerating neurons. Nature 185:541, 1960.
780. Michon J, Moberg E: Traumatic Nerve Lesions of the Upper Limb. Churchill Livingston, London, 1975.
781. Middleton DS: Occupational aneurysms of palmar arteries. Br J Surg 21:215–218, 1933.
782. Miehlke A: Normal and anomalous anatomy of the facial nerve. Trans Am Acad Ophthalmol Otolaryngol 68:1030, 1964.
783. Miehlke A: Surgery of the Facial Nerve. WB Saunders, Philadelphia, 1973.
784. Miehlke A: The results of surgery of the facial nerve. In Miehlke A, ed: Surgery of the Facial Nerve. Urban & Schwarzenberg, Munich, 1973, pp 225–235.
785. Mikhail IK: Median nerve lipoma in the hand. J Bone Joint Surg 46B:726–730, 1964.
786. Millender LH, Nalebuff EA, Holdsworth DE: Posterior interosseous nerve syndrome secondary to rheumatoid synovitis. J Bone Joint Surg 55A:753–757, 1973.
787. Miller RG: Cubital tunnel syndrome: Diagnosis and precise localization. Ann Neurol 6:56–59, 1979.
788. Millesi H: Brachial plexus injuries: Management and results. In Microreconstruction of Nerve Injuries. Terzis JK, ed. W.B. Saunders Co, Philadelphia, 1987, pp 347–360.
789. Millesi H: Founders lecture: Microsurgery of Peripheral Nerves: A Surgical Technique or a Biological Approach. American Society for Surgery of the Hand. San Antonio, Texas, 1987.
790. Millesi H: Indication, technique and results of nerve grafting. Handchirurgie [Suppl] 2:1–24, 1977.
791. Millesi H: Microsurgery of peripheral nerves. Hand 5:157–160, 1973.
792. Millesi H: Nerve grafting. Clin Plast Surg 11:105–120, 1984.
793. Millesi H: Surgical management of brachial plexus injuries. J Hand Surg 2:367–379, 1977.
794. Millesi H: The nerve gap. Hand Clin 2:651–663, 1986.
795. Millesi H, Berger A, Meissl G: Experimentelle Untersuchungen zur Heilung durchtrennter peripherer Nerven. Chir Plast 1:174, 1972.
796. Millesi H: Microsurgery of peripheral nerves: Neurolyses, nerve grafts, brachialplexus injuries. In Bunke HJ, and Furnas DW, eds: Symposium on Clinical Frontiers in Reconstructive Microsurgery. St Louis, CV Mosby, 1984, pp 353–373.
797. Millesi H: Conclusions: Clinical science. In Gorio A, Millesi H, Mingrino S, eds: Posttraumatic Peripheral Nerve Regeneration. Raven Press, New York, 1981. p 626.
798. Millesi H, Meissl G: Consequences of tension at the suture site. In Gorio A, Millesi H, Mingrino S, eds: Posttraumatic Peripheral Nerve Regeneration. Raven Press, New York, 1981, p 277.
799. Millesi H, Meissl G, Berger A: Further experience with interfascicular grafting of the median, ulnar and radial nerves. J Bone Joint Surg 58A:209–218, 1976.

800. Millesi H, Meissl G, Berger A: The interfascicular nerve grafting of the median and ulnar nerves. J Bone Joint Surg 54A:727–750, 1972.
801. Millesi H, Meissl G, Katzer H: Zur behandlung der verletzungen des plexus brachialis. Vorschlag Einer Integrirten therapie burns beitr klin 220:429–446, 1973.
802. Millesi H: Lower extremity nerve lesions. In Terzis JK, ed: Microreconstruction of Nerve Injuries. WB Saunders, Philadelphia, 1987, pp 239–251.
803. Millesi H, Terzis JK: Nomenclature in peripheral nerve surgery. Clin Plast Surg 11:3–8, 1984.
804. Millesi H: Unfallschaden peripherer Nerven. In Zenker R, Deucher F, Schink W, eds: Chirurgie der Gegenwart, vol. 4—Unfallchirurgie. Munchen, Urban & Schwarzenberg, 1975, pp 1–75.
805. Milling MAP, Kinmonth MH: False aneurysm of the ulnar artery. Hand 9:57–59, 1977.
806. Minami M, Ishii S: Satisfactory elbow flexion in complete brachial plexus injuries. Produced by suture of third and fourth intercostal nerves to musculocutaneous nerve. J Hand Surg 12A:1114–1118, 1987.
807. Minami A, Masamichi V, Hiroyuki K, Seiichi J: Thumb reconstruction by free sensory flaps from the foot using microsurgical techniques. J Hand Surg [Br] 9:239–244, 1984.
808. Minami A, Ogino T: Carpal tunnel syndrome in patients undergoing chemodialysis. J Hand Surg 12A:93–97, 1987.
809. Mitchell SW, Morehouse GR, Keen WW: In gunshot wounds and other injuries of nerves. JB Lippincott, Philadelphia, 1864.
810. Miyamoto Y, Tsuge K: Effects of tension on interneural microcirculation in end to end neurorrhaphy. In Gorio A, Millesi H, Mingrino S, eds: Posttraumatic Peripheral Nerve Regeneration. Raven Press, New York, 1981, p 81.
811. Moberg E: Criticism in study of methods for examining sensibility in the hand. Neurology (Minneap) 12:8–19, 1962.
812. Moberg E: Future hopes for the surgical management of peripheral nerve lesions. In Michon J, Moberg E, eds: Traumatic Nerve Lesions. Churchill Livingston, New York, 1975.
813. Moberg E: Methods for examining sensibility in the hand. In Flynn JE, ed: Hand Surgery. Williams & Wilkins, Baltimore, 1966, pp 435–439.
814. Moberg E: Objective methods for determining the functional value of sensibility in the skin. J Bone Joint Surg 40B:454–476, 1958.
815. Molander H, Olsson Y, Engkvist O, et al: Regeneration of peripheral nerve through a polyglactin tube. Muscle Nerve 5:54–57, 1982.
816. Moldauver J: Tourniquet paralysis syndrome. Arch Surg 68:136–144, 1954.
817. Molner W, Paul DJ: Complications of axillary arteriotomies. Radilogy 104:269–276, 1972.
818. Moloney S: Tarsal tunnel syndrome pain abated by operation to relieve pressure. Calif Med 101:378–379, 1964.
819. Moneim MS: Unusually high division of the median nerve. J Hand Surg 7:13–14, 1982.
820. Moon N, Marmor L: Parosteal lipoma of the proximal part of the radius. J Bone Joint Surg 46A:608–614, 1964.
821. Moore JR, Weiland AJ: Bilateral attritional rupture of the ulnar nerve at the elbow. J Hand Surg 5:358–360, 1980.
822. Morain WD, Dellon AL, Mackinnon SE, Colen LB: Reconstructive surgery in the diabetic extremity. Advan Plast Surg 4:1–36, 1987.
823. Morgan RF, Reisman NR, Wilgis EFS: Anatomic localization of sympathetic nerves in the hand. J Hand Surg 8:283–288, 1983.
824. Morley GH: Intraneural lipoma of the median nerve in the carpal tunnel. J Bone Joint Surg 46B:734–735, 1964.
825. Morrey BF, Askew LJ, An KN, Dobyns JH: Rupture of the distal tendon of the biceps brachii. J Bone Joint Surg 67A:418–421, 1985.
826. Morris AH: Irreducible Monteggia lesion with radial-nerve entrapment. J Bone Joint Surg 56A:1744–1746, 1974.
827. Morris H: The rider's sprain. Lancet 2:133, 1982.
828. Morris HH, Peters BH: Pronator syndrome: Clinical and electrophysiologic features in seven cases. J Neurol Neurosurg Psychiatry 39:461–464, 1976.
829. Morris J, Hudson A, Weddell G: A study of degeneration and regeneration in the divided rat sciatic nerve based on electron microscopy. Z Zellforsch Mikrosk Anat 124: 76, 1972.
830. Morton TG: A peculiar and painful affection of the fourth metatarsophalangeal articulation. Am J Med Sci 71:37–45, 1876.
831. Moss SH, Switzer HE: Radial tunnel syndrome: A spectrum of clinical presentations. J Hand Surg 8:414–419, 1983.
832. Moszkowicz LP: Zur Behandlung der schmerzhaften neuroma. Zentralbl Chir 45:547, 1918.
833. Mouchet A: Paralysies tardives du nerf cubital a la suite des fractures du condyle externe de l'humerus. J Chir (Paris) 12:437, 1914.
834. Mountcastle VB, Talbot WH, Darian-Smith I, Kornhuber HH: Neural basis for the sense of flutter-vibration. Science 155:597, 1967.
835. Moyer EK, Kimmel DL: The repair of severed motor and sensory spinal nerve roots by the arterial sleeve method of anastomosis. J Comp Neurol 88:285, 1984.
836. Muburak SJ, Hargens AR, Owen CA, et al: The wick catheter technique for measurement of intramuscular pressure—a new research and clinical tool. J Bone Joint Surg 58A:1016, 1976.
837. Muckart RD: Compression of the common peroneal nerve by intramuscular ganglion from the superior tibiofibular joint. J Bone Joint Surg 58B:241–244, 1976.
838. Muenthaler V, Probst C, Muenthaler A, Weber EG, Schnyder J: Das tarsal tunnel Syndrome. Schweiz Med Wochensehr 94:373–382, 1964.
839. Mulder JD: The causative mechanism in Morton's metatarsalgia. J Bone Joint Surg 33B:94–95, 1951.
840. Mulholland RC: Non-traumatic progressive paralysis of

the posterior interosseous nerve. J Bone Joint Surg 48B:781–785, 1966.

841. Munro D: Prevention of amputation neuromas. Consultant 12:26, 1972.
842. Munro D, Mallory GK: Elimination of the so called amputation neuromas of derivative peripheral nerves. J Med 260:358, 1959.
843. Murphy JB: Cicatrical fixation of ulnar nerve from ancient cubitus valgus—release and transference to new site. Clin John B. Murphy 661–670, 1916.
844. Murphy JB: The clinical significance of cervical ribs. Surg Gynecol Obstet 3:515–520, 1906.
845. Murphy T: Brachial neuritis caused by pressure of the first rib. Aust Med J 15:582, 1910.
846. Murray JF, Carman W, Mackenzie JK: Transmetacarpal amputation of the index finger and clinical assessment of hand strength and complications. J Hand Surg 2:471–481, 1977.
847. Naitziger HC, Grant WT: Neuritis of the brachial plexus. Mechanical in origin: the scalenus anticus syndrome. Surg Gynecol Obstet 67:722–730, 1938.
848. Nakatsuchi Y, Matsui T, Honda Y: Funicular orientation by electrical stimulation and internal neurolysis in peripheral nerve suture. Hand 12:65–73, 1980.
849. Nalebuff EA, Potter TA: Rheumatoid involvement of tendon and tendon sheaths in the hand. Clin Orthop 59:147–159, 1968.
850. Narakas A: Brachial plexus surgery. Ortho Clin Am 12: 303–323, 1981.
851. Narakas A: Indications et resultats du traitement chirurgical direct dans les lesions par elongation du plexus brachial. Rev Chir Orthop 63:88, 1977.
852. Narakas A: Lesions dans les elongations du plexus brachial. Rev Chir Orthop 63:44–55, 1977.
853. Narakas A: Neurotization or nerve transfer for brachial plexus lesions. Ann Chir de la Main 1:101–118, 1982.
854. Narakas A: Surgical treatment of traction injuries of the brachial plexus. Clin Ortho 133:71–90, 1978.
855. Narakas A: Thoughts on neurotization or nerve transfers in irreparable nerve lesions. In Microreconstruction of Nerve Injuries. J.K. Terzis, ed. W.B. Saunders Co., Philadelphia, 1987, pp 447–451.
856. Nashold BS: Current status of the DREZ operation: 1984. Neurosurg 15:942–944, 1984.
857. Nathes A, Chacha PB, Lim P: Acute carpal tunnel syndrome secondary to thrombosis of a persistent median artery. Ann Acad Med Singapore 9:118–121, 1980.
858. Neary D, Eames RA: The pathology of ulnar nerve compression in man. Neuropathol Appl Neurobiol 1:69–88, 1975.
859. Neary D, Ochoa J, Gilliatt RW: Subclinical entrapment neuropathy in man. J Neurol Sci 24:283–298, 1975.
860. Neblett C, Ehni G: Medial epicondylectomy for ulnar palsy. J Neurosurg 32:55–62, 1970.
861. Nelson MR: Effects of elbow position on motor conduction velocity of the ulnar nerve. Phys Ther 60:780–783, 1980.
862. Nelson PM: Implications of the electromyographic examination for hand therapy. Ch 44 In Hunter DA, Schneider R, Mackinnon SE, eds: Rehabilitation of the Hands. CV Mosby, Co., St. Louis, 1984.
863. Nelsen VK, Janetta PJ: Pathophysiology of hemifacial spasm: III: Effects of facial nerve decompression Neurology (Cleve) 34:891–897, 1984.
864. Nichols HM: Anatomic structures of the thoracic outlet. Clin Orthop 207:13–20, 1986.
865. Nicholson OR, Seddon HJ: Nerve repair in civil practice. Br Med J 2:1065–1071, 1957.
866. Nicolle FV, Woolhouse FM: Nerve compression syndromes of the upper limb. J Trauma 5:313–318, 1965.
867. Nielsen HO: Posterior interosseous nerve paralysis caused by fibrous band compression at the supinator muscle. A report of four cases. Acta Orthop Scand 47:304–307, 1976.
868. Nielsen JB, Torup D: Nerve injuries in the upper extremities. Dan Med Bull 11:92–95, 1964.
869. Nirschlel RP, Pettrone FA: Tennis elbow and the surgical treatment of lateral epicondylitis. J Bone Joint Surg 61A:832–839, 1979.
870. Nisenfield FG, Neviaser RJ: Fracture of the hook of the hamate: A diagnosis easily missed. J Trauma 14:612, 1974.
871. Nissen KI: Plantar digital neuritis: Morton's metatarsalgia. J Bone Joint Surg 30B:84–94, 1948.
872. Noble W: Observations on the microcirculation of peripheral nerves. Bibl Anat 10:316, 1968.
873. Nulsen FE, Slade HW: Peripheral nerve regeneration. In Woodhall B, Beebe GW, eds. A follow up study of 3,656 World War II Injuries. Recovery following injury to the brachial plexus. Veterans' Administration Medical Myelograph, pp 389–408, 1956.
874. O'Brien B, Mackinnon SE, Franklin JD, Morrison WA: Cross-facial nerve grafts and microneurovascular free muscle transfer for long-established facial palsy. Br J Plast Surg 33:202, 1980.
875. O'Brien JP, Mackinnon SE, MacLean AR, Dellon AL, Hudson AR, Hunter DA: A model of chronic nerve compression in the rat. Ann Plast Surg 19:430–435, 1987.
876. Ober WB: Mark Akenside, M.D. (1721–1770). Physician and philosophic poet. New York State J Med 68: 3116, 1968.
877. Ochoa J, Danta G, Fowler TJ, Gilliatt RW: Nature of the nerve lesion caused by a pneumatic tourniquet. Nature 233:265, 1971.
878. Ochoa J, Fowler TJ, Gilliatt RW: Anatomical changes in peripheral nerves compressed by a pneumatic tourniquet. J Anat 113:413–433, 1972.
879. Ochoa J, Gilliatt RW, Fowler TJ: Tourniquet paralysis in a baboon. Transam Neurolog Assoc 97:52, 1972.
880. Ochs S: Basic properties of axonplasmic transport. In Dyck PJ, Thomas PK, Lambert EH, Bunge R, eds: Peripheral Neuropathy, 2nd ed. WB Saunders, Philadelphia, 1984.
881. Ochs S: Regeneration of nerve in relation to axoplasmic transport. An analysis. In Gorio A, Millesi H, Mingrino S, eds: Posttraumatic Peripheral Nerve Regeneration. Raven Press, New York, 1981, pp 115–128.
882. Ochsner S, Gage M, DeBakey M: Scalenus anticus (Naffziger's syndrome). Am J Surg 28:669–695, 1935.
883. Oester VT, Davis L: Recovery of sensory functions. In Woodhall B, Beebe GW eds: Peripheral Nerve Regen-

eration. U.S. Government Printing Office, Washington DC, 1956, pp 241–310.
884. Oh SJ, Sarala PK, Kuba T, Elmore RS: Tarsal tunnel syndrome: Electrophysiological study. Ann Neurol 5:327–330, 1979.
885. Ohnishi A, Schilling K, Brimijoin WS, Lambert EH, Fairbanks, VF, Dyck PJ: Lead neuropathy. I. Morphometry, nerve conduction and cholinacetyle transferase transport. New finding of endoneurial edema associated with segmental demyelination. J Neuropathol Exp Neurol 36:499–518, 1977.
886. Olsson Y, Kristensson K, Klatzo J: Permeability of blood vessels in connective tissue sheaths in the peripheral nervous system to exogenous proteins. Acta Neuropathol [Suppl] (Berl) 5:61, 1971.
887. Olsson Y, Reese T: Permeability of vasa nervorum and perineurium in mouse sciatic nerve studies by fluorescence and electronmicroscopy. J Neuropathol Exp Neurol 30:105–119, 1971.
888. Omer GE Jr: Injuries to the nerves of the upper extremities. J Bone Joint Surg 56A:1615–1624, 1974.
889. Omer GE Jr: The results of untreated traumatic injuries. In Omer GE Jr, Spinner M. eds: Management of Peripheral Nerve Problems. WB Saunders, Philadelphia, 1980.
890. Önne L: Recovery of sensibility and sudomotor activity in the hand after nerve suture. Acta Chir Scand (Suppl) 300:1–70, 1962.
891. Orgel MG: Epineurial versus perineurial repair of peripheral nerves. Clin Plast Surg 11:101–104, 1984.
892. Orgel MG, Terzis JK: Epineurial versus perineural repair. An ultrastructural and electrophysiological study of nerve regeneration. Plast Reconstr Surg 60:80–91, 1977.
893. Ortiguela ME, Wood MD, Cahill DR: Anatomy of the sural nerve complex. J Hand Surg [Am] 12:1119–1123, 1987.
894. Ortman JA, Zarife S, Mendell JR: The experimental production of Renaut bodies. J Neurol Sci 62:233–241, 1983.
895. Osborne G: Surgical treatment of tardy ulnar neuritis. J Bone Joint Surg 39B:782, 1957.
896. Osborne G: The elbow and forearm. In Rob C, Smith R, eds: Clinical Surgery. Butterworths, London, 1966, pp 417–454.
897. Osborne G: Ulnar neuritis. Postgrad Med J 35:392–396, 1959.
898. Osborne J: Compression neuritis of the ulnar nerve. Hand 2:10–14, 1970.
899. Otenasek FJ; Progressive paralysis of the nervus dorsalis: Pathological findings in one case. Bull Johns Hopkins Hosp 81:163–167, 1947.
900. Packer JW, Foster RR,.Garcia A, Corantham BA: The humeral fracture with radial nerve palsy: Is exploration warranted? Clin Orthop 88:34–38, 1972.
901. Paget J: Lectures on Surgical Pathology, 2nd ed., Lindsay and Blakiston, Philadelphia, 1854, p 42.
902. Paine EW: Tardy ulnar palsy. Can J Surg 13:255–261, 1970.
903. Paine KWE: The carpal tunnel syndrome. Can J Surg 6:446–449, 1963.
904. Panas J: Sur une cause peu connue de paralysie du nerf cubital. Arch Gen Med 2:5–22, 1878.
905. Pang D, Wessel HB: Thoracic outlet syndrome: Review article. Neurosurg 22:105–121, 1988.
906. Parks BJ: Postoperative peripheral neuropathies. Surgery 74:348–357, 1973.
907. Parr J, Johnson K: Interdigital neuroma treated by neuroma resection. Presented at Foot and Ankle Society Meeting, February, 1988, Atlanta, Georgia.
908. Parry GJG: Mononeuropathy multiplex. Muscle Nerve 8:493–498, 1985.
909. Parsonage MJ, Turner JWA: Neuralgic amyotrophy: The shoulder girdle syndrome. Lancet 1:973–978, 1948.
910. Patrick J: Carpal tunnel syndrome. Br Med J 14:1377–1378, 1965.
911. Pauker SG, Kassier JP; Decision analysis. N Engl J Med 316:250–258, 1987.
912. Payan J: Anterior transposition of the ulnar nerve: An electrophysiological study. J Neurol Neurosurg Psychiatry 33:157–165, 1970.
913. Payr E: Beitrage zur Technik der Blutgefass und Nervennaht nebst Mittheilungen uber die Verevendung eines resorbibaren Metalles in der Chirurgie. Arch Klin Chir 62:67, 1900.
914. Pechan J, Julis I: The pressure measurement in the ulnar nerve: A contribution to the pathophysiology of the cubital tunnel syndrome. J Biomech 8:75–79, 1975.
915. Pecket P, Gloobe H, Nathan H: Variations in the arteries of the median nerve. Clin Orthop 97:144–147, 1973.
916. Peet RM, Hendrickson JD, Anderson TP, Martin GM: Thoracic outlet syndrome: Evaluation of a therapeutic exercise program. Staff Meet Mayo Clinic 31:281–287, 1956.
917. Perrin E, Labry R: La fracture de l'asophyse, styloide, du Peronee. Rev Orthop 13:325–331, 1926.
918. Petropoulos PC, Stefanko S: Experimental observations on the prevention of neurom formation. J Surg Res 1:241, 1961.
919. Petropoulos PC, Stefanko S: Experimental studies of posttraumatic neuroma under various physiologic conditions. J Surg Res 1:235, 1961.
920. Petrucci FS, Morelli A, Raimondi PL: Axillary nerve injuries—21 cases treated by nerve graft and neurolysis. J Hand Surg 7:271–278, 1982.
921. Phalen GS: Calcification adjacent to the pisiform bone. J Bone Joint Surg 34A:579–580, 1952.
922. Phalen GS: The birth of a syndrome, or carpal tunnel revisited. J Hand Surg 6:109–111, 1981.
923. Phalen GS: The carpal tunnel syndrome. Seventeen years experience in diagnosis and treatment of 654 hands. J Bone Joint Surg 48A:211–228, 1966.
924. Phalen GS, Gardner WJ, LaLonda AA: Neuropathy of median nerve due to compression beneath transverse carpal ligament. J Bone Joint Surg 32A:109–112, 1950.
925. Phalen GS, Kendrick JI, Rodriguez JM: Lipomas of the upper extremity. Am J Surg 121:298–306, 1971.
926. Philipeaux JM, Vulpian A: Note sur sa essais de greffe d'un troncon de nerf lingual entre les deux vouts de thypoglose. Arch Physiol Norm Pathol 3:618, 1817.
927. Phillips JE, Mackinnon SE, Dellon AL, Beatty E, O'Brien

J: Vibratory sensory testing in acute compartment syndrome. Clinical and experimental study. Plast Reconstr Surg 79:796–801, 1987.

928. Phor WH, Raszid D: A ganglion causing tarsal tunnel syndrome: Report of a case. Aust NZ J Surg 48:96–97, 1978.

929. Platt H: On the peripheral nerve complications of certain fractures. Surg Gynecol Obstet 47:822–825, 1928.

930. Platt H: On the results of bridging gaps in injured nerve trunks by autogenous fascial tubulization and autogenous nerve grafts. Br J Surg 7:384–389, 1919.

931. Platt H: The pathogenesis and treatment of traumatic neuritis of the ulnar nerve in the post-condylar groove. Br J Surg 13:409–431, 1926.

932. Platt PT: The operative treatment of traumatic ulnar neuritis at the elbow. Surg Gynecol Obstet 47:822–825, 1928.

933. Politis MJ, Ederle K, Spencer PS: Trophism in nerve regeneration. In vivo attraction of regenerating axons by diffusable factors derived from cells in distal nerve stumps of transected peripheral nerve. Brain Res 253:1–12, 1982.

934 Popelka S, Vainio D: Entrapment of the posterior interosseous branch of the radial nerve in rheumatoid arthritis. Acta Orthop Scand 45:370–372, 1974.

935. Popin JL: Atlas of Neurosurgical Techniques. WB Saunders, Philadelphia, 1967.

936. Poppin MK, McCarroll HR Jr, Doyle JR, et al: Recovery of sensibility of the sutured digital nerves. J Hand Surg 4:212–226, 1979.

937. Portmann M, ed: Facial Nerve, Proceedings of the Fifth International Symposium. Masson Publishing USA, New York, 1985.

938. Portmann M: Conclusions (of the Fifth International Symposium on the Facial Nerve regarding A Facial Nerve Grading System). In Portmann M, ed: Facial Nerve. Masson Publishing USA, New York, 1985, pp 43–44.

939. Posch JL, dela Cruz-Saddul F: Nerve repair in trauma surgery: A ten-year study of 231 peripheral injuries. Orthop Rev 9:35–45, 1980.

940. Posch JL, Marcotte DR: Carpal tunnel syndrome: An analysis of 1201 cases. Orthop Rev 5:25–35, 1976.

941. Poth EJ, Bravo-Fernandez E, Dreager GA: Prevention of formation of end-bulb neuromata. Proc Soc Exp Biol Med 60:200–207, 1945.

942. Powell HC: Pathology of diabetic neuropathy: New observations and new hypotheses. Lab Invest 49:515–518, 1983.

943. Powell HC, Meyers RR: Schwann cell changes and demyelination in chronic galactose neuropathy. Muscle Nerve 6:217–218, 1983.

944. Powell HC, Myers RR, Costello ML, et al: Endoneurial fluid pressure in Wallerian degeneration. Ann Neurol 5:550–557, 1979.

945. Pringle RM, Protheroe K, Mukherjee SK: Entrapment neuropathy of sural nerve. J Bone Joint Surg 56B:465–468, 1974.

946. Pulkki T, Vainio K: Compression of the ulnar nerve due to rheumatoid arthritis at the elbow. Ann Chir Gynecol Fenn 51:327–330, 1962.

947. Pulvertaft RG: Unusual tumours of the median nerve. J Bone Joint Surg 46B:731–733, 1964.

948. Purcell FH, Gurdjian ES: Hemangiomata of peripheral nerves. Am J Surg 30:541, 1935.

949. Qvarfordt PG, Ehrenfeld WK, Stoney RJ: Supraclavicular radical scalenectomy and transaxillary first rib resection for the thoracic outlet syndrome. A combined approach. Amer J Surg 148:111–116, 1984.

950. Radinel EL: Tarsal tunnel syndrome. Clin Orthop 181:167–170, 1983.

951. Raff J: Surgery for cervical rib and scalenus anticus syndrome. JAMA 157:219–223, 1955.

952. Raff M, Asbury AK: Ischemic mononeuropathy and mononeuropathy multiplex in diabetes mellitus. N Engl J Med 279:17–22, 1968.

953. Rana NA, Kenwright J, Taylor RG, Rushworth G: Complete lesion of the median nerve associated with dislocation of the elbow joint. Acta Orthop Scand 45:365–369, 1974.

954. Ransford AO, Hughes SPF: Complete brachial plexus lesions—a ten-year follow-up of twenty cases. J Bone Joint Surg 59B:417–420, 1977.

955. Rash MR: Entrapment of the anterior tibial nerve: Report of a case treated surgically. J Neurol Orthop Surg 1:153, 1980.

956. Rask MR: Superficial radial neuritis and deQuervain's disease: Report of three cases. Clin Orthop 131:176–178, 1978.

957. Rasmusson M: Reorganization of racoons somatosensory cortex following removal of the fifth digit. J Compar Neurol 205:313–326, 1982.

958. Rawa Al: Ueber die Nervennaht. Wien Med Wchnschr 35:358, 1885.

959. Rayan GM: Persistent median artery and compression neuropathy. Orthop Rev 40:89–92, 1986.

960. Ramón y Cajal SR: Mechanismo de la degeneracion y regeneration de nervos. Trab Lab Inbest Biol, Madrid 4:119, 1905.

961. Recklinghausen VF: Ueber die multiplen Fibrome per Haut und ihre Beziehung zu den multiplen Neuromen. Verleg v. A. Hirschwald, Berlin, 1982.

962. Reimann AF, Daseler EH, Anson BJ, Beaton LE: The palmaris longus muscle and tendon. The study of 1600 extremities. Anatom Rec 89:495–505, 1944.

963. Reis ND: Anomalous triceps tendon as the cause for snapping elbow in ulnar neuritis. J Hand Surg 5:361–362, 1980.

964. Reisman NR, Dellon AL: The abductor digiti minimi muscle flap: A salvage technique for palmar wrist pain. Plast Reconstr Surg 72:859–863, 1983.

965. Renaut A: Recherches sur quelques points particuliers d'histologie des nerfs. Arch Physiol 8:180–190, 1881.

966. Rengachary SS, Arjunan K: Compression of the ulnar nerve at Guyon's canal by soft tissue giant cell tumor. Neurosurgery 8:400–405, 1981.

967. Rhoades CE, Mowery CA, Gelberman RH: Results of internal neurolysis of the median nerve for severe carpal tunnel syndrome. J Bone Joint Surg 67A:253–256, 1985.

968. Riccardi VM: von Recklinghausen's neurofibromatosis. N Engl J Med 305:1617–1627, 1981.

969. Riccardi VM, Mulvihill JJ: Neurofibromatosis (von Recklinghausen's disease). Adv Neurol 29:1–282, 1981.

970. Richards RL: Traumatic ulnar neuritis: The results of anterior transposition of the ulnar nerve. Edinb Med J 52:14–21, 1945.

971. Richards RR, Waddell JP, Hudson AR: Shoulder arthrodesis for the treatment of brachial plexus palsy. Clin Orthop 198:250–258, 1985.

972. Richardson PM, Issa VMK: Peripheral injury enhances central regeneration of primary sensory neurones. Nature 309:791–793, 1984.

973. Richardson PM, Verge VMK: The induction of a regenerative propensity in sensory neurons following peripheral axonal injury. J Neurocytol 15:585–594, 1986.

974. Riche P: Le Nerf cubital et les muscles de l'eminence thenar. Bull Mem Soc Anat Paris 5:251–252, 1897.

975. Richmond DA: Carpal ganglion with ulnar nerve compression. J Bone Joint Surg 45B:513, 1963.

976. Richmond DA: Lipoma causing a posterior interosseous nerve lesion. J Bone Joint Surg 35B:83, 1953.

977. Rietz KA, Önne L: Analysis of sixty-five operated cases of carpal tunnel syndrome. Acta Chir Scand 133:443–447, 1967.

978. Riley DA, Lang DH: Carbonic anhydrase activity of human peripheral nerves. A possible histochemical aid to nerve repair. J Hand Surg (Am) 9:112–124, 1984.

979. Robertson KB: Electrodiagnosis in neurological rehabilitation. In Umphred DA, ed: Neurological Rehabilitation, CB Mosby, St. Louis, 1985.

980. Roger of Parma, quoted by Henderson HE: Gilbertus Anglicus Medicine of the 13th century, Medical Library Association, Cleveland, 1918.

981. Roles NC, Maudsley RH: Radial tunnel syndrome: Resistant tennis elbow as a nerve entrapment. J Bone Joint Surg 54B:499–508, 1972.

982. Rolfsen L: Snapping triceps tendon with ulnar neuritis. Acta Orthop Scand 41:74–76, 1970.

983. Roos DB: Congenital anomalies associated with thoracic outlet syndrome. Am J Surg 132:771–778, 1976.

984. Roos DB: The place for scalenectomy and first rib resection in thoracic outlet syndrome. Surg 92:1077–1085, 1982.

985. Roos DB, Owens JC: Thoracic outlet syndrome. Arch Surg 93:71–74, 1966.

986. Rorabeck CH, Cassell GS, Hardie R, Logan J: Compartmental pressure measurements—an experimental investigation using the slit catheter. J Trauma 21:446, 1981.

987. Roraback CH, Harris WR: Factors affecting the prognosis of brachial plexus injuries. J Bone Joint Surg 63B:404–407, 1981.

988. Rose EH, Kowalski TA: Vascularized nerve grafts in the dorsum of the foot. J Hand Surg [Am] 10:514–521, 1985.

989. Rose HA, Hood RW, Otis JC, Ranawat CS, Insall JN: Peroneal nerve palsy following total knee arthroplasty. J Bone Joint Surg 64A:347–351, 1982.

990. Rothman HR, Simeone FE: The Spine. Philadelphia, WB Saunders, 1975, pp 387–433.

991. Roussy G, Branche J: Deux cas de paralysies dissociees de la branche posterieure du radial a type de pseudo-griffe cubitale. Rev Neurol (Paris) 24:312–314, 1917.

992. Rowlan SA: Case report–ten year follow-up of lipofibroma of the median nerve in the palm. J Hand Surg 2:316–317, 1977.

993. Rowland SA: Lipofibroma of the median nerve in the palm. J Bone Joint Surg 49A:1309–1313, 1967.

994. Rowntree T: Anomalous innervation of the hand muscles. J Bone Joint Surg 31B:505–510, 1949.

995. Rubin LR: Reanimation of the Paralyzed Face. CV Mosby, St. Louis, 1977.

996. Rubin LR: The anatomy of a smile—its importance in facial paralysis. Plast Reconstr Surg 53:384, 1974.

997. Rubin LR, Lee GW, Simpson RL: Reanimations of the long-standing partial facial paralysis. Plast Reconstr Surg 77:41–49, 1986.

998. Ruby JR, Janetta PJ: Hemifacial spasm. Ultrastructural changes in the facial nerve induced by vascular compression. Surg Neurol 4:369–370, 1975.

999. Ruch TC, Fulton JF, German WJ: Sensory discrimination in monkey, chimpanzee and man after lesions of parietal lobe. Arch Neurol Psychiatry 39:919–938, 1938.

1000. Ruderman MI, Palmer RH, Olarte MR, et al: Tarsal tunnel syndrome caused by hyperlipidemia: Reversal after plasmaphoresis. Arch Neurol 40:124–125, 1983.

1001. Rudge PE; Tourniquet paralysis with prolonged conduction block: Electrophysiological study. J Bone Joint Surg 56B:716–720, 1974.

1002. Rudge P, Ochoa J, Gilliatt RW: Acute peripheral nerve compression in the baboon. Anatomical and physiological findings. J Neurol Sci 23:403, 1974.

1003. Russell DS, Rubinstein LJ: Pathology of Tumors of the Nervous System, 4th ed. Williams & Wilkins, Baltimore, 1977, pp 293–297.

1004. Rydevik B, Lundborg G: Permeability of intraneural microvessels in perineurium following acute graded experimental nerve compression. Scand J Plast Reconstr Surg 11:179, 1977.

1005. Rydevik B, Lundborg G, Bagge U: Effects of graded compression on interneural blood flow. J Hand Surg 6:3, 1981.

1006. Rydevik B, Lundborg G, Nordborg C: Intraneural tissue reactions induced by internal neurolysis. Scand J Plast Reconstr Surg 10:3–8, 1976.

1007. Sade J: Facial nerve reconstruction and its prognosis. Ann Otol Rhinol Laryngol 84:695, 1975.

1008. Saeed MA, Gatens PF: Compound nerve action potential of medial and lateral plantar nerves through the tarsal tunnel. Arch Phys Med Rehabil 63:304–307, 1982.

1009. Sakellaridies H: A follow-up study of 173 peripheral nerve injuries in the upper extremity of civilians. J Bone Joint Surg 44A:140–148, 1962.

1010. Samii M: Facial nerve grafting in acoustic neuroma. Clin Plast Surg 11:221–225, 1984.

1011. Samii M: Intraneurale Neurolyse des Nervus medianus beim Karpaltunnel Syndrom. Handchirurgie 8:117–119, 1976.

1012. Samii M, Kahl RI: Clinische resultate der autologen nerven transplantation. Nelssunger Med Mitteil 46:197–202, 1972.

1013. Sanders FK: Histopathology of nerve grafts. In Seddon

HJ, ed: Peripheral Nerve Injuries. Her Majesty's Printing Office, London, 1954, pp 134–155.
1014. Sanders FK, Young JZ: The influence of peripheral connections on the diameter of regenerating nerve fibres. J Exp Biol 22:203–212, 1946.
1015. Sanders RJ, Raymer S: The supraclavicular approach to scalenectomy and first rib resection: description of technique. J Vasc Surg 2:751–756, 1985.
1016. Sandhu HS, Sandberg BS: Occupational compression of the common peroneal nerve at the neck of the fibula. Aust NZ Surg 46:160–163, 1976.
1017. Saplys R, Mackinnon SE, Dellon AL: The relationship between nerve entrapment versus neuroma complications and the misdiagnosis of deQuervain's disease. Contemp Orthop 15:51–57, 1987.
1018. Sargent P: Lesions of the brachial plexus associated with rudimentary ribs. Brain 44:95–124, 1921.
1019. Sarrafian SK: Anatomy of the Foot and Ankle. JB Lippincott, Philadelphia, 1983.
1020. Sawa S, Iwosak T, Aoki N: Correlation of sensibility evaluation and object recognition in stroke patients. Am J Rehabil Med, 1988. In press.
1021. Schaumburg H, Kaplan J, Windebank A, Vick N, Rasmus S, Pleasure D, Brown MJ: Sensory neuropathy from pyridoxine abuse: A new megavitamin syndrome. N Engl J Med 309:445–448, 1983.
1022. Schjelderup H: Aberrant muscle in the hand causing ulnar nerve compression. (Abstr) J Bone Joint Surg 46B:361, 1964.
1023. Schmidt FO, Dev P, Smith BH: Electronic processing of information by brain cells. Science 193:114–120, 1976.
1024. Schmidt H, Eiken O: The anterior interosseous nerve syndrome. Scand J Plast Reconstr Surg 5:53–56, 1971.
1025. Schmidt FO, Sampson FE: Neuronal fibres proteins. Neurosci Res Program Bull 6:113–219, 1968.
1026. Schuchmann JA, Melvin JL, Duran RJ, Coleman CR: Evaluation of local steroid injection for carpal tunnel syndrome. Arch Phys Med Rehabil 52:253–255, 1971.
1027. Schultz F: Dtsch Z Nervenheilk 3:300, 1893.
1028. Scott FH: On the relation of nerve cells to fatigue of their nerve fibres. J Physiol (Lond) 34:145, 1906.
1029. Seckel BR, Chiu TH, Nyilas E, Sidman RL: Nerve regeneration through synthetic biodegradable nerve guides: Regulation by the target organ. Plast Reconstr Surg 74:173–181, 1984.
1030. Seckel BR, Ryan SE, Gagne RJ, Tin Ho Chiu CST, Watkins E: Target specific nerve regeneration through a nerve guide in the rat. Plast Reconstr Surg 78:793–798, 1986.
1031. Seckel BR, Ryan SE, Simons JE, et al: Vascularized versus nonvascularized nerve grafts. An experimental structural comparison. Plast Reconstr Surg 78:211, 1986.
1032. Sedal L, McLeod JG, Walsh JC: Ulnar nerve lesions associated with the carpal tunnel syndrome. J Neurol Neurosurg Psychiatry 36:118–123, 1973.
1033. Seddon H: Nerve grafting. J Bone Surg 45:447–461, 1963.
1034. Seddon H: Nerve lesions complicating certain closed bone injuries. JAMA 135:691–694, 1947.
1035. Seddon H: Surgical Disorders of the Peripheral Nerves. Williams & Wilkins, Baltimore, 1972.
1036. Seddon HJ: Three types of nerve injury. Brain 66:237, 1943.
1037. Seddon HJ: Carpal ganglion as a cause of paralysis of the deep branch of the ulnar nerve. J Bone Joint Surg 34B:386–390, 1952.
1038. Seddon HJ: Peripheral nerve injuries. Medical Research Council, Special Report Series 282, Her Majesty's Stationery Office, London, 1954.
1039. Seddon HJ: The use of autogenous grafts for repair of large gaps in peripheral nerves. Br J Surg 35:151–167, 1947.
1040. Seddon HJ, Medawar PB: Fibrin suture of human nerves. Lancet 2:87, 1942.
1041. Seddon HJ, Medawar PB, Smiths H: Rate of regeneration of peripheral nerves in man. J Physiol (Lond) 102:191–201, 1943.
1042. Seiler WA, Dellon AL, Mackinnon SE: Correlation of facial muscle anatomy and motor function in Maccaca fascicularis. Peripheral Nerve Repair Regeneration 1:41–48, 1986.
1043. Seiler WA, Schlegel R, Mackinnon SE, Dellon AL: The double crush syndrome: Development of a model. Surg Forum 34:596–598, 1983.
1044. Selig S: Peroneal paralysis due to compression by adhesive plaster. J Bone Joint Surg 20:222–223, 1938.
1045. Seltzer Z, Devor M: Ephaptic transmission in chronically damaged peripheral nerves. Neurology (Minneap) 29:1061–1064, 1974.
1046. Semple JC, Cargill AO: Carpal tunnel syndrome: Results of surgical decompression. Lancet 1:918–919, 1969.
1047. Settergren CR, Wood MB: Comparison of blood flow in free vascularized versus nonvascularized nerve grafts. J Reconstr Microsurg 1:95, 1984.
1048. Seyffarth H: Primary myoses in the M. pronator teres as a cause of lesion of the N. medianus (the pronator syndrome). Acta Psychiat Neurol (Suppl) 74:1, 1951.
1049. Sharma AK, Bajada S, Thomas PK: Influence of Streptozotocin-induced diabetes in myelinated nerve fiber maturation and body growth in the rat. Acta Neuropath (Berl) 53:257–261, 1981.
1050. Sharma AK, Thomas PK, Baker RW: Peripheral nerve abnormalities related to galactose administration in rats. J Neurol Neurosurg Psychiatry 39:794–802, 1976.
1051. Sharrard WJW: Anterior interosseous neuritis. Report of a case. J Bone Joint Surg 50B:804–805, 1968.
1052. Sharrard WJW: Posterior interosseous neuritis. J Bone Joint Surg 48B:777–780, 1966.
1053. Shea JD, McClain EJ: Ulnar nerve compression syndromes at and below the wrist. J Bone Joint Surg 51A: 1095–1103, 1969.
1054. Sheldon WD: Tardy palsy of the ulnar nerve. Med Clin North Am 5:499–509, 1921.
1055. Sherren J: Remarks on chronic neuritis of the ulnar nerve due to deformity in the region of the elbow joint. Edinb Med J 23:500–509, 1908.
1056. Sherren J: Some points in the surgery of peripheral nerves. Edinb Med J 20:297–332, 1906.
1057. Shields RW Jr: Alcoholic polyneuropathy. Muscle Nerve 8:183–187, 1985.
1058. Shizhen Z, Xiangluo T, Muzhil L: The microsurgical anatomy of peripheral nerves. In Shizhen Z, Yongjian

M, Wencyun Y, eds: Microsurgical Anatomy. MTP Press, Lancaster, England, 1985, pp 299–350.

1059. Siivoli J, Sulg I, Pokela R: Somatosensory evoked responses as a diagnostic aid in thoracic outlet syndrome. A preoperative study. Acta Chir (Scand) 148:647–652, 1982.

1060. Silver MA, Gelberman RH, Gellman H, Rhoades CE: Carpal tunnel syndrome: Associated abnormalities in ulnar nerve function and the effect of carpal tunnel release on these abnormalities. J Hand Surg [Am] 10:710–713, 1985.

1061. Silverstein A: Neuropathy in hemophilia. JAMA 190: 534–535, 1964.

1062. Silverstein A: Progressive paralysis of the dorsal interosseous nerve. Report of a case. Arch Neurol Psychiatry 38:885–886, 1937.

1063. Simeone FA: Acute and delayed traumatic peripheral entrapment neuropathies. Surg Clin North Am 51:1329–1336, 1972.

1064. Slingluff CL, Terzis JK, Edgerton MT: The quantitative microanatomy of the brachial plexus in man—reconstructive relevance. In Terzis JK, ed: Microreconstruction of Nerve Injuries. WB Saunders, Philadelphia, 1987, pp 285–324.

1065. Smellie W: A collection of cases and observations in midwifery. Vol 2, 4th ed., London, 1768, pp 446.

1066. Smith BH, Kornblith PL: Axonoplasmic transport and neurological surgery. Neurosurgery 10:268–276, 1982.

1067. Smith JW: True aneurysms of traumatic origin in the palm. Am J Surg 104:7–13, 1962.

1068. Smith MS: Handcuff neuropathy. Ann Emerg Med 10:668, 1981.

1069. Snyder CC: Epineurial repair. Orthop Clin North Am 12:267–276, 1981.

1070. Snyder CC, Knowles RP: Traumatic neuromas J Bone Joint Surg 47A:641–648, 1965.

1071. Snyder CC, Webster H, Pickens JE, et al: Intraneural neurorrhaphy. A preliminary clinical and histological evaluation. Ann Surg 167:691, 1968.

1072. Solieri S: Nevralgia del nervo mediano del processo sopraepitrocleare. Chir Organi Mov 14:171–180, 1929.

1073. Solnitzky O: Pronator syndrome: Compression neuropathy of the median nerve at the level of the pronator teres muscle. Georgetown Med Bull 13:232–238, 1960.

1074. Solomon LR, Hillman RS: Regulation of vitamin B_6 metabolism in human red cells. Am J Clin Nutr 32:1824–1831, 1979.

1075. Spalteholtz W: Hand Atlas of Human Anatomy. Barker LF, Translator of Fourth German edition. JB Lippincott, Philadelphia, 1906, pp 360, 361, 757.

1076. Spencer PS, Sabri MI, Schaumburg HH, et al: Does a defect of energy metabolism in the nerve fiber underlie axonal degeneration in polyneuropathies? Ann Neurol 5:501–507, 1979.

1077. Spencer PS, Schaumberg HH: Central-peripheral distal axonopathy: The pathogenesis of dying back polyneuropathies. In Zimmerman H, ed: Progress in Neuropathology, vol 3. Grune & Stratton, New York, 1976, p 253.

1078. Spencer PS, Schaumberg HH: Classification of neurotoxic disease. In Spencer PS, Schaumberg HH, eds: Experimental and Clinical Neurotoxicology. Williams & Wilkens, Baltimore, 1980, p 92.

1079. Spillane JD: Localized neuritis of the shoulder girdle. Lancet 2:532–534, 1943.

1080. Spindler HA, Dellon AL: Nerve conduction studies and sensibility testing in carpal tunnel syndrome. J Hand Surg 7:260–263, 1982.

1081. Spinner M: Cryptogenic infraclavicular brachial plexus neuritis. Bull Hosp Joint Dis 37:98–104, 1976.

1082. Spinner M: Injuries to the Major Branches of the Peripheral Nerves of the Forearm. WB Saunders, Philadelphia, 1978, pp 245–252.

1083. Spinner M: Management of nerve compression lesions in the upper extremity. In Omer GE Jr, Spinner M, eds: Management of Peripheral Nerve Problems. WB Saunders Co, Philadelphia, 1980.

1084. Spinner M: The anterior interosseous nerve syndrome with special attention to its variations. J Bone Joint Surg 52A:84–94, 1970.

1085. Spinner M: The arcade of Frohse and its relationship to posterior interosseous nerve paralysis. J Bone Joint Surg 50B:809–812, 1968.

1086. Spinner M, Freundlich BD: An important variation of the palmaris longus. Bull Hosp Joint Dis 28:126–130, 1967.

1087. Spinner M, Freundlich BD, Ticher J: Posterior interosseous nerve palsy as a complication of Monteggia fracture in children. Clin Orthop 58:141–145, 1968.

1088. Spinner M, Kaplan EB: The relationship of the ulnar nerve to the medial intermuscular septum in the arm and its clinical significance. Hand 8:239–242, 1976.

1089. Spinner M, Schrieber SN: The anterior interosseous nerve paralysis as a complication of supercondylar fractures in children. J Bone Joint Surg 51A:1584–1590, 1969.

1090. Spinner M, Spencer PS: Nerve compression lesions of the upper extremity: A clinical and experimental review. Clin Orthop 104:46–68, 1974.

1091. Spitzy H: Bemerkung zur Ueberbruckung von Nervendefekten. Munch Med Wochenschr 64:372, 1917.

1092. Sponsel KH, Palm ET: Carpal tunnel syndrome following Colles' fracture. Surg Gynecol Obstet 121:1252, 1965.

1093. Sponseller PD, Engber WD: Double-entrapment of radial tunnel syndrome. J Hand Surg 8:420–423, 1983.

1094. Sprofkin BF: Cheiralgia paresthetica—Wartenberg's disease. Neurology (Minneap) 4:857–862, 1954.

1095. Sprofkin BF, Isom JB: Sensory mononeuropathy. Am Pract Digest Treat 11:745–759, 1960.

1096. Sridhara CR, Izzo KL: Terminal sensory branches of the superficial peroneal nerve: An entrapment syndrome. Arch Phys Med Rehabil 66:789–792, 1985.

1097. Stack HG: Tumours of the hand. Br Med J 1:919–922, 1960.

1098. Stall LA, Van Voorthuisen AE, Van Dijk LM: Neurological complications following arterial catheterization by the axillary approach. Br J Radiol 39:115–116, 1966.

1099. Stalworth JM, Horn JB: Diagnosis and management of thoracic outlet syndrome. Arch Surg 119:1149–1151, 1984.

1100. Stalworth JM, Quinn GJ, Aiken AF: Is first rib resection necessary for relief of thoracic outlet syndrome? Ann Surg 185:581–589, 1979.

1101. Stay EJ, Vawter G: Relationship between nephroblastoma and neurofibromatosis. Cancer 39:2550–2555, 1977.

1102. Stein F, Grabias SL, Deffer PA: Nerve injuries complicating Monteggia lesions. J Bone Joint Surg 53A:1432–1436, 1971.

1103. Steindler A: Operations on the upper extremity problems in kinetics and results. J Bone Joint Surg 9:404, 1927.

1104. Steindler A: Tendon transplantations in the upper extremity. Am J Surg 44:260, 1939.

1105. Stern PJ, Vice M: Compression of the deep branch of the ulnar nerve—a case report. J Hand Surg 8:72–74, 1983.

1106. Stewart HD, Innes AR, Burke FP: The hand complications of Colles' fractures. J Hand Surg [Br] 10:103–106, 1985.

1107. Stewart JD: Focal Peripheral Neuropathies, Chapter 9 Elsevier, New York, 1987.

1108. Stockel K, Schwab M, Thoenen H: Specificity of retrograde transport of nerve growth factor (NGF) and sensory neurons. A biochemical and morphological study. Brain Res 89:1–14, 1975.

1109. Stokes HM: The seriously uninjured hand—weakness of grip. J Occup Med 25:683–684, 1983.

1110. Stookey B: The futility of bridging nerve defects by means of nerve flaps. Surg Gynecol Obstet 29:287–311, 1919.

1111. Stopford JB: Compression of peripheral nerves. Br Med J 1:1027–1028, 1926.

1112. Stopford JSB: Neuritis produced by a wristlet watch. Lancet 1:993–994, 1922.

1113. Stopford JSB: The treatment of large defects in peripheral nerve injuries. Lancet 2:1296–1327, 1920.

1114. Stout AP: The peripheral manifestations of the specific nerve sheath tumour (neurilemmoma). Am J Cancer 24:751–796, 1935.

1115. Stout AP, Laidlaw GF, Haagensen DC: Tumours of the peripheral nerve. Williams & Wilkins, Baltimore, 1937.

1116. Strachan JCH, Ellis BW: Vulnerability of the posterior interosseous nerve during radial head resection. J Bone Joint Surg 53B:320–323, 1971.

1117. Strickland JW, Steichen JB: Nerve tumours of the hand and forearm. J Hand Surg 2:285–291, 1977.

1118. Stromberg WB, McFarlane RM, Bell LL: Injury of the median and ulnar nerves. J Bone Joint Surg 43A:717–730, 1961.

1119. Struthers J: On a peculiarity of the humerus and humeral artery. Monthly J Med Sci 28:264–267, 1848.

1120. Struthers J: On some points in the abnormal anatomy of the arm. Br Foreign Med Chir Rev 14:170–179, 1854.

1121. Sunderland S: A classification of peripheral nerve injuries producing loss of function. Brain 74:491, 1951.

1122. Sunderland S: Nerve and Nerve Injuries, 2nd ed. Churchill Livingstone, Edinburgh, 1978.

1123. Sunderland S: Rate of regeneration of I: sensory nerve fibres and II: motor fibres. Arch Neurol Psychiatry 58:1–14, 251–256, 1947.

1124. Sunderland S: The connective tissues of peripheral nerves. Brain 88:841, 1965.

1125. Sunderland S: The intraneural topography of the radial, median and ulnar nerves. Brain 68:243, 1945.

1126. Sunderland S: Traumatic injuries of peripheral nerves: Simple compression injuries of the radial nerve. Brain 68:56–72, 1945.

1127. Sunderland S, Bradley KC: The cross-sectional area of peripheral nerve trunks devoted to nerve fibres. Brain 72:428–449, 1949.

1128. Sunderland S, Bradley KC: Stress-strain phenomena in human peripheral nerve trunks. Brain 84:102–119, 1961.

1129. Sunderland S, Cossar DF: The structure of the facial nerve. Anat Rec 116:147, 1953.

1130. Sunderland S, Ray LJ: The intraneural topography of the sciatic nerve and its popliteal divisions in man. Brain 71:242–273, 1948.

1131. Suramyi L: Median nerve compression by Struthers' ligament. J Neurol Neurosurg Psychiatry 46:1047–1049, 1983.

1132. Swanson AB, Biddulph SL, Boughman FA, DeGroot G: Ulnar nerve compression due to an anomalous muscle in the canal of Guyon. Clin Orthop 83:64, 1972.

1133. Swanson AB, Boeve NR, Biddulph SL: Silicone-rubber capping of amputation neuromas. Investigational and clinical experience. Interclin Info Bull 11:1, 1972.

1134. Swinson WM, Vigesaa RE, Hieb RE, James EC: Thoracic outlet syndrome: The supraclavicular approach to first rib resection. Surg Rounds, 73–78, Sept. 1986.

1135. Szabo RM, Gelberman RH, Williamson RV, Dellon AL, Yaru NC, Dimick MP: Vibratory sensory testing in acute peripheral nerve compression. J Hand Surg [Am] 9:104–108, 1984.

1136. Szolcsanyi J: A pharmacological approach to lucidation of the role of different nerve fibres and receptor endings in mediation of pain. J Physiol (Paris) 73:251–259, 1977.

1137. Tada K, Nakashima H, Yoshida T, Kitano K: A new treatment of painful amputation neuroma: A preliminary report. J Hand Surg [Br] 12:273–276, 1987.

1138. Takahashi M: Studies of conversion of motor function in intercostal nerves for complete brachial plexus injuries of root avulsion type. J Jpn Orthop Ass 57:1799–1807, 1983.

1139. Taleisnik J: The palmar cutaneous branch of the median nerve and the approach to the carpal tunnel: An anatomic study. J Bone Joint Surg 55:1212–1217, 1973.

1140. Tallas R, Staniforth P, Fisher TR: Neurophysiological studies of autogenous nerve grafts. J Neurol Neurosurg Psychiatry 41:677–683, 1978.

1141. Tamai S, Komatsu S, Sakamoto H, et al: Free muscle transplants in dogs with microsurgical neurovascular anastomoses. Plast Reconstr Surg 46:219, 1970.

1142. Tashima Y, Kimata Y: A case of ganglion causing paralysis of intrinsic muscles innervated by the ulnar nerve. J Bone Joint Surg 43B:153, 1961.

1143. Taylor AS: Brachial birth palsy and injuries of similar types in adults. Surg Gyn Obstet 30:494, 1920.

1144. Taylor AS: Conclusions derived from further experience in the surgical treatment of brachial birth palsy. Am J Med Sci 146:836, 1913.

1145. Taylor AS: Results from the surgical treatment of brachial plexus palsy. JAMA 48:96, 1907.

1146. Taylor EG, Ham FJ: The free vascularized nerve graft. Plast Reconstr Surg 57:413, 1976.

1147. Teece LG: Thrombosis of the ulnar artery. Aust NZ J Surg 19:156–157, 1949.

1148. Tegner R, Brismar T: Experimental uremic neuropathy. Part I (Decreased nerve conduction velocity in rats). J Neurol Sci 65:29–36, 1984.

1149. Telford ED, Mottershead S: Pressure at the cervico-brachial junction: An operative and anatomic study. J Bone Joint Surg 30B:249–263, 1948.

1150. Teneff S: Prevention of amputation neuroma. J Int Coll Surg 12:16, 1949.

1151. Terzis, JK: Microreconstruction of Nerve Injuries. WB Saunders Co, Philadelphia, 1987.

1152. Terzis JK, Dykes RW, Hahstian RW: Electrophysiologic recordings in peripheral nerve surgery—a review. J Hand Surg 1:52–66, 1976.

1153. Terzis J, Faibisoff BA, Williams BH: The nerve gap: Suture under tension versus graft. Plast Reconstr Surg 56:166, 1975.

1154. Terzis JK, Feeker BL, Sismour EN: A computerized study of the intraneural organization of the median nerve. J Hand Surg [Am] 9:605, 1984.

1155. Terzis JK, Manktelow RT: Pectoralis minor: A new concept in facial reanimation. Plast Surg Forum 5, 1982.

1156. Terzis JK, Sweet RC, Dykes RW, Williams HB: Recovery of function in free muscle transplants using microneurovascular anastomoses. J Hand Surg 3:37, 1978.

1157. Thoburn W: Obstetrical paralysis. J Obs Gyn Br Emp 3:454, 1903.

1158. Thomander L, Aldskogius H, Grant G: Motor fiber organization in the intratemporal portion of the cat and rat facial nerves studied with horseradish peroxidase technique. Acta Universitatis Upsaliensis. Abstr of Upsala Dissert Fac Med, #404 iii:1, 1981.

1159. Thomas CG: Clinical manifestations of an accessory palmaris muscle. J Bone Joint Surg 40A:929–930, 1958.

1160. Thomas DF: Kiloh-Nevin syndrome. (Abstr.) J Bone Joint Surg 44B:962, 1962.

1161. Thomas PK, Fullerton PM: Nerve fiber size in the carpal tunnel syndrome. J Neurol Neurosurg Psychiatry 26:520–527, 1963.

1162. Thomas PK, Lascelles RG: Pathology of diabetic neuropathy. Qu J Med 35:449–456, 1966.

1163. Thompson N: Autogenous muscle grafts in the reconstruction of the paralyzed face. In Converse JM, ed: Reconstructive Plastic Surgery, 2nd ed. WB Saunders, Philadelphia, 1977, pp 1841–1848.

1164. Thomson A: A Neuroma and Neurofibromatosis. Turnball and Speers, Edinburgh, 1900.

1165. Tinel J: "The tingling sign in peripheral nerve lesions." Translation by Emanuel B. Kaplan. In Spinner M, ed: Injuries to the Major Branches of Peripheral Nerves of the Forearm, 2nd ed. WB Saunders, Philadelphia, 1978, pp 8–13.

1166. Tobin GR, Schusterman M, Peterson GH, et al: The intramuscular neurovascular anatomy of the latissimus dorsi muscle. The basis for splitting the flap. Plast Reconstr Surg 67:637, 1981.

1167. Tracy JF, Brannon EW: Management of brachial plexus injuries (traction type). J Bone Joint Surg 48:1031, 1958.

1168. Traisman HS, Newcomb AL: Management of Juvenile Diabetes. CV Mosby, St Louis, 1965, pp 1–25.

1169. Tsairis P, Dyck PJ, Molder DW: Natural history of brachial plexus neuropathy. Arch Neurol 27:109–117, 1972.

1170. Tsuge K, Ikuta Y: Macrodactyly and fibrofatty proliferation of the median nerve. Hiroshima J Med Sci 22:83–101, 1973.

1171. Tsuyama N, Hara T: Reconstructive surgery for traumatic brachial plexus injuries. Clin Orthop Surg 3:675–687, 1968.

1172. Tupper JW, Booth DM: Treatment of painful neuromas of sensory nerves in the hand: A comparison of traditional and newer methods. J Hand Surg 1:144–151, 1976.

1173. Turner JWA, Parsonage MJ: Neuralgic amyotrophy (paralytic brachial neuritis). Lancet 2:209–212, 1957.

1174. Turner MS, Caird DM: Anomalous muscles in ulnar nerve compression at the wrist. Hand 9:140–142, 1977.

1175. Tuttle H: Exposure of the brachial plexus with nerve transplantation. JAMA 61:15–17, 1913.

1176. Umphred DA: Neurological Rehabilitation. CV Mosby, St. Louis, 1985.

1177. Upton ARM, McComas AJ: The double crush in nerve entrapment syndromes. Lancet 2:359—362, 1973.

1178. Uriburu IJF, Marchio FJ, Marin JC: Compression syndrome of the deep motor branch of the ulnar nerve. J Bone Joint Surg 58A:145–147, 1976.

1179. Urshel HC, Razzuk MA: Management of the thoracic outlet syndrome. N Engl J Med 286:1140–1143, 1972.

1180. Urshel HC, Razzuk MA, Albers JE, et al: Reoperation for recurrent thoracic outlet syndrome. Ann Thorac Surg 21:1–9, 1976.

1181. Urushidani H: The funicular pattern of the sciatic nerve in Japanese adults. Arch Jpn Chir 43:254–275, 1974.

1182. Uzman BG, Villegas GM: Mouse sciatic nerve regeneration through semipermeable tubes. A quantitative model. J Neurosci Res 9:325, 1983.

1183. Vallois HV: Recherches sur le trajet et les anastomoses du nerf musculo-cutane au niveau du bras. Arch Anat Histol Embryol 1:183, 1922.

1184. Van Beek AL: Electrodiagnostic evaluation of peripheral nerve injuries. Hand Clin 2:747–760, 1986.

1185. Van Buskirk C, Webster C: Prognostic value of sensory defect in rehabilitation of hemiplegics. Neurology (Minneap) 5:407–411, 1955.

1186. Vance RM, Gelberman RH: Acute ulnar neuropathy with fractures at the wrist. J Bone Joint Surg 60A:692–695, 1978.

1187. Vanderpool DW, Chalmers J, Whiston TB: Peripheral compression lesions of the ulnar nerve. J Bone Joint Surg 50B:792–802, 1968.

1188. Vanderput J, Tanner JC, Huypens L: Electrical physiological orientation of the cut ends in primary peripheral nerve repair. Plast Reconstr Surg 44:378–382, 1969.

1189. Vane JR: Prostaglandin Thromboxane Res. 2:791–801, 1976.

1190. Van Hoff MW, Mohn G, eds: Functional Recovery from Brain Damage. Elsevier/North Holland Biomedical Press, Amsterdam, 1981.

1191. Vaughan-Jackson OJ: Rupture of the extensor tendons by attrition at the inferior radioulnar joint. J Bone Joint Surg 30B:528–530, 1948.

1192. Verne J, Iselin M: Reflexions sur deux picels de reparation nerveuse sur l'homme prelevees dix semaines et six mois l'operation. Presse Med 49:789, 1941.

1193. Verocay J: Zur Kenntnis der Neurofibrome. Beitr Pathol Anat 48:1–68, 1910.

1194. Victor M: Polyneuropathy due to nutritional deficiency and alcoholism. In Dyck PJ, Thomas PK, Lambert EH, Bunge R, eds: Peripheral Neuropathy, Vol 1 & 2; 2nd ed. WB Saunders Co., Philadelphia, 1984. pp 1899–1940.

1195. Vinograd A, Taylor E, Grossman S: Sensory retraining of the hemiplegic hand. Am J Occup Ther 5:246–250, 1962.

1196. von Knorring L, Almay BGL, Johansson F: Pain perception and endorphin levels in cerebrospinal fluid. Pain 5:359–365, 1978.

1197. Vulpius O, Stoffel A: Orthopadische Operations-lehre, 2nd ed. Stuttgart Enke, 1920.

1198. Wadsworth TG: The external compression syndrome of the ulnar nerve at the cubital tunnel. Clin Orthop 124:189–204, 1977.

1199. Wadsworth TG, Williams RM: Cubital tunnel external compression syndrome. Nurs Times 73:1357–1359, 1977.

1200. Walker HK: Peripheral neuropathy. In Davidson JK, ed: Clinical Diabetes Mellitus. NY, Thieme, 1986, pp 416–425.

1201. Wall PD: Alterations in the central nervous system after deafferentation connectivity control. Adv Pain Res Ther, 5:677–689, 1983.

1202. Wall PD, Devor M: Sensory afferent impulses originate from dorsal root ganglia as well as from the periphery in normal and nerve injured rats. Pain 17:321, 325, 1983.

1203. Wall PD, Gutnick M: Properties of afferent nerve impulses originating from a neuroma. Nature 248:740, 742, 1974.

1204. Wall PD: In Seigfried J, Zimmerman M, eds: Phantom and Stump Pain. Springer-Verlag, New York, 1981, pp 2–14.

1205. Waller AV: Experiments on the glossopharyngeal and hypoglossal nerves of the frog and observations produced thereby in the structure of their primative fibres. Phil Trans R Soc Lond 140:423, 1850.

1206. Wallin G, Torebjork E, Hallin R: The preliminary observations on the pathophysiology of hyperalgesia in the causalgic pain syndrome. In Zotterman Y, ed: Sensory Functions of the Skin in Primates. Pergamon Press, Elmsford, NY, 1976, 489–499.

1207. Walpin LA: Anomalous tibial nerve innervation of the dorsum of the foot: A factor complicating the diagnosis of tarsal tunnel syndrome. (Abstr.) American Congress of Rehabilitative Medicine, 1984, p 230.

1208. Walsche FMR, Jackson H, Wyburn-Mason R: On some pressure effects not associated with cervical and with rudimentary and "normal" first ribs, and the factors entering into their causation. Brain 67:141–177, 1944.

1209. Walton R, Finseth F: Nerve grafting in the repair of complicated peripheral nerve trauma. J Trauma 17:793–796, 1977.

1210. Warkany J: Friedrich von Recklinghausen and his times. Adv Neurol 29:251–257, 1981.

1211. Warren JD: Anterior interosseous nerve palsies. A complication of forearm fractures. J Bone Joint Surg 45B: 511–513, 1963.

1212. Wartenberg R: Cheiralgia Paresthetica (Isolierte Neuritis des Ramus Superficialis nerve radialis). Z Ges Neurol Psychiatr 141:145–155, 1932.

1213. Wartenberg R: A sign of ulnar palsy. JAMA 112:16–88, 1939.

1214. Watson-Jones R: Carpal semilunar dislocations and other wrist dislocations with associated nerve lesions. Proc R Soc Med 22:1071, 1929.

1215. Weckesser EC: The repair of nerves in the palm and the fingers. Clin Orthop 19:200–207, 1961.

1216. Weinberg HJ, Spencer PS: The fate of Schwann cells isolated from axonal contact. J Neurocytol 7:555–569, 1968.

1217. Weingarden SI, Weingarden HP: Spasmodic torticollis as a cause of ulnar nerve entrapment. Neurosurgery 14:332–334, 1984.

1218. Weisl H, Osborne GV: The pathological changes in rat's nerves subject to moderate compression. J Bone Joint Surg 46B:297–305, 1964.

1219. Weiss P: Damming of axoplasm in constrictive nerve. A sign of perpetual nerve growth in the nerve fibres. Anat Rec 88 [Suppl]:48, 1944.

1220. Weiss P: Evidence of perpetual proximal-distal growth of the nerve fibres. Biol Bull 87:160, 1944.

1221. Weiss P: Nerve reunion with sleeves of frozen dried artery in rabbits, cats and monkeys. Proc Soc Exp Biol Med 54:274, 1943.

1222. Weiss P: Sutureless reunion of severed nerves with cuffs of tantalum. J Neurosurg 1:219, 1944.

1223. Weiss P: The technology of nerve regeneration. A review of sutureless tibulation and related methods of nerve repair. J Neurosurg 1:400, 1944.

1224. Weiss P, Taylor AC: Further experimental evidence against neurotropism in nerve regeneration. J Exp Zool 95:233–257, 1944.

1225. Werner CO, Rosen I, Thorngren KG: Clinical and neurophysiologic characteristics of the pronator syndrome. Clin Orthop 197:231–236, 1985.

1226. Wertsch JJ, Senger JR, Matloub HS: Pseudo-anterior in-

terosseous nerve syndrome. Muscle Nerve 8:68–70, 1985.
1227. Weston B: Prevention of upper limb nerve injuries in Trendelenburg position. Acta Chir Scand 108:61–68, 1954.
1228. White A, Verma PL: Spatial arrangement of facial nerve fibers. J Laryngol Otol 87:957, 1973.
1229. White J: The results of traction injuries to the common peroneal nerve. J Bone Joint Surg 40B:346, 1968.
1230. White NB: Neurilemommas of the extremities. J Bone Joint Surg 49A:1605–1610, 1967.
1231. White WL, Hauna DC: Troublesome lipomata of the upper extremity. J Bone Joint Surg 44A:1353, 1962.
1232. Whitely WH, Alpers BJ: Posterior interosseous palsy with spontaneous neuroma formation. Arch Neurol I:226–229, 1959.
1233. Wilemon WK: Tarsal tunnel syndrome: A fifty year survey of world literature and report of two new cases. Orthop Rev 8:111–117, 1979.
1234. Wiley RG, Blessing WW, Reis DJ: Suicide transport: Destruction of neurons by retrograde transport of ricin abrin and modeccin. Science 216:889, 1982.
1235. Wilgis EFS, Maxwell GP: Distal digital nerve grafts: Clinical and anatomical studies. J Hand Surg 4:439–443, 1979.
1236. Williams HB, Jabaley ME: The importance of internal anatomy of the peripheral nerves to nerve repair in the forearm and hand. Hand Clin 2:689–707, 1986.
1237. Williams HB, Terzis JK: Single fascicular recordings—an intraoperative diagnostic tool for the management of peripheral nerve lesions. Plast Reconstr Surg 57:562–569, 1976.
1238. Willshire WH: Supernumerary first rib: clinical records. Lancet 2:633, 1860.
1239. Wilson DH, Kraut R: Surgery of ulnar neuropathy at the elbow in sixteen cases treated by decompression without transposition. J Neurosurg 38:780–785, 1973.
1240. Wilson PR: In Cousins MJ, Bridenbaugh POD, eds: Neural Blockade in Clinical Assessment and Management of Pain. JB Lippincott, Philadelphia, 1982, pp 557–585.
1241. Wilson RL: Management of pain following peripheral nerve injuries. Orthop Clin North Am 12:343–359, 1981.
1242. Wilson SAK: Proc Soc Med (clin sec), 6:133–141, 1913.
1243. Winckler G: Le nerf peronies accessorie profound: Etude d'anatomie comparee. Arch Anat (Strasbourg) 18:181, 1934.
1244. Windbank AJ, Dyck PJ: Kinetics of 210 Pb and entry into the endoneurium. Brain Res 225:67–73, 1981.
1245. Windbank AJ, McCall JT, Hunder HG, Dyck PJ: The endoneurial content of lead related to the onset and severity of segmental demyelination. J Neuropath Exp Neurol 39:692–699, 1980.
1246. Winkelman NZ, Spinner M: A variant high sensory branch of the median nerve to the third web space. Bull Hosp Joint Dis 34:161–163, 1973.
1247. Wise AJ: A comparative analysis of macro and microsurgical neurorrhaphy techniques. Am J Surg 117:566–572, 1969.
1248. Wolpe J: Systematic desensitization. J Nerv Ment Dis 132:198, 1961.
1249. Woltman HW: Crossing the legs as a factor in the production of peroneal palsy. JAMA 93:670–672, 1929.
1250. Woltman HW: Neuritis associated with acromegaly. Arch Neurol Psychiatry 45:680–682, 1941.
1251. Woltman HW: Pressure as a factor in the development of neuritis of the ulnar and common peroneal nerves in bedridden patients. Am J Med Sci 179:528–532, 1930.
1252. Woltman HW, Kernohan JW: Disease of peripheral nerves. In Baker AB ed: Clinical Neurology. Hoeber-Harper, New York, 1955, p 1629.
1253. Woltman HW, Learmonth JR: Progressive paralysis of the nervus interosseous dorsalis. Brain 57:25–31, 1934.
1254. Woltman HW, Williams HL, Lambert EH: An attempt to relieve hemifacial spasm by neurolysis of the facial nerve: A report of two cases of hemifacial spasm with reflections on the nature of the spasm, the contracture and mass movement. Proc Staff Meet Mayo Clin 26:236–240, 1951.
1255. Wood MB: Discussion, Determination of temporal changes in blood flow in vascularized and nonvascularized nerve grafts in dog by Lux P, Breidenbach W, Firrell J. Plast Reconstr Surg 82:143–144, 1988.
1256. Wood J: On some varieties in human myologies. Proc R Soc Lond 13:299–303, 1864.
1257. Woodall B, Beebe WG: In Peripheral Nerve Regeneration, A follow-up study of 3,656 World War II injuries. VA Medical Monograph, US Government Printing Office, Washington, D.C., 1956.
1258. Woodruff JM, Godwin TA, Erlandson RA, et al: Cellular schwannoma. Am J Surg Pathol 5:733–744, 1981.
1259. Wright EA, McQuillen MP: Hypoexcitability of ulnar nerve in patients with normal motor and nerve conduction studies. Neurology (Minneap) 23:78–83, 1973.
1260. Wright IS: Neurovascular syndrome produced by hyperabduction of the arm. Original communication. Heart J 29:1–19, 1945.
1261. Wynn Parry CB: Brachial plexus lesions. pp 157–177 in Rehabilitation of the Hand 4th ed, 1981.
1262. Wynn Parry CB: Rehabilitation of the Hand, 4th ed. Butterworths, London, 1984.
1263. Wynn Parry CB, Salter M: Sensory re-education after median nerve lesion. Hand 8:250–257, 1976.
1264. Yahr MD, Beebe GW: Recovery of motor function. In Woodhall B, Beebe GW. Peripheral Nerve Regeneration. U.S. Government Printing Office, Washington, DC, 1956, pp 71–202.
1265. Yaksh TL, Hammond DL: Peripheral and central substrates involved in the rostrad transmission of nociceptive information. Pain 13:1–85, 1982.
1266. Yamada KM, Spooner BS, Wessells NK: Ultrastructure and function of the growth cones and axons of cultured nerve cells. J Cell Biol 49:614–635, 1971.
1267. Yamamoto K: A comparative analysis of the process of nerve regeneration following funicular and epineurial suture for peripheral nerve repair. Arch Jpn Chir 43:276–301, 1974.
1268. Yerxa EJ, Barber LM, Diaz O, Black W, Azens P: Development of hand sensitivity test for use in desensitiza-

tion when it presents in the hand. Am J Occup Ther 37:176–181, 1983.

1269. Yoman PM: Fatty infiltration of the median nerve. J Bone Joint Surg 46:737–739, 1964.

1270. Yamano Y: Electrophysiological study of nerve grafting. J Hand Surg 7:588–592, 1982.

1271. Yamano Y, Namba Y, Hino Y, et al: Digital nerve grafts in replanted digits. Hand 4:255–262, 1982.

1272. Young JZ, Medawar PB: Fibrin suture of peripheral nerves. Lancet 2:126, 1940.

1273. Young L, Wray RC, Weeks PM: A randomized prospective comparison of fascicular and epineural digital nerve repairs. Plast Reconstr Surg 68:89–92, 1981.

1274. Young VL, Wray RC, Weeks PM: The results of nerve grafting in the wrist and hand. Ann Plast Surg 5:212–215, 1980.

1275. Yunshao H, Shizhen Z: Acetylcholinesterase: A histochemical identification of motor and sensory fascicles in human peripheral nerve and its use during operation. Plast Reconstr Surg 82:125–130, 1988.

1276. Zachary LS, Dellon AL, Seiler WA: Relationship of intraneural damage in the rat sciatic nerve to the method of injury. Microsurgery 8:182–185, 1987.

1277. Zachary RB: Results of nerve suture. In Seddon HJ, ed: Peripheral Nerve Injuries. Her Majesty's Stationery Office, London. pp 34–388.

1278. Zachary RB: Thenar palsy due to compression of the median nerve in the carpal tunnel. Surg Gynecol Obstet 81:213, 1945.

1279. Zachery RB, Holmes W: Primary suture of nerves. Surg Gynecol Obstet 82:632–651, 1946.

1280. Zahrawi F: Acute compression ulnar neuropathy at Guyon's canal resulting from lipoma. J Hand Surg 9A:238–240, 1984.

1281. Zancolli E, Mitre H: Latissimus dorsi transfer to restore elbow flexion. J Bone Joint Surg [Am] 55:1265–1275.

1282. Zoega H: Fracture of the lower end of the radius with ulnar nerve palsy. J Bone Joint Surg 48B:514–516, 1966.

Index

N

V

W